Review of Basic Physics

ELECTROSTATICS

1. The addition or removal of electrons is called electrification.
2. Like charges repel; unlike charges attract.
3. Coulomb's law of electrostatic force:

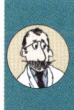
$$F = c\frac{Q_A Q_B}{d^2}$$

4. Only negative charges can move in solids.
5. Electrostatic charge is distributed on the outer surface of conductors.
6. The concentration of charge is greater when the radius of curvature is smaller.

ELECTRODYNAMICS

Ohm's law: $V = IR$

A series circuit:

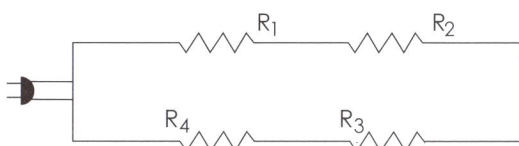

1. $V_t = V_1 + V_2 + V_3 + V_4$
2. I is the same through all elements.
3. $R_t = R_1 + R_2 + R_3 + R_4$

A parallel circuit:

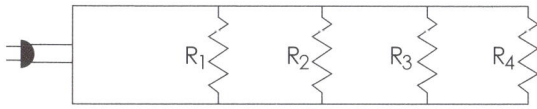

1. V is the same across each circuit element.
2. $I_t = I_1 + I_2 + I_3 + I_4$
3. $\frac{1}{R_t} = \frac{1}{R_1} + \frac{1}{R_2} + \frac{1}{R_3} + \frac{1}{R_4}$

   Electric power: $P = IV = I^2R$ [(A)(V) = W]
   Work: Work = QV [(C)(V) = J]
   Potential: $V = W/Q$ [J/C = V]
   Capacitance: $C = Q/V$ [C/V = F]

MAGNETISM

1. Every magnet has a north pole and a south pole.
2. Like poles repel; unlike poles attract.
3. Gauss's law:

$$F = k\frac{M_1 M_2}{d^2}$$

ELECTROMAGNETISM

1. A magnetic field is always present around a conductor in which a current is flowing.
2. Changing magnetic fields can produce an electric field.
3. Transformer law:

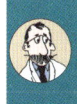
$$\frac{V_p}{V_s} = \frac{N_p}{N_s}$$

CLASSICAL PHYSICS

Linear force: $F = ma$ [(kg)(m/s^2) = N]
Momentum: $p = mv$ [(kg)(m/s)]
Mechanical work (or energy):
Work (or E) = Fs [(N)(m) = J]
Kinetic energy: $E = \frac{1}{2}mv^2$ [(kg)(m^2/s^2) = J]
Mechanical power: $P = Fs/t$ [(N)(m)/s = J/s = W]

Useful Units in Radiology

SI Prefixes

Factor	Prefix	Symbol
10^{18}	Exa	E
10^{15}	Peta	P
10^{12}	Tera	T
10^{9}	Giga	G
10^{6}	Mega	M
10^{3}	Kilo	k
10^{2}	Hecto	h
10^{1}	Deca	da
10^{-1}	Deci	d
10^{-2}	Centi	c
10^{-3}	Milli	m
10^{-6}	Micro	μ
10^{-9}	Nano	n
10^{-12}	Pico	p
10^{-15}	Femto	f
10^{-18}	Atto	a

SI Base Units

Quantity	Name	Symbol
Length	Meter	m
Mass	Kilogram	kg
Time	Second	s
Electric current	Ampere	A

SI Derived Units Expressed in Terms of Base Units

Quantity	Name (SI Unit)	Symbol
Area	Square meter	m^2
Volume	Cubic meter	m^3
Velocity	Meter per second	m/s
Acceleration	Meter per second squared	m/s^2
Mass density	Kilogram per cubic meter	kg/m^3
Current density	Ampere per square meter	A/m^2
Concentration (amount of substance)	Mole per cubic meter	$Mole/m^3$
Specific volume	Cubic meter per kilogram	m^3/kg

Special Quantities of Radiologic Science and Their Associated Special Units

Quantity	Customary Name	Customary Symbol	SI Name	SI Symbol
Exposure	roentgen	R	air kerma	Gy_a
Absorbed dose	rad	rad	gray	Gy_t
Effective dose	rem	rem	sievert	Sv
Radioactivity	curie	Ci	becquerel	Bq
Multiply	R	by 0.01	to obtain	Gy_a
Multiply	rad Gy	by 0.01	to obtain	Gy_t
Multiply	rem	by 0.01	to obtain	Sv
Multiply	Ci	by 3.73×10^{10}	to obtain	Bq
Multiply	R	by 2.583×10^{-4}	to obtain	C/kg

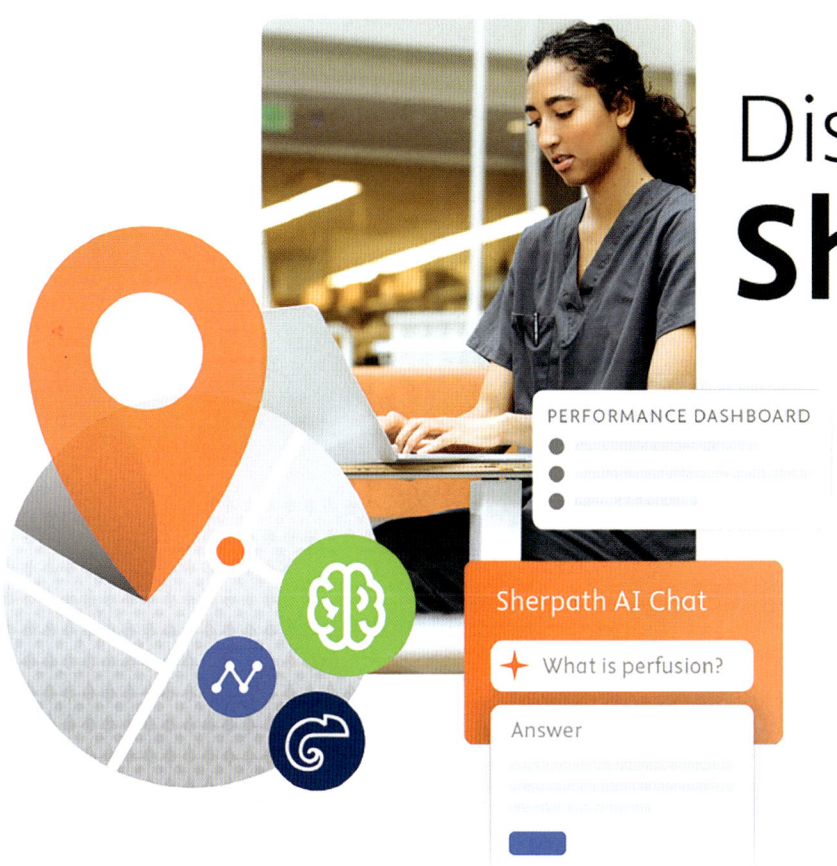

Discover Sherpath®

The digital teaching and learning technology built specifically for healthcare education.

Sherpath's all-in-one course delivery solution powers your textbook with innovative resources, including the following:

Digital lessons aligned with learning objectives create an interactive experience with multimedia, adaptive remediation, assignment assessments, and more. *Only available for select collections.*

Elsevier Adaptive Quizzing customizes quizzes based on performance and allows you to choose relevant quiz topics.

Sherpath AI conversational AI tool generates personalized answers to questions, sourced solely from Elsevier's vast library of trusted, evidence-based content.

eBook and resources are seamlessly accessible within Sherpath for quick access to relevant course materials, activities, and reading recommendations.

Performance dashboard offers a holistic view of course progress and areas of strength and weakness.

Enhanced test banks provide all-in-one access to your test bank from your Sherpath courses. *Only available for select collections.*

STUDENTS — Ask your instructor about enhancing your course experience with Sherpath!

INSTRUCTORS — Scan code or visit myevolve.us/sphp to learn more!

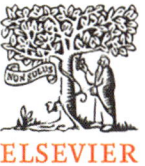

24-0461 TM/AF

BUSHONG'S
RADIOLOGIC SCIENCE FOR TECHNOLOGISTS
PHYSICS, BIOLOGY, AND PROTECTION

BUSHONG'S
RADIOLOGIC SCIENCE FOR TECHNOLOGISTS
PHYSICS, BIOLOGY, AND PROTECTION

THIRTEENTH EDITION

STEWART CARLYLE BUSHONG, ScD, FAAPM, FACR
Professor of Radiologic Science
Baylor College of Medicine
Houston, Texas

ELIZABETH S. SHIELDS, MHA, RT(R)
Program Director, Radiologic
Technology Program
Novant Health Presbyterian
Medical Center
Charlotte, North Carolina

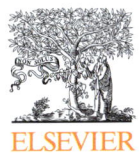

Elsevier
3251 Riverport Lane
St. Louis, Missouri 63043

BUSHONG'S RADIOLOGIC SCIENCE FOR TECHNOLOGISTS: ISBN: 978-0-323-76536-7
PHYSICS, BIOLOGY, AND PROTECTION, THIRTEENTH EDITION

Copyright © 2026 Elsevier Inc. All rights are reserved, including those for text and data mining, AI training, and similar technologies.

For accessibility purposes, images in electronic versions of this book are accompanied by alt-text descriptions provided by Elsevier. For more information, see https://www.elsevier.com/about/accessibility.

Publisher's note: Elsevier takes a neutral position with respect to territorial disputes or jurisdictional claims in its published content, including in maps and institutional affiliations.

No part of this publication may be reproduced or transmitted in any form or by any means, electronic or mechanical, including photocopying, recording, or any information storage and retrieval system, without permission in writing from the publisher. Details on how to seek permission, further information about the Publisher's permissions policies and our arrangements with organizations such as the Copyright Clearance Center and the Copyright Licensing Agency, can be found at our website: www.elsevier.com/permissions.

This book and the individual contributions contained in it are protected under copyright by the Publisher (other than as may be noted herein).

Notice

Practitioners and researchers must always rely on their own experience and knowledge in evaluating and using any information, methods, compounds or experiments described herein. Because of rapid advances in the medical sciences, in particular, independent verification of diagnoses and drug dosages should be made. To the fullest extent of the law, no responsibility is assumed by Elsevier, authors, editors or contributors for any injury and/or damage to persons or property as a matter of products liability, negligence or otherwise, or from any use or operation of any methods, products, instructions, or ideas contained in the material herein.

Previous editions copyrighted 2021, 2017, 2013, 2008, 2004, 2001, 1997, 1993, 1988, 1984, 1980, and 1975.

Content Strategist: Meg Benson/ Luke Held
Content Development Manager: Danielle Frazier
Content Development Specialist: Sarah Vora
Publishing Services Manager: Deepthi Unni
Project Manager: Beula Christopher
Design Direction: Ryan Cook

Printed in India

Last digit is the print number: 9 8 7 6 5 4 3 2 1

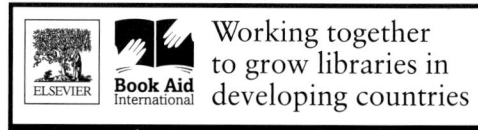

BCM
Baylor College of Medicine

I wrote the first edition of this textbook in 1974, not expecting anyone to read it, much less buy it! I wrote it to get promoted. My academic chairman explained to me that to be promoted to tenured full professor at Baylor College of Medicine, one had to write a textbook. (Bushong SC. A Book Report. *Radiologic Technology*, 84 (4), pp 405–409, March/April 2013.)

The greatest reward I have received in writing this Golden Anniversary edition is the many new friends I now have because of this textbook. So, I dedicate this edition to you, my friends in radiology education. Many have contributed to this textbook, and many have shared with me the speaking platform at educational meetings. Thank you very much for your friendship, and I apologize to those I have left out because I have now made it to double overtime and I can't remember!

Kenneth Abramovitch, University of Texas
James Adams, Jefferson Community & Technical College
Nancy Adams, Louisiana State University
Arlene M. Adler, Indiana University Northwest
Christian Allard, Universidat de Arica
Carla Allen, University of Missouri
Keith Allen, College of DuPage
Felipe Allende, Universidad Centrale, Chile
Kelly Angel, Kaiser Permanente
Richard S. Angulo, Pima Medical Institute, Chula Vista, California
Nathan Annenberg, Fordham University
Sebastian Arancibia, Universidad Centrale, Chile
Maria Ayers, Health Care Imaging, Australia
Matt Ayers, Health Care Imaging, Australia
Alex Backus, Gateway Community College
Philip Ballinger, Ohio State University
Stephen Balter, Columbia University
Ed Barnes, Medical Technology Management Institute
Gary Barnes, University of Alabama
Marcy Barnes, Lexington Community College
Cecilia Munoz Barsbino, University of Peru
Shirley A. Bartley, Hillyard Technical Center
Tammy Bauman, Banner Thunderbird Medical Center
Richard Bayless, University of Montana
Chris Beaudry, Yakima Valley Community College
Rochel Becker, Johns Hopkins School of Medical Imaging
Theresa Beland, Kaiser Permanente

Alberto Bello, Jr., Danville Area Community College
Bobbie Lynnette Biglane, US Air Force
Melanie Billmeier, North Central Texas College
Clinton Bishop, South Plains College,
Nathaniel L. Bishop, Jefferson College of Health Sciences
George Bissett, Texas Children's Hospital
Christy Foster Bollman, Gurnick Academy of Medical Arts
Christie Bolton, Jefferson State College
Denise Bowman, Community Hospital of Monterrey Peninsula
Colleen Brady, Minnesota State College
Jeffrey Brown, Kaiser Permanente
Karen Brown, Gateway Community College
Norman L. Burgess, Brookhaven College
Barry Burns, University of North Carolina
Cheryl Burtle, Logan University, Chesterfield, Missouri
Deanna Butcher, St. Cloud Hospital
Priscilla Butler, American College of Radiology
Cisca Bye, Montgomery County Community College
James Byrne, Houston Community College
Andres Cabezas Cabrera, Universidad Centrale, Chile
Robert Cahalan, Iowa SRT
Donna L. Caldwell, Arkansas State University
Shaun T. Caldwell, UT MD Anderson Cancer Center
William J. Callaway, Lincoln Land Community College
Claudia Calo, Universidad Abierta Interamericana, Argentina
Richard R. Carlton, Arkansas State University

Mary Ellen Carpenter, Essex County College
Quinn Carroll, Midland College
Richard Carson, Oregon Institute of Technology
Christi Carter, Brookhaven College
Alejandro Cerda, Clinicas las Condes, Chile
Tammy Chaffee, Dona Ana Community College
Timothy C. Chapman, Gateway Community College
Christian Chavez, Universidat de Arica
Jean Christensen, Mercy Medical Center
Valerie Christensen, Association of Educators in Radiologic Science
Katie Christopher, Southside College of Health Sciences, Colonial Heights, Virginia
Carolyn L. Cianciosa, Niagara County Community College
David Clayton, UT MD Anderson Cancer Center
Jennifer Clayton, Linn Benton Community College
Brent Colby, Sanford Health School of Radiography, North Dakota
Brenda M. Coleman, Columbia State Community College
Edgar Colon, Universidad Central del Carribian
Judy Cook, Tarrant County College
Cathy Cooper, Alabama SRT
Charles Coulston, Bluegrass Community & Technical College
Annja Cox, Dona Ana Community College
Tracy Crandall, Atlanta SRT
Russell Crank, Rockingham Memorial Hospital Healthcare
Suzanne E. Crandall, Iowa Methodist Medical Center
Angela Culliton, Mercy Medical Center
Cheryl V. Cunningham, Virginia Western Community College
Geoffrey Currie, Charles Sturt University, Australia
Jacklynn Scott Darling, Morehead State University
Rob Davidson, Canberra University, Australia
Lynne Davis, Houston Community College
Tavia DeFazio, United Hospital Center, West Virginia
Denise DeGennaro, Lone Star College
Jomar DeGuzman, Good Samaritan College, Philippines
Ann Delaney, University of Montana
Jenny Delawalla, Gwinnett Technical College
Tammy Delker, Indian Hills Community College, Ottumwa, Iowa
Lois Depouw, Rasmussen College
Steve Deutsch, Spencer Hospital
Keith Diehl, Santa Rosa Junior College
Randall D. Dings, Pima Community College
Martha Dollar, Columbus Technical College
Sarajane Doty, Kentucky Community and Technical College
Mary Doucette, Great Basin College
Marsha Dougherty, Lone Star College
Eric Douglas, St. Luke's Episcopal Hospital

Cheryl DuBose, Arkansas State University
Pat Duffy, Roxbury Community College
Andrea Guillen Dutton, Chaffey College
Ursula Dyer, Kilgore College
Hamed Ebrahimnejad, Kerman University, Iran
John W. Eichinger, Technical College of the Low Country
Karen Emory, Grady Memorial Healthcare
Venessa Engelbrecht, Charles Stuart University, Australia
Michael A. Enriquez, Merced Community College
Rodrigo Espinoza, Universidad Centrale, Chile
Lisa S. Fanning, Massachusetts College of Health Sciences
Shanna Farish, Medical RT Board of Examiners
Terri Fauber, Virginia Commonwealth University
Bill Faulkner, University of Tennessee
Scott Flamm, Texas Heart Institute
Kae Brock Fleming, Columbia State Community College
Gwen Faber, Grand Rapids Community College, Grand Rapids, Michigan
Geneva Flexon, Southside College of Health Sciences, Colonial Heights, Virginia
Sherry Floerchinger, Dixie State College of Utah
M. Ella Flores, Blinn College
Mike Frain, Northern New Mexico College
Eugene Frank, Riverland Community College
Dawn Fucillo, Washington State University
Richard Fucillo, Burlington Community College
Michael Fugate, University of Florida
Merryl Fulmer, Huntingdon Valley, Pennsylvania
Federico Furtado, Medica Uruguaya y Sanatorio Americano
Rodrigo Antonio Galaz, University of Santiago, Chile
Marcelo Galvez, Clinica las Condes, Chile
Ismael Garcia, Del Mar College
Sandra Garcia, Fort Sam Houston
Andrew Gardner, Atlanta Technical College
Joe Garza, Lone Star College
Rudy Garza, Austin Community College
Camille Gaudet, Hospital Regional Dr-Georges-L-Dumont
Pamela Gebhart-Cline, Riverside School
Diane George, Jackson State College
Susan Giboney, Kaiser Permanente
Tim Gienapp, Apollo College
Julia A. Gill, Virginia SRT
Laci Giroir, Beaumont Baptist Hospital
Yvonne Grant, Iowa SRT
Joel Gray, Medical Physics Consulting
Mark Greco, Charles Stuart University, Australia
Susan Green, Jefferson State Community College, Alabama
Ginger Griffin, Jacksonville Community College
Olga Grisak, Colorado Mesa University

Bob Grossman, Keiser University, Lakeland, Florida
LaVern Gurley, Shelby State Community College
Jennyfer Gutierrez, University of Peru
Dick Gwilt, Indian Health Service
Jeff Hamzeh, Keiser University
Loretta Hanset, Harris County Hospital District
Michael D. Harpin, University of South Alabama
Wendell Harris, Southwest Virginia Community College
Nancy Harvey, University of Iowa
Kenya Haugen, Baptist Health System
Art Haus, Ohio State University
Nancy Hawking, University of Arkansas
Joyce O. Hawkins, Bon Secours Richmond Health System
John Hazle, UT MD Anderson Cancer Center
Clyde R. Hembree, University of Tennessee
Ed Hendrick, Northwestern University
Chad Hensley, University of Nevada-Las Vegas
Tracy Herrmann, University of Cincinnati
Don Hessel, Research Medical Center, Kansas City, Missouri
Victoria Holas, Arizona Western College
Peggy Hoosier, Advanced Health Education Center
James Ibaviosa, Mercy Hospital
Miguel Iglesias, Colegio Technologo Medico del Peru
Keith Indeck, Norwalk Radiology Center
Janie Jackson, Tarrant County College
Donald Jacobson, Medical College of Wisconsin
Brad Jenkins, National Polytechnic College
Jeniesa Johnson, Tarrant County College
Nancy Johnson, Gateway Community College
Starla Jones, Medical College of Georgia
Linda Joppe, Rasmussen College
Helen Schumpert Kauchak, Asheville MRI
Dianne M. Kawamura, Weber State University
Leslie E. Kendrick, Boise State University
Cheryl Kerr, San Diego Naval Station
April D. Kidd, USFDA/CDRH
Jeannie Kilgore, Clovis Community College
Jeffery B. Killian, Midwestern State University
Kelly Kocis, Boise State University, Idaho
Cindy Kramer, Delta College, University Center, Michigan
Paul A. Kusber, Mills-Peninsula School
Ruth Kusterer, Virginia SRT
Kent Lambert, Drexel University
Tim Lambrecht, Baylor Grapevine Diagnostic Imaging
John P. Lampignano, Gateway Community College
Traci B. Lang, Virginia SRT
Dustin Latner, Polk State College
Paul Laudicina, College of DuPage
Gary Leach, Memorial Hermann Hospital
Jonathan Lee, Cape Fear Community College, North Carolina
Lois Lehman, Texas Scottish Rite Hospital for Children
Richard Lehrer, Santa Rosa Junior College
Deborah Leighty, Hillsborough Community College
Patricia Lenza, Concord's Community College
Theresa Levitsky, St. Francis Medical Center
Kurt Loveland, Southern Illinois University
Michelle Luciano, UNE Puerto Rico
Peachy S. Luna, Philippine Association of Deans and Faculty of Colleges of Radiologic Technology, Inc.
Eileen M. Maloney, American Registry of Radiologic Technologists
Jacob Manning, Keiser University, Lakeland, Florida
Rodrigo Marchant, Central University of Chile
Victor Ruiz Marquez, University of Peru
Mark J. Martone, Massachusetts College of Health Sciences
Ron Marker, Wheaton Franciscan Healthcare
Chris B. Martin, Oklahoma Health Sciences Center
Valerie Martin, Brookhaven College
Starla Mason, Laramie County Community College
Allyson Matheaus, Wharton County Junior College
LeAnn Maupin, Oregon Institute of Technology
William May, Mississippi State University
Kelly McCowan, Rowan Cabarrus Community College, Salisbury, North Carolina
Cynthia McCullough, Mayo Clinic
Dave McLaren, Polk State College
Joy Mason, WVU Medicine
Robert Meisch, Indiana State University
Francisco Mena, Clinicas las Condes, Chile
Darrly Mendoza, Mills-Peninsula School
Joy Menser, Owensboro Community College
Maria Messner, Tower Health, Pennsylvania
Kim Metcalf, George Washington University
Massimo Midiri, University of Palermo
Becky Miller, Horry-Georgetown Technical College
Debbie K. Miller, Spokane Community College
Jacob Miller, Western Suffolk BOCES School of Radiologic Technology, New York
Fabian Monforte, Universidad del Salvador, Argentina
Ruby Montgomery, Marion County Community College
Dawn Moore, Atlanta SRT
Fernando A. Morales, Universidad Diego Portales
Christopher Morris, Gadsden State Community College, Gadsden, Alabama
Jose Rafael Moscoso, Universidad Central Del Caribe, Puerto Rico
C. William Mulkey, Midlands Technical College
Cecilia Barabino Munoz, Universidad Mayor de San Marcos, Peru
Mindy Mutschler, Mercy Medical Center
Glenna Neumann, Atlanta SRT
Charles Newell, University of South Alabama
Mary Ellen Newton, St. Francis School

Edward Nickoloff, Columbia University
Jon Nissenbaum, Massachusetts Eye and Ear Infirmary
Tanya Nolan, Weber State University
Larry Norris, Lone Star College
Juan Luis Nunovero, Universidad Nacional Mayor de San Marcos, Peru
Sandra Ochoa, Del Mar College
Cyndee Oliver, Lone Star College
Erica O'Quinn, East Tennessee State University
Stephen Osborne, East Tennessee State University
Lori Oswalt, Covenant School of Radiography
Francis Ozor, Lone Star College
George Pales, University of Nevada
Paula Pate-Schloder, Misericordia University
Brenda L. Pfeiffer, Loma Linda University
Rob Posteraro, Texas Tech University
Chase Poulsen, Jefferson College of Health Sciences
Jerilyn J. Powell, Rapid City Regional Hospital
Valerie J.H. Powell, Robert Morris University
Kevin J. Powers, Virginia SRT
Perri Preston, University of Florida
Roger A. Preston, Reid Hospital & Health Services
Cheryl Pressly, Grady Health School of Imaging Technology
James Pronovost, Naugatuck Valley Community College
Barbara Smith Pruner, Portland Community College
John Radtke, Louisiana State University
Eytan Raz, University of Rome
Rolly Reyes, El Camino College, Torrance, California
Roland Rhymus, Loma Linda University
Teresa Rice, Houston Community College
Jennifer A. Rigsby, Austin Community College
Ted Roberson, Washoe Medical Center
Cynthia Robertson, Lone Star College
Rita Robinson, Memorial Hermann Hospital
Jeannean Rollins, Arkansas State University
Veronica Rosales, University Centrale, Chile
Lil Rossidilla, Pima Medical Institute
Donna Rufsholm, South Peninsula Hospital
Bonnie Rush, Educational Enterprise
Francesca Russo, Santa Marcia Dilicodia
Loren A. Sachs, Orange Coast College
Marilyn Sackett, Advanced Health Education Center
Dorothy Saia, Stamford Hospital
Ehsan Samei, Duke University
Beatriz Sanchez, Pontifica Universidad Catolica de Chile
Thomas Sandridge, University of Illinois
Natalia dos Santos, Medica Uruguaya y Santorio Americano
Jim Sass, Gwinnett Technical College
Bette Schans, Colorado Mesa University
Lana Scherer, Covenant Health
Martin Schotten, Yuma Medical Center
Jill Schulz, Covenant Medical Center
Euclid Seeram, British Columbia Institute of Technology
Victor Seghers, Texas Children's Hospital
Kim Seigman, Covenant Health
Joseph Shackelford, Jackson Community College
Eric J. Shepard, Fort Sam Houston
Elizabeth Shields, Presbyterian Hospital
Linda Shields, El Paso Community College
Anthony Siebert, University of California, Davis
Marcelo Zenteno Silva, Central University of Chile
Mark A. Sime, Mercy Medical Center
Taffi Simone, Riverside Health System
Kathryn M. Slagle, University of Alaska-Anchorage
Dawn Stark, Mississippi State University
Katrina Lynn Steinsultz, Lansing Community College
Mike Stewart, Dona Ana Community College
Rees Stuteville, Oregon Institute of Technology
Donald Summers, Gwinnet Technical College
Raquel Tapia, Del Mar College
Christl Thompson, El Paso Community College
Kyle Thornton, City College of San Francisco
Gina Tice, Gadsden State Community College
Kimberly Todd, Jackson State Community College
Renee Tossell, Pima Community College
Brenna Travis, Tarrant County College
Alfred Traylor, The Johns Hopkins Hospital
Mark Trifunovic, Macquarie Medical Imaging, Australia
Shayne Trotter, Health Care Imaging, Australia
Pete Tually, Telemed, Australia
William Tyler, Savannah Technical Institute
Virginia Vanderford, Portland Community College
Beth L. Veale, Midwestern State University
Michele Patricia Muller Mansur Vieira, Brazil
Natalia Viera, Medica Uruguaya y Sanatorio Americano
Susan Sprinkle Vincent, Advanced Health Education Center
Donna Vitetta, White Plains College
Matt von Hippel, Niels Bohr Institute, Copenhagen, Denmark
Louis Wagner, University of Texas Medical School
Jeff Walmsley, Lorain Community College
Steven D. Walters, Regional Medical Center of San Jose
Cheryl Dutton Walton, Huntsville Hospital
Patti Ward, Colorado Mesa University
Lynette K. Watts, Midwestern State University
Laurie Weaver, Casper College
Stephanie A. Wells, Brookhaven College
Diana S. Werderman, Trinity College
Amy D. Westbury, Orangeburg-Calhoun Technical College
Rhonda Wever, Atrium Health, North Carolina
Mark White, University of Nebraska
Tracey B. White, Arkansas State University

Erica K. Wight, University of Alaska-Anchorage
Raymond Wilenzek, Tulane University
Christine Wiley, North Shore Community College
Carla Williams, Carteret Community College
Judy Williams, Grady Memorial Hospital
Charles Willis, UT MD Anderson Cancer Center
Bettye G. Wilson, American Registry of Radiologic Technologists
Robert Wilson, University of Tennessee
Ken Wintch, Colorado Mesa University
Leslie F. Winter, Joint Review Committee on Education in Radiologic Technology
Ray Winters, Arkansas State University
Mary E. Wolfe, Catholic Medical Center
Tom Wolfe, Baptist College of Health Sciences, Memphis
Andrew Woodward, Wor-Wic Community College
Amber Wooten, Arkansas State University
Melinda Wren, Del Mar College
Donna Lee Wright, Midwestern State University
Jennifer Yates, Merritt College
Brad York, Houston Community College
Suin You, Charles Stuart University, Australia
Brian Zawislak, Northwestern University Medical School
Marcelo Zentano, Universidad Centrale, Chile
Xie Nan Zhu, Guangzhou Medical College
Kelly J. Zuniga, Houston Community College

This Book Is Also Dedicated To My Dog Friends Here and Gone

Abby Carlyle Kuramoto
Abigale Rose Spencer
Ally Carlyle Myers
Anabella Carlyle Lartique
Apple Marie Orr
Arlo Carlyle Hopkinson
Atlas Jamma Holmes*
Baily Schroth (†)
Baily Spaulding
Bandit Davidson (†)
Belle Carlyle Frick*
Bella Bushong
Bello Carlyle Jacobson
Bently Carlyle Conrad
Biscuit Carlyle Martin
Boef Kuipers (†)
Bridget Carlyle Kendrigan
Brittney Prominski
Brownie Hindman (†)
Brutus Payne (†)
Bucky Carlyle Jacobson
Buffy Jackson (†)
Butterscotch Bushong (†)
Buttons Carlyle Fountain*
Buzz Carlyle Cochran
Casey Carlyle White
Casper Miller (†)
Cassie Kronenberger (†)
Chandon Davis (†)
Charlie Brown Phenicie*
Charley Carlyle Butler
Charlie Carlyle Bushong
Charlie Carlyle Lartique
Chester Chase (†)
Choco Walker (†)
Clifford Carlyle Devor
Coco Winsor
Cody Carlyle Brady (†)
Cookie Lake (†)
Cuddle-Bug Sims*
Daisey Carlyle Kronenberger
Daisey Carlyle Smith
Daisy Carlyle Brady
Daizy Carlyle Jacobson
Desi Lohrenz
Dilly Carlyle Tallant*
Doxie Carlyle Robinson
Dually Jackson
Dude Schwartz
Duke Carlyle McMullin
Duncan Hindman (†)

Dwight Eisenhower (Ike) DWIC Green*
Ebony Bushong (†)
Emme Carlyle Couch
Flap Maly
Fonzie Schroth (†)
Frank Edlund
Gemma Louise Henley*
George Carlyle Snodgrass Jacobson
Geraldine Bushong (†)
Ginger Chase (†)
Gipper Carlyle Kendrigan
Gracie Pauline Holmes*
Grayton Friedlander
Gretchen Scharlach (†)
Griffin Carlyle Conrad
Guadalupe Tortilla Holmberg
Gus Carlyle Robinson
Harley Hunt Weiss*
Hedgington Bova MacFarlane Esq.
Heidi Carlyle Couch
Huckleberry (Huck) Carlyle Elliott
Hugo MutzvCheyneWalk Morris
Ivy Carlyle Kuramoto*
Jemimah Bushong (†)
Jenn Sheba Jacobson
Jessie Carlyle Jacobson
Jessie Jackson Jacobson
Jody Carlyle Rogers
Joy Carlyle Alexander *
Kalli Carlyle Fields
Kate Davidson (†)
Katie Carlyle Fields
Katie Carlyle Robinson
Kelsie Carlyle Mase*
Kermit Carlyle Chase
Kokopelli Carlyle Hames
Lacy Carlyle Haskins*
Latte Carlyle Stewart
Leo Carlyle Sanders
Lily Carlyle Klotman*
Linus Black (†)
Lizzie Carlyle Bryan
Lizzy Prominski
Lo Phoebe Holmes*
Loftus Meadows
Louie Carlyle Edlund
Lucky Carlyle Craig
Lucy Spaulding (†)
Luna Carlyle Cochran
Maddie Bushong

Marley Carlyle Sanders
Marlo Carlyle Racke
Max Velcro Dykes
Maxwell Carlyle McMullin
Maxwell Haus (†) and my lenses
Mazy Carlyle Bushong*
Metoo Carlyle Bertrand
Miabella Allure's Ohh La La Burleson*
Micky Carlyle Chadwick*
Midnight Lunsford (†)
Milou Baily Bertrand*
Mimi Hana (Indian Princess)
Mocha Carlyle Stewart
Molly Carlyle Jacobson
Molly Holmberg (†)
Mrs. Jones Carlyle Bush
Murphy Carlyle Sanders
Muttly Chase (†)
Nugget Carlyle Devor
Old Dog Walker
Pancho Villa Holmberg (†)
Peanut Schroth (†)
Penny Carlyle Friedlander
Pepper Carlyle Miller
Percy Lohrenz
Petra Chase (†)
Pippa Albin Selinger*
Powers Jackson
Prissy Carlyle Myers
Queenie Carlyle Reed
Reagan Carlyle Coutant*
Recon Carlyle Garza*
Rita Carlyle Kronenberger
Sadie Bell Brady
Sadie Carlyle Burdick
Sadie Carlyle Reed
Sage Carlyle Foye
Sammie Chase
Sapphire Miller (†)
Sasha Carlyle Dyk*
Scotty Leigh Strax
Sebastian Miller (†)
Sedona Carlyle Dennis
Sheba Carlyle Jacobson
Skyla Carlyle Schroth
Sophe Carlyle Archer
Susi Bueso
Taco Carlyle Mashek
Tater Tot Castleberry
Teddy Carlyle Ellis

Teddy Schroth (†)
Tessa Carlyle Robinson
Thelma Carlyle Edlund
Theodore Carlyle Watson
Thomas Davis Noble*
Tigger Carlyle Brice
Tiggy Carlyle Plant (†)
Toby Schroth (†)

Toto Walker (†)
Travis Chase (†)
Tuffy Beman
Woody Carlyle Hindman
Zoe Carlyle Craft
Beau Carlyle Shields*
Bijou Carlyle Shields*
Bubba Carlyle Shields*

Junior Carlyle Shields

(†) = R.I.P.

Bold* = Dogs whose pictures were submitted for the Golden Anniversary Edition. Some pictures are featured at the end of selected chapters.

Dedicated to the ETFS AIP Chapter

In May 2023 my wife, Bettie, and I moved to an Eagle's Trace Retirement Community even though I have not retired. Much reduced pay, time, talent, and cognition but still not retired.

I identify Eagle's Trace as a finishing school (ETFS) in memory of my high school girlfriends who attended a finishing school to learn etiquette. It took me three attempts to pass an entrance examination to ETFS which had only two questions: (1) How much money do you have? (2) When can you send it?

Shortly after enrolling, one of my classmates noticed my bumper sticker.

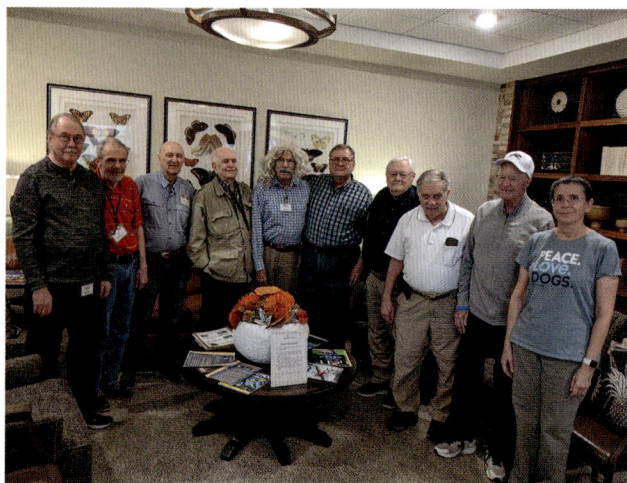

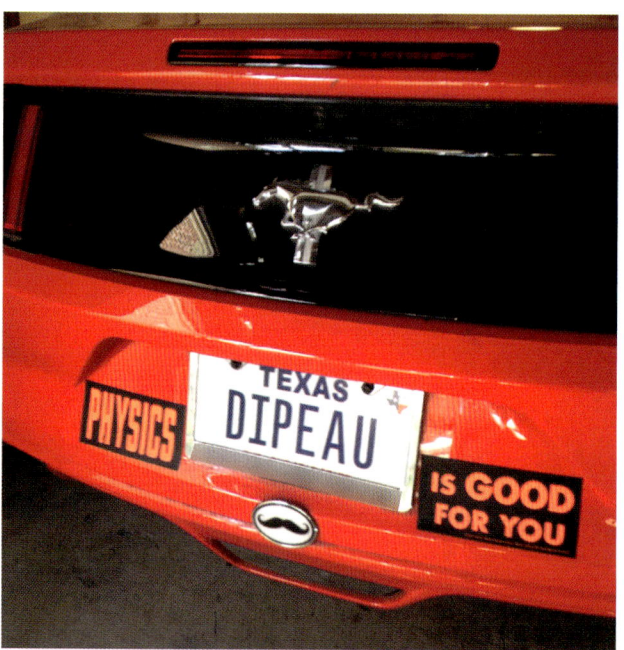

This is a photo of some of our chapter members who are from left to right: Mark Andersen, 1980, Johns Hopkins University; Robert Boyd, 1975, Warwick University; Hugh Scott, 1962, Manchester University; Joe Lovett, University of Pennsylvania; Stewart Bushong, 1966, University of Pittsburgh; Rich Weber, 1972, Carnegie Mellon University; Tom Thomas, 1959, University Kansas; Robert Hesse, 1969, St. Louis University; Edward Mercado, 1963, Rensselaer Polytechnique Institute; Ivanna Albertin, 1987, UC Berkeley.

I want to recognize and thank Rich Weber and Joe Lovette who were particularly helpful in drafting the new material of Part VI of this Golden Anniversary edition.

That resulted in the formation of the ETFS AIP Chapter. AIP is the American Institute of Physics, and there are now 23 members of our chapter.

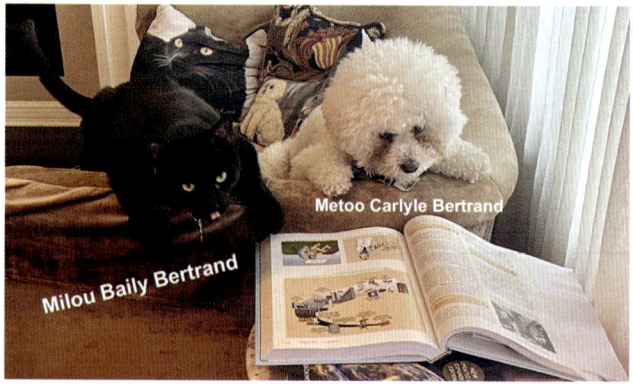

Preface

PURPOSE AND CONTENT

The purpose of *Bushong's Radiologic Science for Technologists: Physics, Biology, and Protection* is threefold: to convey a working knowledge of radiologic physics to prepare radiography students for the certification examination by the American Registry of Radiologic Technologists (ARRT) and to provide a base of knowledge from which practicing radiologic technologists can make informed decisions about technical factors, diagnostic image quality, and radiation management for both patients and personnel.

This textbook provides a solid presentation of radiologic science, including the fundamentals of radiologic physics, diagnostic imaging, radiobiology, and radiation management. The fundamentals of radiologic science cannot be removed from mathematics. The few mathematical equations presented here are always followed by sample problems with direct clinical application. As a further aid to learning, all mathematical formulas are highlighted with their own icon which follows:

Likewise, the most important ideas under discussion are presented with their own Penguin icon as follows:

This Golden Anniversary edition improves the popular feature of informational bullets by including even more key concepts and definitions in each chapter. This edition also presents learning objectives and chapter summaries that encourage students and make the texts user-friendly for all. Challenge Questions at the end of each chapter include definition exercises, short answer questions, and a few calculations. Answers to all questions are provided on the Elsevier site at http://evolve.elsevier.com.

HISTORICAL PERSPECTIVE

For decades after Roentgen's discovery of x-rays in 1895, diagnostic radiology remained a relatively stable field of study and practice. Truly great changes during that time can be counted on one hand: the Crookes tube, the radiographic grid, radiographic intensifying screens, and image intensification.

Since the publication of the first edition of this textbook in 1975, however, newer systems for diagnostic x-ray imaging have come into routine use: multislice helical computed tomography, tomosynthesis, digital radiography, and digital fluoroscopy. Truly spectacular advances in computer technology and image receptors have made these innovations possible.

NEW TO THIS EDITION

The chapters of this edition have been reorganized, consolidated, and updated to reflect the current educational and medical imaging environments, and manufacturer images have been updated.

Such updates involve descriptions of subjects that promise incredible acceleration of medical imaging—tomosynthesis, artificial intelligence (AI), quantum computing (qubits), and changes in radiation management. The expansion of the universe is accelerating and so is the expansion of radiologic science. The 13th edition includes new chapters on AI and quantum computing.

Preparing for this Golden Anniversary edition has been a very educational experience for me. I know the purpose of composing this textbook is to help you, the student, to understand this very difficult subject of physics and its application to imaging.

When I questioned the usefulness of a Summary at the end of each chapter, many reasons were given for not abandoning it. The most compelling reason that the Summary remains is to have you page to the end of each chapter first and read the Summary. That will give you a quick look and review of the deeper material you will encounter in the chapter.

For the first time, in this edition the glossary will appear on the Evolve website at http://evolve.elsevier.com.

ANCILLARIES

Workbook

This resource has been updated to reflect the changes in the text and their rapid advancements in the field of radiologic science, and it offers a complete selection of worksheets organized by textbook chapter.

Evolve Resources

Instructor ancillaries including an Exam Review test bank of over 900 questions, a collection of the images in the text, a PowerPoint presentation, and the glossary for the text are all available at http://evolve.elsevier.com.

Sherpath

Designed for the way students learn today, Sherpath is Elsevier's digital-first, personalized teaching and learning technology that delivers interconnected course content and tools in a single interface. Sherpath integrates into existing learning management systems and fully includes the ebook version of this text. Featuring adaptive quizzing, the Sherpath AI chat tool, customized remediation, assessments, and more, Sherpath's interactive environment boosts student engagement and appeals to all types of learners. A comprehensive performance dashboard will save you time and help you gauge student progress throughout the course to gain a holistic view of any topics of misconception or students who are struggling.

A NOTE ON THE TEXT

All scientific and radiological organizations have now formally adopted the international system of units (SI units) and they are used in this Golden Anniversary edition. With this system comes the corresponding units of radiation and radioactivity. The roentgen and the rad are replaced by the gray (Gy_a and Gy_t, respectively) and the rem by the sievert (Sv). I distinguish the measurement of radiation exposure from tissue dose by applying a subscript a or t to mGy. A summary of special quantities and units in radiologic science can be found on the inside covers of this textbook.

ACKNOWLEDGMENTS

For the preparation of this Golden Anniversary edition, I am indebted to the many readers of the previous editions who submitted criticisms, corrections, suggestions, and compliments.

I continue to be particularly indebted to the many educators identified earlier in this Golden Anniversary edition. Their suggestions for changes and clarifications were always right on target. Many of the recent responding educators supplied illustrations and suggestions for significant improvement, which you will see in this Golden Anniversary edition.

I am particularly indebted and thankful to Elizabeth Shields (Betsy to me) at the Novant Presbyterian Medical Center in Charlotte, North Carolina. Betsy and I were first acquainted many years ago when she suggested changes to slides that I used in an annual meeting of the North Carolina Society of Radiologic Technologists. Following that conversation, I asked for her continuous help in producing the graphical material for many of my presentations such as … To Shield or not To Shield (radiation protection), Are You a Robot (artificial intelligence), Medical Imaging Trifecta (protection, imaging, future), Build the Wall (radiation protection), and The Galloping Pace of Digital Imaging (imaging).

It was quickly apparent to me that an educator like Betsy, not a medical physicist, should be my coauthor positioned to continue this effort. Done, as you see on the cover of this Golden Anniversary edition. Betsy has much help in the physics of radiologic science at her institution and I am pleased that officially she has joined me in this effort.

Hopefully you will get another 50 years out of this project but I doubt it. There are incredible changes in education at every level at this time. The changes are not simply increasing, but accelerating. There is no hint of where we will be at the time of preparing the next edition.

As you, the student or educator, use this textbook as an educational tool and have questions or comments. Betsy invites you to e-mail her at esshields@novanthealth.org. Together you and she can continue to strive to make this very difficult material easier to learn and "Make Physics Fun." Thank you to so many, especially Betsy, for years of contribution to this book.

Stewart Carlyle Bushong

Contents

PART I
RADIOLOGIC PHYSICS, 1
1. Essential Concepts of Radiologic Science, 2
2. Basic Physics Primer, 17
3. The Structure of Matter, 34
4. Electromagnetic Energy, 53
5. Electricity, Magnetism, and Electromagnetism, 69

PART II
X-RADIATION, 91
6. The X-ray Imaging System, 92
7. The X-ray Tube, 111
8. X-ray Production, 129
9. X-ray Emission, 142
10. X-ray Interaction With Matter, 153

PART III
X-RAY IMAGING, 169
11. Computed Radiography, 170
12. Digital Radiography, 182
13. Digital Radiographic Technique, 189
14. Image Acquisition, 202
15. Scatter Radiation, 213
16. Digital Image Descriptors and Evaluation, 233
17. Radiographic Artifacts, 247

PART IV
ADVANCED MEDICAL IMAGING, 259
18. Mammography, 260
19. Fluoroscopy, 274
20. Interventional Radiology, 288
21. Computed Tomography, 305
22. Tomosynthesis, 331

PART V
MEDICAL IMAGE DISPLAY, 343
23. Patient-Image Optimization, 344
24. Viewing the Medical Image, 350
25. Medical Image Informatics, 360
26. Digital Display Device, 368

PART VI
THE MEDICAL IMAGE, 377
27. Imaging Science, 378
28. Artificial Intelligence, 395
29. Quantum Computing, 406
30. Image Perception, 417

PART VII
RADIOBIOLOGY, 427
31. Human Biology, 428
32. Fundamental Principles of Radiobiology, 441
33. Molecular Radiobiology, 449
34. Cellular Radiobiology, 456
35. Deterministic Effects of Radiation, 465
36. Stochastic Effects of Radiation, 481

PART VIII
RADIATION PROTECTION, 499
37. Health Physics, 500
38. Designing for Radiation Protection, 510
39. Radiography/Fluoroscopy Patient Radiation Dose, 527
40. Computed Tomography Patient Radiation Dose, 538
41. Patient Radiation Dose Management, 548
42. Occupational Radiation Dose Management, 559

Index, 576

PART I

RADIOLOGIC PHYSICS

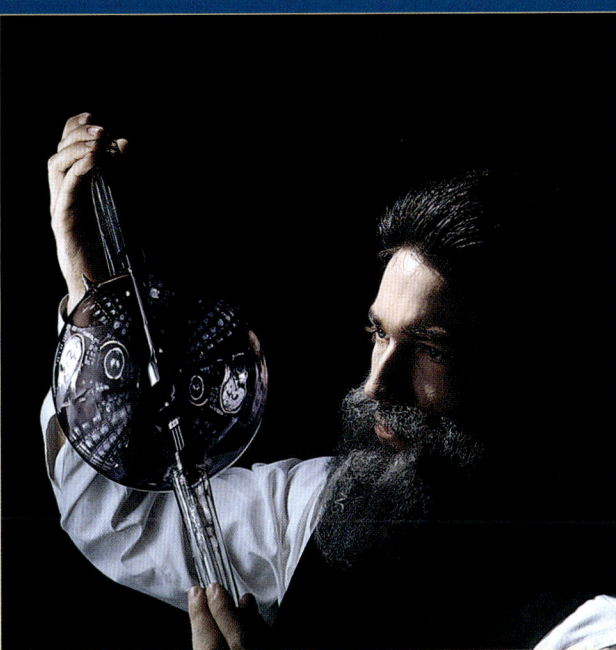

CHAPTER 1

Essential Concepts of Radiologic Science

OBJECTIVES

At the completion of this chapter, the student should be able to do the following:
1. Describe the characteristics of matter and energy.
2. Identify the various forms of energy.
3. Define electromagnetic radiation and ionizing radiation.
4. State the relative intensity of ionizing radiation from various sources.
5. List the concepts of basic radiation protection.
6. Discuss the derivation of scientific systems of measurement.
7. List and define units of radiation and radioactivity.

OUTLINE

Nature of Our Surroundings 3
Matter and Energy 3
Sources of Ionizing Radiation 5
Discovery of X-rays 6
Development of Medical
   Imaging 8
Reports of Radiation Injury 10
Basic Radiation Protection 10
   Protective Apparel 12
   Gonadal Shielding 12
Protective Barriers 12
Filtration 13
Collimation 13
Terminology for Radiologic
   Science 13
   Numeric Prefixes 13
   Radiologic Units 13
The Medical Imaging Team 15
Summary 15
Challenge Questions 15

THIS CHAPTER explores the basic concepts of the science and technology of x-ray imaging. These include the study of matter, energy, the electromagnetic spectrum, and ionizing radiation. The production and use of ionizing radiation as a diagnostic tool serve as the basis for radiography. Radiographers are healthcare professionals who deal specifically with x-ray imaging. Radiographers have a great responsibility to perform x-ray examinations in accordance with established radiation protection standards for the safety of patients and medical personnel.

The instant an x-ray tube produces x-rays, all the laws of physics are evident. The projectile electron from the cathode hits the target of the anode, producing x-rays. Some x-rays interact with tissue, and other x-rays interact with the image receptor, forming an image. The physics of radiography deals with the production and interaction of x-rays.

Radiography is a career choice with great opportunities in several diverse fields. Welcome to the field of medical imaging!

NATURE OF OUR SURROUNDINGS

In a physical analysis, all things can be classified as **matter** or **energy**. Matter is anything that occupies space and has **mass**. It is the material substance of which physical objects are composed. All matter is composed of fundamental building blocks called **atoms**, which are arranged in various complex ways. These atomic arrangements are considered at great length in Chapter 3.

A primary distinguishing characteristic of matter is **mass**, the quantity of matter contained in any physical object. We generally use the term **weight** when describing the mass of an object, and, for our purposes, we may consider mass and weight to be the same. Remember, however, that in the strictest sense they are not the same. Mass is actually described by its energy equivalence, whereas weight is the force exerted on a body under the influence of gravity.

Mass is measured in kilograms (kg). For example, on Earth, a 200-lb (91-kg) male weighs more than a 120-lb (55-kg) female. This occurs because of the mutual attraction, called **gravity**, between Earth's mass and the mass of the male and female. On the Moon, a person would weigh only about one-sixth of what they weigh on Earth because the mass of the Moon is much less than that of the Earth. However, the mass of the male and female remains unchanged at 91 and 55 kg, respectively.

 Mass is the quantity of matter as described by its energy equivalence.

MATTER AND ENERGY

Matter is anything that occupies space. It is the material substance having mass of which physical objects are composed. The fundamental complex building blocks of matter are atoms and molecules. The **kilogram**, the International System (SI) unit of mass, is unrelated to gravitational effects. The prefix kilo stands for 1000; a kilogram (kg) is equal to 1000 g.

Although mass, the quantity of matter, remains unchanged regardless of its state, it can be transformed from one size and shape into another. Consider a 1-kg

 A PENGUIN TALE BY BENJAMIN RIPLEY ARCHER, PHD

In the vast expanse of the Antarctic region, there was once a great, beautiful, isolated iceberg floating in the serene sea. Because of its location and accessibility, the great iceberg became a mecca for penguins from the entire area. As more and more penguins flocked to their new home and began to cover the slopes of the ice field, the iceberg began to sink farther and farther into the sea. Penguins kept climbing on, forcing others off the iceberg and back into the ocean. Soon the iceberg became nearly submerged owing to the sheer number of penguins that attempted to take up residence there.

Moral: The **Penguin** represents an important fact or bit of information that we must learn to understand a subject. The brain, similar to the iceberg, can retain only so much information before it becomes overloaded. When this happens, concepts begin to become dislodged, like penguins from the sinking iceberg. So, the key to learning is to reserve space for true "penguins" to fill the valuable and limited confines of our brains. Thus key points in this book are highlighted and referred to as "**Penguins**."

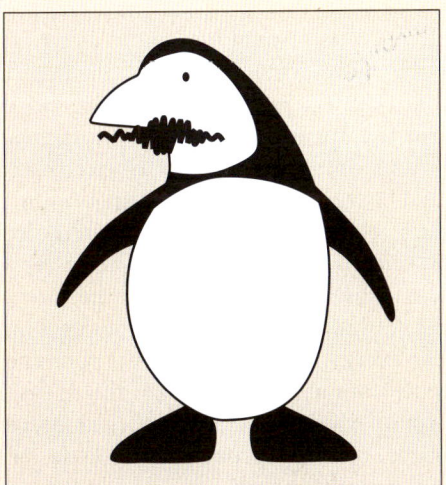

block of ice, whose shape changes as the block of ice melts into a puddle of water. If the puddle is allowed to dry, the water apparently disappears entirely. However, we know that the ice is transformed from a solid state to a liquid state and that liquid water becomes water vapor suspended in air. If we could gather all the molecules that make up the ice, the water, and the water vapor and measure their masses, we would find that each form has the same mass.

Similar to matter, energy can exist in several forms. The SI unit for energy is **joule (J)**. In radiology, the unit electron volt (eV) is often used.

Potential energy is the ability to do work by virtue of position. A guillotine blade held aloft by a rope and pulley is an example of an object that possesses potential energy (Fig. 1.1). If the rope is cut, the blade will descend and do its ghastly task. Work is required to get the blade to its high position, and because of this position, the blade is said to possess potential energy. Other examples of objects that possess potential energy include a rollercoaster on top of an incline and the stretched spring of an open screen door.

 Energy is the ability to do work.

Kinetic energy is the energy of motion. It is possessed by all matter in motion: a moving automobile, a turning windmill wheel, and a falling guillotine blade. These systems can all do work because of their motion.

Chemical energy is the energy released by a chemical reaction. An important example of this type of energy is that which is provided to our bodies through chemical reactions involving the foods we eat. At the molecular level, this area of science is called **biochemistry**. The energy released when dynamite explodes is a more dramatic example of chemical energy.

Electrical energy represents the work that can be done when an electron moves through an electric potential difference (voltage). The most familiar form of electrical energy is normal household electricity, which involves the movement of electrons through a copper wire by an electric potential difference of 110 volts (V). All electric apparatus, such as motors, heaters, and blowers, function through the use of electrical energy.

Thermal energy (heat) is the energy of motion at the molecular level. It is the kinetic energy of molecules and is closely related to temperature. The faster the molecules of a substance are vibrating, the more thermal energy the substance has and the higher its temperature.

Nuclear energy is the energy that is contained within the nucleus of an atom. We control the release and use of this type of energy in electric nuclear power plants. An example of the uncontrolled release of nuclear energy is the atomic bomb.

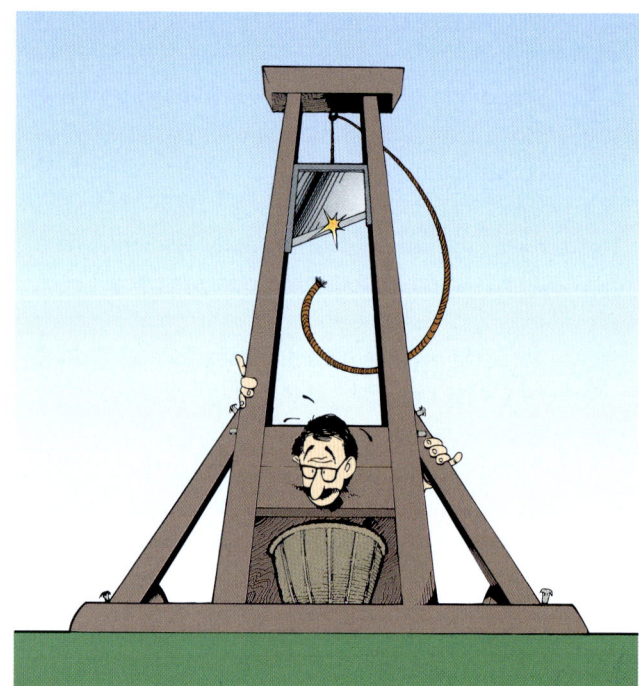

FIG. 1.1 The blade of a guillotine offers a dramatic example of both potential and kinetic energy. When the blade is pulled to its maximum height and locked into place, it has potential energy. When the blade is allowed to fall, the potential energy is released as kinetic energy.

Electromagnetic energy is perhaps the least familiar form of energy. However, it is the most important for our purposes because it is the type of energy that is used in x-ray imaging. The energy traveling through space is a combination of electric and magnetic fields. In addition to x-rays and gamma rays, electromagnetic energy includes radio waves; microwaves; and ultraviolet, infrared, and visible light. Electromagnetic energy does not include sound or diagnostic ultrasound.

Just as matter can be transformed from one size, shape, and form to another, energy can be transformed from one type to another. In radiology, for example, electrical energy in the x-ray imaging system is used to produce electromagnetic energy (the x-ray), which is then converted to an electrical signal in a digital image receptor (IR).

Reconsider now the statement that all things can be classified as matter or energy. Look around you and think of absolutely anything, and you should be convinced of this statement. You should be able to classify anything as matter, energy, or both. Frequently, matter and energy exist side by side—a moving automobile has mass and kinetic energy; boiling water has mass and thermal energy; the Leaning Tower of Pisa has mass and potential energy.

Perhaps the strangest property associated with matter and energy is that they are interchangeable, a characteristic first described by Albert Einstein in his famous theory of relativity. Einstein's **mass-energy** equivalence equation is a cornerstone of that theory.

This mass-energy equivalence serves as the basis for the atomic bomb, nuclear power plants, and certain nuclear medicine imaging modalities.

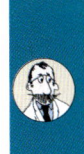

MASS-ENERGY
$E = mc^2$
where E is energy, m is mass, and c is the velocity (speed) of electromagnetic radiation (light) in a vacuum.

The energy emitted and transferred through space is called **radiation**. When a piano string vibrates, it is said to radiate sound; the sound is a form of radiation. Ripples or waves radiate from the point where a pebble is dropped into a still pond. Visible light, a form of electromagnetic energy, is radiated by the Sun and is called **electromagnetic radiation**. Electromagnetic energy is usually referred to as electromagnetic radiation or, simply, **radiation**.

Matter that intercepts radiation and absorbs part or all of it is said to be exposed or **irradiated**. Spending a day at the beach exposes you to ultraviolet light. Ultraviolet light is the type of radiation that causes sunburn. During a radiographic examination, the patient is exposed to x-rays. The patient is said to be irradiated.

Radiation is the transfer of energy.

Ionizing radiation is a special type of radiation that includes x-rays. Ionizing radiation is any type of radiation that is capable of removing an orbital electron from the atom with which it interacts (Fig. 1.2). This type of interaction between radiation and matter is called **ionization**. Ionization occurs when an x-ray passes close to an orbital electron of an atom and transfers sufficient energy to the electron to remove it from the atom. The ionizing radiation may interact with and ionize additional atoms. The orbital electron and the atom from which it was separated are called an **ion pair**. The electron is a negative ion, and the remaining atom is a positive ion.

Ionization is the removal of an electron from an atom.

Thus any type of energy capable of ionizing matter is known as ionizing radiation. X-rays, gamma rays, and ultraviolet light are the only forms of electromagnetic radiation with sufficient energy to ionize. Some fast-moving particles (particles with high kinetic energy) are also capable of ionization. Examples of particle-type ionizing radiation are alpha and beta particles (see Chapter 3). Although alpha and beta particles are sometimes called rays, this designation is incorrect.

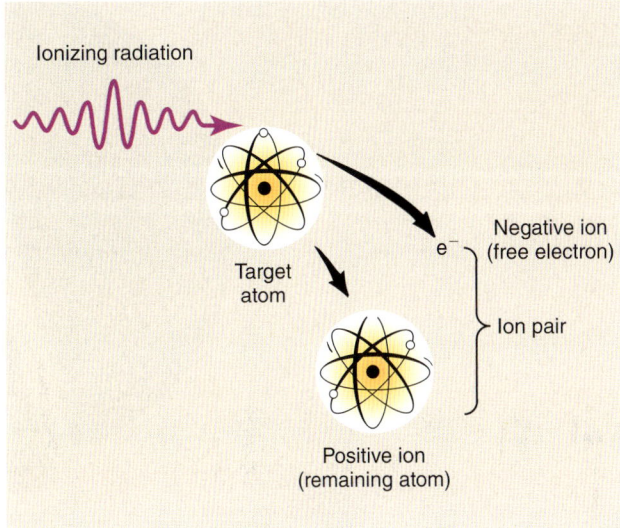

FIG. 1.2 Ionization is the removal of an electron from an atom. The ejected electron and the resulting positively charged atom together are called an ion pair.

SOURCES OF IONIZING RADIATION

Many types of radiation are harmless, but ionizing radiation can injure humans. We are exposed to many sources of ionizing radiation. The sources are divided into two broad categories: **ubiquitous background radiation** and **human-made radiation**. Annually, a US citizen is exposed to an average radiation dose of 6.2 millisieverts (mSv).

Ubiquitous background radiation consists of four subcategories: **cosmic rays, terrestrial radiation, internally deposited radionuclides**, and **radon**. Ubiquitous background radiation results in an annual dose of approximately 3.1 mSv. The mSv is the SI unit of effective dose. It is used to express the radiation exposure of populations and radiation risk in those populations. Fig. 1.3 depicts the distribution of ubiquitous background radiation doses. Cosmic rays are particulate and electromagnetic radiation emitted by the Sun and stars. On Earth, the intensity of cosmic radiation increases with altitude and latitude. Terrestrial radiation results from deposits of uranium, thorium, and other radionuclides on the Earth. The intensity is highly dependent on the geology of the local area. Internally deposited radionuclides, mainly potassium-40 (^{40}K), are natural metabolites. They have always been with us and contribute an equal dose to each of us.

The largest source of ubiquitous background radiation is radon. Radon is a radioactive gas that is produced by the natural radioactive decay of uranium,

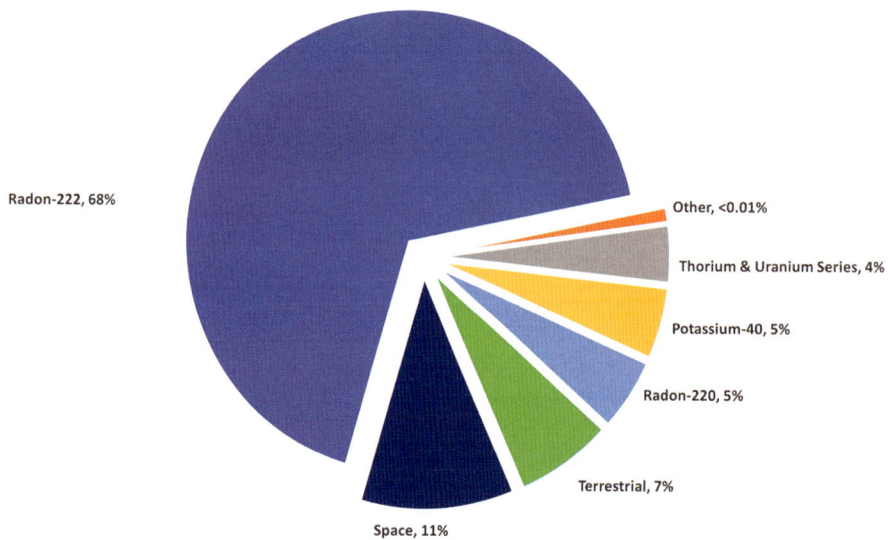

FIG. 1.3 Source distribution of ubiquitous background radiation dose to the US population. (With permission of the National Council on Radiation Protection and Measurements. http://NCRPonline.org.)

which is present in trace quantities on Earth. All Earth-based materials, such as concrete, bricks, and gypsum wallboard, contain radon. Radon emits alpha particles, which are not penetrating and therefore contribute radiation dose only to the lung.

Humans have existed for several hundred thousand years in the presence of this ubiquitous background radiation, and human evolution undoubtedly has been influenced by this radiation. Some geneticists contend that evolution is influenced primarily by ionizing radiation. If this is so, then we must indeed be concerned with the control of unnecessary radiation exposure because over the past century, with increasing medical applications of radiation, the average annual exposure of our population to radiation has increased significantly.

Human-made radiation sources include medical radiation; consumer products; industrial, security, educational, or research facilities using radioactive material; and occupational sources to certain categories of workers. Consumer product sources include smoke detectors, lantern mantles, fluorescent lamp starters, tritium gun sights and watches, tobacco, televisions, and building materials.

By far, the most significant source of human-made radiation is diagnostic and interventional medical radiation. Like ubiquitous background radiation, this dose is not evenly distributed across the population. People with health issues receive the majority of doses. The US annual individual effective dose from diagnostic and interventional medical radiation was estimated at 0.53 mSv in the 1980s and ~3.0 mSv in 2006. These estimates were made by the National Council on Radiation Protection and Measurements (NCRP). The sixfold increase between the 1980s and 2006 was principally attributable to the increased use of computed tomography (CT).

In 2019, the NCRP published an update on the diagnostic and interventional medical radiation exposure in the US from 2006 to 2016. The update reported there was a substantial reduction, ~15% to 20% in the annual dose to the US population in the decade, to ~2.3 mSv. Technological advances in imaging equipment, as well as awareness campaigns, Image Gently and Image Wisely, have led to this drop. Fig. 1.4 depicts the percentage of annual effective dose from different modalities of diagnostic and interventional medical radiation from 2006 to 2016.

The benefits derived from the application of x-rays in medicine are indisputable; however, such applications must be made with prudence and with care taken to reduce unnecessary exposure of patients and personnel. This responsibility falls primarily on radiographers because they usually control the operation of x-ray imaging systems during radiologic examinations.

DISCOVERY OF X-RAYS

X-rays were not developed; they were discovered quite by accident. During the 1870s and 1880s, physics laboratories from many universities were investigating the conduction of cathode rays through a large, partially evacuated glass tube known as a Crookes tube. Sir William Crookes was an Englishman from a relatively

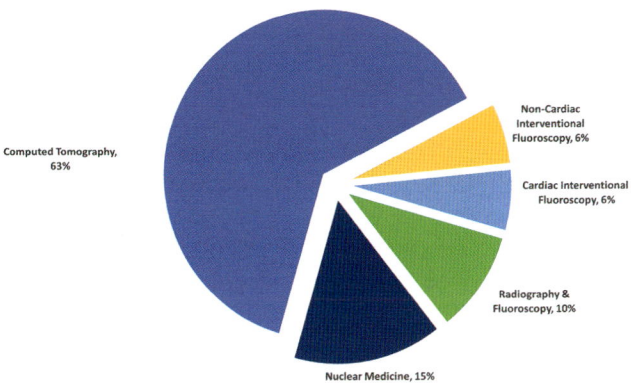

FIG. 1.4 Percentage of diagnostic and interventional medical radiation dose from different modalities. (With permission of the National Council on Radiation Protection and Measurements, http://NCRPonline.org.)

humble background who was a self-taught genius.

The tube that bears his name was the forerunner of modern fluorescent lamps and x-ray tubes. There were many different types of Crookes tubes, most of which were capable of producing x-rays. Wilhelm Roentgen was experimenting with a type of Crookes tube when he discovered x-rays (Fig. 1.5).

On November 8, 1895, Roentgen was working in his physics laboratory at Würzburg University in Germany. He had darkened his laboratory and completely enclosed his Crookes tube with black photographic paper so he could better visualize the effects of the cathode rays in the tube. A plate coated with **barium platinocyanide**, a fluorescent material, was lying on a bench top several meters from the Crookes tube.

No visible light escaped from the Crookes tube because of the black paper that enclosed it, but Roentgen noted that the barium platinocyanide glowed. The intensity of the glow increased as the plate was brought closer to the tube; consequently, there was little doubt about the origin of the stimulus of the glow. This glow is called **fluorescence**.

Roentgen's immediate approach to investigating this "X-light," as he called it, was to interpose various materials—wood, aluminum, his hand!—between the Crookes tube and the fluorescing plate. The "X" was for unknown. He feverishly continued these investigations for several weeks.

Roentgen's initial investigations were extremely thorough, and he was able to report his experimental results to the scientific community before the end of 1895 (Table 1.1). For this work, he received the first Nobel Prize in Physics in 1901.

Roentgen recognized the value of his discovery in medicine. He produced and published the first x-ray image in early 1896. It was an image of his wife's hand (Fig. 1.6). Fig. 1.7 is a photograph of what is reported to be the first medical x-ray examination in the United States, conducted in early February 1896, in the physics laboratory at Dartmouth College.

The discovery of x-rays is characterized by many amazing features, and this causes it to rank high among

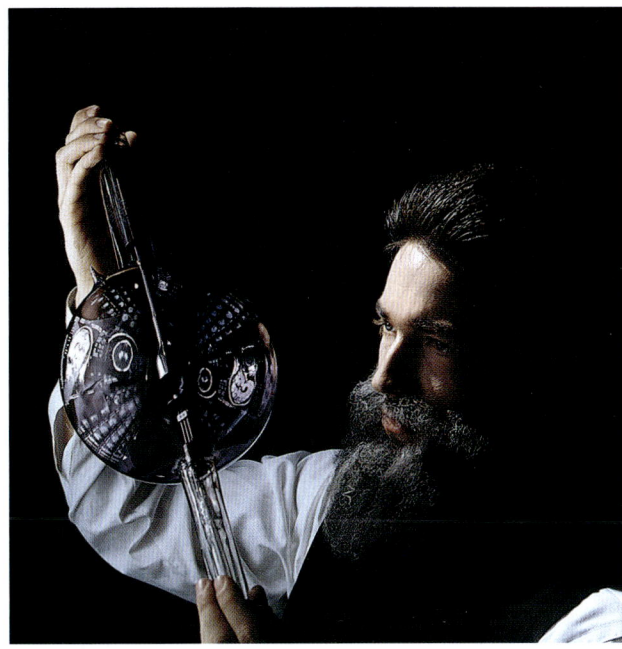

FIG. 1.5 The type of Crookes tube Roentgen used when he discovered x-rays. Cathode rays (electrons) leaving the cathode are attracted by high voltage to the anode, where they produce x-rays and fluorescent light. (Courtesy Gary Leach, Memorial Hermann Hospital.)

TABLE 1.1	Roentgen's Original Properties of X-rays
1.	X-rays are highly penetrating invisible rays that are a form of electromagnetic radiation.
2.	X-rays are electrically neutral and therefore not affected by either electric or magnetic fields.
3.	X-rays can be produced over a wide variety of energies and wavelengths.
4.	X-rays release very small amounts of heat when passing through matter.
5.	X-rays travel in straight lines.
6.	X-rays travel at the speed of light, 3×10^8 m/s, in a vacuum.
7.	X-rays can ionize matter.
8.	X-rays cause fluorescence of certain crystals.
9.	X-rays cannot be focused by a lens.
10.	X-rays affect photographic film.
11.	X-rays produce chemical and biological changes in matter through ionization and excitation.
12.	X-rays produce secondary and scattering radiation.

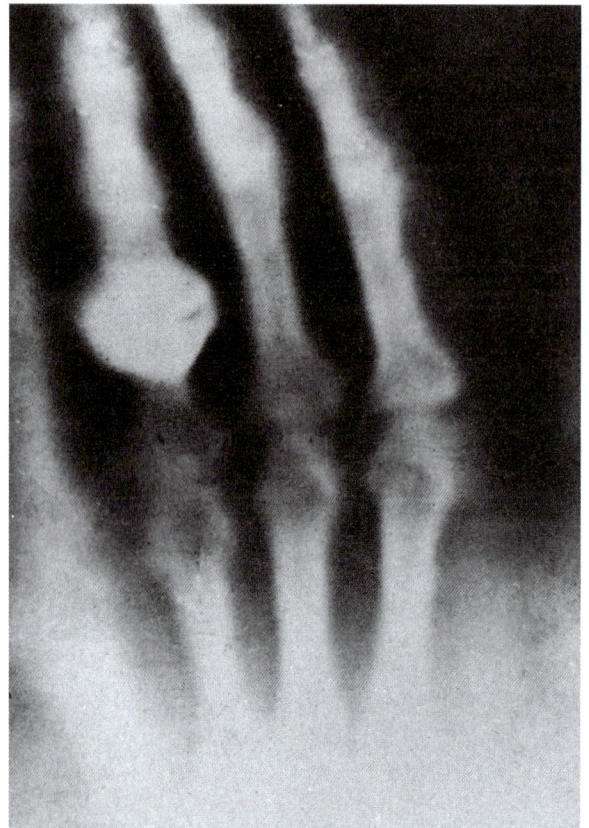

FIG. 1.6 The hand shown in this radiograph belongs to Mrs. Roentgen. This first indication of the possible medical applications of x-rays was made within a few days of the discovery. (Courtesy Deutsches Roentgen Museum.)

the events in human history. First, the discovery was accidental. Second, probably no fewer than a dozen contemporaries of Roentgen had previously observed x-radiation, but none of these other physicists had recognized its significance or investigated it. Third, Roentgen followed his discovery with such scientific vigor that within little more than 1 month, he had described x-radiation with nearly all of the properties we currently recognize.

DEVELOPMENT OF MEDICAL IMAGING

There are three general types of x-ray examinations: radiography, fluoroscopy, and computed tomography (CT). Radiography uses a solid-state image receptor (IR) and usually an x-ray tube mounted from the ceiling on a track that allows the tube to be moved in any direction. Such examinations provide the radiologist with fixed images.

Fluoroscopy is usually conducted with an x-ray tube located under the examination table supporting the patient. The radiologist is provided with moving images on a digital display device.

CT uses a rotating x-ray source and detector array. A volume of data is acquired so that fixed images can be reconstructed in any anatomic plane—coronal, sagittal, transverse, or oblique.

There are many variations of these three basic types of examinations, but in general, x-ray imaging equipment is similar.

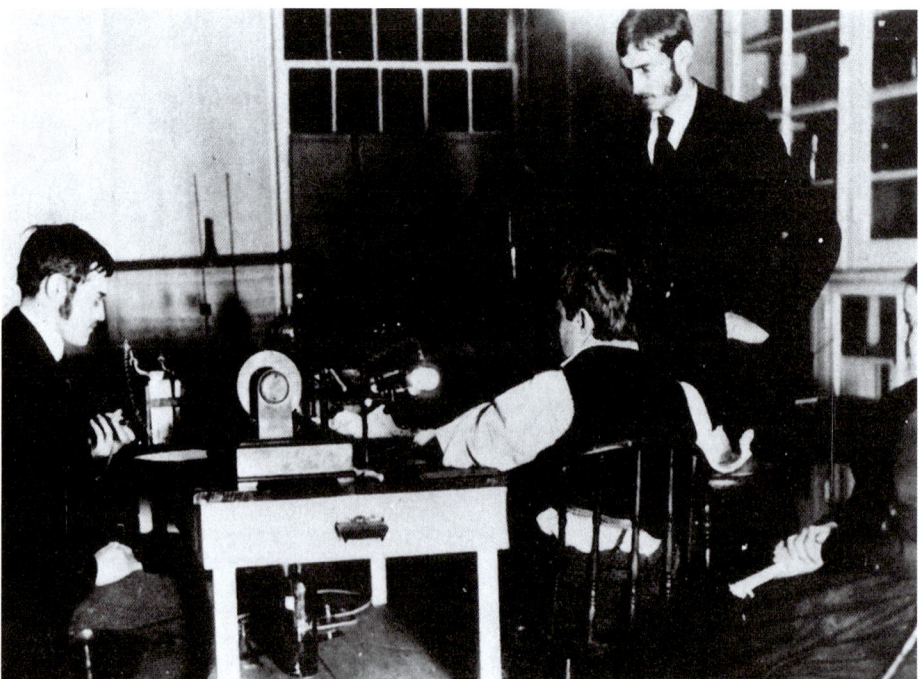

FIG. 1.7 This photograph records the first medical x-ray examination in the United States. A young patient, Eddie McCarthy, broke his wrist while skating on the Connecticut River and submitted to having it photographed by the "X-light." With him are (*left to right*) Professor E.B. Frost, Dartmouth College, and his brother, Dr. G.D. Frost, Medical Director, Mary Hitchcock Hospital. The apparatus was assembled by Professor F.G. Austin in his physics laboratory at Reed Hall, Dartmouth College, on February 3, 1896. (Courtesy Mary Hitchcock Hospital.)

To provide an x-ray beam that is satisfactory for imaging, you must supply the x-ray tube with a high voltage and an electric current.

X-ray voltages are measured in kilovolt peak (**kVp**). One kilovolt (**kV**) is equal to 1000 V of electric potential. X-ray currents are measured in milliamperes (**mA**), where the ampere (A) is a measure of electric current. The prefix **milli** stands for 1/1000 or 0.001.

Question: The usual x-ray source-to-image receptor distance during radiography is 1 m. How many millimeters is that?
Answer: 1 mm = 1/1000 m or 10^{-3} m; therefore 1 m = 1000 mm.

Currently, voltage and current are supplied to an x-ray tube through rather complicated electric circuits, but in Roentgen's time, only simple static generators were available. These units could provide currents of only a few milliamperes and voltages up to 50 kVp. Currently, 1000 mA and 150 kVp are commonly used.

Early radiographic procedures often required exposure times of 30 minutes or longer. Long exposure time resulted in image blur. One development that helped reduce this exposure time was the use of a fluorescent intensifying screen in conjunction with glass photographic plates.

Michael Pupin is said to have demonstrated the use of a radiographic intensifying screen in 1896, but only many years later did it receive adequate recognition and use. Radiographs during Roentgen's time were made by exposing a glass plate with a layer of photographic emulsion coated on one side.

Charles L. Leonard found that by exposing two glass x-ray plates with the emulsion surfaces together, the exposure time was halved, and the image was considerably enhanced. This demonstration of double-emulsion radiography was conducted in 1904, but **double-emulsion film** did not become commercially available until 1918.

Much of the high-quality glass used in radiography came from Belgium and other European countries. This supply was interrupted during World War I; therefore radiologists began to make use of film rather than glass plates.

The demands of the US Army for increased radiologic services made a substitute for the glass plate necessary. The substitute was **cellulose nitrate**, and it quickly became apparent that the substitute was better than the original glass plate. Fire hazards associated with the storage of cellulose nitrate film led to the development of cellulose acetate film, known as "safety film," in the 1920s. Polyester plastic, with dimensional stability, replaced cellulose acetate as the base for x-ray film in 1960.

The **fluoroscope** was developed in 1898 by the American inventor Thomas A. Edison (Fig. 1.8). Edison's original fluorescent material was barium platinocyanide, a

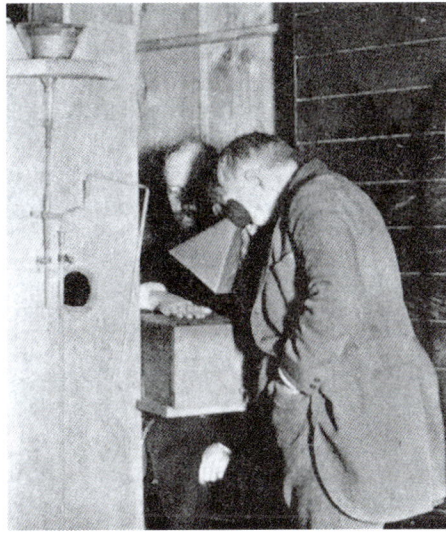

FIG. 1.8 Thomas Edison is seen viewing the hand of his unfortunate assistant, Clarence Dally, through a fluoroscope of his own design. Dally's hand rests on the box that contains the x-ray tube.

widely used laboratory material. He investigated the fluorescent properties of more than 1800 other materials, including **zinc cadmium sulfide** and **calcium tungstate**—two materials currently in use.

There is no telling what additional inventions Edison might have developed had he continued his x-ray research, but he abandoned it when his assistant and long-time friend, Clarence Dally, experienced a severe x-ray burn that eventually required amputation of both arms. Dally died in 1904 and is counted as the first x-ray fatality in the United States.

Two devices designed to reduce the exposure of patients to x-rays and thereby minimize the possibility of x-ray burn were introduced before the turn of the 20th century by a Boston dentist, William Rollins. Rollins used x-rays to image teeth and found that restricting the x-ray beam with a sheet of lead with a hole in the center, a **diaphragm**, and inserting a leather or aluminum filter improved the diagnostic quality of radiographs.

This first application of **collimation** and **filtration** was followed very slowly by the general adoption of these techniques. It was later recognized that these devices reduce the hazard associated with x-rays.

Two developments that occurred at approximately the same time transformed the use of x-rays from a novelty in the hands of a few physicists into a valuable, large-scale medical specialty. In 1907 H.C. Snook introduced a substitute high-voltage power supply, an interrupterless **transformer**, for the static machines and induction coils then in use.

Although the Snook transformer was far superior to these other devices, its capability greatly exceeded the capability of the Crookes tube. It was not until the introduction of the Coolidge tube that the Snook transformer was widely adopted.

The type of Crookes tube that Roentgen used in 1895 had existed for several years. Although some modifications were made by x-ray workers, it remained essentially unchanged into the second decade of the 20th century.

After considerable clinical testing, William D. Coolidge unveiled his hot-cathode x-ray tube to the medical community in 1913. It was immediately recognized as far superior to the Crookes tube. It was a vacuum tube that allowed x-ray intensity and energy to be selected separately and with great accuracy. This had not been possible with gas-filled tubes, which made standards for techniques difficult to obtain. X-ray tubes in use today are refinements of the **Coolidge tube**.

Radiology emerged as a medical specialty because of the Snook transformer and the Coolidge x-ray tube.

The era of modern radiography dates back to the matching of the Coolidge tube with the Snook transformer; only then did acceptable kVp and mA levels become possible. Few developments since then have had such a major influence on medical imaging.

In 1913, Gustav Bucky (German) invented the stationary **grid** ("Glitterblende"); 2 months later, he applied for a second patent for a moving grid. In 1915 Hollis Potter (American), probably unaware of Bucky's patent because of World War I, also invented a moving grid. To his credit, Potter recognized Bucky's work, and the Potter-Bucky grid was introduced in 1921.

In 1946 the light amplifier tube was demonstrated at Bell Telephone Laboratories. This device was adapted for fluoroscopy by 1950 as an image intensifier tube. Currently, image-intensified fluoroscopy is being replaced by solid-state IRs.

Each recent decade has seen remarkable improvements in medical imaging. Diagnostic ultrasonography appeared in the 1960s, as did the gamma camera. Positron emission tomography and x-ray CT were developed in the 1970s. Magnetic resonance imaging (MRI) became an accepted modality in the 1980s, and currently digital radiography and digital fluoroscopy have replaced screen-film radiography and image-intensified fluoroscopy. Table 1.2 chronologically summarizes some of the more important developments.

REPORTS OF RADIATION INJURY

The first x-ray fatality in the United States occurred in 1904. Unfortunately, radiation injuries occurred rather frequently in the early years. These injuries usually took the form of skin damage (sometimes severe), loss of hair, and anemia. Physicians and, more commonly, patients were injured, primarily because the low energy of radiation then available resulted in the necessity for long exposure times to obtain acceptable images.

By about 1910, these acute injuries began to be controlled as the biological effects of x-rays were scientifically investigated and reported. With the introduction of the Coolidge tube and the Snook transformer, the frequency of reports of injuries to superficial tissues decreased.

Years later, it was discovered that blood disorders such as aplastic anemia and leukemia were occurring in radiologists at a much higher rate than in others. Because of these observations, protective devices and apparel, such as lead gloves and aprons, were developed for use by radiologists. X-ray workers were routinely observed for any effects of their occupational exposure and were provided with personnel radiation monitoring devices. This attention to radiation safety in radiology has been effective.

Because of effective radiation protection practices, radiology is now considered a safe occupation.

BASIC RADIATION PROTECTION

Today, the emphasis on radiation control in diagnostic radiology has shifted back to the protection of patients. Current studies suggest that even the low doses of x-rays used in routine diagnostic procedures may result in a small incidence of latent harmful effects. It is also well established that human fetuses are sensitive to x-rays early in pregnancy.

It is hoped that this introduction has emphasized the importance of providing adequate protection for both radiographers and patients. As you progress through your training in radiologic technology, you will quickly learn how to operate your x-ray imaging systems safely, with minimal radiation exposure, by following standard radiation protection procedures.

One caution is in order early in your training—after you have worked with x-ray imaging systems, you will become so familiar with your work environment that you may become complacent about radiation control. Do not allow yourself to develop this attitude because it can lead to unnecessary radiation exposure. Radiation protection must be an important consideration during each x-ray procedure. Table 1.3 reports the Ten Commandments of Radiation Protection.

Always practice ALARA. Keep radiation exposures **A**s **L**ow **A**s **R**easonably **A**chievable.

Minimizing radiation exposure to radiographers and patients is easy if the x-ray imaging systems designed for this purpose are recognized and understood. A brief description of some of the primary radiation protection devices follows.

TABLE 1.2 Important Dates in the Development of Modern Radiology

Date	Event
1895	Roentgen discovers x-rays.
1896	First medical applications of x-rays in diagnosis and therapy are made.
1900	The American Roentgen Society, the first American radiology organization, is founded.
1901	Roentgen receives the first Nobel Prize in Physics.
1905	Einstein introduces his theory of relativity and the famous equation $E = mc^2$.
1907	The Snook interrupterless transformer is introduced.
1913	Bohr theorizes his model of the atom, featuring a nucleus and planetary electrons.
1913	The Coolidge hot-filament x-ray tube is developed.
1917	The cellulose nitrate film base is widely adopted.
1920	Several investigators demonstrate the use of soluble iodine compounds as contrast media.
1920	The American Society of Radiologic Technologists is founded.
1921	The Potter-Bucky grid is introduced.
1922	Compton describes the scattering of x-rays.
1923	Cellulose acetate "safety" x-ray film is introduced (Eastman Kodak).
1925	The First International Congress of Radiology is convened in London.
1928	The roentgen is defined as the unit of x-ray intensity.
1929	Forssmann demonstrates cardiac catheterization … on himself!
1929	The rotating anode x-ray tube is introduced.
1930	Tomographic devices are shown by several independent investigators.
1932	Blue tint is added to x-ray film (DuPont).
1932	The US Committee on X-Ray and Radium Protection (now the National Council on Radiation Protection and Measurements [NCRP]) issues the first dose limits.
1942	Morgan exhibits an electronic photo-timing device.
1942	The first automatic film processor (Pako) is introduced.
1948	Coltman develops the first fluoroscopic image intensifier.
1951	Multidirectional tomography (polytomography) is introduced.
1953	The rad is officially adopted as the unit of absorbed dose.
1956	Xeroradiography is demonstrated.
1956	First automatic roller transport film processing (Eastman Kodak) is introduced.
1960	Polyester base film is introduced (DuPont).
1963	Kuhl and Edwards demonstrate single-photon emission computed tomography.
1965	Ninety-second rapid processor is introduced (Eastman Kodak).
1966	Diagnostic ultrasonography enters routine use.
1973	Hounsfield completes the development of first computed tomography (CT) imaging system Electric and Musical Industries (EMI).
1973	Damadian and Lauterbur produce the first magnetic resonance image (MRI).
1974	Rare earth radiographic intensifying screens are introduced.
1977	Mistretta demonstrates digital subtraction fluoroscopy.
1979	The Nobel Prize in Physiology or Medicine is awarded to Allan Cormack and Godfrey Hounsfield for CT.
1980	The first commercial superconducting MRI system is introduced.
1981	Slot-scan chest radiography is demonstrated by Barnes.
1981	The International System of Units (SI) is adopted by the International Commission on Radiation Units and Measurements.
1982	Picture Archiving and Communication System becomes available.
1984	Laser-stimulable phosphors for computed radiography appear (Fuji).
1988	A superconducting quantum interference device for magnetoencephalography is first used.
1989	The SI is adopted by the NCRP and most scientific and medical societies.
1990	Helical CT is introduced (Toshiba).
1991	Twin-slice CT is developed (Elscint).
1992	The Mammography Quality Standard Acts is passed.
1996	Digital radiography that uses thin-film transistors is developed.
1997	Charge-coupled device digital radiography is introduced by Swissray.
1997	Amorphous selenium flat panel image receptor is demonstrated by Rowlands.
1998	Multislice CT is introduced (General Electric).
1998	Amorphous silicon-CsI image receptor is demonstrated for digital radiography.
2000	The first direct digital mammographic imaging system is made available (General Electric).
2002	Sixteen-slice helical CT is introduced.
2002	Positron emission tomography is placed into routine clinical service.
2003	The Nobel Prize in Physiology or Medicine is awarded to Paul Lauterbur and Sir Peter Mansfield for MRI.
2003	Digital radiographic tomosynthesis is demonstrated.
2004	The 64-slice helical CT is introduced.
2005	Dual-source CT is announced (Siemens).
2007	The 320-slice helical CT is introduced (Toshiba).
2009	NCRP Report No. 160, *Ionizing radiation exposure of the population of the United States: 2006*, is published.
2011	Digital mammographic tomosynthesis is clinically approved.
2012	The Nobel Prize in Physics is awarded for superposition and entanglement.
2017	3D printers and segmentation algorithms expand CT and MRI applications.
2018	Artificial intelligence appears in special journals and meetings.
2023	Open AI releases the first Large Language Model, ChatGPT.
2023	The Nobel Prize in Physics is awarded for attosecond quantum tunneling.

TABLE 1.3	The Ten Commandments of Radiation Protection

1. Understand and apply the cardinal principles of radiation control: time, distance, and shielding.
2. Do not allow familiarity to result in false security.
3. Never stand in the primary beam.
4. Always wear protective apparel when not behind a protective barrier.
5. Always wear an occupational radiation monitor and position it outside the protective apron at the collar.
6. Never hold a patient during a radiographic examination. Use mechanical restraining devices when possible. Otherwise, have family or friends hold the patient.
7. The person who is holding the patient must always wear a protective apron and, if possible, protective gloves.
8. Use gonadal shields on all people of childbearing age or younger when such use will not interfere with the examination.
9. Examination of the pelvis and lower abdomen of pregnant patients should be avoided whenever possible, especially during the first trimester.
10. Always collimate to the smallest field size appropriate for the examination.

Protective Apparel
Lead-impregnated material is used to make aprons and gloves worn by radiologists and radiographers during fluoroscopy and some radiographic procedures.

Gonadal Shielding
The same lead-impregnated material used in aprons and gloves is used to fabricate gonadal shields. Gonadal shields should be used with all persons of childbearing age or younger when the gonads are near the useful x-ray beam and when the use of such shielding will not interfere with the diagnostic value of the examination.

Protective Barriers
The radiographic or CT control console is always located behind a protective barrier. Often, the barrier is lead lined and is equipped with a leaded glass window. Under normal circumstances, personnel remain behind the barrier during x-ray examination. Fig. 1.9 is a rendering of a radiographic and fluoroscopic examination room. Many radiation safety features are illustrated.

Other procedures should be followed. Abdominal and pelvic x-ray examinations of expectant mothers should not be conducted during the first trimester unless absolutely necessary. Every effort should be made to ensure that an examination will not have

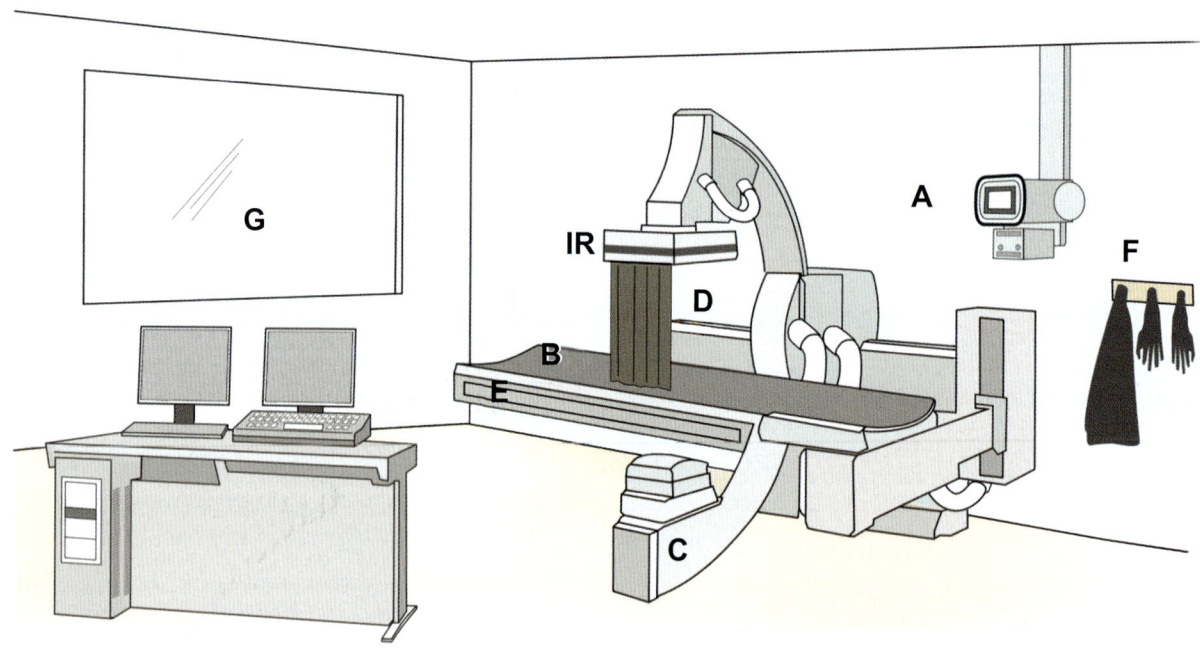

FIG. 1.9 The general purpose radiographic and fluoroscopic imaging system includes an overhead radiographic tube (A) and a fluoroscopic examining table (B) with an x-ray tube under the table (C). Some of the more common radiation protection devices are the lead curtain (D), the Bucky slot cover (E), a lead apron and gloves (F), and the protective viewing window (G). The location of the image receptor (IR) and associated imaging equipment is shown.

to be repeated because of technical errors. Repeat examinations subject the patient to twice the necessary radiation. The benefits of exposing patients should far outweigh any risks.

Except for appropriate screening, x-ray examination of asymptomatic patients is not acceptable.

Patients who require assistance during examination should never be held by x-ray personnel. Mechanical immobilization devices should be used. When necessary, a member of the patient's family, appropriately shielded, should provide the necessary assistance.

Filtration

Metal filters, usually aluminum or copper, are inserted into the x-ray tube housing so that low-energy x-rays are absorbed before they reach the patient. These x-rays have little diagnostic value.

Collimation

Collimation restricts the useful x-ray beam to that part of the body to be imaged and thereby spares adjacent tissue from unnecessary radiation exposure. Collimators take many different forms. Adjustable light-locating collimators are the most frequently used collimating devices. Collimation also reduces scatter radiation and thus improves image contrast.

TERMINOLOGY FOR RADIOLOGIC SCIENCE

Every profession has its own language. Radiologic science is no exception. Several words and phrases characteristic of radiologic science already have been identified; many more will be defined and used throughout this book. For now, an introduction to this terminology should be sufficient.

Numeric Prefixes

Often in radiologic science, we must describe very large or very small multiples of standard units. Two units, the mA and kVp, have already been discussed. By writing 70 kVp instead of 70,000 V peak, we can understandably express the same quantity with fewer characters. For such an economy of expression, scientists have devised a system of prefixes and symbols (Table 1.4).

Question: How many kilovolts equal 37,000 V?
Answer: $37{,}000\,V = 37 \times 10^3\,V$
$\quad\quad\quad = 37\,kV$

Question: The diameter of a blood cell is approximately 10 μm. How many meters is that?
Answer: $10\,\mu m = 10 \times 10^{-6}\,m$
$\quad\quad\quad = 10^{-5}\,m$
$\quad\quad\quad = 0.00001\,m$

TABLE 1.4	Standard Scientific Prefixes	
Multiple	Prefix	Symbol
10^{18}	exa-	E
10^{15}	peta-	P
10^{12}	**tera-**	**T**
10^{9}	**giga-**	**G**
10^{6}	**mega-**	**M**
10^{3}	**kilo-**	**k**
10^{2}	hecto-	h
10	deka-	da
10^{-1}	deci-	d
10^{-2}	**centi-**	**c**
10^{-3}	**milli-**	**m**
10^{-6}	**micro-**	**μ**
10^{-9}	**nano-**	**n**
10^{-12}	pico-	p
10^{-15}	femto-	f
10^{-18}	atto-	a

Boldfaced prefixes and symbols are those most used in radiologic science.

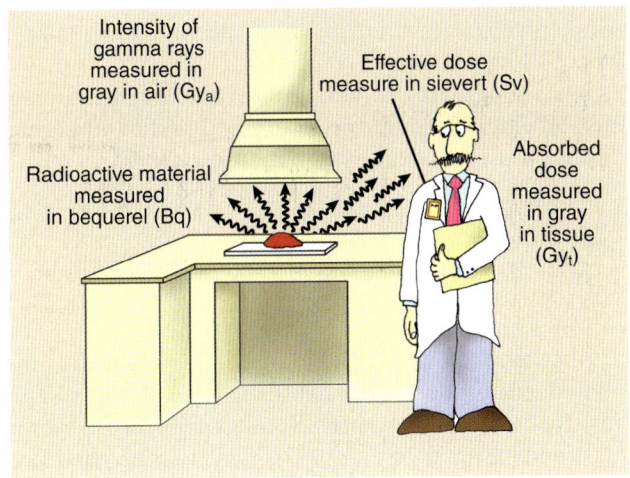

FIG. 1.10 Radiation is emitted by radioactive material. The quantity of radioactive material is measured in becquerel. Radiation quantity is measured in gray or sievert, depending on the precise use.

Radiologic Units

The four units used to measure radiation should become a familiar part of your vocabulary. Fig. 1.10 relates them to a hypothetical situation in which they would be used. Table 1.5 shows the relationship of the earlier radiologic units to their SI equivalents.

TABLE 1.5 Special Quantities of Radiologic Science and Their Associated Special Units

Quantity	CUSTOMARY UNIT Name	Symbol	INTERNATIONAL SYSTEM OF UNITS (SI) Name	Symbol
Exposure	Roentgen	R	air kerma	Gy_a
Absorbed dose	rad	rad	Gray	Gy_t
Effective dose	rem	rem	Sievert	Sv
Radioactivity	Curie	Ci	Becquerel	Bq
Multiply	R	by 0.01	to obtain	Gy_a
Multiply	rad	by 0.01	to obtain	Gy_t
Multiply	rem	by 0.01	to obtain	Sv
Multiply	Ci	by 3.7×10^{10}	to obtain	Bq

In 1981 the International Commission on Radiation Units and Measurements issued standard units based on SI that have since been adopted by all countries except the United States. The NCRP and all US scientific and medical societies adopted the SI units by the early 1990s. It was not until 2017 that the American Registry of Radiologic Technologists (ARRT) adopted SI units in their examinations.

Air Kerma (Kinetic Energy Released in Matter) (Gy_a). Air kerma is the kinetic energy transferred from photons to electrons during ionization and excitation. Air kerma is measured in joules per kilogram (J/kg), where 1 J/kg is 1 gray (Gy_a).

In keeping with the adoption of the Wagner/Archer method described in the preface, the SI unit of air kerma (mGy_a) is used to express radiation exposure.

Air kerma (Gy_a) is the SI unit of radiation exposure.

Absorbed Dose (Gy_t) Biologic effects usually are related to the **r**adiation **a**bsorbed **d**ose (rad). The absorbed dose is the radiation energy absorbed per unit mass and has units of J/kg or Gy_t. The units Gy_a and Gy_t refer to radiation dose in air and tissue, respectively. For a given air kerma (radiation exposure), the absorbed dose depends on the type of tissue being irradiated. More about this is found in Chapter 39.

The gray (Gy_t) is the SI unit of **r**adiation **a**bsorbed **d**ose (rad).

Effective Dose: Sievert (Sv) Occupational radiation monitoring devices are analyzed in terms of sievert, which is used to express the quantity of radiation received by radiation workers and population. The sievert also expresses a patient dose that accounts for partial-body irradiation.

Some types of radiation produce more damage than x-rays. The sievert accounts for these differences in biologic effectiveness. This is particularly important for people working near nuclear reactors or particle accelerators. More about effective dose is discussed in Chapter 37.

Fig. 1.11 summarizes the conversion from the traditional units of occupational radiation exposure to SI units.

The sievert (Sv) is the SI unit of occupational radiation exposure and effective dose.

Radioactivity: Becquerel (Bq) The becquerel is the unit of quantity of radioactive material, not the radiation emitted by that material. One becquerel is the quantity of radioactivity in which a nucleus disintegrates every second (1 d/s = 1 Bq). Megabecquerels (MBq) are common quantities of radioactive material. The traditional unit of radioactivity was the curie (Ci), where $1\,Ci = 3.7 \times 10^{10}\,Bq$.

Radioactivity and the becquerel have nothing to do with x-rays.

The becquerel (Bq) is the SI unit of radioactivity.

Question: 0.05 µCi iodine-125 is used for radioimmunoassay. What is this radioactivity in becquerels?

Answer: $0.05\,\mu Ci = 0.05 \times 10^{-6}\,Ci$
$= (0.05 \times 10^{-6}\,Ci)(3.7 \times 10^{10}\,Bq/Ci)$
$= 0.185 \times 10^4\,Bq = 1850\,Bq$

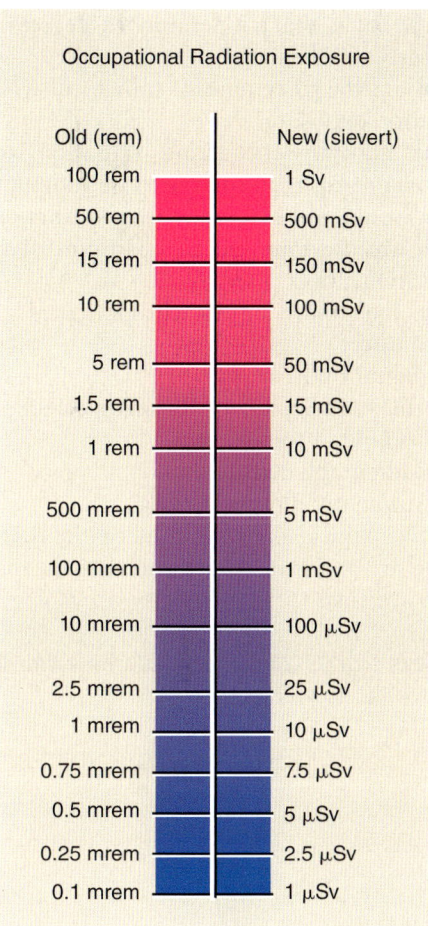

FIG. 1.11 Scales for effective dose.

THE MEDICAL IMAGING TEAM

To become part of this exciting profession, a student must complete the prescribed academic courses, obtain clinical experience, and pass the national certification examination given by the ARRT. Both academic expertise and clinical skills are required of radiographers. The ARRT Task Inventory (https://www.arrt.org/pages/arrt-reference-documents/by-document-type/task-inventories) lists the job responsibilities typically required for entry-level radiographers.

Radiologic science programs accredited by the Joint Review Committee on Education in Radiologic Technology (JRCERT) must follow a JRCERT-adopted curriculum. One such curriculum is the latest American Society of Radiologic Technologists (ASRT) *Radiography Curriculum* (https://www.asrt.org/educators/asrt-curricula/radiography), which outlines a common body of knowledge essential for entry-level radiographers.

The national certification examination for radiographers is administered by the ARRT. The primary purpose of ARRT examinations is to assess the knowledge and cognitive skills entry-level radiographers need to perform their jobs. The ARRT *Content Specifications for Radiography Examination* (https://www.arrt.org/pages/earn-arrt-credentials/credential-options/radiography) outlines the topics covered on the examination.

Every medical profession has a scope of practice that delineates parameters and identifies boundaries for their respected practice and is formatted as lists of tasks appropriate as part of the work of the individual who is educated and clinically competent for that profession. The scope of practice for radiographers is outlined in *The ASRT Practice Standards for Medical Imaging and Radiation Therapy* (https://www.asrt.org/main/standards-and-regulations/professional-practice). Additionally, federal and state laws and accreditation standards are necessary for participation in medical imaging as a radiographer.

SUMMARY

Radiology offers a career in many areas of medical imaging, and it requires knowledge of medicine, biology, and physics. This first chapter weaves the history and development of radiography with an introduction to medical physics.

Medical physics includes the study of matter, energy, and the electromagnetic spectrum of which x-rays are a part. The production of x-radiation and its safe diagnostic use serve as the basis of medical imaging. Along with emphasizing the importance of radiation safety, this chapter presents a detailed list of clinical and patient care skills required for radiographers.

This chapter also introduces the various standards of measurement and applies them to concepts associated with several areas within radiologic science. The technical aspects of radiologic science require the identification and proper use of the units of radiation measurements.

CHALLENGE QUESTIONS

1. Define or otherwise identify the following:
   a. Energy
   b. Derived quantity
   c. Ionizing radiation
   d. Air kerma
   e. The average level of ubiquitous environmental radiation
   f. The Coolidge tube
   g. Fluoroscopy
   h. Electromagnetic radiation
   i. Ionization
   j. Barium platinocyanide
2. Match the following dates with the appropriate event:

   a. 1901   1. Roentgen discovers x-rays.
   a. 1907   2. Roentgen wins the first Nobel Prize in Physics.
   i. 1913   3. The Snook transformer is developed.
   i. 1895   4. The Coolidge hot-cathode x-ray tube is introduced.

3. In accordance with ALARA, describe how a patient requiring assistance should be immobilized during a radiographic examination.
4. Name four examples of electromagnetic radiation.
5. How is x-ray interaction different from that seen in other types of electromagnetic radiation?
6. What is the purpose of x-ray beam filtration?
7. Describe the process that results in the formation of a negative ion and a positive ion.
8. What the largest source of ubiquitous background radiation?
9. What is the velocity of the mobile x-ray imaging system if the hospital elevator travels 20 m to the next floor in 30 s?
10. A radiographer has a mass of 58 kg. What is their weight on Earth? On the Moon?
11. The acronym ALARA stands for what?
12. Name devices designed to minimize radiation exposure to the patient and the operator.
13. Liquid hydrogen with a boiling temperature of 77 K is used to cool some superconducting magnets. What is this temperature in degrees Celsius? In degrees Fahrenheit?
14. What are the three natural sources of whole-body radiation exposure?
15. What naturally occurring radiation source is responsible for the radiation dose to lung tissue?
16. How would you define the term "radiation"?
17. What are the four special quantities of radiation measurement?
18. Place the following in chronological order of appearance:
    a. Digital fluoroscopy
    b. American Society of Radiologic Technologists
    c. Computed tomography
    d. Radiographic grids
    e. Automatic film processing
19. List five clinical skills required by the ARRT.
20. What are the three units common to the SI and MKS systems?

The answers to the Challenge Questions can be found at http://evolve.elsevier.com.

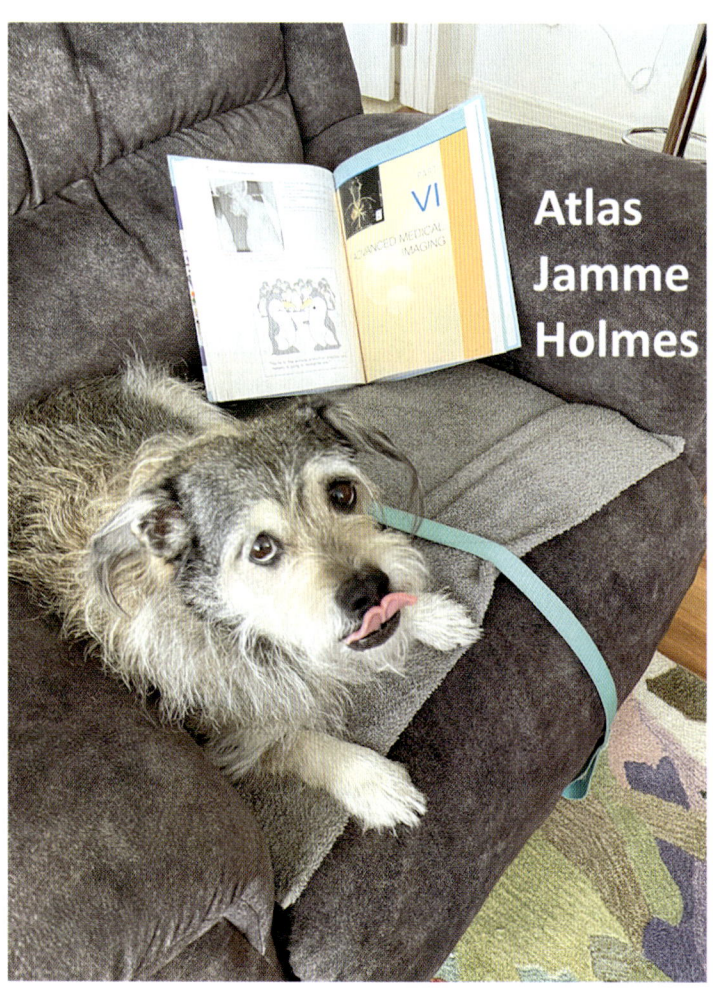

Basic Physics Primer

CHAPTER 2

OBJECTIVES

At the completion of this chapter, the student should be able to do the following:

1. Perform mathematical problems using fractions, decimals, and exponents.
2. Determine significant digits in the answer to a mathematic problem.
3. Solve for the unknown (x) using the rules of algebra.
4. Identify scientific exponential notation and the associated prefixes.
5. Properly construct and interpret a graph.
6. Define base quantities, derived quantities, and special quantities used in radiologic science and their International System of Units (SI) of measure.
7. State Newton's three fundamental laws of motion.
8. Define the properties of mechanics.

OUTLINE

Mathematics for Radiologic Science 18
   Fractions 18
   Decimals 19
   Significant Figures 19
   Algebra 20
   Number Systems 21
   Rules for Exponents 22
   Graphing 22
Standard Units of Measurement 23
   Length 24
   Mass 24
   Time 25
   Units 25
Mechanics 26
   Velocity 26
   Acceleration 27
   Newton's Laws of Motion 27
   Weight 28
   Momentum 29
   Work 29
   Power 29
   Energy 29
   Heat 30
Summary 32
Challenge Questions 32

Having considered the historic events of the application of ionizing radiation in the form of x-rays, this chapter examines the important characteristics of some basic physics concepts that impact your understanding of x-ray physics. In 1976, the US Congress passed the Metrification Act of America, which gave us 20 years to abandon the traditional English units for the International System of Units (SI). We are still not there!

The instant an x-ray tube produces x-rays, all of the laws of physics are evident. The projectile electron from the cathode hits the target of the anode, producing x-rays. Some x-rays interact with tissue, and other x-rays interact with the image receptor, forming an image. The physics of radiography deals with the production and interaction of x-rays.

Every field of science involves taking measurements, understanding them, and communicating them to others. This chapter presents a brief review of the mathematics essential to radiologic science and introduces standard units of measurement all radiographers should use to ensure accuracy.

MATHEMATICS FOR RADIOLOGIC SCIENCE

Physics owes a great deal of its certainty to mathematics, and accordingly, most of the concepts of physics can be expressed mathematically. It is therefore important in the study of radiologic science to have a solid foundation in the basic concept of mathematics. The following sections review fundamental mathematics. You should become proficient at working each type of problem presented in this review.

Fractions

A fraction is a numeric value expressed by dividing one number by another. Such division results in the **quotient** of the two numbers. A fraction has a numerator and a denominator.

> Fraction = x/y = numerator/denominator = a value called the quotient

If the quotient of the numerator divided by the denominator is less than 1, the value is a proper fraction. Improper fractions have values greater than 1.

Question: Give examples of a proper fraction.
Answer: 1/2, 3/5, 5/7, 9/10
Question: Give examples of an improper fraction.
Answer: 3/2, 6/5, 10/7, 13/10

> **ADDITION AND SUBTRACTION**
> First, find a common denominator, then add or subtract.
> x/y + a/b = xb/yb + ay/yb = (xb + ay)/yb

Question: What is the value of 2/3 + 4/5?
Answer: 2/3 + 4/5 = 10/15 + 12/15 = 22/15, which is an improper fraction, or 1 7/15, which is a proper fraction.
Question: What is the value of 4/5 − 2/3?
Answer: 4/5 − 2/3 = 12/15 − 10/15 = 2/15, which is a proper fraction.

> **MULTIPLICATION**
> To multiply fractions, simply multiply numerators and denominators.
> x/y × a/b = xa/yb

Question: What is the value of 2/5 × 7/4?
Answer: 2/5 × 7/4 = 14/20 = 7/10, which is a proper fraction.
Question: What is the value of 9/8 × 12/7?
Answer: 9/8 × 12/7 = 108/56 = 27/14, which is an improper fraction, or 1 13/14, which is a proper fraction.

> **DIVISION**
> To divide fractions, invert the second fraction and multiply.
> x/y ÷ a/b = x/y × b/a = xb/ya

Question: What is the value of 5/2 ÷ 7/4?
Answer: 5/2 ÷ 7/4 = 5/2 × 4/7 = 20/14 = 10/7, which is an improper fraction, or 1 3/7, which is a proper fraction.
Question: What is the value of 3/10 ÷ 7/2?
Answer: 3/10 ÷ 7/2 = 3/10 × 2/7 = 6/70 = 3/35, which is a proper fraction.

A special application of fractions in medical imaging is the ratio. Ratios express the mathematical relationship between similar quantities, such as feet to the mile or pounds to the kilogram.

Question:	What is the ratio of feet to a mile?
Answer:	There are 5280 ft in a mile; therefore the ratio is 5280 ft/mi.
Question:	What is the ratio of the pound to the kilogram?
Answer:	There are 2.2 pounds in a kilogram; therefore the ratio is 2.2 lb/kg.

These ratios can also be used when converting units from one system to another. Dimensional analysis is a problem-solving technique that uses the fact that any quantity can be multiplied by one without changing its value.

Question:	How many feet are in 81 miles?
Answer:	81 mi × 5280 ft/1 mi = 42,680 ft
Question:	How many kilograms are in 185 pounds?
Answer:	185 lb × 1 kg/2.2 lb = 84 kg

Decimals

Fractions in which the denominator is a power of 10 may easily be converted to decimals.

> **CONVERTING FRACTIONS TO DECIMALS**
> 3/10 = 0.3
> 3/1000 = 0.003
> 161/10,000 = 0.0161
> 1527/10,000 = 0.1527
> If the denominator is not a power of 10, the decimal equivalent can be found by division or with a calculator.
>
> 5/12 = 5 ÷ 12
>   = 0.41$\overline{6}$
>
> The bar above the 6 indicates that this digit is repeating. When one divides 5 by 12 using a calculator, the answer is 0.416666….

Rarely do we convert fractions to decimals without a calculator, computer, or smartphone. Depending on the calculator, it is simply a matter of keying numbers in the proper sequence.

Question:	What is the decimal equivalent of the proper fraction 3/7?
Answer:	3/7 = 0.429
Question:	What is the decimal equivalent of the improper fraction 123/69?
Answer:	123/69 = 1.78

Significant Figures

Students often wonder how many decimal places to report in an answer. For example, suppose you were asked to find the area of a circle.

Question:	What is the area of a circle with a radius of 1.25 cm?
Answer:	$A = \pi r^2$
	$= 3.14 \times (1.25 \text{ cm})^2$
	$= 3.14 \times 1.5625 \text{ cm}^2$
	$= 4.90625 \text{ cm}^2$

This answer is unsuitable because it implies much greater precision in the measurement of the area than we actually have. This result must be rounded off according to specific rules.

> In addition and subtraction, round to the same number of decimal places as the entry with the least number of digits to the right of the decimal point.

Question:	Add 5.0631, 117.2, and 21.42, and round off the answer.
Answer:	5.0631
	117.2
	+21.42
	143.6831

Because 117.2 has one digit to the right of the decimal point, the answer is 143.7.

Question:	Solve the following and round off the answer. 42.83 − 7.6147
Answer:	42.83
	−7.6147
	35.2153

Because 42.83 has two digits to the right of the decimal point, the answer is 35.22.

> In multiplication and division, round to the same number of digits as the entry with the least number of significant digits.

Question: What is the product of 17.24 and 0.382?

Answer:
$$17.24 \\ \times 0.382 \\ \overline{6.58568}$$

Because 0.382 has three significant digits (the zero is not significant) and 17.42 has four digits, the answer must have three digits: the answer is 6.59.

Question: How would you report the area of the circle discussed previously?
Answer: 4.91 cm^2

Question: What is the quotient of 3.1416 divided by 1.05?
Answer: 3.1416/1.05 = 2.992

Because 1.05 has three significant digits (in this case, the zero is significant because it is followed by a number greater than zero) and 3.1416 has five significant digits, the answer must have three digits. The answer is 2.99.

Algebra

Rules of algebra provide definite ways to manipulate fractions and equations to solve for unknown quantities. Usually the unknowns are designated by an alphabetic symbol such as x, y, or z. Three principal rules of algebra are used in the solution of problems in medical imaging.

> When an unknown, x, is multiplied by a number, divide both sides of the equation by that number.
> ax = c, ax/a = c/a, x = c/a

Question: Solve the equation 5x = 10 for x.
Answer:
5x = 10
5x/5 = 10/5
x = 2

> When numbers are added to an unknown, x, subtract that number from both sides of the equation.
> xa = b, xa − a = b − a, x = b − a

Question: Solve the equation x + 7 = 10.
Answer:
x + 7 − 7 = 10−7
x = 3

> When an equation is presented in the form of a proportion, cross-multiply and then solve for the unknown, x.
> x/a = b/c, $\frac{x}{a} \times \frac{b}{c}$, cx = ab, x = ab/c

The crossed arrows (x) show the direction of cross-multiplication.

Question: Solve the equation x/5 = 3/8.
Answer:
x/5 = 3/8
8x = 3 × 5
8x = 15
8x/8 = 15/8
x = 17/8

Often, all three rules may be necessary to solve a particular problem.

Question: Solve 6x + 3 = 15 for the value of x.
Answer:
6x + 3 = 15
6x + 3−3 = 15−3
6x = 12
6x/6 = 12/6
x = 2

Question: Solve 4/x = (3/4)^2 for the value of x.
Answer:
4/x = (3/4)2
4/x = 9/16
64 = 9x
9x = 64
9x/9 = 64/9
x = 7.1

Question: Solve ABx + C = D for x.
Answer:
ABx + C = D
ABx + C − C = D − C
ABx = D − C
ABx/AB = (D − C)/ABx = (D − C)/AB

Note that the first and third of the previous examples are nearly identical in form. Symbols are often used in physics equations instead of numbers.

A special application of fractions and rules of algebra to medical imaging is the proportion. A proportion expresses the equality of two ratios. The ratio of a radiographic grid is directly proportional to the quotient of the height of the grid strips to the interspace between grid strips.

Question: If the grid height is 800 μm, and the interspace 80 μm, what is the grid ratio?
Answer: 800 μm/80 μm = 10/1.
The grid ratio = 10/1.

Usually this is written 10:1 and is expressed as a "ten to one ratio grid."

The statement "gas mileage is inversely proportional to automobile weight" can be used as a numeric proportion to solve for an unknown quantity.

Question: A 1650-pound compact car gets 34 mpg. What is the expected mileage for a 3600-pound luxury car?
Answer: Set up the inverse proportion as follows: x/1650 lb = 34 mpg/3600 lb and use the rules of algebra to solve for x. x = (34 mpg) (1650 lb)/3600 lb; x = 15.6 mpg.

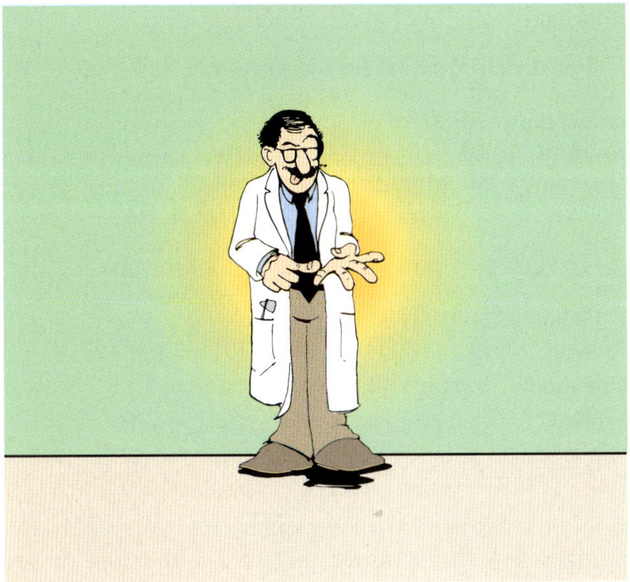

FIG. 2.1 The probable origin of the decimal number system.

TABLE 2.1		Various Ways to Represent Numbers in the Decimal System	
Fractional Form	Decimal Form	Exponential Form	Logarithmic Form
10,000	10,000	10^4	4.000
1000	1000	10^3	3.000
100	100	10^2	2.000
10	10	10^1	1.000
1	1	10^0	0.000
1/10	0.1	10^{-1}	−1.000
1/100	0.01	10^{-2}	−2.000
1/1000	0.001	10^{-3}	−3.000
1/10,000	0.0001	10^{-4}	−4.000

Radiation intensity is directly proportional to the mAs of a radiographic imaging system.

Question: At 50 mAs, the entrance skin exposure (ESE) is 2.4 mGy$_a$. What will be the ESE if the technique is increased to 60 mAs?

Answer: x/60 mAs = 2.4 mGy$_a$/50 mAs

x = (2.4 mGy$_a$)(60 mAs)/50 mAs

x = 2.88 mGy$_a$

An understanding of algebraic relationships is important to many concepts in radiography. For directly proportional relationships, when one variable changes, the other variable changes in the same direction by the same factor. Given k is constant, A = kB, then if A doubles, B doubles. For directly related relationships, a change in one variable results in a change in the other variable in the same direction, but not by the same factor. When A increases, B increases but not by the same factor.

For inversely proportional relationships, when one variable changes, the other variable changes in the opposite direction by the reciprocal factor. Given k is constant, A = k/B, then if A doubles, B is halved. For inversely related relationships, a change in one variable results in a change in the other variable in the opposite direction, but not by the reciprocal factor. When A increases, B decreases but not by the reciprocal factor.

Number Systems

We use a system of numbers that is based on multiples of 10, called the **decimal system**. The origin of this decimal system is unknown, but theories have been proposed (Fig. 2.1). Numbers in this system can be represented in various ways, four of which are shown in Table 2.1.

The superscript on "10" in the exponential form of Table 2.1 is called the **exponent**. The exponential form, also referred to as scientific notation, is particularly useful in medical imaging.

Note that very large and very small numbers are difficult to write in decimal and fractional forms. In medical imaging, many numbers are very large or very small. Exponential form allows these numbers to be written and manipulated with relative ease.

To express a number in exponential form, first write the number in decimal form. If there are digits to the left of the decimal point, the exponent will be positive.

To determine the value of this positive exponent, position the decimal point after the first digit, and count the number of digits the decimal point was moved. For example, the national debt of the United States was approximately $30 trillion on April 25, 2022. Coincidentally, April 25 just happens to be World Penguin Day.

To express this in scientific notation, we must position the decimal point after the first digit, 2, and count the number of digits that the decimal point was moved. The result of this exercise shows that the exponent will be +13.

US national debt =
$30,420,895,865,073.55 = $3.04 × 10^{13}

The exponent is found by positioning the decimal point to the right of the first nonzero digit and counting the number of digits the decimal point was moved.

A string on Robert Earl Keen's guitar has a diameter of 0.00075 m. What is its diameter in exponential notation? First, position the decimal point between the 7 and the 5. Next, count the number of digits the decimal point has moved and express this quantity as a negative exponent.

0.00075 m = 7.5 × 10^{-4} m

Another example from physics is a number called **Planck's constant**, symbolized by **h**. Planck's constant is related to the energy of an x-ray. Its decimal form is as follows:

$$h = 0.000000000000000000000000000000000663 \, J \cdot s$$

Obviously, this form is too cumbersome to write each time. Thus Planck's constant is always written in exponential form:

$$h = 6.63 \times 10^{-34} \, J \cdot s$$

Question: Express 4050 in exponential form.
Answer: $4050 = 4.05 \times 10^3$

Question: Express 1/2000 in exponential form.
Answer: First convert to decimal form.
$1/2000 = 0.0005$
$0.0005 = 5 \times 10^{-4}$

Question: X-rays have a velocity of 300,000,000 m/s. Express this in exponential form.
Answer: $300,000,000 \, m/s = 3 \times 10^8 \, m/s$

Question: If a dedicated chest x-ray imaging system has a source-to-image receptor distance (SID) of 10 ft, what is the SID in centimeters (cm)? Express the answer in exponential form.
Answer: $10 \, ft \times 12 \, in/ft \times 2.54 \, cm/in = 304.8 \, cm$.
$304.8 \, cm = 3.048 \, m \times 10^2 \, cm$

Rules for Exponents

Another advantage of handling numbers in exponential form is evident in operations other than addition and subtraction. The general rules for these types of numeric operations are shown in Table 2.2.

The following examples should sufficiently emphasize the principles involved. For multiplication, add the exponents.

Question: Simplify $10^6 \times 10^8$
Answer: $10^6 \times 10^8 = 10^{(6+8)} = 10^{14}$
Question: Simplify $2^8 \times 2^{12}$
Answer: $2^8 \times 2^{12} = 2^{(8+12)} = 2^{20}$

For division, subtract the exponents.

Question: $10^{10}/10^2$
Answer: $10^{10}/10^2 = 10^{(10-2)} = 10^8$
Question: Simplify $2^3/3^5$
Answer: $2^3/3^5 = 2^{(3-5)} = 2^{-2} = 1/2^2 = 1/4$

To raise to a power, multiply the exponents.

Question: Simplify $(3 \times 10^{10})^2$
Answer: $(3 \times 10^{10})^2 = 3^2 \times (10^{10})^2 = 9 \times 10^{20}$
Question: Simplify $(2.718 \times 10^{-4})^3$
Answer: $(2.718 \times 10^{-4})^3 = 20.08 \times 10^{-12}$
$= 2.008 \times 10^{-11}$

Note that the rules for exponents apply only when the numbers raised to a power are raised to the same power.

Question: Given $a = 6.62 \times 10^{-27}$ and $b = 3.766 \times 10^{12}$, what is $a \times b$?
Answer: $a \times b = (6.62 \times 10^{-27}) \times (3.766 \times 10^{12})$
$a \times b = (6.62 \times 3.766) \times (10^{-27} \times 10^{12})$
$= 24.931 \times 10^{(-27+12)}$
$= 24.93 \times 10^{-15}$
$= 2.49 \times 10^{-14}$

Graphing

Knowledge of graphing is essential to the study of radiologic science. It is important not only to be able to read information from graphs but to graph data obtained from measurements or observations.

Most graphs are based on two axes: a horizontal or x-axis, and a vertical or y-axis. The point where the

TABLE 2.2	Rules for Handling Numbers in Exponential Form	
Operation	Rule	Example
Multiplication	$10^x \times 10^y = 10^{(x+y)}$	$10^2 \times 10^3 = 10^{(2+3)} = 10^5$
Division	$10^x / 10^y = 10^{(x-y)}$	$10^6 - 10^4 = 10^{(6-4)} = 10^2$
Raising to a Power	$(10^x)^y$	$(10^5)^3 = 10^{(5\times3)} = 10^{15}$
Inverse	$10^{-x} = 1/10^x$	$10^{-3} = 1/10^3 = 1/1000$
Unity	$10^0 = 1$	$3.7 \times 10^0 = 3.7$

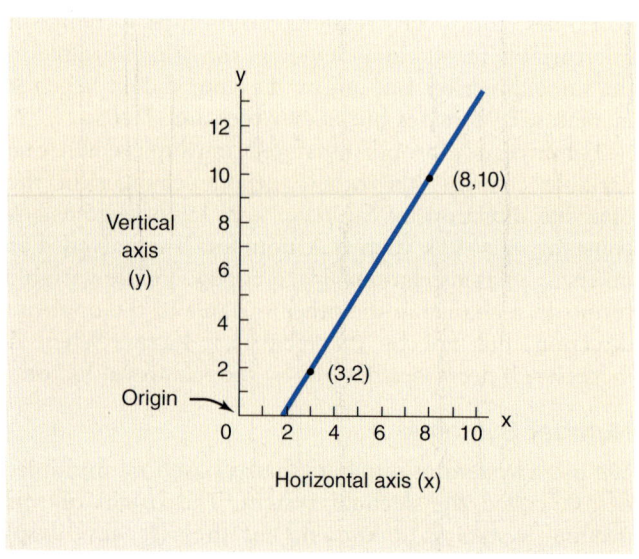

FIG. 2.2 The principal features of any graph are x- and y-axes that intersect at the origin. Points of data are entered as ordered pairs.

two axes meet is called the origin, labeled 0 in Fig. 2.2. Coordinates are points on a graph. Coordinates have the form of ordered pairs (x,y), where the first number of the pair represents a distance along the x-axis and the second number represents a distance up the y-axis.

The ordered pair (3,2) represents a point 3 units along the x-axis and 2 units up the y-axis. This point is plotted in Fig. 2.2. If the value of one additional ordered pair is known, say (8,10), a straight-line graph can be constructed.

In radiologic science, the axes of graphs are not usually labeled x and y. Usually, the relationship between two specific quantities is desired. Suppose, for example, that after a week of camping in the hill country west of Austin, Texas, you arrived home with enough caged opossums to conduct a radiation lethality experiment.

The results of your experimental opossum irradiation are given in Table 2.3. You now plot the percent radiation lethality as a function of radiation dose and that results in Fig. 2.3. You want to estimate the opossum lethal dose (LD)$_{50/60}$, which is that dose of radiation that will kill half of the opossums, 50%, within 60 days.

Question: Plot the data from Table 2.3 and estimate the opossum lethal dose (LD)$_{50/60}$.

Answer: View Fig. 2.3, which shows the plot of the data from Table 2.3. Draw a horizontal line at the 50% lethality level on the y-axis and, when it intersects the smooth curve, drop down to the radiation dose on the x-axis. The LD$_{50/60}$ for the opossums in this experiment is 5.1 Gy$_t$.

If the data to be plotted are in exponential form and therefore extend over a very large range of values, a linear scale is not adequate. In such situations, a logarithmic scale, as shown in Fig. 2.4 must be used.

Radiologic data frequently require a semilogarithmic graph, as shown in Fig. 2.5. The y-axis is a logarithmic scale and the x-axis is a linear scale.

Question: One half-life of uranium-235 is 7.038 × 10^8 years. How much time, in units of half-life, is required for uranium-235 to decay to less than 1% of its original?

Answer: From the semilogarithmic graph in Fig. 2.5, it is easier to estimate the answer of 7 half-lives.

STANDARD UNITS OF MEASUREMENT

Physics is the study of interactions of matter and energy in all their diverse forms. Similar to all scientists, physicists strive for exactness or certainty in describing these interactions. They try to remove the uncertainties by eliminating subjective descriptions of events. Assuming that all measurements are made correctly, all observers who use the methods of physics will obtain exactly the same results.

TABLE 2.3	Observations of Opossum Response to Radiation Used to Estimate LD$_{50/60}$		
Radiation Dose (Gy$_t$)	Number Irradiated	Number Dead	Percent Lethality
1.3	12	0	0
3.2	8	1	9
3.8	9	2	21
4.7	10	4	42
5.6	11	6	58
6.5	6	5	86
8.7	10	9	93
10.5	7	7	100

LD, Lethal dose.

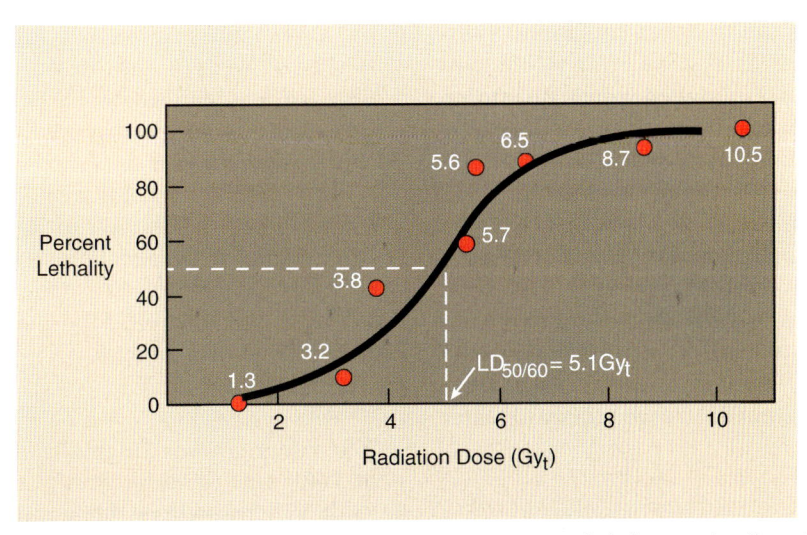

FIG. 2.3 The data from Table 2.3 are plotted as percent opossum lethality as a function of radiation dose.

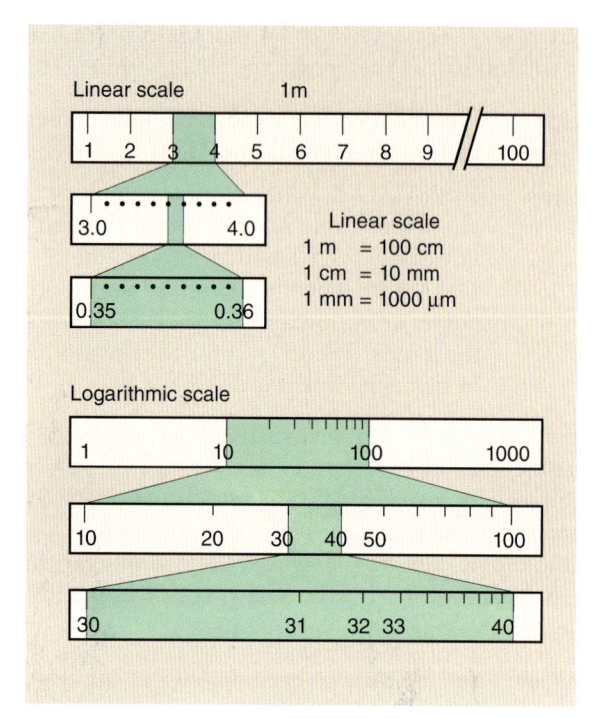

FIG. 2.4 Equal lengths of linear scale have equal value. The logarithmic scale allows a large range of values to be plotted.

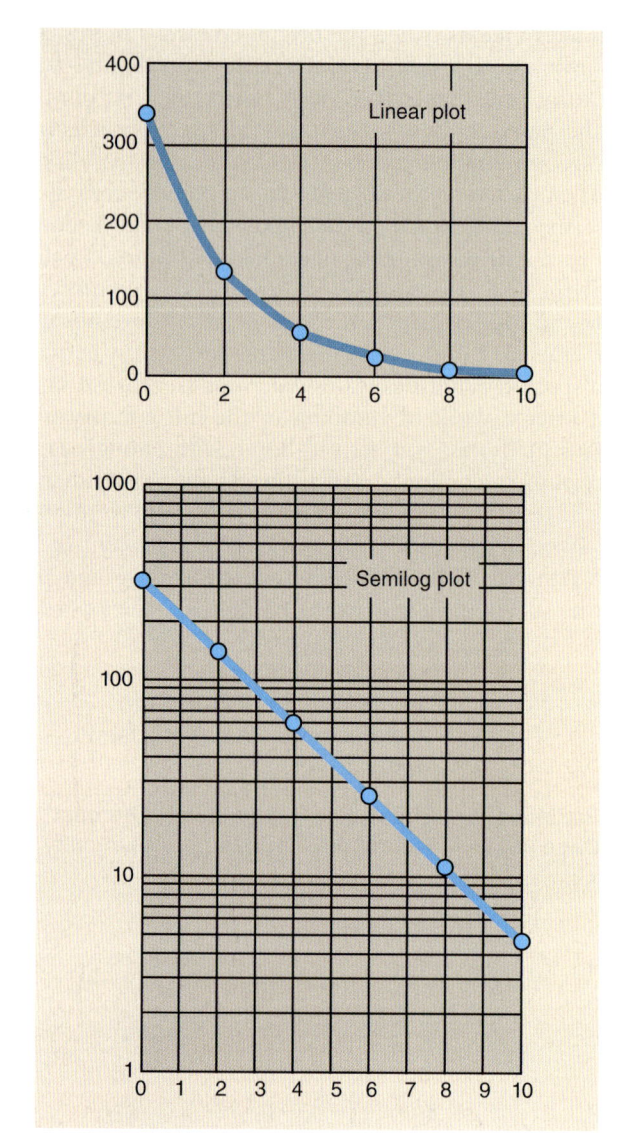

FIG. 2.5 Semilogarithmic graph paper is often used to plot radiologic data.

In addition to seeking certainty, physicists strive for simplicity; therefore only three measurable quantities are considered base quantities. These **base quantities** are length, mass, and time, and they are the building blocks of all other quantities. Fig. 2.6 indicates the role these base quantities play in supporting some of the other quantities used in radiologic science.

The secondary quantities are called **derived quantities** because they are derived from a combination of one or more of the three base quantities. For example, volume is length cubed (l^3), mass density is mass divided by volume (m/l^3), and velocity is length divided by time (l/t).

Additional quantities are designed to support measurement in specialized areas of science and technology. These additional quantities are called **special quantities**. In radiologic science, special quantities are those of exposure, dose, effective dose, and radioactivity.

Whether a physicist is studying something large, such as the universe, or something small, such as an atom, meaningful measurements must be reproducible. Therefore after the fundamental quantities have been established, it is essential that they be related to a well-defined and invariable standard. Standards are normally defined by international organizations and usually are redefined when the progress of science requires greater precision.

Length

For many years, the standard unit of length was accepted to be the distance between two lines engraved on a platinum-iridium bar kept at the International Bureau of Weights and Measures in Paris, France. This distance was defined to be exactly 1 **meter** (m). The English-speaking countries also base their standards of length on the meter.

In 1960 the need for a more accurate standard of length led to redefinition of the meter in terms of the wavelength of orange light emitted from an isotope of krypton (krypton-86). One meter is now defined as the distance traveled by that light in a vacuum in 1/299,792,458 second (s).

Mass

The kilogram was originally defined to be the mass of 1000 cm^3 of water at 4° Celsius (°C). In the same vault in Paris where the standard meter was kept, a platinum-iridium cylinder represents the standard unit of mass—the **kilogram** (kg), which has the same mass

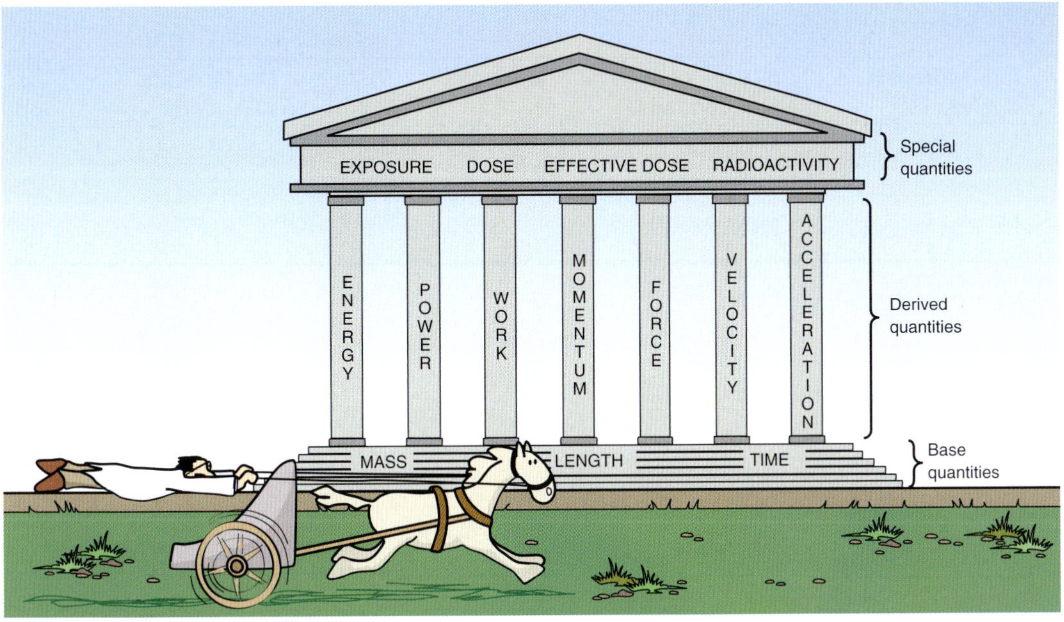

FIG. 2.6 Base quantities support derived quantities, which in turn support the special quantities of radiologic science.

as 1000 cm³ of water. The kilogram is a unit of mass, and the **newton** (**N**) and the **pound** (**lb**), a British unit, are units of weight.

Time

The standard unit of time is the **second** (**s**). Originally, the second was defined in terms of the rotation of the Earth on its axis—the mean solar day. In 1956 it was redefined as a certain fraction of the tropical year 1900. In 1964 the need for a better standard of time led to another redefinition.

Now, time is measured by an atomic clock and is based on the vibration of cesium atoms. The atomic clock is capable of keeping time correctly to approximately 1 second in 5000 years.

> The second (s) is based on the vibration of cesium atoms.

Units

Every measurement has two parts: a **magnitude** and a **unit**. For example, the SID is 100 cm. The magnitude, 100, is not meaningful unless a unit is also designated. Here, the unit of measurement is the centimeter.

Table 2.4 shows four **systems of units** that represent base quantities. The SI system (Le Système International d'Unités), an extension of the MKS (meters, kilograms, and seconds) system, represents the current state of units. SI includes the three base units of the MKS system plus an additional four. Derived units and special units of SI represent derived quantities and special quantities of radiologic science (Table 2.5).

> The same system of units must always be used when one is working on problems or reporting answers.

The following would be unacceptable because of inconsistent units: mass density = 8.1 g/ft³ and pressure = 700 lb/cm².

Mass density should be reported with units of kilograms per cubic meter (kg/m³). Pressure should be given in newtons per square meter (N/m²).

Question: The dimensions of a box are 30 cm × 86 cm × 4.2 m. Find the volume.

Answer: Formula for the volume of an object: V = length × width × height or V = lwh. However, because the dimensions are given in different systems of units, we must choose only one system. Therefore V = (0.3 m) (0.86 m) (4.2 m) = 1.1 m³.

Note that the units are multiplied also: m × m × m = m³.

TABLE 2.4 System of Units

	International System (SI)[a]	System of Meters, Kilograms, and Seconds	System of Centimeters, Grams, and Seconds	British
Length	Meter (m)	Meter (m)	Centimeter (cm)	Foot (ft)
Mass	Kilogram (kg)	Kilogram (kg)	Gram (g)	Pound (lb)[b]
Time	Second (s)	Second (s)	Second (s)	Second (s)

[a]The SI includes four additional base units.
[b]The pound is actually a unit of force that is related to mass.

TABLE 2.5 Special Quantities of Radiologic Science and Their Units

Radiographic Quantities	Special Units	International System (SI) Units
Exposure	C/kg	Air kerma (Gy_a)
Dose	J/kg	$Gray_t$ (Gy_t)
Effective Dose	J/kg	Sievert (Sv)
Radioactivity	s^{-1}	Becquerel (Bq)

Question: Find the mass density of a solid box 10 cm on each side with a mass of 0.4 kg.

Answer: D = mass/volume (change 10 cm to 0.1 m)
= 0.4 kg/(0.1 m × 0.1 m × 0.1 m)
= 0.4 kg/0.001 m³
= 400 kg/m³

Question: A 9-in.-thick patient has a coin placed on the skin. The source-to-image receptor distance (SID) is 100 cm. What will be the magnification of the coin?

Answer: The formula for magnification is:

$$M = \frac{SID}{SOD} = \frac{\text{source-to-image receptor distance}}{\text{source-to-object receptor distance}}$$

$$M = \frac{SID}{SOD} = \frac{100 \text{ cm}}{100 \text{ cm} - 9 \text{ in.}}$$

The 9 in. must be converted to centimeters so that the units are consistent.

$$M = \frac{SID}{SOD} = \frac{100 \text{ cm}}{100 \text{ cm} - (9 \text{ in.} \times 2.54 \text{ cm/in.})}$$

$$= \frac{100 \text{ cm}}{100 \text{ cm} - (23 \text{ cm})}$$

$$= \frac{100 \text{ cm}}{77 \text{ cm}}$$

M = 1.3

The image of the coin will be 1.3 times the size of the coin.

MECHANICS

Mechanics is a segment of physics that deals with objects at rest and objects in motion. Objects at rest are static. Objects in motion are dynamic.

Velocity

The motion of an object can be described with the use of two terms: **velocity** and **acceleration**. Velocity, sometimes called speed, is a measure of how fast something is moving or, more precisely, the rate of change of its position with time.

The velocity of a car is measured in kilometers per hour (miles per hour). Units of velocity in SI are meters per second (m/s). The equation for velocity (v) is as follows:

VELOCITY

$$v = \frac{d}{t}$$

where d represents the distance traveled in time, t.

Question: What is the velocity of a ball that travels 60 m in 4 s?

Answer: $v = \frac{d}{t}$

$v = \frac{60 \text{ m}}{4 \text{ s}}$

v = 15 m/s

Question: Light is capable of traveling 669 million miles in 1 hour. What is its velocity in SI units?

Answer: $v = \frac{d}{t}$

$= \frac{6.69 \times 10^8 \text{ mi}}{\text{h}} \times \frac{1609 \text{ m/mi}}{3600 \text{ s/h}}$

$= 2.99 \times 10^8$ m/s

Often, the velocity of an object changes as its position changes. For example, a dragster at the Charlotte Motor Speedway starts from rest and finishes with a velocity of 80 m/s. The **initial velocity**, designated by v_o, is 0 (Fig. 2.7). The **final velocity**, represented by v_f, is

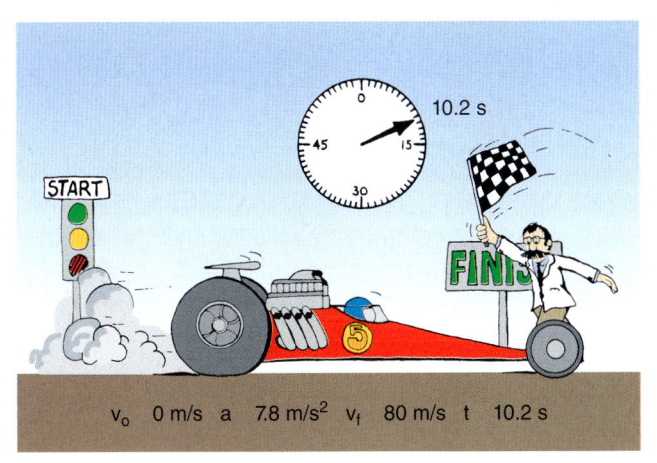

FIG. 2.7 Drag racing provides a familiar example of the relationships among initial velocity, final velocity, acceleration, and time.

80 m/s. The **average velocity** can be calculated from the following expression:

> **AVERAGE VELOCITY**
> $$\bar{v} = \frac{v_o + v_f}{2}$$
> where the bar over the v represents average velocity.

Question: What is the average velocity of the dragster?

Answer:
$$\bar{v} = \frac{0 \text{ m/s} + 80 \text{ m/s}}{2}$$
$$= 40 \text{ m/s}$$

> The velocity of light is constant and is symbolized by c: $c = 3 \times 10^8$ m/s.

Acceleration

The rate of change of velocity with time is acceleration. It is how "quickly or slowly" the velocity is changing. Because acceleration is velocity divided by time, the unit is meters per second squared (m/s²).

If velocity is constant, acceleration is zero. On the other hand, a constant acceleration of 2 m/s² means that the velocity of an object increased by 2 m/s each second. The defining equation for acceleration is given by the following:

> **ACCELERATION**
> $$a = \frac{v_f - v_o}{t}$$

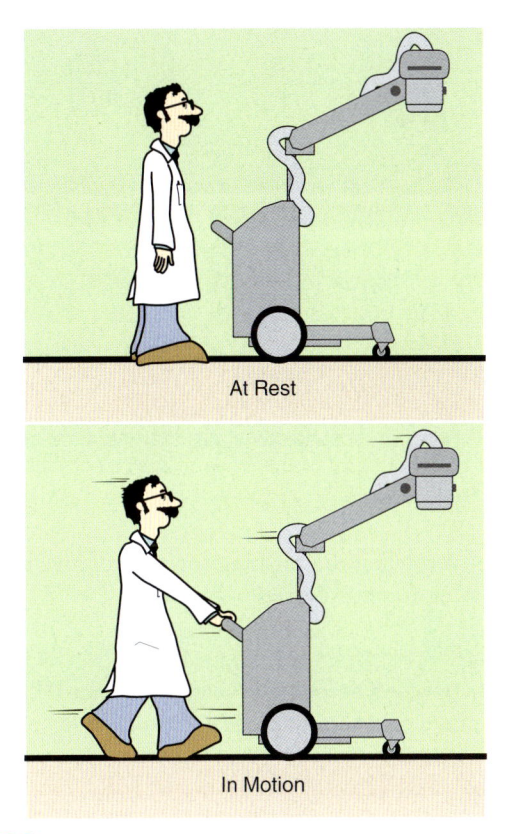

FIG. 2.8 Newton's first law states that a body at rest will remain at rest and a body in motion will continue in motion until acted on by an outside force.

Question: What is the acceleration of the dragster?

Answer:
$$a = \frac{80 \text{ m/s} - 0 \text{ m/s}}{10.2 \text{ s}}$$
$$= 7.8 \text{ m/s}^2$$

Newton's Laws of Motion

In 1686 the English scientist Isaac Newton presented three principles that even today are recognized as fundamental laws of motion.

> Newton's first law: Inertia—A body will remain at rest or will continue to move with constant velocity in a straight line unless acted on by an external force.

Newton's first law states that if no force acts on an object, there will be no acceleration. The property of matter that acts to resist a change in its state of motion is called **inertia**. Newton's first law is thus often referred to as the law of inertia (Fig. 2.8). A mobile x-ray imaging system obviously will not move until forced by a push. Once in motion, however, it will continue to move

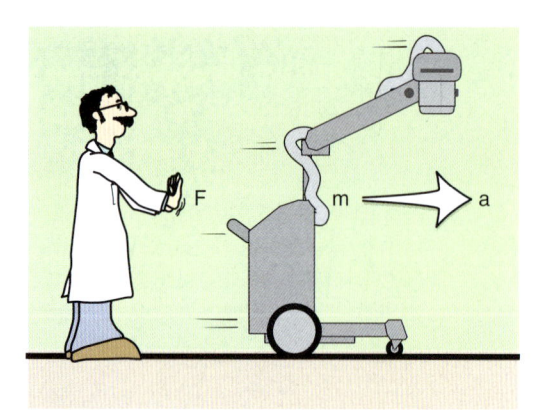

FIG. 2.9 Newton's second law states that the force applied to move an object is equal to the mass of the object multiplied by the acceleration.

forever, even when the pushing force is removed, unless an opposing force is present—friction.

> Newton's second law: Force—The force (F) that acts on an object is equal to the mass (m) of the object multiplied by the acceleration (a) produced.

Newton's second law is a definition of the concept of **force**. Force can be thought of as a push or pull on an object. If a body of mass (m) has an acceleration (a), then the force (F) on it is given by the mass times the acceleration. Newton's second law is illustrated in Fig. 2.9. Mathematically, this law can be expressed as follows:

> **FORCE**
> F = ma
> The SI unit of force is the newton (N).

Question: Find the force on a 55-kg mass accelerating at 14 m/s².
Answer: F = ma
F = (55 kg)(14 m/s²) = 770 N

Question: For a 3600-lb (1636-kg) Ford Mustang to accelerate at 15 m/s², what force is required?
Answer: F = ma
F = (1636 kg)(15 m/s²) = 24,540 N

Newton's third law of motion states that for every action, there is an equal and opposite reaction. Action was Newton's word for force. According to this law, if you push on a heavy block, the block will push back on you with the same force that you apply. On the other hand, if you were the physics professor illustrated in Fig. 2.10, whose crazed students had tricked him into

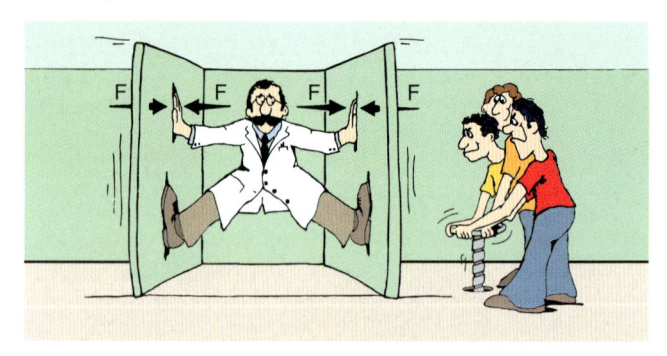

FIG. 2.10 Crazed student technologists performing a routine physics experiment to prove Newton's third law.

the clamp room, no matter how hard you pushed, the walls would continue to close.

> Newton's third law: Action/reaction—For every action, there is an equal and opposite reaction.

Weight

Weight (Wt) is a force on a body caused by the pull of gravity on it. Experiments have shown that objects that fall to Earth accelerate at a constant rate. This rate, termed the **acceleration due to gravity** and represented by the symbol g, is 9.8 m/s² on the Earth and 1.6 m/s² on the Moon.

Weightlessness observed in outer space is attributable to the absence of gravity. Thus the value of gravity in outer space is zero. The weight of an object is equal to the product of its mass and the acceleration of gravity.

Question: A student radiographer has a mass of 75 kg. What is their weight on the Earth? On the Moon?
Answer: Earth: g = 9.8 m/s²
Wt = mg
= 75 kg (9.8 m/s²)
= 735 N
Moon: g = 1.6 m/s²
Wt = mg
= 75 kg (1.6 m/s²)
= 120 N

> **WEIGHT**
> Wt = mg
> Weight is the product of mass and the acceleration of gravity on the Earth: 1 lb = 4.5 N.
> The unit of weight is the same as that for force, the newton (N).

This example displays an important concept. The weight of an object can vary according to the value of gravity acting on it. However, note that the mass of an object does not change, regardless of its location. The student's 75-kg mass remains the same on the Earth, on the Moon, or in space.

Momentum

The product of the mass of an object and its velocity is called **momentum**, represented by **p**. The greater the velocity of an object, the more momentum the object possesses. For example, a truck accelerating down a hill gains momentum as its velocity increases.

> **MOMENTUM**
> p = mv
> Momentum is the product of mass and velocity.

The total momentum before any interaction is equal to the total momentum after the interaction. Imagine a billiard ball colliding with two other balls at rest (Fig. 2.11). The total momentum before the collision is the mass times the velocity of the cue ball. After the collision, this momentum is shared by the three balls. Thus the original momentum of the cue ball is conserved after the interaction.

Work

Work, as used in physics, has specific meaning. The work done on an object is the force applied to that object times the distance over which it is applied. In mathematical terms, the unit of work is the joule (J). When you lift an image receptor, you are doing work. However, when the image receptor is merely held motionless, no work (in the physics sense) is being performed, even though considerable effort is being expended.

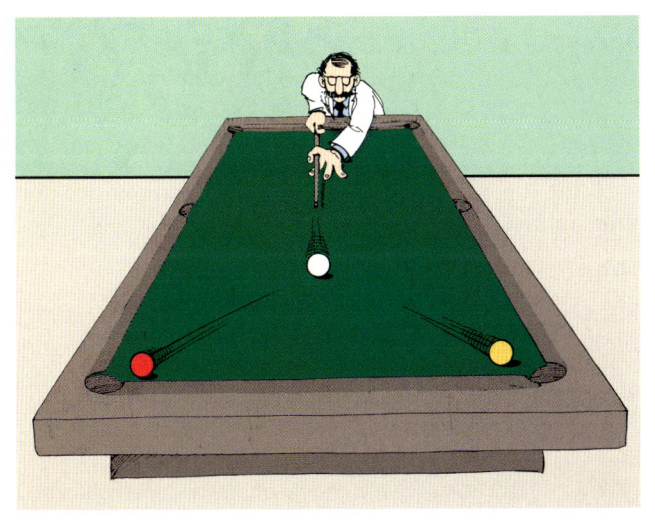

FIG. 2.11 The conservation of momentum occurs with every billiard shot.

> **WORK**
> W = Fd
> Work is the product of force and distance.

Question: Find the work done in lifting an infant patient weighing 90 N (20 lb) to a height of 1.5 m.

Answer:
Work = Fd
= (90 N)(1.5 m)
= 135 J

Power

Power is the rate of doing work. The same amount of work is required to lift an image receptor to a given height, whether it takes 1 second or 1 minute to do so. Power gives us a way to include the time required to perform the work.

> **POWER**
> P = Work/t = Fd/t
> Power is the quotient of work by time.

The SI unit of power is the joule/second (J/s), which is a **watt (W)**. The British unit of power is the **horsepower (hp)**.

Question: A radiographer lifts a 0.8-kg image receptor from the floor to the top of a 1.5-m table with an acceleration of 3 m/s^2. What is the power exerted if it takes 1.0 s?

Answer: This is a multistep problem. We know that P = work/t; however, the value of work is not given in the problem. Recall that work = Fd and F = ma. First, find F.

F = ma
= (0.8 kg)(3 m/s^2)
= 2.4 N.

Next, find work:

Work = Fd
= (2.4 N)(1.5 m)
= 3.6 J

Now, P can be determined:

P = Work/t
= 3.6 J/1.0 s
= 3.6 W

Energy

There are many forms of energy, as previously discussed. The law of conservation of energy states that energy may be transformed from one form to another, but it cannot be created or destroyed. The total amount of energy is constant. For example, electrical energy is converted into light energy and heat energy in an electric light bulb. The unit of energy and of work is the same, the joule.

> Energy is the ability to do work.

Two forms of mechanical energy often are used in radiologic science: kinetic energy and potential energy. Kinetic energy is the energy associated with the motion of an object as expressed by the following:

> **KINETIC ENERGY**
> $KE = \frac{1}{2}mv^2$
> Kinetic energy depends on the mass of the object and on the square of its velocity.

Question: Consider two rodeo chuckwagons, A and B, with the same mass. If B has twice the velocity of A, verify that the kinetic energy of chuckwagon B is four times that of chuckwagon A.

Answer: Chuck wagon A: $KE_A = \frac{1}{2}mv_A^2$

Chuck wagon B: $KE_B = \frac{1}{2}mv_B^2$

However, $m_A = m_B$, $v_B = 2v_A$.

Therefore $KE_B = \frac{1}{2}m_A(2v_A)^2$
$= \frac{1}{2}m_A(4v_A^2)$

$KE_B = 2mv_A^2$
$= 4\left(\frac{1}{2}mv_A^2\right)$
$= 4\,KE_A$

Potential energy is the stored energy of position or configuration. A textbook on a desk has potential energy because of its height above the floor ... and the potential for a better job if it is read. It has the ability to do work by falling to the ground. Gravitational potential energy is given by the following:

> **POTENTIAL ENERGY**
> $PE = mgh$
> where h is the distance above the Earth's surface.

A skier at the top of a jump, a coiled spring, and a stretched rubber band are examples of other systems that have potential energy because of their position or configuration.

If a scientist held a ball in the air atop the Leaning Tower of Pisa (Fig. 2.12), the ball would have only potential energy, no kinetic energy. When it is released

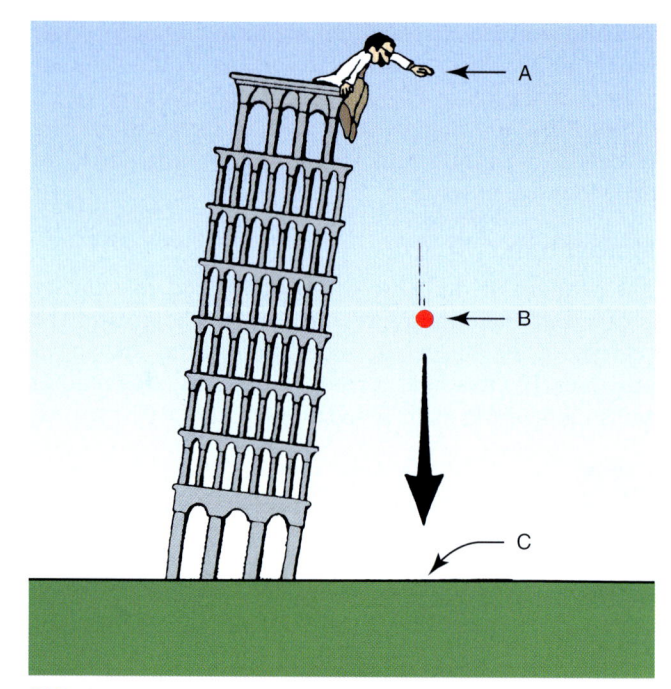

FIG. 2.12 Potential energy results from the position of an object. Kinetic energy is the energy of motion. (A) Maximum potential energy, no kinetic energy. (B) Potential energy and kinetic energy. (C) Maximum kinetic energy, no potential energy.

and begins to fall, the potential energy decreases as the height decreases. At the same time, the kinetic energy is increasing as the ball accelerates. Just before impact, the kinetic energy of the ball becomes maximum as its velocity reaches maximum. Because it now has no height, the potential energy becomes zero. All the initial potential energy of the ball has been converted into kinetic energy during the fall.

Question: A radiographer holds a 6-kg x-ray tube 1.5 m above the ground. What is its potential energy?

Answer: Potential energy = mgh
$= 6\,kg \times 9.8\,m/s^2 \times 1.5\,m$
$= 88\,kg \cdot m^2/s^2$
$= 88\,J$

Table 2.6 presents a summary of the quantities and units in mechanics.

Heat

Heat is a form of energy that is very important to radiographers. Excessive heat, a deadly enemy of an x-ray tube, can cause permanent damage. For this reason, the radiographer should be aware of the properties of heat.

> Heat is the kinetic energy of the random motion of molecules.

TABLE 2.6	Summary of Quantities, Equations, and Units Used in Mechanics			
Quantity	Symbol	Defining Equation	International System (SI)	
Velocity	V	v = d/t	m/s	
Average velocity			m/s	
Acceleration	a		m/s^2	
Force	F	F = ma	N	
Weight	Wt	Wt = mg	N	
Momentum	p	p = mv	kg-m/s	
Work	W	W = Fd	J	
Power	P	P = W/t	W	
Kinetic energy	KE	KE = mv^2	J	
Potential energy	PE	PE = mgh	J	

The more rapid and disordered the motion of molecules, the more heat an object contains. The unit of heat, the **calorie**, is defined as the heat necessary to raise the temperature of 1 g of water by 1°C. The same amount of heat will have different effects on different materials. For example, the heat required to change the temperature of 1 g of silver by 1°C is approximately 0.05 calorie.

> Heat is transferred from one location to another by conduction, convection, and radiation.

Conduction is the transfer of heat through a material or by touching. Molecular motion from a high-temperature object that touches a lower-temperature object equalizes the temperature of both.

Conduction is easily observed when a hot object and a cold object are placed in contact. After a short time, heat conducted to the cooler object results in equal temperatures of the two objects. Heat is conducted from an x-ray tube anode through the rotor to the insulating oil.

Convection is the mechanical transfer of "hot" molecules in a gas or liquid from one place to another. A steam radiator or forced-air furnace warms a room by convection. The air around the radiator is heated, causing it to rise, while cooler air circulates in and takes its place.

Thermal radiation is the transfer of heat by the emission of **infrared radiation**. The reddish glow emitted by hot objects is evidence of heat transfer by radiation. An x-ray tube cools primarily by radiation.

A forced-air furnace blows heated air into the room, providing forced circulation to complement the natural convection. Heat is convected from the housing of an x-ray tube to air.

Temperature normally is measured with a thermometer. A thermometer is usually calibrated at two reference points—the freezing and boiling points of water. The three scales that have been developed to measure temperature are Celsius (°C), Fahrenheit (°F), and Kelvin (K) (Fig. 2.13).

These scales are interrelated as follows:

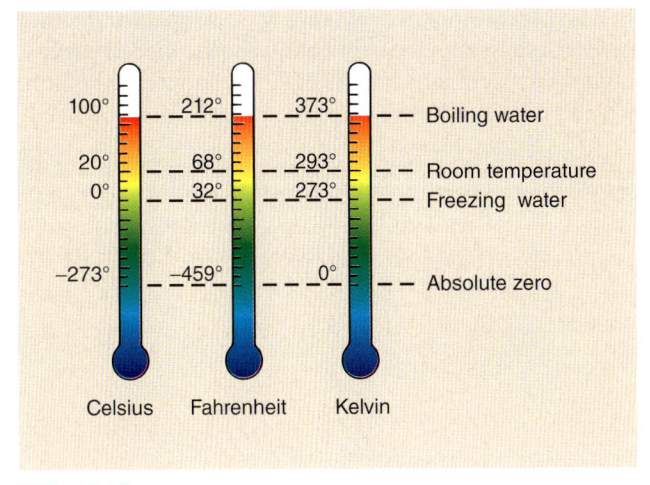

FIG. 2.13 Three scales are used to represent temperature. Celsius is the adopted scale for weather reporting everywhere except the United States. Kelvin is the scientific scale.

> **TEMPERATURE SCALES**
>
> $T_C = \frac{5}{9} T_F - 32$
>
> $T_F = \frac{9}{5} T_C + 32$
>
> $T_K = T_C + 273$
>
> $T_C = T_K - 273$
>
> $T_F = \frac{9}{5} T_K - 273 + 32$
>
> $T_K = \frac{5}{9} T_F - 32 + 273$
>
> The subscripts C, F, and K refer to Celsius, Fahrenheit, and Kelvin, respectively.

Question: Convert 77°F to °C.
Answer:
$T_C = \frac{5}{9}(T_F - 32)$
$= \frac{5}{9}(77 - 32)$
$= \frac{5}{9}(45) = 25°C$

One can use the following for easy, approximate conversion:

> **APPROXIMATE TEMPERATURE CONVERSION**
> From °F to °C, subtract 30 and divide by 2.
> From °C to °F, double and then add 30.

Magnetic resonance imaging with a superconducting magnet requires extremely cold liquids called **cryogens**. Liquid nitrogen, which boils at 77°K, and liquid helium, which boils at 4°K, are the two cryogens that are used.

Question: Liquid helium is used to cool superconducting wire in magnetic resonance imaging systems. What is its temperature in °F?

Answer:
$T_K = T_C + 273$
$T_C = T_K - 273$
$T_C = 4 - 273$
$T_C = -269°C$
$T_F = \frac{9}{5}T_C + 32$
$T_F = -484 + 32$
$T_F = -452°F$

The relationship between temperature and energy is often represented by an energy thermometer (Fig. 2.14). We consider x-rays to be energetic, although on the cosmic scale, they are rather ordinary.

SUMMARY

This chapter introduces primary mathematics, physics, and standards of measurement as necessary for radiologic science.

Basic algebra and the use of fractions, decimals, and significant figures are presented. The various number systems are introduced, as well as the rules for significant figures and exponents. Graphing, as it is required for radiologic science, is illustrated.

Mass, length, and time are the basic units of physics, and it is shown here how these units are used to describe the special units of radiologic science.

Newton's laws of motion are described as they relate to medical imaging. Newton was first to properly describe the concepts of mechanics each of which are discussed here.

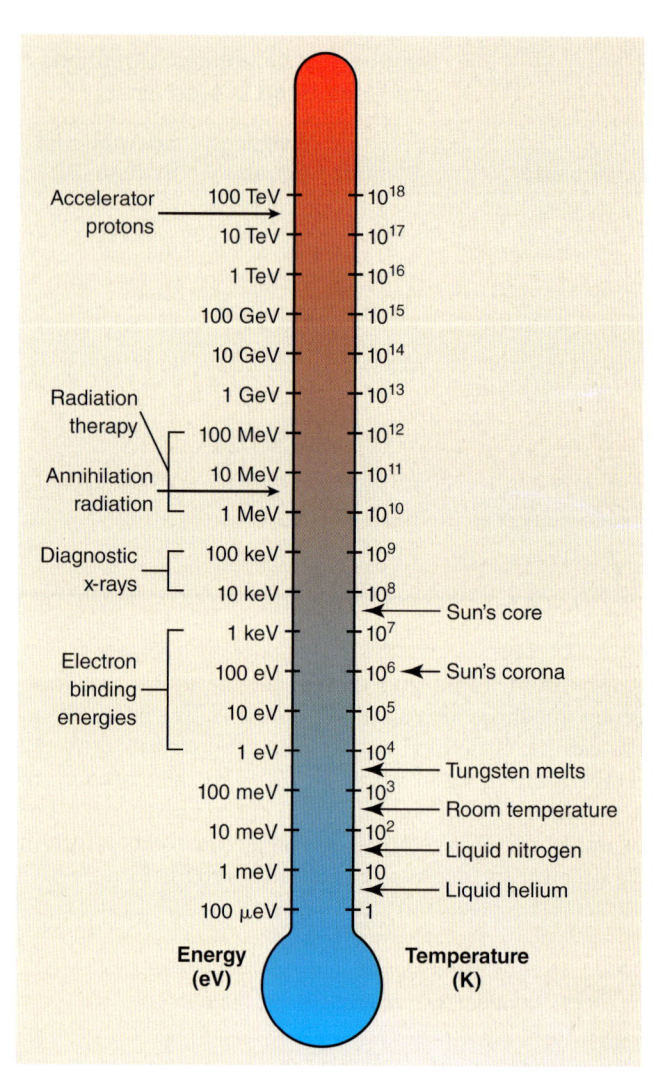

FIG. 2.14 The energy thermometer scales temperature and energy together.

CHALLENGE QUESTIONS

1. Perform the following mathematic problems with fractions. Express each answer in a proper fraction.
   a. 1/2 + 2/3 =
   b. 7/8 − 1/4 =
   c. 1/6 × 1/2 =
   d. 3/4 ÷ 1/8 =
2. Using the ratio 2.54 cm/in, convert 72 into cm. Round the answer to the correct number of significant digits.
3. Convert the following fractions to decimals.
   a. 3/10
   b. 53/100
   c. 40/1000
4. Perform the following mathematic problems with decimals. Round each answer to the correct number of significant digits.
   a. 3.0045 + 2.25 + 8.002 =
   b. 124.78 − 6.5 =
   c. 3.14 × 0.0115 =
   d. 75.25 ÷ 3.11 =
5. Solve using the rules of algebra.
   a. Given: mA × time in seconds = mAs
   b. 200 mA × _____ seconds = 8 mAs
   c. $\dfrac{x}{877\ \mu Gy_a} = \dfrac{200\ mAs}{400\ mAs}$
   d. Given grid ratio = $\dfrac{\text{Height of lead strips}}{\text{Interspace between lead strips}}$

If the lead strip height of a given grid is 2 mm and the interspace distance is 0.25 mm, what is the grid ratio?
6. Convert to exponential form.
    a. 625,000,000
    b. 820
    c. 5/1000
    d. 0.000125

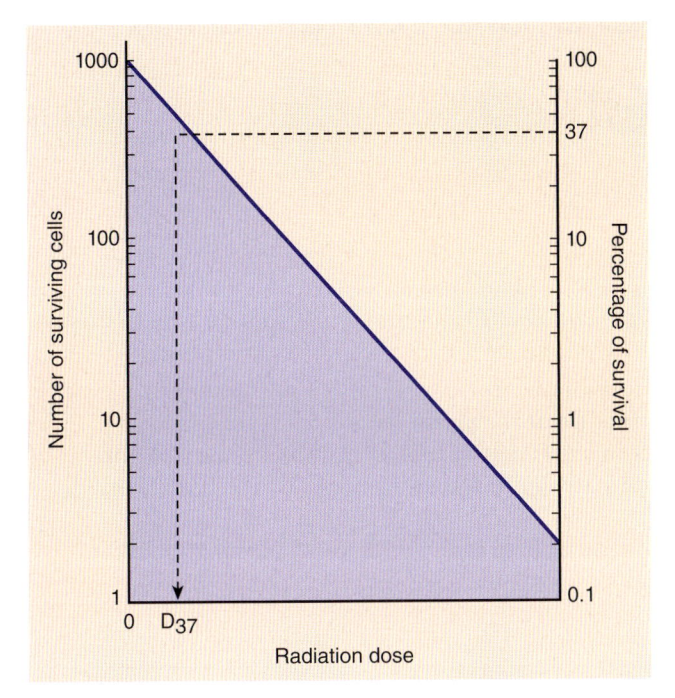

7. In the dose-response graph above, showing the results of the irradiation of 1000 cells, the y-axis is a _____ (linear, logarithmic) scale.
8. The dose-response graph above demonstrates a(n) _____ (inverse, direct) relationship between radiation dose and the number of surviving cells. 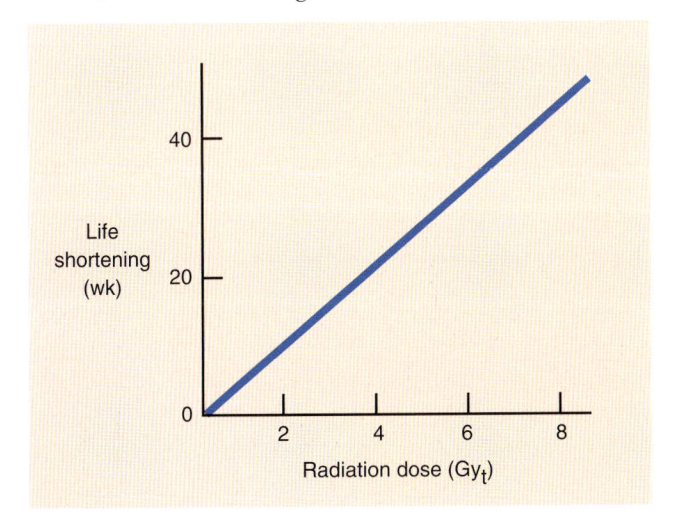
9. In the previous dose-response graph, showing the results of life shortening after chronic irradiation, the y-axis is a _____ (liner, logarithmic) scale.
10. The dose-response graph above demonstrates a(n) _____ (inverse, direct) relationship between chronic radiation dose and life shortening. 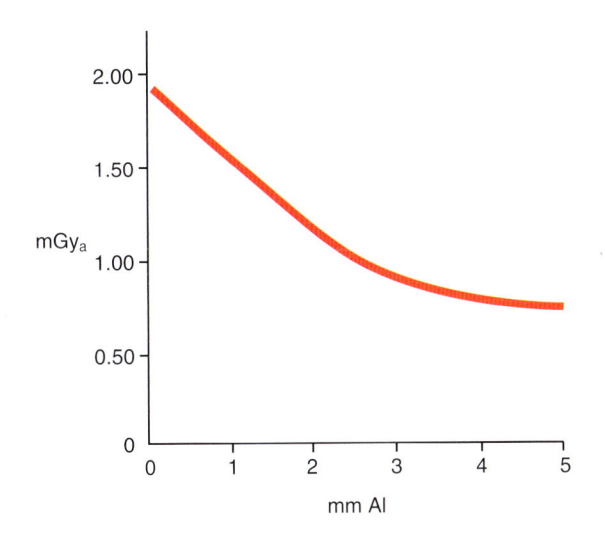
11. In the previous graph of added filtration (mm Al) on beam intensity (mGy_a), _____ mm Al is required to reduce the beam intensity to 1.00 mGy_a.
12. State the three base quantities and the SI unit of measure for each base quantity.
13. What are the four special quantities of radiation measurement?
14. State Newton's three laws of motion.
15. Define power.
16. Define energy.
17. State the law of conservation of energy.
18. Define kinetic energy and potential energy.
19. _____ is the kinetic energy of the random motion of molecules.
20. List the three methods of heat transfer systems.

The answers to the Challenge Questions can be found by logging on to our website at http://evolve.elsevier.com.

CHAPTER 3

The Structure of Matter

OBJECTIVES

At the completion of this chapter, the student should be able to do the following:

1. Relate the history of the atom.
2. Identify the structure of the atom.
3. Describe electron shells and instability within atomic structure.
4. Discuss radioactivity and the characteristics of alpha and beta particles.
5. Explain the difference between two forms of ionizing radiation: particulate and electromagnetic.

OUTLINE

Centuries of Discovery 35
   Greek Atom 35
   Dalton Atom 35
   Thomson Atom 36
   Bohr Atom 37
Fundamental Particles 37
Atomic Structure 38
   Electron Arrangement 39
   Electron-Binding Energy 41
Atomic Nomenclature 43

Combinations of Atoms 45
Radioactivity 45
   Radioisotopes 46
   Radioactive Half-Life 47
Types of Ionizing Radiation 49
   Particulate Radiation 49
   Electromagnetic Radiation 50
Summary 51
Challenge Questions 51

CHAPTER 3 The Structure of Matter

THIS CHAPTER moves from the study of energy and force to the basis of matter itself. What composes matter? What is the magnitude of matter?

From the inner space of the atom to the outer space of the universe, there is an enormous range in the size of matter. More than 40 orders of magnitude are needed to identify objects as small as the atom and as large as the universe. Because matter spans such a large magnitude, exponential form is used to express the measurements of objects. Fig. 3.1 shows the orders of magnitude and illustrates how matter in our surroundings varies in size.

The atom is the building block of the radiographer's understanding of the interaction between ionizing radiation and matter. This chapter explains what happens when energy in the form of an x-ray interacts with tissue. Although tissue has an extremely complex structure, it is made up of atoms and combinations of atoms. By examining the structure of atoms, we can learn what happens when the structure is changed.

CENTURIES OF DISCOVERY

Greek Atom

One of civilization's most pronounced continuing scientific investigations has sought to determine precisely the structure of matter. The earliest recorded reference to this investigation comes from the Greeks several hundred years BC.

Pythagoras, sixth century BC, and Archimedes three centuries later thought that matter was composed of four substances: earth, water, air, and fire. According to them, all matter could be described as combinations of these four basic substances in various proportions, modified by four basic essences: wet, dry, hot, and cold. Fig. 3.2 shows how this theory of matter was represented at that time.

The Greeks used the term **atom**, meaning "indivisible" [a (not) + temon (cut)] to describe the smallest part of the four substances of matter. Each type of atom was represented by a symbol (Fig. 3.3A). Currently, 118 substances or **elements** have been identified; 92 are naturally occurring, and the additional 26 have been artificially produced in high-energy particle accelerators.

We now know that the atom is the smallest particle of matter that has the properties of an element. Many particles are much smaller than the atom; these are called subatomic particles.

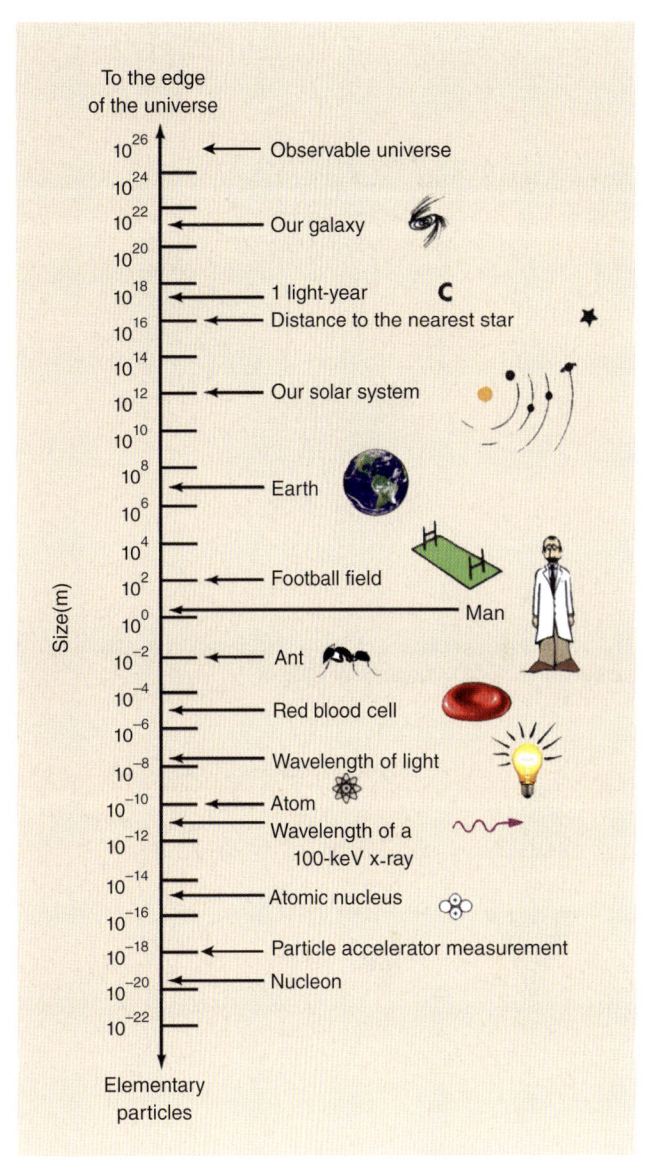

FIG. 3.1 The size of objects varies enormously. The range of sizes in nature requires that scientific notation be used because more than 40 orders of magnitude are necessary.

> An atom is the smallest particle that has all the properties of an element.

Dalton Atom

The Greek description of the structure of matter persisted for hundreds of years. In fact, it formed the theoretical basis for the vain efforts by medieval alchemists to transform lead into gold. It was not until the 19th century that the foundation for modern atomic theory was laid. In 1808 John Dalton, an English schoolteacher, published a book summarizing his experiments, which showed that the elements could be classified according to integral values of atomic mass.

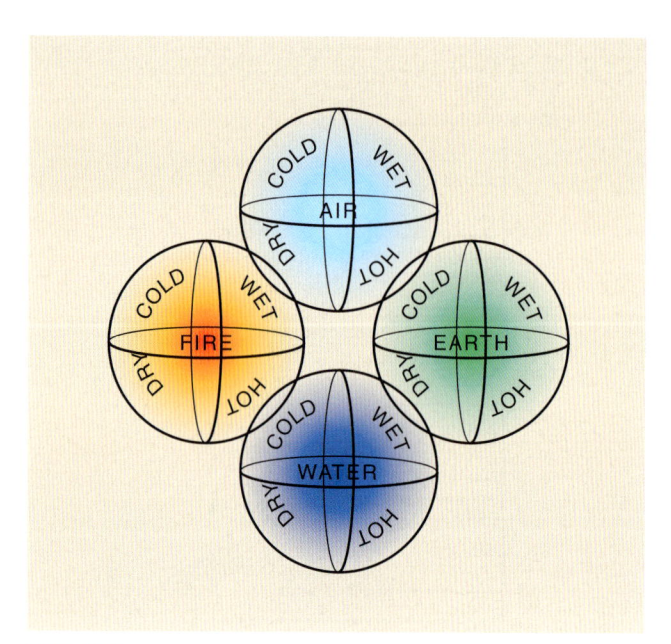

FIG. 3.2 Representation of the substances and essences of matter as viewed by the ancient Greeks.

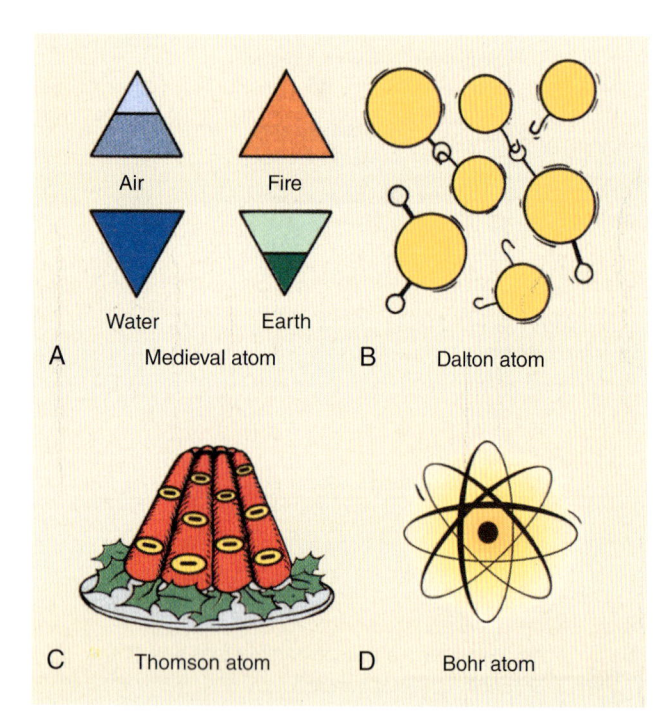

FIG. 3.3 Through the years, the atom has been represented by many symbols. (A) The Greeks envisioned four different atoms, representing air, fire, earth, and water. These triangular symbols were adopted by medieval alchemists. (B) Dalton's atoms had hooks and eyes to account for chemical combination. (C) Thomson's model of the atom has been described as a plum pudding, with the plums representing the electrons. (D) The Bohr atom has a small, dense, positively charged nucleus surrounded by electrons at precise energy levels.

According to Dalton, an element was composed of identical atoms that reacted the same way chemically. For example, all oxygen atoms were alike. They looked alike, they were constructed alike, and they reacted alike. However, they were very different from atoms of any other element.

The physical combination of one type of atom with another was visualized as being an eye-and-hook affair (see Fig. 3.3B). The size and number of the eyes and hooks were different for each element.

Some 50 years after Dalton's work, a Russian scholar, Dmitri Mendeleev, showed that if the elements were arranged in order of increasing atomic mass, a periodic repetition of similar chemical properties occurred. At that time, approximately 65 elements had been identified. Mendeleev's work resulted in the first periodic table of the elements. Although there were many holes in Mendeleev's table, it showed that all the then-known elements could be placed in one of eight groups.

Fig. 3.4 is a rendering of the periodic table of elements. Each block represents an element. The superscript is the atomic number. The subscript is the elemental mass.

> All elements are arranged into eight groups, as shown in the periodic table of elements.

All elements in the same group (i.e., column) react chemically in a similar fashion and have similar physical properties. Except for hydrogen, the elements of group I, called the alkali metals, are all soft metals that combine readily with oxygen and react violently with water. The elements of group VII, called halogens, are easily vaporized and combine with metals to form water-soluble salts. Group VIII elements, called the noble gases, are highly resistant to reaction with other elements.

These elemental groupings are determined by the placement of electrons in each atom. This is considered more fully later.

Thomson Atom

After the publication of Mendeleev's periodic table, additional elements were separated and identified, and the periodic table slowly filled. However, knowledge of the structure of atoms remained scanty.

Before the turn of the 20th century, atoms were considered indivisible. The only difference between the atoms of one element and the atoms of another was their mass. Through the efforts of many scientists, it slowly became apparent that there was an electrical nature to the structure of an atom.

In the late 1890s, while investigating the physical properties of cathode rays (electrons), J.J. Thomson concluded that electrons were an integral part of all atoms. He described the atom as looking something like a plum pudding, in which the plums represented negative electric charges (electrons) and the pudding was a shapeless mass of uniform positive electrification (see Fig. 3.3C). The number of electrons was thought to

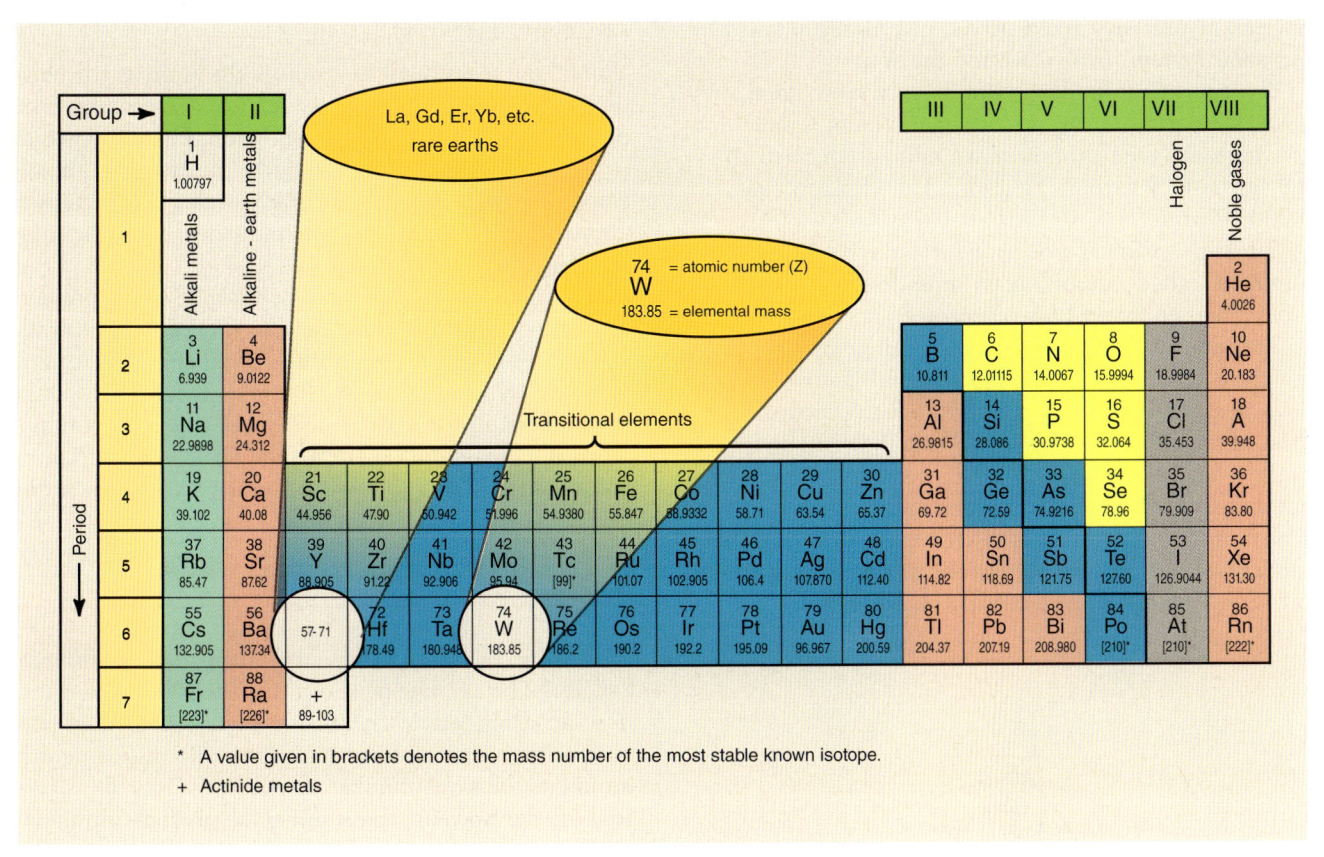

FIG. 3.4 Periodic table of elements.

equal the quantity of positive electrification because the atom was known to be electrically neutral.

Through a series of ingenious experiments, Ernest Rutherford in 1911 disproved Thomson's model of the atom. Rutherford introduced the nuclear model, which described the atom as containing a small, dense, positively charged center surrounded by a negative cloud of electrons. He called the center of the atom the **nucleus**.

Bohr Atom

In 1913 Niels Bohr improved Rutherford's description of the atom. Bohr's model was a miniature solar system in which the electrons revolved about the nucleus in prescribed orbits or energy levels. For our purposes, the Bohr atom (see Fig. 3.3D) represents the best way to picture the atom, although the details of atomic structure are more accurately described by a newer model, called **quantum chromodynamics**.

Simply put, the Bohr atom contains a small, dense, positively charged nucleus surrounded by negatively charged electrons that revolve in fixed, well-defined orbits about the nucleus. In the normal atom, the number of electrons is equal to the number of positive charges in the nucleus. (protons)

FUNDAMENTAL PARTICLES

Our understanding of the atom today is essentially that which Bohr presented a century ago. With the development of high-energy particle accelerators, the structure of the atomic nucleus is slowly being mapped and identified. More than 100 subatomic particles have been detected and described by physicists working with particle accelerators. Several Nobel Prizes in Physics have been awarded in recent years because of this work; the Higgs Boson is a good example.

Nuclear structure is now well defined (Fig. 3.5). Nucleons—protons and neutrons—are composed of quarks that are held together by gluons. However, these particles are of little consequence to radiologic science. Only the three primary constituents of an atom, the electron, the proton, and the neutron, are considered here. They are the fundamental particles (Table 3.1).

> The fundamental particles of an atom are the electron, the proton, and the neutron.

The atom can be viewed as a miniature solar system whose sun is the nucleus and whose planets are the electrons. The arrangement of electrons around the nucleus determines the manner in which atoms interact.

Electrons are very small particles that carry one unit of negative electric charge. Their mass is only 9.1×10^{-31} kg. They can be pictured as revolving about the nucleus in precisely fixed orbits, just as the planets in our solar system revolve around the Sun.

Because an atomic particle is extremely small, its mass is expressed in atomic mass units (amu) for convenience. One atomic mass unit is equal to 1/12 the mass of a carbon-12 atom. The electron mass is 0.000549 amu.

When precision is not necessary, a system of whole numbers called atomic mass numbers is used. The atomic mass number of an electron is 0.

The nucleus contains particles called nucleons, of which there are two types: protons and neutrons. Both have nearly 2000 times the mass of an electron. The mass of a proton is 1.673×10^{-27} kg; the neutron is just slightly heavier at 1.675×10^{-27} kg. The atomic mass number of each is 1. The primary difference between a proton and a neutron is electric charge. The proton carries one unit of positive electric charge. The neutron carries no charge; it is electrically neutral.

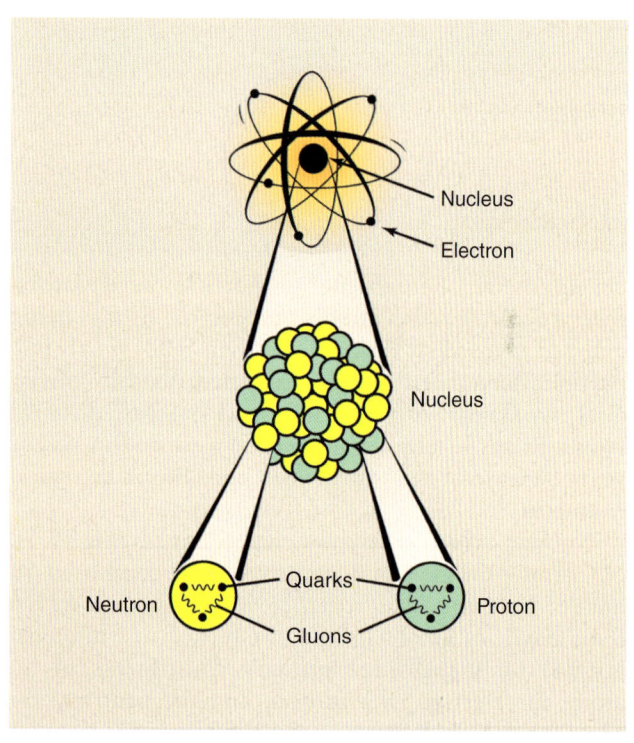

FIG. 3.5 The nucleus consists of protons and neutrons, which are made of quarks bound together by gluons.

ATOMIC STRUCTURE

You might be tempted to visualize the atom as a beehive of subatomic activity because classical representations of it usually appear like that shown in Fig. 3.3D, which is greatly oversimplified. In fact, the atom is mostly empty space, similar to our solar system. The nucleus of an atom is very small but contains nearly all the mass of the atom.

If a basketball, whose diameter is 23 cm, represents the size of the uranium nucleus, the largest naturally occurring atom, the path of the orbital electrons is more than 12 km (7.2 mi) away. Because it contains all the neutrons and protons, the nucleus of the atom contains most of its mass. For example, the nucleus of a uranium atom contains 99.998% of the entire mass of the atom.

> The atom is essentially empty space.

Possible electron orbits are grouped into different "shells." The arrangement of these shells helps to reveal how an atom reacts chemically (i.e., how it combines with other atoms to form molecules). Because a neutral atom has the same number of electrons in orbit as protons in the nucleus, the number of protons ultimately determines the chemical behavior of an atom.

The number of protons determines the chemical element. Atoms that have the same number of protons but differ in the number of neutrons are isotopes; they behave in the same way during chemical reactions.

The periodic table of the elements (see Fig. 3.4) lists matter in order of increasing complexity, beginning with hydrogen (H). An atom of hydrogen contains one proton in its nucleus and one electron outside the nucleus. Helium (He), the second atom in the table, contains two protons, two neutrons, and two electrons.

The third atom, lithium (Li), contains three protons, four neutrons, and three electrons. Two of these electrons are in the same shell, the K shell, as are the electrons of hydrogen and helium. The third electron is in the next farther shell from the nucleus, the L shell.

Electrons can exist only in certain shells, which represent different electron-binding energies. For identification purposes, electron orbital shells are given the

TABLE 3.1	Important Characteristics of the Fundamental Particles						
					MASS		
Particle	Location	Charge	Symbol	Relative	Kilograms	amu	Number
Electron	Shells	−1	−	1	9.109×10^{-31}	0.000549	0
Proton	Nucleus	+1	+	1836	1.673×10^{-27}	1.00728	1
Neutron	Nucleus	0	O	1838	1.675×10^{-27}	1.00867	1

amu, Atomic mass units.

CHAPTER 3 The Structure of Matter   39

The total number of electrons in the orbital shells is exactly equal to the number of protons in the nucleus. If an atom has an extra electron or has had an electron removed, it is said to be *ionized*. An ionized atom is not electrically neutral but carries a charge equal in magnitude to the difference between the numbers of electrons and protons.

You might assume that atoms can be ionized by changing the number of positive charges as well as the number of negative charges. However, atoms cannot be ionized by the addition or subtraction of protons because they are bound very strongly together, and that action would change the type of atom. An alteration in the number of neutrons does not ionize an atom because the neutron is electrically neutral.

Fig. 3.7 represents the interaction between an x-ray and a carbon atom, a primary constituent of tissue. The x-ray transfers its energy to an orbital electron and ejects that electron from the atom. This process requires approximately 34 eV of energy. The x-ray may cease to exist, and an ion pair is formed. The remaining atom is now a positive ion because it contains one more positive charge than negative charge.

> Ionization is the removal of an orbital electron from an atom.

In all except the lightest atoms, the number of neutrons is always greater than the number of protons. The larger the atom, the greater the abundance of neutrons over protons.

Electron Arrangement

The maximum number of electrons that can exist in each shell (Table 3.2) increases with the distance of the shell from the nucleus. These numbers need not be memorized because the electron limit per shell can be calculated from the expression:

> **MAXIMUM ELECTRONS PER SHELL**
> $2n^2$
> where n is the shell number.

Question: What is the maximum number of electrons that can exist in the O shell?

Answer: The O shell is the fifth shell from the nucleus; therefore n = 5

$$2n^2 = 2(5)^2$$
$$= 2(25)$$
$$= 50 \text{ electrons}$$

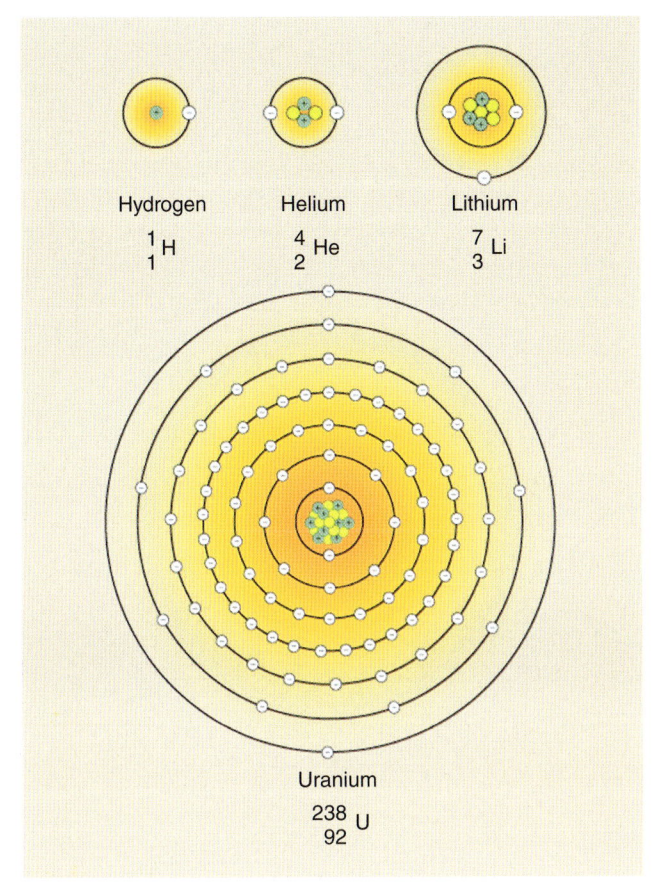

FIG. 3.6 Atoms are composed of neutrons and protons in the nucleus and electrons in specific orbits surrounding the nucleus. Shown here are the three smaller atoms and the largest naturally occurring atom, uranium.

names K, L, M, N, and so forth, to represent the relative binding energies of electrons from closest to the nucleus to farthest from the nucleus. The closer an electron is to the nucleus, the greater is its binding energy.

The next atom in the periodic table, beryllium (Be), has four protons and five neutrons in the nucleus. Two electrons are in the K shell, and two are in the L shell.

The complexity of the electron configuration of atoms increases as one progresses through the periodic table to the most complex naturally occurring element, uranium (U). Uranium has 92 protons and 146 neutrons. The electron distribution is as follows: 2 in the K shell, 8 in the L shell, 18 in the M shell, 32 in the N shell, 21 in the O shell, 9 in the P shell, and 2 in the Q shell.

Fig. 3.6 shows a schematic representation of four atoms. Although these atoms are mostly empty space, they have been diagrammed on one page. If the actual size of the helium nucleus were that in Fig. 3.6, the K-shell electrons would be several city blocks away.

> In their normal state, atoms are electrically neutral; the electric charge on the atom is zero.

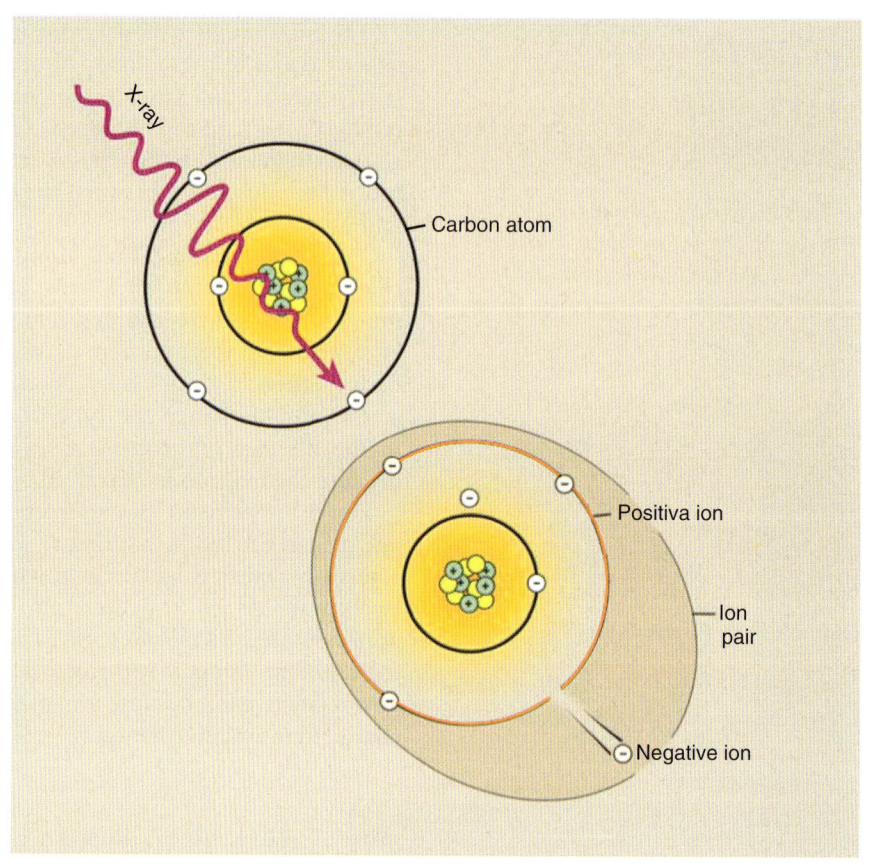

FIG. 3.7 Ionization of a carbon atom by an x-ray leaves the atom with a net electric charge of +1. The ionized atom and the released electron are called an ion pair.

TABLE 3.2	Maximum Number of Electrons That Can Occupy Each Electron Shell	
Shell Number	Shell Symbol	Number of Electrons
1	K	2
2	L	8
3	M	18
4	N	32
5	O	50
6	P	72
7	Q	98

This answer, 50 electrons, is a theoretical value. Even the largest atom does not completely fill shell O or higher.

Physicists call the shell number *n* the **principal quantum number**. Every electron in every atom can be precisely identified by four quantum numbers, the most important of which is the principal quantum number. The other three quantum numbers represent the existence of subshells, which are not important to radiologic science.

The observant reader may have noticed a relationship between the number of shells in an atom and its position in the periodic table of the elements. Oxygen has eight electrons; two occupy the K shell and six occupy the L shell. Oxygen is in the second period (row) and the sixth group (column) of the periodic table (see Fig. 3.4).

Aluminum has the following electron configuration: K shell, two electrons; L shell, eight electrons; M shell, three electrons. Therefore, aluminum is in the third period (M shell) and third group (three electrons) of the periodic table.

> **ELECTRON ARRANGEMENT**
> The number of electrons in the outermost shell:
> …is equal to its group in the periodic table.
> …determines the valence of an atom.
> The number of the outermost electron shell:
> …is equal to its period in the periodic table.

Question: What are the period and group for the gastrointestinal contrast agent barium (refer to Fig. 3.4)?

Answer: Period 6 and group II.

> No outer shell can contain more than eight electrons.

Why does the periodic table show elements repeating similar chemical properties in groups of eight? In addition to the limitation on the maximum number of electrons allowed in any shell, the outer shell is always limited to eight electrons.

All atoms that have one electron in the outer shell lie in group I of the periodic table; atoms with two electrons in the outer shell fall in group II, and so forth. When eight electrons are in the outer shell, the shell is filled. Atoms with filled outer shells lie in group VIII, the noble gases, and are very stable chemically.

The orderly scheme of atomic progression from smallest to largest atom is interrupted in the fourth period. Instead of simply adding electrons to the next outer shell, electrons are added to an inner shell.

The atoms associated with this phenomenon are called the **transitional elements**. Even in these elements, no outer shell ever contains more than eight electrons. The chemical properties of the transitional elements depend on the number of electrons in the two outermost shells.

The shell notation of the electron arrangement of an atom not only identifies the relative distance of an electron from the nucleus but also indicates the relative energy by which the electron is attached to the nucleus.

You might expect that an electron would spontaneously fly off from the nucleus, just as a ball twirling on the end of a string would do if the string were cut. The type of force that prevents this from happening is called **centripetal force** or "center-seeking" force, which results from a basic law of electricity that states that opposite charges attract one another and like charges repel (Fig. 3.8).

> The force that keeps an electron in orbit is the centripetal force.

You might therefore expect that the electrons would drop into the nucleus because of the strong electrostatic attraction. In the normal atom, the centripetal force just balances the force created by the electron velocity, the centrifugal force or flying-out-from-the-center force, so that electrons maintain their distance from the nucleus while traveling in a circular or an elliptical path.

Fig. 3.8 is a representation of this state of affairs for a small atom. In more complex atoms, the same balance of forces exists and each electron can be considered separately.

Electron-Binding Energy

The strength of attachment of an electron to the nucleus is called the **electron-binding energy**. The closer an electron is to the nucleus, the more tightly it is bound. K-shell electrons have higher binding energies than L-shell electrons, L-shell electrons are more tightly bound to the nucleus than M-shell electrons, and so forth.

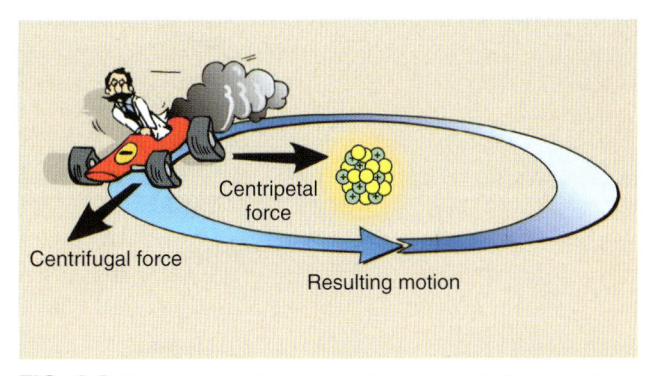

FIG. 3.8 Electrons revolve around the nucleus in fixed orbits or shells. Electrostatic attraction results in a specific electron path around the nucleus.

Not all K-shell electrons of all atoms are bound with the same binding energy. The greater the total number of electrons in an atom, the more tightly each is bound.

To put it differently, the larger and more complex the atom, the higher is the binding energy for electrons in any given shell. Because electrons of atoms with many protons are more tightly bound to the nucleus than those of small atoms, it generally takes more energy to ionize a large atom than to ionize a small atom.

Fig. 3.9 represents the binding energy of electrons of several atoms of radiologic importance. The metals tungsten (W) and molybdenum (Mo) are used as targets in an x-ray tube. Barium (Ba) and iodine (I) are used as radiographic and fluoroscopic contrast agents.

Question: How much energy is required to ionize tungsten through removal of a K-shell electron?

Answer: The minimum energy must equal the binding energy or 69 keV; with less than that, the atom cannot be ionized by the removal of a K-shell electron.

Carbon (C) is an important element in human tissue. As with other tissue atoms, the binding energy for the outer shell electrons is only approximately 10 eV. Yet approximately 34 eV is necessary to ionize tissue atoms. The value 34 eV is called the **ionization potential**. The difference, 24 eV, causes multiple electron excitations, which ultimately result in heat. The concept of ionization potential is important to the description of linear energy transfer, which is discussed in Chapter 32.

Question: How much more energy is necessary to ionize barium than to ionize carbon by removal of K-shell electrons?

Answer: Barium binding energy = 37,400 eV.
Carbon-binding energy = 300 eV.
Difference = 37,100 eV
= 37.1 keV

42　PART I　Radiologic Physics

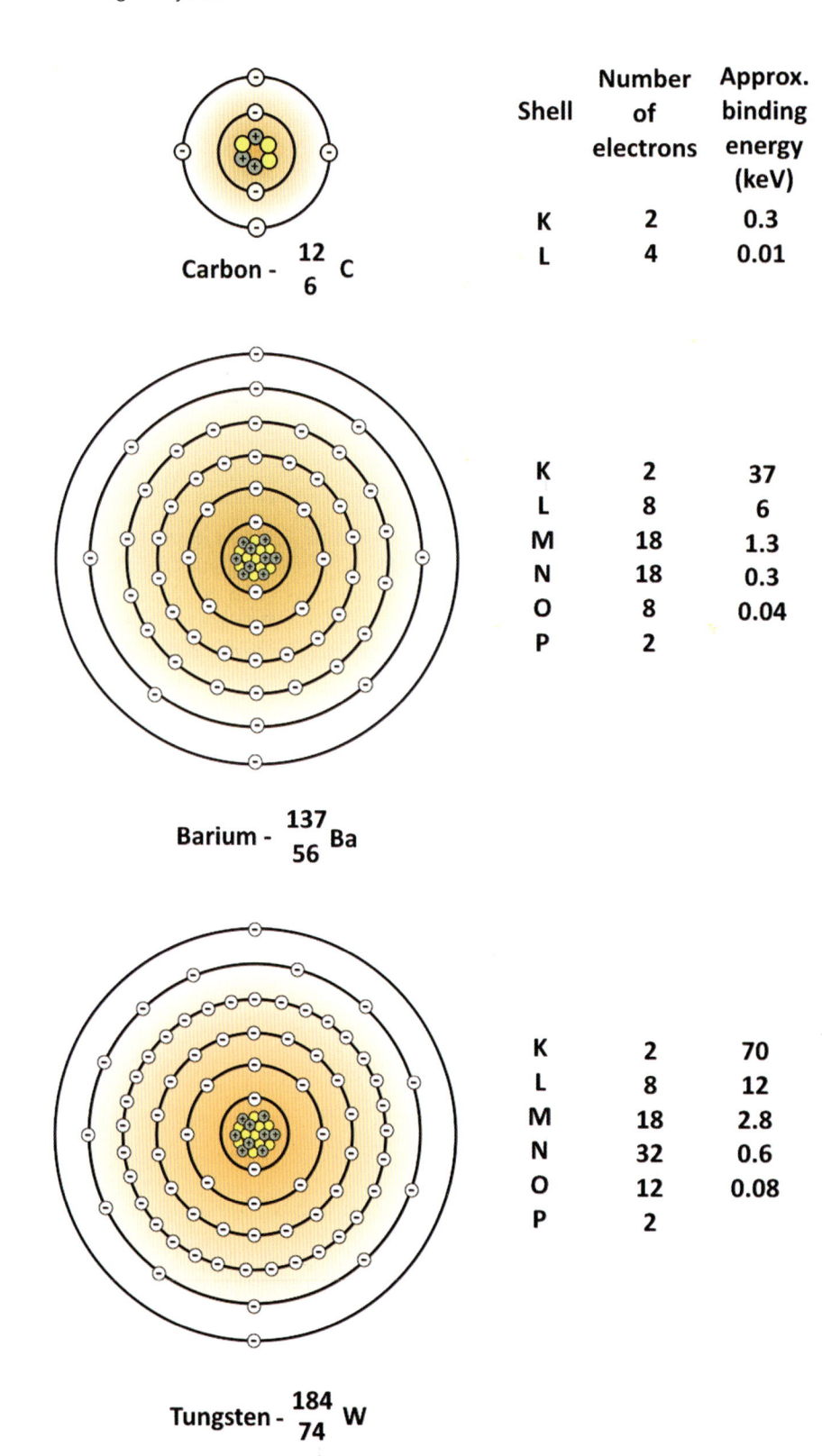

Shell	Number of electrons	Approx. binding energy (keV)
K	2	0.3
L	4	0.01

Carbon - $^{12}_{6}$C

Shell	Number of electrons	Approx. binding energy (keV)
K	2	37
L	8	6
M	18	1.3
N	18	0.3
O	8	0.04
P	2	

Barium - $^{137}_{56}$Ba

Shell	Number of electrons	Approx. binding energy (keV)
K	2	70
L	8	12
M	18	2.8
N	32	0.6
O	12	0.08
P	2	

Tungsten - $^{184}_{74}$W

FIG. 3.9 Atomic configurations and approximate electron-binding energies for three radiologically important atoms. As atoms get bigger, electrons in a given shell become more tightly bound.

ATOMIC NOMENCLATURE

Often an element is indicated by an alphabetic abbreviation. Such abbreviations are called **chemical symbols**. Table 3.3 lists some of the important elements in radiologic science and their chemical symbols.

The chemical properties of an element are determined by the number and arrangement of electrons. In the neutral atom, the number of electrons equals the number of protons. The number of protons is called the atomic number, represented by Z. Table 3.3 shows that the atomic number of barium is 56, thus indicating that 56 protons are in the barium nucleus.

The number of protons plus the number of neutrons in the nucleus of an atom is called the atomic mass number, symbolized by A. The atomic mass number is always a whole number. The use of atomic mass numbers is helpful in many areas of radiologic science.

> The atomic mass number and the precise mass of an atom are not equal.

An atom's atomic mass number is a whole number that is equal to the number of nucleons in the atom. The actual atomic mass of an atom is determined by measurement and rarely is a whole number. For example, ^{135}Ba has A = 135 because its nucleus contains 56 protons and 79 neutrons. The atomic mass of ^{135}Ba is 134.91 amu.

Only one atom, ^{12}C, has an atomic mass equal to its atomic mass number. This occurs because the ^{12}C atom is the arbitrary standard for atomic measure.

Many elements in their natural state are composed of atoms with different atomic mass numbers and different atomic masses but identical atomic numbers. The characteristic mass of an element is determined by the relative abundance of isotopes and their respective atomic masses.

For example, barium has an atomic number of 56. The atomic mass number of its most abundant isotope is 138. However, natural barium consists of seven different isotopes with atomic mass numbers of 130, 132, 134, 135, 136, 137, and 138; the elemental mass is determined by calculating the average of all these isotopes.

TABLE 3.3 Characteristics of Some Elements Important to Radiologic Science

Element	Chemical Symbol	Atomic Number (Z)	Atomic Mass Number (A)[a]	Number of Naturally Occurring Isotopes	Elemental Mass (amu)[b]	K-Shell Electron-Binding Energy (keV)
Beryllium	Be	4	9	1	9.012	0.11
Carbon	C	6	12	3	12.01	0.28
Oxygen	O	8	16	3	15	0.53
Aluminum	Al	13	27	1	26.98	1.56
Calcium	Ca	20	40	6	40.08	4.04
Iron	Fe	26	56	4	55.84	7.11
Copper	Cu	29	63	2	63.54	8.98
Molybdenum	Mo	42	98	7	95.94	20
Rhodium	Rh	45	103	5	102.9	23.2
Ruthenium	Ru	44	102	7	101	22.1
Silver	Ag	47	107	2	107.9	25.7
Tin	Sn	50	120	10	118.6	29.2
Iodine	I	53	127	1	126.9	33.2
Barium	Ba	56	138	7	137.3	37.4
Tungsten	W	74	184	5	183.8	69.5
Rhenium	Re	75	186	2	185.9	71.7
Gold	Au	79	197	1	196.9	80.7
Lead	Pb	82	208	4	207.1	88
Uranium	U	92	238	3	238	116

amu, Atomic mass units; *keV*, kiloelectron volts.
[a]Most abundant isotope.
[b]Average of naturally occurring isotopes.

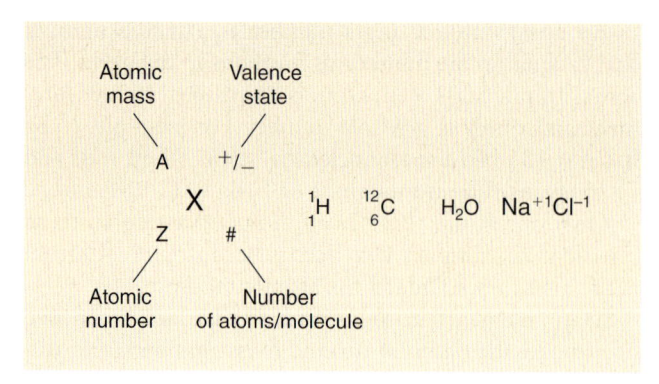

FIG. 3.10 Protocol for representing elements in a molecule.

| TABLE 3.4 | Characteristics of Various Nuclear Arrangements |

Arrangement	Atomic Number	Atomic Mass Number	Neutron Number
Isotope	Same	Different	Different
Isobar	Different	Same	Different
Isotone	Different	Different	Same
Isomer	Same	Same	Same

With the protocol described in Fig. 3.10, the atoms of Fig. 3.6 would have the following symbolic representation:

$$^{1}_{1}H, \ ^{4}_{2}He, \ ^{7}_{3}Li, \ ^{238}_{92}U$$

Because the chemical symbol also indicates the atomic number, the subscript is often omitted.

$$^{1}H, \ ^{4}He, \ ^{7}Li, \ ^{238}U$$

> Atoms that have the same atomic number but different atomic mass numbers are isotopes.

Isotopes of a given element contain the same number of protons but varying numbers of neutrons. Most elements have more than one stable isotope. The seven natural isotopes of barium are as follows:

$$^{130}Ba, \ ^{132}Ba, \ ^{134}Ba, \ ^{135}Ba, \ ^{136}Ba, \ ^{137}Ba, \ ^{138}Ba$$

The term **isotope** describes all atoms of a given element. Such atoms have different nuclear configurations but nevertheless react the same way chemically.

Question: How many protons and neutrons are in each of the seven naturally occurring isotopes of barium?

Answer: The number of protons in each isotope is 56. The number of neutrons is equal to A−Z. Therefore:
^{130}Ba: 130−56 = 74 neutrons
^{132}Ba: 132−56 = 76 neutrons
^{134}Ba: 134−56 = 78 neutrons, and so forth.

> Atomic nuclei that have the same atomic mass number but different atomic numbers are isobars.

Isobars are atoms that have different numbers of protons and different numbers of neutrons but the same total number of nucleons. Isobaric radioactive transitions from parent atom to daughter atom result from the release of a beta particle or a positron. The parent and the daughter are atoms of different elements.

> Atoms that have the same number of neutrons but different numbers of protons are isotones.

Isotones are atoms with different atomic numbers and different mass numbers but a constant value for the quantity A−Z. Consequently, isotones are atoms with the same number of neutrons in the nucleus.

The final category of atomic configuration is the **isomer**.

> Isomers have the same atomic number and the same atomic mass number.

In fact, isomers are identical atoms except that they exist at different energy states because of differences in nucleon arrangement. Technetium 99m decays to technetium 99 with the emission of a 140-keV gamma ray, which is very useful in nuclear medicine. Table 3.4 presents a summary of the characteristics of these nuclear arrangements.

Question: From the following list of atoms, pick out those that are isotopes, isobars, and isotones.
$$^{131}_{54}Xe, \ ^{130}_{53}I, \ ^{132}_{55}Cs, \ ^{131}_{53}I$$

Answer: ^{130}I and ^{131}I are isotopes. ^{131}I and ^{131}Xe are isobars. ^{130}I, ^{131}Xe, and ^{132}Cs are isotones.

One method of association to help with these iso-definitions is: isotope, same proton; isobar, same A; isotone, same neutron; and isomer, metastable.

CHAPTER 3　The Structure of Matter　45

COMBINATIONS OF ATOMS

> Atoms of various elements may combine to form structures called molecules.

Four atoms of hydrogen (H_2) and two atoms of oxygen (O_2) can combine to form two molecules of water ($2H_2O$). The following equation represents this atomic combination:

$$2H_2 + O_2 \rightarrow 2H_2O$$

An atom of sodium (Na) can combine with an atom of chlorine (Cl) to form a molecule of sodium chloride (NaCl), which is common table salt:

$$Na + Cl \rightarrow NaCl$$

Both of these molecules are common in the human body. Molecules, in turn, may combine to form even larger structures: cells and tissues.

> A chemical compound is any quantity of one type of molecule.

Although more than 100 different elements are known, most elements are rare. Approximately 95% of Earth and its atmosphere consists of only a dozen elements. Similarly, hydrogen, oxygen, carbon, and nitrogen compose more than 95% of the human body. Water molecules make up approximately 80% of the human body.

There is an organized scheme for representing elements in a molecule (Fig. 3.10). The shorthand notation that incorporates the chemical symbol with subscripts and superscripts is used to identify atoms.

The chemical symbol (X) is positioned between two subscripts and two superscripts. The subscript and superscript to the left of the chemical symbol represent the atomic number and atomic mass, respectively. The subscript and superscript to the right are values for the number of atoms per molecule and the valence state of the atom, respectively.

The formula NaCl represents one molecule of the compound sodium chloride. Sodium chloride has properties that are different from those of sodium or chlorine. Atoms combine with each other to form compounds in two main ways. The examples of H_2O and NaCl can be used to describe these two types of chemical bonds.

Oxygen and hydrogen combine into water through covalent bonds. Oxygen has six electrons in its outermost shell. It has room for two more electrons, so in a water molecule, two hydrogen atoms share their single electrons with the oxygen. The hydrogen electrons orbit the H and the O, thus binding the atoms together. This covalent bonding is characterized by the sharing of electrons.

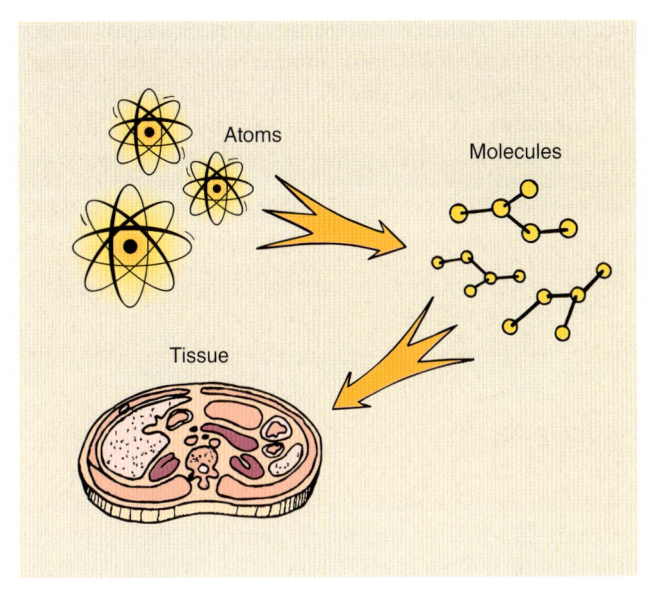

FIG. 3.11 Matter has many levels of organization. Atoms combine to make molecules and molecules combine to make tissues.

Sodium and chlorine combine into salt through ionic bonds. Sodium has one electron in its outermost shell. Chlorine has space for one more electron in its outermost shell. The sodium atom will give up its electron to the chlorine. When it does, it becomes ionized because it has lost an electron and now has an imbalance of electric charges.

The chlorine atom also becomes ionized because it has gained an electron and now has more electrons than protons. The two atoms are attracted to each other, resulting in an ionic bond because they have opposite electrostatic charges.

Sodium, hydrogen, carbon, and oxygen atoms can combine to form a molecule of sodium bicarbonate ($NaHCO_3$). A measurable quantity of sodium bicarbonate constitutes a chemical compound commonly called baking soda.

> The smallest particle of an element is an atom; the smallest particle of a compound is a molecule.

The interrelations between atoms, elements, molecules, and compounds are orderly. This organizational scheme is what the ancient Greeks were trying to describe by their substances and essences. Fig. 3.11 is a diagram of this current scheme of matter.

RADIOACTIVITY

Some atoms exist in an abnormally excited state characterized by an unstable nucleus. To reach stability, the nucleus spontaneously emits particles and energy and transforms itself into another atom. This process is called **radioactive decay**. The atoms involved are **radionuclides**. Any nuclear arrangement is called a **nuclide**; only nuclei that undergo radioactive decay are radionuclides.

> Radioactivity is the spontaneous emission of particles and energy to become stable.

Radioisotopes

Many factors affect nuclear stability. Perhaps the most important is the number of neutrons. When a nucleus contains too few or too many neutrons, the atom can disintegrate radioactively, bringing the number of neutrons and protons into a stable ratio.

In addition to stable isotopes, many elements have **radioactive isotopes** or **radioisotopes**. These may be artificially produced in particle accelerators or nuclear reactors.

Many radioisotopes of barium have been discovered, all of which are artificially produced. In the following list of barium isotopes, the nine radioisotopes are boldface:

$$^{127}Ba, \,^{128}Ba, \,^{129}Ba, \,^{130}Ba, \,^{131}Ba, \,^{132}Ba, \,^{133}Ba$$

$$^{134}Ba, \,^{135}Ba, \,^{136}Ba, \,^{137}Ba, \,^{138}Ba, \,^{139}Ba, \,^{140}Ba$$

Artificially produced radioisotopes have been identified for nearly all elements. A few elements have naturally occurring radioisotopes as well.

There are two primary sources of naturally occurring radioisotopes. Some originated at the time of Earth's formation and are still decaying very slowly. An example is uranium, which ultimately decays to radium, which in turn decays to radon. These and other decay products of uranium are radioactive. Others, such as ^{14}C, are continuously produced in the upper atmosphere through the action of cosmic radiation.

Radioisotopes can decay to stability in many ways, but two, **beta emission** and **alpha emission**, are important here for descriptive purposes. Radioactive decay by **positron emission** is important for some nuclear medicine imaging.

During beta emission, an electron created in the nucleus is ejected from the nucleus with considerable kinetic energy and escapes from the atom. The result is the loss of a small quantity of mass and one unit of negative electric charge from the nucleus of the atom. Simultaneously, a neutron undergoes conversion to a proton.

The result of beta emission therefore is to increase the atomic number by one ($Z \rightarrow Z + 1$), while the atomic

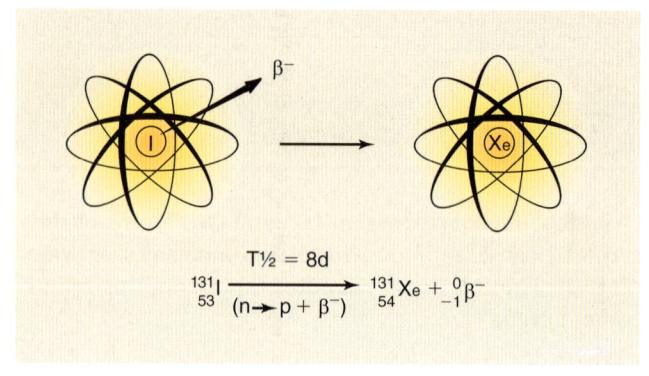

FIG. 3.12 ^{131}I decays to ^{131}Xe with the emission of a beta particle.

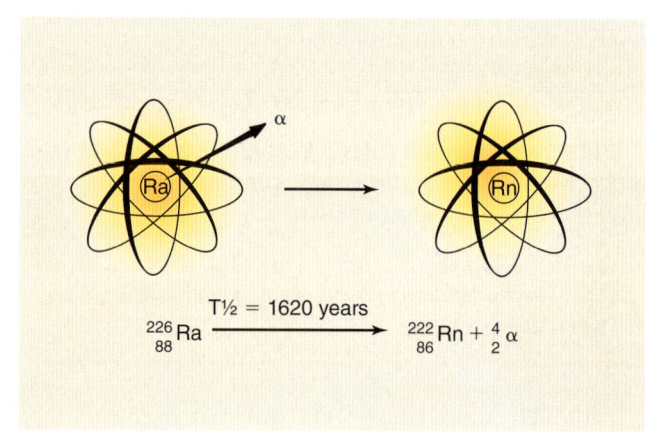

FIG. 3.13 The decay of ^{226}Ra to ^{222}Rn is accompanied by alpha emission.

mass number remains the same (A = constant). This nuclear transformation results in the changing of an atom from one type of element to another (Fig. 3.12).

Radioactive decay by alpha emission is a much more violent process. The alpha particle consists of two protons and two neutrons bound together; its atomic mass number is 4. A nucleus must be extremely unstable to emit an alpha particle, but when it does, it loses two units of positive charge and four units of mass. The transformation is significant because the resulting atom is not only chemically different but is also lighter by 4 amu (Fig. 3.13).

> Radioactive decay results in emission of alpha particles, beta particles, and usually gamma rays.

Beta emission occurs much more frequently than alpha emission. Virtually all radioisotopes are capable of transformation by beta emission, but only heavy radioisotopes are capable of alpha emission. Some radioisotopes are pure beta emitters or pure alpha emitters, but most emit gamma rays simultaneously with the particle emission.

Question: ^{139}Ba is a radioisotope that decays by beta emission. What will be the values of A and Z for the atom that results from this emission?

Answer: In beta emission, a neutron is converted to a proton and a beta particle: n → p + β, therefore $^{139}_{56}$Ba → $^{139}_{57}$?
Lanthanum is the element with Z = 57; thus $^{139}_{57}$La is the result of the beta decay of $^{139}_{56}$Ba.

Radioactive Half-Life

Radioactivity is not here one day and gone the next. Rather, radioisotopes disintegrate into stable isotopes of different elements at a decreasing rate so that the quantity of radioactive material never quite reaches zero.

Remember from Chapter 1 that radioactive material is measured in becquerels and that 1 Bq is equal to the disintegration of 1 atom each second.

The rate of radioactive decay and the quantity of material present at any given time are described mathematically by a formula known as the **radioactive decay law**. From this formula, we obtain a quantity known as **radioactive half-life** (T½). Radioactive half-lives of radioisotopes vary from less than a second to many years. Each radioisotope has a unique and characteristic radioactive half-life.

> The radioactive half-life of a radioisotope is the time required for a quantity of radioactivity to be reduced to one-half its original value.

The radioactive half-life of ^{131}I is 8 days (Fig. 3.14). If 10 MBq of ^{131}I was present on January 1 at noon, then at noon on January 9, only 5 MBq would remain. On January 17, 2.5 MBq would remain, and on January 25, 1.25 MBq would remain. A plot of the radioactive decay of ^{131}I allows one to determine the amount of radioactivity remaining after any given length of time (see Fig. 3.14).

After approximately 24 days, or three half-lives, the linear-linear plot of the decay of ^{131}I becomes very difficult to read and interpret. Consequently, such graphs are usually presented in semilogarithmic form (Fig. 3.15). With a presentation such as this, one can estimate radioactivity after a very long time.

Question: On Monday at 8 AM, 10 MBq of ^{131}I is present. How much will remain on Friday at 5 PM?

Answer: The time of decay is 4 days. According to Fig. 3.15, at 4 days, approximately 63% of the original activity will remain. Therefore 6.3 MBq will be present on Friday at 5 PM.

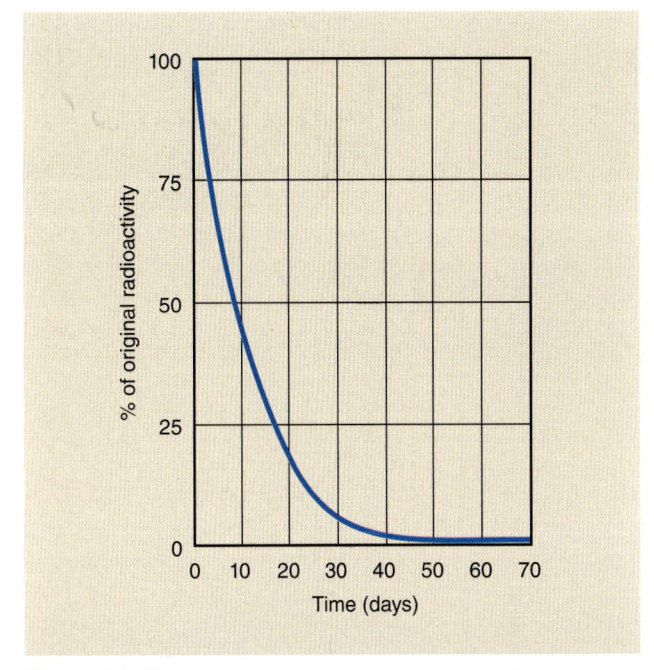

FIG. 3.14 ^{131}I decays with a radioactive half-life of 8 days. This linear graph allows estimation of radioactivity only for a short time.

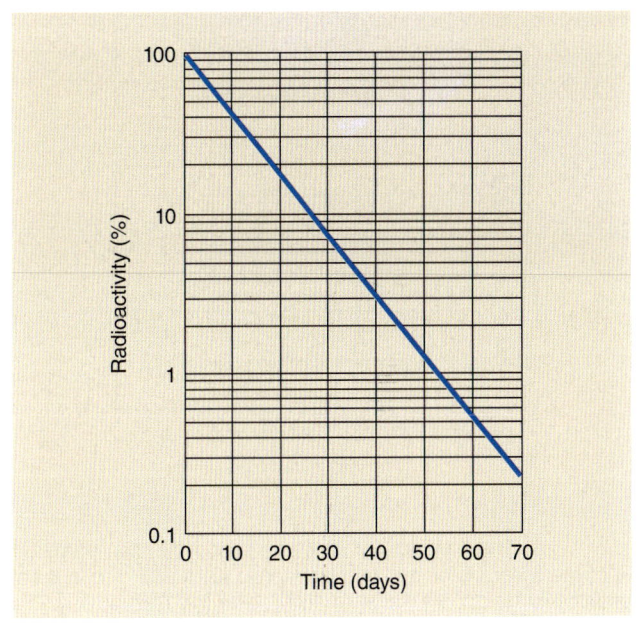

FIG. 3.15 This semilogarithmic graph is useful for estimating the radioactivity of ^{131}I at any given time.

Theoretically, all the radioactivity of a radioisotope never disappears. After each period of time equivalent to one radioactive half-life, one-half the activity present at the beginning of that time will remain. Therefore although the quantity of a radioisotope progressively decreases, it never quite reaches zero.

Fig. 3.16 shows two similar graphs used to estimate the quantity of any radioisotope remaining after any length of time. In these graphs, the percentage of original radioactivity remaining is plotted against time, measured

48   PART I   Radiologic Physics

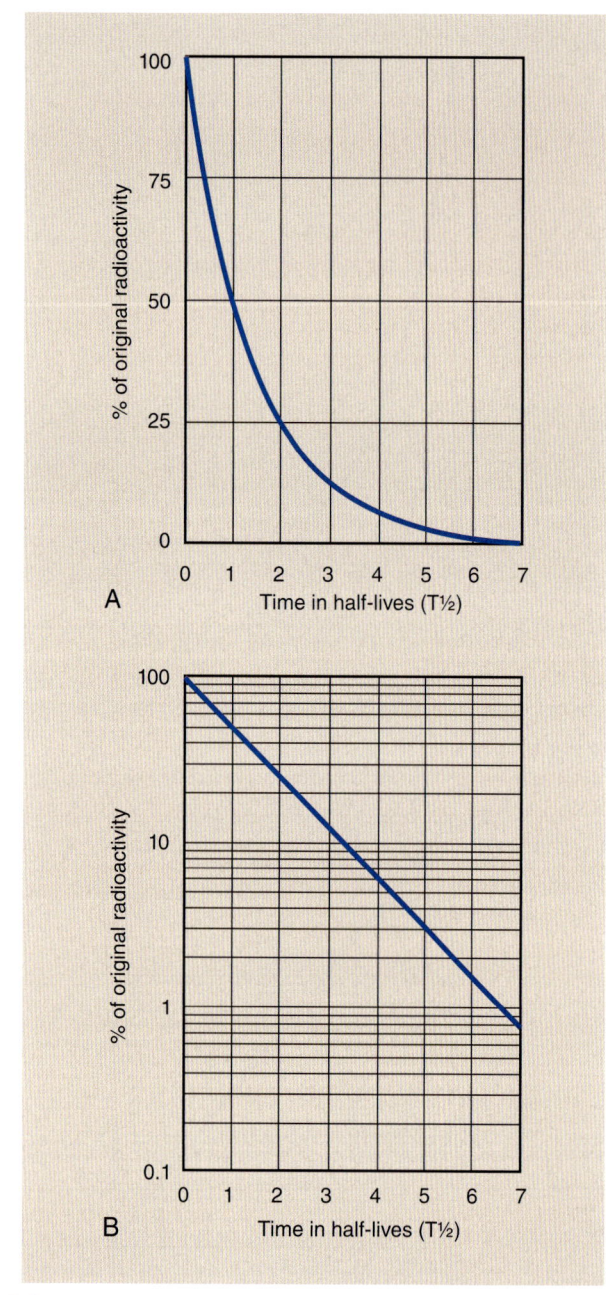

FIG. 3.16 The radioactivity after any period can be estimated from the linear (A) or the semilogarithmic (B) graph. The original quantity is assigned a value of 100%, and the time of decay is expressed in units of radioactive half-life.

in units of radioactive half-life. To use these graphs, one must express the initial radioactivity as 100% and convert the time of interest into units of radioactive half-life. For decay times exceeding three radioactive half-lives, the semilogarithmic form is easier to use.

Question: 6.5 MBq of ^{131}I is present at noon on Wednesday. How much will remain 1 week later?
Answer: Fig. 3.16 shows that at 0.875 T½, approximately 55% of the initial radioactivity will remain; 55% × 6.5 MBq = 0.55 × 6.5 = 3.6 MBq.

^{14}C is a naturally occurring radioisotope with T½ = 5730 years. The concentration of ^{14}C in the environment is constant, and ^{14}C is incorporated into living material at a constant rate. Trees of the petrified forest contain less ^{14}C than living trees because the ^{14}C of living trees is in equilibrium with the atmosphere. The carbon in a petrified tree was fixed many thousands of years ago, and that fixed ^{14}C is reduced over time by radioactive decay (Fig. 3.17).

Question: If a piece of petrified wood contains 25% of the ^{14}C that a tree living today contains, how old is the petrified wood?
Answer: The ^{14}C in living matter remains constant as long as the matter is alive because it is constantly exchanged with the environment. In this case, the petrified wood has been dead long enough for the ^{14}C to decay to 25% of its original value. That time period represents two radioactive half-lives. Consequently, we can estimate that the petrified wood sample is approximately 2 × 5730 = 11,460 years old.
Question: How many radioactive half-lives are required before a quantity of radioactive material has decayed to less than 1% of its original value?
Answer: A simple approach to this type of problem is to count radioactive half-lives.

Radioactive Half-Life Number	Radioactivity Remaining (%)
1	50
2	25
3	12.5
4	6.25
5	3.12
6	1.56
7	0.78

A simpler approach finds the answer more precisely in Fig. 3.16: 6.5 radioactive half-lives. Another approach is to use the following relationship:

> **RADIOACTIVE DECAY**
> Activity remaining = Original activity (0.5)^n
> where n = number of radioactive half-lives.

The concept of radioactive half-life is essential to radiologic science. It is used daily in nuclear medicine and has an exact parallel in x-ray terminology, the **half-value layer**. The better you understand radioactive half-life now, the better you will understand the meaning of half-value layer later.

> 3.3 radioactive half-lives = 1 radioactive tenth life

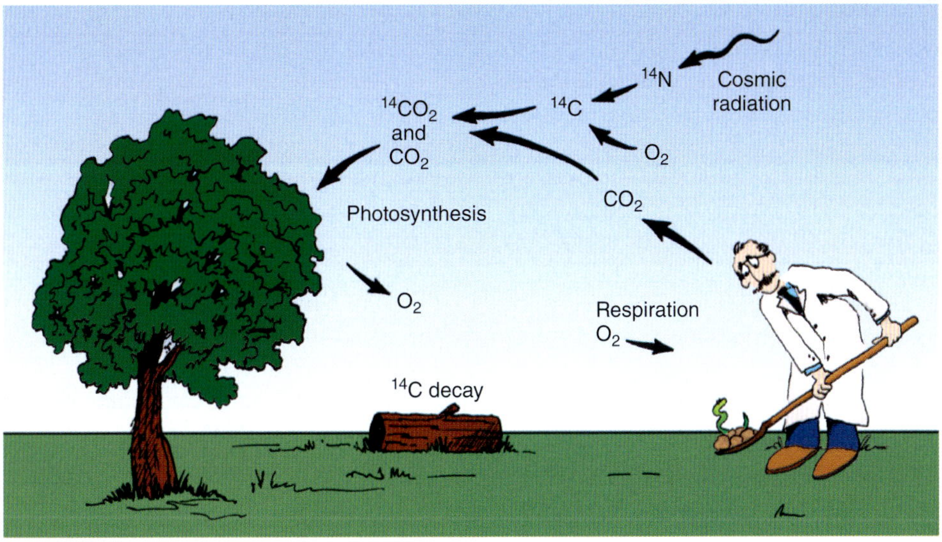

FIG. 3.17 Carbon is a biologically active element. A small fraction of all carbon is the radioisotope ^{14}C. As a tree grows, ^{14}C is incorporated into the wood in proportion to the amount of ^{14}C in the atmosphere. When the tree dies, further exchange of ^{14}C with the atmosphere does not take place. If the dead wood is preserved by petrification, the ^{14}C content diminishes as it radioactively decays. This phenomenon serves as the basis for radiocarbon dating.

TABLE 3.5 General Classification of Ionizing Radiation

Type of Radiation	Symbol	Atomic Mass Number	Charge	Origin
PARTICULATE				
Alpha radiation	α	4	+2	Nucleus
Beta radiation	β⁻	0	−1	Nucleus
	β⁺	0	+1	Nucleus
ELECTROMAGNETIC				
Gamma rays	γ	0	0	Nucleus
X-rays	X	0	0	Electron cloud

TYPES OF IONIZING RADIATION

All ionizing radiation can be conveniently classified into two categories: **particulate radiation** and **electromagnetic radiation** (Table 3.5). The types of radiation used in diagnostic ultrasonography and in magnetic resonance imaging are nonionizing radiation.

Although all ionizing radiation acts on biologic tissue in the same manner, there are fundamental differences between various types of radiation. These differences can be analyzed according to five physical characteristics: mass, energy, velocity, charge, and origin.

Particulate Radiation

Many subatomic particles are capable of causing ionization. Consequently, electrons, protons, and even rare nuclear fragments all can be classified as particulate ionizing radiation if they are in motion and possess sufficient kinetic energy. At rest, they cannot cause ionization.

There are two main types of particulate radiation: **alpha particles** and **beta particles**. Both are associated with radioactive decay.

The alpha particle is equivalent to a helium nucleus. It contains two protons and two neutrons. Its mass is approximately 4 amu, and it carries two units of positive electric charge. Compared with an electron, the alpha particle is large and exerts great electrostatic force. Alpha particles are emitted only from the nuclei of heavy elements. Light elements cannot emit alpha particles because they do not have enough excess mass.

> An alpha particle is a helium nucleus that contains two protons and two neutrons.

After being emitted from a radioactive atom, the alpha particle travels with high velocity through matter. However, because of its great mass and charge, it easily transfers this kinetic energy to orbital electrons of other atoms.

Ionization accompanies alpha radiation. The average alpha particle possesses 4 to 7 MeV of kinetic energy and ionizes approximately 40,000 atoms for every centimeter of travel through air.

Because of this amount of ionization, the energy of an alpha particle is quickly lost. It has a very short range in matter. Whereas in air, alpha particles can travel approximately 5 cm, in soft tissue, the range may be less than 100 μm. Consequently, alpha radiation from an external source is nearly harmless because the radiation energy is deposited in the superficial layers of the skin.

With an internal source of radiation, just the opposite is true. If an alpha-emitting radioisotope is deposited in the body, it can intensely irradiate the local tissue. Radon gas irradiating lung tissue is an important example.

Beta particles differ from alpha particles in terms of mass and charge. They are light particles with an atomic mass number of 0, and they carry one unit of negative or positive charge. The only difference between electrons and negative beta particles is their origin. Beta particles originate in the nuclei of radioactive atoms and electrons exist in shells outside the nuclei of all atoms.

Positive beta particles are **positrons**. They have the same mass as electrons and are considered to be antimatter. We will see positrons again when we discuss pair production.

> A beta particle is an electron emitted from the nucleus of a radioactive atom.

After being emitted from a radioisotope, beta particles traverse air, ionizing several hundred atoms per centimeter. The beta particle range is longer than that for the alpha particle. Depending on its energy, a beta particle may traverse 10 to 100 cm of air and approximately 1 to 2 cm of soft tissue.

Electromagnetic Radiation

X-rays and gamma rays are forms of electromagnetic ionizing radiation. This type of radiation is covered more completely in the next chapter; the discussion here is brief.

X-rays and gamma rays are often called **photons**. Photons have no mass and no charge. They travel at the speed of light ($c = 3 \times 10^8$ m/s) and are considered energy disturbances in space.

Just as the only difference between beta particles and electrons is their origin, so too the only difference between x-rays and gamma rays is their origin. Gamma rays are emitted from the nucleus of a radioisotope and are usually associated with alpha or beta emission. X-rays are produced outside the nucleus in the electron shells.

> Gamma rays come from the nucleus. X-rays come from the electron cloud.

X-rays and gamma rays exist at the speed of light or not at all. After being emitted, they have an ionization rate in air of approximately 100 ion pairs/cm, approximately equal to that for beta particles. In contrast to beta particles, x-rays and gamma rays have an unlimited range in matter.

Photon radiation loses intensity with distance but theoretically never reaches zero. In contrast, particulate radiation has a finite range in matter, and that range depends on the particle's energy.

Table 3.6 summarizes the more important characteristics of each of these types of ionizing radiation. In nuclear medicine, beta and gamma radiation are most important. In radiography, only x-rays are important. The penetrability and low ionization rate of x-rays make them particularly useful for medical imaging (Fig. 3.18).

TABLE 3.6 Characteristics of Several Types of Ionizing Radiation

Type of Radiation	Approximate Energy (MeV)	Approximate Range In Air	Approximate Range In Soft Tissue	Origin
PARTICULATE				
Alpha particles	4–7	1–10 cm	≤0.1 mm	Heavy radioactive nuclei
Beta particles	0–7	0–10 m	0–2 cm	Radioactive nuclei
ELECTROMAGNETIC				
X-rays	0–25	0–100 m	0–30 cm	Electron cloud
Gamma rays	0–5	0–100 m	0–30 cm	Radioactive nuclei

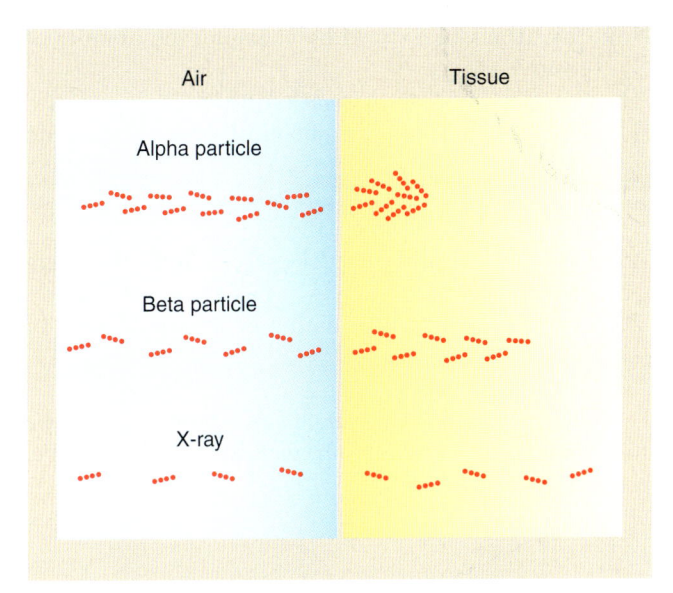

FIG. 3.18 Different types of radiation ionize matter with different degrees of efficiency. Alpha particles represent highly ionizing radiation with a very short range in matter. Beta particles do not ionize so readily and have a longer range. X-rays have a low ionization rate and a very long range.

SUMMARY

As a miniature solar system, the Bohr atom set the stage for the modern interpretation of the structure of matter. An atom is the smallest part of an element, and a molecule is the smallest part of a compound.

The three fundamental particles of the atom are the electron, proton, and neutron. Electrons are negatively charged particles that orbit the nucleus in shells held in place by electrostatic forces. Chemical reactions occur when outermost orbital electrons are shared or given up to other atoms. Nucleons, neutrons, and protons each have nearly 2000 times the mass of electrons. Protons are positively charged, and neutrons have no charge.

Elements are grouped in a periodic table in order of increasing complexity. The groups on the table indicate the number of electrons in the outermost shell. The elements in the periods on the periodic table have the same number of orbital shells.

Some atoms have the same number of protons and electrons as other elements but a different number of neutrons, giving the element a different atomic mass. These are isotopes.

Some atoms, which contain too many or too few neutrons in the nucleus, undergo radioactive decay. This is called radioactivity. Two types of particulate emission that occur after radioactive decay are alpha and beta particles. The radioactive half-life of a radioisotope is the time required for the quantity of radioactivity to be reduced to one-half its original value.

Ionizing radiation consists of particulate and electromagnetic radiation. Alpha and beta particles produce particulate radiation. Alpha particles have four atomic mass units, are positive in charge, and originate from the nucleus of heavy elements. Beta particles have an atomic mass number of zero and have one unit of negative charge. Beta particles originate in the nucleus of radioactive atoms.

X-rays and gamma rays are forms of electromagnetic radiation called photons. These rays have no mass and no charge. X-rays are produced in the electron shells, and gamma rays are emitted from the nucleus of a radioisotope.

CHALLENGE QUESTIONS

1. Define or otherwise identify the following:
   a. Photon
   b. The Rutherford atom
   c. Positron
   d. Nucleons
   e. The arrangement of the periodic table of the elements
   f. Radioactive half-life
   g. W (chemical symbol for what element?)
   h. Alpha particle
   i. K shell
   j. Chemical compound
2. Fig. 3.1 shows the following approximate sizes: an atom, 10^{-10} m; Earth, 10^7 m. By how many orders of magnitude do these objects differ?
3. How many protons, neutrons, electrons, and nucleons are found in the following?

   $^{17}_{8}$O, $^{27}_{13}$Al, $^{60}_{27}$Co, $^{226}_{88}$Ra

4. Using the data in Table 3.1, determine the mass of ^{99}Tc in atomic mass units and in kilograms.
5. Diagram the expected electron configuration of ^{40}Ca.
6. If atoms large enough to have electrons in the T shell existed, what would be the maximum number allowed in that shell?
7. How much more tightly bound are K-shell electrons in tungsten than (1) L-shell electrons, (2) M-shell electrons, and (3) free electrons? (Refer to Fig. 3.9.)
8. From the following list of nuclides, identify sets of isotopes, isobars, and isotones.

   $^{60}_{28}$Ni $^{61}_{28}$Ni $^{62}_{28}$Ni

   $^{59}_{27}$Co $^{60}_{27}$Co $^{61}_{27}$Co

   $^{58}_{26}$Fe $^{59}_{26}$Fe $^{60}_{26}$Fe

9. $^{90}_{38}$Sr has a radioactive half-life of 29 years. If 10 MBq were present in 1960, approximately how much would remain in 2020?

10. Complete the following table with relative values.

Type of Radiation	Mass	Energy	Charge	Origin
α				
β				
β⁺				
γ				
X				

11. For what is Mendeleev remembered?
12. Who developed the concept of the atom as a miniature solar system?
13. List the fundamental particles within an atom.
14. What property of an atom does binding energy describe?
15. Can atoms be ionized by changing the number of positive charges?
16. Describe how ion pairs are formed.
17. What determines the chemical properties of an element?
18. Why does an electron not spontaneously fly away from the nucleus of an atom?
19. Describe the difference between alpha and beta emission.
20. How does carbon-14 dating determine the age of petrified wood?

The answers to the Challenge Questions can be found by logging on to our website at http://evolve.elsevier.com.

Sasha Carlyle Dyk

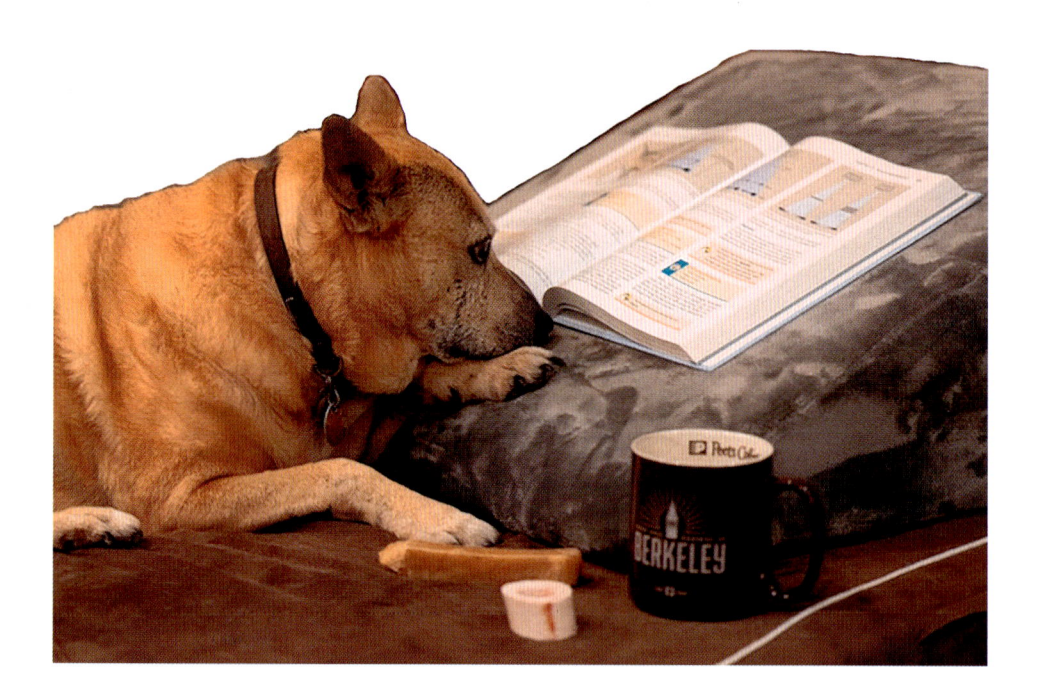

Electromagnetic Energy

CHAPTER 4

OBJECTIVES

At the completion of this chapter, the student should be able to do the following:

1. Identify the properties of photons.
2. Explain the inverse square law.
3. Define wave theory and quantum theory.
4. Discuss the electromagnetic spectrum.
5. Recognize the differences and similarities between matter and energy.

OUTLINE

Photons 54
   Velocity and Amplitude 54
   Frequency and Wavelength 55
Electromagnetic Spectrum 57
   Visible Light 58
   Radiofrequency 59
   Ionizing Radiation 60
Waves and Particles 60
   Wave Model: Visible Light 61
   Inverse Square Law 62
   Particle Model: Quantum Theory 65
Matter and Energy 66
Summary 67
Challenge Questions 67

PHOTONS WERE first described by the ancient Greeks. Today, photons are known as electromagnetic energy; however, these designations are commonly used interchangeably. Electromagnetic energy is present everywhere and exists over a wide energy range. X-rays, visible light, and radiofrequencies are examples of electromagnetic energy.

The properties of electromagnetic energy include frequency, wavelength, velocity, and amplitude. In this chapter, discussions of visible light, radiofrequency (RF), and ionizing radiation highlight these properties and the importance of electromagnetic energy in medical imaging. The wave equation and the inverse square law are mathematical formulas that further describe how electromagnetic energy behaves.

The wave-particle duality of electromagnetic energy is introduced as wave theory and quantum theory. Matter and energy, as well as their importance to medical imaging, are summarized.

PHOTONS

Ever present all around us is a state of energy called **electromagnetic energy**. This energy exists over a wide range, sometimes identified as an energy continuum. A continuum is a continuous, ordered sequence. Examples of continuums are free-flowing rivers and sidewalks. If the river is dammed or the sidewalk curbed, then the continuum is interrupted. Only an extremely small segment of the electromagnetic energy continuum—the visible light segment—is naturally apparent to us.

The ancient Greeks recognized the unique nature of light. It was not one of their four basic essences, but light was given an entirely separate status. They called an atom of light a **photon**. Today, many types of electromagnetic energy, in addition to visible light, are recognized, but the term *photon* is still used.

A photon is the smallest quantity of any type of electromagnetic energy, just as an atom is the smallest quantity of an element. A photon may be pictured as a small bundle of energy, sometimes called a *quantum*, which travels through space at the speed of light. We speak of x-ray photons, light photons, and other types of electromagnetic energy as photon radiation.

> An x-ray photon is a quantum of electromagnetic energy.

The physics of visible light has always been a subject of investigation, set apart from other areas of science. Nearly all of the classical laws of optics were described hundreds of years ago. Late in the 19th century, James Clerk Maxwell showed that visible light has both electric and magnetic properties—hence the term *electromagnetic energy*.

By the beginning of the 20th century, other types of electromagnetic energy had been described, and a uniform theory evolved. Electromagnetic energy is best explained by reference to a model, in much the same way that the atom is best described by the Bohr model.

Velocity and Amplitude

Photons are energy disturbances that move through space at the speed of light (c). Some sources give the speed of light as 186,000 m/s, but in the SI system of units, it is 3×10^8 m/s.

Question: What is the value of c in miles per second, given $c = 3 \times 10^8$ m/s?

Answer:
$$C = \frac{3 \times 10^8 \text{ m}}{\text{s}} \times \frac{\text{mi}}{5280 \text{ ft}} \times \frac{3.2808 \text{ ft}}{\text{m}}$$
$$= \frac{3 \times 10^8 \times 3.2808 \text{ m} - \text{mi} - \text{ft}}{5.280 \times 10^3 \text{ s} - \text{ft} - \text{m}}$$
$$= \frac{9.8424 \times 10^8 \text{ m} - \text{mi} - \text{ft}}{5.280 \times 10^3 \text{ s} - \text{ft} - \text{m}}$$
$$= 1.864 \times 10^5 \text{ mi/s}$$
$$= 186,400 \text{ mi/s}$$

Although photons have no mass and therefore no identifiable form, they do have electric and magnetic fields that are continuously changing in a sinusoidal fashion. Physicists use the term *field* to describe interactions among different energies, forces, or masses that can otherwise be described only mathematically. For instance, we can understand the gravitational field even though we cannot see it. We know the gravitational field exists because we are held to the Earth by it.

> The velocity of all electromagnetic radiation is 3×10^8 m/s.

The gravitational field governs the interaction of different masses. Similarly, the electric field governs the interaction of electrostatic charges, and the magnetic field governs the interaction of magnetic poles.

Fig. 4.1 shows three examples of a sinusoidal variation. This type of variation is usually called a **sine wave**. Sine waves can be described by a mathematical formula and therefore have many applications in physics.

Sine waves exist in nature and are associated with many familiar objects (Fig. 4.2). Simplistically, sine waves are variations of amplitude over time.

Alternating electric current consists of electrons moving back and forth sinusoidally through a conductor. A long rope fastened at one end vibrates as a sine wave

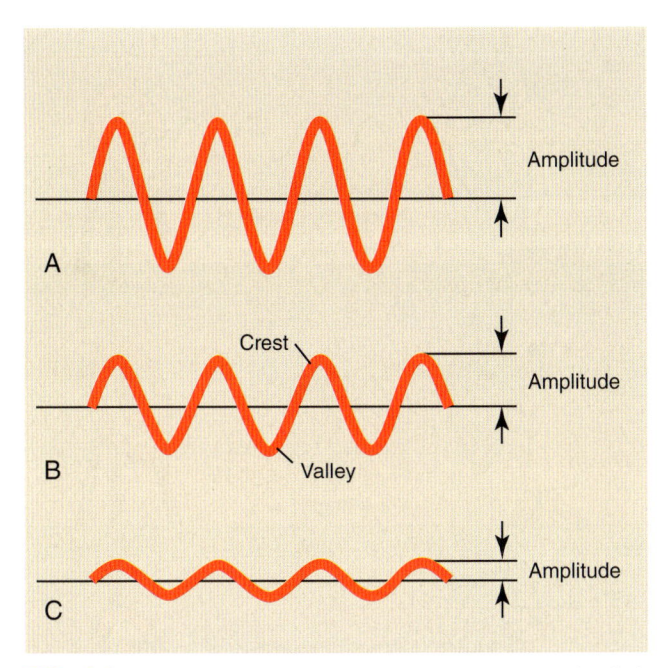

FIG. 4.1 These three sine waves are identical except for their amplitudes.

if the free end is moved up and down in a whiplike fashion.

The arms of a tuning fork vibrate sinusoidally after being struck with a hard object. The weight on the end of a coil spring varies sinusoidally up and down after the spring has been stretched.

The sine waves in Fig. 4.1 are identical except for their amplitude; sine wave A has the largest amplitude, and sine wave C has the smallest. Sine wave amplitude is discussed later in connection with high-voltage generation and rectification in an x-ray imaging system.

> **Amplitude** is one-half the range from crest to valley over which the sine wave varies.

Frequency and Wavelength

The sine wave model of electromagnetic energy describes variations in the electric and magnetic fields as the photon travels with velocity c. The important properties of this model are **frequency, represented by f,** and **wavelength, represented by the Greek letter lambda (λ).**

Another interpretation of the vibrating rope in Fig. 4.2 is the Texas roadside critter observing the motion of the rope from a point midway between the fastened end and the scientist (Fig. 4.3).

What does the critter see? If he moves his field of view along the rope, he will observe the crest of the sine wave traveling along the rope to the end. If he fixes his attention on one segment of the rope such as point A, he will see the rope rise and fall harmonically as the waves pass. The more rapidly the scientist holding the

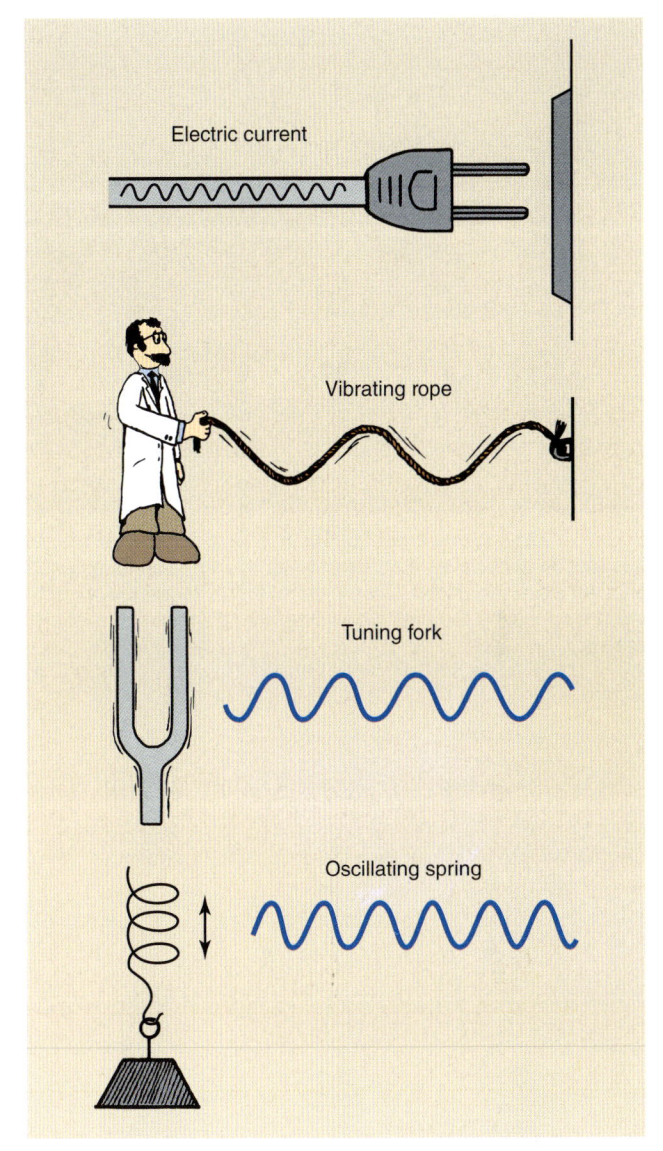

FIG. 4.2 Sine waves are associated with many naturally occurring phenomena in addition to electromagnetic energy.

loose end moves the rope up and down, the faster the sequence of the rise and fall.

The rate of rise and fall is frequency. It is usually identified as cycles per second. The unit of measurement is the hertz (Hz). One hertz is equal to 1 cycle per second. The frequency is equal to the number of crests or the number of valleys that pass the point of an observer per unit of time.

If the critter used a stopwatch and counted 20 crests passing in 10 seconds, then the frequency would be 20 cycles in 10 seconds, or 2 Hz. If the scientist doubles the rate at which he moves the rope up and down, then the critter would count 40 crests passing in 10 seconds and the frequency would be 4 Hz.

> **Frequency** is the number of wavelengths that pass a point of observation per second.

56   PART I   Radiologic Physics

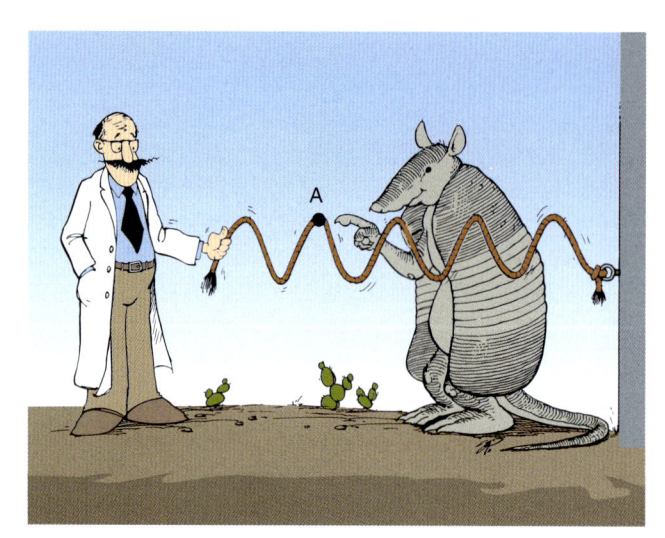

FIG. 4.3 Moving one end of a rope in a whiplike fashion will set into motion sine waves that travel down the rope to the fastened end. An observer, midway, can determine the frequency of oscillation by counting the crests or valleys that pass point A per unit of time.

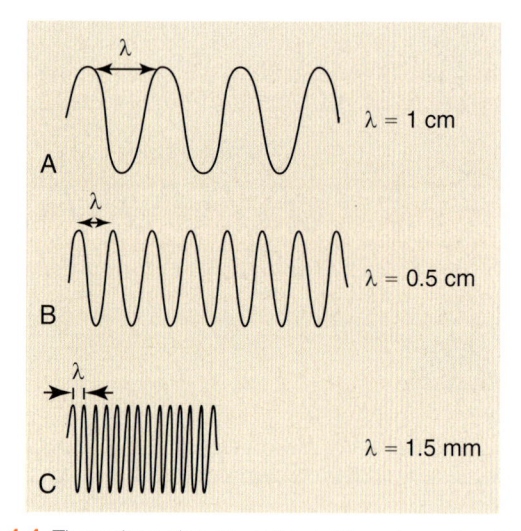

FIG. 4.4 These three sine waves have different wavelengths. The shorter the wavelength (λ), the higher the frequency.

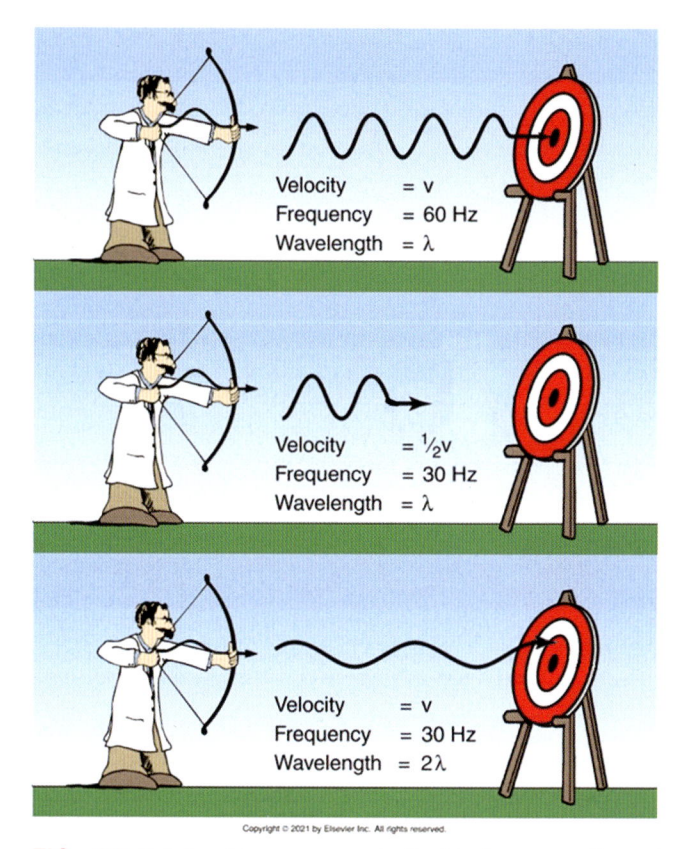

FIG. 4.5 Relationships among velocity (v), frequency (f), and wavelength (λ) for any sine wave.

The wavelength is the distance from one crest to another, from one valley to another, or from any point on the sine wave to the next corresponding point. Fig. 4.4 shows sine waves of three different wavelengths. With a meter rule, you can verify that wave A repeats every 1 cm and therefore has a wavelength of 1 cm. Similarly, wave B has a wavelength of 0.5 cm, and wave C has a wavelength of 1.5 mm. Clearly, then, as the frequency is increased, the wavelength is reduced. The wave amplitude is not related to wavelength or frequency.

Three wave parameters—velocity, frequency, and wavelength—are needed to describe electromagnetic energy. The relationship among these parameters is important. A change in one affects the value of the others. Velocity is constant.

Suppose a radiographer is positioned to observe the flight of the sine wave arrows to determine their frequency (Fig. 4.5). The first sine wave is measured and is found to have a frequency of 60 Hz, which signifies 60 wavelengths of the sine wave every second.

The archer now puts an identical sine wave arrow into his bow and shoots it with less force so that this second arrow has only half the velocity of the first arrow. The observer correctly measures the frequency at 30 Hz, even though the wavelength of the second arrow was the same as that of the first arrow. In other words, as the velocity decreases, the frequency decreases proportionately.

Now the archer shoots a third sine wave arrow with precisely the same velocity as the first but with a wavelength twice as long as that of the first. What should be the observed frequency? The correct answer is 30 Hz.

> At a given velocity, wavelength and frequency are inversely proportional.

This brief analogy demonstrates how the three parameters associated with a sine wave are interrelated.

A simple mathematical formula, called the **wave equation**, expresses this interrelationship:

> **THE WAVE EQUATION**
> Velocity = Frequency × Wavelength
> or
> $v = f\lambda$

The wave equation is used for both sound and electromagnetic energy. However, keep in mind that sound waves are very different from electromagnetic photons. The sources of sound are different. They are propagated in different ways, and their velocities vary greatly. The velocity of sound depends on the density of the material through which it passes. Sound cannot travel through a vacuum.

Question: The speed of sound in air is approximately 340 m/s. The highest treble tone that a person can hear is about 20 kHz. What is the wavelength of this sound?

Answer:
$$c = f\lambda$$
$$\lambda = \frac{v}{f}$$
$$= \frac{340 \text{ m/s}}{20 \text{ kHz}}$$
$$= \frac{3.40 \times 10^2 \text{ m}}{\text{s}} \times \frac{\text{s}}{2 \times 10^4 \text{ cycle}}$$
$$= 1.7 \times 10^{-2} \text{ m}$$
$$= 1.7 \text{ cm}$$

When dealing with electromagnetic energy, we can simplify the wave equation because all such energy travels with the same velocity.

> **ELECTROMAGNETIC WAVE EQUATION**
> $c = f\lambda$

The product of frequency and wavelength always equals the velocity of light for electromagnetic energy. Stated differently, for electromagnetic energy, frequency and wavelength are inversely proportional. The following are alternative forms of the electromagnetic wave equation.

> **ELECTROMAGNETIC WAVE EQUATION**
> $f = \frac{c}{\lambda}$ and $\lambda = \frac{c}{f}$

As the frequency of electromagnetic energy increases, the wavelength decreases and vice versa.

Question: Yellow light has a wavelength of 580 nm. What is the frequency of a photon of yellow light?

Answer:
$$f = \frac{c}{\lambda}$$
$$= \frac{3 \times 10^8 \text{ m/s}}{580 \text{ nm}}$$
$$= \frac{3 \times 10^8 \text{ m}}{\text{s}} \times \frac{1}{580 \times 10^{-9} \text{ m}}$$
$$= \frac{3 \times 10^8 \text{ m}}{\text{s}} \times \frac{1}{5.8 \times 10^{-7} \text{ m}}$$
$$= 0.517 \times 10^{15} \text{ cycles/s}$$
$$= 5.17 \times 10^{14} \text{ Hz}$$

Question: The highest energy x-ray produced at 100 kVp (100 keV) has a frequency of 2.42×10^{19} Hz. What is its wavelength?

Answer:
$$\lambda = \frac{c}{f}$$
$$= \frac{3 \times 10^8 \text{ m}}{\text{s}} \times \frac{\text{s}}{2.42 \times 10^{19} \text{ cycles/s}}$$
$$= 1.24 \times 10^{-11} \text{ m}$$
$$= 12.4 \text{ pm}$$

ELECTROMAGNETIC SPECTRUM

The frequency range of electromagnetic energy extends from approximately 10^2 to 10^{24} Hz. The photon wavelengths associated with these radiations are approximately 10^7 to 10^{-16} m, respectively. This wide range of values covers many types of electromagnetic energy, most of which are familiar to us. Grouped together, these types of energy make up the **electromagnetic spectrum**.

> The electromagnetic spectrum includes the entire range of electromagnetic energy.

The known electromagnetic spectrum has three regions most important to radiologic science: visible light, x-ray and gamma radiation, and RF. Other portions of the spectrum include ultraviolet light, infrared light, and microwave radiation.

With all of these various types of energy, the photons are essentially the same. Each can be represented as a bundle of energy consisting of varying electric and magnetic fields that travel at the speed of light. The photons of these various portions of the electromagnetic spectrum differ only in frequency and wavelength.

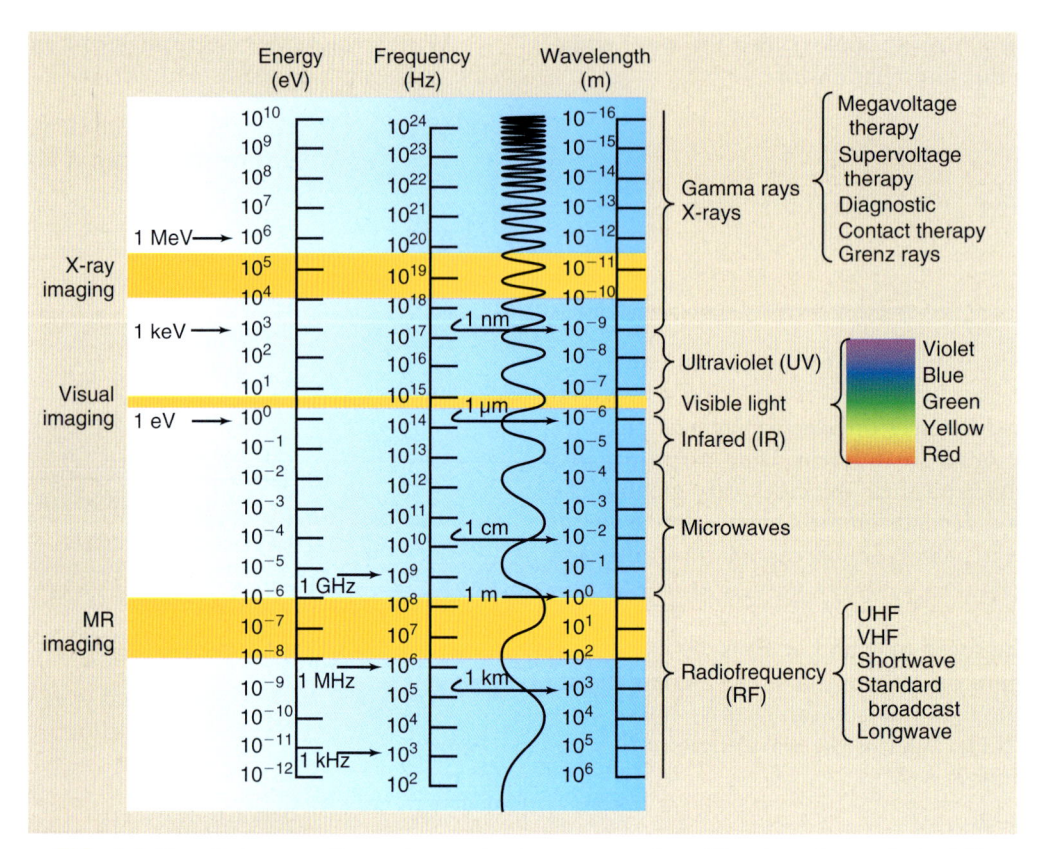

FIG. 4.6 The electromagnetic spectrum extends over more than 25 orders of magnitude. *MR,* Magnetic resonance; *UHF,* ultra high frequency; *VHF,* very high frequency.

Ultrasound is not produced in photon form and does not have a constant velocity. Ultrasound is a wave of moving molecules. Ultrasound requires matter; electromagnetic energy can exist in a vacuum.

> Diagnostic ultrasound is not a part of the electromagnetic spectrum.

The electromagnetic spectrum shown in Fig. 4.6 contains three different scales, one each for energy, frequency, and wavelength. Because the velocity of all electromagnetic energy is constant, the wavelength and frequency are inversely related.

Although segments of the electromagnetic spectrum are often given precise ranges, these ranges actually overlap because of production methods and detection techniques. For example, by definition, ultraviolet light has a shorter wavelength than violet light and cannot be sensed by the eye. What is visible violet light to one observer, however, may be ultraviolet light to another. Similarly, microwaves and infrared light are indistinguishable in their common region of the spectrum.

The earliest investigations focused on visible light. Studies of reflection, refraction, and diffraction showed light to be wavelike. Consequently, visible light is described by wavelength, measured in nanometers (nm).

In the 1880s, some scientists began to experiment with the radio, which required the oscillation of electrons in a conductor. Consequently, the unit of frequency, the hertz, is used to describe radio waves.

Finally, in 1895, Roentgen discovered x-rays by applying an electric potential (kilovolts) across a Crookes tube. Consequently, x-rays are described in terms of a unit of energy, the electron volt (eV).

> The energy of a photon is directly proportional to its frequency.

It should be clear that these three scales are directly related mathematically. If you know the value of electromagnetic energy on one scale, you can easily compute its value on the other two.

The electromagnetic spectrum has been scientifically investigated for longer than a century. Scientists working with energy in one portion of the spectrum were often unaware of others investigating another portion. Consequently, there is no generally accepted single dimension for measuring electromagnetic energy.

Visible Light

An optical physicist describes visible light in terms of wavelength. When sunlight passes through a prism

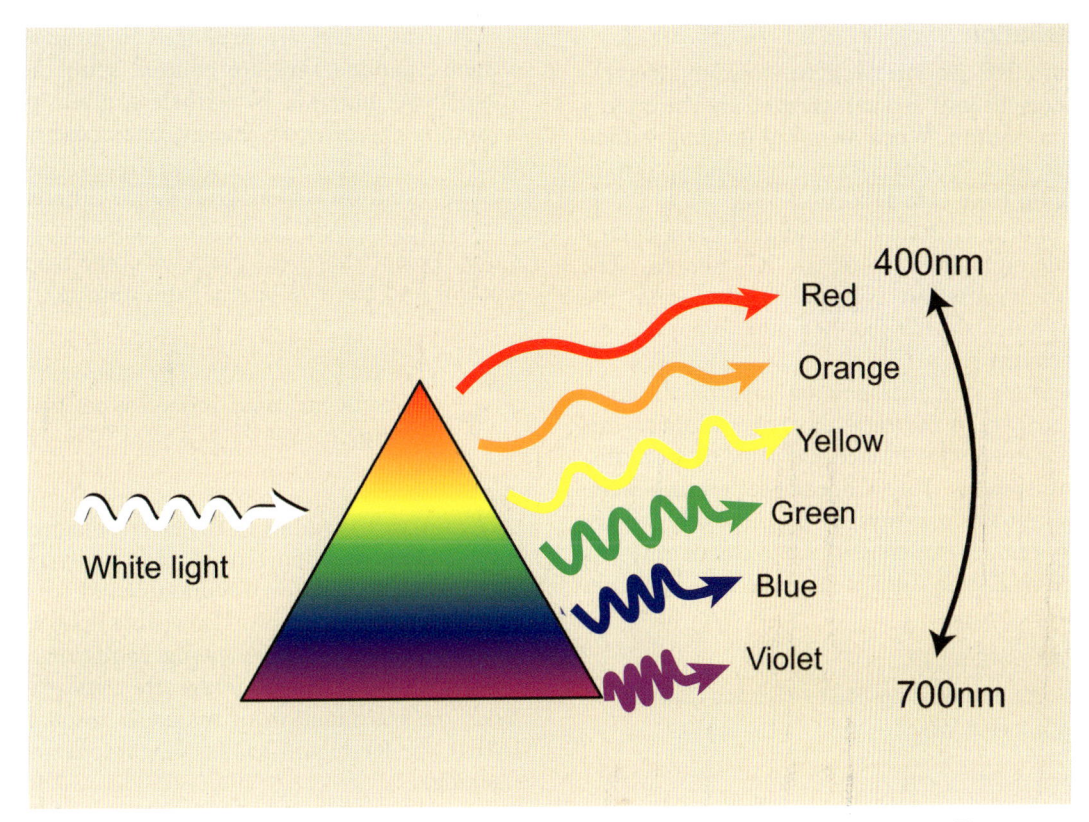

FIG. 4.7 When it passes through a prism, white light is refracted into its component colors. These colors have wavelengths that extend from approximately 400 to 700 nm.

(Fig. 4.7), it emerges not as white sunlight but as the colors of the rainbow.

Although photons of visible light travel in straight lines, their course can deviate when they pass from one transparent medium to another. This deviation in line of travel, called **refraction**, is the cause of many peculiar but familiar phenomena, such as a rainbow or the apparent bending of a straw in a glass of water.

White light is composed of photons of a range of wavelengths, and the prism acts to separate and group the emerging light into colors because different wavelengths are refracted through different angles. The component colors of white light have wavelength values ranging from approximately 400 nm for violet to 700 nm for red.

Visible light occupies the smallest segment of the electromagnetic spectrum, and yet it is the only portion that we can sense directly. Sunlight also contains two types of invisible light: infrared and ultraviolet.

Infrared light consists of photons with wavelengths longer than those of visible light but shorter than those of microwaves. Infrared light heats any substance on which it shines. It may be considered radiant heat.

Ultraviolet light is located in the electromagnetic spectrum between visible light and ionizing radiation. It is responsible for molecular interactions that can result in sunburn.

Radiofrequency

A radio or television engineer describes radio waves in terms of their frequency. For example, radio station WIMP might broadcast at 960 kHz, and its associated television station WIMP-TV might broadcast at 63.7 MHz. Communication broadcasts are usually identified by their frequency of transmission and are called **radiofrequency** (**RF**) emissions.

RF covers a considerable portion of the electromagnetic spectrum. RF has relatively low energy and a relatively long wavelength. Ham radio operators speak of broadcasting on the 10-m band or the 30-m band; these numbers refer to the approximate wavelength of emission.

Standard AM radio broadcasts have a wavelength of about 100 m. Television and FM broadcasting both occur at much shorter wavelengths. Because microwaves are also used for communication, RF and microwave emissions overlap considerably.

Very-short-wavelength RF is **microwave** radiation. Microwave frequencies vary according to use but are always higher than broadcast RF and lower than infrared. Microwaves have many uses, such as cellular telephone communication, highway speed monitoring, medical diathermy, and hotdog preparation.

Ionizing Radiation

Different from RF or visible light, ionizing electromagnetic energy usually is characterized by the energy contained in a photon. When an x-ray imaging system is operated at 80 kVp, the x-rays it produces contain energies ranging from 0 to 80 keV.

An x-ray photon contains considerably more energy than a visible light photon or an RF photon. The frequency of x-radiation is much higher and the wavelength is much shorter than for other types of electromagnetic energy.

It is sometimes said that gamma rays have higher energy than x-rays. In the early days of radiology, this was true because of the limited capacity of available x-ray imaging systems. Today, linear accelerators make it possible to produce x-rays of considerably higher energies than gamma-ray emissions. Consequently, it is inappropriate to distinguish between the two based on their respective energies.

> The only difference between x-rays and gamma rays is their origin.

X-rays are emitted from the electron cloud of an atom that has been stimulated artificially (Fig. 4.8). Gamma rays, on the other hand, come from inside the nucleus of a radioactive atom (Fig. 4.9).

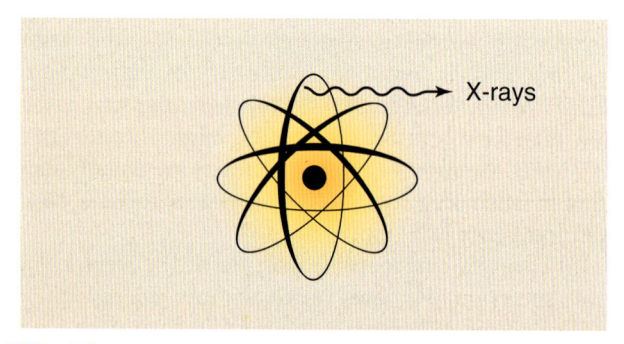

FIG. 4.8 X-rays are produced outside the nucleus of excited atoms.

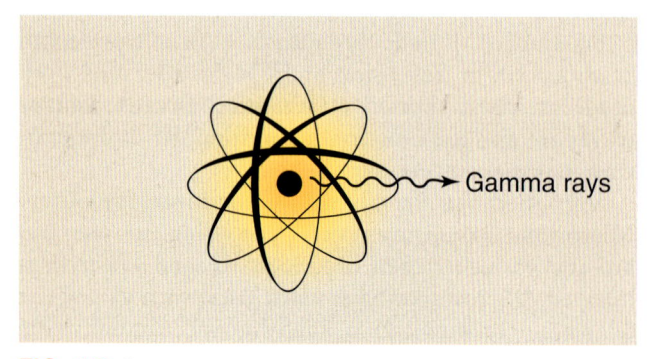

FIG. 4.9 Gamma rays are produced inside the nucleus of radioactive atoms.

Whereas x-rays are produced in diagnostic imaging systems, gamma rays are emitted spontaneously from radioactive material. Nevertheless, given an x-ray and a gamma ray of equal energy, one could not tell them apart.

This situation is analogous to the difference between beta particles and electrons. These particles are the same, except that beta particles come from inside the nucleus and electrons come from outside the nucleus.

> Visible light is identified by wavelength, RF is identified by frequency, and x-rays are identified by energy.

Again, three regions of the electromagnetic spectrum are particularly important to radiologic science. Naturally, the x-ray region is fundamental to producing a high-quality radiograph. The visible light region is also important because the viewing conditions of a radiographic or fluoroscopic image are critical to diagnosis. With the introduction of magnetic resonance imaging (MRI), the RF region has become important in medical imaging.

The electromagnetic relationship triangle (Fig. 4.10) can be helpful in relating each scale to the other two.

WAVES AND PARTICLES

A photon of x-radiation and a photon of visible light are fundamentally the same, except that x-radiation has a much higher frequency, and hence a shorter wavelength, than visible light. These differences result in differences in the way these photons interact with matter.

Visible-light photons tend to behave more like waves than particles. The opposite is true of x-ray photons, which behave more like particles than waves. In fact,

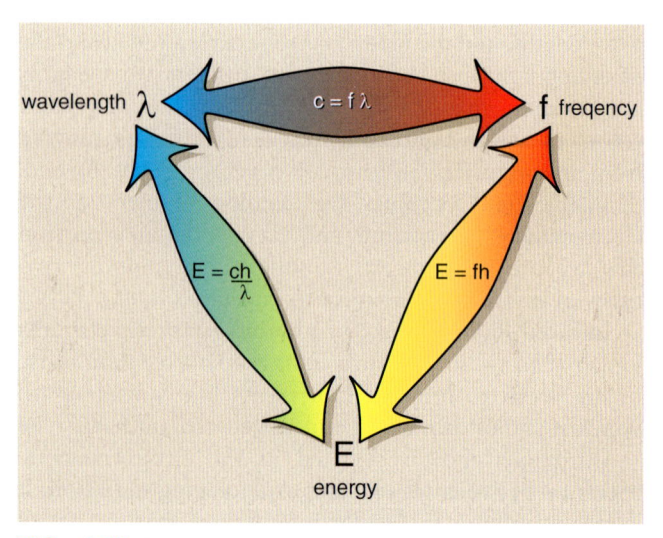

FIG. 4.10 The electromagnetic relationship triangle. Planck's constant is h and is defined later in this chapter.

both types of photons exhibit both types of behavior—a phenomenon known as the **wave-particle duality** of electromagnetic energy.

> Photons interact with matter most easily when the matter is approximately the same size as the photon wavelength.

Another general way to consider the interaction of electromagnetic radiation with matter is as a function of wavelength. Radio and TV waves, whose wavelengths are measured in meters, interact with metal rods or wires called **antennas**.

Microwaves, whose wavelengths are measured in centimeters, interact most easily with objects of the same size, such as hotdogs and hamburgers.

The wavelength of visible light is measured in nanometers (nm); visible light interacts with living cells, such as the rods and cones of the eye. Ultraviolet light interacts with molecules, and x-rays interact with electrons and atoms. All radiation with a wavelength longer than those of x-radiation interacts primarily as a wave phenomenon.

> X-rays behave as though they are particles.

Wave Model: Visible Light

One of the unique features of animal life is the sense of vision. It is interesting that we have developed organs that sense only a very narrow portion of the enormous spread of the electromagnetic spectrum. This narrow portion is called **visible light**.

The visible-light spectrum extends from short-wavelength violet radiation through green and yellow to long-wavelength red radiation. On either side of the visible-light spectrum are ultraviolet light and infrared light. Neither can be detected by the human eye, but they can be detected by other means, such as a photographic emulsion.

Visible light interacts with matter very differently from x-rays. When a photon of light strikes an object, it sets the object's molecules into vibration. The orbital electrons of some atoms of certain molecules are excited to an energy level that is higher than normal. This energy is immediately re-emitted as another photon of light; it is reflected.

The atomic and molecular structures of any object determine which wavelengths of light are reflected. A leaf in the sunlight appears green because nearly all of the visible-light photons are absorbed by the leaf. Only photons with wavelengths in the green region are reflected. Similarly, a balloon may appear red by absorbing all visible light photons except long-wavelength red photons, which are reflected.

Many familiar phenomena of light, such as reflection, absorption, and transmission, are most easily explained by using the wave model of electromagnetic energy. When a pebble is dropped into a still pond, ripples radiate from the center of the disturbance like miniature waves.

This situation is similar to the wave nature of visible light. Fig. 4.11 shows the difference in the water waves between an initial disturbance caused by a small object and one caused by a large object. The distance between the crests of waves is much greater with the large object than with the small object.

> Visible light behaves like a wave.

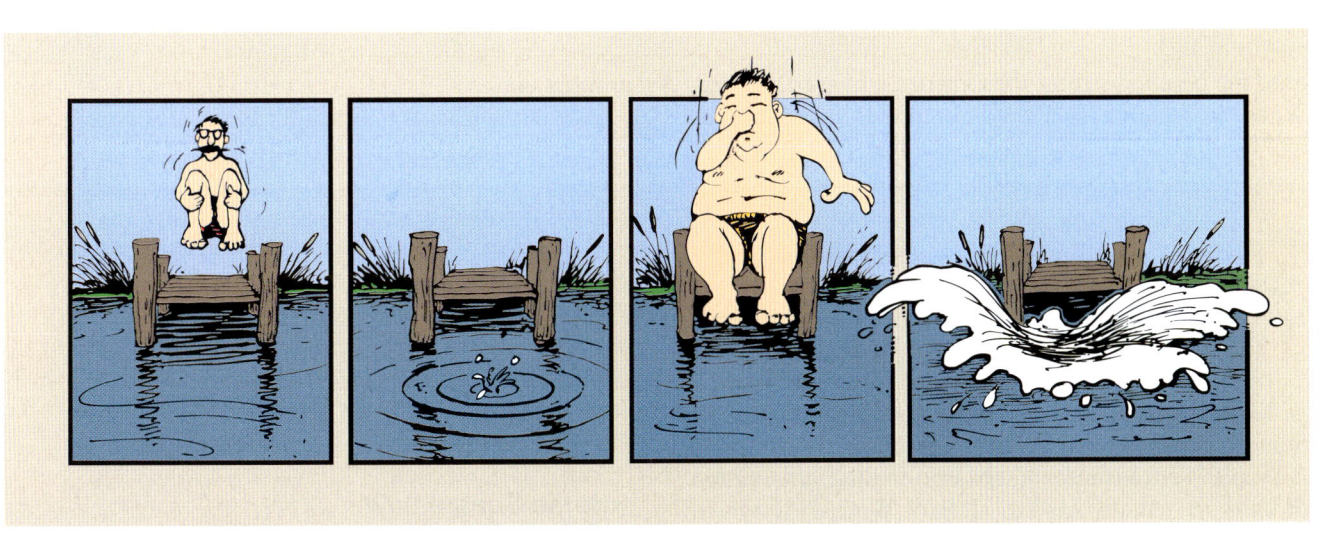

FIG. 4.11 A small object dropped into a smooth pond creates waves of short wavelength. A large object creates waves of much longer wavelength.

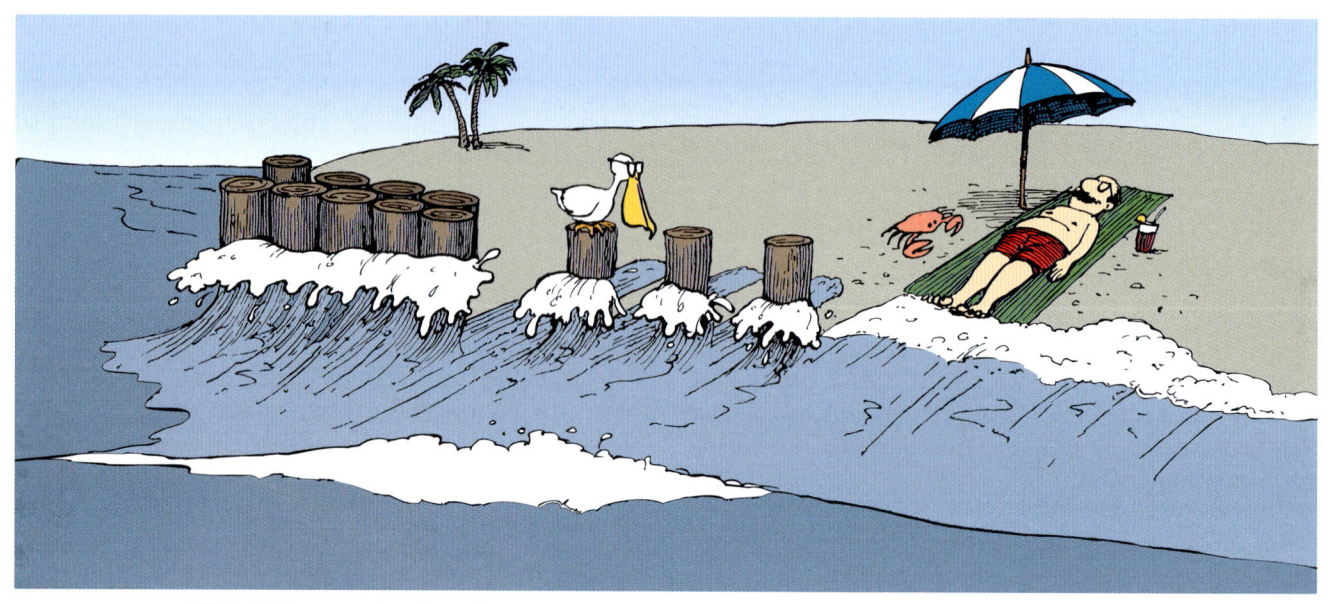

FIG. 4.12 Energy is reflected when waves crash into a bulkhead. It is absorbed by a beach. It is partially absorbed or attenuated by a line of pilings. Light is also reflected, absorbed, or attenuated, depending on the composition of the surface on which it is incident.

With these water waves, the difference in wavelength is proportional to the energy introduced into the system. With light, the opposite is true: The shorter the photon wavelength, the higher the photon energy.

If the analogy of the pebble in the pond is extended to a continuous succession of pebbles dropped into a smooth ocean, then at the edge of the ocean, the waves will appear straight rather than circular. Light waves behave as though they were straight rather than circular because the distance from the source is so great. The manner in which light is reflected from or transmitted through a surface is a consequence of this straight, wavelike motion.

When the waves of the ocean crash into a vertical bulkhead (Fig. 4.12), the reflected waves scatter from the bulkhead at the same angle at which the incident waves struck it. When the bulkhead is removed and replaced with a beach, the water waves simply crash onto the beach, dissipate their energy, and are absorbed. When an intermediate condition exists in which the bulkhead has been replaced by a line of pilings, the energy of the waves is scattered and absorbed.

> Electromagnetic energy attenuation is the reduction in intensity that results from scattering and absorption.

Visible light can similarly interact with matter. **Reflection** from the silvered surface of a mirror is common. Examples of **transmission, absorption,** and **attenuation** of light are equally easy to identify. When light waves are absorbed, the energy deposited in the absorber reappears as heat. A black asphalt road reflects very little visible light but absorbs a considerable amount. In so doing, the road surface can become quite hot.

Just a slight modification can change how some materials transmit or absorb light. There are three degrees of interaction between light and an absorbing material: transparency, translucency, and opacity (Fig. 4.13).

Window glass is transparent; it allows light to be transmitted almost unaltered. One can see through glass because the surface is smooth and the molecular structure is tight and orderly. Incident light waves cause molecular and electronic vibrations within the glass. These vibrations are transmitted through the glass and are re-irradiated almost without change.

When the surface of the glass is roughened with sandpaper, light is still transmitted through the glass but is greatly scattered and reduced in intensity. Instead of seeing clearly, one sees only blurred forms. Such glass is translucent.

When the glass is painted black, the characteristics of the pigment in the paint are such that no light can pass through. Any incident light is totally absorbed in the paint. Such glass is opaque to visible light.

The terms **radiopaque** and **radiolucent** are used routinely in x-ray diagnosis to describe the visual appearance of anatomical structures. Structures that absorb x-rays are called *radiopaque*. Structures that transmit x-rays are called *radiolucent* (Fig. 4.14). Whereas bone is radiopaque, lung tissue and, to some extent, soft tissue are radiolucent.

Inverse Square Law

When light is emitted from a source such as the sun or a light bulb, the intensity decreases rapidly with

CHAPTER 4 Electromagnetic Energy   63

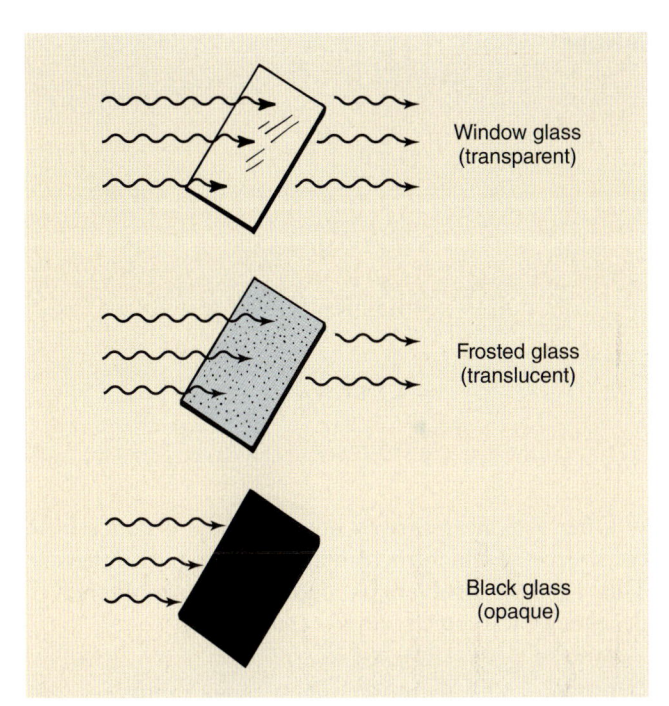

FIG. 4.13 Objects absorb light in three degrees: not at all (transmission), partially (attenuation), and completely (absorption). The objects associated with these degrees of absorption are called transparent, translucent, and opaque, respectively.

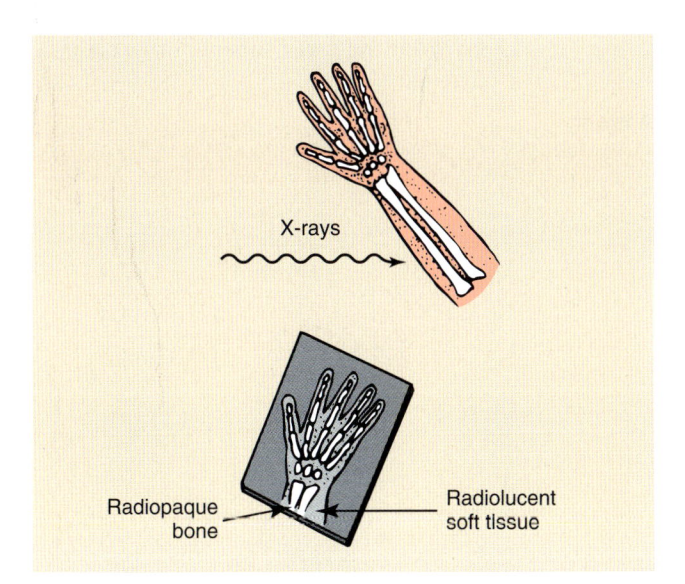

FIG. 4.14 Structures that attenuate x-rays are described as radiolucent or radiopaque, depending on the relative degree of x-ray transmission or absorption, respectively.

the distance from the source. X-rays exhibit precisely the same property. Fig. 4.15 shows that as a book is moved farther from a light source, the intensity of light falls.

This decrease in intensity is inversely proportional to the square of the distance of the object from the source.

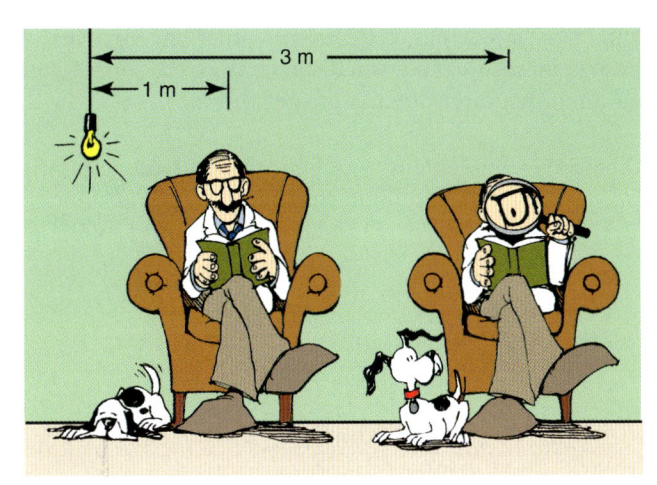

FIG. 4.15 The inverse square law describes the relationship between radiation intensity and distance from the radiation source.

INVERSE SQUARE LAW

$$\frac{I_1}{I_1} = \frac{d_2^2}{d_1^2}$$

or

$$\frac{I_1}{I_2} = \left(\frac{d_2}{d_1}\right)^2$$

where I_1 is the intensity at distance d_1 from the source and I_2 is the intensity at distance d_2 from the source.

The reason for the rapid decrease in intensity with increasing distance is that the total light emitted is spread out over an increasingly larger area. The equivalent of this phenomenon in the water wave analogy is the reduction of wave amplitude with distance from the source. The wavelength remains fixed.

> The intensity of electromagnetic radiation is inversely related to the square of the distance from the source.

If the source of electromagnetic radiation is not a point but rather a line, such as a fluorescent lamp, the inverse square law does not hold at distances close to the source. At great distances from the source, the inverse square law can be applied.

> The inverse square law can be applied to distances greater than seven times the longest dimension of the source.

To apply the inverse square law, you must know three of the four parameters, which consist of two distances and two intensities. The usual situation involves a known intensity at a given distance from the source and an unknown intensity at a greater distance.

Question: The intensity of light from a reading lamp is 100 millilumens (mlm), I_2, at a distance of 1 m, d_2. (The lumen is a unit of light intensity.) What is the intensity, I_1, of this light at 3 m, d_1?

Answer:
$$\frac{I_1}{I_2} = \frac{d_2^2}{d_1^2}$$
$$\frac{I_1}{100 \text{ mlm}} = \frac{1 \text{ m}^2}{3 \text{ m}^2}$$
$$I = (100 \text{ mlm})\left(\frac{1 \text{ m}}{3 \text{ m}}\right)^2$$
$$= (100 \text{ mlm})(1/9)$$
$$= 11 \text{ mlm}$$

This relationship between electromagnetic radiation intensity and distance from the source applies equally well to x-ray intensity.

Question: The exposure from an x-ray tube operated at 70 kVp, 200 mAs is 4 mGy$_a$ at 90 cm. What will the exposure be at 180 cm?

Answer:
$$\frac{I_1}{I_2} = \left(\frac{d_2}{d_1}\right)^2$$
$$I_1 = I_2\left(\frac{d_2}{d_1}\right)^2$$
$$= (4 \text{ mGy}_a)\frac{90 \text{ cm}^2}{180 \text{ cm}}$$
$$= (4 \text{ mGy}_a)\left(\frac{1}{2}\right)^2$$
$$= (4 \text{ mGy}_a)\left(\frac{1}{4}\right)^2$$
$$= 1 \text{ mGy}_a$$

This example illustrates that when the distance from the source is doubled, the intensity of radiation is reduced to one-fourth; conversely, when the distance is halved, the intensity is increased by a factor of four.

Question: For a given technique, the x-ray intensity at 1 m is 4.5 mGy$_a$. What is the intensity at the edge of the control booth, a distance of 3 m, if the useful beam is directed at the booth? (This, of course, should never be done!)

Answer:
$$\frac{I_1}{I_2} = \left(\frac{d_2}{d_1}\right)^2$$
$$I_1 = I_2\left(\frac{d_2}{d_1}\right)^2$$
$$= (4.5 \text{ mGy}_a)\frac{1 \text{ cm}^2}{3 \text{ cm}} = 4.5 \text{ mGy}_a\left(\frac{1}{3}\right)^2$$
$$= 4.5 \text{ mGy}_a\left(\frac{1}{9}\right)^2$$
$$= 0.5 \text{ mGy}_a$$

Often it is necessary to determine the distance from the source at which the radiation has a given intensity. This type of problem is commonly encountered in designing radiologic facilities.

Question: A temporary chest radiographic imaging system is to be set up in a large hall. The technique used results in an exposure of 0.25 mGy$_a$ at 180 cm. The area behind the chest stand in which the exposure intensity exceeds 0.01 mGy$_a$ is to be cordoned off. How far from the x-ray tube will this area extend?

Answer:
$$\frac{I_1}{I_2} = \frac{d_2^2}{d_1^1}$$
$$\frac{0.25 \text{ mGy}_a}{0.01 \text{ mGy}_a} = \frac{(d_2)^2}{(180 \text{ cm})^2}$$
$$(d_2)^2 = (180 \text{ cm})^2\left(\frac{0.25 \text{ mGy}_a}{0.01 \text{ mGy}_a}\right)$$
$$d_2 = \left[(180 \text{ cm})^2\left(\frac{0.25}{0.01}\right)\right]^{\frac{1}{2}}$$
$$= (180)(0.25)\frac{1}{2}$$
$$= (180)(5)$$
$$= 900 \text{ cm}$$
$$= 9 \text{ m}$$

In the previous exercises, the intensity of the x-ray beam is calculated at a distance that assumes that the source is constant. In practical radiography, it is typical to work the other way around. One must calculate what the intensity of the beam should be at the source (i.e., the x-ray focal spot), so that exposure at the distance to the image receptor will remain constant. Thus later we will use the above formula, but with one side inverted, and we will call it the **square law**.

CHAPTER 4 Electromagnetic Energy

TABLE 4.1	Examples of the Wide Range of X-rays Produced by Application in Medicine, Research, and Industry	
Type of X-ray	**Approximate kVp**	**Application**
Diffraction	<10	Research: structural and molecular analysis
Grenz rays[a]	10–20	Medicine: dermatology
Superficial	50–100	Medicine: therapy of superficial tissues
Diagnostic	30–150	Medicine: imaging anatomical structures and tissues
Orthovoltage[a]	200–300	Medicine: therapy of deep-lying tissues
Supervoltage[a]	300–1000	Medicine: therapy of deep-lying tissues
Megavoltage	>1000 (1 MV)	Medicine: therapy of deep-lying tissues
		Industry: checking the integrity of welded metals

[a]These radiation therapy modalities are no longer in use.

Particle Model: Quantum Theory

In contrast to other portions of the electromagnetic spectrum, x-rays are usually identified by their energy, measured in electron volts (eV). X-ray energy ranges from approximately 10 keV to 50 MeV. The associated wavelength for this range of x-radiation is approximately 10^{-10} to 10^{-14} m. The frequency of these photons ranges from approximately 10^{18} to 10^{22} Hz.

Table 4.1 describes the various types of x-rays produced and the general use that is made of each. We are interested primarily in the diagnostic range of x-radiation, although what is said for that range holds equally well for other types of x-radiation.

An x-ray photon can be thought of as containing an electric field and a magnetic field that vary sinusoidally at right angles to each other with a beginning and an end that have diminishing amplitude (Fig. 4.16). The wavelength of an x-ray photon is measured similarly to that of any electromagnetic energy: It is the distance from any position on the sine wave to the corresponding position of the next wave. The frequency of an x-ray photon is calculated similarly to the frequency of any electromagnetic photon, with use of the wave equation.

> The x-ray photon is a discrete bundle of energy.

X-rays exist with the speed of light (c), or they do not exist at all. That is one of the substantive statements of **Planck's quantum theory**. Max Planck was a German physicist whose mathematical and physical theories synthesized our understanding of electromagnetic radiation into a uniform model; for this work, he received the Nobel Prize in Physics in 1918.

> The energy of a photon is directly proportional to its frequency.

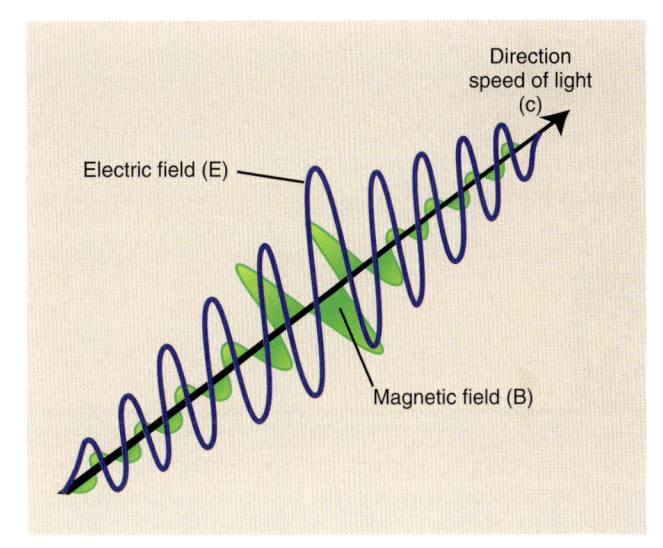

FIG. 4.16 All electromagnetic radiation, including x-rays, can be visualized as two perpendicular sine waves that travel in a straight line at the speed of light. One of the sine waves represents an electric field and the other a magnetic field.

Another important consequence of this theory is the relationship between energy and frequency: Photon energy is directly proportional to photon frequency. The constant of proportionality, known as **Planck's constant** and symbolized by h, has a numeric value of 4.15×10^{-15} eVs or 6.63×10^{-34} Js. Mathematically, the relationship between energy and frequency is expressed as follows:

> **PLANCK'S QUANTUM EQUATION**
>
> $E = hf$
>
> where E is the photon energy, h is Planck's constant, and f is the photon frequency in hertz.

Question: What is the frequency of a 70 keV x-ray?

Answer:
$$E = hf$$
$$f = \frac{E}{h}$$
$$= \frac{7 \times 10^4 \text{ eV}}{4.15 \times 10^{-15} \text{ eV}}$$
$$= 1.69 \times 10^{19}/\text{s}$$
$$= 1.69 \times 10^{19} \text{ Hz}$$

Question: What is the energy in one photon of radiation from radio station WIMP-AM, which has a broadcast frequency of 960 kHz?

Answer:
$$E = hf$$
$$= (4.15 \times 10^{-15} \text{ eVs})(9.6 \times 10^5/\text{s})$$
$$= 3.98 \times 10^{-9} \text{ eV}$$

An extension of Planck's equation is the relationship between photon energy and photon wavelength; this relationship is useful in computing equivalent wavelengths of x-rays and other types of radiation.

EQUIVALENT PLANCK'S EQUATION

$E = hf$, $f = E/h$, $E = \dfrac{hc}{\lambda}$

In other words, photon energy is inversely proportional to photon wavelength. In this relationship, the constant of proportionality is a combination of two constants: Planck's constant and the speed of light. The longer the wavelength of electromagnetic energy, the lower the energy of each photon.

Question: What is the energy in one photon of green light whose wavelength is 550 nm?

Answer:
$$E = \frac{hc}{\lambda}$$
$$= \frac{(4.15 \times 10^{-15} \text{ eVs})(3 \times 10^8/\text{s})}{500 \times 10^{-9} \text{ m}}$$
$$= \frac{12.45 \times 10^{-7} \text{ eVm}}{5.5 \times 10^{-7} \text{ m}}$$
$$= 2.26 \text{ eV}$$

MATTER AND ENERGY

We began Chapter 1 with the statement that everything in existence can be classified as matter or energy. We further stated that matter and energy are really manifestations of each other.

According to classical physics, matter can be neither created nor destroyed, a law known as the **law of conservation of matter**. A similar law, the **law of conservation of energy**, states that energy can be neither created nor destroyed.

Einstein and Planck greatly extended these theories. According to quantum physics and the physics of relativity, matter can be transformed into energy and vice versa. Nuclear fission, the basis for generating electricity, is an example of converting matter into energy. In radiology, a process known as **pair production** (see Chapter 10) is an example of the conversion of energy into mass.

A simple relationship introduced in Chapter 1 allows for the calculation of the energy equivalence of mass and the mass equivalence of energy. This equation is a consequence of Einstein's theory of relativity and is familiar to all.

Similar to the electron volt, the joule (J) is a unit of energy. One joule is equal to 6.24×10^{18} eV.

RELATIVITY

$E = mc^2$

where E is the energy measured in joules, m is the mass measured in kilograms, and c is the velocity of light measured in meters per second.

Question: What is the energy equivalence of an electron (mass = 9.109×10^{-31} kg), as measured in joules and in electron volts?

Answer:
$$E = mc^2$$
$$= (9.109 \times 10^{-15} \text{ kg})(3 \times 10^8 \text{ m/s})^2$$
$$= 81.972 \times 10^{-15} \text{ J}$$
$$= (8.1972 \times 10^{-15} \text{ J})\left(\frac{6.24 \times 10^{18} \text{ eV}}{\text{J}}\right)$$
$$= 51.15 \times 10^4 \text{ eV}$$
$$= 511.5 \text{ keV}$$

The problem might be stated in the opposite direction as follows:

Question: What is the mass equivalent of a 70 keV x-ray?

Answer:
$$E = mc^2$$
$$m = \frac{E}{c^2}$$
$$= \frac{(70 \times 10^3 \text{ eV})\left(\frac{\text{J}}{6.24 \times 10^{18} \text{eV}}\right)}{(3.8 \times 10^8 \text{ m/s})^2}$$
$$= \frac{11.2 \times 10^{-15} \text{ J}}{9 \times 10^{-16} \text{ m}^2/\text{s}^2}$$
$$= 1.25 \times 10^{-31} \text{ kg}$$

By using the relationships reported earlier, one can calculate the mass equivalence of a photon when only the photon wavelength or photon frequency is known.

Question: What is the mass equivalence of one photon of 1000 MHz microwave radiation?

Answer:
$$E = hf = mc^2$$
$$m = \frac{hf}{c^2}$$
$$= \frac{(6.626 \times 10^{-34}\text{ J})(1000 \times 10^6 \times \text{Hz})}{(3 \times 10^8 \text{ m/s})^2}$$
$$= 0.736 \times 10^{-41} \text{ kg}$$
$$= 7.36 \times 10^{-42} \text{ kg}$$

Question: What is the mass equivalence of a 330-nm photon of ultraviolet light?

Answer:
$$E = \frac{hc}{\lambda} = mc^2$$
$$m = \left(\frac{hc}{\lambda}\right)\left(\frac{1}{c^2}\right) = \frac{h}{\lambda c}$$
$$= \frac{6.626 \times 10^{-34} \text{ J}}{(3 \times 10^{-9}\text{ m})(3 \times 10^8 \text{ m/s})}$$
$$= 0.00669 \times 10^{-33} \text{ kg}$$
$$= 6.69 \times 10^{-36} \text{ kg}$$

Calculations of this type can be used to set up a scale of mass equivalence for the electromagnetic spectrum (Fig. 4.17). This scale can be used to check the answers to the previous examples and to some of the problems in the companion Workbook.

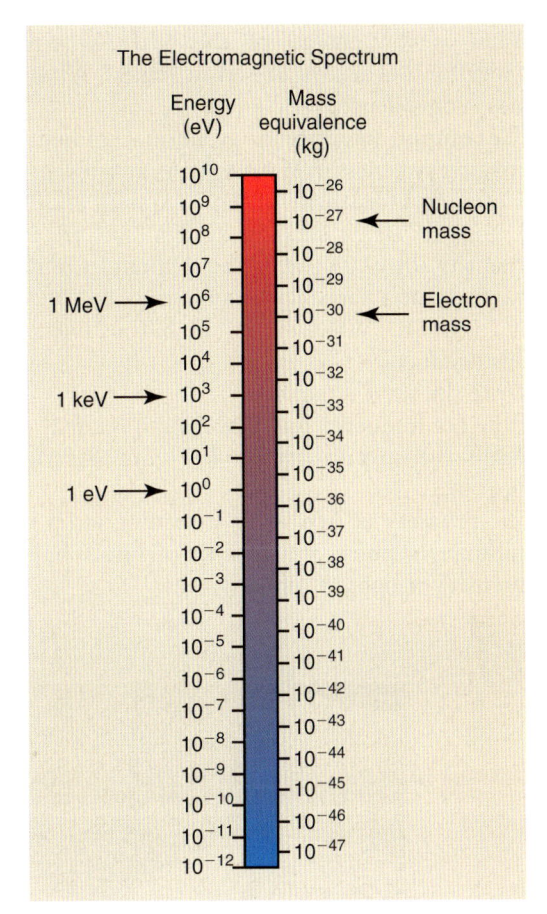

FIG. 4.17 Mass and energy are two forms of the same medium. This scale shows the equivalence of mass measured in kilograms to energy measured in electron volts.

SUMMARY

Although matter and energy are interchangeable, x-ray imaging is based on energy in the form of x-ray photons that interact with tissue and an image receptor.

X-rays are one type of photon of electromagnetic energy. Frequency, wavelength, velocity, and amplitude are used to describe the various imaging regions of the electromagnetic spectrum. These characteristics of electromagnetic energy determine how such radiation interacts with matter.

CHALLENGE QUESTIONS

1. Define or otherwise identify the following:
   a. Photon
   b. Radiolucency
   c. The inverse square law
   d. Frequency
   e. The law of conservation of energy
   f. Gamma ray
   g. Electromagnetic spectrum
   h. Sinusoidal variation
   i. Quantum
   j. Visible light
2. Accurately diagram one photon of orange light ($\lambda = 620$ nm) and identify its velocity, electric field, magnetic field, and wavelength.
3. A thunderclap associated with lightning has a frequency of 800 Hz. If its wavelength is 50 cm, what is its velocity? How far away is the thunder if the time interval between seeing the lightning and hearing the thunder is 6 s?
4. What is the frequency associated with a photon of microwave radiation that has a wavelength of 10^{-4} m?
5. Radio station WIMP-FM broadcasts at 104 MHz. What is the wavelength of this radiation?
6. In mammography, 26 keV x-rays are used. What is the frequency of this radiation?
7. Radiography of a barium-filled colon calls for high-kVp technique. These x-rays can have energy of 110 keV. What is the frequency and wavelength of this radiation?

8. What is the energy of the 110 keV x-ray in Question 7 when expressed in joules? What is its mass equivalence?
9. The output intensity of a normal radiographic imaging system is 0.05 mGy$_a$/mAs at 100 cm. What is the output intensity of such a system at 200 cm?
10. A mobile x-ray imaging system has an output intensity of 0.04 mGy$_a$ at 100 cm. Conditions require that a particular examination be conducted at 75 cm SID. What will be the output intensity at this distance?
11. Write the wave equation.
12. How are frequency and wavelength related?
13. Write the inverse square law and describe its meaning.
14. The intensity of light from a reading lamp is 200 millilumens (mlm) at a distance of 2 m. What is the intensity of light at 3 m?
15. What are the three imaging windows of the electromagnetic spectrum, and what unit of measure is applied to each?
16. What is the energy range of diagnostic x-rays?
17. What is the difference between x-rays and gamma rays?
18. Some regions of the electromagnetic spectrum behave like waves, and some regions behave like particles in their interaction with matter. What is this phenomenon called?
19. Define attenuation.
20. What is the frequency of a 70-keV x-ray photon?

The answers to the Challenge Questions can be found by logging on to our website at http://evolve.elsevier.com.

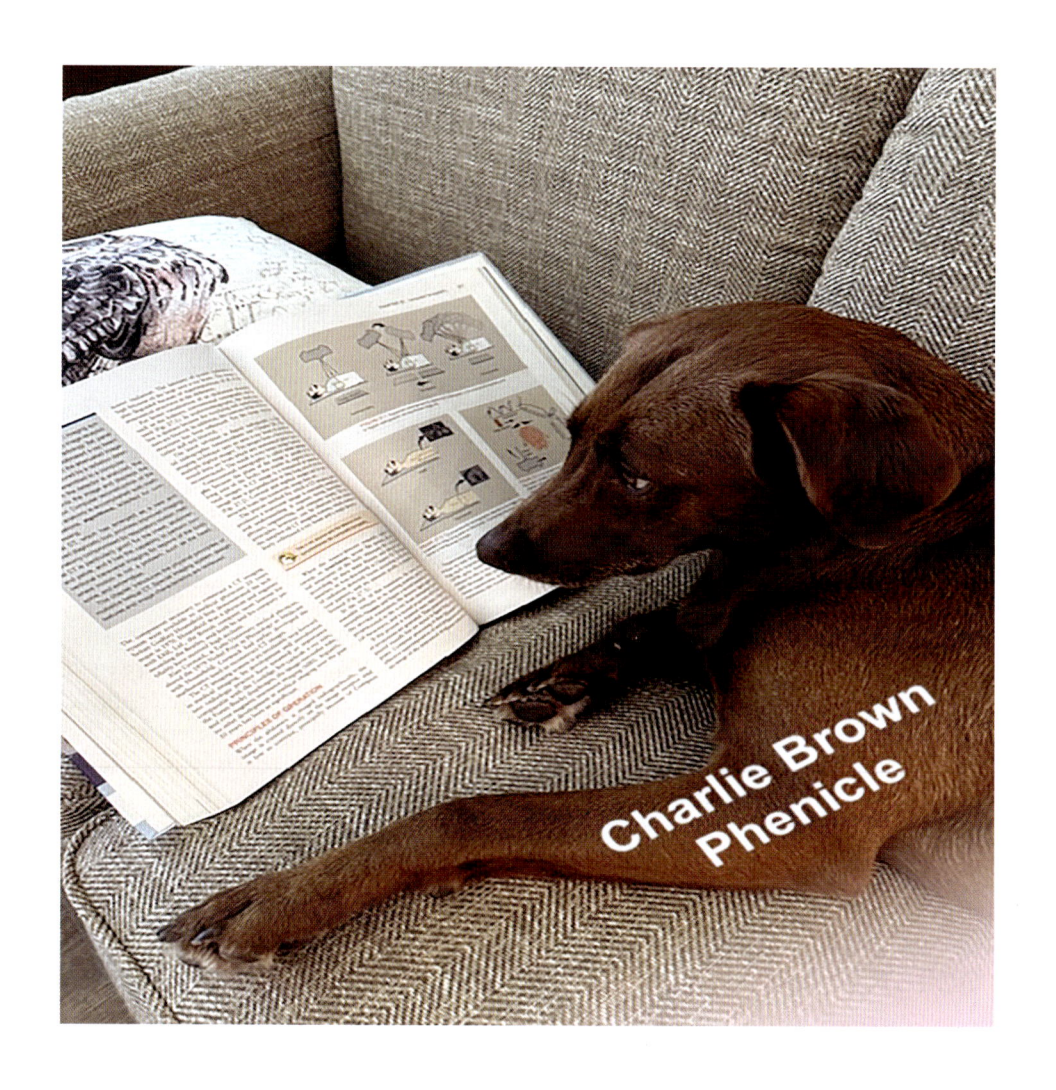

CHAPTER 5

Electricity, Magnetism, and Electromagnetism

OBJECTIVES

At the completion of this chapter, the student should be able to do the following:

1. Define electrification and provide examples.
2. List the laws of electrostatics.
3. Identify units of electric current, electric potential, and electric power.
4. Identify the interactions between matter and magnetic fields.
5. Discuss the four laws of magnetism.
6. Relate the experiments of Oersted, Lenz, and Faraday in defining the relationships between electricity and magnetism.
7. Identify the laws of electromagnetic induction.

OUTLINE

Electrostatics 70
   Electrostatic Laws 71
   Electric Potential 74
Electrodynamics 74
   Electric Circuits 75
   Electric Power 77
Magnetism 77
   Magnetic Laws 81
   Magnetic Induction 82
Electromagnetism 83
   Electromagnetic Induction 86
   Electromechanical Devices 86
   The Transformer 88
Summary 90
Challenge Questions 90

THIS CHAPTER on electricity, magnetism, and electromagnetism briefly introduces the basic concepts needed for further study of the x-ray imaging system and its various components.

Because the primary function of the x-ray imaging system is to convert electric energy into electromagnetic energy—x-rays—the study of electricity, magnetism, and electromagnetism is particularly important.

This chapter begins by introducing some examples of familiar devices that convert electricity into other forms of energy. Electrostatics is the science of stationary electric charges. Electrodynamics is the science of electric charges in motion. Electromagnetism describes how electrons are given electric potential energy (voltage) and how electrons in motion create magnetism.

Magnetism has become increasingly important in diagnostic imaging with the application of magnetic resonance imaging (MRI). This chapter describes the nature of magnetism by discussing the laws that govern magnetic fields. These laws are similar to those that govern electric fields; knowing them is essential to understanding the function of several components of the x-ray imaging system.

Electromagnetic induction is a means of transferring electric potential energy from one position to another, as in a transformer.

The primary function of an x-ray imaging system (Fig. 5.1) is to convert electric energy into electromagnetic energy. Electric energy is supplied to the x-ray imaging system in the form of well-controlled electric current. A conversion takes place in the x-ray tube, where most of this electric energy is transformed into heat—some of it into x-rays.

Fig. 5.2 shows other, more familiar examples of electric energy conversion. When an automobile battery runs down, an electric charge restores the chemical energy of the battery. Electric energy is converted into mechanical energy with a device known as an electric motor, which can be used to drive a circular saw. A kitchen toaster or electric range converts electric energy into thermal energy. There are, of course, many other examples of converting electric energy into other forms of energy.

ELECTROSTATICS

Electric charge comes in discrete units that are **positive** or **negative**. Electrons and protons are the smallest units of electric charge. The electron has one unit of negative charge; the proton has one unit of positive charge. Thus the electric charges associated with an electron and a proton have the same magnitude but opposite signs.

> **Electrostatics** is the study of stationary electric charges.

Because of the way atoms are constructed, electrons often are free to travel from the outermost shell of one atom to another atom. Protons, on the other hand, are fixed inside the nucleus of an atom and are not free to move. Consequently nearly all discussions of electric charge deal with negative electric charge—that associated with the electron.

Upon touching a metal doorknob after walking across a deep-pile carpet in winter, you get a shock (by contact). Such a shock occurs because electrons are rubbed off the carpet onto your shoes (by friction), causing you to become electrified. An object is said to be **electrified** if it has too few or too many electrons.

> Electrification can be created by contact, friction, or induction.

However, the outer shell electrons of some types of atoms are loosely bound and can be removed easily. Removal of these electrons electrifies the substances from which they were removed and results in static electricity.

If you run a comb through your hair, electrons are removed from the hair and deposited on the comb. The comb becomes electrified with too many negative charges. An electrified comb can pick up tiny pieces of paper as though the comb were a magnet (Fig. 5.3). Because of its excess electrons, the comb repels some electrons in the paper, causing the closest end of the paper to become slightly positively charged. This results in a small electrostatic attractive force. Similarly, hair is electrified because it has an abnormally low number of electrons and may stand on end because of mutual repulsion.

One object that is always available to accept electric charges from an electrified object is the Earth. The Earth behaves as a huge reservoir for stray electric charges. In this capacity, it is called an **electric ground**.

During a thunderstorm, wind and cloud movement can remove electrons from one cloud and deposit them on another (by induction). Both such clouds become electrified, one negatively and one positively.

If the electrification becomes sufficiently intense, a discharge can occur between the clouds; in this case, electrons are rapidly transported back to the cloud that is deficient. This phenomenon is called **lightning**.

CHAPTER 5 Electricity, Magnetism, and Electromagnetism

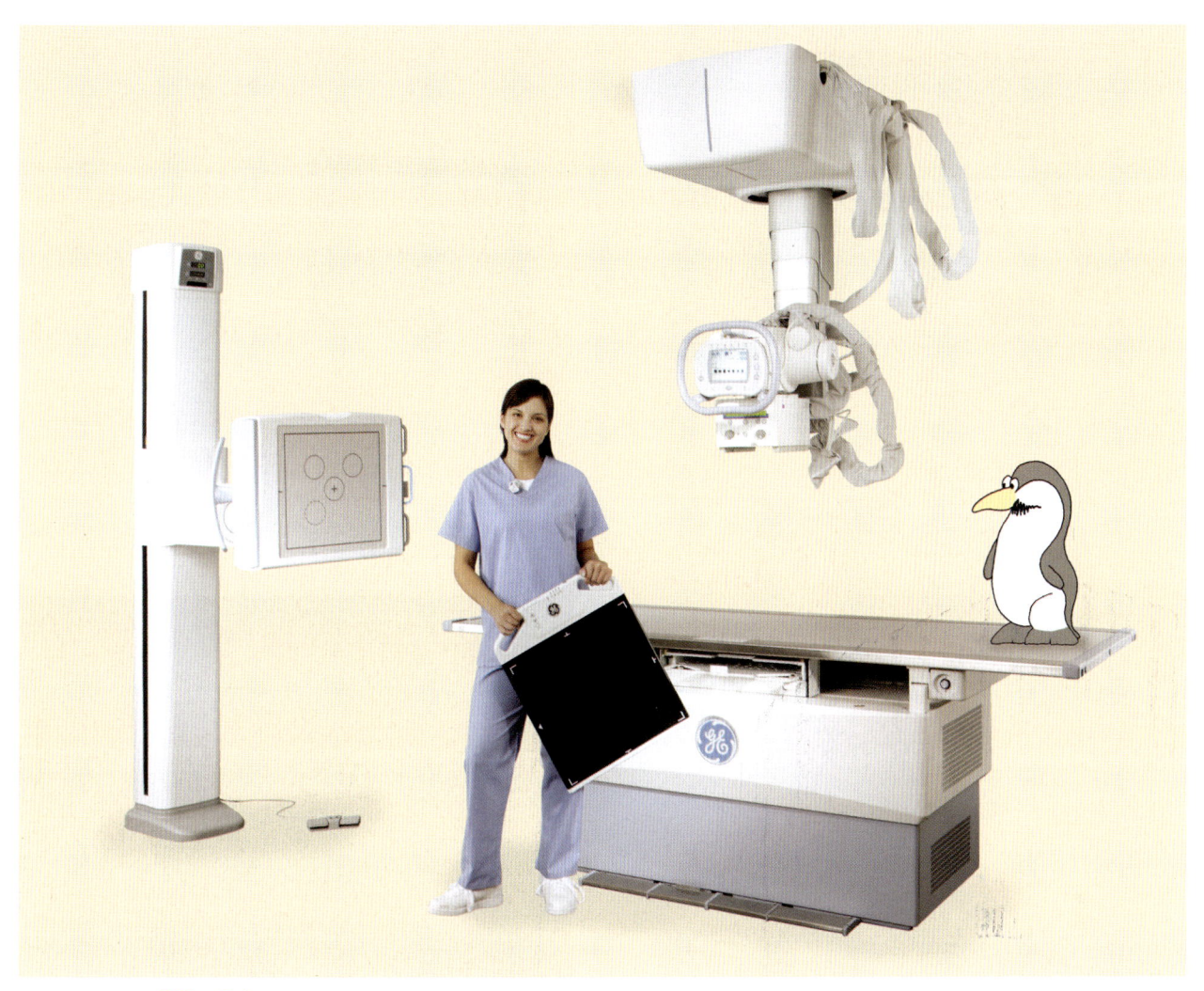

FIG. 5.1 The x-ray imaging system converts electrical energy into electromagnetic energy. (Courtesy Heidi Seerden, GE Healthcare.)

Although lightning can occur between clouds, it most frequently occurs between an electrified cloud and the Earth (Fig. 5.4).

Another familiar example of electrification is seen in every *Frankenstein* movie. Usually Dr. Frankenstein's laboratory is filled with electric gadgets, wire, and large steel balls with sparks flying in every direction (Fig. 5.5). These sparks are created because the various objects—wires, steel balls, and so forth—are highly electrified.

The smallest unit of electric charge is the electron. This charge is much too small to be useful, so the fundamental unit of electric charge is the coulomb (C): $1\,C = 6.3 \times 10^{18}$ electron charges.

Question: What is the electrostatic charge of one electron?

Answer: One coulomb (C) is equivalent to 6.3×10^{18} electron charges; therefore

$$\frac{1\,C}{6.3 \times 10^{18}\ \text{electron charges}}$$

$= 1.6 \times 10^{-19}$ C/electron charges

Question: The electrostatic charge transferred between two people after one has scuffed his feet across a nylon rug is 1 microcoulomb. How many electrons are transferred?

Answer: $1\,C = 6 \times 10^{18}$ electrons
$1\,\mu C = 6 \times 10^{12}$ electrons transferred

Question: One ampere is the flow of 1 coulomb per second; therefore "mAs" is a measure of what quantity?

Answer: $mAs = m\frac{C}{s}s = mC$, which is electrostatic charge

Electrostatic Laws

Four general laws of electrostatics describe how electric charges interact with each other and with neutral objects.

Unlike charges attract; like charges repel.

72   PART I   Radiologic Physics

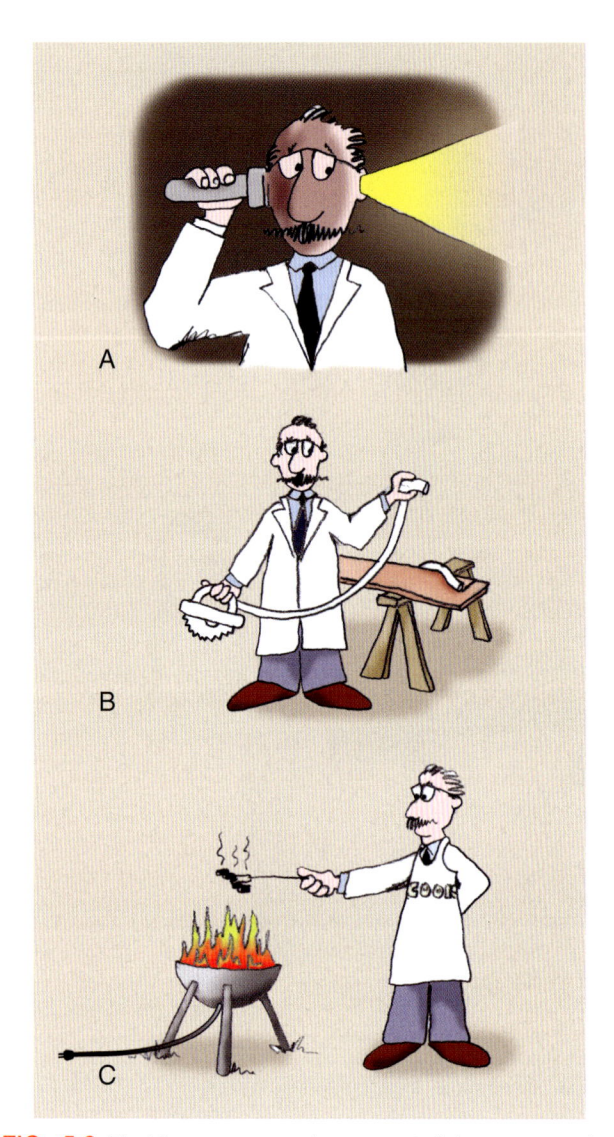

FIG. 5.2 Electric energy can be converted from or to other forms by various devices, such as the battery (A) from chemical energy, the motor (B) to mechanical energy, and the barbecue (C) to thermal energy.

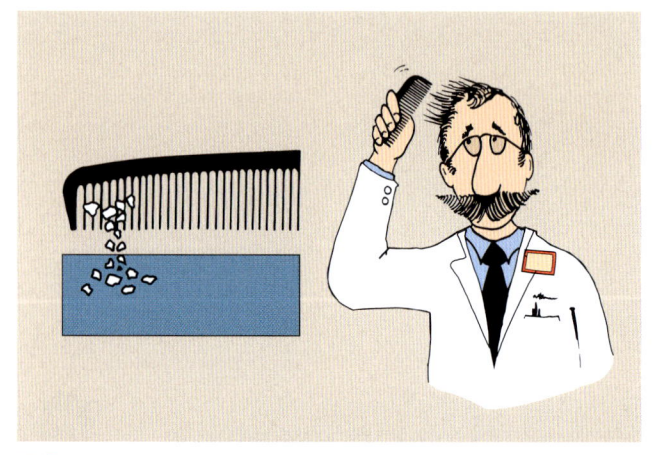

FIG. 5.3 Running a comb briskly through your hair may cause both your hair and the comb to become electrified through the transfer of electrons from the hair to the comb. The electrified condition may make it possible to pick up small pieces of paper with the comb and may cause one's hair to stand on end.

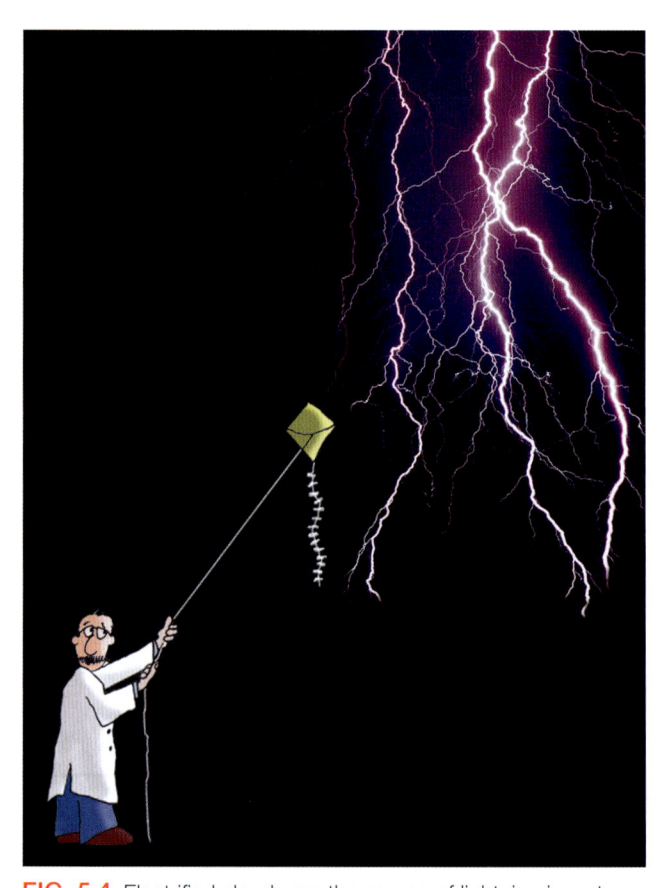

FIG. 5.4 Electrified clouds are the source of lightning in a storm.

An electric field is associated with each electric charge. The electric field points outward from a positive charge and inward to a negative charge. Uncharged particles do not have an electric field. In Fig. 5.6, lines associated with each charged particle illustrate the intensity of the electric field.

When two similar electric charges—negative and negative or positive and positive—are brought close together, their electric fields are in opposite directions, which cause the electric charges to repel each other.

When unlike charges—one negative and one positive—are close to each other, the electric fields radiate in the same direction and cause the two charges to attract each other. The force of attraction between unlike charges or repulsion between like charges is attributable to the electric field. It is called an **electrostatic force**.

The magnitude of the electrostatic force is given by Coulomb's law as follows:

COULOMB'S LAW

$$F = k\frac{Q_a Q_b}{d^2}$$

where F is the electrostatic force (newton), Q_a and Q_b are electrostatic charges (coulomb), d is the distance between the charges (meter), and k is a constant of proportionality.

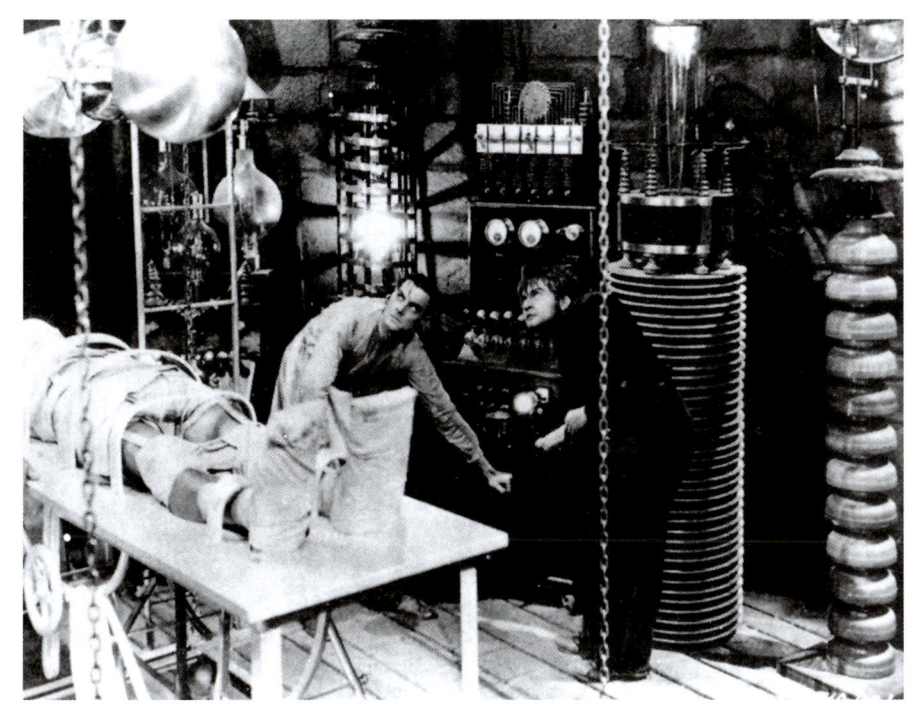

CHAPTER 5 Electricity, Magnetism, and Electromagnetism 73

FIG. 5.5 Early radiographers are shown in this scene from the original *Frankenstein* movie (1931). (Courtesy Bettmann/Corbis.)

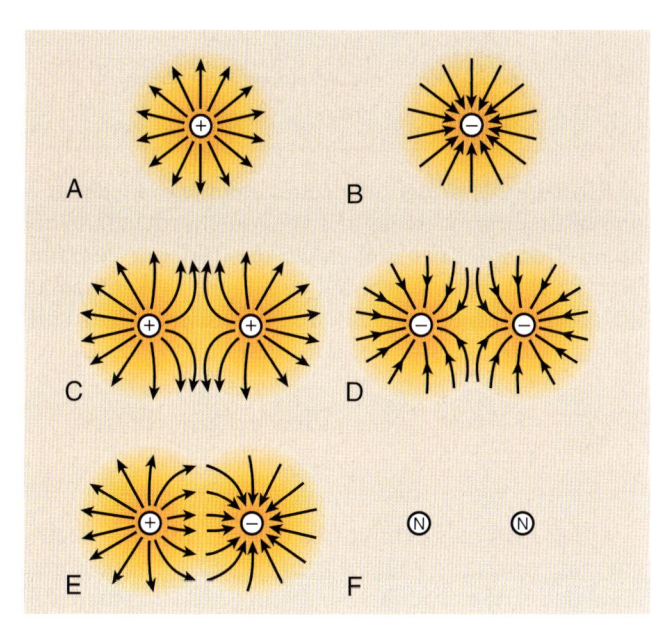

FIG. 5.6 Electric fields radiate out from a positive charge (A) and toward a negative charge (B). Like charges repel one another (C and D). Unlike charges attract one another (E). Uncharged particles do not have an electric field (F).

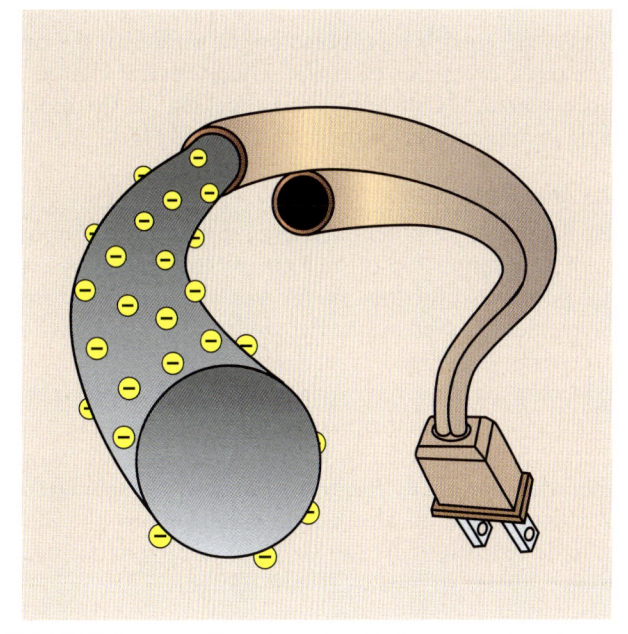

FIG. 5.7 Cross-section of an electrified copper wire, showing that the surface of the wire has excessive electrostatic charges.

The electrostatic force is very strong when objects are close but decreases rapidly as objects separate. This **inverse square** relationship for electrostatic force is the same as that for x-ray intensity (see Chapter 4). The electrostatic force between two charges is directly proportional to the product of their magnitudes and inversely proportional to the square of the distance between them.

When a diffuse nonconductor such as a thunder cloud becomes electrified, the electric charges are distributed rather uniformly throughout. With electrified copper wire, excess electrons are distributed on the outer surface (Fig. 5.7).

> The electric charge of a conductor is concentrated along the sharpest curvature of the surface.

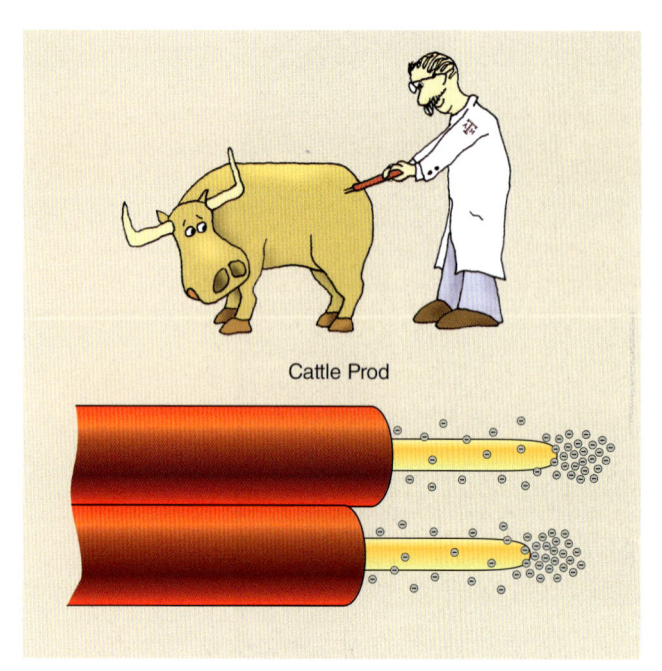

FIG. 5.8 Electrostatic charges are concentrated on surfaces of sharpest curvature. The cattle prod is a device that takes advantage of this electrostatic law.

With an electrified cattle prod (Fig. 5.8), electric charges are equally distributed on the surface of the two electrodes, except at each tip, where electric charge is concentrated. ("Our business is shocking" is the motto of the manufacturer of the leading cattle prod.)

Electric Potential

The discussion of potential energy in Chapter 1 emphasized the relationship of such energy to work. A system that possesses potential energy is a system with stored energy. Such a system has the ability to do work when this energy is released.

Electric charges have potential energy. When positioned close to each other, like electric charges, have electric potential energy because they can do work when they fly apart. Electrons bunched up at one end of a wire create an electric potential because the electrostatic repulsive force causes some electrons to move along the wire so that work can be done.

> The unit of electric potential is the volt (V).

Electric potential is sometimes called *voltage*; the higher the voltage, the greater the potential to do work. In the United States, the voltage in homes and offices is 110 V. X-ray imaging systems and your clothes dryer usually require 220 V or higher. The volt is potential energy/unit charge, or joule/coulomb (1 V = 1 J/C).

ELECTRODYNAMICS

We recognize electrodynamic phenomena as electricity. If an electric potential is applied to objects such as copper wire, then electrons move along the wire. This electron movement is an electric current, or **electricity**.

Electricity occurs in many types of objects and ranges from the very small electric currents of the human body (e.g., those measured by electrocardiograms) to the very large currents of 440,000-V cross-country electric transmission lines.

> Electrodynamics is the study of electric charges in motion.

The direction of electric current is important. In his early classic experiments, Benjamin Franklin assumed that positive electric charges were conducted on his kite string. The unfortunate result was the convention that the direction of electric current is always opposite that of electron flow. Whereas electrical engineers work with electric current, physicists are usually concerned with electron flow.

A section of conventional household electric wire consists of a metal conducting wire, usually copper, coated with a rubber or plastic insulating material. The insulator confines the electron flow to the conductor. Touching the insulator does not result in a shock; touching the conductor does.

> A conductor is any substance through which electrons easily flow.

Most metals are good electric conductors; copper is one of the best. Water is also a good electric conductor because of the salts and other impurities it contains. That is why everyone should avoid water when operating power tools. Glass, clay, and other earthlike materials are usually good electric insulators.

> An insulator is any material that does not allow electron flow.

Other materials exhibit two entirely different electric characteristics. In 1946, William Shockley demonstrated semiconduction. The principal semiconductor materials are silicon (Si) and germanium (Ge). This development led to microchips and thus the explosive rise of computer technology.

> A semiconductor is a material that under some conditions behaves as an insulator and in other conditions behaves as a conductor.

At room temperature, all materials resist the flow of electricity. Resistance decreases as the temperature of the material is reduced (Fig. 5.9). **Superconductivity** is the property of some materials to exhibit no resistance below a critical temperature (Tc).

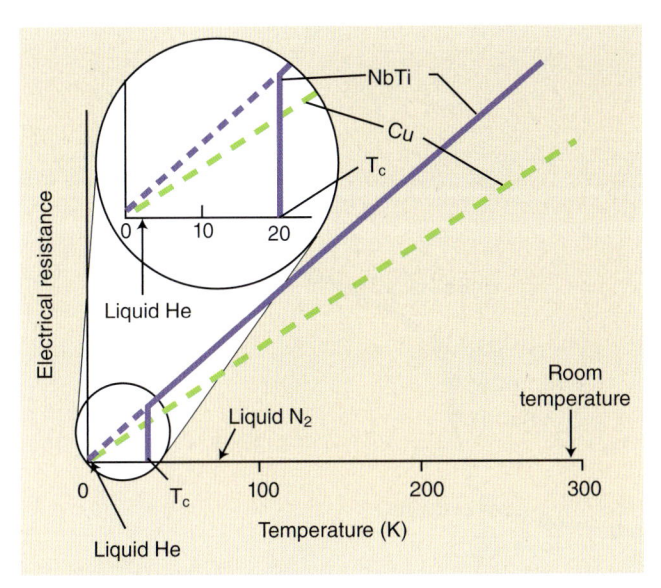

FIG. 5.9 The electrical resistance of a conductor (Cu) and a superconductor (NbTi) as a function of temperature.

Superconductivity was discovered in 1911 but was not developed commercially until the early 1960s. Scientific investigation into superconductivity has grown in recent years and now focuses on high-temperature superconductivity (Fig. 5.10).

Superconducting materials such as niobium and titanium allow electrons to flow without resistance. Ohm's law, described in the next section, does not hold true for superconductors. A superconducting circuit can be viewed as one in perpetual motion because electricity exists without voltage. For material to behave as a superconductor, however, it must be made very cold, which requires energy.

Table 5.1 summarizes the four electric states of matter.

Electric Circuits

Modifying a conducting wire by reducing its diameter (wire gauge) or inserting different devices (circuit elements) can increase its resistance. When this resistance is controlled and the conductor is made into a closed path, the result is an **electric circuit**.

> Increasing electric resistance results in a reduced electric current.

Electric current is measured in amperes (A). The ampere is proportional to the number of electrons flowing in the electric circuit. One ampere is equal to an electric charge of 1 C flowing through a conductor each second.

Electric potential is measured in volts (V), and electric resistance is measured in ohms (Ω). Electrons at high voltage have high potential energy and high capacity to do work. If electron flow is inhibited, the electric circuit resistance is high.

The manner in which electric currents behave in an electric circuit is described by a relationship known as *Ohm's law*.

> The voltage across the total circuit or any portion of the circuit is equal to the current times the resistance.

OHM'S LAW

$V = IR$

where V is the electric potential in volts, I is the electric current in amperes, and R is the electric resistance in ohms. Variations of this relationship are expressed as follows:

$R = \dfrac{V}{I}$

and

$I = \dfrac{V}{R}$

Question: If a current of 0.5 A passes through a conductor that has a resistance of 6 Ω, what is the voltage across the conductor?

Answer:
$V = IR$
$= (0.5 \text{ A})(6 \text{ }\Omega)$
$= 3 \text{ V}$

Question: A kitchen sliced-bread toaster draws a current of 2.5 A. If the household voltage is 110 V, what is the electric resistance of the toaster?

Answer:
$R = \dfrac{V}{I}$
$= \dfrac{110 \text{ V}}{2.5 \text{ A}}$
$= 44 \text{ }\Omega$

Most electric circuits, such as those used in radios, televisions, and other electronic devices, are very complicated. X-ray circuits are also complicated and contain a number of different types of circuit elements. Table 5.2 identifies some of the important types of circuit elements, the functions of each, and their symbols.

Electric current is the flow of electrons through a conductor. These electrons can be made to flow in one direction along the conductor, in which case the electric current is called **direct current** (DC).

Most applications of electricity require that the electrons be controlled so that they flow first in one direction and then in the opposite direction. Current in which electrons oscillate back and forth is called **alternating current** (AC).

76   PART I   Radiologic Physics

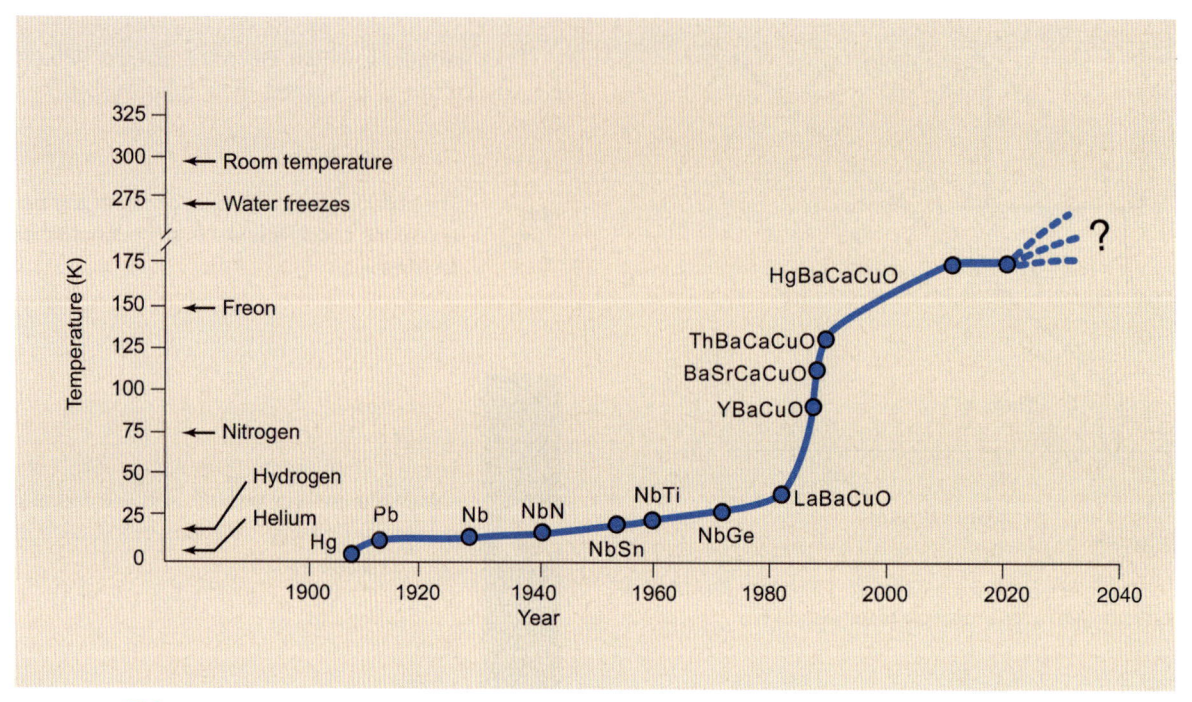

FIG. 5.10 Recent years have seen a dramatic rise in the critical temperature for superconducting materials.

TABLE 5.1	Four Electric States of Matter	
State	**Material**	**Characteristics**
Superconductor	Niobium	No resistance to electron flow
	Titanium	No electric potential required
		Must be very cold
Conductor	Copper	Variable resistance
	Aluminum	Obeys Ohm's law
		Requires a voltage
Semiconductor	Silicon	Can be conductive
	Germanium	Can be resistive
		Basis for computers
Insulator	Rubber	Does not permit electron flow
	Glass	Extremely high resistance
		Necessary with high voltage

TABLE 5.2	Symbol and Function of Electric Circuit Elements	
Circuit Element	**Symbol**	**Function**
Resistor	⏦	Inhibits flow of electrons
Battery	+|||−	Provides electric potential
Capacitor	⊣⊢	Momentarily stores electric charge
Transformer	⫞⫞	Increases or decreases voltage by a fixed amount (AC only)
Diode	▸⊣	Allows electrons to flow in only one direction

> Electrons that flow in only one direction constitute DC; electrons that flow alternately in opposite directions constitute AC.

Fig. 5.11 diagrams the phenomenon of DC and shows how it can be described by a graph called a **voltage waveform**. The horizontal axis, or x-axis, of the voltage waveform represents time; the vertical axis, or y-axis, represents the amplitude of the voltage waveform. For DC, the electrons always flow in the same direction; therefore DC is represented by a horizontal

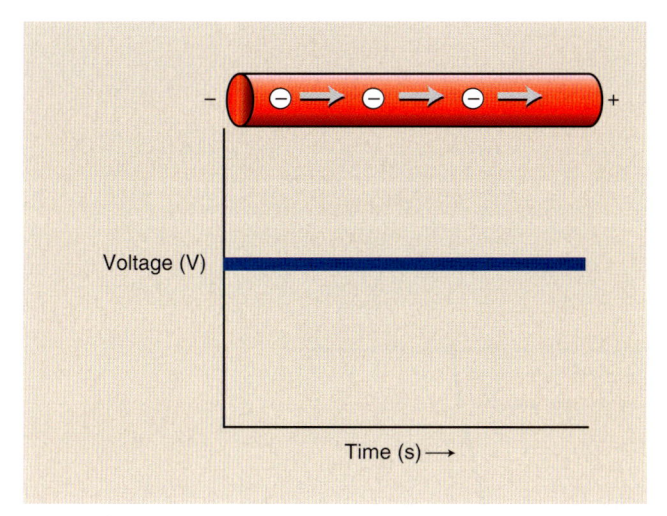

FIG. 5.11 Representation of direct current. Electrons flow in one direction only. The graph of the associated electric waveform is a straight line.

line. The vertical separation between this line and the time axis represents the magnitude of the current or the voltage.

The voltage waveform for AC is a sine curve (Fig. 5.12). Electrons flow first in a positive direction and then in a negative direction. At one instant in time (points 0, 2 in Fig. 5.12), all electrons are at rest. Then they move, first in the positive direction with increasing voltage. When they reach maximum flow number, represented by the vertical distance from the time axis (point 1), the electric voltage is reduced. They come to zero again momentarily (point 2) and then reverse motion and flow in the negative direction, increasing in negative electric voltage to maximum (point 3). Next the electric voltage is reduced again to zero.

This oscillation in electron direction occurs sinusoidally, with each requiring 1/60 second, or 16.7 ms. Consequently, thanks principally to George Westinghouse, AC is identified as a 60-Hz current (50 Hz in Europe and in much of the rest of the world).

Electric Power

Electric power is measured in **watts** (**W**). Common household electric appliances, such as toasters, blenders, mixers, and radios, generally require 500 to 1500 W of electric power. Lightbulbs require 30 to 150 W of electric power. An x-ray imaging system requires 20 to 150 kW of electric power.

> One watt is equal to 1 A of current flowing through an electric potential of 1 V. Power (W) = voltage (V) × current (A).

> **ELECTRIC POWER**
> P = IV
> where P is the power in watts, I is the current in amperes, and V is the electric potential in volts.

Question: If the cost of electric power is 10 cents per kilowatt-hour (kW-h), how much does it cost to operate a 100-W lightbulb for an average of 5 hours per day for 1 month?

Answer: Total on time = (30 days/mo)(5 h/day)
= 150 h/mo
Total power consumed
= (150 h/mo)(100/W)
= 15,000 W − h/mo
= 15 kW−h/mo
Total cost = (15 kW−h/mo)
(10 cents/kW−h)
= $1.50/mo

Question: An x-ray imaging system that draws a current of 80 A is supplied with 220 V. What is the power consumed?

Answer: P = IV
= (80 A)(220 V)
= 17,600 W
= 17.6 kW

Question: The overall resistance of a mobile x-ray imaging system is 10 Ω. When plugged into a 110-V receptacle, how much current does it draw and how much power is consumed?

Answer: P = IV
= (11 A)(110 V)
= 1210 W
or P = I²R
= (11 A)² 10
= 1210 W

MAGNETISM

Around 1000 BC, shepherds and dairy farmers near the village of Magnesia (what is now western Turkey) discovered magnetite, an oxide of iron (Fe_3O_4). This rodlike stone, when suspended by a string, would rotate back and forth; when it came to rest, it pointed the way to water. It was called a **lodestone** or leading stone.

Of course, if you walk toward the North Pole from any spot on the Earth, you will find water. So the word **magnetism** comes from the name of that ancient village where the cows were very ancient also. When milked, they produced milk of magnesia (Fig. 5.13)!

Magnetism is a fundamental property of some forms of matter. Ancient observers knew that lodestones would attract iron filings. They also knew that rubbing an amber rod with fur caused it to attract small, lightweight objects such as paper. They considered these

78 PART I Radiologic Physics

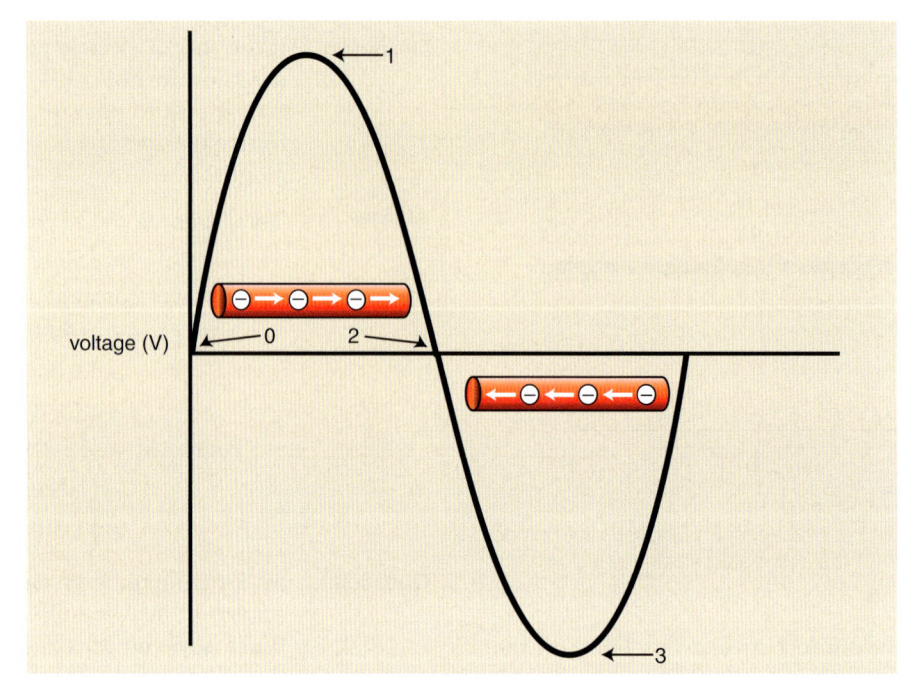

FIG. 5.12 Representation of alternating current. Electrons flow alternately in one direction and then the other. Alternating current is represented graphically by a sinusoidal electric waveform.

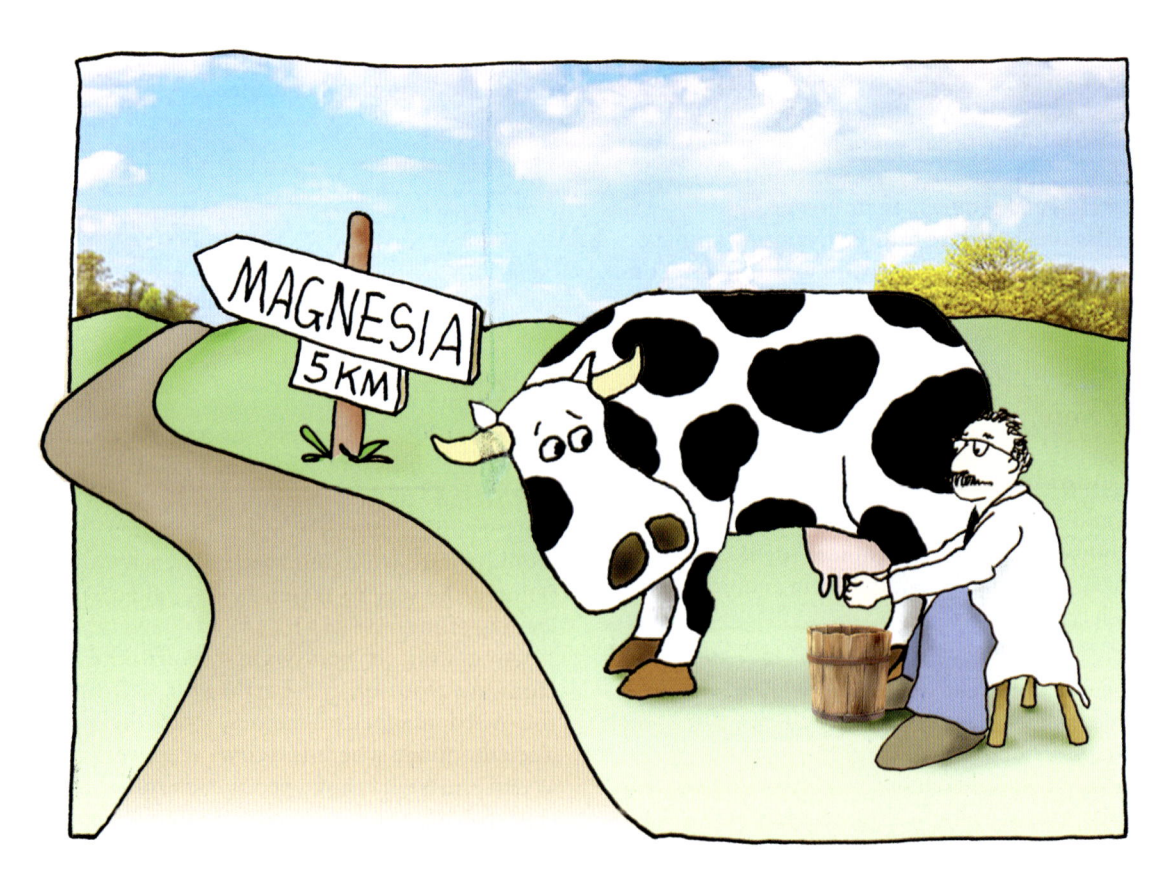

FIG. 5.13 Ancient cows of Magnesia, Turkey, produced milk of magnesia when milked.

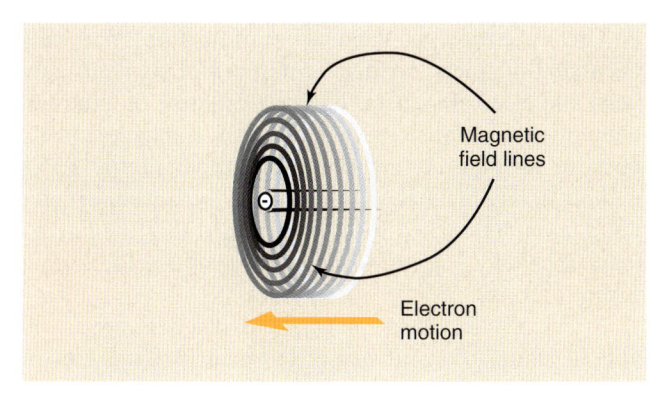

FIG. 5.14 A moving charged particle induces a magnetic field in a plane perpendicular to its motion.

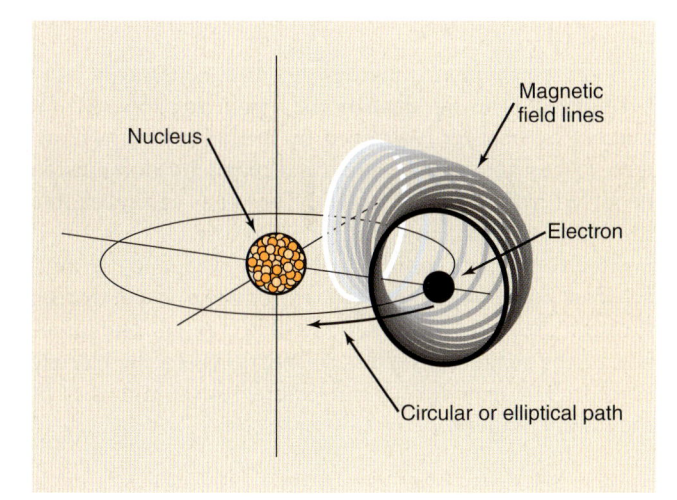

FIG. 5.15 When a charged particle moves in a circular or elliptical path, the perpendicular magnetic field moves with the charged particle.

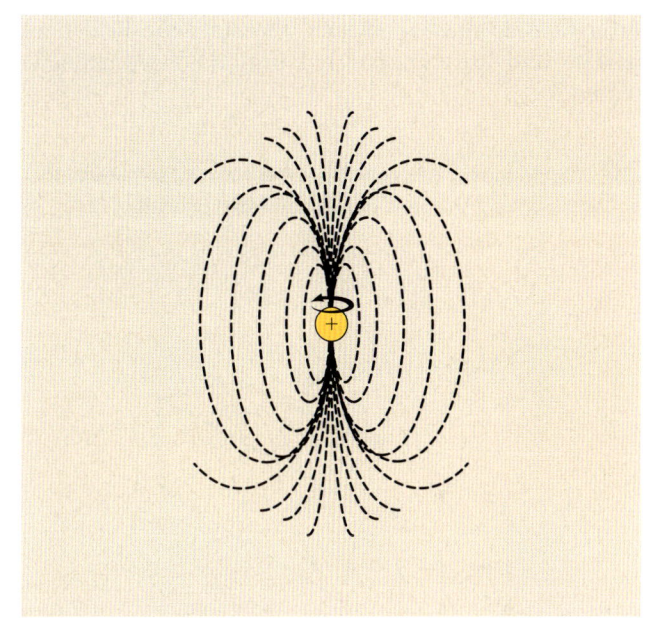

FIG. 5.16 A spinning charged particle will induce a magnetic field along the axis of spin.

phenomena to be different. We know them as magnetism and electrostatics, respectively; both are manifestations of the electromagnetic force.

Magnetism is perhaps more difficult to understand than other characteristic properties of matter, such as mass, energy, and electric charge, because magnetism is difficult to detect and measure. We can feel mass, visualize energy, and be shocked by electricity, but we cannot sense magnetism.

> Any charged particle in motion creates a magnetic field.

The magnetic field of a charged particle, such as an electron in motion, is perpendicular to the motion of that particle. The intensity of the magnetic field is represented by imaginary lines (Fig. 5.14).

If the electron's motion is a closed loop, as with an electron circling a nucleus, magnetic field lines will be perpendicular to the plane of motion (Fig. 5.15).

Electrons behave as if they rotate on an axis clockwise or counterclockwise. This rotation creates a property called **electron spin**. The electron spin creates a magnetic field, which is neutralized in electron pairs. Therefore, atoms that have an odd number of electrons in any shell exhibit a very small magnetic field.

Spinning electric charges also induce a magnetic field (Fig. 5.16). The proton in a hydrogen nucleus spins on its axis and creates a nuclear magnetic dipole called a **magnetic moment**. This forms the basis of MRI.

> The imaginary lines of a magnetic field are always closed loops.

The lines of a magnetic field do not start or end as the lines of an electric field do. Such a field is called **dipolar**; it always has a north and a south pole. The small magnet created by the electron orbit is called a **magnetic dipole**.

An accumulation of many atomic magnets with their dipoles aligned creates a **magnetic domain**. If all the magnetic domains in an object are aligned, it acts like a magnet. Under normal circumstances, magnetic domains are randomly distributed (Fig. 5.17A).

When acted on by an external magnetic field, however, such as the Earth in the case of naturally occurring ores or an electromagnet in the case of artificially induced magnetism, randomly oriented dipoles align with the magnetic field (see Fig. 5.17B). This is what happens when ferromagnetic material is made into a permanent magnet.

The magnetic dipoles in a bar magnet can be thought of as generating imaginary lines of the magnetic field (Fig. 5.18). If a nonmagnetic material is brought near such a magnet, these field lines are not disturbed. However, if ferromagnetic material such as soft iron is

80 PART I Radiologic Physics

brought near the bar magnet, the magnetic field lines deviate and are concentrated into the ferromagnetic material.

> Magnetic permeability is the ability of a material to attract the lines of magnetic field intensity.

There are three principal types of magnets: naturally occurring magnets, artificially induced permanent magnets, and electromagnets. The best example of a **natural magnet** is the Earth itself. Earth has a magnetic field because it spins on an axis. Lodestones in the Earth exhibit strong magnetism presumably because they have remained undisturbed for a long time within the Earth's magnetic field. Lightning can also produce lodestones when it strikes.

Artificially produced **permanent magnets** are available in many sizes and shapes but principally as bar- or horseshoe-shaped magnets, usually made of iron. A compass is a prime example of an artificial permanent magnet. Permanent magnets are typically produced by aligning their domains in the field of an electromagnet (Fig. 5.19).

Such permanent magnets do not necessarily stay permanent. One can destroy the magnetic property of a magnet by heating it or even by hitting it with a hammer. Either act causes individual magnetic domains to be jarred from their alignment. They thus again become randomly aligned, and magnetism is lost.

Electromagnets consist of wire wrapped around an iron core. When an electric current is conducted through the wire, a magnetic field is created. The intensity of the magnetic field is proportional to the electric current. The iron core greatly increases the intensity of the magnetic field.

> All matter can be classified according to either of four interactions with an external magnetic field.

Many materials are unaffected when brought into a magnetic field. Such materials are **nonmagnetic** and include substances such as wood and glass.

Diamagnetic materials are weakly repelled by either magnetic pole. They cannot be artificially magnetized, and they are not attracted to a magnet. Examples of such diamagnetic materials are water and plastic.

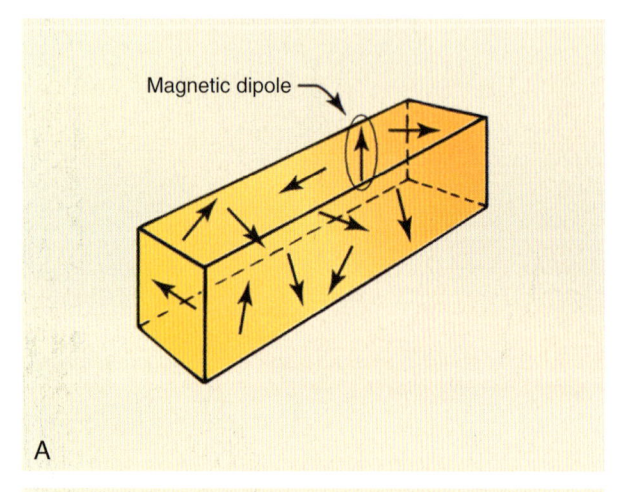

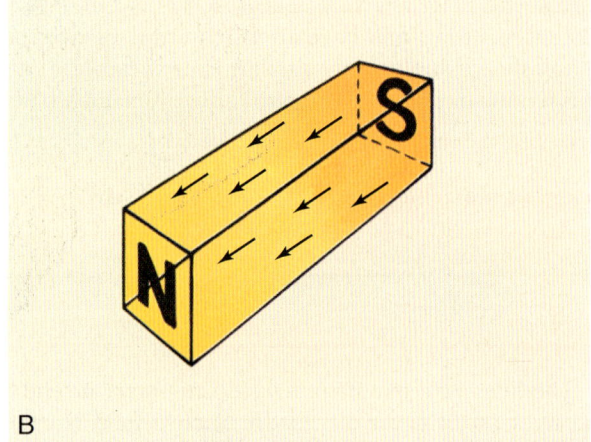

FIG. 5.17 (A) In ferromagnetic material, the magnetic dipoles are randomly oriented. (B) This changes when the dipoles are brought under the influence of an external magnetic field.

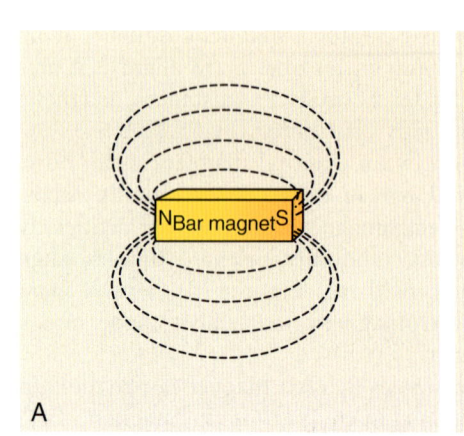

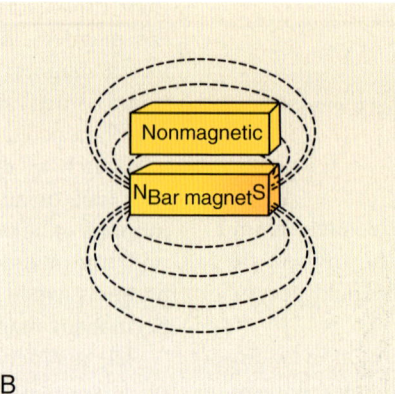

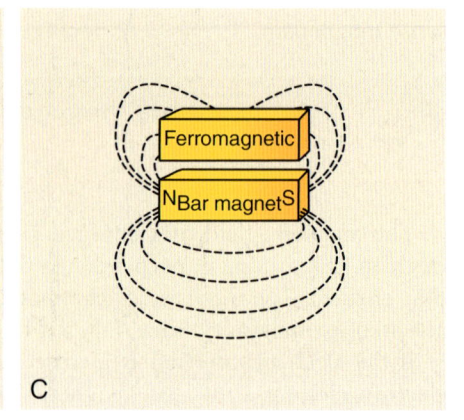

FIG. 5.18 (A) Imaginary lines of force. (B) These lines of force are undisturbed by nonmagnetic material. (C) They are deviated by ferromagnetic material.

Ferromagnetic materials include iron, cobalt, and nickel. These are strongly attracted by a magnet and usually can be permanently magnetized by exposure to a magnetic field. An alloy of aluminum, nickel, and cobalt called **alnico** is one of the more useful magnets produced from ferromagnetic material. Rare earth ceramics have been developed recently and are considerably stronger magnets (Fig. 5.20).

Paramagnetic materials lie somewhere between ferromagnetic and nonmagnetic. They are very slightly attracted to a magnet and are loosely influenced by an external magnetic field. Contrast agents used in MRIs are paramagnetic.

> The degree to which a material can be magnetized is its magnetic susceptibility.

When wood is placed in a strong magnetic field, it does not increase the strength of the field: Wood has low magnetic susceptibility. On the other hand, when iron is placed in a magnetic field, it greatly increases the strength of the field: Iron has high magnetic susceptibility.

This phenomenon is used in transformers when the core of the transformer greatly enhances its efficiency. These four magnetic states of matter are summarized in Table 5.3.

Magnetic Laws

The physical laws of magnetism are similar to those of electrostatics and gravity. The forces associated with these three fields are fundamental.

The equations of force and the fields through which they act have the same form. Much work in theoretical physics involves the attempt to combine these fundamental forces with two others—the strong nuclear force and the weak interaction—to formulate a grand unified field theory.

In contrast to the case with electricity, there is no smallest unit of magnetism. Dividing a magnet simply creates two smaller magnets, which when divided again and again make baby magnets (Fig. 5.21).

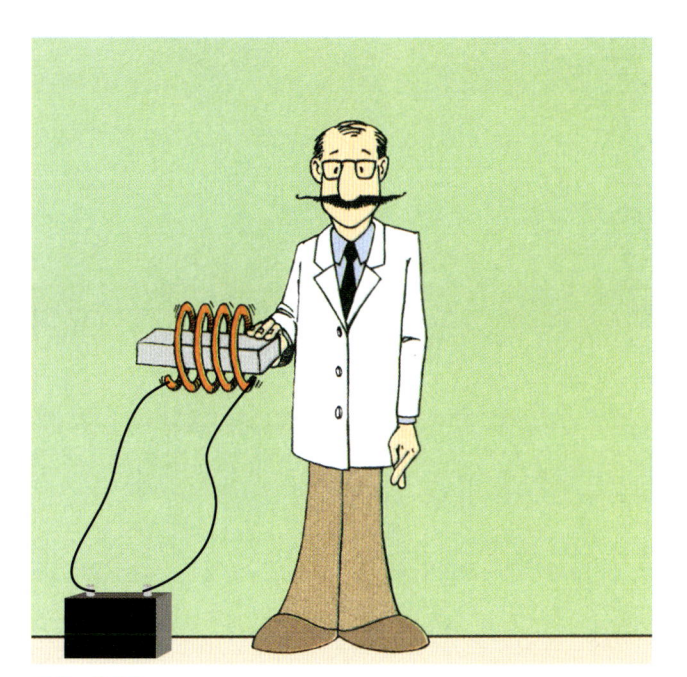

FIG. 5.19 A method for using an electromagnet to render ceramic bricks magnetic.

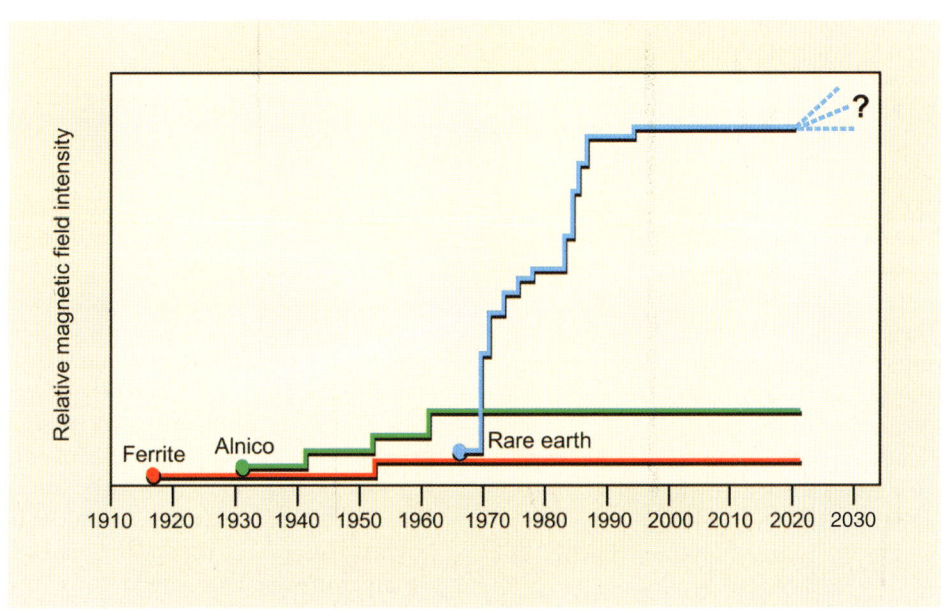

FIG. 5.20 Developments in permanent magnet design have resulted in a great increase in magnetic field intensity.

TABLE 5.3 Four Magnetic States of Matter

State	Material	Characteristics
Nonmagnetic	Wood, glass	Unaffected by a magnetic field
Diamagnetic	Water, plastic	Weakly repelled from both poles of a magnetic field
Paramagnetic	Gadolinium	Weakly attracted to both poles of a magnetic field
Ferromagnetic	Iron, nickel, cobalt	Can be strongly magnetized

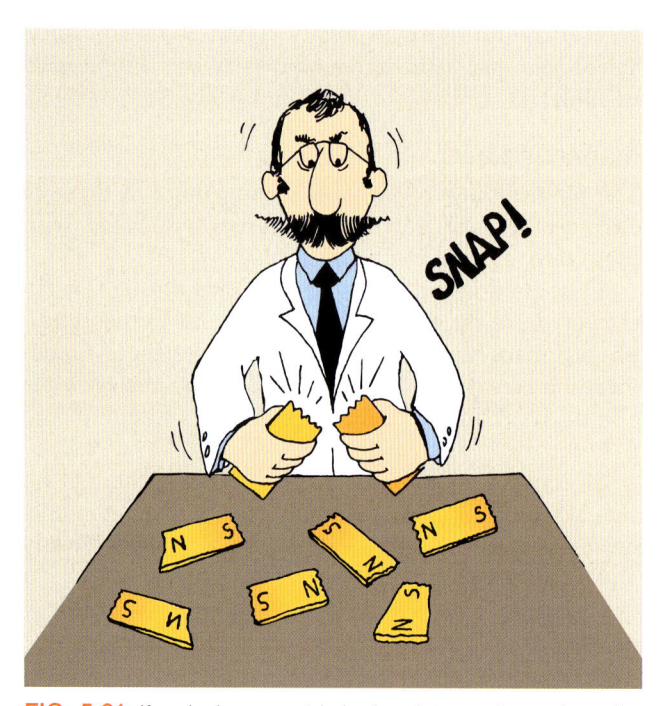

FIG. 5.21 If a single magnet is broken into smaller and smaller pieces, baby magnets result.

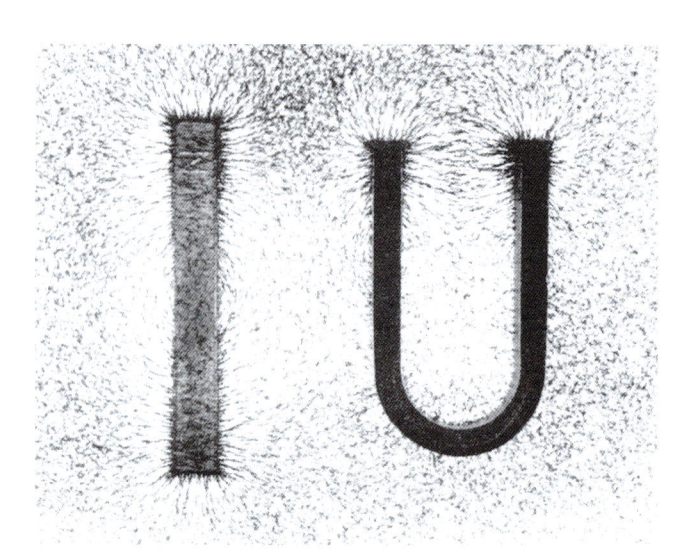

FIG. 5.22 Demonstration of magnetic lines of force with iron filings.

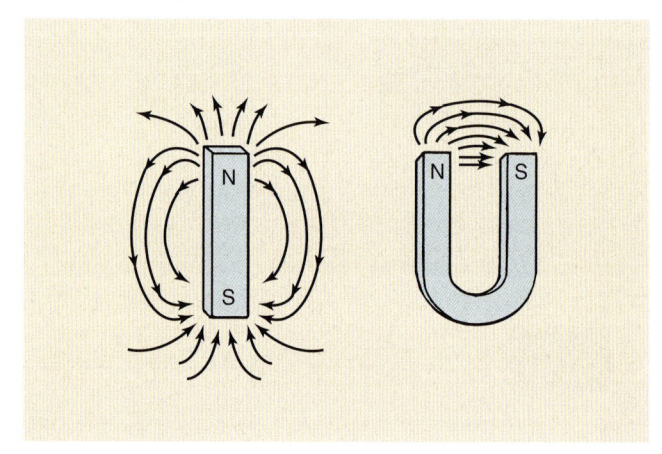

FIG. 5.23 The imaginary lines of the magnetic field leave the north pole and enter the south pole.

How do we know that these imaginary lines of the magnetic field exist? They can be demonstrated by the action of iron filings near a magnet (Fig. 5.22).

If a magnet is placed on a surface with small iron filings, the filings attach most strongly and with greater concentration to the ends of the magnet. These ends are called **magnetic poles**, and every magnet has two magnetic poles, a north pole and a south pole, analogous to positive and negative electrostatic charges.

As with electric charges, like magnetic poles repel, and unlike magnetic poles attract. Also by convention, the imaginary lines of the magnetic field leave the north pole of a magnet and return to the south pole (Fig. 5.23).

Magnetic Induction

Just as an electrostatic charge can be induced from one material to another, so too some materials can be made magnetic by **induction**. The imaginary magnetic field lines just described are called *magnetic lines of induction*, and the density of these lines is proportional to the intensity of the magnetic field.

> Ferromagnetic objects can be made into magnets by induction.

When ferromagnetic material, such as a piece of soft iron, is brought into the vicinity of an intense magnetic field, the lines of induction are altered by attraction to the soft iron and the iron is made temporarily magnetic (Fig. 5.24). If copper, a diamagnetic material, were to replace the soft iron, there would be no such effect.

This principle is used with many MRI systems that use an iron magnetic shield to reduce the level of the fringe magnetic field. Ferromagnetic material acts as a magnetic sink by drawing the lines of the fringe magnetic field into it.

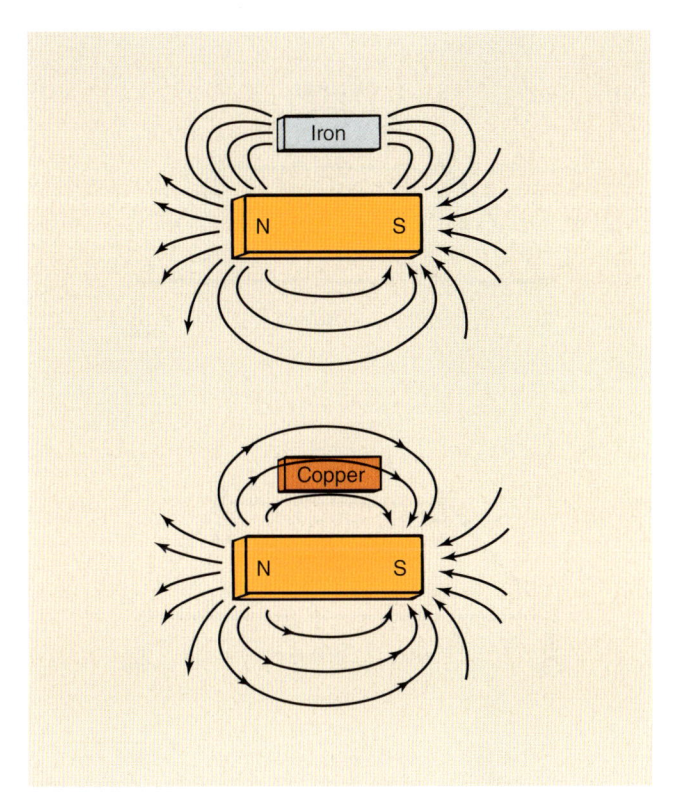

FIG. 5.24 Ferromagnetic material such as iron attracts magnetic lines of induction, whereas nonmagnetic material such as copper does not.

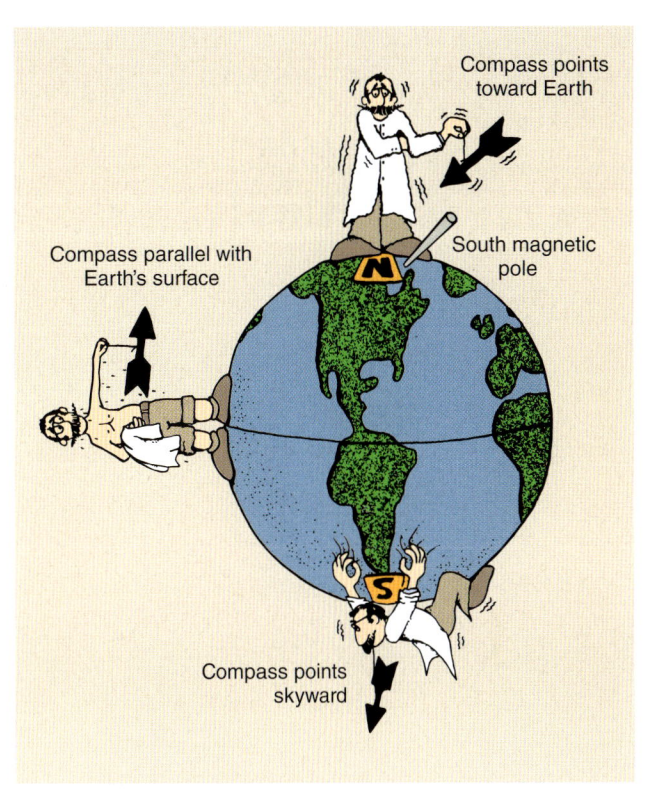

FIG. 5.25 A compass reacts with the Earth as though it were a bar magnet seeking the North Pole.

When ferromagnetic material is removed from the magnetic field, it usually does not retain its strong magnetic property. Soft iron, therefore, makes an excellent temporary magnet. It is a magnet only while its magnetism is being induced. If properly tempered by heat or exposed to an external field for a long period, however, some ferromagnetic materials retain their magnetism when removed from the external magnetic field and become permanent magnets.

The electric and magnetic forces were joined by Maxwell's field theory of electromagnetic radiation. The force created by a magnetic field and the force of the electric field behave similarly. This magnetic force is similar to electrostatic and gravitational forces that are also inversely proportional to the square of the distance between the objects under consideration. If the distance between two bar magnets is halved, the magnetic force increases by four times.

> The magnetic force is proportional to the product of the magnetic pole strengths divided by the square of the distance between them.

The Earth behaves as though it has a large bar magnet embedded in it. The polar convention of magnetism actually has its origin in the compass. At the equator, the north pole of a compass seeks the Earth's North Pole.

As one travels toward the North Pole, the attraction of the compass becomes more intense until the compass needle points directly into the Earth, not at the geographic North Pole but at a region in northern Canada—the magnetic pole (Fig. 5.25). The magnetic pole in the Southern Hemisphere is in Antarctica. There, the north end of the compass would point toward the sky.

> The SI unit of magnetic field strength is the tesla. An older unit is the gauss. One Tesla (T) = 10,000 gauss (G).

The use of a compass might suggest that the Earth has a strong magnetic field, but it does not. The Earth's magnetic field is approximately 50 µT at the equator and 100 µT at the poles. This is far less than the magnet on a cabinet door latch, which is approximately 100 mT, or the magnet of an MRI system, which is 3 T.

ELECTROMAGNETISM

Until the 19th century, electricity and magnetism were viewed as separate effects. Although many scientists suspected that the two were connected, research was hampered by the lack of any convenient way of producing and controlling electricity.

Thus the early study of electricity was limited to the investigation of static electricity, which could be

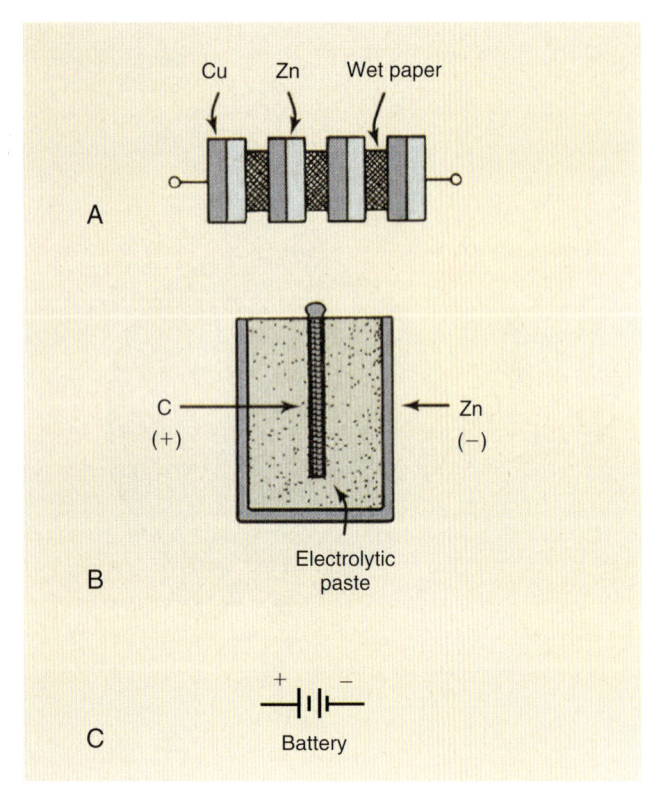

FIG. 5.26 (A) Original Voltaic pile. (B) A modern dry cell. (C) Symbol for a battery.

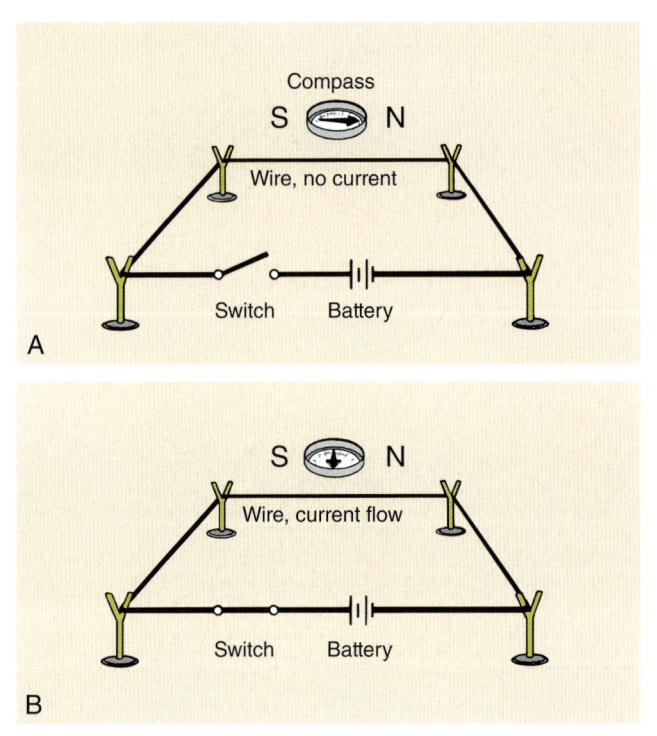

FIG. 5.27 Oersted's experiment. (A) With no electric current in the wire, the compass points north. (B) With electric current, the compass points toward the wire.

produced by friction (e.g., the effect produced by rubbing fur on a rubber rod). Charges could be induced to move but only in a sudden discharge, as with a spark jumping a gap.

The development of methods for producing a steady flow of charges (i.e., an electric current) during the 19th century stimulated investigations of both electricity and magnetism. These investigations led to an enhanced understanding of electromagnetic phenomena and ultimately led to the electronic revolution on which today's technology is largely based.

In the late 1700s, an Italian anatomist, Luigi Galvani, made an accidental discovery. He observed that a dissected frog leg twitched when touched by two different metals, just as if it had been touched by an electrostatic charge. This prompted Alessandro Volta, an Italian physicist of the same era, to question whether an electric current might be produced when two different metals are brought into contact.

Using zinc and copper plates, Volta succeeded in producing a feeble electric current. To increase the current, he stacked the copper-zinc plates like a Dagwood sandwich to form what was called the **Voltaic pile**, a precursor of the modern battery. Each zinc-copper sandwich is called a **cell** of the battery.

Modern dry cells use a carbon rod as the positive electrode, surrounded by an electrolytic paste housed in a negative zinc cylindrical can. Fig. 5.26 shows the Voltaic pile, the modern battery, and the symbol for a battery.

These devices are examples of sources of electric potential. Any device that converts some form of energy directly into electric energy is said to be a source of electric potential.

> Electric potential is measured in units of joule per coulomb, or volt.

Now that they finally had a source of constant electric current, scientists began extensive investigations into the possibility of a link between electric and magnetic forces. Hans Oersted, a Danish physicist, discovered the first such link in 1820.

Oersted fashioned a long, straight wire, supported near a free-rotating magnetic compass (Fig. 5.27). With no current in the wire, the magnetic compass pointed north as expected. When a current was passed through the wire, however, the compass needle swung to point straight at the wire. Here we have evidence of a direct link between electric and magnetic phenomena. The electric current evidently produced a magnetic field strong enough to overpower the Earth's magnetic field and cause the magnetic compass to point toward the wire.

CHAPTER 5   Electricity, Magnetism, and Electromagnetism   85

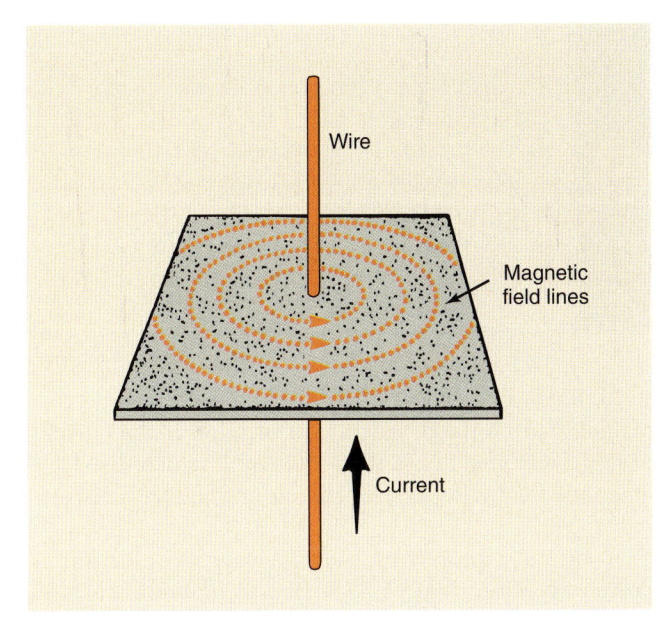

FIG. 5.28 Magnetic field lines form concentric circles around the current-carrying wire.

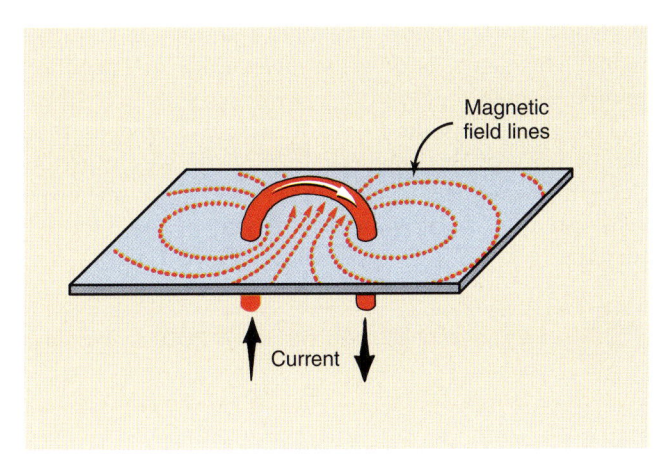

FIG. 5.29 Magnetic field lines are concentrated on the inside of the loop.

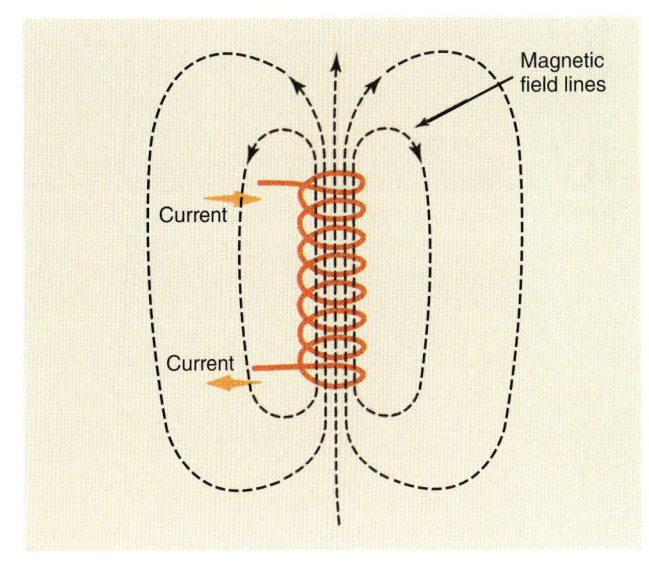

FIG. 5.30 Magnetic field lines of a solenoid.

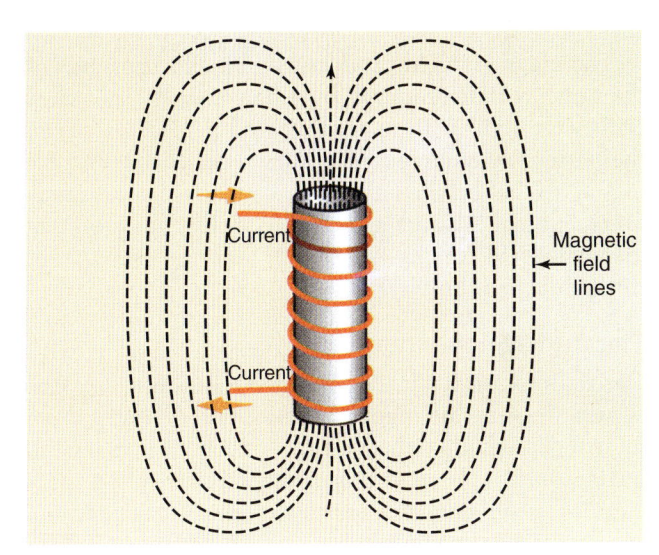

FIG. 5.31 Magnetic field lines of an electromagnet.

> Any charge in motion induces a magnetic field.

A charge at rest produces no magnetic field. Electrons that flow through a wire produce a magnetic field about that wire. The magnetic field is represented by imaginary lines that form concentric circles centered on the wire (Fig. 5.28).

Magnetic field lines form concentric circles around each tiny section of a loop of the wire. Because the wire is curved, however, these magnetic field lines overlap inside the loop. In particular, at the very center of the loop, all of the field lines come together, making the magnetic field strong (Fig. 5.29).

Stacking more loops on top of each other increases the intensity of the magnetic field running through the center or axis of the stack of loops. The magnetic field of a solenoid is concentrated through the center of the coil (Fig. 5.30).

> A coil of wire is called a *solenoid*.

The magnetic field can be intensified further by wrapping the coil of wire around ferromagnetic material, such as iron. The iron core intensifies the magnetic field. In this case, almost all of the magnetic field lines are concentrated inside the iron core, escaping only near the ends of the coil. This type of device is called an **electromagnet** (Fig. 5.31).

> An electromagnet is a current-carrying coil of wire wrapped around an iron core.

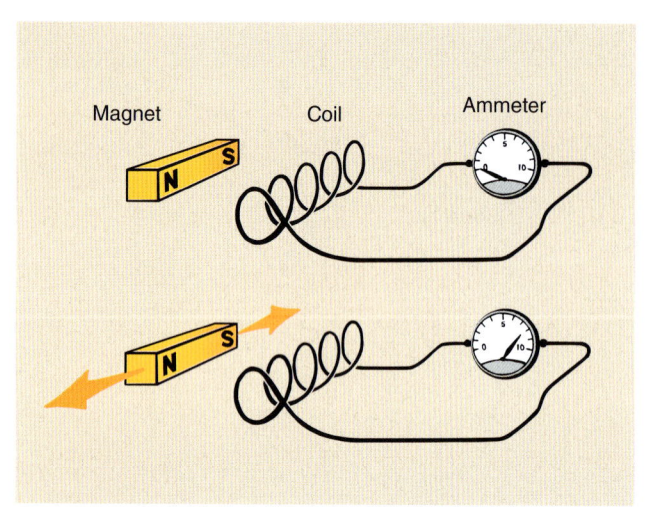

FIG. 5.32 Schematic description of Faraday's experiment shows how a moving magnetic field induces an electric current.

> **FARADAY'S LAW**
> The magnitude of the induced electric current depends on four factors:
> 1. The strength of the magnetic field
> 2. The velocity of the magnetic field as it moves past the conductor
> 3. The angle of the conductor to the magnetic field
> 4. The number of turns in the conductor

The magnetic field produced by an electromagnet is the same as that produced by a bar magnet. That is, if both were hidden from view behind a piece of paper, the pattern of magnetic field lines revealed by iron filings sprinkled on the paper surface would be the same. Of course, the advantage of the electromagnet is that its magnetic field can be adjusted by varying the current through its coil of wire.

Electromagnetic Induction

Oersted's experiment demonstrated that electricity can be used to generate magnetic fields. It is obvious, then, to wonder whether the reverse is true: Can magnetic fields somehow be used to generate electricity? Michael Faraday, a self-educated British experimenter, found the answer to that question.

From a series of experiments, Faraday concluded that an electric current cannot be induced in a circuit merely by the presence of a magnetic field. For example, consider the situation illustrated in Fig. 5.32. A coil of wire is connected to a current-measuring device called an **ammeter**. If a bar magnet were set next to the coil, the meter would indicate no current in the coil.

However, Faraday discovered that when the magnet is moved, the coil wire does have a current, as indicated by the ammeter. Therefore to induce a current with the use of a magnetic field, the magnetic field cannot be constant but must be changing.

> Electromagnetic induction: An electric current is induced in an electric circuit if some part of that circuit is in a changing magnetic field.

This observation is summarized in what is called **Faraday's law**.

Actually, no physical motion is needed. An electromagnet can be fixed near a coil of wire. If the current in the electromagnet is then increased or decreased, its magnetic field will likewise change and induce a current in the coil.

A prime example of electromagnetic induction is radio reception (Fig. 5.33). Radio emission consists of waves of electromagnetic radiation. Each wave has an oscillating electric field and an oscillating magnetic field. The oscillating magnetic field induces motion in electrons in the radio antennae, resulting in a radio signal. This signal is detected and decoded to produce sound.

The essential point in all of these examples is that the intensity of the magnetic field at the wire must be changing to induce an electric current. If the magnetic field intensity is constant, there will be no induced current.

> Varying magnetic field intensity induces an electric current.

Electromechanical Devices

Electric motors and electric generators are practical applications of Oersted's and Faraday's experiments. In one experiment, an electric current produces a mechanical motion (the motion of the compass needle). This is the basis of the electric motor.

In the other experiment, mechanical motion (the motion of a magnet near a coil of wire) induces electricity in a coil of wire. This is the principle on which the electric generator operates.

In an electric generator, a coil of wire is placed in a strong magnetic field between two magnetic poles. The coil is rotated by mechanical energy. The mechanical energy can be supplied by hand, by water flowing over a water wheel, or by steam flowing past the vanes of a turbine blade in a nuclear power plant. Because the coil of wire is moving in the magnetic field, a current is induced in the coil of wire.

The net effect of an electric generator is to convert mechanical energy into electrical energy. The conversion process is, of course, not 100% efficient because

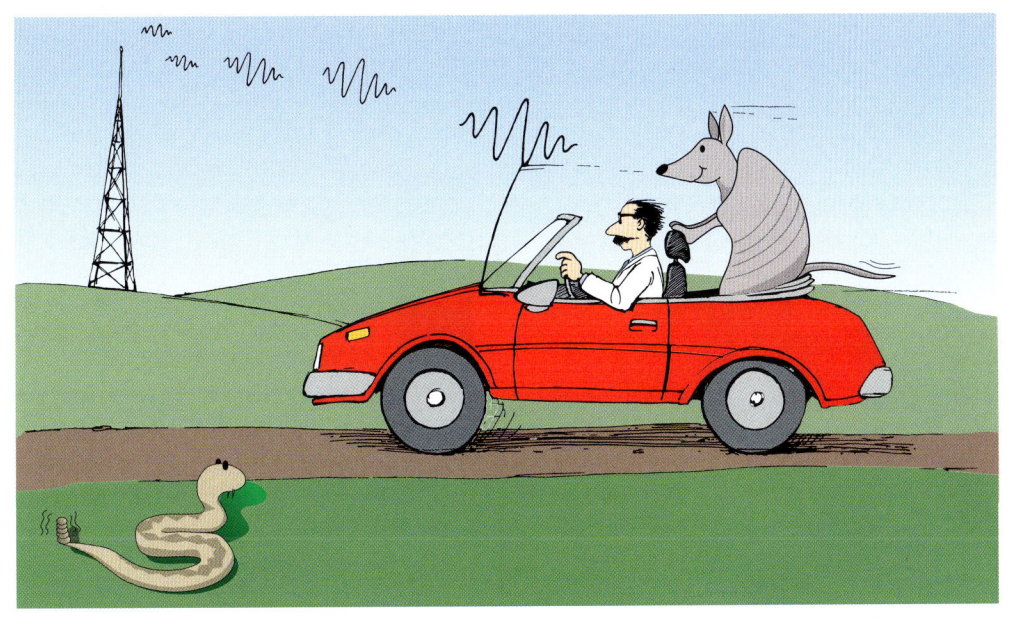

FIG. 5.33 Radio reception is based on the principles of electromagnetic induction.

of frictional losses in the mechanical moving parts and heat losses caused by resistance in the electrical components.

An electric motor has basically the same components as an electric generator. In this case, however, electric energy is supplied to the current loop to produce a mechanical motion—that is, a rotation of the loop in the magnetic field.

A practical electric motor uses many turns of wire for the current loop and many bar magnets to create the external magnetic field. The principle of operation, however is the same.

The type of motor used with x-ray tubes is an induction motor (Fig. 5.34). In this type of motor, the rotating rotor is a shaft made of bars of copper and soft iron fabricated into one mass; however, the external magnetic field is supplied by several fixed electromagnets called **stators**.

> An induction motor powers the rotating anode of an x-ray tube.

No electric current is passed to the rotor. Instead, current is produced in the rotor windings by induction. The electromagnets surrounding the rotor are energized in sequence, producing a changing magnetic field. The induced current produced in the rotor windings generates a magnetic field.

Just as in a conventional electric motor, this magnetic field attempts to align itself with the magnetic field of the external electromagnets. Because these electromagnets are being energized in sequence, the rotor begins to rotate, trying to bring its magnetic field into alignment.

The result is the same as in a conventional electric motor; that is, the rotor rotates continuously. The difference, however, is that the electrical energy is supplied to the external magnets rather than the rotor.

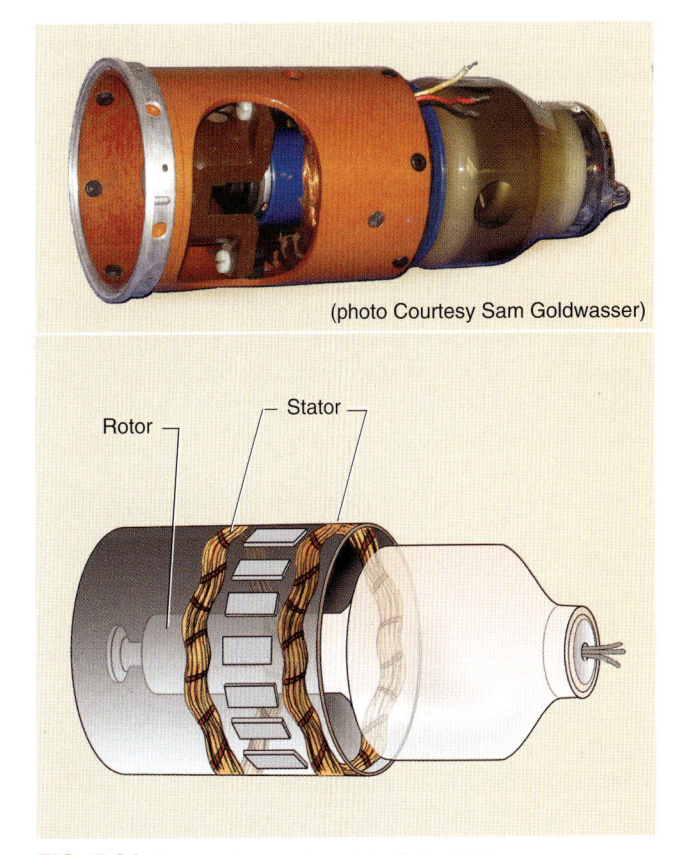

(photo Courtesy Sam Goldwasser)

FIG. 5.34 Principal parts of an induction motor.

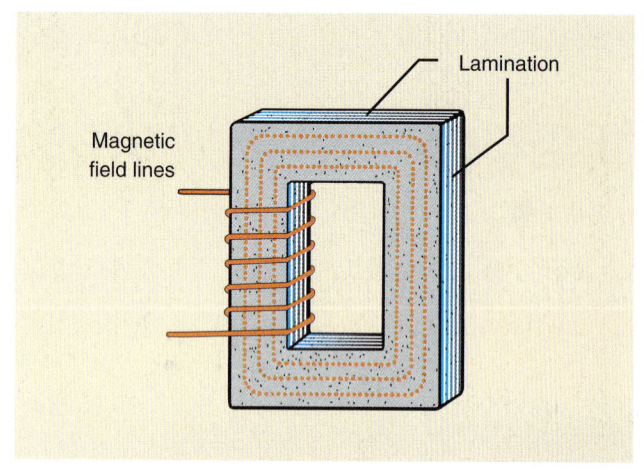

FIG. 5.35 An electromagnet that incorporates a closed iron core produces a closed magnetic field that is primarily confined to the core.

The Transformer

Another device that uses the interacting magnetic fields produced by changing electric currents is the **transformer**. However, the transformer does not convert one form of energy to another but rather transforms electric potential and electric current into higher or lower intensity.

> A transformer changes the intensity of alternating voltage and current.

Consider an electromagnet with a ferromagnetic core bent around so that it forms a continuous loop (Fig. 5.35). There are no end surfaces from which ferromagnetic field lines can escape. Therefore the magnetic field tends to be confined to the loop of the magnetic core material.

If a secondary coil is then wound around the other side of this loop of core material, almost all of the magnetic field produced by the primary coil also passes through the center of the secondary coil. Thus there is a good coupling between the magnetic field produced by the primary coil and the secondary coil. A changing electric current in the primary coil induces a changing current in the secondary coil. This type of device is a transformer.

A transformer will operate only with a changing electric current (AC). A direct current (DC) applied to the primary coil will induce no current in the secondary coil.

The transformer is used to change the magnitude of voltage and current in an AC circuit. The change in voltage is directly proportional to the ratio of the number of turns (windings) of the secondary coil (N_s) to the number of turns in the primary coil (N_p). If there are 10 turns on the secondary coil for every turn on the primary coil, then the voltage generated in the secondary circuit (V_s) will be 10 times the voltage supplied to the primary circuit (V_p). Mathematically, the transformer law is represented as follows:

> **TRANSFORMER LAW**
>
> $$\frac{V_s}{V_p} = \frac{N_s}{N_p}$$
>
> The quantity N_s/N_p is known as the **turns ratio** of the transformer.

Question: The secondary side of a transformer has 300,000 turns; the primary side has 600 turns. What is the turns ratio?

Answer: $N_s = 300,000$
$N_p = 600$
Turns ratio = 300,000/600
= 500 : 1

The voltage change across the transformer is proportional to the turns ratio. A transformer with a turns ratio greater than 1 is a **step-up transformer** because the voltage is increased or stepped up from the primary side to the secondary side. When the turns ratio is less than 1, the transformer is a **step-down transformer**.

As the voltage changes across a transformer, the electric current changes also; the transformer law may also be written as follows.

> **EFFECT OF TRANSFORMER LAW ON CURRENT**
>
> $$\frac{I_s}{I_p} = \frac{N_p}{N_s}$$
>
> or
>
> $$\frac{I_s}{I_p} = \frac{V_p}{V_s}$$

Question: The turns ratio of a filament transformer is 0.125. What is the filament current if the current through the primary winding is 0.8 A?

Answer:
$$\frac{I_s}{I_p} = \frac{N_p}{N_s}$$

$$I_s = I_p \left(\frac{N_p}{N_s}\right)$$

$$= (0.8 \text{ A})\left(\frac{1}{0.125}\right)$$

$$= 6.4 \text{ A}$$

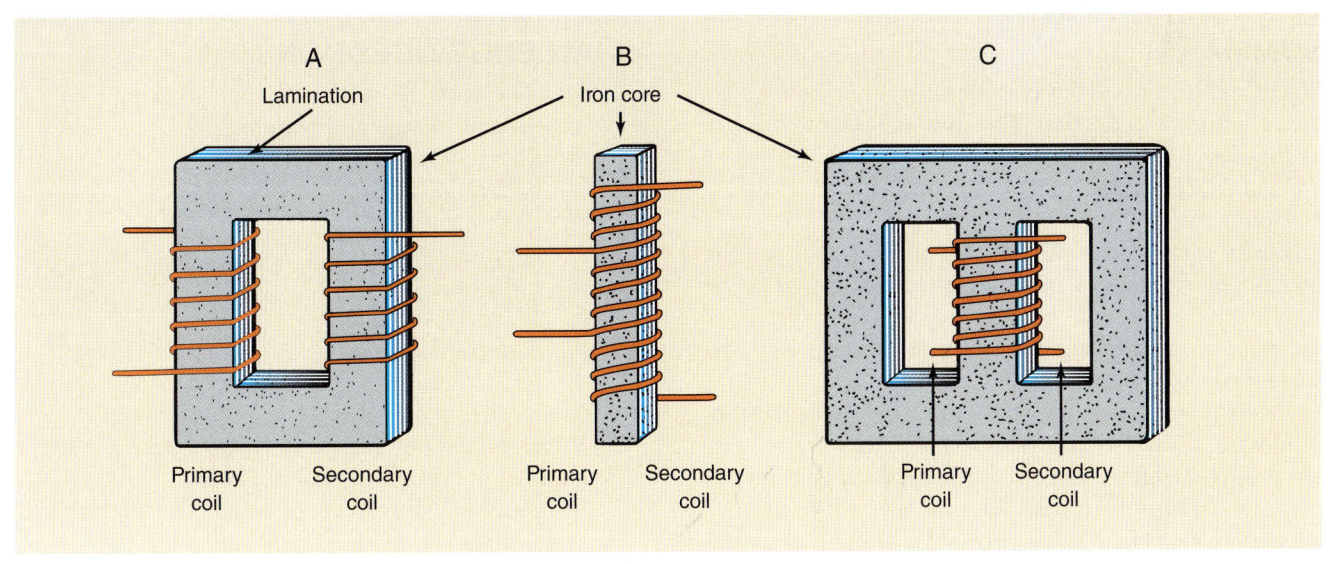

FIG. 5.36 Type of transformers. (A) Closed-core transformer. (B) Autotransformer. (C) Shell-type transformer.

The change in electric current across a transformer is in the opposite direction from the voltage change but in the same proportion: an inverse relationship. For example, if the voltage is doubled, the current is halved.

In a step-up transformer, the current on the secondary side (I_s) is smaller than the current on the primary side (I_p). In a step-down transformer, the secondary current is larger than the primary current.

Question: There are 125 turns on the primary side of a transformer and 90,000 turns on the secondary side. If 110 V AC is supplied to the primary winding, what is the voltage induced in the secondary winding?

Answer:
$$\frac{V_s}{V_p} = \frac{N_s}{N_p}$$
$$V_s = V_p \left[\frac{N_s}{N_p}\right]$$
$$= (110 \text{ V})\left(\frac{90,000}{125}\right)$$
$$= (110)(720) \text{ V}$$
$$= 79,200 \text{ V}$$
$$= 79.2 \text{ kV}$$

There are many ways to construct a transformer (Fig. 5.36). The type of transformer discussed thus far, built around a square core of ferromagnetic material, is called a **closed-core transformer** (see Fig. 5.36A).

The ferromagnetic core is not a single piece but rather is built out of laminated layers of iron. This layering helps reduce energy losses, resulting in greater efficiency.

Another type of transformer is the autotransformer (see Fig. 5.36B). It consists of an iron core with only one winding of wire about it. This single winding acts as both the primary and the secondary windings. Connections are made at different points on the coil for both the primary and the secondary sides.

> The autotransformer has one winding and varies both voltage and current.

An autotransformer is generally smaller, and because the primary and the secondary sides are connected to the same wire, its use is generally restricted to cases in which only a small step up or step down in voltage is required. Thus an autotransformer would not be suitable for use as the high-voltage transformer in an x-ray imaging system.

The third type of transformer is the **shell-type transformer** (see Fig. 5.36C). This type of transformer confines even more of the magnet field lines of the primary winding because the secondary is wrapped around it and there are essentially two closed cores. This type is more efficient than the closed-core transformer. Most currently used transformers are shell type.

The practical applications of the laws of electromagnetism appear in the electric motor (electric current produces mechanical motion), the electric generator (mechanical motion produces electric current), and the transformer (alternating electric current and electric potential are transformed in intensity). The transformer law describes how electric current and voltage change from the primary coil to the secondary coil.

SUMMARY

Electrons can flow from one object to another by contact, friction, or induction. The laws of electrostatics are as follows:
- Like charges repel.
- Unlike charges attract.

Electrostatic force is directly proportional to the product of the charges and inversely proportional to the square of the distance between them. Electric charges are concentrated along the sharpest curvature of the surface of the conductor.

Electrodynamics is the study of electrons in motion, otherwise known as electricity. Conductors are materials through which electrons flow easily. Insulators are materials that inhibit the flow of electrons. Electric current is measured in amperes (A), electric potential is measured in volts (V), and electric resistance is measured in ohms (Ω).

Electric power is energy produced or consumed per unit time. One watt of power is equal to 1 A of electricity flowing through an electric potential of 1 V.

Matter has magnetic properties because some atoms have an odd number of electrons in the outer shells. The unpaired spin of these electrons produces a net magnetic field within the atom. Natural magnets get their magnetism from the Earth, permanent magnets are artificially induced magnets, and electromagnets are produced when current-carrying wire is wrapped around an iron core.

Every magnet, no matter how small, has two poles: north and south. Like magnetic poles repel, and unlike magnetic poles attract. Ferromagnetic material can be made magnetic when placed in an external magnetic field. The force between poles is proportional to the product of the magnetic pole strengths divided by the square of the distance between them.

Alessandro Volta's development of the battery as a source of electric potential energy prompted additional investigations of electric and magnetic fields. Hans Oersted demonstrated that electricity can be used to generate magnetic fields. Michael Faraday observed the current produced in the presence of a changing magnetic field.

Practical applications of the laws of electromagnetism appear in the electric motor (electric current produces mechanical motion), the electric generator (mechanical motion produces electric current), and the transformer (alternating electric current and electric potential are transformed in intensity). The transformer law describes how electric current and voltage change from the primary coil to the secondary coil.

CHALLENGE QUESTIONS

1. Define or otherwise identify the following:
   a. Electric charge and its unit
   b. Electrodynamics
   c. Electric power
   d. Electrostatics
   e. Dipole
   f. Induction
   g. Magnetic domain
   h. Autotransformer
   i. Gauss; Tesla
   j. Electric potential
2. What is the difference between a conductor, a semiconductor, and a superconductor?
3. Diagram the difference between an electric field and a magnetic field.
4. A radiographic exposure requires 100 mAs. How many electrons is this?
5. Describe three types of transformers.
6. What are the three ways to electrify an object?
7. List the four laws of electrostatics.
8. Why is electrification easier in dry Phoenix than in humid Houston?
9. A mobile x-ray imaging system operates on 110 V AC power. Its maximum capacity is 110 kVp and 100 mA. What is the turns ratio of the high-voltage transformer?
10. What should be the primary current in the previous question to produce a secondary current of 100 mA?
11. Magnetic fields in excess of 5 G can interfere with cardiac pacemakers. How many mT is this?
12. What is the role of magnetism in the study of x-ray imaging?
13. List the three principal types of magnets.
14. Describe an electromagnet.
15. Explain how a magnetic domain can cause an object to behave like a magnet.
16. State Ohm's law and describe its effect on electric circuits.
17. What happens when a bar magnet is heated to a very high temperature?
18. List three diamagnetic materials.
19. Where in everyday life might one find an electromagnet?
20. What is the range in intensity of the Earth's magnetic field?

The answers to the Challenge Questions can be found by logging on to our website at http://evolve.elsevier.com.

PART II

X-RADIATION

CHAPTER 6

The X-ray Imaging System

OBJECTIVES

At the completion of this chapter, the student should be able to do the following:

1. Identify the components of the x-ray imaging system operating console.
2. Explain the operation of the high-voltage generator.
3. Relate the differences among single-phase, three-phase, and high-frequency power.
4. Discuss the importance of voltage ripple to x-ray intensity and quality.
5. Define the power rating of an x-ray imaging system.

OUTLINE

Operating Console 94
Autotransformer 95
   Adjustment of Kilovolt Peak 96
   Control of Milliamperage 97
   Filament Transformer 98
Exposure Timers 98
   Synchronous Timers 99
   Electronic Timers 99
   Milliampere-Second Timers 99
   Automatic Exposure Control 99
High-Voltage Generator 100
   High-Voltage Transformer 100
Voltage Rectification 101
Single-Phase Power 104
Three-Phase Power 104
High-Frequency Generator 105
Capacitor Discharge
   Generator 106
Falling Load Generator 106
Voltage Ripple 106
Power Rating 108
X-ray Circuit 109
Summary 109
Challenge Questions 109

CHAPTER 6 The X-ray Imaging System

WHEN FAST-MOVING electrons slam into a metal object, x-rays are produced. The kinetic energy of the electrons is transformed into electromagnetic energy. The function of the x-ray imaging system is to provide a controlled flow of electrons intense enough to produce an x-ray beam appropriate for imaging.

The three main components of an x-ray imaging system are (1) the operating console, (2) the x-ray tube, and (3) the high-voltage generator. The x-ray tube is discussed in Chapter 7. This chapter describes the components of the operating console that are used to control the voltage applied to the x-ray tube, the current through the x-ray tube, and the exposure time.

This chapter also discusses the high-voltage generator in its many forms. The high-voltage generator contains the high-voltage step-up transformer and the rectification circuit. The final section of this chapter combines all components into a single complete circuit diagram.

The many different types of x-ray imaging systems are usually identified according to the energy of the x-rays they produce or the purpose for which the x-rays are intended. Diagnostic x-ray imaging systems come in many different shapes and sizes, two of which are shown in Fig. 6.1. These systems are usually operated at voltages of 25 to 150 kVp and at tube currents of 100 to 1200 mA.

The general purpose x-ray examination room contains a radiographic imaging system and a fluoroscopic imaging system. The fluoroscopic x-ray tube is usually located under the examination table; the radiographic x-ray tube is attached to an overhead movable crane assembly that permits easy positioning of the x-ray tube and aiming of the x-ray beam.

This type of equipment can be used for nearly all radiographic and fluoroscopic examinations. Rooms with a fluoroscope and two or more overhead radiographic tubes are used for special interventional procedures.

Regardless of the type of x-ray imaging system used, a patient-supporting examination couch is required. This examination couch may be flat or curved but must be uniform in thickness and as transparent to x-rays as possible. Carbon fiber couches are strong and absorb little x-radiation.

> Carbon fiber couches contribute to reduced patient radiation dose.

Most patient couches are floating—easily unlocked and moved by the radiographer—or motor driven. Table controls are table side or remote controlled (Figs. 6.2 and 6.3). Just under the couch is an opening to hold a thin tray for a cassette and Potter-Bucky grid. If the couch is used for fluoroscopy, the tray must move to the foot of the couch, and the opening must be automatically shielded for radiation protection with a Bucky slot cover. Fluoroscopic couches tilt and are identified by their degrees of tilt. For example, a table would tilt 90 degrees to the foot side and 30 degrees to the head side (Fig. 6.4).

Question: How far below horizontal will a patient's head go on a fluoroscopic couch?

Answer: 30 degrees below horizontal

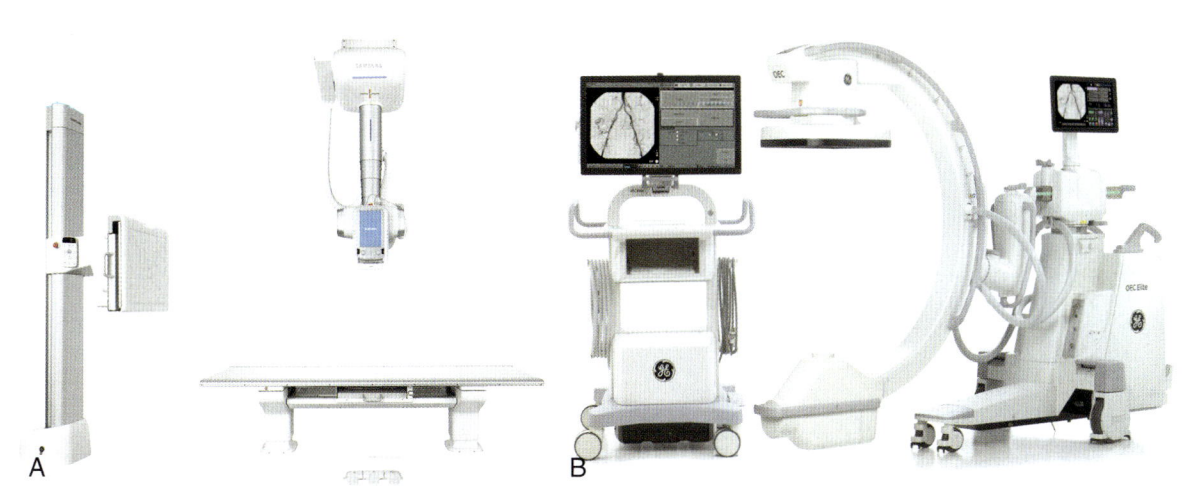

FIG. 6.1 There are several types of x-ray imaging systems. (A) Radiographic. (B) Mobile C-arm system. (A, Courtesy Samsung Healthcare; B, Courtesy GE Healthcare.)

Regardless of its design, every x-ray imaging system has three principal parts: the **x-ray tube**, the **operating console**, and the **high-voltage generator**. However, with most systems, the x-ray tube is located in the examination room, and the operating console is located in an adjoining room with a protective barrier separating the two.

> With dental and mobile x-ray imaging systems, the three components are housed very compactly.

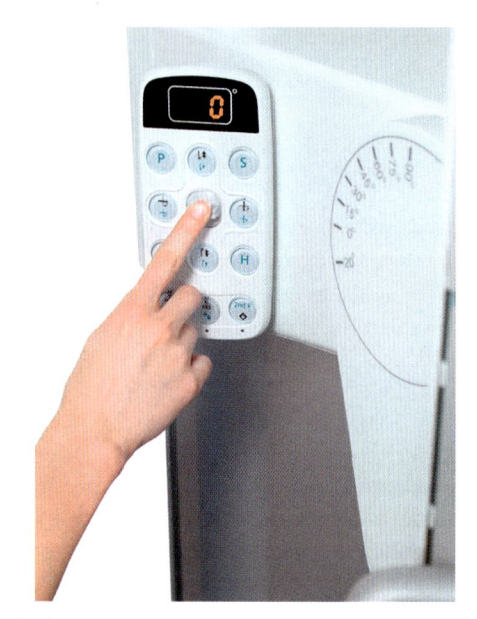

FIG. 6.2 Table side and wall stand control operates table and wall stand movements. (Courtesy Samsung Healthcare.)

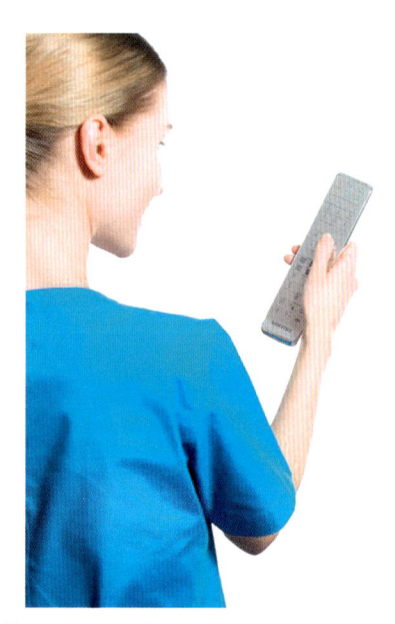

FIG. 6.3 Remote control used to operate overhead radiographic imaging system. Remote control also controls movements to automatically set table and overhead tube to preprogrammed position. (Courtesy Samsung Healthcare.)

The protective barrier must have a window for viewing the patient during the examination. Ideally, the room should be designed so that it is possible to reach the operating console without having to enter the examination room.

The high-voltage generator is always close to the x-ray tube, usually in the examination room. A few installations take advantage of false ceilings and place these generators out of sight above the examination room.

Newer generator designs that use high-frequency circuits require even less space. (Fig. 6.5) is a plan drawing of a conventional, general-purpose x-ray examination room.

OPERATING CONSOLE

The part of the x-ray imaging system most familiar to radiographers is the operating console. The operating console allows radiographers to control the x-ray tube current and voltage so that the useful x-ray beam is of proper intensity and quality.

> X-ray intensity describes quantity; x-ray penetrability describes quality.

Radiation intensity refers to the number of x-rays in an x-ray beam. Radiation intensity is usually expressed in milligray (mGy_a) or milligray/milliampere-second (mGy_a/mAs). Radiation quality refers to the energy of the x-ray beam and is expressed in kilovolt peak (kVp) or, more precisely, half-value layer (see Chapter 9).

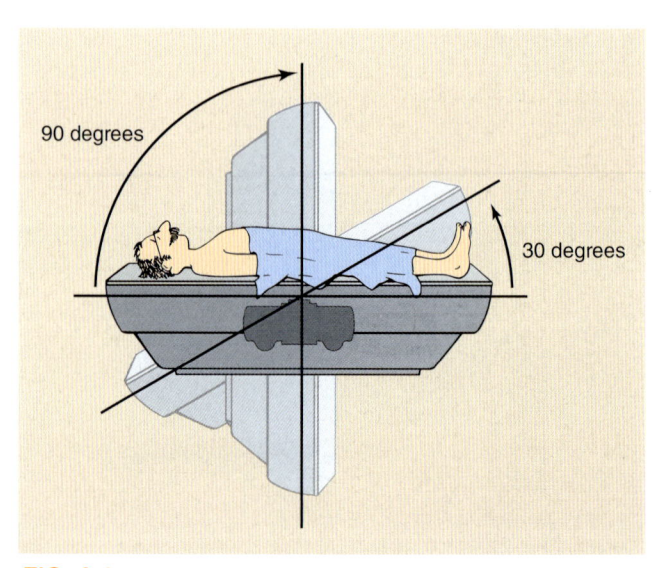

FIG. 6.4 A fluoroscopic couch is identified by its head and foot tilt.

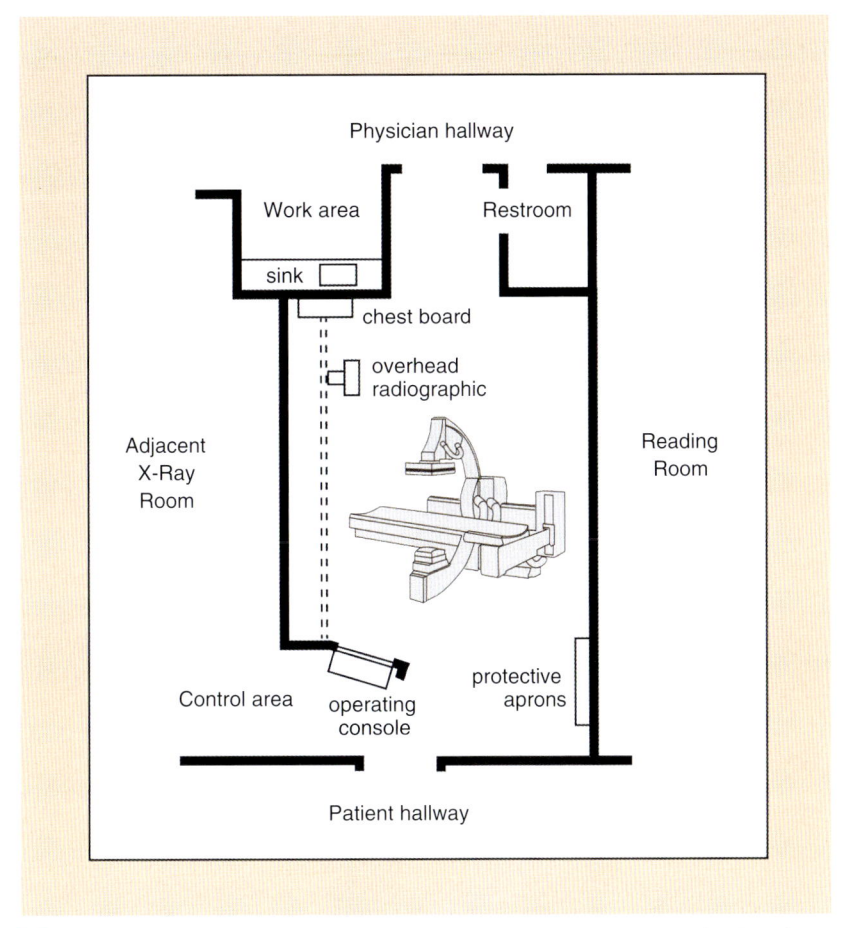

FIG. 6.5 Plan drawing of a general purpose x-ray examination room, showing locations of the various x-ray apparatus items.

The operating console usually provides for control of line compensation, kVp, mA, and exposure time. Meters are provided for monitoring kVp, mA, and exposure time. Many operating consoles also provide a meter for mAs. Imaging systems that incorporate automatic exposure control (AEC) have separate controls for mAs.

All of the electric circuits that connect the meters and controls on the operating console are at low voltage to minimize the possibility of hazardous shock. Fig. 6.6 is a simplified schematic diagram for a typical operating console. A look inside an operating console will indicate how simplified this schematic drawing is!

Operating consoles are digital, and techniques are selected with a touch screen. Numeric technique selection is often replaced by icons indicating the body part, size, and shape. Many of the features are automatic, but the radiographer must know their purpose and their proper use.

Most x-ray imaging systems are designed to operate on 220 V of power, although some can operate on 110 or 440 V. Unfortunately, electric power companies are not capable of providing 220 V accurately and continuously.

Because of variations in power distribution to the hospital and in power consumption by various sections of the hospital, the voltage provided to an x-ray unit easily may vary by as much as 5%. Such variation in supply voltage results in a large variation in the x-ray beam, which is inconsistent with the production of high-quality images.

The **line compensator** measures the voltage provided to the x-ray imaging system and adjusts that voltage to precisely 220 V. Older units required radiographers to adjust the supply voltage while observing a line voltage meter. Currently, x-ray imaging systems have automatic line compensation and hence have no meter.

AUTOTRANSFORMER

The power supplied to the x-ray imaging system is delivered first to the autotransformer. The voltage supplied from the autotransformer to the high-voltage transformer is variable but controlled. It is much safer and easier to control a low voltage and then increase it than to increase a low voltage to the kilovolt level and then control the kilovolt magnitude.

> The autotransformer has a single winding and is designed to supply a precise voltage to the filament circuit and to the high-voltage circuit of the x-ray imaging system.

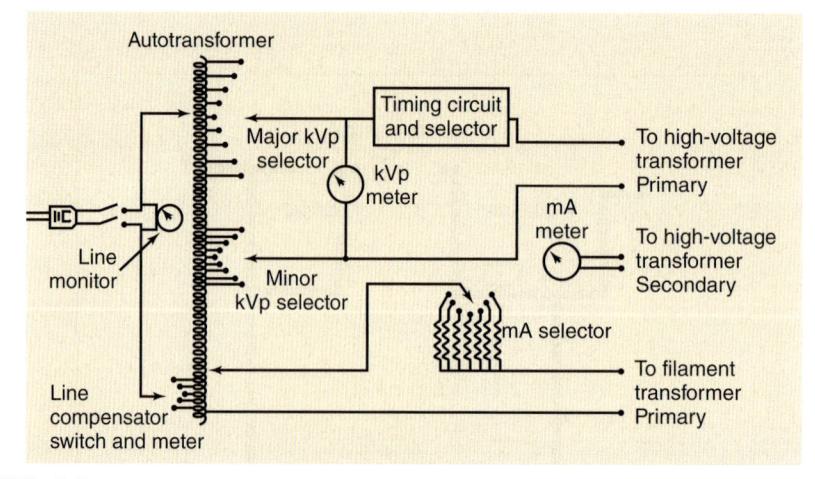

FIG. 6.6 Circuit diagram of the operating console, with controls and meters identified.

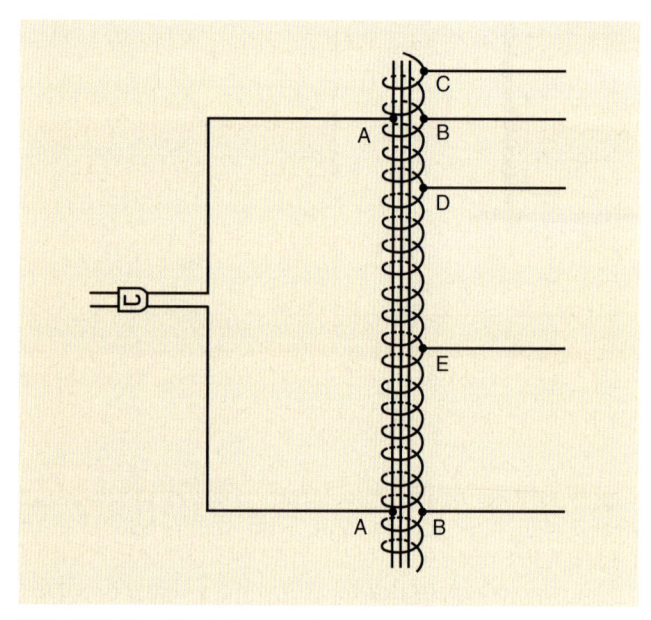

FIG. 6.7 Simplified diagram of an autotransformer.

The autotransformer works on the principle of electromagnetic induction but is very different from the conventional transformer. It has only one winding and one core. This single winding has a number of connections along its length (Fig. 6.7). Two of the connections, A and A' as shown in the figure, conduct the input power to the autotransformer and are called primary connections.

Some of the secondary connections, such as C in Fig. 6.7, are located closer to one end of the winding than are the primary connections. This allows the autotransformer to increase voltage. Other connections, such as D and E in Fig. 6.7, allow a decrease in voltage. The autotransformer can be designed to step up voltage to approximately twice the input voltage value.

Because the autotransformer operates as an induction device, the voltage it receives (the primary voltage) and the voltage it provides (the secondary voltage) are related directly to the number of turns of the transformer enclosed by the respective connections. The autotransformer law is the same as the transformer law.

> **AUTOTRANSFORMER LAW**
>
> $$\frac{V_s}{V_p} = \frac{N_s}{N_p}$$
>
> where V_p is the primary voltage, V_s is the secondary voltage, N_p is the number of windings enclosed by primary connections, and N_s is the number of windings enclosed by secondary connections.

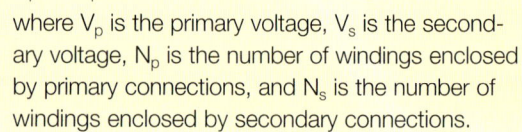

Question: If the autotransformer in Fig. 6.7 is supplied with 220 V to the primary connections AA', which enclose 500 windings, what is the secondary voltage across BB' (500 windings), CB' (700 windings), and DE (200 windings)?

Answer:
BB: $V_s = V_p \left(\dfrac{N_s}{N_p} \right)$

$= (220 \text{ V}) \left(\dfrac{500}{500} \right) = 220 \text{ V}$

CB: $V_s = (220 \text{ V})(1.4) = 308 \text{ V}$
$= (220 \text{ V})(1.4) = 308 \text{ V}$

DE: $V_s = (220 \text{ V}) \left(\dfrac{200}{500} \right)$

$= (220 \text{ V})(0.4) = 88 \text{ V}$

Adjustment of Kilovolt Peak

Some older x-ray operating consoles have adjustment controls labeled **major kVp** and **minor kVp**; by selecting a combination of these controls, radiographers can provide precisely the required kilovolt peak. The minor kilovolt peak adjustment "fine tunes" the selected technique. The major kilovolt peak adjustment and the minor kilovolt peak adjustment represent two separate series of connections on the autotransformer.

> kVp determines the quality of the x-ray beam.

Appropriate connections can be selected with an adjustment knob, a push button, or a touch screen. If the primary voltage to the autotransformer is 220 V, the output of the autotransformer is usually controllable from approximately 100 to 400 V. This low voltage from the autotransformer becomes the input to the high-voltage step-up transformer that increases the voltage to the chosen kilovolt peak.

Question: An autotransformer connected to a 440-V supply contains 4000 turns, all of which are enclosed by the primary connections. If 2300 turns are enclosed by secondary connections, what voltage is supplied to the high-voltage generator?

Answer:
$$V_s = V_p \left(\frac{N_s}{N_p}\right)$$
$$= (440 \text{ V})\left(\frac{2300}{4000}\right)$$
$$= (440 \text{ V})(0.575)$$
$$= 253 \text{ V}$$

The kVp meter is placed across the output terminals of the autotransformer and therefore actually reads voltage, not kVp. However, the scale of the kVp meter registers kilovolts because of the known multiplication factor of the turns ratio.

On most operating consoles, the kVp meter registers, even though no exposure is being made and the circuit has no current. This type of meter is known as a **prereading kVp meter**. It allows the kilovoltage to be monitored before an exposure.

Control of Milliamperage

The x-ray tube electric current, crossing from cathode to anode, is measured in milliamperes (mA). The number of electrons emitted by the filament is determined by the temperature of the filament.

The filament temperature is in turn controlled by the filament current, which is measured in amperes (A). As the filament current increases, the filament becomes hotter, and more electrons are released by thermionic emission. Filaments normally operate at currents of 3 to 6 A.

A correction circuit has to be incorporated to counteract the **space charge effect**. As the kVp is raised, the anode becomes more attractive to the electrons that would not have enough energy to leave the filament area. These electrons also join the electron stream, which effectively increases the mA with kVp.

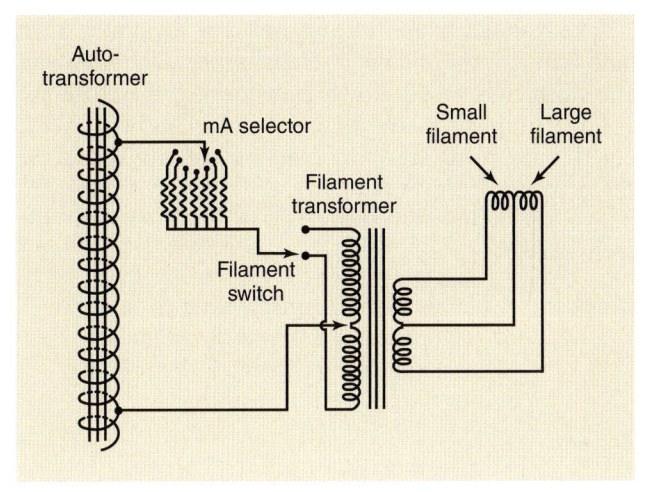

FIG. 6.8 Filament circuit for dual-filament x-ray tube.

> Thermionic emission is the release of electrons from a heated filament.

X-ray tube current is controlled through a separate circuit called the **filament circuit** (Fig. 6.8). Connections on the autotransformer provide voltage for the filament circuit. Precision resistors are used to reduce this voltage to a value that corresponds to the selected milliamperage.

X-ray tube current normally is not continuously variable. Precision resistors result in fixed stations that provide x-ray tube currents of 100, 200, or 300 mA, and higher.

The **falling load generator** constitutes an exception. In a falling load generator, the exposure begins at maximum mA, and the mA drops as the anode heats. The result is minimum exposure time.

> The product of x-ray tube current (mA) and exposure time(s) is mAs, which is also electrostatic charge (C).

Question: An image is made at 400 mA and an exposure time of 100 ms. Express this in mAs and as the total number of electrons.

Answer:
100 ms = 0.1 s
(400 mA)(0.1 s) = 40 mAs
40 mAs = (40 mC/s)(s)
(remember, 1 A = 1 C/s)
   = 40 mC
   = $(40 \times 10^{-3} \text{C})(6.3 \times 10^{18} \text{ e}^-/\text{C})$
   = $2.52 \times 10^{15} \text{e}^-$
   = 2.52×10^{17} electrons

The voltage from the mA selector switch is then delivered to the filament transformer. The filament transformer is a step-down transformer; therefore the voltage supplied to the filament is lower (by a factor equal to the turns ratio) than the voltage supplied to the filament transformer. Similarly, the current is increased across the filament transformer in proportion to the turns ratio.

Question: A filament transformer with a turns ratio of 1/10 provides 6.2 A to the filament. What is the current through the primary coil of the filament transformer?

Answer: $\frac{I_p}{I_s} = \frac{N_s}{N_p}$ where I_p = primary current,

I_s = secondary current, and $\frac{N_s}{N_p}$ = turns ratio

$I_p = I_s \left(\frac{N_s}{N_p}\right)$

$= (6.2)\left(\frac{1}{10}\right)$

$= 0.62$ A

X-ray tube electric current is monitored with an mA meter that is placed in the tube circuit. The mA meter is connected at the center of the secondary winding of the high-voltage step-up transformer. The secondary voltage is alternating at 60 Hz such that the center of this winding is always at zero volts (Fig. 6.9).

In this way, no part of the meter is in contact with the high voltage, and the meter may be safely put on the operating console. Sometimes this meter allows that mAs can be monitored in addition to mA.

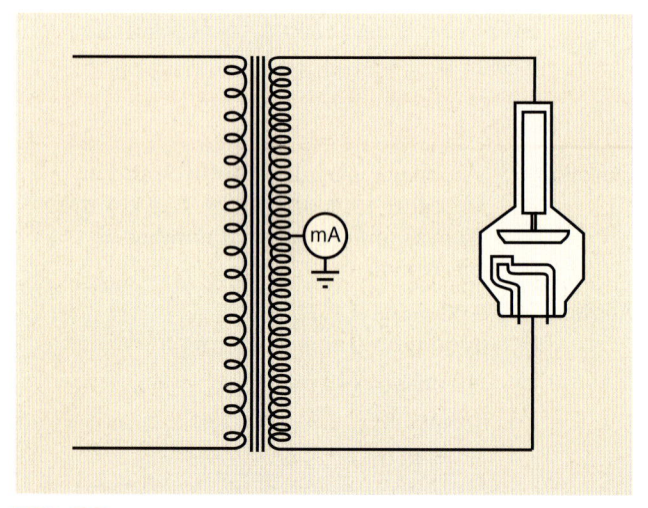

FIG. 6.9 The mA meter is in the x-ray tube circuit at a center tap on the output of the high-voltage step-up transformer. This ensures electrical safety.

Filament Transformer

The full title for this transformer is the filament heating isolation step-down transformer. It steps down the voltage to approximately 12 V and provides the current to heat the filament. Because the secondary windings are connected to the high-voltage supply for the x-ray tube, the secondary windings are heavily insulated from the primary.

In the filament transformer, the primary windings are of thin copper and carry a current of 0.5 to 1 A and approximately 150 V. The secondary windings are thick and, at approximately 12 V electric potential, carry a current of 5 to 8 A (not mA!).

EXPOSURE TIMERS

For any given radiographic examination, the number of x-rays that reach the image receptor is directly related to both the x-ray tube electric current and the time that the x-ray tube is energized. X-ray operating consoles provide a wide selection of x-ray beam-on times and, when used in conjunction with the appropriate mA station, provide an even wider selection of values for mAs.

Question: A KUB examination (radiography of the kidneys, ureters, and bladder) calls for 70 kVp, 40 mAs. If the radiographer selects the 200-mA station, what exposure time should be used?

Answer: $\frac{40 \text{ mAs}}{200 \text{ mAs}} = 0.20$ s $= 200$ ms

Question: A lateral cerebral angiogram calls for 74 kVp, 20 mAs. If the generator has a 1000-mA capacity, what is the shortest exposure time possible?

Answer: $\frac{20 \text{ mAs}}{1000 \text{ mA}} = 0.02$ s $= 20$ ms

Paramount in the design of all timing circuits is that the radiographer starts the x-ray exposure and the timer stops it. During fluoroscopy, if the radiographer releases the exposure switch or the fluoroscopic foot switch, the exposure is terminated immediately.

As an additional safety feature, another timing circuit is activated on every radiographic exposure. This timer, called a **guard timer**, will terminate an exposure after a prescribed time, usually six seconds. Thus it is not possible for any timing circuit to continuously irradiate a patient for an extensive period.

The timer circuit is separate from the other main circuits of the x-ray imaging system. It consists of an electronic device whose action is to "make" and "break" the high voltage across the x-ray tube. This is nearly always done on the **primary side** of the high-voltage transformer, where the voltage is lower.

There are four types of timing circuits. Three are controlled by the radiographer, and one is automatic. After studying this section, try to identify the types of timers on the imaging systems you use.

Synchronous Timers

In the United States, electric current is supplied at a frequency of 60 Hz. In Europe, Latin America, and other parts of the world, the frequency is 50 Hz. A special type of electric motor, known as a synchronous motor, is a precision device designed to drive a shaft at precisely 60 revolutions per second (rps). In some x-ray imaging systems, synchronous motors are used as timing mechanisms.

X-ray imaging systems with synchronous timers are recognizable because the minimum exposure time possible is 1/60 seconds (17 ms), and timing intervals increase by multiples thereof, such as, 1/30, 1/20, and so on. Synchronous timers cannot be used for serial exposures because they must be reset after each exposure.

Electronic Timers

Electronic timers are the most sophisticated, most complicated, and most accurate of the x-ray exposure timers. Electronic timers consist of rather complex circuitry based on the time required to charge a capacitor through a variable resistance.

Electronic timers allow a wide range of time intervals to be selected and are accurate to intervals as small as 1 ms. Because they can be used for rapid serial exposures, they are particularly suitable for interventional radiology procedures.

> Most exposure timers are electronic and are controlled by a microprocessor.

Milliampere-Second Timers

Most x-ray apparatus is designed for accurate control of x-ray tube electric current and exposure time. However, the product of mA and time—mAs—determines the total number of x-rays emitted and therefore the exposure of the image receptor. A special kind of electronic timer, called an mAs timer, monitors the product of mA and exposure time and terminates exposure when the desired mAs value is attained.

The mAs timer is usually designed to provide the highest safe tube current for the shortest exposure for any mAs selected. Because the mAs timer must monitor the actual tube current, it is located on the secondary side of the high-voltage transformer.

> mAs timers are used on falling load and capacitor discharge imaging systems.

Automatic Exposure Control

The automatic exposure control (AEC) requires a special understanding on the part of the radiographer.

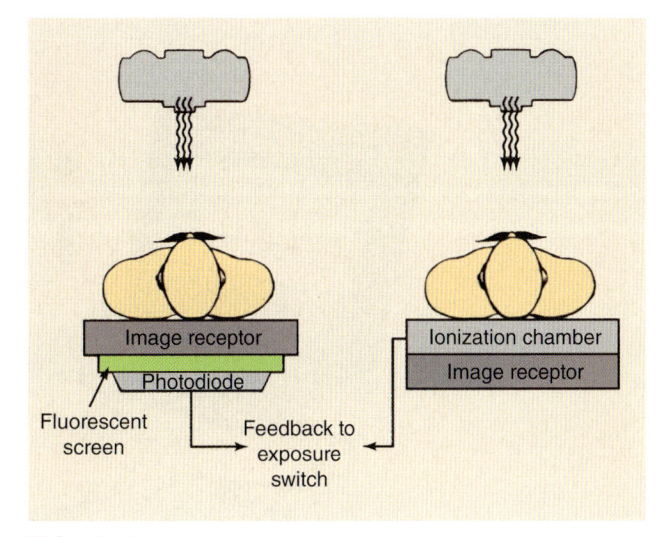

FIG. 6.10 Automatic exposure control terminates the x-ray exposure at the desired image receptor signal intensity. This is done with an ionization chamber or a photodiode detector assembly.

The AEC is a device that measures the quantity of radiation that reaches the image receptor. It automatically terminates the exposure when the image receptor has received the required radiation intensity. Fig. 6.10 shows two approaches to the design of an AEC device.

The type of AEC used by most manufacturers incorporates a flat, parallel plate ionization chamber positioned between the patient and the image receptor. This chamber is made radiolucent so that it will not interfere with the radiographic image. Ionization within the chamber creates a charge. When the appropriate charge has been reached, the exposure is terminated.

When an AEC x-ray imaging system is installed, it must be calibrated. This calls for making exposures of a test object and adjusting the AEC for the range of x-ray intensities required for quality images. The service engineer usually takes care of this calibration.

After the AEC is in clinical operation, the radiographer selects the type of examination, which then sets the appropriate mA and kVp. At the same time, the exposure timer is set to the backup time. When the electric charge from the ionization chamber reaches a preset level, a signal is returned to the operating console, where the exposure is terminated.

The AEC is currently widely used and often is provided in addition to an electronic timer. The AEC mode requires particular care, especially in examinations that use low kVp, such as mammography. Because of varying tissue thickness and composition, the AEC may not respond properly at low kVp.

When radiographs are taken in the AEC mode, the electronic timer should be set to 1.5 times the expected exposure time as a backup timer in case the AEC fails to terminate. This precaution should be followed for the protection of the patient and the x-ray tube. Many units automatically set this precaution.

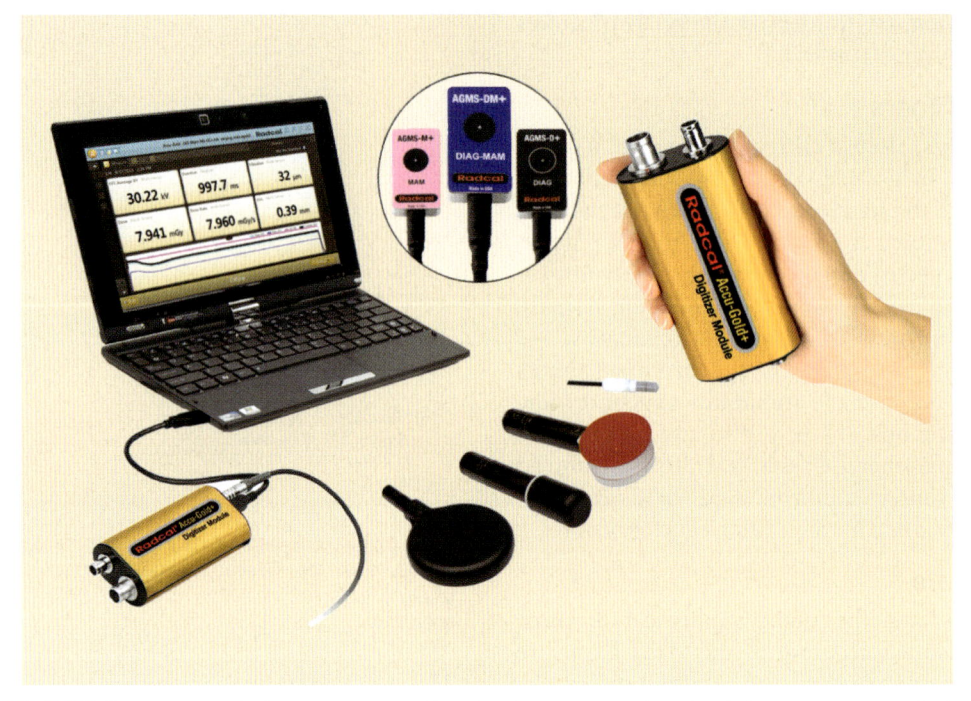

FIG. 6.11 Solid-state radiation detectors and ion chambers are used to check timer accuracy and a host of other imaging system specifications. (Courtesy Vicky Chen, Radcal Corporation.)

If specific area shielding, such as a gonad shield, is a part of the examination, be sure that the x-ray beam is properly collimated. Should a portion of the uncollimated useful x-ray beam intercept the specific area shield, the patient radiation dose will be increased.

> Never allow the useful x-ray beam to include a specific area shield!

Solid-state radiation detectors are currently used for exposure-timer checks (Fig. 6.11). These devices operate with a very accurate internal clock based on a quartz-crystal oscillator. They can measure exposure times as short as 1 ms and, when used with an oscilloscope, can display the radiation waveform.

HIGH-VOLTAGE GENERATOR

The high-voltage generator of an x-ray imaging system is responsible for increasing the output voltage from the autotransformer to the kVp necessary for x-ray production. A cutaway view of a typical high-voltage generator is shown in Fig. 6.12. Although some heat is generated in the high-voltage section, the heat is conducted to oil. The oil is used primarily for electrical insulation.

> The high-voltage generator contains three primary parts: the high-voltage transformer, the filament transformer, and rectifiers.

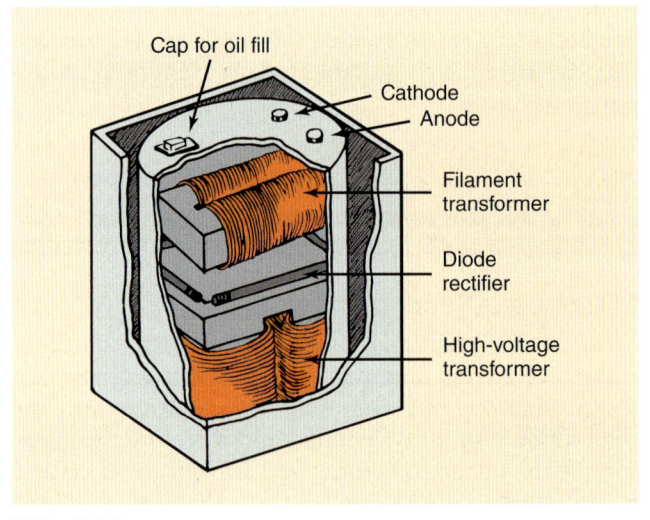

FIG. 6.12 Cutaway view of a typical high-voltage generator showing oil-immersed diodes and transformers.

High-Voltage Transformer

The high-voltage transformer is a step-up transformer; that is, the secondary voltage is higher than the primary voltage because the number of secondary windings is greater than the number of primary windings. The ratio of the number of secondary windings to the number of primary windings is called the **turns ratio** (see Chapter 5). The voltage increase is proportional to the turns ratio, according to the transformer law. In addition, the current is reduced proportionately.

The turns ratio of a high-voltage transformer is usually between 500:1 and 1000:1. Because transformers

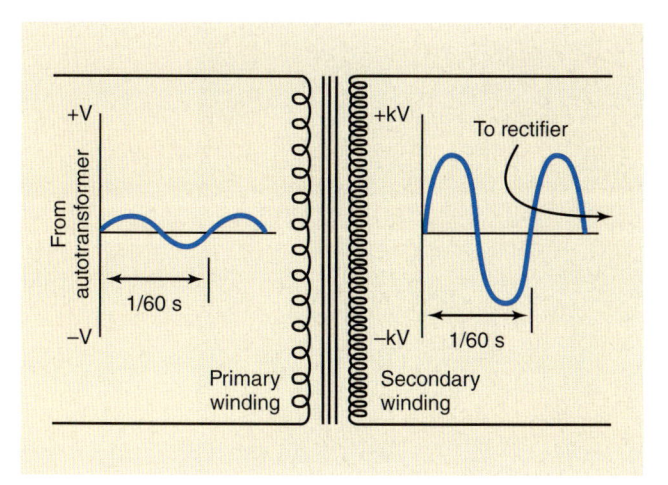

FIG. 6.13 Voltage induced in the secondary winding of a high-voltage step-up transformer is alternating like the primary voltage but has a higher value.

operate only on alternating current (AC), the voltage waveform on both sides of a high-voltage transformer is sinusoidal (Fig. 6.13).

The only difference between the primary and secondary waveforms is their **amplitude**. The primary voltage is measured in volts (V), and the secondary voltage is measured in kilovolts (kV). The primary current is measured in amperes (A), and the secondary current is measured in milliamperes (mA).

Question: The turns ratio of a high-voltage transformer is 700:1, and the supply voltage is peaked at 120 V. What is the secondary voltage supplied to the x-ray tube?

Answer: $(120\ Vp)(700:1) = 84,000\ Vp$
$= 84\ kVp$

Voltage Rectification

The current from a common wall plug is 60-Hz AC. The current changes direction 120 times each second. However, an x-ray tube requires a direct current (DC); that is, electron flows in only one direction. Therefore some means must be provided for converting AC to DC.

Radiographers outside the United States may use a frequency of 50 Hz. In the case of 50-Hz power, there are 100 half-cycles per second, each lasting 10 ms. In all other respects, the rectification process is the same.

> Rectification is the process of converting AC to DC.

The electronic device that allows current flow in only one direction is a **rectifier**. Although transformers operate with alternating electric current, x-ray tubes must be provided with DC. X-rays are produced by the acceleration of electrons from the cathode to the anode and cannot be produced by electrons flowing in the reverse direction, from anode to cathode.

Reversal of electron flow would be disastrous for the x-ray tube. The construction of the cathode assembly is such that it could not withstand the tremendous heat generated by such an operation even if the anode could emit electrons thermionically. If the electron flow is to be only in the cathode-to-anode direction, the secondary voltage of the high-voltage transformer must be rectified.

> Voltage rectification is required to ensure that electrons flow from x-ray tube cathode to anode only.

Rectification is accomplished with diodes. A diode is an electronic device that contains two electrodes. Originally, all diode rectifiers were vacuum tubes called **valve tubes**; these have been replaced by solid-state rectifiers made of silicon (Fig. 6.14).

It has long been known that metals are good conductors of electricity and that some other materials, such as glass and plastic, are poor conductors of electricity, called insulators.

A third class of materials, called **semiconductors**, lies between the range of insulators and conductors in the ability to conduct electricity. Tiny crystals of these semiconductors have some useful electrical properties and allow semiconductors to serve as the basis for solid-state microprocessor marvels nowadays.

Semiconductors are classified into two types: n type and p type. N-type semiconductors have loosely bound electrons that are relatively free to move. P-type semiconductors have spaces, called **holes**, where there are no electrons. These holes are similar to the space between cars in heavy traffic. Holes are as mobile as electrons.

Consider a tiny crystal of n-type material placed in contact with a p-type crystal to form what is called a p-n junction (Fig. 6.15). If a higher potential is placed on the p side of the junction, then the electrons and holes will both migrate toward the junction and wander across it. This flow of electrons and holes constitutes an electric current.

If, however, a positive potential is placed on the n side of the junction, both the electrons and the holes will be swept away from the junction, and no electrons will be available at the junction surface to form a current. Thus in this case, no electric current passes through the p-n junction.

Therefore a solid-state p-n junction tends to conduct electricity in only one direction. This type of p-n junction is called a solid-state diode. Solid-state diodes are rectifiers because they conduct electric current in

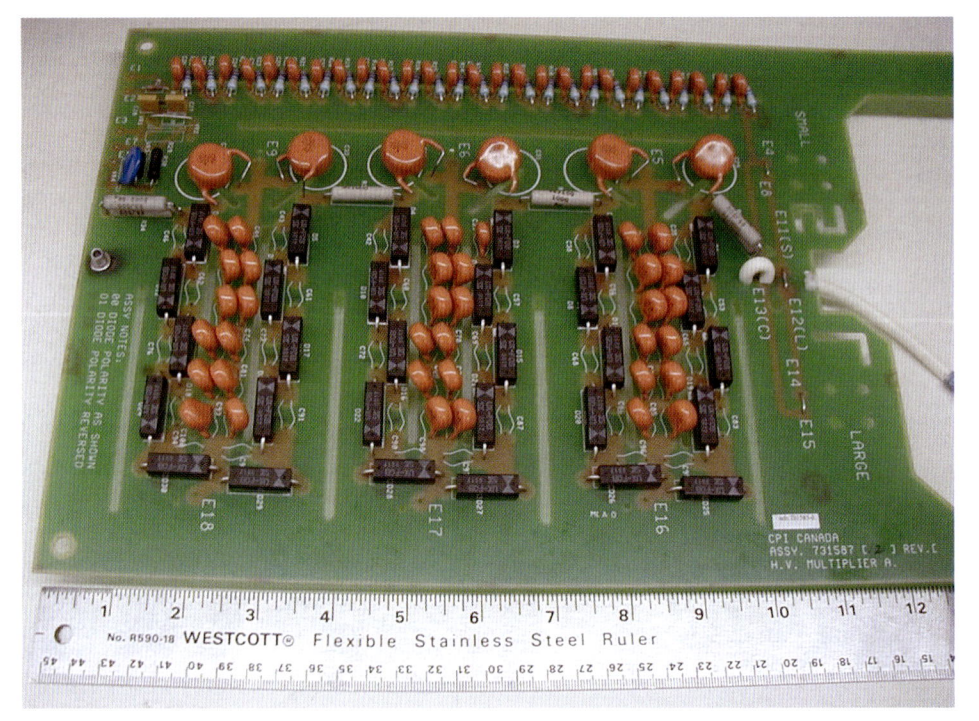

FIG. 6.14 Rectifiers in most modern x-ray generators are the silicon, semiconductor type.

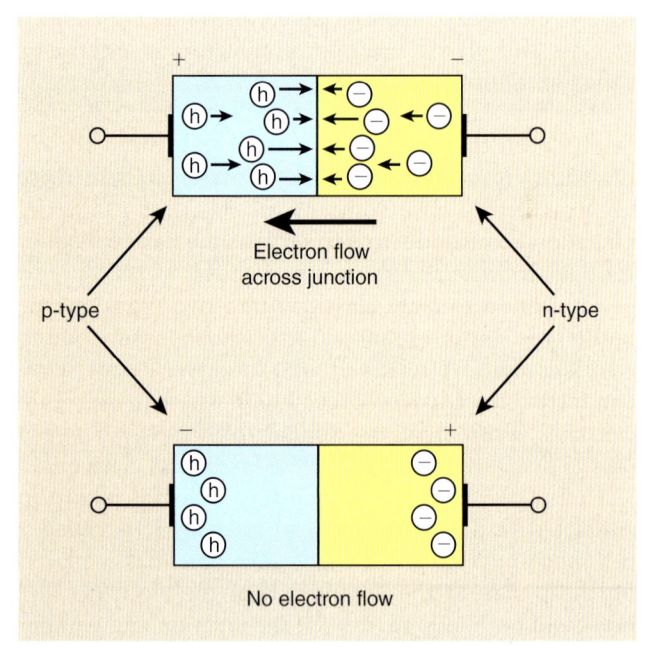

FIG. 6.15 A p-n junction semiconductor shown as a solid-state diode.

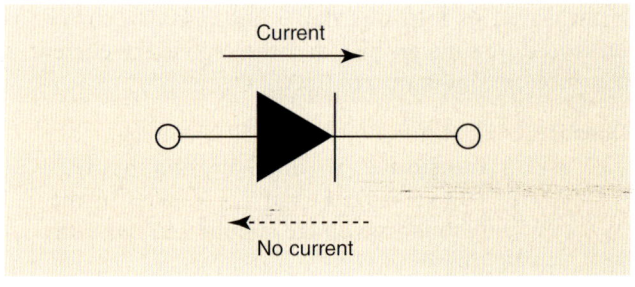

FIG. 6.16 The electronic symbol for a solid-state diode.

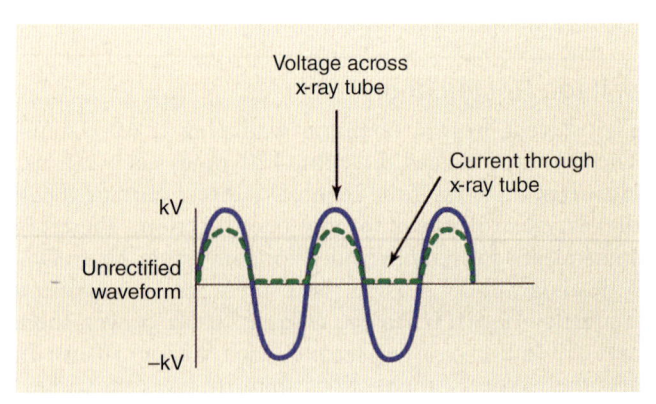

FIG. 6.17 Unrectified voltage and current waveforms on the secondary side.

only one direction. The arc in the symbol for a diode indicates the direction of conventional electric current, which is opposite to the flow of electrons (Fig. 6.16). Electron flow is used when medical imaging systems are described.

> Rectifiers are located in the high-voltage section.

Rectification is essential for the safe and efficient operation of the x-ray tube. The unrectified voltage at the secondary side of the high-voltage step-up transformer is shown in Fig. 6.17. This voltage waveform appears as the voltage waveform supplied to the

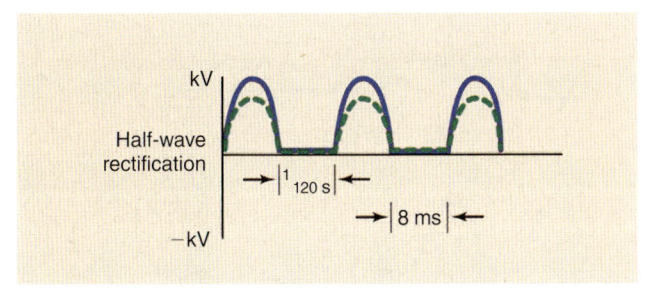

FIG. 6.18 Half-wave rectification.

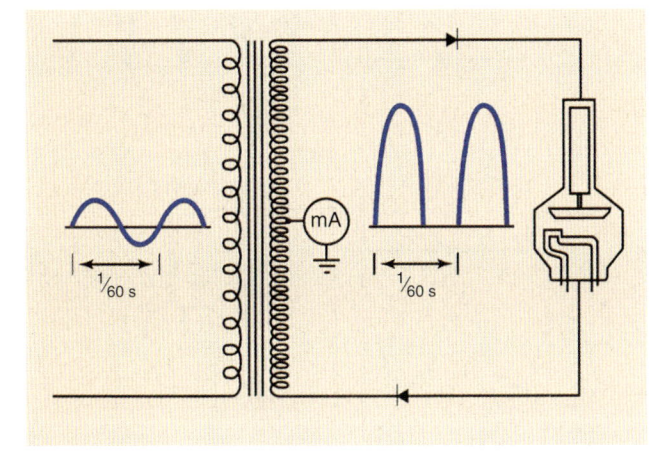

FIG. 6.19 A half-wave–rectified circuit contains one or more diodes.

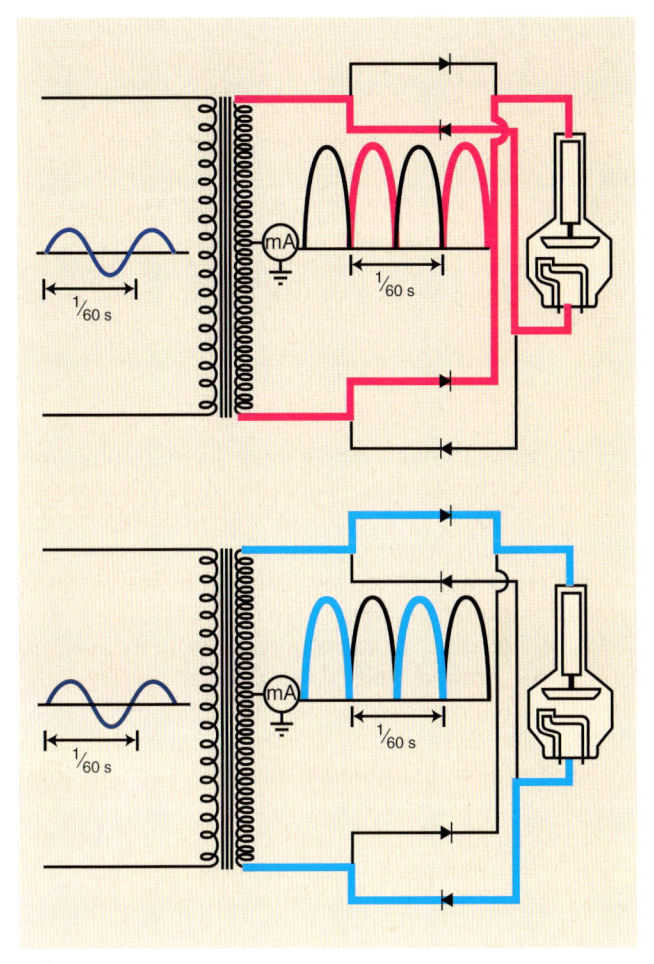

FIG. 6.20 A full-wave–rectified circuit contains at least four diodes. Current is passed through the tube at 120 pulses per second.

primary side of the high-voltage transformer, except its amplitude is much greater.

However, the current that passes through the x-ray tube exists only during the positive half of the cycle when the anode is positive and the cathode is negative. During the negative half of the cycle, current can flow only from anode to cathode, but this does not occur because the anode is not constructed to emit electrons.

The inverse voltage is removed from the supply to the x-ray tube by rectification. **Half-wave rectification** (Fig. 6.18) is a condition in which the voltage is not allowed to swing negatively during the negative half of its cycle.

Rectifiers are assembled into electronic circuits to convert AC into the DC necessary for the operation of an x-ray tube (Fig. 6.19). During the positive portion of the AC waveform, the rectifier allows electric current to pass through the x-ray tube.

However, during the negative portion of the AC waveform, the rectifier does not conduct, and thus no electric current is allowed. The resultant electric current is a series of positive pulses separated by gaps when the negative current is not conducted.

This resultant electric current is a rectified current because electrons flow in only one direction. This form of rectification is called **half-wave rectification** because only one-half of the AC waveform appears in the output.

In some portable and dental x-ray imaging systems, the x-ray tube serves as the vacuum tube rectifier. Such a system is said to be **self-rectified**, and the resulting waveform is the same as that of half-wave rectification.

Half-wave–rectified circuits contain zero, one, or two diodes. The x-ray output from a half-wave high-voltage generator pulsates, producing 60 x-ray pulses each second.

One shortcoming of half-wave rectification is that it wastes half the supply of power. It also requires twice the exposure time. However, it is possible to devise a circuit that rectifies the entire AC waveform. This form of voltage rectification is called **full-wave rectification**.

Full-wave–rectified x-ray imaging systems contain at least four diodes in the high-voltage circuit, usually arranged as shown in Fig. 6.20. In a full-wave–rectified circuit, the negative half-cycle corresponding to the inverse voltage is reversed so that the anode is always positive (Fig. 6.21).

> The main advantage of full-wave rectification is that the exposure time for any given technique is cut in half.

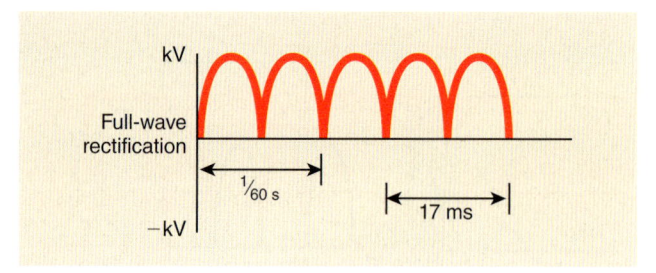

FIG. 6.21 Voltage across a full-wave–rectified circuit is always positive.

The current through the circuit is shown during both the positive and the negative phases of the input waveform. Note that in both cases, the output voltage across the x-ray tube is positive. In addition, there are no gaps in the output waveform. All of the input waveform is rectified into usable output.

Fig. 6.22 helps to explain full-wave rectification. During the positive half-cycle of the secondary voltage waveform, electrons flow from the negative side to diodes C and D. Diode C is unable to conduct electrons in that direction, but diode D can. The electrons flow through diode D and the x-ray tube.

The electrons then butt into diodes A and B. Only diode A is positioned to conduct them, and they flow to the positive side of the transformer, thus completing the circuit.

During the negative half-cycle, diodes B and C are pressed into service, and diodes A and D block electron flow. Note that the polarity of the x-ray tube remains unchanged. The cathode is always negative and the anode is always positive, even though the induced secondary voltage alternates between positive and negative.

The half-wave–rectified x-ray tube emits x-rays only half of the time. The pulsed x-ray output of a full-wave–rectified machine occurs 120 times each second instead of 60 times per second as with half-wave rectification.

Single-Phase Power

All of the voltage waveforms discussed so far are produced by single-phase electric power. Single-phase power results in a pulsating x-ray beam. This is caused by the alternate swing in voltage from zero to a maximum potential 120 times each second under full-wave rectification.

The x-rays produced when the single-phase voltage waveform has a value near zero are of little diagnostic value because of their low energy; such x-rays have low penetrability. One method of overcoming this deficiency is to use some sophisticated electrical engineering principles to generate three simultaneous voltage waveforms that are out of step with one another. Such a manipulation results in three-phase electric power.

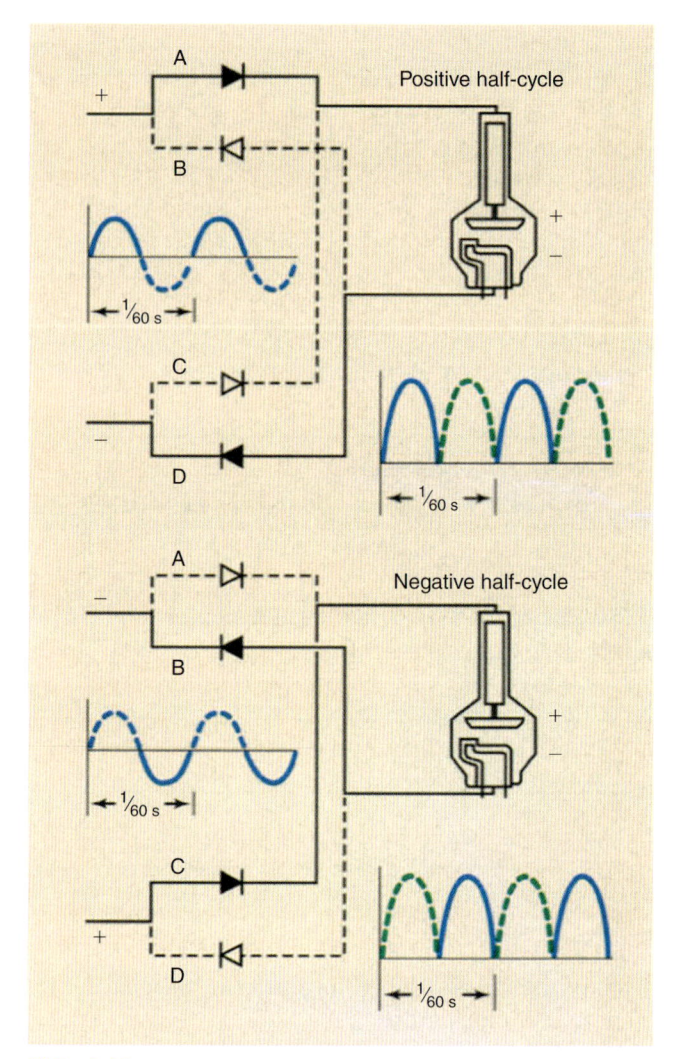

FIG. 6.22 In a full-wave–rectified circuit, two diodes (A and D) conduct during the positive half-cycle, and two (B and C) conduct during the negative half-cycle.

Three-Phase Power

The engineering required to produce three-phase power involves the manner in which the high-voltage step-up transformer is wired into the circuit, the details of which are beyond the scope of this discussion. Fig. 6.23 shows the voltage waveforms for single-phase power, three-phase power, and full-wave–rectified three-phase power.

With three-phase power, multiple voltage waveforms are superimposed on one another, resulting in a waveform that maintains a nearly constant high voltage. There are six pulses per 1/60 second compared with the two pulses characteristic of single-phase power.

> The voltage applied to the x-ray tube is nearly constant when using three-phase power.

There are limitations to the speed of starting an exposure—**initiation time**—and ending an exposure—**extinction time**. Additional electronic circuits are necessary to correct this deficiency; this adds to the additional size and cost of the three-phase voltage generator.

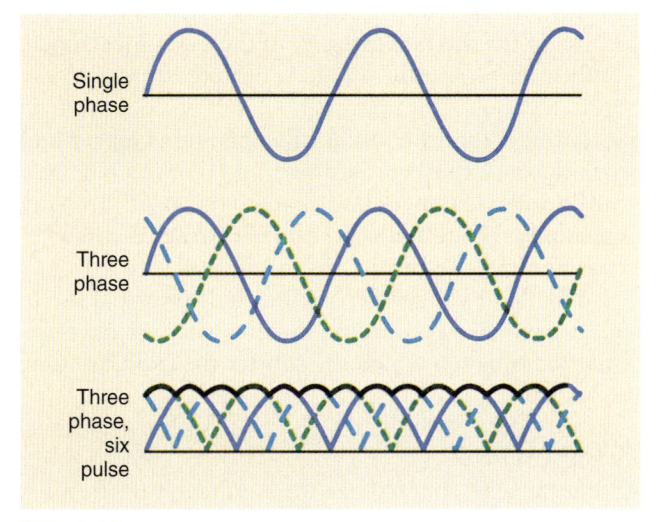

FIG. 6.23 Three-phase power is a more efficient way to produce x-rays than is single-phase power. Shown are the voltage waveforms for unrectified single-phase power, unrectified three-phase power, and rectified three-phase power.

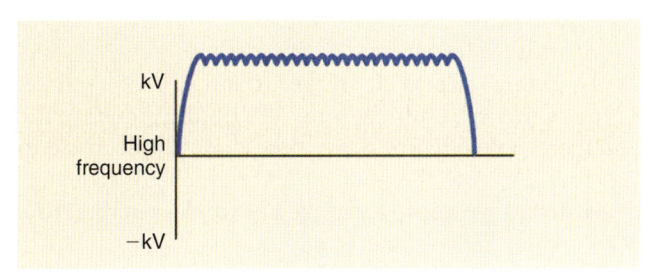

FIG. 6.24 High-frequency voltage waveform.

High-Frequency Generator

High-frequency circuits are finding increasing application in generating high voltage for many x-ray imaging systems. Full-wave–rectified power at 60 Hz is converted to a higher frequency, from 500 to 25,000 Hz, and then is transferred to high voltage (Fig. 6.24).

One advantage of the high-frequency generator is its size. They are very much smaller than 60-Hz high-voltage generators. High-frequency generators produce a nearly constant potential voltage waveform, improving image quality at a lower patient radiation dose.

This technology was first used with portable x-ray imaging systems. Now, all mammography and computed tomography systems use high-frequency circuits.

High-frequency voltage generation uses inverter circuits (Fig. 6.25). Inverter circuits are high-speed switches, or choppers, that convert DC into a series of square pulses.

Many portable x-ray high-voltage generators use storage batteries and silicon-controlled rectifiers to generate square waves at 500 Hz; this becomes the input to the high-voltage step-up transformer. The high-voltage step-up transformer operating at 500 Hz is approximately the size of a 60-Hz transformer, which is rather large and heavy.

High-frequency x-ray generators are sometimes grouped by frequency (Table 6.1). The principal differences are found in the electric components designed as the inverter module. The real advantage of such circuits is that they are much smaller, less costly, and more efficient than 60-Hz high-voltage generators.

> Full-wave rectification or high-frequency voltage generation is used in almost all stationary x-ray imaging systems.

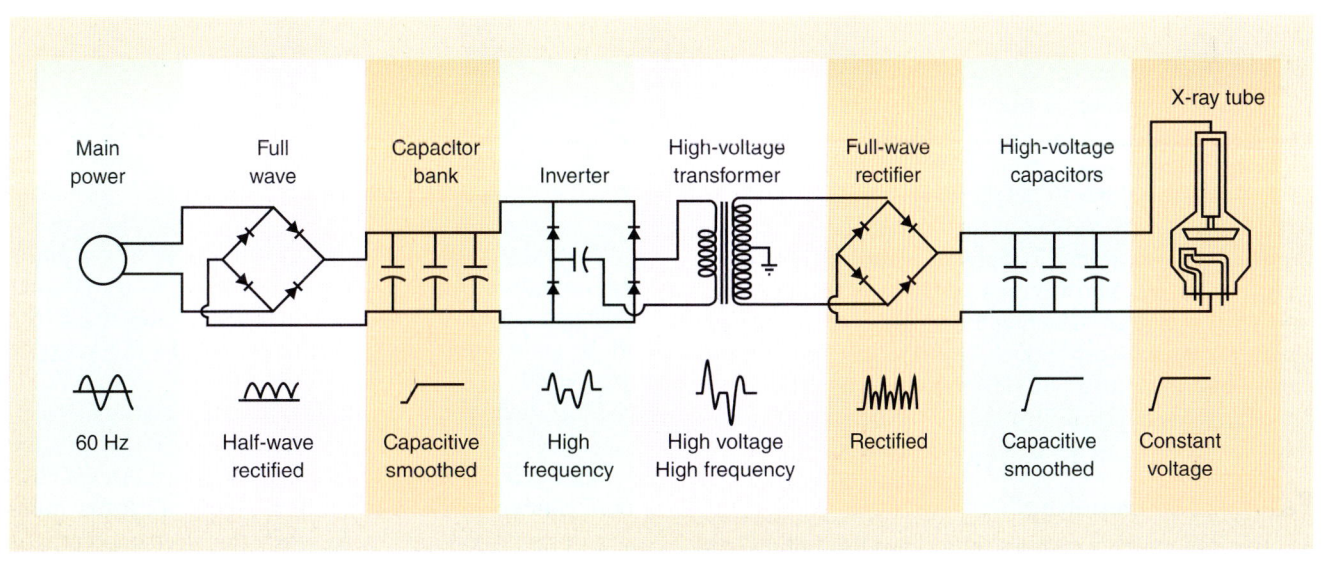

FIG. 6.25 Inverter circuit of a high-voltage generator.

TABLE 6.1	Characteristics of High-Frequency X-ray Generators
Frequency Range (kHz)	**Inverter Features**
<1	Thyristors
1–10	Large silicon-controlled rectifier
10–100	Power field effect transistors

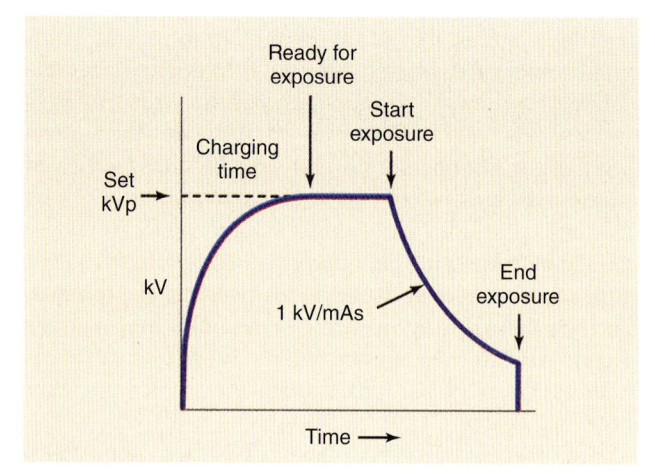

FIG. 6.26 X-ray tube voltage falls during exposure with a capacitor discharge generator.

Capacitor Discharge Generator

Some portable x-ray imaging systems still use a high-voltage generator, which operates by charging a series of SCRs from the DC voltage of a nickel-cadmium battery. By stacking (in an electric sense) the SCRs, the charge is stored at very high voltage. During exposure, the charge is released (discharged) to form the x-ray tube current needed to produce x-rays (Fig. 6.26).

> During capacitor discharge, the voltage falls approximately 1 kV/mAs.

This falling voltage limits the available x-ray tube current and causes kVp to fall during exposure. The result is the need for precise radiographic technique charts.

After a given exposure time, the capacitor bank continues to discharge, which could cause continued x-ray emission. Such x-ray emission is stopped by a grid-controlled x-ray tube, an automatic lead beam stopper, or both. A grid-controlled x-ray tube has a specially designed cathode to control x-ray tube current.

Falling Load Generator

Many x-ray imaging systems today engage a falling load technique to ensure the shortest possible exposure time. The x-ray tube anode can accommodate only a limited heat level, as we shall see in Chapter 7.

Supposing the limit on exposure time, and therefore x-ray intensity, for an interventional radiology imaging system at the 1000 mA station is 500 ms and therefore 500 mAs, as shown in Fig. 6.27. At the selected kVp and 1000 mA, the shortest exposure time allowed is 500 ms because of the thermal capacity of the x-ray tube anode.

When an x-ray tube anode is heated, it immediately begins to cool. The approach of falling load voltage generation is that the initial tube loading is higher and drops during exposure, as shown in Fig. 6.28. The rate of drop follows the cooling characteristics of the x-ray tube anode. The result is the same 500 mAs at a shorter exposure time; 300 ms in this example.

Falling load voltage generation finds principal use in high-capacity x-ray imaging systems such as interventional radiology in which the shorter the exposure time the better.

Voltage Ripple

Another way to characterize these voltage waveforms is by **voltage ripple**. Single-phase power has 100% voltage ripple: The voltage varies from zero to its maximum value. Three-phase, six-pulse power produces voltage with only approximately 14% ripple; consequently, the voltage supplied to the x-ray tube never decreases to less than 86% of the maximum value.

A further improvement in three-phase power results in 12 pulses per cycle rather than 6. Three-phase, 12-pulse power results in only 4% ripple; therefore the voltage supplied to the x-ray tube does not decrease to less than 96% of the maximum value. High-frequency generators have approximately 1% ripple and therefore even greater x-ray quantity and quality.

Fig. 6.29 shows these various power sources and the resultant voltage waveforms they provide to the x-ray tube, as well as the approximate voltage ripple. The most efficient method of x-ray production also involves the waveform with the lowest voltage ripple.

> Less voltage ripple results in higher radiation intensity and quality.

An x-ray tube voltage with less ripple offers many advantages. The principal advantage is the higher radiation intensity and quality that result from the more constant voltage supplied to the x-ray tube (Fig. 6.30).

The radiation intensity is greater because the efficiency of x-ray production is higher when the x-ray tube voltage is high. Stated differently, for any projectile electron emitted by the x-ray tube filament, a greater number of x-rays are produced when the electron energy is high than when it is low.

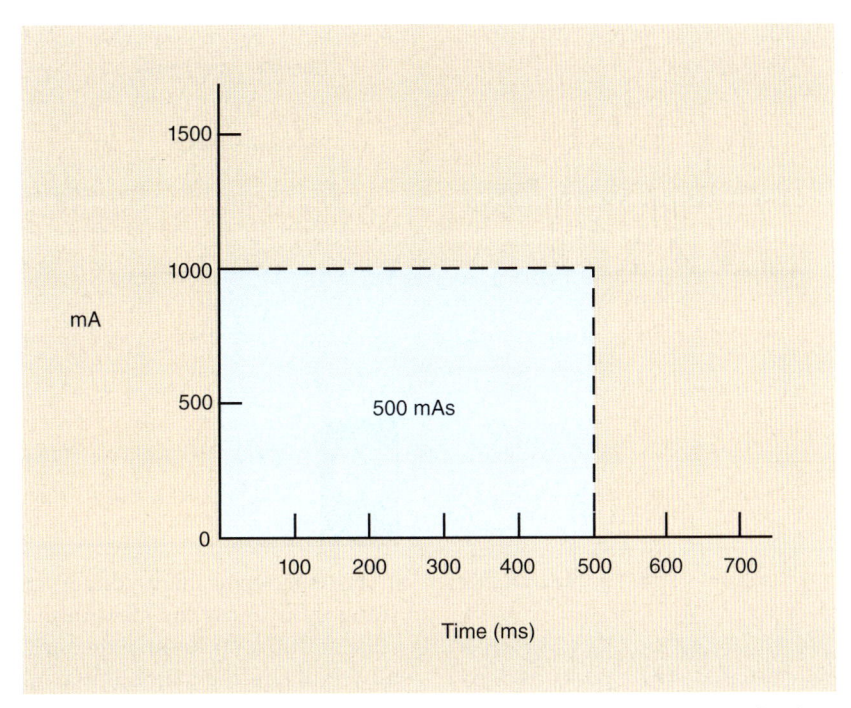

FIG. 6.27 A fixed radiographic technique of 1000 mA, 500 ms results in 500 mAs, the area of the box.

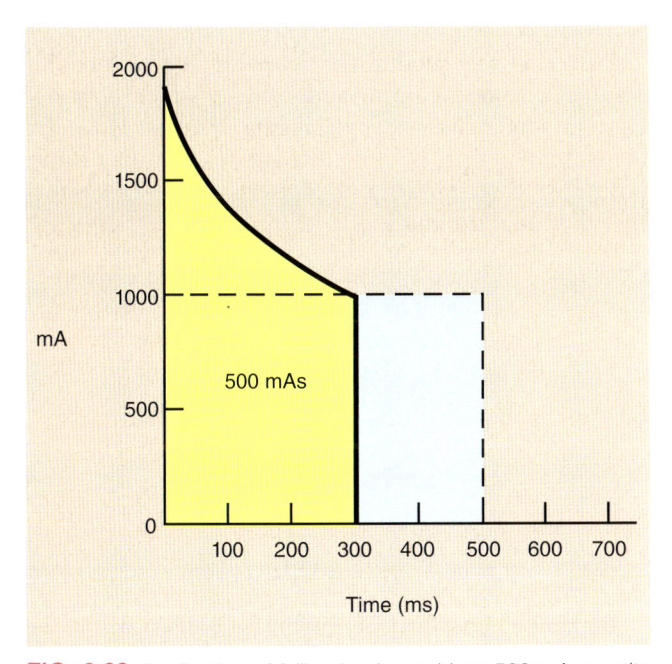

FIG. 6.28 Application of falling load to achieve 500 mAs results in a much shorter exposure time, 300 ms.

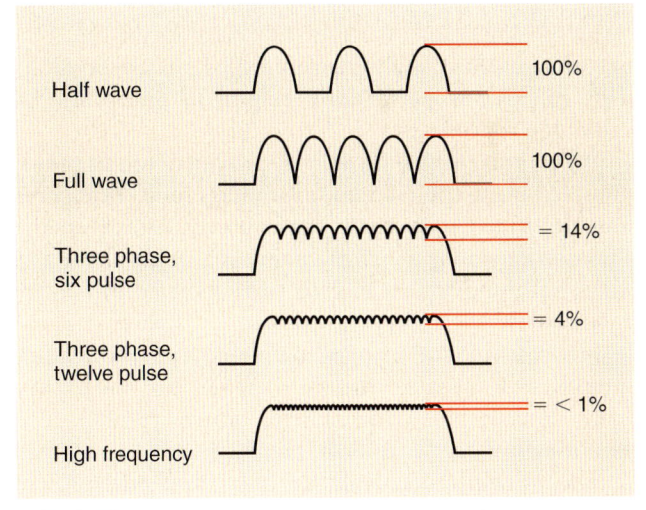

FIG. 6.29 Voltage waveforms resulting from various power supplies. The ripple of the kilovoltage is indicated as a percentage for each waveform.

Low-voltage ripple increases radiation quality because fewer low-energy projectile electrons pass from cathode to anode to produce low-energy x-rays. Consequently, the average x-ray energy is greater than that resulting from high-voltage ripple modes.

Because the x-ray beam intensity and penetrability are greater for less voltage ripple than for single-phase power, technique charts developed for one cannot be used on the other. New technique charts with three-phase or high-frequency x-ray imaging systems are needed.

Three-phase operation may require as much as a 10-kVp reduction to produce the same image receptor exposure when operated at the same mAs as single-phase operation. A high-frequency generator may require a 12-kVp reduction.

Three-phase radiographic equipment is manufactured with tube currents as high as 1200 mA; therefore

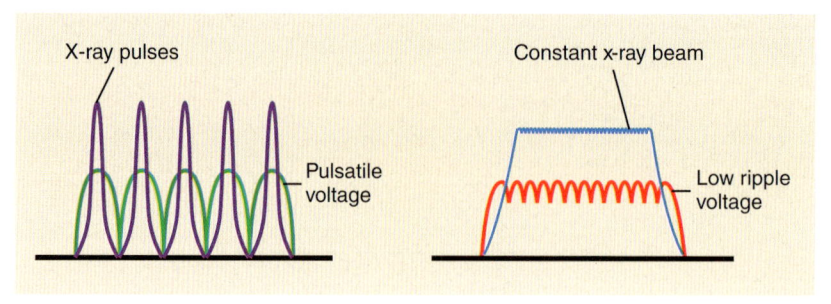

FIG. 6.30 Both the number of x-rays and the x-ray energy increase as the voltage waveform increases.

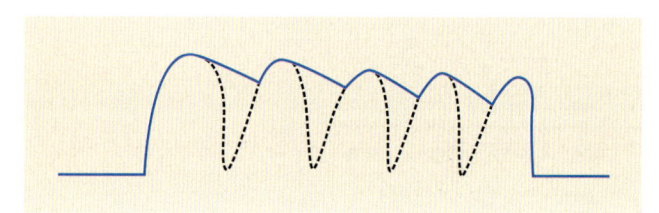

FIG. 6.31 Voltage waveform is smoothed by the capacitance of long high-voltage cables. Illustration shows peaks followed by slanting declining lines, where half peaks are completed by dashed lines to show five consecutive positive peaks.

exceedingly short, high-intensity exposures are possible. This capacity is particularly helpful in interventional radiology procedures.

When three-phase power is provided for a radiographic/fluoroscopic room, all radiographic exposures are performed with three-phase power. However, the fluoroscopic mode usually remains as a single phase and takes advantage of the electric capacitance of the x-ray tube cables.

Fluoroscopic mA is very low compared with radiographic mA. Because the x-ray cables are long, they have considerable capacitance, which results in a smoother voltage waveform (Fig. 6.31).

The principal disadvantage of a three-phase x-ray apparatus is its initial cost. However, the costs of installation and operation can be lower than those associated with single-phase equipment. The cost of high-frequency generators is moderate. Low-ripple generators have greater overall capacity and flexibility compared with single-phase equipment.

Power Rating

Transformers and high-voltage generators usually are identified by their power rating in kilowatts (kW). Electric power for any device is specified in watts. A high-voltage generator for a basic radiographic unit is rated at 30 to 50 kW. Generators for interventional radiology have power ratings up to approximately 150 kW. Electric power for any device is specified in watts, as shown in the following equations.

> Power = Current × Potential
> Watts = Amperes × Volts

For specifying high-voltage generators, the industry standard is to use the maximum tube current (mA) possible at 100 kVp for an exposure of 100 ms. This generally results in the maximum available power.

> High-voltage generator power (kW) = maximum x-ray tube current (mA) at 100 kVp and 100 ms.

Power is the product of amperes and volts. This assumes constant current and voltage, which does not exist in single-phase x-ray imaging systems. However, the actual power is close enough to the low-ripple power of three-phase and high-frequency generators that the equation holds.

Question: When a system with low-voltage ripple is energized at 100 kVp, 100 ms, the maximum possible tube current is 800 mA. What is the power rating?

Answer:
Power rating = Current (A) × Potential (V)
= 800 mA × 100 kVp
= 80,000 mA × kVp
= 80,000 W
= 80 kW

Because the product of amperes × volts = watts, the product of milliamperes × kilovolts = watts. However, power rating is expressed in kilowatts, so the defining equation for three-phase and high-frequency power is as follows.

Question: An interventional radiology imaging system is capable of 1200 mA when operated in 100 kVp, 100 ms. What is the power rating?

Answer:
$$\text{Power rating (kW)} = \frac{1200 \text{ mA} \times 100 \text{ kVp}}{1000}$$
$$= 120 \text{ kW}$$

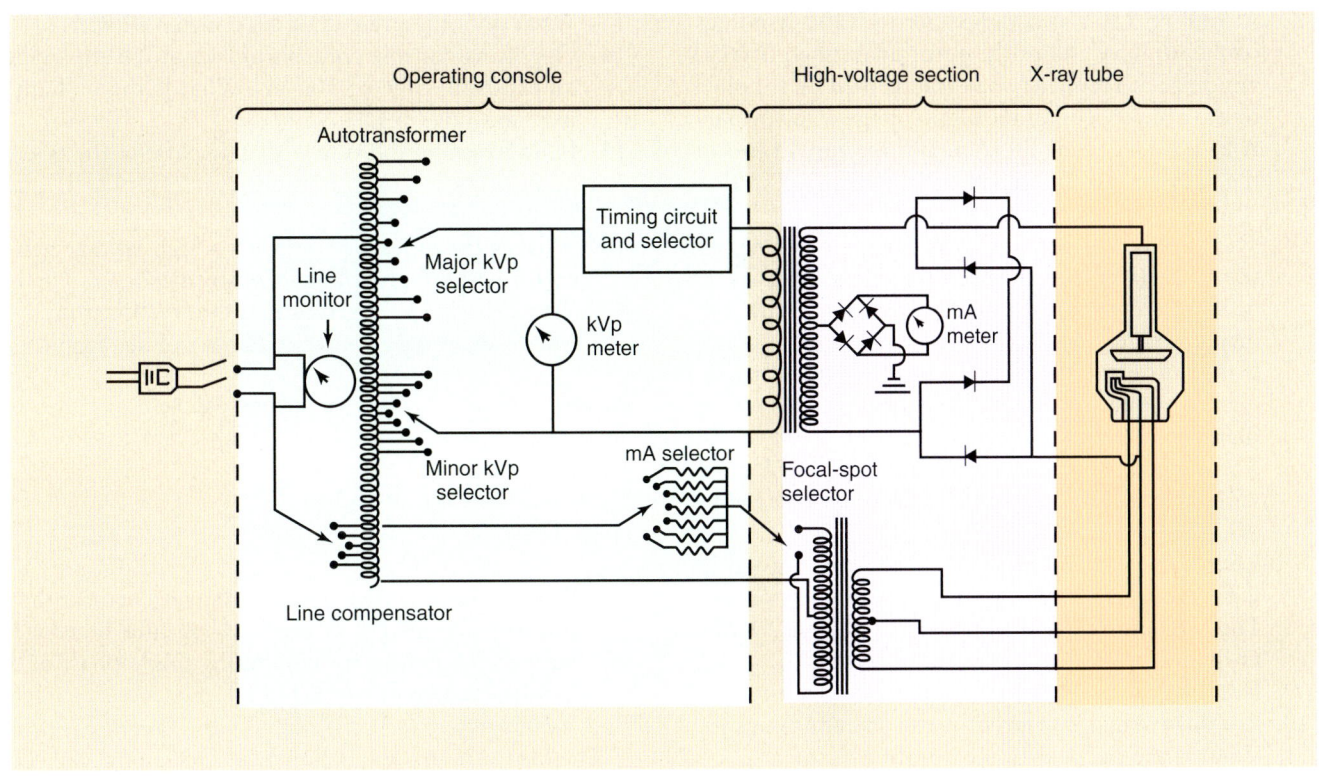

FIG. 6.32 The schematic circuit of an x-ray imaging system.

Single-phase generators have 100% voltage ripple and are less efficient x-ray generators. Consequently, the single-phase expression of power rating is as follows.

Question: A single-phase radiographic unit installed in a private office reaches maximum capacity at 100 ms of 120 kVp and 500 mA. What is its power rating?

Answer: Power rating (kW)
$$= (0.7)\frac{(500 \text{ mA})(120 \text{ kVp})}{1000}$$
$$= 42 \text{ kW}$$

X-ray Circuit

Fig. 6.32 is a simplified schematic diagram of the three main sections of the x-ray imaging system: the x-ray tube, the operating console, and the high-voltage generator. This figure also shows the locations of all meters, controls, and important components.

SUMMARY

The x-ray imaging system has three principal sections: (1) the operating console, (2) the x-ray tube, and (3) the high-voltage generator. The design and operation of the x-ray tube are discussed in Chapter 7.

The operating console consists of an on/off control and controls to select kVp, mA, and time or mAs. The AECs are also located on the operating console.

The high-voltage generator provides power to the x-ray tube in three possible ways: single-phase power, three-phase power, and high-frequency power. The difference between single- and three-phase power involves the manner in which the high-voltage step-up transformer is electrically positioned. With three-phase power, the voltage across the x-ray tube is nearly constant during exposure and never drops to zero, as does the voltage for single-phase power.

The components of an x-ray imaging system are sometimes identified by their power rating in kilowatts (kW). Maximum available power for high-voltage generators equals the maximum tube current (mA) at 100 kVp for an exposure of 100 ms.

CHALLENGE QUESTIONS

1. Define or otherwise identify the following:
    a. Semiconductor
    b. Automatic exposure control (AEC)
    c. Line compensation
    d. Capacitor
    e. mA meter location
    f. Diode
    g. Voltage ripple
    h. Rectification
    i. Autotransformer
    j. Power

2. A total of 220 V is supplied across 1200 windings of the primary coil of the autotransformer. If 1650 windings are tapped, what voltage will be supplied to the primary coil of the high-voltage transformer?
3. A kVp meter reads 86 kVp, and the turns ratio of the high-voltage step-up transformer is 1200. What is the true voltage across the meter?
4. The supply voltage from the autotransformer to the filament transformer is 60 V. If the turns ratio of the filament transformer is 1/2, what is the filament voltage?
5. If the current in the primary of the filament transformer in question 4 were 0.5 A, what would be the filament current?
6. The supply to a high-voltage step-up transformer with a turns ratio of 550 is 190 V. What is the voltage across the x-ray tube?
7. Locate the various meters and controls shown in Fig. 6.32 on an x-ray imaging system you operate.
8. The radiographic table must be radiolucent. Define radiolucent.
9. Describe the movements of a patient couch.
10. List the five major controls on the operating console.
11. What is the purpose of the autotransformer?
12. How does primary voltage relate to secondary voltage in an autotransformer?
13. What does the prereading kVp meter allow?
14. Operating console controls are set at 200 mA with an exposure time of 100 ms. What is the milliampere-seconds (mAs)?
15. In an examination of a pediatric patient, the operating console controls are set at 600 mA/30 ms. What is the mAs?
16. What is the difference between a high-voltage generator and a high-voltage transformer?
17. Why does the x-ray circuit require rectification?
18. Match the power source with the voltage ripple.

Power	% Voltage Ripple
Single phase	14
Three phase, six pulse	100
Three phase, 12 pulse	14
High frequency	1

19. What is the only type of high-voltage generator that can be positioned in or on the x-ray tube housing?
20. State the equations for computing single-phase and high-frequency power rating.

The answers to the Challenge Questions can be found by logging on to our website at http://evolve.elsevier.com.

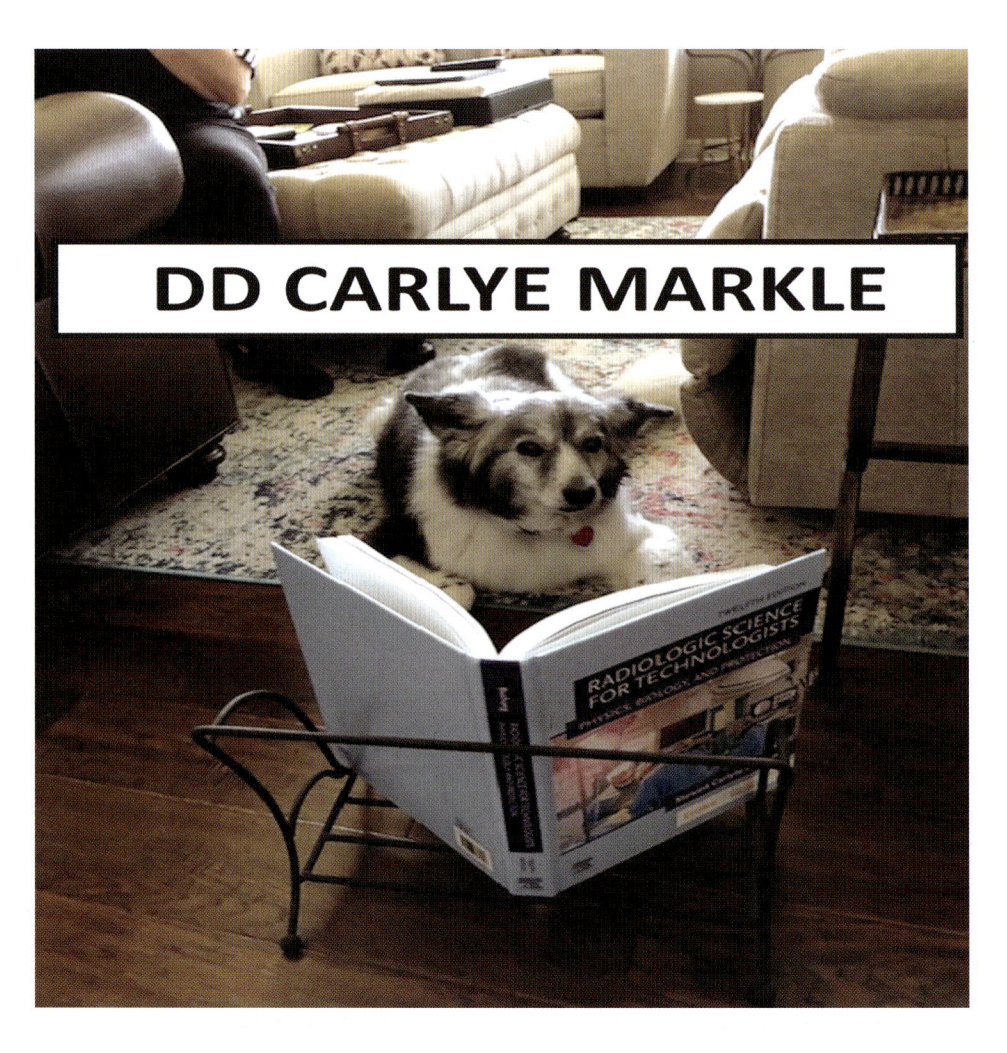

The X-ray Tube

CHAPTER 7

OBJECTIVES

At the completion of this chapter, the student should be able to do the following:

1. Describe the general design of an x-ray tube.
2. List the external components that house and protect the x-ray tube.
3. Discuss the cathode and filament currents.
4. Describe the parts of the anode and the induction motor.
5. Define the line-focus principle.
6. What is the heel effect, and how does it affect image quality?
7. Explain and interpret x-ray tube rating charts.

OUTLINE

External Components 112
   Ceiling Support System 112
   Floor-to-Ceiling Support System 112
   C-Arm Support System 112
   Protective Housing 113
   Glass or Metal Enclosure 113
Internal Components 114
   Cathode 114
   Anode 116
X-ray Tube Failure 123
Rating Charts 125
   Radiographic Rating Chart 125
   Anode Cooling Chart 126
   Housing Cooling Chart 127
Summary 127
Challenge Questions 128

THE X-RAY tube is a component of the x-ray imaging system rarely seen by radiographers. It is contained in a protective housing and therefore is inaccessible. Fig. 7.1 is a schematic diagram of a rotating anode diagnostic x-ray tube. Its components are considered separately, but it should be clear that there are two primary parts: the cathode and the anode. Each of these is an electrode, and any electronic tube with two electrodes is a diode. An x-ray tube is a special type of diode.

The external structure of the x-ray tube consists of three parts: the support structure, the protective housing, and the glass or metal enclosure. The internal structures of the x-ray tube are the anode and the cathode.

An explanation of the external components of the x-ray tube and the internal structure of the x-ray tube follows. The causes and prevention of x-ray tube failure are discussed.

With proper use, an x-ray tube used in general radiography should last many years. X-ray tubes used in computed tomography (CT) and interventional radiology generally have a shorter life.

EXTERNAL COMPONENTS

The x-ray tube and housing assembly are quite heavy; therefore they require a support mechanism so the radiographer can position them.

Ceiling Support System

The ceiling support system is probably the most frequently used. It consists of two perpendicular sets of ceiling-mounted rails. This allows for both longitudinal and transverse travel of the x-ray tube.

A telescoping column attaches the x-ray tube housing to the rails, allowing for variable source-to-image receptor distance (SID). When the x-ray tube is centered above the examination table at the standard SID, the x-ray tube is in a preferred **detent position**.

Other positions can be chosen and locked by the radiographer. Some ceiling-supported x-ray tubes have a single control that removes all locks, allowing the tube to "float." This lock should be used only for minor adjustments and should not be used to move the tube farther than about 1 m because arm and shoulder strain can occur.

Floor-to-Ceiling Support System

The floor-to-ceiling x-ray tube support system has a single column with rollers at each end: one attached to a ceiling-mounted rail and the other attached to a floor-mounted rail. The x-ray tube slides up and down the column as the column rotates. A variation of this type of support system has the column positioned on a single floor support system with one or two floor-mounted rails.

C-Arm Support System

Interventional radiology suites often are equipped with C-arm support systems (Fig. 7.2), so called because the system is shaped like a C. These systems are ceiling mounted or mobile and provide for very flexible x-ray tube positioning. The image receptor is attached to the other end of the C-arm from the x-ray tube. Variations called L-arm or U-arm support are also common.

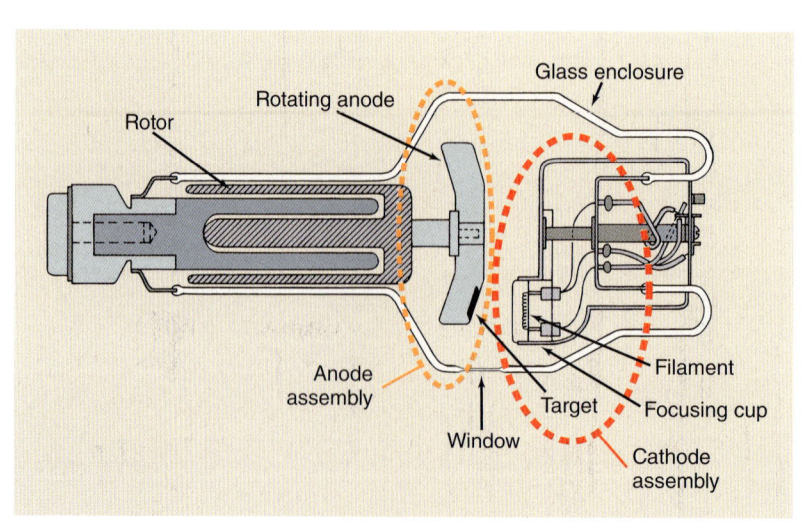

FIG. 7.1 Principal parts of a rotating anode x-ray tube.

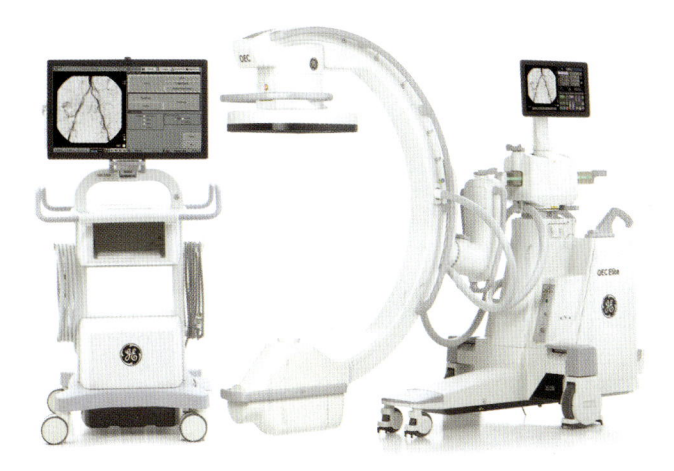

FIG. 7.2 Mobile C-arm support; one method of supporting an x-ray tube. (Courtesy GE Healthcare.)

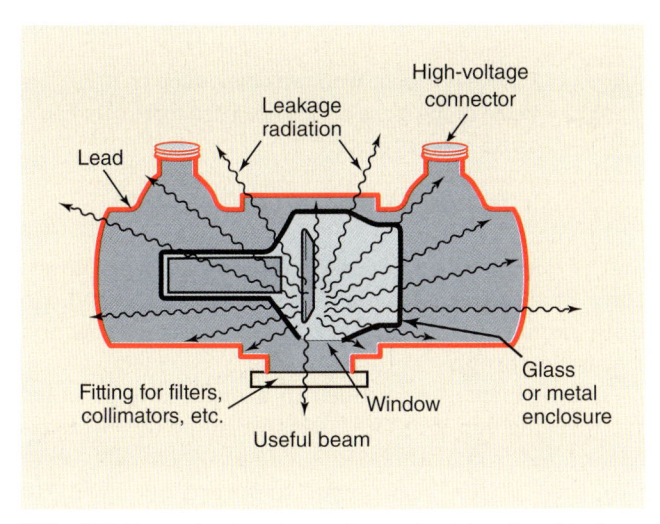

FIG. 7.3 Protective housing reduces the intensity of leakage radiation to less than 1 mGy$_a$/h at 1 m.

Protective Housing

When x-rays are produced, they are emitted **isotropically**—that is, with equal intensity in all directions. We use only x-rays emitted through the special section of the x-ray tube housing called the **window** (Fig. 7.3). The x-rays emitted through the window are called the **useful beam**.

X-rays that escape through the protective housing are called **leakage radiation**; they contribute nothing in the way of diagnostic information and result in unnecessary exposure of the patient and the radiographer. Properly designed protective housing reduces the level of leakage radiation to less than 1 mGy$_a$/h at 1 m when operated at maximum conditions.

> Protective housing guards against excessive radiation exposure and electric shock.

The protective housing incorporates specially designed high-voltage receptacles to protect against accidental electric shock. Death by electrocution was a very real hazard for early radiographers. The protective housing also provides **mechanical support** for the x-ray tube and protects the tube from damage caused by rough handling.

The protective housing around some x-ray tubes contains oil that serves as both an insulator against electric shock and as a thermal cushion to dissipate heat. Some protective housings have a cooling fan to air cool the tube or the oil in which the x-ray tube is immersed. A bellows-like device allows the oil to expand when heated. If the expansion is too great, a microswitch is activated, so the tube cannot be used until it cools.

Glass or Metal Enclosure

An x-ray tube is an electronic vacuum tube with components contained within a glass or metal enclosure. The x-ray tube, however, is a special type of vacuum tube that contains two electrodes: the cathode and the anode. It is relatively large, perhaps 30 to 50 cm long and 20 cm in diameter. The glass enclosure is made of Pyrex glass to enable it to withstand the tremendous heat that is generated.

> X-ray tubes are designed with a glass or a metal enclosure.

The enclosure maintains a vacuum inside the x-ray tube. This vacuum allows for more efficient x-ray production and a longer tube life. When just a little gas is in the enclosure, the electron flow from the cathode to anode is reduced, fewer x-rays are produced, and more heat is generated.

Early x-ray tubes, modifications of the Crookes tube, were not vacuum tubes but rather contained controlled quantities of gas within the enclosure. The modern x-ray tube, the Coolidge tube, is a vacuum tube. If it becomes gassy, x-ray production falls and the tube can fail.

An improvement in x-ray tube design incorporates metal rather than glass as part or all of the enclosure. As a glass enclosure tube ages, some tungsten vaporizes and coats the inside of the glass enclosure. This alters the electrical properties of the tube, allowing tube electric current to stray and interact with the glass enclosure; the result is arcing and tube failure.

Metal enclosure x-ray tubes maintain a constant electric potential between the electrons of the tube electric current and the enclosure. Therefore they have a longer life and are less likely to fail. Virtually all high-capacity x-ray tubes now use metal enclosures.

The x-ray tube window is an area of the glass or metal enclosure, approximately 5 cm^2, that is thin and through which the useful beam of x-rays is emitted.

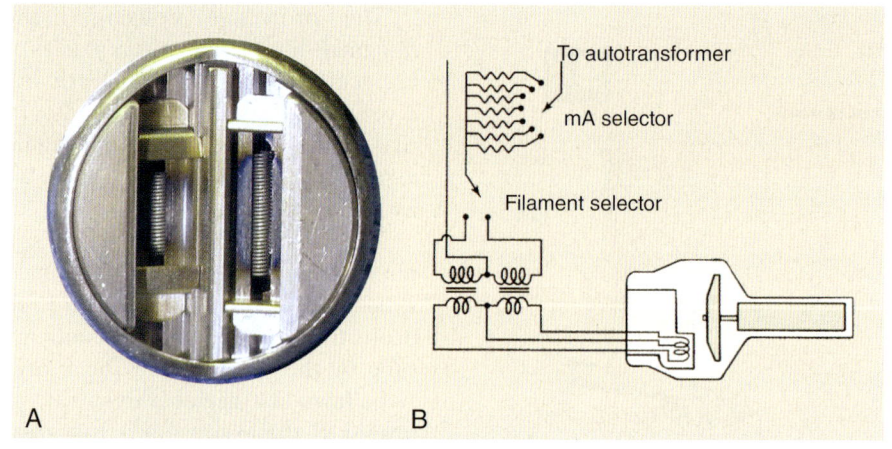

FIG. 7.4 (A) Dual-filament cathode designed to provide focal spots of 0.5 mm and 1.5 mm. (B) Schematic for a dual-filament cathode.

INTERNAL COMPONENTS
Cathode

Such a window allows for the maximum emission of x-rays with minimum absorption.

Fig. 7.4 shows a photograph of a dual-filament cathode and a schematic drawing of its electric supply. The two filaments supply separate electron beams to produce two focal spots.

> The cathode is the negative side of the x-ray tube. It has two primary parts: a filament and a focusing cup.

The **filament** is a coil of wire similar to that in a kitchen toaster, but it is much smaller. The filament is approximately 2 mm in diameter and 1 or 2 cm long. In the kitchen toaster, an electric current is conducted through the coil, causing it to glow and emit a large quantity of heat.

An x-ray tube filament emits electrons when it is heated. When the current through the filament is sufficiently high, the outer-shell electrons of the filament atoms are "boiled off" and ejected from the filament. This phenomenon is known as **thermionic emission**.

Filaments are usually made of **thoriated tungsten**. Tungsten provides for higher thermionic emission than other metals. Its melting point is 3410°C; therefore it is not likely to burn out like the filament of a light bulb. Also, tungsten does not vaporize easily. If it did, the tube would become gassy quickly, and its internal parts would be coated with tungsten. The addition of 1% to 2% thorium to the tungsten filament enhances the efficiency of thermionic emission and prolongs tube life.

> Tungsten vaporization, with deposition on the inside of the glass enclosure, is the most common cause of tube failure.

Ultimately, however, tungsten metal does vaporize and is deposited on internal components. This upsets some of the electric characteristics of the tube and can cause arcing and lead to tube failure. Such malfunction is usually abrupt.

The filament is embedded in a metal shroud called the **focusing cup** (Fig. 7.5). Because all of the electrons accelerated from cathode to anode are electrically negative, the electron beam tends to spread out owing to electrostatic repulsion. Some electrons can even miss the anode completely.

The focusing cup is negatively charged so that it electrostatically confines the electron beam to a small area of the anode (Fig. 7.6). The effectiveness of the focusing cup is determined by its size and shape, its charge, the filament size and shape, and the position of the filament in the focusing cup.

Most rotating anode x-ray tubes have two filaments mounted in the cathode assembly "side by side," creating large and small focal spot sizes. Filaments in biangular x-ray tubes have to be placed "end to end," with the small focus filament above the large filament.

Certain types of x-ray tubes called **grid-controlled** tubes are designed to be turned on and off very rapidly. Grid-controlled tubes are used in portable capacitor discharge imaging systems, interventional radiology, and cineradiography, each of which requires multiple exposures for precise exposure time.

The term **grid** is borrowed from vacuum tube electronics and refers to an element in the x-ray tube that acts as the switch. In a grid-controlled x-ray tube, the focusing cup is the grid and therefore the exposure switch.

CHAPTER 7 The X-ray Tube 115

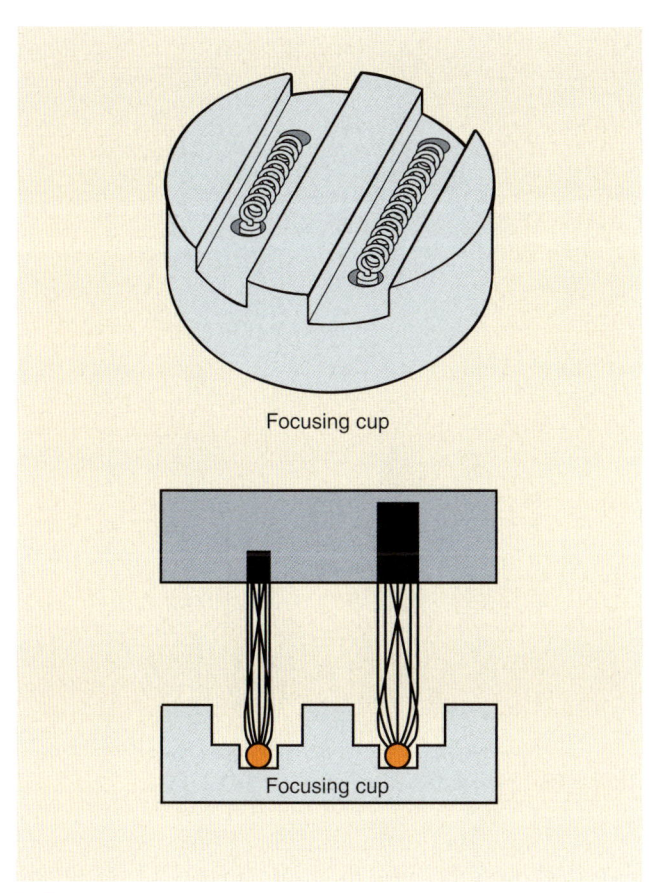

FIG. 7.5 The focusing cup is a metal shroud that surrounds the filament.

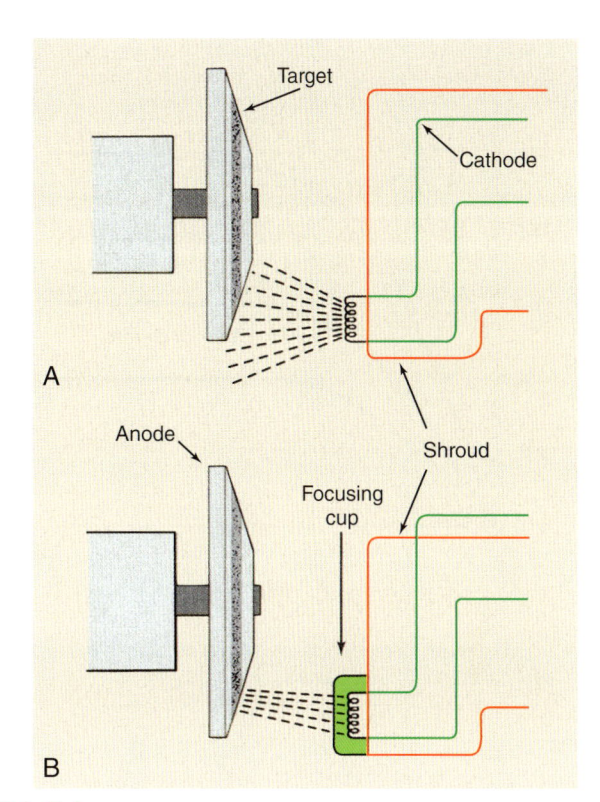

FIG. 7.6 (A) Without a focusing cup, the electron beam is spread beyond the anode because of mutual electrostatic repulsion among the electrons. (B) With a focusing cup that is negatively charged, the electron beam is condensed and directed to the target.

When the x-ray imaging system is first turned on, a low current passes through the filament to warm it and prepare it for the thermal jolt necessary for x-ray production. At low filament current, there is no tube current because the filament does not get hot enough for thermionic emission. When the filament current is high enough for thermionic emission, a small increase in filament current results in a large increase in x-ray tube current.

> The x-ray tube current is adjusted by controlling the filament current.

This relationship between filament current and x-ray tube current depends on the tube voltage (Fig. 7.7). Fixed stations of 100, 200, 300 mA, and so forth usually correspond to discrete connections on the filament transformer or to precision resistors.

When emitted from the filament, electrons are in the vicinity of the filament before they are accelerated to the anode. Because these electrons carry negative charges, they repel one another and tend to form a cloud around the filament.

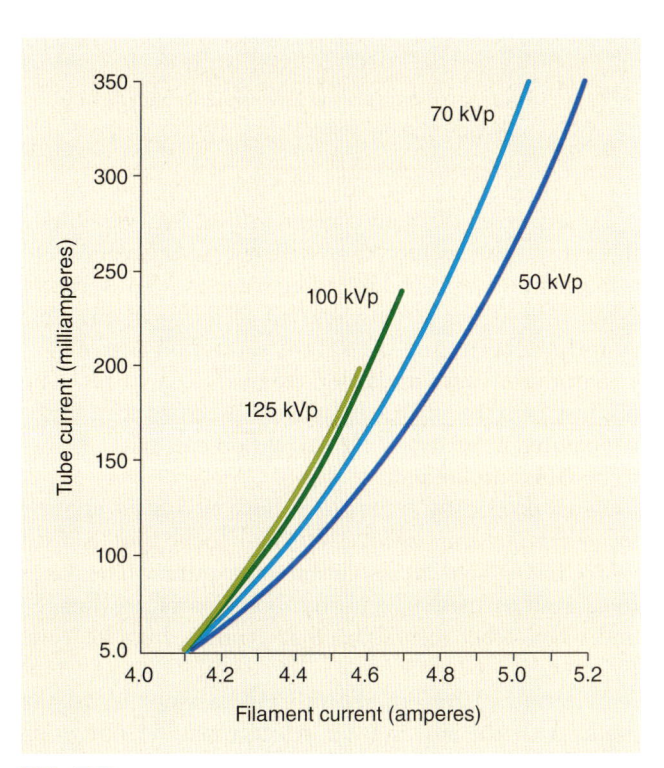

FIG. 7.7 The x-ray tube current is actually controlled by changing the filament current. Because of thermionic emission, a small change in filament current results in a large change in tube current.

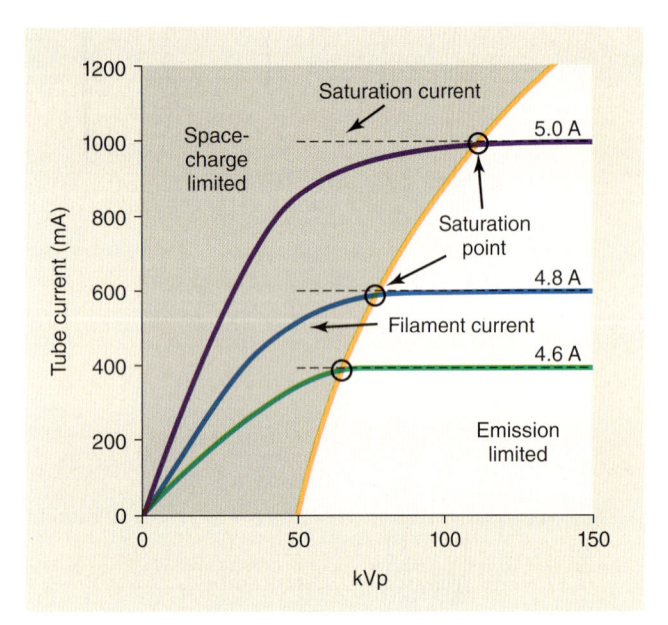

FIG. 7.8 At a given filament current, tube current reaches a maximum level called saturation current.

This cloud of electrons, called a space charge, makes it difficult for subsequent electrons to be emitted by the filament because of electrostatic repulsion. This phenomenon is called the **space charge effect**. A major obstacle in producing x-ray tubes with currents that exceed 1000 mA is the design of adequate space charge–compensating devices.

> Thermionic emission at low kVp and high mA can be space charge limited.

At any given filament current—say, 4.8 A (Fig. 7.8)—the x-ray tube current rises with increasing voltage to a maximum value. A further increase in kVp does not result in a higher mA because all of the available electrons have been used. This is the **saturation current**.

Saturation current is not reached at a lower kVp because of space charge limitation. When an x-ray tube is operated at or below the saturation current, it is said to be **emission limited**.

Most diagnostic x-ray tubes have two focal spots—termed *large* and *small*. The small focal spot is used when better spatial resolution is required. The large focal spot is used when large body parts are imaged and when other techniques that produce high heat are required.

Selection of one or the other focal spot is usually made with the mA station selector on the operating console. Normally, either filament can be used with the lower mA stations—approximately 300 mA or less. At approximately 400 mA and higher, only the larger focal

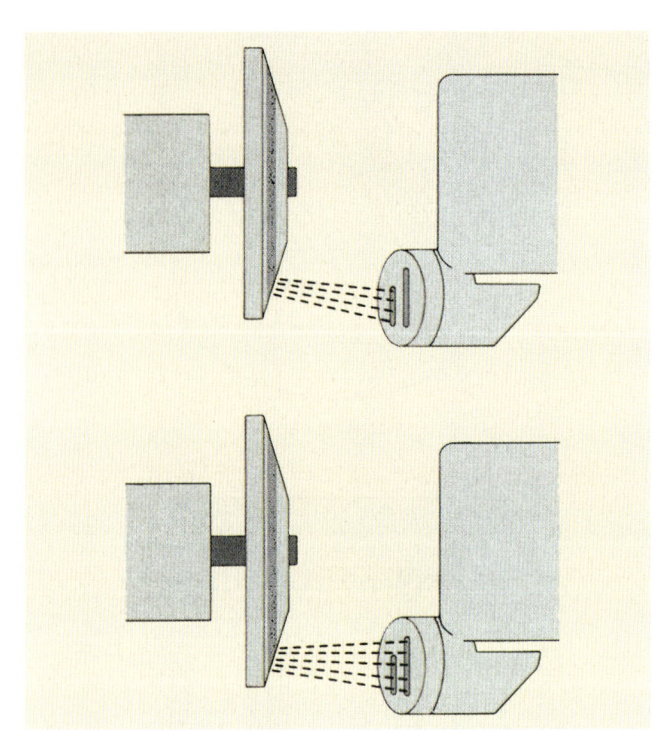

FIG. 7.9 In a dual-focus x-ray tube, focal spot size is controlled by heating one of the two filaments.

spot is allowed because the heat capacity of the anode could be exceeded if the small focal spot were used.

Small focal spots range from 0.1 to 1 mm; large focal spots range from 0.3 to 2 mm. Each filament of a dual-filament cathode assembly is embedded in the focusing cup (Fig. 7.9). The small focal spot size is associated with the small filament, and the large focal spot size is associated with the large filament. An electric current is directed through the appropriate filament.

Anode

The anode is the positive side of the x-ray tube. There are two types of anodes, **stationary** and **rotating** (Fig. 7.10). Stationary anode x-ray tubes are used in dental x-ray imaging systems, some portable imaging systems, and other special-purpose units in which high tube current and power are not required. General-purpose x-ray tubes use the rotating anode because they must be capable of producing high-intensity x-ray beams in a short time.

> The anode is the positive side of the x-ray tube; it conducts electricity and radiates heat and x-rays from the target.

The anode serves three functions in an x-ray tube. The anode is an electrical conductor. It receives electrons emitted by the cathode and conducts them

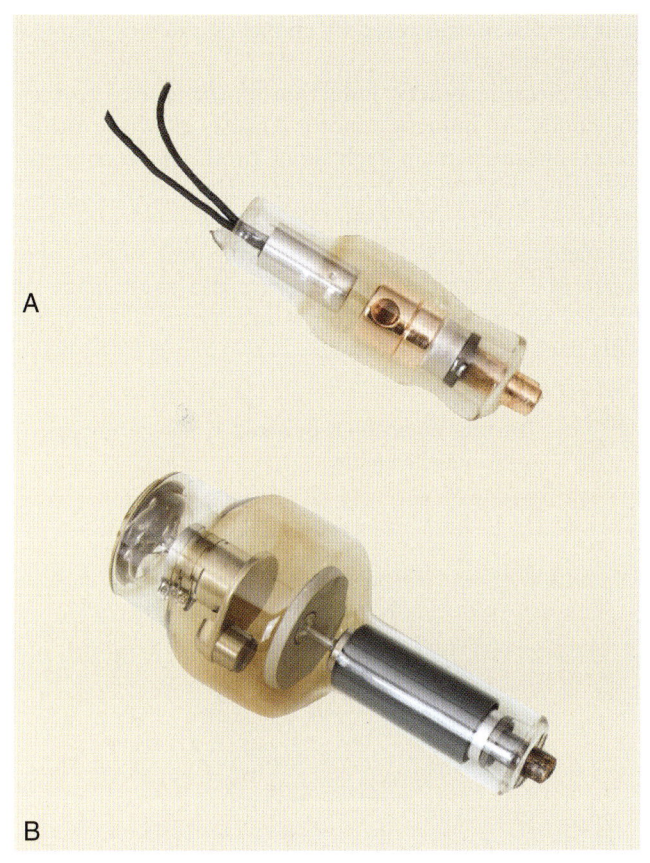

FIG. 7.10 All diagnostic x-ray tubes can be classified according to the type of anode. (A) Stationary anode. (B) Rotating anode.

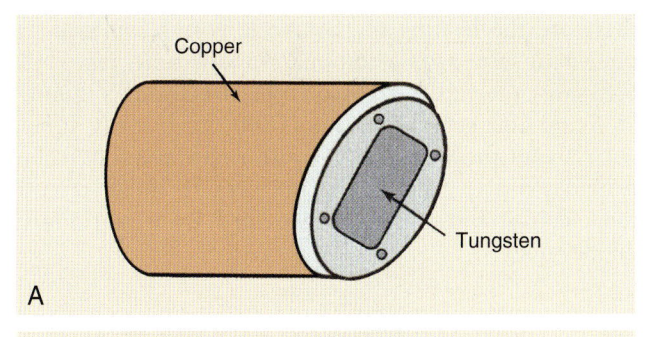

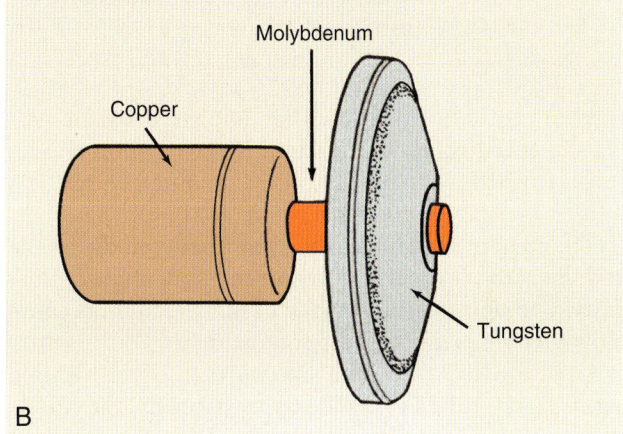

FIG. 7.11 (A) In a stationary anode tube, the target is embedded in the anode. (B) In a rotating anode tube, the target is the rotating disc.

through the tube to the connecting cables and back to the high-voltage generator. The anode also provides mechanical support for the target.

The anode also must be a good thermal dissipator. When the projectile electrons from the cathode interact with the anode, more than 99% of their kinetic energy is converted into heat. This heat must be dissipated quickly. Copper, molybdenum, and graphite are the most common anode materials. Adequate heat dissipation is the major engineering hurdle in designing higher capacity x-ray tubes.

The **target** is the area of the anode struck by the electrons from the cathode. In stationary anode tubes, the target consists of a tungsten alloy embedded in the copper anode (Fig. 7.11A). In rotating anode tubes, the entire rotating disc is the target (Fig. 7.11B).

Alloying the tungsten (usually with rhenium) gives it added mechanical strength to withstand the stresses of high-speed rotation and the effects of repetitive thermal expansion and contraction. High-capacity x-ray tubes have molybdenum or graphite layered under the tungsten target (Fig. 7.12). Both molybdenum and graphite have lower mass density than tungsten, making the anode lighter and easier to rotate.

> **THE TUNGSTEN TARGET**
> Tungsten is the target material of choice for general radiography for three main reasons:
> 1. **Atomic number**—Tungsten's high atomic number, 74, results in high-efficiency x-ray production and in high-energy x-rays. The reason for this is discussed more fully in Chapter 8.
> 2. **Thermal conductivity**—Tungsten has a thermal conductivity nearly equal to that of copper. It is thus an efficient metal for dissipating the heat produced.
> 3. **High melting point**—Any material, if heated sufficiently, will melt and become liquid. Tungsten has a high melting point (3400°C, compared with 1100°C for copper) and therefore can stand up under high tube electric current without pitting or bubbling.

Specialty x-ray tubes for mammography have molybdenum or rhodium targets principally because of their low atomic number and low K-characteristic x-ray energy. This concept is discussed fully in Chapter 8. Table 7.1 summarizes the properties of these target materials.

The rotating anode x-ray tube allows the electron beam to interact with a much larger target area;

therefore the heating of the anode is not confined to one small spot, as in a stationary anode tube. Fig. 7.13 compares the target areas of typical stationary anode (4 mm²) and rotating anode (1800 mm²) x-ray tubes with 1-mm focal spots. Thus the rotating anode tube provides nearly 500 times more area to interact with the electron beam than is provided by a stationary anode tube.

> Higher x-ray tube currents and shorter exposure times are possible with the rotating anode.

Heat capacity can be further improved by increasing the speed of anode rotation. Most rotating anodes revolve at 3400 rpm (revolutions per minute). The anodes of high-capacity x-ray tubes rotate at 10,000 rpm.

The stem of the anode is the shaft between the anode and the rotor. It is narrow to reduce its thermal conductivity. The stem is usually made of molybdenum because molybdenum is a poor heat conductor.

Occasionally, the rotor mechanism of a rotating anode x-ray tube fails. When this happens, the anode becomes overheated and pits or cracks, causing tube failure (Fig. 7.14).

How does the anode rotate inside an enclosure with no mechanical connection to the outside? Most things that revolve are powered by chains or axles or gears of some sort.

An electromagnetic **induction motor** is used to turn the anode. An induction motor consists of two principal parts separated from each other by the glass or metal enclosure (Fig. 7.15). The part outside the glass or metal enclosure, called the **stator**, consists of a series of electromagnets equally spaced around the neck of the tube. Inside the glass or metal enclosure is a shaft made of bars of copper and soft iron fabricated into one mass. This part is called the **rotor**.

> The rotating anode is powered by an electromagnetic induction motor.

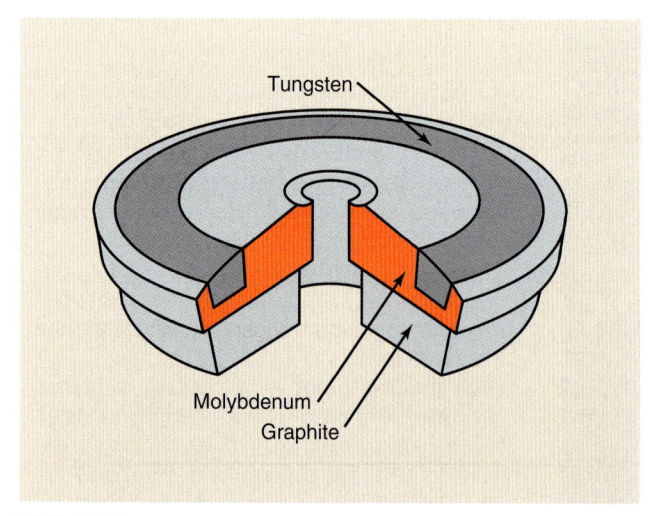

FIG. 7.12 A layered anode consists of a target surface backed by one or more layers to increase heat capacity.

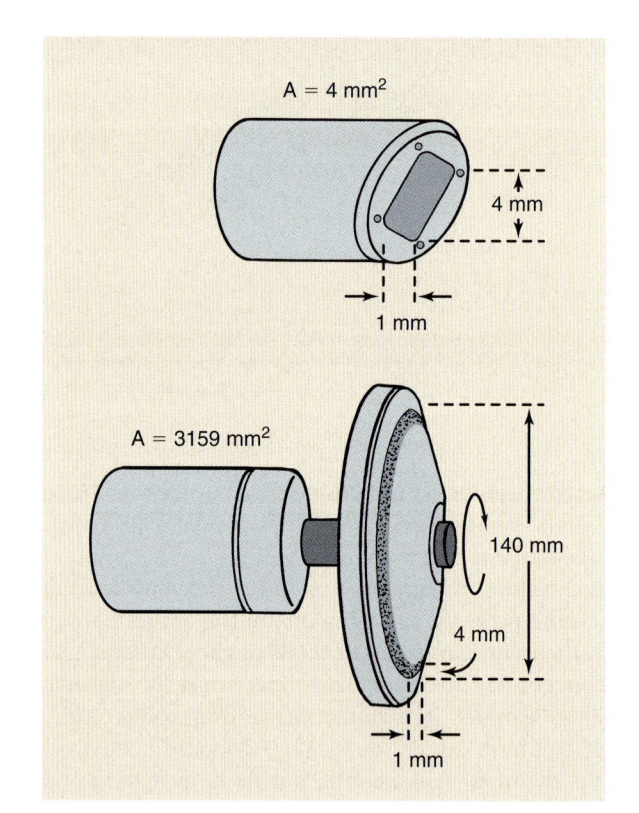

FIG. 7.13 Stationary anode tube with a 1-mm focal spot may have a target area of 4 mm². A comparable 15-cm diameter rotating anode tube can have a target area of approximately 1800 mm², which increases the heating capacity of the tube by a factor of nearly 500.

TABLE 7.1	Characteristics of X-ray Targets			
Element	Chemical Symbol	Atomic Number	K X-ray Energy (keV)[a]	Melting Temperature (°C)
Tungsten	W	74	69	3400
Molybdenum	Mo	42	19	2600
Rhodium	Rh	45	23	3200

[a]X-rays resulting from electron transitions into the K shell.

CHAPTER 7 The X-ray Tube 119

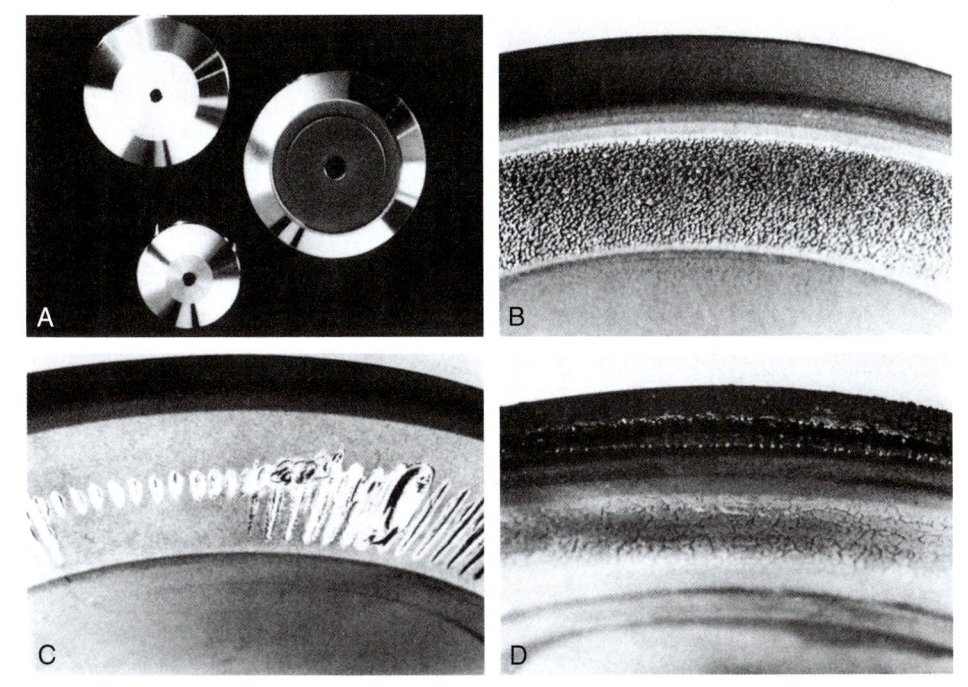

FIG. 7.14 Comparison of smooth, shiny appearances of rotating anodes when new (A) versus their appearance after failure (B, C, and D). Examples of anode separation and surface melting shown were caused by slow rotation caused by bearing damage (B), repeated overload (C), and exceeding maximum heat storage capacity (D). (Courtesy Philips Medical Systems.)

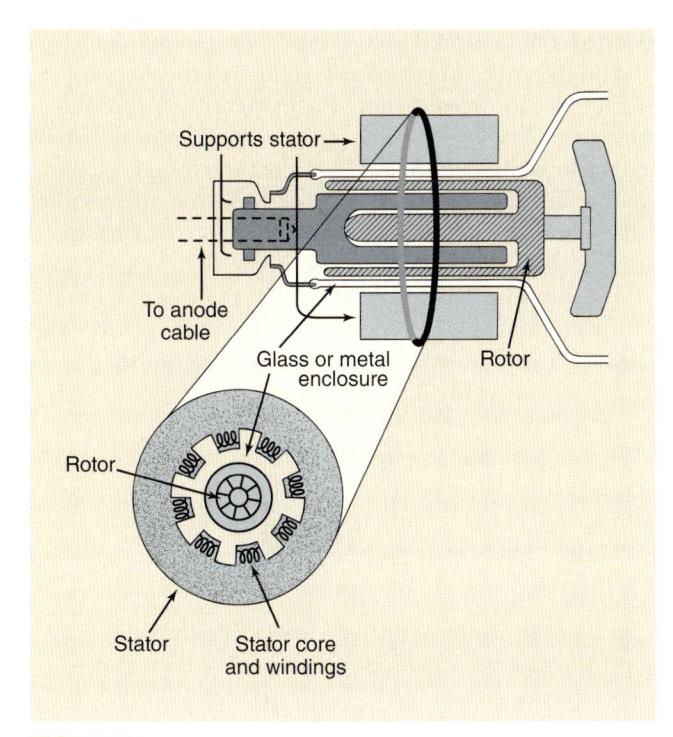

FIG. 7.15 The target of a rotating anode tube is powered by an induction motor, the principal components of which are the stator and the rotor.

The induction motor works through electromagnetic induction, similar to a transformer. Current in each stator winding induces a magnetic field that surrounds the rotor. The stator windings are energized sequentially so that the induced magnetic field rotates on the axis of the stator. This magnetic field interacts with the ferromagnetic rotor, causing it to rotate synchronously with the activated stator windings.

When the radiographer pushes the exposure button of a radiographic imaging system, there is a short delay before an exposure is made. This allows the rotor to accelerate to its designated rpm while the filament is heated. Only then is the kVp applied to the x-ray tube.

During this time, filament current is increased to provide the correct x-ray tube current. When a two-position exposure switch is used, the switch should be pushed to its final position in one motion. This minimizes the time that the filament is heated and prolongs tube life.

When the exposure is completed on imaging systems equipped with high-speed rotors, one can hear the rotor slow down and stop within approximately 1 minute. The high-speed rotor slows down as quickly as it does because the induction motor is put into reverse. The rotor is a precisely balanced, low-friction device that, if left alone, might take many minutes to coast to rest after use.

In a new x-ray tube, the coast time is approximately 60 seconds. With age, the coast time is reduced because of wear of the rotor bearings.

One design that allows for massive anodes uses a shaft fixed at each end (Fig. 7.16). In this x-ray tube, the anode is attached to the enclosure and the whole insert rotates. The cathode is positioned on the axis, and the electron beam is deflected electromagnetically onto the anode.

120   PART II   X-Radiation

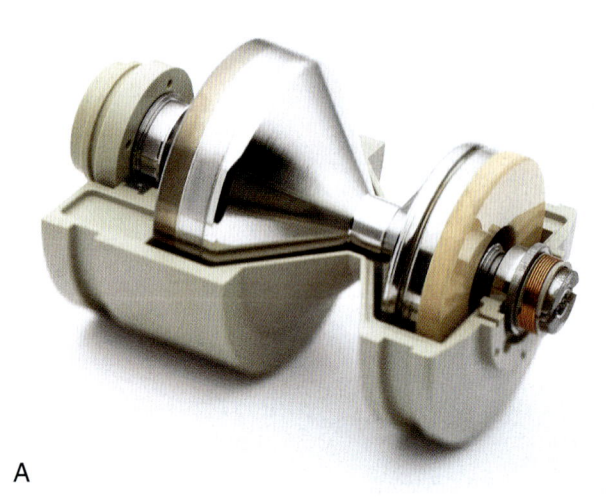

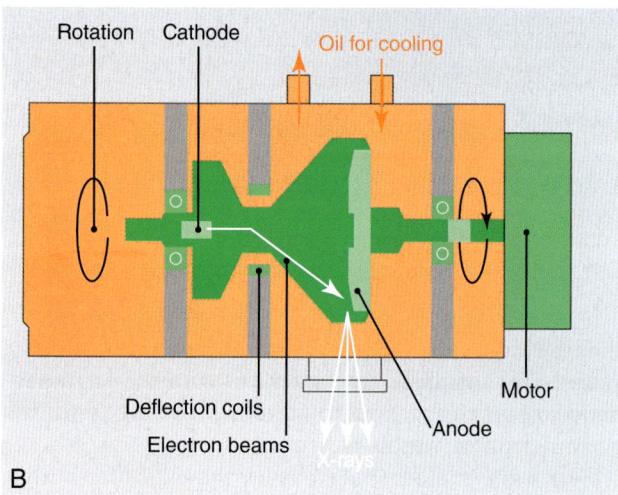

FIG. 7.16 (A) This very high-capacity x-ray tube revolves in a bath of oil for complete heat dissipation. (B) The cooling capacity is greater than any heat load. (Courtesy Siemens Medical Systems.)

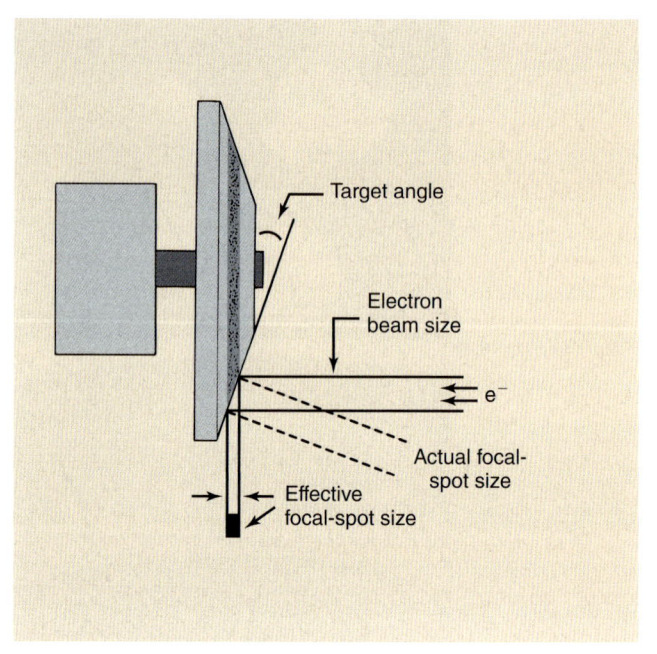

FIG. 7.17 The line-focus principle allows high anode heating with small effective focal spots. As the target angle decreases, so too does the effective focal spot size.

Because the disc is part of the enclosure, the cooling oil is in contact with the back of the anode, allowing optimum cooling. The principal advantages are improved heat dissipation and greater capacity.

> The focal spot is the actual x-ray source.

The focal spot is the area of the target from which x-rays are emitted. X-ray imaging requires small focal spots because the smaller the focal spot, the better the spatial resolution of the image. Unfortunately, as the size of the focal spot decreases, the heating of the target is concentrated onto a smaller area. This is one limiting factor in focal spot size.

Before the rotating anode was developed, another design was incorporated into x-ray tube targets to allow a large area for heating while maintaining a small focal spot. This design is known as the **line-focus principle**. By angling the target (Fig. 7.17), one makes the effective area of the target much smaller than the actual area of electron interaction.

The effective target area, or effective focal spot size, is the area projected onto the patient and the image receptor. This is the value given when large or small focal spots are identified. When the target angle is made smaller, the effective focal spot size is also made smaller. Diagnostic x-ray tubes have target angles that vary from approximately 5 to 20 degrees.

The limiting factor in the target angle is the ability of the cone of x-rays produced to adequately cover the largest field size used. In general radiography, this is usually taken as the diagonal of a 35-cm × 43-cm image receptor, which is approximately 55 cm.

When a smaller image receptor is used, the anode angle can be steeper. The advantage of the line-focus principle is that it simultaneously improves spatial resolution and heat capacity.

> The line-focus principle results in an effective focal spot size much less than the actual focal spot size.

Biangular targets are available that produce two focal spot sizes because of two different target angles on the anode (Fig. 7.18). Combining biangular targets with different-length filaments results in a very flexible combination.

A circular effective focal spot is preferred. Usually, however, it has a shape characterized as a double

CHAPTER 7 The X-ray Tube 121

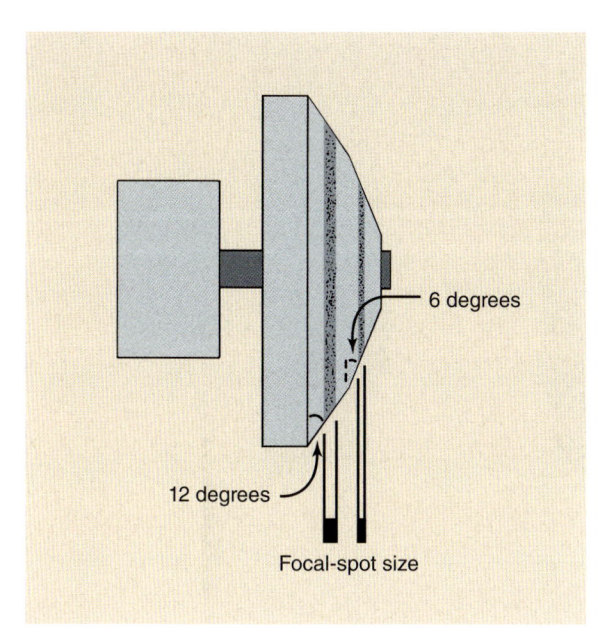

FIG. 7.18 Some targets have two angles to produce two focal spots. To achieve this, the filaments must be placed one above the other.

TABLE 7.2	Nominal Focal Spot Size Compared with Maximum Acceptable Dimensions				
NOMINAL FOCAL SPOT SIZE (MM)			**ACCEPTABLE MEASURED FOCAL SPOT SIZE (MM)**	
Width	×	Length	Width	×	Length
0.1	×	0.1	0.15	×	0.15
0.3	×	0.3	0.45	×	0.65
0.4	×	0.4	0.6	×	0.85
0.5	×	0.5	0.75	×	1.1
1.0	×	1.0	1.4	×	2.0
2.0	×	2.0	2.6	×	3.7

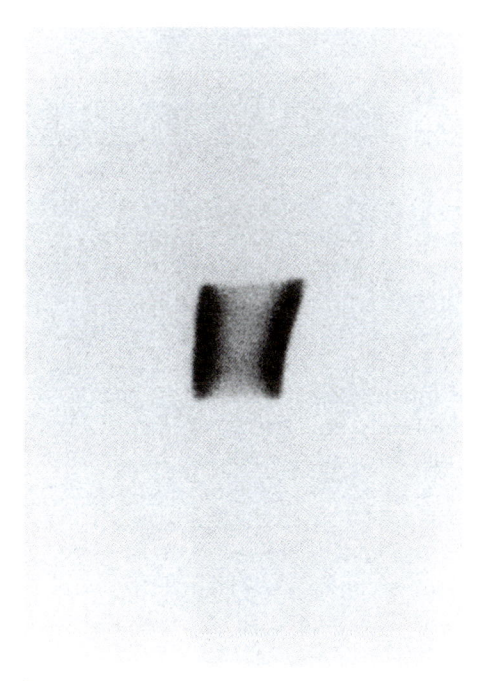

FIG. 7.19 The usual shape of a focal spot is the double banana. (Courtesy Donald Jacobson, Medical College of Wisconsin.)

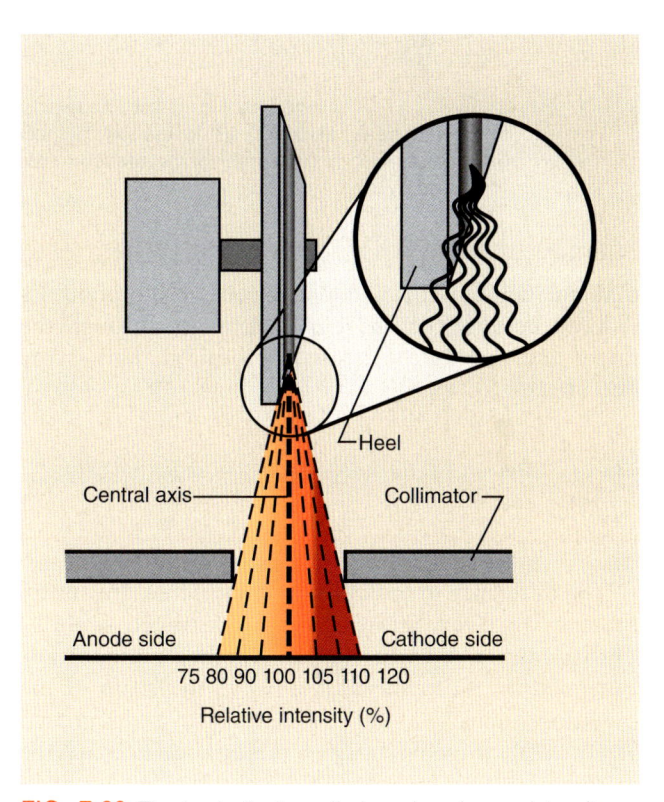

FIG. 7.20 The heel effect results in reduced x-ray intensity on the anode side of the useful beam caused by absorption in the "heel" of the target.

banana (Fig. 7.19). These differences in x-ray intensity across the focal spot are controlled principally by the design of the filament and the focusing cup and by the voltage on the focusing cup.

The National Electrical Manufacturers Association has established standards and variances for focal spot sizes. When a manufacturer states a focal spot size, that is its nominal size. Table 7.2 shows the maximum measured size permitted that is still within the standard.

One unfortunate consequence of the line-focus principle is that the radiation intensity on the cathode side of the x-ray field is greater than that on the anode side. Electrons emitted from the cathode interact with atoms of the anode at various depths into the target.

The x-rays that constitute the useful beam emitted toward the anode side must traverse a greater thickness of anode material than the x-rays emitted toward the cathode direction (Fig. 7.20). The intensity of x-rays

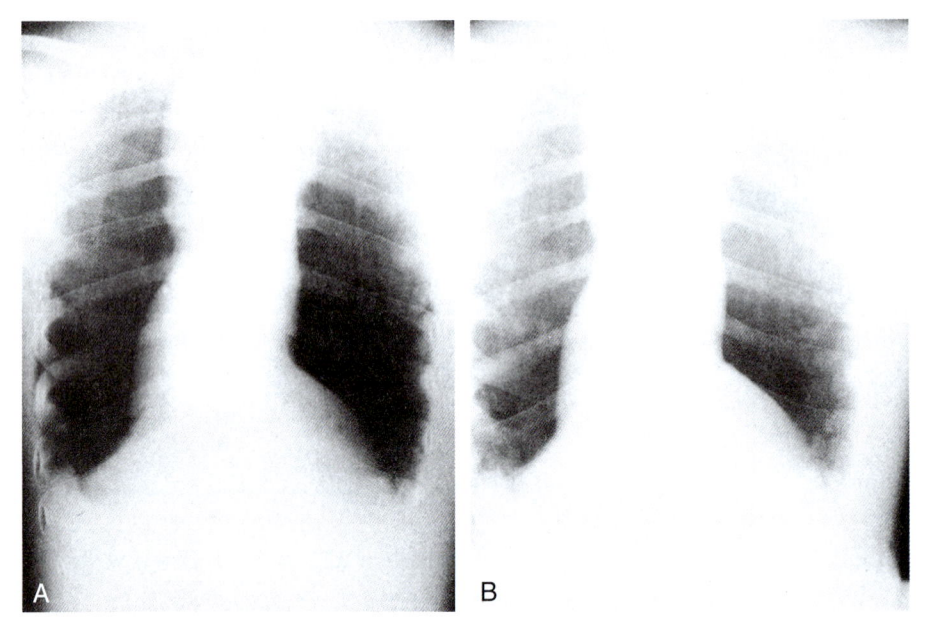

FIG. 7.21 Posteroanterior chest images demonstrate the heel effect. (A) Image taken with the cathode up (superior). (B) Image with cathode down (inferior). More uniform radiographic density is obtained with the cathode positioned to the thicker side of the anatomy, as in (A). (Courtesy Pat Duffy, Roxbury Community College.)

that are emitted through the "heel" of the anode is reduced because they have a longer path through the target and therefore increased absorption. This is the **heel effect**.

> The smaller the anode angle, the larger the heel effect.

The difference in radiation intensity across the useful beam of an x-ray field can vary by as much as 45%. The **central ray** of the useful beam is the imaginary line generated by the centermost x-ray in the beam. If the radiation intensity along the central ray is designated as 100%, then the intensity on the cathode side may be as high as 120%, and that on the anode side may be as low as 75%.

The heel effect is important when one is imaging anatomical structures that differ greatly in thickness or mass density. In general, positioning the cathode side of the x-ray tube over the thicker part of the anatomy provides more uniform x-ray exposure of the image receptor. The cathode and anode directions are usually indicated on the protective housing, sometimes near the cable connectors.

In chest radiography, for example, the cathode should be inferior. The lower thorax in the region of the diaphragm is considerably thicker than the upper thorax and therefore requires higher radiation intensity if x-ray exposure of the image receptor is to be more uniform.

In abdominal imaging, on the other hand, the cathode should be superior. The upper abdomen is thicker than the lower abdomen and pelvis, requiring greater x-ray intensity for more uniform x-ray exposure.

Fig. 7.21 shows two posteroanterior chest images—one taken with the cathode down and the other with the cathode up. Can you tell the difference? Which do you think represents better radiographic quality? Resolve the difference before looking at the figure legend.

In mammography, the x-ray tube is designed so that the more intense side of the x-ray beam, the cathode side, is positioned toward the chest wall. With angling of the x-ray tube, advantage can be taken of the foreshortening that occurs to the focal spot size, resulting in an even smaller effective focal spot size.

Another important consequence of the heel effect is the changing focal spot size. The effective focal spot is smaller on the anode side of the x-ray field than on the cathode side (Fig. 7.22). Some manufacturers of mammography equipment take advantage of this property by angling the x-ray tube to produce the smaller focal spot along the chest wall.

> The heel effect results in a smaller effective focal spot and less radiation intensity on the anode side of the x-ray beam.

X-ray tubes are designed so that projectile electrons from the cathode interact with the target only at the actual focal spot. However, some of the electrons

CHAPTER 7 The X-ray Tube   123

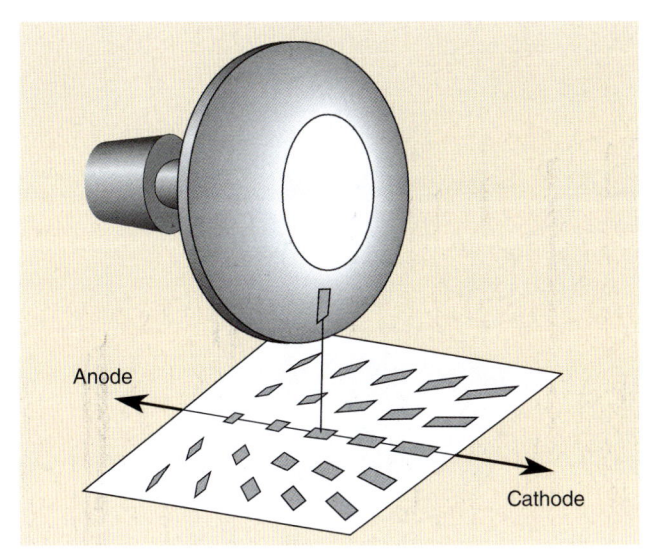

FIG. 7.22 The effective focal spot changes size and shape across the projected x-ray field.

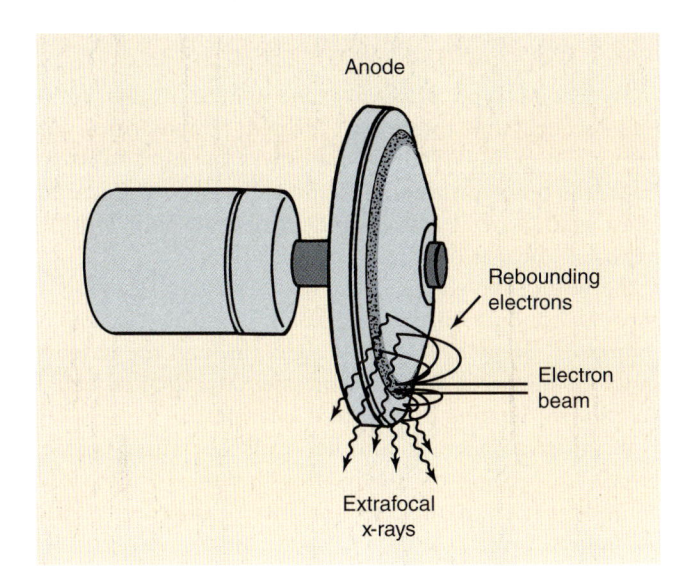

FIG. 7.23 Extrafocal x-rays result from the interaction of electrons with the anode off of the focal spot.

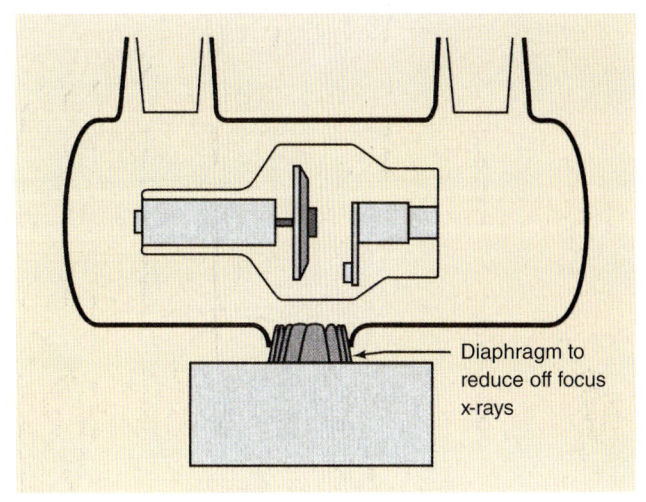

FIG. 7.24 An additional diaphragm is positioned close to the focal spot to reduce extrafocal radiation.

bounce off the focal spot and then land on other areas of the target, causing x-rays to be produced from outside the focal spot (Fig. 7.23).

These x-rays are called **off-focus radiation**. This is similar to squirting a water pistol at concrete pavement: Some of the water splashes off the pavement and lands in a larger area.

Off-focus radiation is undesirable because it extends the size of the focal spot. The additional x-ray beam area increases skin dose modestly but unnecessarily. Off-focus radiation can significantly reduce image contrast.

Finally, off-focus radiation can image patient tissue that was intended to be excluded by the variable-aperture collimators. Examples of such undesirable images are the ears in a skull examination, the soft tissue beyond the cervical spine, and the lungs beyond the borders of the thoracic spine.

Off-focus radiation is reduced by designing a fixed diaphragm in the tube housing near the window of the x-ray tube (Fig. 7.24). This is a geometric solution.

Another effective solution is the metal enclosure x-ray tube. Electrons reflected from the focal spot are extracted by the metal enclosure and conducted away. Therefore they are not available to be attracted to the target outside of the focal spot. The use of a grid does not reduce off-focus radiation.

X-RAY TUBE FAILURE

With careful use, x-ray tubes can provide many years of service. With inconsiderate use, x-ray tube life may be shortened substantially.

The length of x-ray tube life is primarily under the control of the radiographer. Basically, x-ray tube life is extended by using the minimum radiographic factors of mA, kVp, and exposure time that are appropriate for each examination. The use of faster image receptors results in longer tube life.

X-ray tube failure has several causes, most of which are related to the thermal characteristics of the x-ray tube. Enormous heat is generated in the anode of the x-ray tube during x-ray exposure. This heat must be dissipated for the x-ray tube to continue to function.

This heat can be dissipated in one of three ways: radiation, conduction, or convection (Fig. 7.25). **Radiation** is the transfer of heat by the emission of infrared radiation. Heat lamps emit not only visible light but also infrared radiation.

Conduction is the transfer of energy from one area of an object to another. The handle of a heated iron skillet becomes hot because of conduction. **Convection** is the

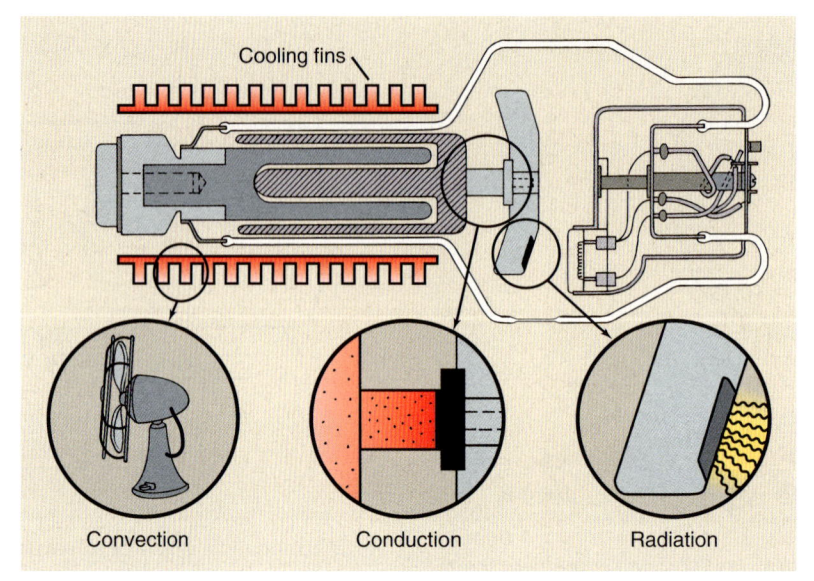

FIG. 7.25 Heat from an anode is dissipated by radiation, conduction, or convection, most often radiation.

transfer of heat by the movement of a heated substance from one place to another. Many homes and offices are heated by the convection of hot air.

> Excessive heat results in reduced x-ray tube life.

All three modes of heat transfer occur in an x-ray tube. Most of the heat is dissipated by radiation. The anode may glow red hot. It always emits infrared radiation.

Unfortunately, some heat is conducted through the neck of the anode to the rotor and glass enclosure. The heated glass enclosure raises the temperature of the oil bath; this convects the heat to the tube housing and then to the room air.

When the temperature of the anode is excessive during a single exposure, localized surface melting and pitting of the anode can occur. These surface irregularities result in variable and reduced radiation output. If surface melting is sufficiently severe, the tungsten can be vaporized and can plate the inside of the glass enclosure. This can cause filtering of the x-ray beam and interference with electron flow from the cathode to the anode.

If the temperature of the anode increases too rapidly, the anode may crack, becoming unstable in rotation and rendering the tube useless. If maximum techniques are required for a particular examination, the anode should first be warmed by low-technique operation.

> Maximum radiographic techniques should never be applied to a cold anode.

A second type of x-ray tube failure results from maintaining the anode at elevated temperatures for prolonged periods. During exposures lasting 1 to 3 seconds, the temperature of the anode may be sufficient to cause it to glow like an incandescent light bulb. During exposure, heat is dissipated by radiation.

Between exposures, heat is dissipated, primarily through conduction, to the oil bath in which the tube is immersed. Some heat is conducted through the narrow molybdenum neck to the rotor assembly; this can cause subsequent heating of the rotor bearings.

Bearing damage is another cause of tube failure. Excessive heating of the bearings results in increased rotational friction and an imbalance of the rotor anode assembly.

If thermal stress on the x-ray tube anode is maintained for prolonged periods, such as during fluoroscopy, the thermal capacity of the anode system and of the x-ray tube housing is the limitation to operation. During fluoroscopy, the x-ray tube current is usually less than 5 mA, rather than hundreds of mA as in radiography.

Under such fluoroscopic conditions, the rate of heat dissipation from the rotating target attains equilibrium with the rate of heat input, and this rate, rarely, is sufficient to cause surface defects in the target. However, the x-ray tube can fail because of the continuous heat delivered to the rotor assembly, the oil bath, and the x-ray tube housing. Bearings can fail, the glass enclosure can crack, and the tube housing can fail.

A final cause of tube failure involves the filament. Because of the high temperature of the filament, tungsten atoms are vaporized slowly and plate the inside of the glass or metal enclosure, even with normal use.

This tungsten, along with that vaporized from the anode, can disturb the electric balance of the x-ray tube, causing abrupt, intermittent changes in tube current, which often lead to arcing and tube failure.

> The most frequent cause of abrupt tube failure is electron arcing from the filament to the enclosure because of vaporized tungsten.

With excessive heating of the filament caused by high mA operation for prolonged periods, more tungsten is vaporized. The filament wire becomes thinner and eventually breaks, producing an **open filament**. This same type of failure occurs when an incandescent light bulb burns out.

In the same way that the life of a light bulb is measured in hours—2000 hours is standard—that of an x-ray tube is measured in tens of thousands of exposures. Most CT x-ray tubes are now guaranteed for 50,000 exposures.

Question: A 7-MHU helical CT x-ray tube is guaranteed for 50,000 scans, each scan limited to 5 seconds. What is the x-ray tube life in terms of hours?

Answer: Guaranteed tube life = (50,000 scans)
(5 s/scan)
= 250,000 s
= 69 hours

RATING CHARTS

Radiographers are guided in the use of x-ray tubes by **x-ray tube rating charts**. It is essential that radiographers be able to read and understand these charts, even though most of these charts are now digitally stored in the operating console.

The following material is principally for instruction purposes. Today radiographers do not get clinically involved with x-ray tube rating charts. Service engineers, on the other hand, must be well aware of such charts. Three types of x-ray tube rating charts are particularly important: the radiographic rating chart, the anode cooling chart, and the housing cooling chart.

Radiographic Rating Chart

Of the three rating charts, the radiographic rating chart is the most important because it conveys which radiographic techniques are safe and which techniques are unsafe for x-ray tube operation. Each chart shown in Fig. 7.26

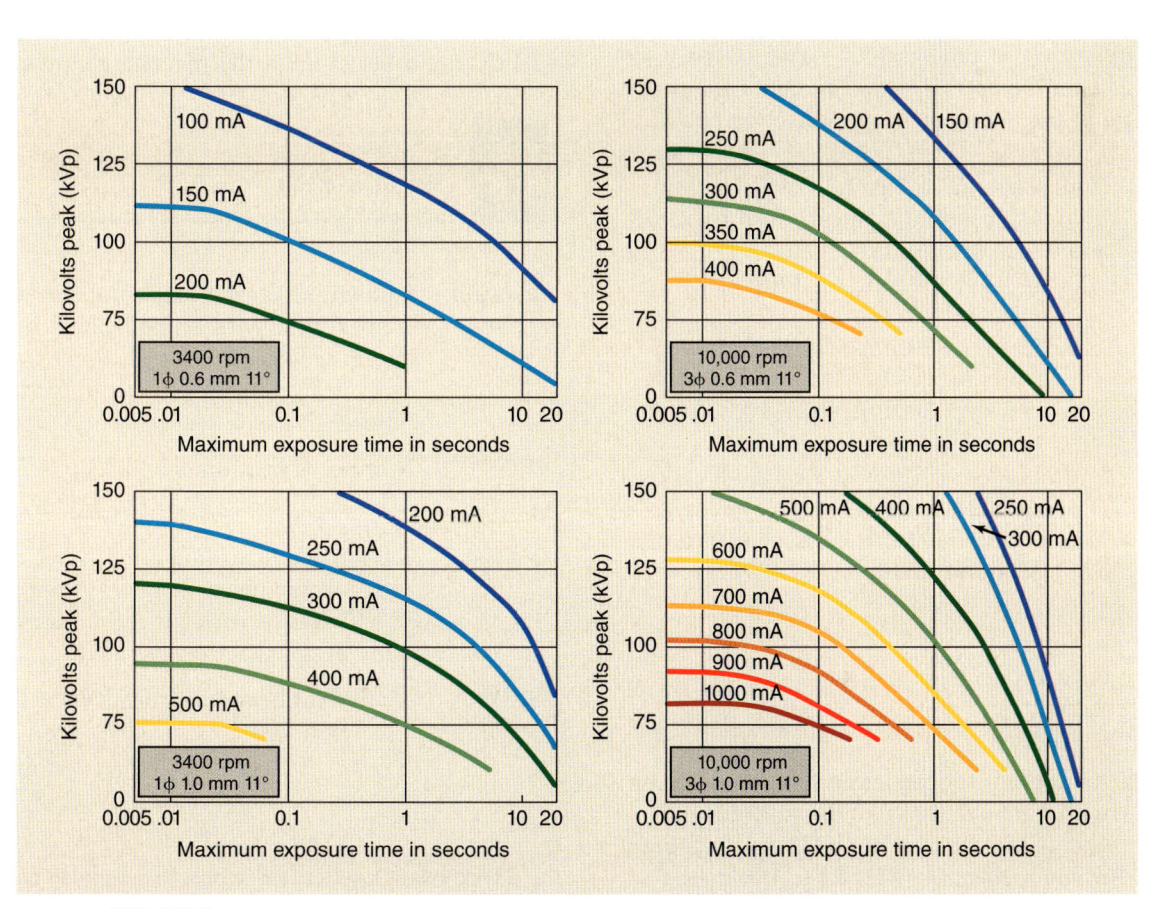

FIG. 7.26 Representative radiographic rating charts for a given x-ray tube. Each chart specifies the conditions of operation under which it applies. (Courtesy GE Healthcare.)

contains a family of curves representing the various tube currents in mA. The x-axis and the y-axis show scales of the two other radiographic parameters: time and kVp.

For a given mA, any combination of kVp and time that lies below the mA curve is safe. Any combination of kVp and time that lies above the curve representing the desired mA is unsafe. If an unsafe exposure was made, the tube might fail abruptly.

> Most x-ray imaging systems have a microprocessor control that does not allow for an unsafe exposure.

A series of radiographic rating charts accompanies every x-ray tube. There are different charts for the filament in use (large or small focal spot), the speed of anode rotation (3400 or 10,000 rpm), the target angle, and the voltage rectification (half-wave, full-wave, three-phase, high frequency).

Be sure to use the proper radiographic rating chart with each tube. This is particularly important after x-ray tubes have been replaced. An appropriate radiographic rating chart is supplied with each replacement x-ray tube and can be different from that of the original tube.

The application of radiographic rating charts is not difficult and can be used as a tool to check the proper functioning of the microprocessor protection circuit.

Question: With reference to Fig. 7.26, which of the following conditions of exposure are safe, and which are unsafe?
    a. 95 kVp, 150 mA, 1 s; 3400 rpm; 0.6-mm focal spot
    b. 85 kVp, 400 mA, 0.5 s; 3400 rpm; 1-mm focal spot
    c. 125 kVp, 500 mA, 0.1 s; 10,000 rpm; 1-mm focal spot
    d. 75 kVp, 700 mA, 0.3 s; 10,000 rpm; 1-mm focal spot
    e. 88 kVp, 400 mA, 0.1 s; 10,000 rpm; 0.6-mm focal spot

Answer:
    a. Unsafe
    b. Unsafe
    c. Safe
    d. Safe
    e. Unsafe

Question: Radiographic examination of the abdomen with a tube that has a 0.6-mm focal spot and anode rotation of 10,000 rpm requires technique factors of 95 kVp, 150 mAs. What is the shortest possible exposure time for this examination?

Answer: Locate the proper radiographic rating chart (upper right in Fig. 7.26) and the 95-kVp line (horizontal line the near middle of the chart). Beginning from the left (shorter exposure times), determine the mAs for the intersection of each mA curve with the 95-kVp level.
1. The first intersection is approximately 350 mA at 0.03 s = 10.5 mAs. This is not enough.
2. The next intersection is approximately 300 mA at 0.2 s = 60 mAs. This is not enough.
3. The next intersection is approximately 250 mA at 0.6 s = 150 mAs. This is sufficient. Consequently, 0.6 s is the minimum possible exposure time.

Anode Cooling Chart

The anode has a limited capacity for storing heat. Although heat is dissipated to the oil bath and x-ray tube housing, it is possible through prolonged use or multiple exposures to exceed the heat storage capacity of the anode.

In x-ray applications, thermal energy is measured in heat units (HUs) or joules (J). One heat unit is equal to the product of 1 kVp, 1 mA, and 1 second. One heat unit is also equal to 1.4 J. Calories and British thermal units (BTUs) are other familiar thermal energy units.

> **SINGLE PHASE**
> HU = kVp × mA × s = 0.7 J

Question: Radiographic examination of the lateral lumbar spine with a single-phase imaging system requires 98 kVp, 120 mAs. How many heat units are generated by this exposure?

Answer: Number of heat units = 98 kVp × 120 mAs
    = 11,760 HU

Question: A fluoroscopic examination is performed with a single-phase imaging system at 76 kVp and 1.5 mA for 3.5 minutes. How many heat units are generated?

Answer: Number of heat units = 75 kVp × 1.5 mA
    × 3.5 min
    × 60 s/min
    = 23,940 HU

More heat is generated when three-phase equipment and high-frequency equipment are used than when single-phase equipment is used. A modification factor

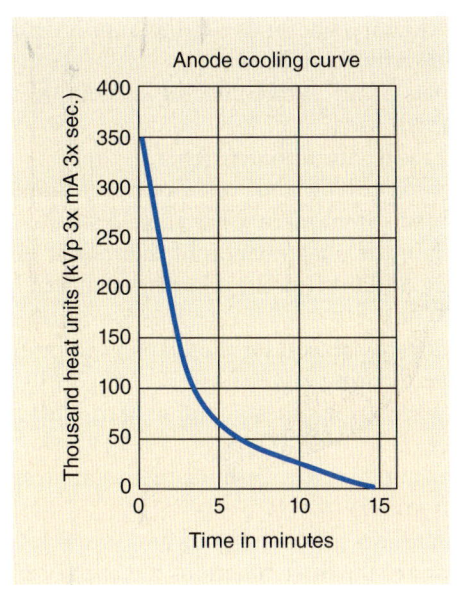

FIG. 7.27 Anode cooling chart shows the time required for a heated anode to cool. (Courtesy GE Healthcare.)

of 1.4 is necessary for calculating three-phase or high-frequency heat units.

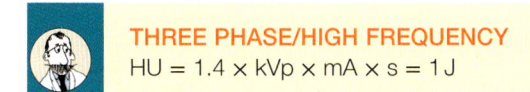

> **THREE PHASE/HIGH FREQUENCY**
> HU = 1.4 × kVp × mA × s = 1 J

Question: Six sequential skull films are exposed with a three-phase generator operated at 82 kVp, 120 mAs. What is the total heat generated?

Answer: Number of heat units/film = 1.4 × 82 kVp × 120 mAs
= 13,776 HU
Total HU = 6 × 13,776 HU
= 82,656 HU

The thermal capacity of an anode and its heat dissipation characteristics are contained in a rating chart called an **anode cooling chart** (Fig. 7.27). Different from the radiographic rating chart, the anode cooling chart does not depend on the filament size or the speed of rotation.

The tube represented in Fig. 7.27 has a maximum anode heat capacity of 350,000 HU. The chart shows that if the maximum heat load were attained, it would take 15 minutes for the anode to cool completely.

The rate of cooling is rapid at first and slows as the anode cools. In addition to determining the maximum heat capacity of the anode, the anode cooling chart is used to determine the length of time required for complete cooling after any level of heat input.

Question: A particular examination results in the delivery of 50,000 HU to the anode in a matter of seconds. How long will it take the anode to cool completely?

Answer: The 50,000-HU level intersects the anode cooling curve at approximately 6 minutes. From that point on, the curve to complete cooling requires an additional 9 minutes (15 − 6 = 9). Therefore 9 minutes is required for complete cooling.

Although the heat generated in producing x-rays is expressed in heat units, joules are the equivalent. By definition:

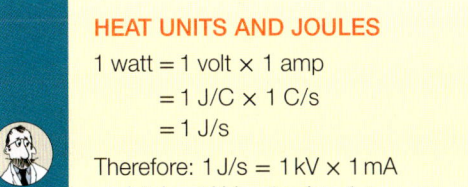

> **HEAT UNITS AND JOULES**
> 1 watt = 1 volt × 1 amp
> = 1 J/C × 1 C/s
> = 1 J/s
> Therefore: 1 J/s = 1 kV × 1 mA
> and 1 J = 1 kV × 1 mA × 1 s
> and because 1 HU = 1 kVp × 1 mA × 1 s
> 1 HU = 1.4 J (3Ø, HF)
> 1 J = 0.7 HU (3Ø, HF)

Question: How much heat energy (in joules) is produced during a single high-frequency mammographic exposure of 25 kVp, 200 mAs?

Answer: 25 kVp × 200 mAs = 5000 HU
5000 HU × 1.4 J/HU = 7000 J = 7 kJ

Housing Cooling Chart

The cooling chart for the housing of the x-ray tube has a shape similar to that of the anode cooling chart and is used in precisely the same way. Radiographic x-ray tube housings usually have maximum heat capacities in the range of several million heat units. Complete cooling after maximum heat capacity requires from 1 to 2 hours.

SUMMARY

The primary support structure for the x-ray tube, which allows the greatest ease of movement and range of position, is the ceiling support system. A protective housing covers the x-ray tube and provides the following three functions: it (1) reduces leakage radiation to less than 1 mGy$_a$/h at 1 m, (2) provides mechanical support, thereby protecting the tube from damage, and (3) serves as a way to conduct heat away from the x-ray tube target.

The glass or metal enclosure surrounds the cathode (−) and the anode (+), which are the electrodes of the vacuum tube. The cathode contains the tungsten filament, which is the source of electrons. The rotating anode is the tungsten–rhenium disc, which serves as a target for electrons accelerated from the cathode. The line-focus principle results from angled targets. The heel effect is the variation in x-ray intensity across the x-ray beam that results from the absorption of x-rays in the heel of the target.

Safe operation of the x-ray tube is the responsibility of the radiographer. X-ray tube failure can be prevented. The causes of tube failure are threefold:

- A single excessive exposure causes pitting or cracking of the anode.
- Long exposure time causes excessive heating of the anode, resulting in damage to the bearings in the rotor assembly. Bearing damage causes warping and rotational friction of the anode.
- Even with normal use, vaporization of the filament causes tungsten to coat the glass or metal enclosure; this eventually causes arcing.

Tube rating charts printed by manufacturers of x-ray tubes aid in the use of acceptable exposure levels to maximize x-ray tube life. All such charts are now embedded electronically on the console of new x-ray imaging systems.

CHALLENGE QUESTIONS

1. Define or otherwise identify the following:
   a. Housing cooling chart
   b. Leakage radiation
   c. Heat unit (HU)
   d. Focusing cup
   e. Anode rotation speed
   f. Thoriated tungsten
   g. X-ray tube current
   h. Grid-controlled x-ray tube
   i. Convection
   j. Space charge
2. List the three methods used to support x-ray tubes and briefly describe each.
3. Where in an x-ray imaging system is thoriated tungsten used?
4. What is a saturation current?
5. Why are arcing and tube failure no longer major problems in modern x-ray tube design?
6. Explain the phenomenon of thermionic emission.
7. What addition to the filament material prolongs tube life?
8. What is the reason for the filament to be embedded in the focusing cup?
9. Why are x-ray tubes manufactured with two focal spots?
10. Is the anode or the cathode the negative side of the x-ray tube?
11. List and describe the two types of anodes.
12. What are the three functions the anode serves in an x-ray tube?
13. How do atomic number, thermal conductivity, and melting point affect the selection of anode target material?
14. Draw diagrams of a stationary and a rotating anode.
15. How does the anode rotate inside a glass enclosure with no mechanical connection to the outside?
16. Draw the difference between the actual focal spot and the effective focal spot.
17. Define the heel effect and describe how it can be used advantageously.
18. Explain the three causes of x-ray tube failure.
19. What happens when an x-ray tube is space charge limited?
20. What is a detent position?

The answers to the Challenge Questions can be found by logging on to our website at http://evolve.elsevier.com.

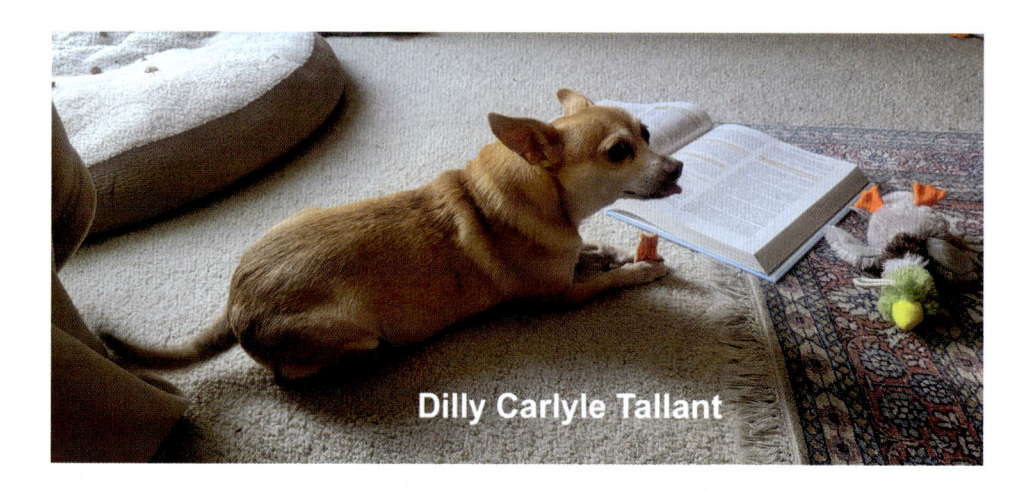

X-ray Production

CHAPTER 8

OBJECTIVES

At the completion of this chapter, the student should be able to do the following:

1. Discuss the interactions between projectile electrons and the x-ray tube target.
2. Identify characteristic and bremsstrahlung x-rays.
3. Describe the x-ray emission spectrum.
4. Explain how mAs, kVp, added filtration, target material, and voltage ripple affect the x-ray emission spectrum.

OUTLINE

Electron-Target Interactions 130
  Anode Heat 131
  Characteristic Radiation 131
  Bremsstrahlung Radiation 133
X-ray Emission Spectrum 134
  Characteristic X-ray Emission Spectrum 135
  Bremsstrahlung X-ray Spectrum 135
Factors Affecting the X-ray Emission Spectrum 136
  Effect of mA and mAs 136
  Effect of kVp 137
  Effect of Added Filtration 138
  Effect of Target Material 138
  Effect of Voltage Waveform 139
Summary 140
Challenge Questions 140

CHAPTER 7 DISCUSSED the internal components of the x-ray tube—the cathode and the anode—within the evacuated glass or metal enclosure. This chapter explains the interactions of the projectile electrons that are accelerated from the cathode to the x-ray tube target.

These electron-target interactions produce two types of x-rays—characteristic and bremsstrahlung. These are described by the x-ray emission spectrum, which helps in understanding x-ray emission. Various conditions that affect the x-ray emission spectrum are discussed.

ELECTRON-TARGET INTERACTIONS

The x-ray imaging system description in Chapter 6 emphasizes that its primary function is to accelerate electrons from the cathode to the anode in the x-ray tube. The three principal parts of an x-ray imaging system—the operating console, the x-ray tube, and the high-voltage generator—are designed to provide a large number of electrons with high kinetic energy focused onto a small spot on the anode.

> Kinetic energy is the energy of motion.

Stationary objects have no kinetic energy; objects in motion have kinetic energy proportional to their mass and to the square of their velocity. The kinetic energy equation follows.

> **KINETIC ENERGY**
> $$KE = \frac{1}{2}mv^2$$
> where m is the mass in kilograms, v is velocity in meters per second, and KE is kinetic energy in joules.

For example, a 1000-kg automobile has four times the kinetic energy of a 250-kg motorcycle traveling at the same speed (Fig. 8.1). However, if the motorcycle were to double its velocity, it would have the same kinetic energy as the automobile.

In determining the magnitude of the kinetic energy of a projectile, velocity is more important than mass. In an x-ray tube, the projectile is the electron. All electrons have the same mass; therefore electron kinetic energy is increased by raising the kilovolt peak (kVp). As electron kinetic energy is increased, both the intensity (quantity) and the energy (quality) of the x-ray beam are increased.

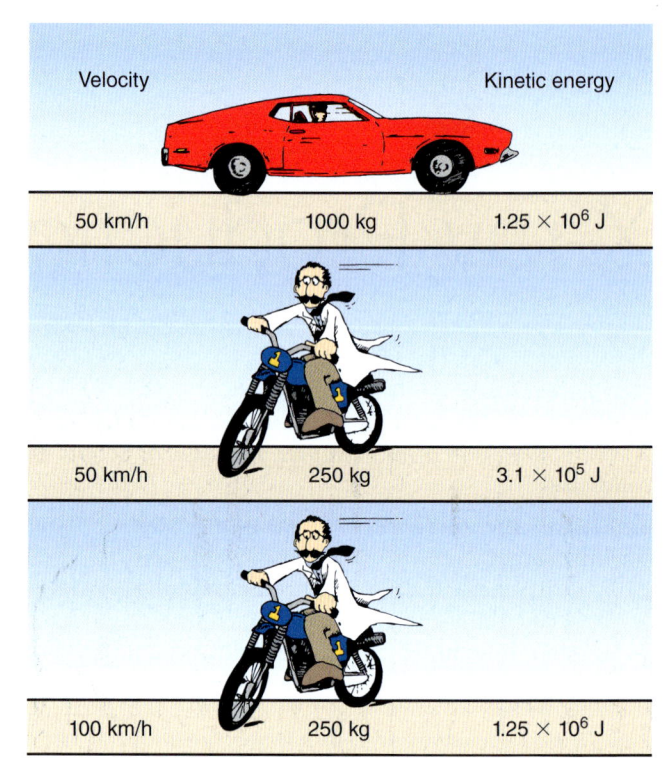

Velocity		Kinetic energy
50 km/h	1000 kg	1.25×10^6 J
50 km/h	250 kg	3.1×10^5 J
100 km/h	250 kg	1.25×10^6 J

FIG. 8.1 Kinetic energy is proportional to the product of mass and velocity squared.

The modern x-ray imaging system is remarkable. It conveys to the x-ray tube target an enormous number of electrons at a precisely controlled kinetic energy. For example, at 100 mA, 6×10^{17} electrons travel from the cathode to the anode of the x-ray tube every second.

In an x-ray imaging system operating at 70 kVp, each electron arrives at the target with a maximum kinetic energy of 70 keV. Because there are 1.6×10^{-16} J per keV, this energy is equivalent to the following:

> $(70 \text{ keV})(1.6 \times 10^{-16} \text{ J/keV}) = 1.12 \times 10^{-14}$ J

When this energy is inserted into the expression for kinetic energy and calculations are performed to determine the velocity of the electrons, the result is as follows:

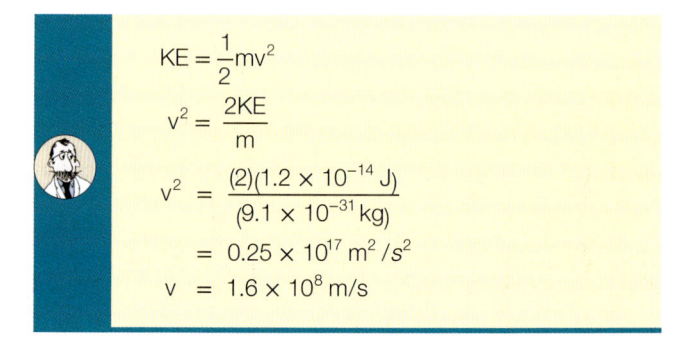

> $$KE = \frac{1}{2}mv^2$$
> $$v^2 = \frac{2KE}{m}$$
> $$v^2 = \frac{(2)(1.2 \times 10^{-14} \text{ J})}{(9.1 \times 10^{-31} \text{ kg})}$$
> $$= 0.25 \times 10^{17} \text{ m}^2/\text{s}^2$$
> $$v = 1.6 \times 10^8 \text{ m/s}$$

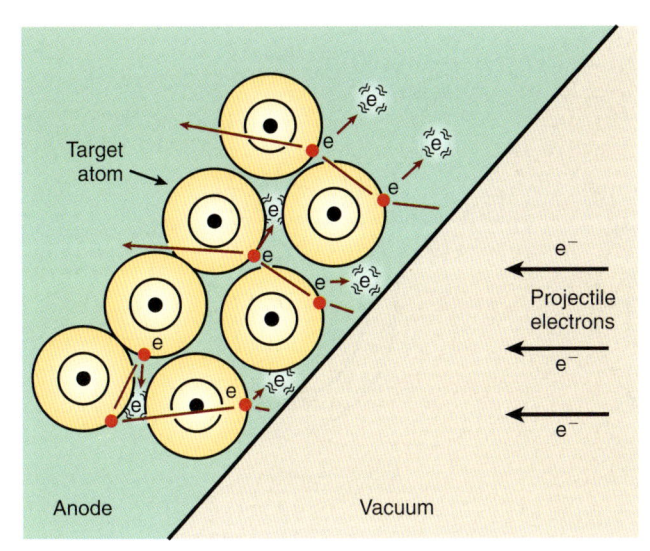

FIG. 8.2 Most of the kinetic energy of projectile electrons is converted to heat by interactions with outer-shell electrons of target atoms. These interactions are primarily excitations rather than ionizations.

Question: At what fraction of the velocity of light do 70-keV electrons travel?

Answer: $\dfrac{v}{c} = \dfrac{1.6 \times 10^8 \,\text{m/s}}{3.0 \times 10^8 \,\text{m/s}} = 0.53$

The distance between the filament and the x-ray tube target is only approximately 1 cm. It is not difficult to imagine the intensity of the accelerating force required to raise the velocity of electrons from zero to half the speed of light over such a short distance.

Electrons traveling from the cathode to the anode constitute the x-ray tube current. When these electrons hit the heavy metal atoms of the x-ray tube target, they transfer their kinetic energy to the target atoms.

These interactions occur within a very small depth of penetration into the target. As they occur, the projectile electrons slow down and finally come nearly to rest, at which time they are conducted through the x-ray anode assembly and out into the associated electronic circuitry.

The electron from the cathode interacts with the orbital electrons or the nuclear field of target atoms. These interactions result in the conversion of electron kinetic energy into thermal energy (heat) and electromagnetic energy in the form of infrared radiation (also heat) and x-rays.

Anode Heat

Most of the kinetic energy of electrons is converted into heat (Fig. 8.2). The electrons interact with the outer-shell electrons of the target atoms but do not transfer sufficient energy to these outer-shell electrons to ionize them. Rather, the outer-shell electrons are simply raised to an excited, or higher, energy level.

The outer-shell electrons immediately drop back to their normal energy level with the emission of infrared radiation. The constant excitation and return of outer-shell electrons are responsible for most of the heat generated in the anodes of x-ray tubes.

> Approximately 99% of the kinetic energy of electrons from the cathode is converted to heat.

Only approximately 1% of electron kinetic energy is used for the production of x-radiation. Therefore, sophisticated as it is, the x-ray imaging system is not very efficient.

The production of heat in the anode increases directly with increasing x-ray tube current. Doubling the x-ray tube current doubles the heat produced.

Heat production also increases directly with increasing kVp, at least in the diagnostic range. Although the relationship between varying kVp and varying heat production is approximate, it is sufficiently exact to allow the computation of heat units for use with anode cooling charts.

The efficiency of x-ray production is independent of the tube current. Consequently, regardless of what mA is selected, the efficiency of x-ray production remains constant.

The efficiency of x-ray production increases with increasing kVp. At 60 kVp, only 0.5% of the electron kinetic energy is converted to x-rays. At 100 kVp, approximately 1% is converted to x-rays, and at 20 MV, 70% is converted.

Characteristic Radiation

If the projectile electron interacts with an inner-shell electron of the target atom rather than with an outer-shell electron, **characteristic x-rays** can be produced. Characteristic x-rays result when the interaction is sufficiently violent to ionize the target atom through total removal of an inner-shell electron.

> Characteristic x-rays are emitted when an outer-shell electron fills an inner-shell void.

Fig. 8.3 illustrates how characteristic x-rays are produced. When the projectile electron from the cathode ionizes a target atom by removing a K-shell electron, a temporary electron void is produced in the K shell. This is an unnatural state for the target atom, and it is corrected when an outer-shell electron falls into the void in the K shell.

The transition of an orbital electron from an outer shell to an inner shell is accompanied by the emission

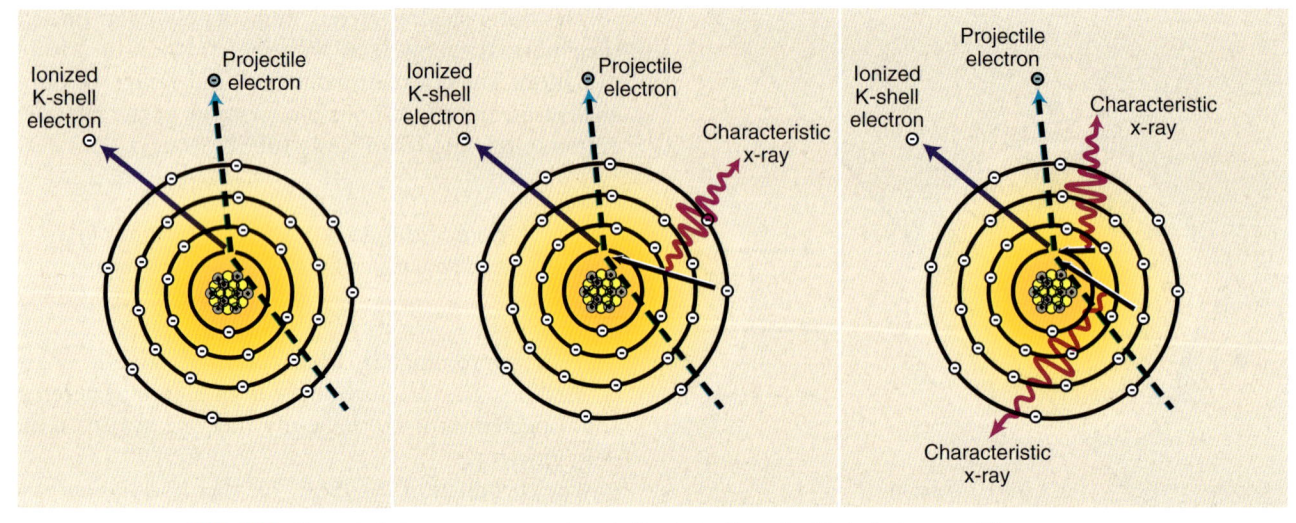

FIG. 8.3 Characteristic x-rays are produced after ionization of a K-shell electron. When an outer shell electron fills the vacancy in the K shell, an x-ray is emitted.

of an x-ray. The x-ray has energy equal to the difference in the binding energies of the orbital electrons involved.

Question: A K-shell electron is removed from a tungsten atom and is replaced by an L-shell electron. What is the energy of the characteristic x-ray that is emitted?

Answer: Reference to Fig. 8.4 shows that for tungsten, K-shell electrons have binding energies of 69 keV, and L-shell electrons are bound by 12 keV. Therefore the characteristic x-ray emitted has energy of 69 − 12 = 57 keV.

By the same procedure, the energy of x-rays resulting from M-to-K, N-to-K, O-to-K, and P-to-K transitions can be calculated. For example, tungsten has electrons in shells out to the P shell, and when a K-shell electron is ionized, its position can be filled with electrons from any of the outer shells.

All of these x-rays are called K x-rays because they result from outer shell electron transitions into the K shell. The 69-keV K-shell binding energy is why we have to set 70 kVp or higher on the control panel to get K-characteristic x-rays.

Similar characteristic x-rays are produced when the target atom is ionized by removal of electrons from shells other than the K shell. Note that Fig. 8.3 does not show the production of x-rays resulting from ionization of an L-shell electron.

Such a diagram would show the removal of an L-shell electron by the projectile electron. The vacancy in the L shell would be filled by an electron from any of the outer shells. X-rays resulting from electron transitions to the L shell are called L x-rays and have much less energy than K x-rays because the binding energy of an L-shell electron is much lower than that of a K-shell electron.

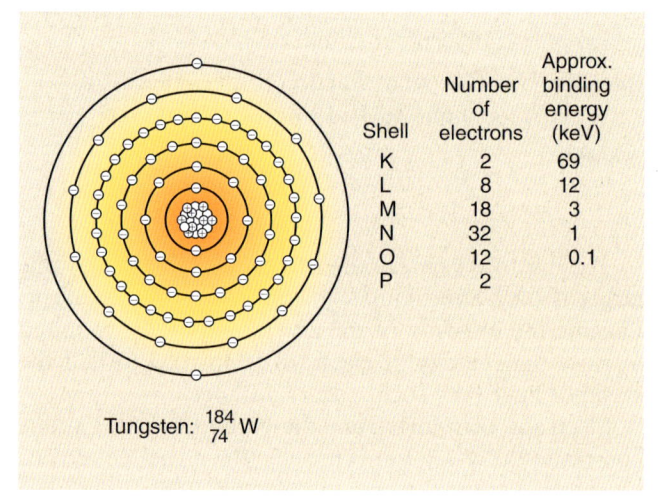

Shell	Number of electrons	Approx. binding energy (keV)
K	2	69
L	8	12
M	18	3
N	32	1
O	12	0.1
P	2	

Tungsten: $^{184}_{74}$W

FIG. 8.4 Atomic configuration and electron-binding energies for tungsten.

Only the K-characteristic x-rays of tungsten are useful for imaging.

Similarly, M-characteristic x-rays, N-characteristic x-rays, and even O-characteristic x-rays can be produced in a tungsten target. Fig. 8.4 illustrates the electron configuration and Table 8.1 summarizes the production of characteristic x-rays in tungsten.

Although many characteristic x-rays can be produced, these can be produced only at specific energies, equal to the differences in electron-binding energies for the various electron transitions.

Except for K x-rays, all of the characteristic x-rays have very low energy. The L x-rays, with approximately 12 keV of energy, penetrate only a few centimeters into soft tissue. Consequently, they are useless

TABLE 8.1 Characteristic X-rays of Tungsten and Their Effective Energies

Characteristic	L Shell	M Shell	N Shell	O Shell	P Shell	Effective Energy of X-ray
K	57.4	66.7	68.9	69.4	69.5	69
L		9.3	11.5	12.0	12.1	12
M			2.2	2.7	2.8	3
N				0.52	0.6	0.6
O					0.08	0.1

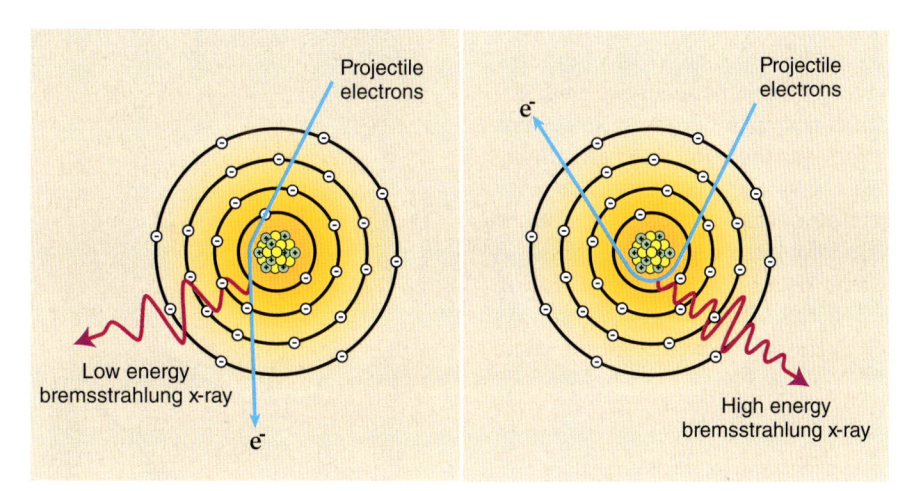

FIG. 8.5 Bremsstrahlung x-rays result from the interaction between a projectile electron and a target nucleus. The electron is slowed, and its direction is changed.

as diagnostic x-rays, as are all the other low-energy characteristic x-rays. The last column in Table 8.1 shows the effective energy for each of the characteristic x-rays of tungsten.

> This type of x-radiation is called characteristic because it is characteristic of the target element.

Because the electron-binding energy for every element is different, the energy of characteristic x-rays produced in the various elements is also different. The effective energy of characteristic x-rays increases with increasing atomic number of the target element.

Bremsstrahlung Radiation

The production of heat and characteristic x-rays involves interactions between the projectile electrons and the electrons of x-ray tube target atoms. A third type of interaction in which the projectile electron can lose its kinetic energy is an interaction with the nuclear field of a target atom. In this type of interaction, the kinetic energy of the projectile electron is also converted into electromagnetic energy.

A projectile electron that completely avoids the orbital electrons as it passes through a target atom may come sufficiently close to the nucleus of the atom to come under the influence of its electric field (Fig. 8.5). Because the electron is negatively charged and the nucleus is positively charged, there is an electrostatic force of attraction between them.

The closer the projectile electron gets to the nucleus, the more it is influenced by the electric field of the nucleus. This field is very strong because the nucleus contains many protons and the distance between the nucleus and projectile electron is very small.

As the projectile electron passes by the nucleus, it is slowed down and changes its course, leaving with reduced kinetic energy in a different direction. This loss of kinetic energy reappears as an x-ray.

> Bremsstrahlung x-rays are produced when a projectile electron is slowed by the nuclear field of a target atom nucleus.

These types of x-rays are called **bremsstrahlung** x-rays. Bremsstrahlung is a German word that means "braking radiation." Bremsstrahlung x-rays can be considered radiation that results from the slowing of projectile cathode electrons by the nucleus.

A projectile electron can lose any amount of its kinetic energy in an interaction with the nucleus of a target atom, and the bremsstrahlung x-ray associated with the loss can take on corresponding values. For example, when an x-ray imaging system is operated at 70 kVp, electrons from the cathode have kinetic energies from zero to 70 keV.

An electron with kinetic energy of 70 keV can lose all, none, or any intermediate level of that kinetic energy in a bremsstrahlung interaction. Therefore the bremsstrahlung x-ray produced can have any energy up to 70 keV.

This is different from the production of characteristic x-rays, which have very specific energies. Fig. 8.5 illustrates how one can consider the production of such a wide range of energies through the bremsstrahlung interaction.

A low-energy bremsstrahlung x-ray results when the electron is barely influenced by the nucleus. A maximum-energy x-ray occurs when the electron loses all its kinetic energy. Bremsstrahlung x-rays with energies between these two extremes occur more frequently.

> In the diagnostic energy range, most x-rays are bremsstrahlung x-rays.

Bremsstrahlung x-rays can be produced at any projectile electron energy. K-characteristic x-rays require an x-ray tube potential of at least 70 kVp. For example, at 65 kVp, no useful characteristic x-rays are produced; therefore the x-ray beam is all bremsstrahlung. At 100 kVp, approximately 15% of the x-ray beam is characteristic, and the remaining is bremsstrahlung.

X-RAY EMISSION SPECTRUM

Most people have seen or heard of pitching machines (the devices used by baseball teams for batting practice so that pitchers do not get worn out). Similar machines are used to automatically eject bowling balls, tennis balls, and even ping-pong balls.

Suppose there was a device that could eject all of these types of balls randomly. The most straightforward way to determine how often each type of ball was ejected on average would be to catch each ball as it was ejected and then identify it and drop it into a basket; at the end of the observation period, the total number of each type of ball could be counted.

Let us suppose that the results obtained for a given period are those shown in Fig. 8.6. A total of 600 balls were ejected. Perhaps the easiest way to represent these

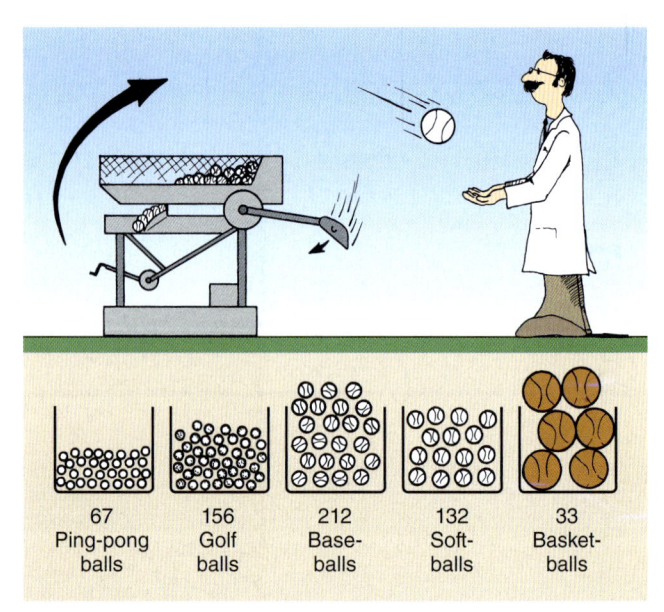

FIG. 8.6 Over a given period, an automatic ball-throwing machine might eject 600 balls, distributed as shown.

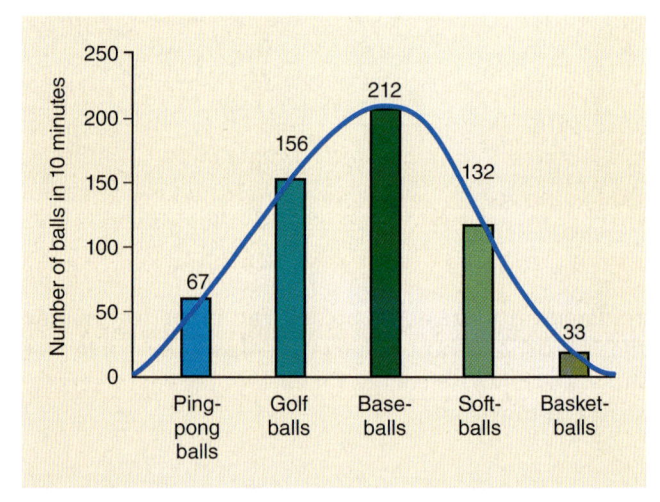

FIG. 8.7 Bar graph representing the results of observation of balls ejected by the automatic pitching machine shown in Fig. 8.6. When the height of each bar is joined, a smooth emission spectrum is created.

results graphically would be to plot the total number of each type of ball emitted during the observation period and represent each total by a bar (Fig. 8.7).

Such a bar graph can be described as a discrete ball ejection spectrum that is representative of the automatic pitching machine. It is a plot of the number of balls ejected as a function of the type of ball. It is called discrete because only five distinct types of balls are involved.

> A discrete spectrum contains only specific values.

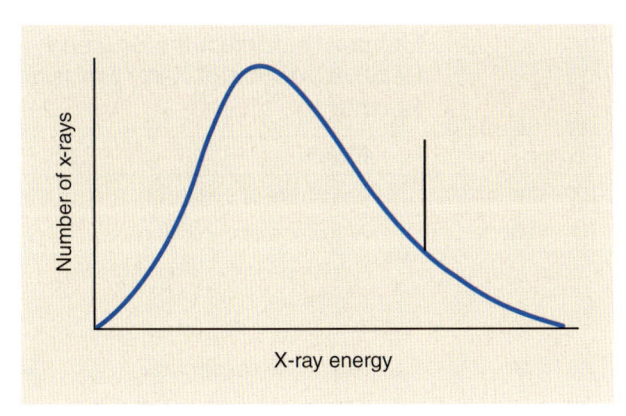

FIG. 8.8 General form of an x-ray emission spectrum.

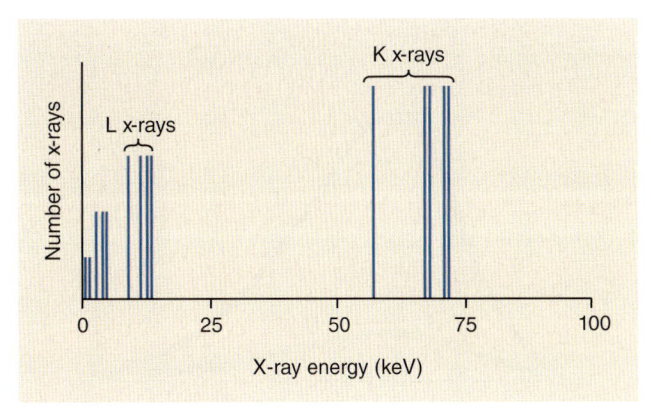

FIG. 8.9 Characteristic x-ray emission spectrum for tungsten contains 15 different x-ray energies.

Connecting the bars with a curve as shown would indicate a large number of different types of balls. Such a curve is called a continuous ejection spectrum. The word **spectrum** refers to the range of types of balls or values of any quantity, such as x-rays. The total number of balls ejected is represented by the sum of the areas under the bars in the case of the discrete spectrum and the area under the curve in the case of the continuous spectrum. The height of the curve is the amplitude.

> A continuous spectrum contains all possible values.

Without regard for the absolute number of balls emitted, Fig. 8.7 also could be identified as a relative ball ejection spectrum because at a glance, one can tell the relative frequency with which each type of ball was ejected. Relatively speaking, baseballs are ejected most frequently and basketballs least frequently.

This type of relationship is fundamental to describing the radiation output of an x-ray tube. If one could stand in the middle of the useful x-ray beam, catch each individual x-ray, and measure its energy, one could describe what is known as the **x-ray emission spectrum** (Fig. 8.8).

Here, the relative number of x-rays emitted is plotted as a function of the energy of each individual x-ray. X-ray energy is the variable that is considered.

Although we cannot catch and identify each individual x-ray, instruments are available that allow us to do essentially that. X-ray emission spectra have been measured for all types of x-ray imaging systems. Data on x-ray emission spectra are needed if one is to gain an understanding of how changes in kVp, mA, and added filtration affect the quality of an image.

Characteristic X-ray Emission Spectrum

The discrete energies of characteristic x-rays are characteristic of the differences between electron-binding energies in a particular element. For example, a characteristic x-ray from tungsten can have 1 of 15 different energies (see Table 8.1) and no others. A plot of the frequency with which characteristic x-rays are emitted as a function of their energy would look similar to that shown for tungsten in Fig. 8.9.

Such a plot is called the characteristic x-ray emission spectrum. Five vertical lines representing K x-rays and four vertical lines representing L x-rays are included. The lower energy lines represent characteristic emissions from the outer electron shells.

> Characteristic x-rays have precisely fixed energies and form a discrete emission spectrum.

The relative intensity of the K x-rays is greater than that of the lower energy characteristic x-rays because of the nature of the interaction process. K x-rays are the only characteristic x-rays of tungsten with sufficient energy to be of value in diagnostic x-ray imaging. Although there are five K x-rays, it is customary to represent them as one, as has been done in Fig. 8.10 with a single vertical line, at 69 keV. Only this line will be shown in later graphs.

Bremsstrahlung X-ray Spectrum

If it were possible to measure the energy contained in each bremsstrahlung x-ray emitted from an x-ray tube, one would find that these energies range from the peak electron energy all the way down to zero. In other words, when an x-ray tube is operated at 90 kVp, bremsstrahlung x-rays with energies up to 90 keV are emitted. A typical bremsstrahlung x-ray emission spectrum is shown in Fig. 8.10.

> Bremsstrahlung x-rays have a range of energies and form a continuous emission spectrum.

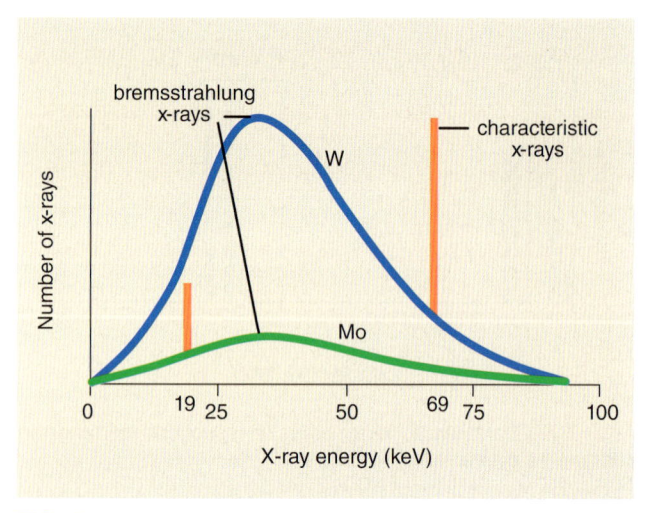

FIG. 8.10 The bremsstrahlung x-ray emission spectrum extends from zero to maximum projectile electron energy, with the highest number of x-rays having approximately one-third the maximum energy. The characteristic x-ray emission spectrum for tungsten (W) is represented by a line at 69 keV. That for molybdenum (Mo) is represented by a line at 19 keV.

TABLE 8.2	Factors That Affect the Size and Relative Position of X-ray Emission Spectra
Factor	**Effect**
Tube current	Amplitude of spectrum
Tube voltage	Amplitude and position
Added filtration	Amplitude; most effective at low energy
Target material	Amplitude of spectrum and position of line spectrum
Voltage waveform	Amplitude; most effective at high energy

Question: At what kVp was the x-ray imaging system presented in Fig. 8.10 operated?

Answer: Because the bremsstrahlung spectrum intersects the energy axis at approximately 90 keV, the imaging system must have been operated at approximately 90 kVp.

The general shape of the bremsstrahlung x-ray spectrum is the same for all x-ray imaging systems. The maximum energy (keV) of a bremsstrahlung x-ray is numerically equal to the kVp of operation.

The greatest number of x-rays is emitted with energy approximately one-third of the maximum energy. The number of x-rays emitted decreases rapidly at very low energies.

Question: What would be the expected emission spectrum for an x-ray imaging system with a pure molybdenum (Mo) target (effective energy of K x-ray = 19 keV) operated at 90 kVp?

Answer: The spectrum should look something like Fig. 8.8. The curve intersects the energy axis at 0 and 90 keV and has the general shape shown in Fig. 8.10. The bremsstrahlung spectrum is much lower because the atomic number of Mo is low (Z = 42), and x-ray production is much less efficient. A line extends above the curve at 19 keV to represent the K-characteristic x-rays of molybdenum.

As described in Chapter 4, the energy of an x-ray is equal to the product of its frequency (f) and Planck's constant (h). X-ray energy is inversely proportional to its wavelength. As x-ray wavelength increases, x-ray energy decreases.

> Maximum x-ray energy is associated with the minimum x-ray wavelength (λ_{min}).

The minimum wavelength of x-ray emission corresponds to the maximum x-ray energy, and the maximum x-ray energy is numerically equal to the kVp.

FACTORS AFFECTING THE X-RAY EMISSION SPECTRUM

The total number of x-rays emitted from an x-ray tube could be determined by adding together the number of x-rays emitted at each energy over the entire spectrum, a process called **integration**. Graphically, the total number of x-rays emitted is equivalent to the area under the curve of the x-ray emission spectrum.

The general shape of an emission spectrum is always the same, but its relative position along the energy axis can change. The farther to the right a shift of the amplitude is, the higher the effective energy or quality of the x-ray beam.

The larger the height of the amplitude, the higher the x-ray intensity or quantity. A number of factors under the control of the radiographer influence the size and shape of the x-ray emission spectrum and therefore the effective energy and intensity of the x-ray beam. These factors are summarized in Table 8.2.

Effect of mA and mAs

If one changes the x-ray tube electric current from 200 to 400 milliamperes (mA) while all other conditions remain constant, twice as many electrons will flow from the cathode to the anode, and the mAs will be doubled. This operating change will produce twice as many x-rays at every energy. In other words, the x-ray emission spectrum will be changed in amplitude but not in shape (Fig. 8.11).

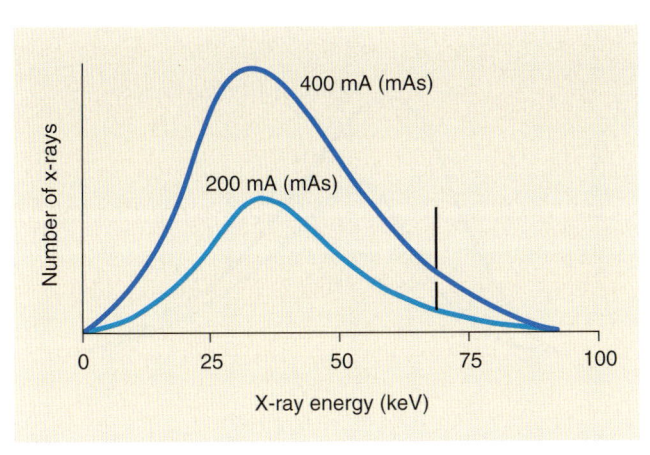

FIG. 8.11 Change in mA or mAs results in a proportionate change in the amplitude of the x-ray emission spectrum at all energies.

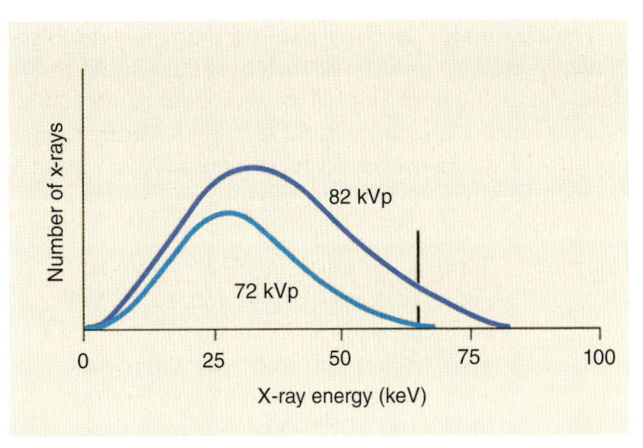

FIG. 8.12 Change in kVp results in an increase in the amplitude of the emission spectrum at all energies but a greater increase at high energies than at low energies. Therefore the spectrum is shifted to the right, or high-energy, side.

> A change in mA or mAs results in a proportional change in the amplitude of the x-ray emission spectrum at all energies.

Each point on the curve labeled 400 mA or 400 mAs is precisely two times higher than the associated point on the 200 mA or 200 mAs curve. Thus the area under the x-ray emission spectrum varies in proportion to changes in mA or mAs, as does the x-ray intensity.

FOUR PRINCIPAL FACTORS INFLUENCING THE SHAPE OF AN X-RAY EMISSION SPECTRUM

1. The projectile electrons accelerated from cathode to anode do not all have peak kinetic energy. Depending on the types of rectification and high-voltage generation, many of these electrons may have very low energies when they strike the target. Such electrons can produce only heat and low-energy x-rays.
2. The target of a diagnostic x-ray tube is relatively thick. Consequently, many of the bremsstrahlung x-rays emitted result from multiple interactions of the projectile electrons, and for each successive interaction, a projectile electron has less energy.
3. Low-energy x-rays are more likely to be absorbed in the target.
4. External filtration is always added to the x-ray tube assembly. This added filtration serves selectively to remove low-energy x-rays from the beam.

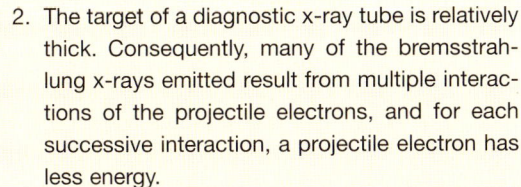

Question: Suppose the area under the 200-mA (200 mAs) curve in Fig. 8.11 totals 4.2 cm² and the x-ray quantity is 3 mGy$_a$. What would the area under the curve and the x-ray quantity be if the tube current were increased to 400 mA (400 mAs) while other operating factors remain constant?

Answer: In going from 200 to 400 mA or mAs, the tube current has been increased by a factor of 2. The area under the curve and the x-ray quantity are increased proportionately:
Area = 4.2 cm² × 2 = 8.4 cm²
Intensity = 3 mGy$_a$ × 2 = 6 mGy$_a$

Effect of kVp

As the kVp is raised, the area under the curve increases to an area approximating the square of the factor by which kVp was increased. Accordingly, the x-ray quantity increases with (kVp_2^2 / kVp_1^2).

When kVp is increased, the relative distribution of emitted x-ray energy shifts to the right to a higher average x-ray energy. The maximum energy of x-ray emission always remains numerically equal to the kVp.

> A change in kVp affects both the amplitude and the position of the x-ray emission spectrum.

Fig. 8.12 demonstrates the effect of increasing the kVp while other factors remain constant. The lower spectrum represents x-ray operation at 72 kVp, and the upper spectrum represents operation at 82 kVp—a 10-kVp (or 15%) increase.

The area under the curve has approximately doubled, while the relative position of the curve has shifted to the right, the high-energy side. More x-rays are emitted at all energies during operation at 82 kVp than during operation at 72 kVp. However, the increase is relatively greater for high-energy x-rays than for low-energy x-rays.

Question: Suppose the curve labeled 72 kVp in Fig. 8.12 covers a total area of 3.6 cm² and represents an x-ray quantity of 1.25 mGy$_a$. What area under the curve and x-ray quantity would be expected for operations at 82 kVp?

Answer: The area under the curve and the output intensity are proportional to the square of the ratio of the kVp change. A ratio can be established.

$$\left(\frac{82}{72}\right)^2 (3.6 \text{ cm}^2) = (1.3)(3.6 \text{ cm}^2) = 4.7 \text{ cm}^2$$

and

$$(1.3)(1.25 \text{ mGy}_a) = 1.63 \text{ mGy}_a$$

This example partially explains the rule of thumb used by radiographers to relate the kVp and mAs changes necessary to produce a constant signal on an image receptor. The rule states that a 15% increase in kVp is equivalent to doubling the mAs. At low kVp, such as 50 to 60 kVp, approximately a 7-kVp increase is equivalent to doubling the mAs. At tube potentials greater than approximately 100 kVp, a 15-kVp change may be necessary.

> In the diagnostic range, a 15% increase in kVp is equivalent to doubling the mAs.

A 15% increase in kVp does not double the x-ray intensity but is equivalent to doubling the mAs to the image receptor. To double the output intensity by increasing kVp, one would have to raise the kVp by as much as 40%.

Radiographically, only a 15% increase in kVp is necessary because with increased kVp, the penetrability of the x-ray beam is increased. Therefore less radiation is absorbed by the patient, leaving a proportionately greater number of x-rays to expose the image receptor.

Effect of Added Filtration

Adding filtration to the useful x-ray beam reduces x-ray beam intensity while increasing the average energy. This effect is shown in Fig. 8.13, where an x-ray tube is operated at 95 kVp with 2-mm aluminum (Al) added filtration compared with the same operation with 4-mm Al added filtration.

Added filtration more effectively absorbs low-energy x-rays than high-energy x-rays; therefore the

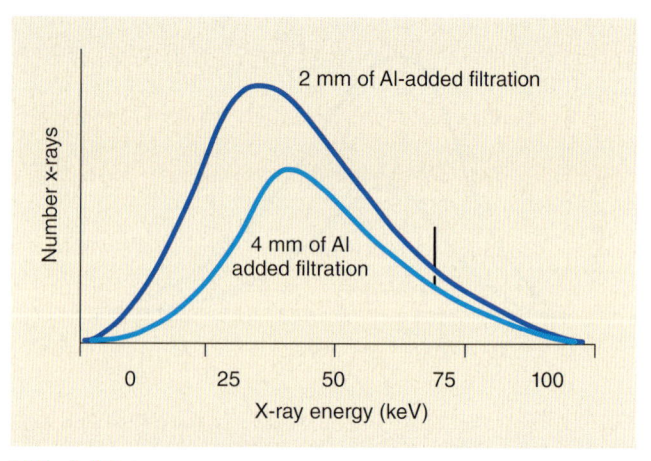

FIG. 8.13 Adding filtration to an x-ray tube results in reduced x-ray intensity but increased effective energy. The emission spectra represented here resulted from operation at the same mA and kVp but with different filtration.

bremsstrahlung x-ray emission spectrum is reduced further on the left than on the right.

> The result of added filtration is an increase in the average energy of the x-ray beam with an accompanying reduction in x-ray intensity.

Adding filtration is sometimes called **hardening** the x-ray beam because of the relative increase in average energy. The characteristic spectrum is not affected, nor is the maximum energy of x-ray emission. There is no simple method for calculating the precise changes that occur in x-ray energy and intensity with a change in added filtration.

Effect of Target Material

The atomic number of the target affects both the intensity and the effective energy of x-rays. As the atomic number of the target material increases, the efficiency of the production of bremsstrahlung radiation increases, and high-energy x-rays increase in number to a greater extent than low-energy x-rays.

The change in the bremsstrahlung x-ray spectrum is not nearly as pronounced as the change in the characteristic spectrum. After an increase in the atomic number of the target material, the characteristic spectrum is shifted to the right, representing the higher energy characteristic radiation. This phenomenon is a direct result of the higher electron-binding energies associated with increasing atomic number.

> Changing target atomic number is the only factor that will change the discrete x-ray emission spectrum.

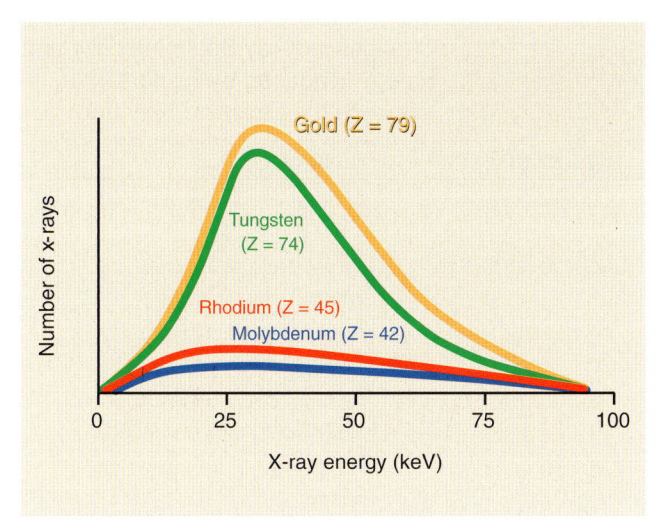

FIG. 8.14 Discrete emission spectrum shifts to the right with an increase in the atomic number of the target material. The continuous spectrum increases slightly in amplitude, particularly to the high-energy side, with an increase in target atomic number.

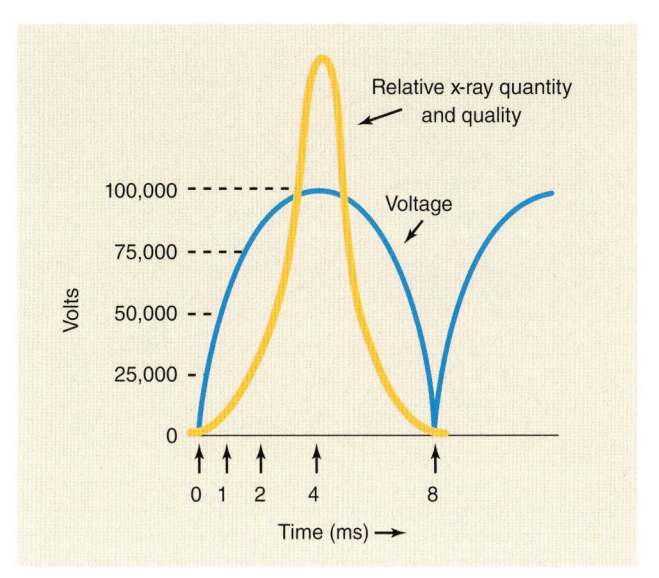

FIG. 8.15 As the voltage across the x-ray tube increases from zero to its peak value, x-ray intensity and energy increase slowly at first and then rapidly as peak voltage is obtained.

These changes are shown schematically in Fig. 8.14. Tungsten is the primary component of x-ray tube targets, but some specialty x-ray tubes use gold as target material. The atomic numbers for tungsten and gold are 74 and 79, respectively.

Molybdenum (Z = 42) and rhodium (Z = 45) are target elements used for mammography. In many dedicated mammography imaging systems, these elements are incorporated separately into the anode as different targets.

The x-ray quantity from such mammography target material is low owing to the inefficiency of x-ray production. This occurs because of the low atomic number of these target elements. Elements of low atomic number also produce low-energy characteristic x-rays.

Effect of Voltage Waveform

There are five voltage waveforms: half-wave-rectified, full-wave-rectified, three-phase/six-pulse, three-phase/12-pulse, and high-frequency waveforms.

Half-wave-rectified and full-wave-rectified voltage waveforms are the same except for the frequency of x-ray pulse repetition. There are twice as many x-ray pulses per cycle with full-wave rectification as with half-wave rectification.

The difference between three-phase/six-pulse and three-phase/12-pulse power is simply the reduced ripple obtained with 12-pulse generation compared with six-pulse generation. High-frequency generators are based on fundamentally different electrical engineering principles. They produce the lowest voltage ripple of all high-voltage generators.

Fig. 8.15 shows an exploded view of a full-wave-rectified voltage waveform for an x-ray imaging system operated at 100 kVp. Recall that the amplitude of the waveform corresponds to the applied voltage and that the horizontal axis represents time.

At t = 0, the voltage across the x-ray tube is zero, indicating that at this instant, no electrons are flowing and no x-rays are being produced. At t = 1 ms, the voltage across the x-ray tube has increased from 0 to approximately 60,000 V. The x-rays produced at this instant are of relatively low intensity and energy; none exceeds 60 keV.

At t = 2 ms, the tube voltage has increased to approximately 80,000 V and is rapidly approaching its peak value.

At t = 4 ms, the maximum tube voltage is obtained, and the maximum energy and intensity of x-ray emission are produced. For the following one-quarter cycle between 4 and 8 ms, the x-ray intensity and energy decrease again to zero.

The number of x-rays emitted at each instant through a cycle is not proportional to the voltage. The number is low at lower voltages and increases at higher voltages. The quantity of x-rays is much greater at peak voltages than at lower voltages. Consequently, voltage waveforms of three-phase or high-frequency operation result in considerably more intense x-ray emission than those of single-phase operation.

The relationship between x-ray intensity and type of high-voltage generator provides the basis for another rule of thumb used by radiographers. If a radiographic technique calls for 72 kVp on single-phase equipment, then on three-phase equipment, approximately 64 kVp—a 12% reduction—will produce similar results. High-frequency generators produce approximately the equivalent of a 16% increase in kVp, or slightly more than a doubling of mAs over single-phase power.

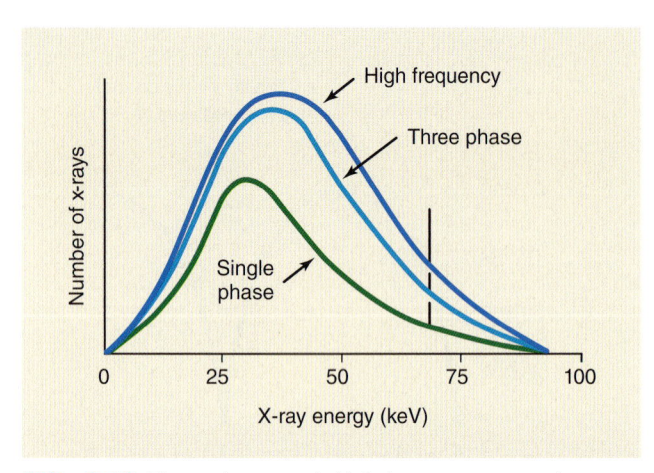

FIG. 8.16 Three-phase and high-frequency operations are considerably more efficient than single-phase operation. Both the x-ray intensity (area under the curve) and the effective energy (relative shift to the right) are increased. Shown are representative spectra for 92-kVp operation at constant mAs.

> Because of reduced ripple, operation with three-phase power or high frequency is equivalent to an approximate 12% increase in kVp, or almost a doubling of mAs over single-phase power.

This discussion is summarized in Fig. 8.16, where an x-ray emission spectrum from a full-wave-rectified unit is compared with that from a three-phase, 12-pulse generator and a high-frequency generator, all operated at 92 kVp and at the same mAs. The x-ray emission spectrum that results from high-frequency operation is more efficient than that produced with a single-phase or a three-phase generator. The area under the curve is considerably greater, and the x-ray emission spectrum is shifted to the high-energy side.

The characteristic x-ray emission spectrum remains fixed in its position on the energy axis but increases slightly in magnitude as a result of the increased number of projectile electrons available for K-shell electron interactions.

Question: What would be the difference in the x-ray emission spectra between full-wave-rectified operation and half-wave-rectified operation if the kVp and the mAs were held constant?

Answer: Under constant conditions of kVp and mAs, there should be no difference in the x-ray emission spectra. The x-ray intensity and energy will remain the same for both modes of operation. Exposure time will double for the half-wave-rectified operation.

TABLE 8.3 Changes in X-ray Beam Intensity and Energy Produced by Factors That Influence the Emission Spectrum

By Increasing	Results
Current (mAs)	An increase in intensity; no change in energy
Voltage (kVp)	An increase in intensity and energy
Added filtration	A decrease in intensity and an increase in energy
Target atomic number (Z)	An increase in intensity, energy and characteristic x-radiation
Voltage ripple	A decrease in intensity and energy

Table 8.3 presents a summary of the effect on x-ray intensity and energy produced by each of the factors that influence the x-ray emission spectrum. Although five factors are listed, only the first two, mAs and kVp, are routinely controlled by radiographers. Occasionally, the added filtration is changed if the imaging system design permits.

SUMMARY

When electrons are accelerated from the cathode to the target of the anode, three effects take place: the production of heat, the formation of characteristic x-rays, and the formation of bremsstrahlung x-rays.

Characteristic x-rays are produced when an electron ionizes an inner-shell electron of a target atom. As the inner-shell void is filled, a characteristic x-ray is emitted.

Bremsstrahlung x-rays are produced by the slowing down of an electron by the target atom's nuclear field. Most x-rays in the diagnostic range (20–150 kVp) are bremsstrahlung x-rays.

X-ray emission spectra can be graphed as the number of x-rays for each increment of energy in keV. Characteristic x-rays of tungsten have a discrete energy of 69 keV. Bremsstrahlung x-rays have a range of energies up to X keV, where X is the kVp.

CHALLENGE QUESTIONS

1. Define or otherwise identify the following:
    a. Projectile electron
    b. Binding energy
    c. Characteristic x-rays
    d. Bremsstrahlung x-rays
    e. X-ray intensity
    f. X-ray energy

g. Effective energy
   h. Added filtration
   i. Emission spectrum
   j. Molybdenum
2. Calculate the energy and wavelength of the characteristic x-ray produced when a K-shell electron is replaced by an M-shell electron in tungsten.
3. At what fraction of the velocity of light do 90-keV electrons travel?
4. What does the discrete x-ray spectrum represent?
5. Draw the x-ray emission spectrum for an x-ray imaging system with a tungsten-targeted x-ray tube operated at 90 kVp.
6. When an x-ray imaging system is operated at 80 kVp, its emission spectrum represents an output intensity of 35 μGya/mAs. What will be the output intensity if the voltage is increased to 90 kVp? How will the emission spectrum change?
7. Discuss the effect on the x-ray emission spectrum if a single-phase x-ray imaging system is changed to a three-phase system.
8. Explain the effect the addition of filtration to an x-ray tube has on the discrete and continuous x-ray emission spectra.
9. How is the kinetic energy of the projectile electrons streaming from cathode to anode of the x-ray tube increased?
10. At 80 kVp, what is the energy in joules of electrons arriving at the x-ray tube target?
11. Why is the x-ray tube considered an inefficient device?
12. Draw the diagram and write a description of the formation of characteristic radiation.
13. What is the importance of K-characteristic x-rays in forming a diagnostic radiograph?
14. What is the range of energies of bremsstrahlung x-rays?
15. What is the minimum wavelength associated with x-rays emitted from an x-ray tube operated at 90 kVp?
16. List three factors that affect the shape of the x-ray emission spectrum, and briefly describe each.
17. Define and explain the 15% kVp rule.
18. What is the diagnostic range of x-rays?
19. What type of x-radiation is useful for mammography but not for general diagnostic imaging?
20. In your clinical setting, observe or ask what filtration is used on the x-ray tubes. Why is filtration important?

The answers to the Challenge Questions can be found by logging on to our website at http://evolve.elsevier.com.

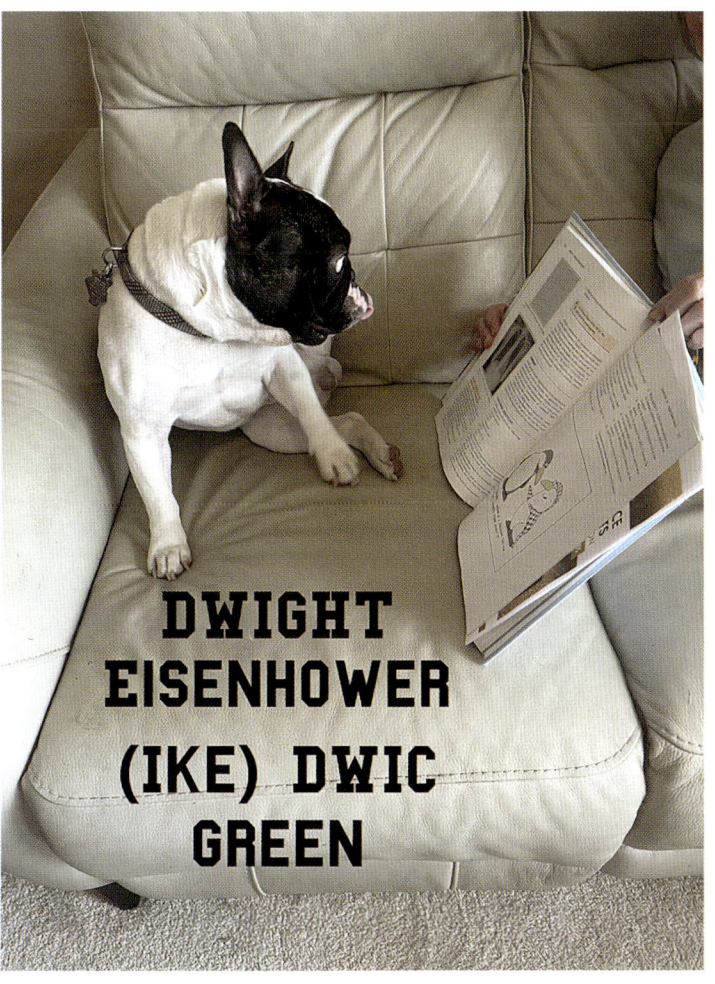

CHAPTER 9

X-ray Emission

OBJECTIVES

On completion of this chapter, the student should be able to do the following:

1. Define and understand x-ray radiation intensity.
2. List and discuss the factors that affect the intensity of the x-ray beam.
3. Explain x-ray energy and its relation to penetrability.
4. List and discuss the factors that affect the energy of the x-ray beam.

OUTLINE

X-ray Intensity 143
   mAs and X-ray Intensity 143
   kVp and X-ray Intensity 144
   Distance and X-ray Intensity 145
   Filtration and X-ray Intensity 146
X-ray Energy 146
   Penetrability and X-ray Energy 146
   Half-Value Layer and X-ray Energy 146
   Factors That Affect X-ray Energy 147
Types of Filtration 148
Summary 150
Challenge Questions 151

X-RAYS ARE emitted through a window in the glass or metal enclosure of the x-ray tube in the form of a spectrum of energies. The x-ray beam is characterized by the number of x-rays in the beam and the average energy of the beam. This chapter discusses the numerous factors that affect the intensity and energy of the x-ray beam.

The intensity of the x-ray beam of an x-ray imaging system is measured in milligray in air (mGya) and is the **air kerma** (**k**inetic **e**nergy **r**eleased in **ma**tter). Other terms, such as x-ray quantity and radiation exposure, are also often used. All have somewhat the same meaning, and all are measured in mGy_a.

X-RAY INTENSITY

The mGy_a is a measure of the number of ion pairs produced in air by a beam of x-rays. Ionization of air increases as the number of x-rays in the beam increases. The relationship between the x-ray intensity as measured in mGy_a and the number of x-rays in the beam is not always one to one.

Radiation exposure **rate** expressed as mGy_a/s, mGy_a/min, or mGy_a/mAs can also be used to express x-ray intensity.

> X-ray intensity is the number of x-rays in the useful beam.

Small variations are related to the effective x-ray energy. These variations are unimportant over the x-ray energy range used in medical imaging, and we can therefore assume that the number of x-rays in the useful beam is the radiation intensity. Most general purpose x-ray tubes, when operated at approximately 70 kVp, produce x-ray intensities of approximately 50 μGy_a/mAs at a 100-cm source-to-image receptor distance (SID).

Fig. 9.1 is a nomogram for estimating x-ray intensity for a wide range of techniques. These curves apply only for single-phase, full-wave-rectified apparatus.

Several factors affect x-ray intensity. Most were discussed briefly in Chapter 8; consequently, this section may serve primarily as a review. The factors that affect x-ray intensity affect x-ray exposure of the image receptor similarly. These relationships are summarized in Table 9.1.

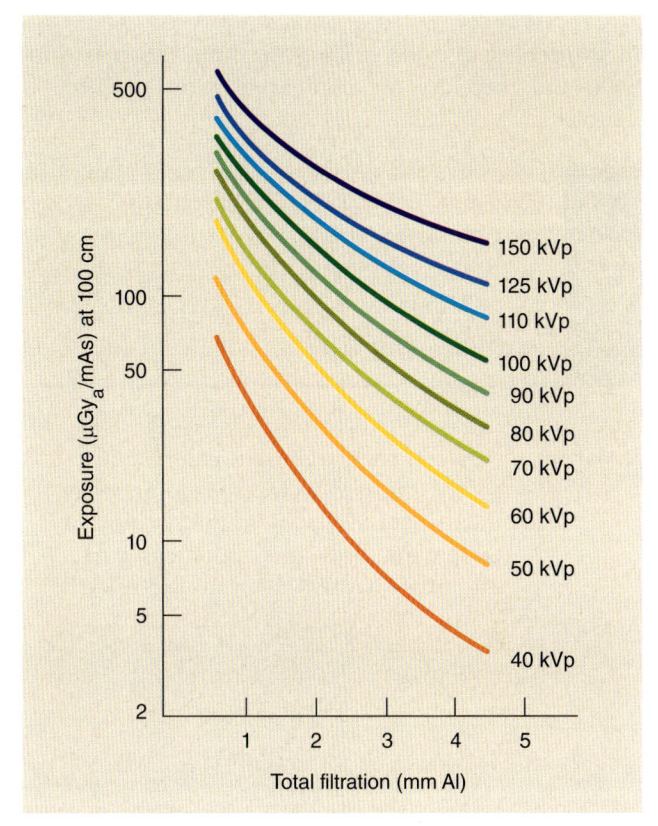

FIG. 9.1 Nomogram for estimating the intensity of x-ray beams. From the position on the *x*-axis corresponding to the filtration of the imaging system, draw a vertical line until it intersects with the appropriate voltage (kVp). A horizontal line from that point will intersect the *y*-axis at the approximate x-ray intensity for the imaging system. (Courtesy Edward McCullough, University of Wisconsin.)

TABLE 9.1 Factors That Affect X-ray Intensity and Image Receptor Exposure

The Effect of Increasing	X-ray Intensity Is	Image Receptor Exposure Is
mAs	Increased proportionately	Increased
kVp	Increased by $\left(\frac{kVp_2}{kVp_1}\right)^2$	Increased by $\left(\frac{kVp_2}{kVp_1}\right)^5$
Distance	Reduced by $\left(\frac{d_1}{d_2}\right)^2$	Reduced by $\left(\frac{d_1}{d_2}\right)^2$
Filtration	Reduced	Reduced

kVp, Kilovolt peak; *mAs*, milliampere seconds.

mAs and X-ray Intensity

X-ray intensity is directly proportional to milliampere seconds (mAs). When mAs is doubled, the number of projectile electrons striking the tube target is doubled, and therefore the number of x-rays emitted is doubled.

> **MAS AND X-RAY INTENSITY**
>
> $$\frac{I_1}{I_2} = \frac{mAs_1}{mAs_2}$$
>
> where I_1 and I_2 are the x-ray intensities at mAs_1 and mAs_2, respectively.

Question: A lateral chest technique calls for 110 kVp, 10 mAs, which results in an x-ray intensity of 320 µGy$_a$ at the position of the patient. If the mAs is increased to 20 mAs, what will the x-ray intensity be?

Answer:
$$\frac{x}{320\ \mu Gy_a} = \frac{20\ mAs_1}{10\ mAs_2}$$
$$x = \frac{(320\ \mu Gy_a)(20\ mAs)}{10\ mAs}$$
$$= 640\ \mu Gy_a$$

> X-ray intensity is directly proportional to mAs.

Question: The radiographic technique for a kidney, ureter, and bladder examination uses 60 mAs at 74 kVp. The result is an x-ray intensity of 2.5 mGy$_a$. What will be the x-ray intensity if the mAs can be reduced to 45 mAs?

Answer:
$$\frac{x}{2.5\ mGy_a} = \frac{45\ mAs_1}{60\ mAs_2}$$
$$x = \frac{(2.5\ \mu Gy_a)(45\ mAs)}{60\ mAs}$$
$$= 1.9\ mGy_a$$

> Remember that mAs is just a measure of the total number of projectile electrons that travel from the cathode to the anode to produce x-rays.
>
> mAs = mA × s
> = mC/s × s
> = mC
>
> where C (coulomb) is a measure of electrostatic charge and 1 C = 6.25 × 10^{18} electrons.

kVp and X-ray Intensity

X-ray intensity varies rapidly with changes in **kilovolt peak (kVp)**. The change in x-ray intensity is proportional to the square of the ratio of the kVp; in other words, if the kVp were doubled, the x-ray intensity would increase by a factor of 4. Mathematically, this is expressed as follows:

> **KVP AND X-RAY INTENSITY**
>
> $$\frac{I_1}{I_2} = \left(\frac{kVp_1}{kVp_2}\right)^2$$
>
> where I_1 and I_2 are the x-ray intensities at kVp_1 and kVp_2, respectively.

Question: A lateral chest technique calls for 10 mAs at 110 kVp and results in an x-ray intensity of 0.32 mGy$_a$. What will be the intensity if the kVp is increased to 125 kVp and the mAs remains fixed?

Answer:
$$\frac{0.32\ mGy_a}{I_2} = \left(\frac{110\ kVp}{125\ kVp}\right)^2$$
$$I_2 = (0.32\ mGy_a)\left(\frac{125\ kVp}{110\ kVp}\right)^2$$
$$= (0.32\ mGy_a)(1.14)^2$$
$$= (0.32\ mGy_a)(1.29)$$
$$= 0.41\ mGy$$

> X-ray intensity is proportional to kVp^2.

Question: An extremity is examined using a technique of 8 mAs at 58 kVp, which results in an entrance skin exposure (ESE) of 240 µGy$_a$. If the technique is changed to 8 mAs at 54 kVp to improve contrast, what will be the x-ray intensity?

Answer:
$$\frac{I}{240\ \mu Gy_a} = \left(\frac{54\ kVp}{58\ kVp}\right)^2$$
$$I = (240\ \mu Gy_a)\left(\frac{54\ kVp}{58\ kVp}\right)^2$$
$$= (240\ \mu Gy_a)(0.93)^2$$
$$= (240\ \mu Gy_a)(0.867)$$
$$= 208\ \mu Gy$$

In practice, a slightly different situation prevails. Radiographic technique factors must be selected from a relatively narrow range of values, from approximately 50 to 120 kVp. Theoretically, doubling the x-ray intensity by kVp manipulation alone requires an increase of 40% in kVp.

This relationship is not adopted clinically because as kVp is increased, the penetrability of the x-ray beam is increased and relatively fewer x-rays are absorbed in the patient. More x-rays are transmitted through the patient and interact with the image receptor.

Consequently, to maintain a constant exposure of the image receptor, an increase of 15% in kVp should be accompanied by a reduction of one-half in mAs. Such an increase in kVp results in doubling the x-ray intensity.

Increasing kVp and reducing mAs so that image receptor exposure remains constant significantly reduces the patient's radiation dose. The disadvantage of such a technique adjustment was reduced image contrast when screen film was the image receptor. There is little change in image contrast as we now use digital image receptors.

Distance and X-ray Intensity

X-ray intensity varies inversely with the square of the distance from the x-ray tube target. This relationship is known as the **inverse square law** (see Chapter 4).

> **DISTANCE AND X-RAY INTENSITY**
>
> $$\frac{I_1}{I_2} = \left(\frac{d_2}{d_1}\right)^2$$
>
> where I_1 and I_2 are the x-ray intensities at distances d_1 and d_2, respectively.

Question: Mobile radiography is conducted at 100 cm SID and results in an exposure at the image receptor of 0.13 mGy$_a$. If 91 cm is the maximum SID that can be obtained for a particular examination, what will be the image receptor exposure?

Answer:
$$\frac{0.12 \text{ mGy}_a}{I_2} = \left(\frac{91 \text{ cm}}{100 \text{ cm}}\right)^2$$

$$I_2 = (0.13 \text{ mGy}_a)\left(\frac{100 \text{ cm}}{91 \text{ cm}}\right)^2$$

$$= (0.13 \text{ mGy}_a)(1.1)^2$$

$$= (0.13 \text{ mGy}_a)(1.1)$$

$$= 0.16 \text{ mGy}_a$$

> X-ray intensity is inversely proportional to the square of the distance from the source.

Question: A posteroanterior (PA) chest examination (120 kVp/3 mAs) with a dedicated x-ray imaging system is taken at an SID of 300 cm. The x-ray exposure at the image receptor is 0.12 mGy$_a$. If the same technique is used at an SID of 100 cm, what will be the image receptor exposure?

Answer:
$$\frac{I}{0.12 \text{ mGy}_a} = \left(\frac{300 \text{ cm}}{100 \text{ cm}}\right)^2$$

$$I = 0.12 \text{ mGy}_a \left(\frac{300 \text{ cm}}{100 \text{ cm}}\right)^2$$

$$= (0.12 \text{ mGy}_a)(3)^2$$

$$= (0.12 \text{ mGy}_a)(9)$$

$$= 1.08 \text{ mGy}_a$$

> When SID is increased, mAs must be increased by SID^2 to maintain constant exposure to the image receptor.

Compensating for a change in SID by changing mAs by the factor SID^2 is known as the **square law**, a corollary to the inverse square law.

> **THE SQUARE LAW**
>
> $$\frac{\text{mAs}_1}{\text{mAs}_2} = \frac{\text{SID}_1^2}{\text{SID}_2^2}$$
>
> where mAs$_1$ is the technique at d_1 and mAs$_2$ is the technique at d_2.

In practical terms, this can be rewritten as follows:

$$\frac{\text{Old mAs}}{\text{New mAs}} = \frac{\text{Old distance squared}}{\text{New distance squared}}$$

Question: What should be the new mAs in the previous question to reduce the x-ray intensity to 0.12 mGy$_a$ at 100 cm?

Answer:
$$\frac{x \text{ mAs}}{3 \text{ mAs}} = \frac{0.12 \text{ mGy}_a}{1.08 \text{ mGy}_a}$$

$$x \text{ mAs} = (3 \text{ mAs}) \left(\frac{0.12 \text{ mGy}_a}{1.08 \text{ mGy}_a} \right)$$

$$= (3 \text{ mAs})(0.111) = 0.3 \text{ mAs}$$

Filtration and X-ray Intensity

X-ray imaging systems have metal filters, usually 1 to 5 mm of aluminum (Al), positioned in the useful beam. The purpose of x-ray beam filtration is to reduce the number of low-energy x-ray incidents in the patient.

Low-energy x-rays contribute nothing useful to the image. They only increase the patient ESE unnecessarily because they are absorbed in superficial tissues and do not penetrate through the patient to reach the image receptor.

> Adding filtration to the useful x-ray beam reduces the patient radiation dose.

When filtration is added to the x-ray beam, the patient radiation dose is reduced because fewer low-energy x-rays are in the useful beam. Calculation of the reduction in exposure requires knowledge of half-value layer (HVL), which is discussed in the following section.

An estimate of exposure reduction can be made from the nomogram in Fig. 9.1, where it is shown that the reduction is not proportional to the thickness of the added filter but is related in a complex way. The disadvantage of x-ray beam filtration is reduced image contrast caused by x-ray beam hardening. X-ray beam hardening increases the number of high-energy x-rays in the beam by removing the lower-energy nonpenetrating x-rays.

X-RAY ENERGY

There are many descriptors for the energy of a diagnostic x-ray beam, and all are useful as they are applied to different situations. Energy in this sense determines the manner in which the diagnostic x-ray beam interacts with the patient and therefore is a principal factor in producing a diagnostic image.

Penetrability and X-ray Energy

As the energy of an x-ray beam is increased, the penetrability of the beam through the patient or shielding material is also increased. Penetrability refers to the ability of x-rays to penetrate deeper in tissue and be transmitted through the patient to the image receptor. High-energy x-rays are able to penetrate tissue more deeply than low-energy x-rays.

X-rays with high penetrability sometimes are termed high-quality x-rays. Those with low penetrability are low-quality x-rays.

Factors that affect x-ray beam energy also influence image contrast. The principal factors influencing x-ray beam energy are kVp and added filtration. Distance, mA, and mAs do not affect radiation energy; they do affect radiation intensity.

Half-Value Layer and X-ray Energy

X-rays are attenuated exponentially; high-energy x-rays are more penetrating than low-energy x-rays. Although 100-keV x-rays are attenuated at the rate of approximately 3%/cm of soft tissue, 10-keV x-rays are attenuated at approximately 15%/cm of soft tissue. X-rays of any given energy are more penetrating in materials of low atomic number than in material of high atomic number.

> Attenuation is the reduction in x-ray intensity that results from absorption and scattering.

In radiography, the energy of x-rays is usually measured by the HVL because such measurement is relatively easy. Therefore the HVL is an energy characteristic of the useful x-ray beam. The HVL of an x-ray beam is the thickness of absorbing material necessary to reduce the x-ray intensity to half of its original value.

The absorbing material used to measure the HVL of a diagnostic x-ray beam is Al. A diagnostic x-ray beam usually has an HVL in the range of 3 to 5 mm Al. The HVL in soft tissue is 3 to 6 cm.

The HVL is determined experimentally, with a setup similar to that shown in Fig. 9.2. This setup consists of three principal parts: the x-ray tube; a radiation detector; and graded thicknesses of filters, usually Al.

First, a radiation measurement is made with no filter between the x-ray tube and the radiation detector. Then, measurements of radiation intensity are made for successively thicker sections of filter. The thickness of filtration that reduces the x-ray intensity to half of its original value is the HVL.

Several methods can be used to determine the HVL of an x-ray beam. Perhaps the most straightforward way is to graph the results of x-ray intensity measurements made with an experimental setup, like that in Fig. 9.2. The graph in Fig. 9.3 shows how this can be done when the following steps are completed.

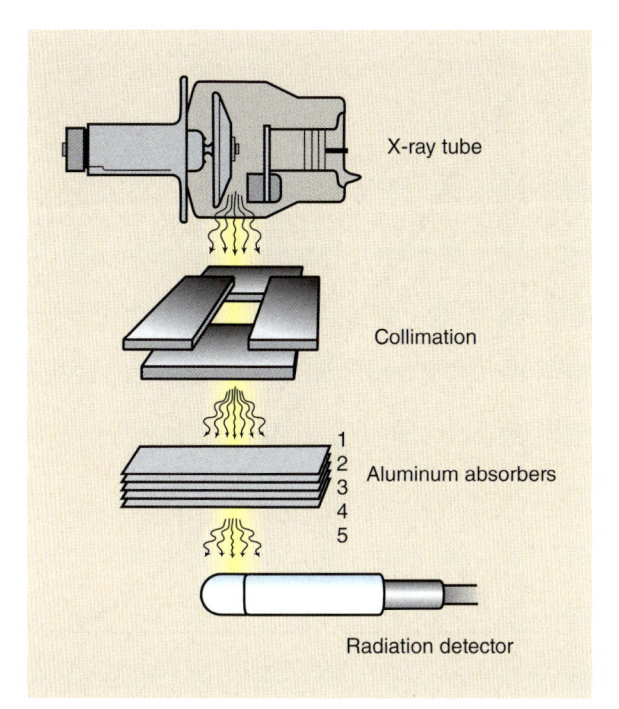

FIG. 9.2 Typical experimental arrangement for the determination of half-value layer.

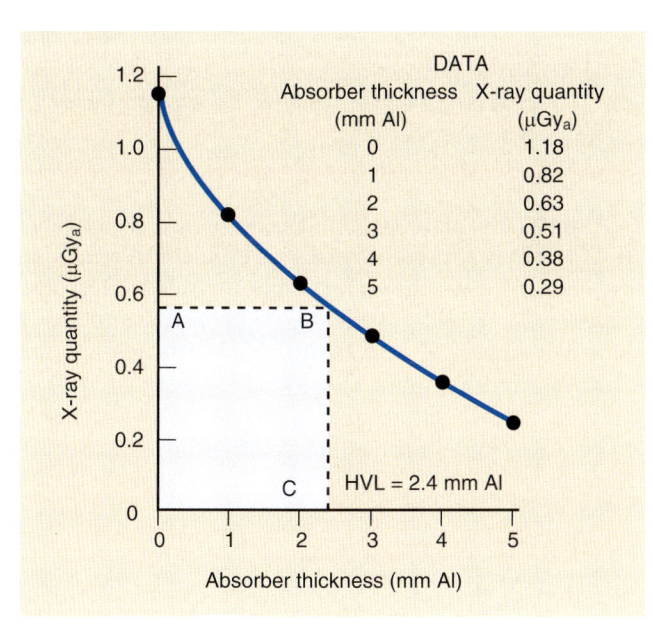

FIG. 9.3 Data in the table are typical for half-value layer (HVL) determination. The plot of these data shows an HVL of 2.4 mm Al.

Question: The following data were obtained with the x-ray tube operated at 70 kVp, while the radiation detector was positioned 100 cm from the target with 1.0 mm Al filters inserted between the target and the detector. Estimate the HVL from observation of these data. Then plot the data to see how close you were.

mm Al	0	1.0	2.0	3.0	4.0	5.0
µGy$_a$	1.18	0.82	0.63	0.51	0.38	0.29

Answer: One-half of 1.18 µGy$_a$ is 0.59 µGy$_a$; therefore the HVL must be between 2 and 3 mm of Al. A plot of the data shows the HVL to be 2.4 mm Al.

STEPS TO DETERMINE THE HALF-VALUE LAYER
1. Determine the x-ray beam intensity with no absorbing material in the beam and then with different known thicknesses of an absorber.
2. Plot the ordered pairs of data (thickness of absorber, x-ray intensity).
3. Determine the x-ray intensity equal to half the original intensity and locate this value on the y- or vertical axis of the graph in Fig. 9.3.
4. Draw a horizontal line parallel to the x-axis from point A in step 3 until it intersects the curve (B).
5. From point B, drop a vertical line to the x-axis.
6. On the x-axis, read the thickness of the absorber required to reduce the x-ray intensity to half of its original value point (C). This is the HVL.

Question: The data of Fig. 9.3 were plotted from measurements designed to estimate HVL. What does this graph suggest the HVL to be?

Answer: At zero filtration, x-ray quantity is 1.18 mGy$_a$. One-half of 1.18 mGy$_a$ is 0.59 mGy$_a$. At the level of 0.59 mGy$_a$, a horizontal line is drawn from the y-axis until it intersects the plotted curve. From that intersection, a vertical line is dropped to the x-axis, where it intersects at 2.4 mm Al, the HVL.

X-ray beam penetrability changes in a complex way with variations in kVp and filtration. Different combinations of added filtration and kVp can result in the same x-ray beam HVL. For example, measurements may show that a single x-ray imaging system has the same HVL when operated at 90 kVp with 2 mm Al total filtration as when operated at 70 kVp with 4 mm Al total filtration. In this case, x-ray penetrability remains constant, as does the HVL.

X-ray beam energy can be identified by kVp or filtration, but HVL is most appropriate.

Factors That Affect X-ray Energy

Some of the factors that affect x-ray intensity have no effect on x-ray energy. Other factors affect both x-ray intensity and energy. These relationships are summarized in Table 9.2.

| TABLE 9.2 | Factors That Affect X-ray Energy and Intensity |

| | EFFECT ON | |
An Increase in	X-ray Energy	X-ray Intensity
mAs	None	Increased
kVp	Increased	Increased
Distance	None	Reduced
Filtration	Increased	Reduced

kVp, Kilovolt peak; *mAs*, milliampere seconds.

| TABLE 9.3 | Approximate Relationship Between the Kilovolt Peak and Half-Value Layer |

Kilovolt Peak	Half-Value Layer (mm Al)
50	1.9
75	2.8
100	3.7
125	4.6
150	5.4

Al, Aluminum.

As the **kilovolt peak (kVp)** is increased, so too is x-ray beam energy and, therefore, so too is the HVL. An increase in kVp results in a shift of the x-ray emission spectrum toward the high-energy side, indicating an increase in the effective energy of the x-ray beam. The result is a more penetrating x-ray beam.

> Increasing kVp increases the energy of an x-ray beam.

Table 9.3 shows the measured change in HVL as kVp is increased from 50 to 150 kVp for a representative x-ray imaging system. The total filtration of the beam is 2.5 mm of Al.

The primary purpose of adding **filtration** to an x-ray beam is to selectively remove low-energy x-rays that have little chance of getting to the image receptor. Fig. 9.4 shows the emission spectrum of an unfiltered x-ray beam and an x-ray beam with normal filtration.

The ideally filtered x-ray beam would be monoenergetic because such a beam would further reduce the patient's radiation dose. It is desirable to remove all x-rays below a certain energy level determined by the type of x-ray examination. To improve image contrast, it is also desirable to remove x-rays with energies above a certain level. Unfortunately, such removal of regions of an x-ray beam is not normally possible.

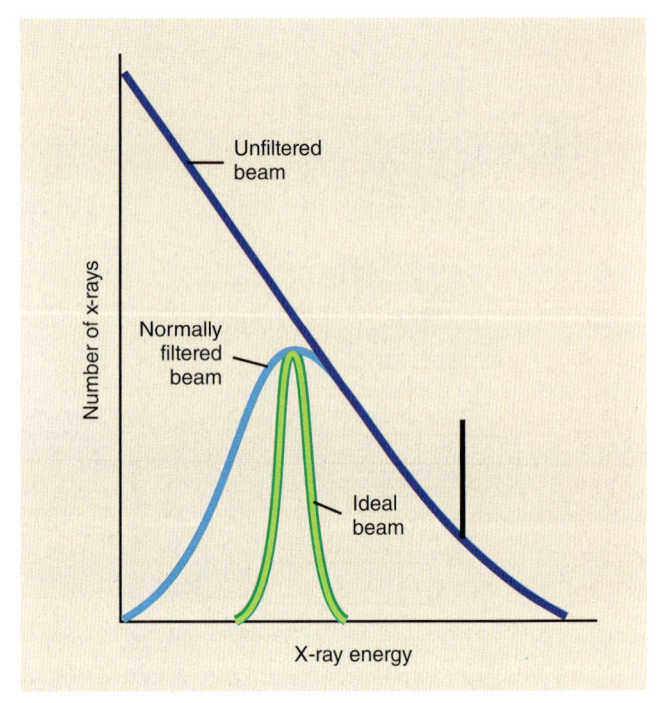

FIG. 9.4 Filtration is used selectively to remove low-energy x-rays from the useful beam. Ideal filtration would remove all low-energy x-rays.

> Increasing filtration increases the average energy of an x-ray beam.

Almost any material could serve as an x-ray filter. Al (Z = 13) is chosen because it is efficient in removing low-energy x-rays through the photoelectric effect and because it is readily available, inexpensive, and easily shaped. Copper (Z = 29), tin (Z = 50), gadolinium (Z = 64), and holmium (Z = 67) have been used sparingly in special situations. As filtration is increased, so too is x-ray beam energy, but x-ray intensity is decreased.

TYPES OF FILTRATION

Filtration of diagnostic x-ray beams has two components: inherent filtration and added filtration.

The glass or metal enclosure of an x-ray tube filters the emitted x-ray beam. This type of filtration is called **inherent filtration**. Inspection of an x-ray tube reveals that the part of the glass or metal enclosure through which x-rays are emitted—the **window**—is very thin. This provides for low inherent filtration.

The inherent filtration of a general-purpose x-ray tube is approximately 0.5 mm Al equivalent. With age, inherent filtration tends to increase because some of the tungsten metal of both the target and filament is vaporized and is deposited on the inside of the window.

Special-purpose x-ray tubes, such as those used in mammography, have very thin windows. They are sometimes made of beryllium (Z = 4) rather than glass and have an inherent filtration of approximately 0.1 mm Al.

A thin sheet of Al positioned between the protective x-ray tube housing and the x-ray beam collimator is the usual form of **added filtration**.

> Added filtration results in increased HVL.

The addition of a filter to an x-ray beam attenuates x-rays of all energies emitted, but it attenuates a greater number of low-energy x-rays than high-energy x-rays. This shifts the x-ray emission spectrum to the high-energy side, resulting in an x-ray beam with higher energy and greater penetrability. The HVL increases, but the extent of the increase in the HVL cannot be predicted even when the thickness of the added filter is known.

Because added filtration attenuates the x-ray beam, it affects x-ray intensity. This value can be predicted if the HVL of the beam is known. The addition of filtration equal to the beam HVL reduces the beam intensity to half its prefiltered value and results in a higher x-ray beam energy.

Question: An x-ray imaging system has an HVL of 2.2 mm Al. The exposure rate is 20 μGy_a/mAs at 100 cm SID. If 2.2 mm Al is added to the beam, what will be the x-ray exposure rate?

Answer: This is an addition of one HVL; therefore the x-ray exposure will be 10 μGy_a/mAs.

Added filtration usually has two sources. First, 1 mm or more sheets of Al are permanently installed in the port of the x-ray tube between the housing and the collimator.

With a conventional light-localizing variable-aperture collimator, the collimator contributes an additional 1 mm Al equivalent added filtration. This filtration results from the silver surface of the mirror in the collimator (Fig. 9.5).

One of the most difficult tasks facing radiographers is producing an image with uniform intensity when a body part that varies greatly in thickness or tissue composition is examined. When a filter is used in this fashion, it is called a **compensating filter** because it compensates for differences in subject radiopacity.

Compensating filters can be fabricated for many procedures; therefore they come in various sizes and shapes. They are nearly always constructed of Al, but plastic materials also can be used. Fig. 9.6 shows some common compensating filters.

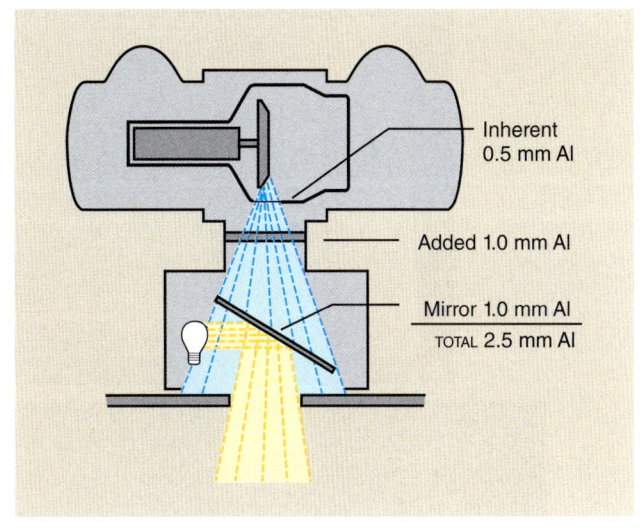

FIG. 9.5 Total filtration consists of the inherent filtration of the x-ray tube, an added filter, and filtration by the mirror of the light-localizing collimator.

During PA chest radiography, for instance, if the left chest is relatively radiopaque because of fluid, consolidation, or mass, the image would appear with a very low signal on the left side of the chest and a very high signal on the right side of the chest. One could compensate for this signal variation by inserting a wedge filter so that the thin part of the wedge is positioned over the left side of the chest. Such use of a wedge filter results in more uniform x-ray exposure of the image receptor.

The wedge filter is principally used during radiography of a body part, such as the foot, that varies considerably in thickness (Fig. 9.7). During an anteroposterior projection of the foot, the wedge would be positioned with its thick portion shadowing the toes and the thin portion toward the heel.

A bilateral wedge filter, or a trough filter, is sometimes used in chest radiography (Fig. 9.8). The thin central region of the wedge is positioned over the mediastinum, and the lateral thick portions shadow the lung fields. The result is a more uniform radiation exposure of the image receptor. Specialty compensating wedges of this type are usually used with dedicated apparatus, such as an x-ray imaging system used exclusively for chest radiography.

Special "bow-tie"–shaped filters are used with computed tomography imaging systems to compensate for the shape of the head or body. Conic filters, either concave or convex, find application in digital fluoroscopy, in which an image receptor like the image intensifier tube is round.

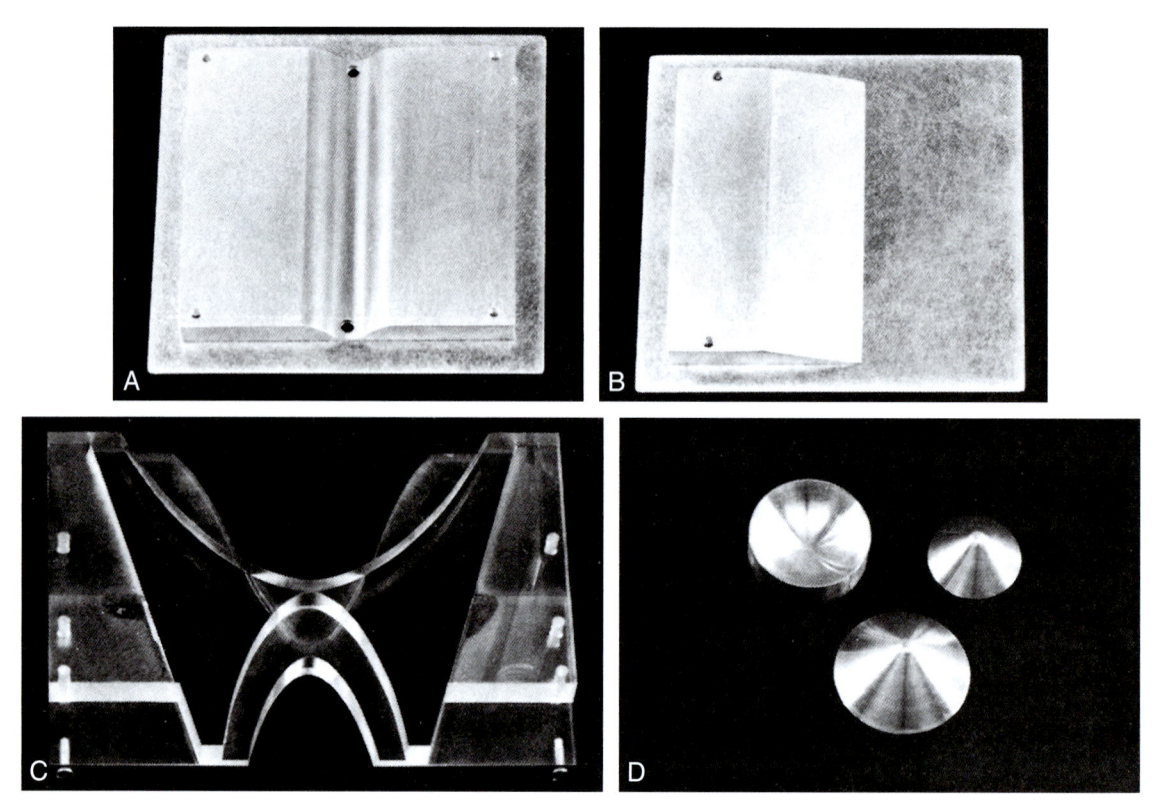

FIG. 9.6 Compensating filters. (A) Trough filter. (B) Wedge filter. (C) "Bow-tie" filter for use in computed tomography. (D) Conic filters for use in digital fluoroscopy.

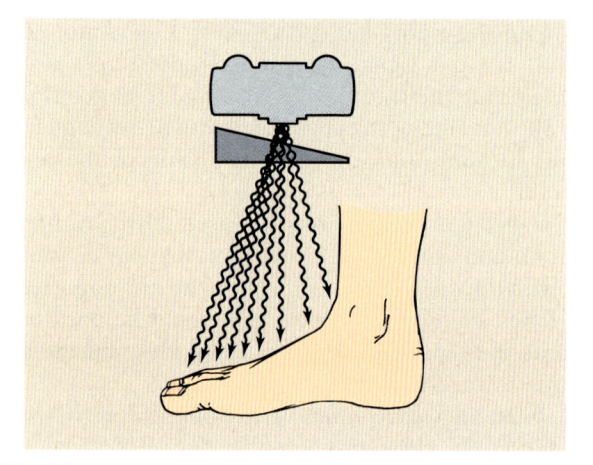

FIG. 9.7 Use of a wedge filter for examination of the foot.

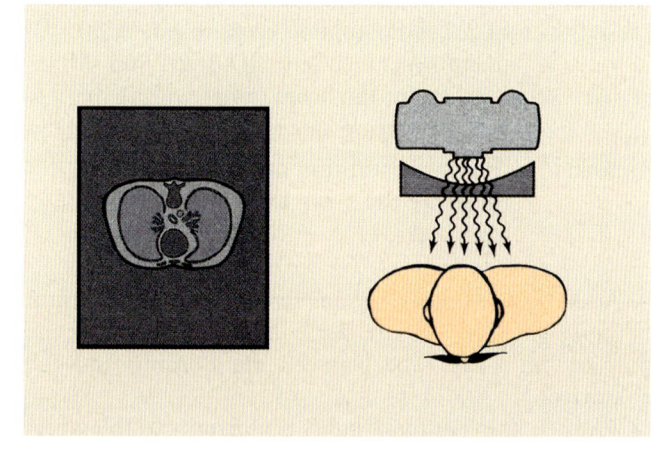

FIG. 9.8 Use of a trough filter for examination of the chest.

A step-wedge filter is an adaptation of the wedge filter (Fig. 9.9). It is used in some interventional radiology procedures, usually when long sections of the anatomy are imaged with the use of two or three separate image receptors.

A common application of a step-wedge filter involves a three-step Al wedge and three 35- × 43-cm image receptors for translumbar and femoral arteriography and venography. These procedures call for a careful selection of radiographic techniques.

Compensating filters are useful for producing quality radiographic images. They are not patient radiation protection devices.

SUMMARY

Radiation intensity is the number of x-rays in the useful beam. Factors that affect radiation intensity include the following:
- mAs: x-ray intensity is directly proportional to mAs.
- kVp: x-ray intensity is proportional to the square of the kVp.
- Distance: x-ray intensity varies inversely with distance from the source.
- Filtration: x-ray intensity is reduced by filtration, which preferentially absorbs low-energy x-rays in the beam.

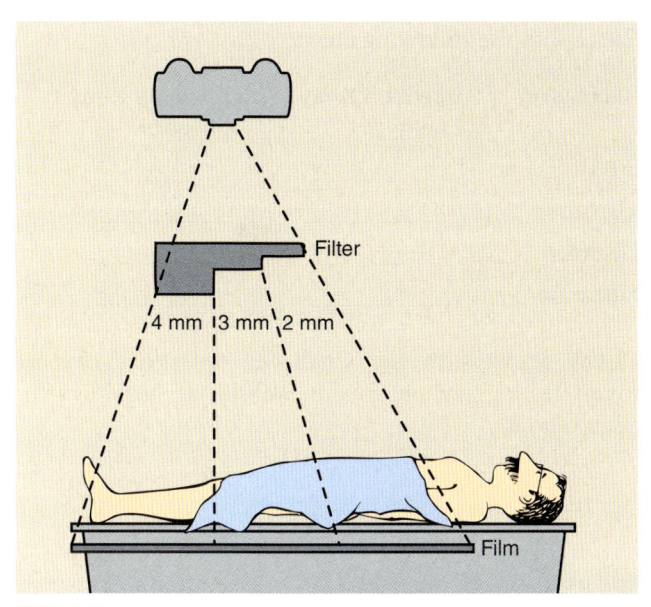

FIG. 9.9 Arrangement of apparatus with the use of an aluminum step-wedge filter for serial radiography of the abdomen and lower extremities.

Radiation energy determines the penetrating power of the x-ray beam. The penetrability is represented by the HVL, which is the thickness of additional filtration that reduces x-ray intensity to half its original value. Factors that affect x-ray beam energy or penetrability include the following:
- kVp: x-ray energy is increased as kVp is increased.
- Filtration: x-ray energy is increased when filtration is added to the beam.

There are three types of filtration: (1) inherent filtration of the glass or metal enclosure, (2) added filtration in the form of Al sheets, and (3) compensating filters, which provide variation in intensity across the x-ray beam.

CHALLENGE QUESTIONS

1. Define or otherwise identify the following:
    a. Inherent filtration
    b. The unit describing x-ray intensity
    c. A filtered x-ray spectrum
    d. A kVp change equal to twice the mAs
    e. Three filter materials used with diagnostic x-ray beams
    f. Half-value layer
    g. Wedge filter
    h. The description of x-ray energy
    i. The approximate HVL of your x-ray imaging system
    j. X-ray penetrability
2. Graph the change in HVL with changing kVp (from 50 to 120 kVp) for an x-ray imaging system that has total filtration of 2.5 mm Al. Check your answer by plotting the data in Table 9.3.
3. An abdominal radiograph taken at 84 kVp, 150 mAs results in patient radiation exposure of 6.5 mGy_a. The image is repeated at 84 kVp, 250 mAs. What is the new radiation exposure?
4. An image of the lateral skull was taken at 68 kVp, 20 mAs and is repeated. If the kVp is increased to 78 kVp, what should be the new mAs?
5. A chest radiograph taken at 180-cm SID results in an exposure of 120 μGy_a. What would the exposure be if the same radiographic factors were used at 100-cm SID?
6. The following data were obtained with a fluoroscopic x-ray tube operated at 80 kVp: The exposure levels were measured 50 cm above the patient couch with Al absorbers positioned on the surface of the couch. Estimate the HVL through visual inspection of the data; then plot the data and determine the precise value of the HVL.

Added mm Al	μGy_a
None	650
1	480
3	300
5	210
7	160
9	130

7. When operated at 74 kVp, 100 mAs with 2.2 mm Al added filtration and 0.6 mm Al inherent filtration, the HVL of an x-ray imaging system is 3.2 mm Al and its output intensity at 100-cm SID is 3.5 mGy_a. How much additional filtration is necessary to reduce the x-ray intensity to 1.75 mGy_a?
8. The following technique factors have been shown to produce good-quality radiographs of the cervical spine with an x-ray imaging system that has 3 mm Al total filtration. Refer to Fig. 9.1, and estimate the x-ray intensity at 100-cm SID for each.
    a. 62 kVp, 70 mAs
    b. 70 kVp, 40 mAs
    c. 78 kVp, 27 mAs
9. A radiographic exposure is 80 kVp at 50 mAs. How many electrons will interact with the target?
10. An extremity is radiographed at 60 kVp, 10 mAs, resulting in an x-ray intensity of 280 μGy_a. If the technique is changed to 55 kVp, 10 mAs, what is the resultant x-ray intensity?
11. What is the square law and how is it used?

12. What is the primary purpose of x-ray beam filtration?
13. The kVp is reduced from 78 to 68 kVp. What, if anything, should be done with mAs to maintain exposure of the image receptor constant?
14. What is the relationship between x-ray intensity and mAs?
15. Define half-value layer.
16. List the two ways an x-ray beam can be shifted to a higher average energy.
17. Why is Al used for x-ray beam filtration?
18. Describe the use of a wedge filter during radiography of a foot.
19. Does adding filtration to the x-ray beam affect the intensity of x-rays reaching the image receptor?
20. Fill in the following chart:

Increasing	Effect on X-ray Energy	Effect on X-ray Intensity
mAs	_____	_____
kVp	_____	_____
Distance	_____	_____
Filtration	_____	_____

The answers to the Challenge Questions can be found by logging on to our website at http://evolve.elsevier.com.

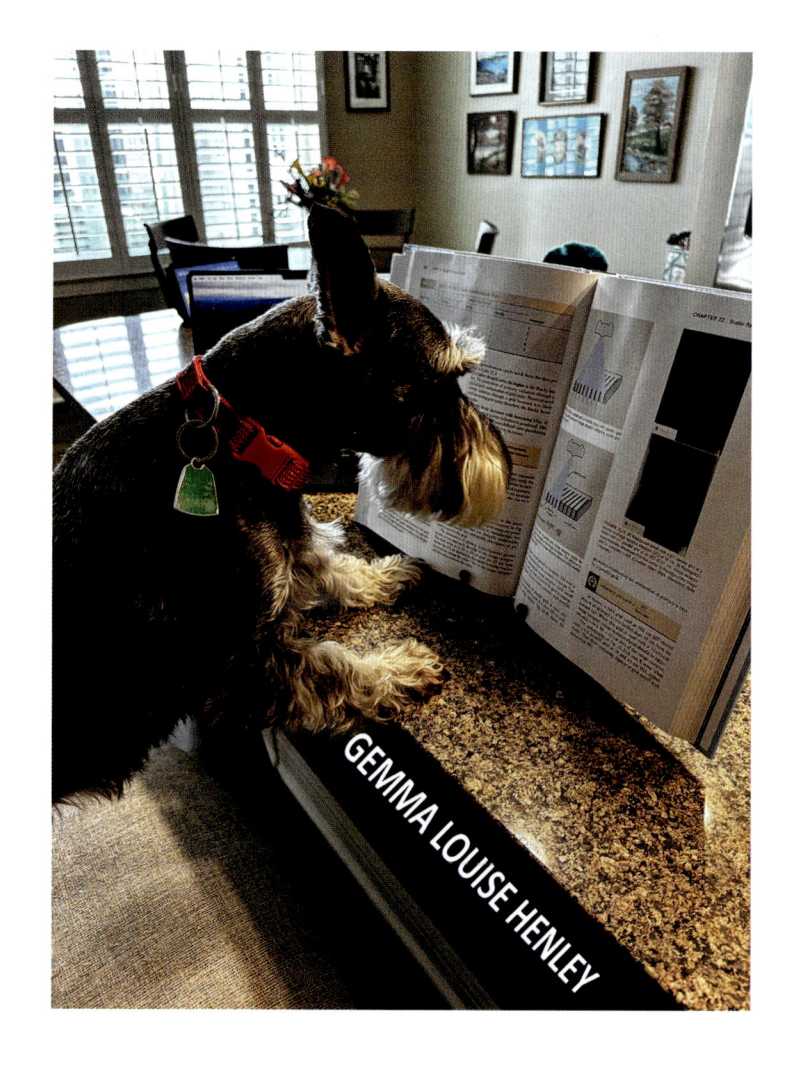

CHAPTER 10

X-ray Interaction With Matter

OBJECTIVES

At the completion of this chapter, the student should be able to do the following:

1. Describe each of the five x-ray interactions with matter.
2. Define differential absorption, and describe its effect on image contrast.
3. Explain the effect of atomic number and mass density of tissue on differential absorption.
4. Discuss why radiologic contrast agents are used to image some tissues and organs.
5. Explain the difference between absorption and attenuation.

OUTLINE

Five X-ray Interactions 154
   Coherent Scattering 154
   Compton Scattering 155
   Photoelectric Effect 156
   Pair Production 159
   Photodisintegration 159
Differential Absorption 160
   Dependence on Atomic Number 161
   Dependence on Mass Density 162
Contrast Examinations 164
Exponential Attenuation 164
Summary 165
Challenge Questions 166

X-RAYS INTERACT with matter in the following five ways: (1) coherent scattering, (2) Compton scattering, (3) photoelectric effect, (4) pair production, and (5) photodisintegration. Only Compton scattering and photoelectric effect are important in making an x-ray image. The conditions that govern these two interactions control differential absorption, which determines the degree of contrast of an x-ray image.

FIVE X-RAY INTERACTIONS

In Chapter 4, the interaction between electromagnetic radiation and matter was described briefly. This interaction was said to have wave-like and particle-like properties. Electromagnetic radiation interacts with structures that are similar in size to the wavelength of the radiation.

X-rays have very short wavelengths, approximately 10^{-8} to 10^{-9} m. The higher the energy of an x-ray, the shorter its wavelength. Consequently, low-energy x-rays tend to interact with whole atoms, which have diameters of approximately 10^{-9} to 10^{-10} m; moderate-energy x-rays generally interact with electrons, and high-energy x-rays generally interact with nuclei.

X-rays interact at these various structural levels through five mechanisms: coherent scattering, Compton scattering, photoelectric effect, pair production, and photodisintegration. Two of these—Compton scattering and photoelectric effect—are of particular importance to diagnostic x-ray imaging. They are discussed in some detail here.

Coherent Scattering

X-rays with energies below approximately 10 keV interact with matter by coherent scattering, sometimes called classical scattering or Thompson scattering (Fig. 10.1). J.J. Thompson was the physicist to first identify the electron in 1897 and describe coherent scattering. He received the 1908 Nobel Prize in Physics.

In coherent scattering, the incident x-ray interacts with a target atom, causing the atom to become excited. The target atom immediately releases this excess energy as a scattered x-ray with wavelength equal to that of the incident x-ray ($\lambda = \lambda'$) and therefore of equal energy. However, the direction of the scattered x-ray is different from that of the incident x-ray.

The result of coherent scattering is a change in direction of the x-ray without a change in its energy. There is no energy transfer and, therefore, no ionization. Most coherently scattered x-rays are scattered in the forward direction.

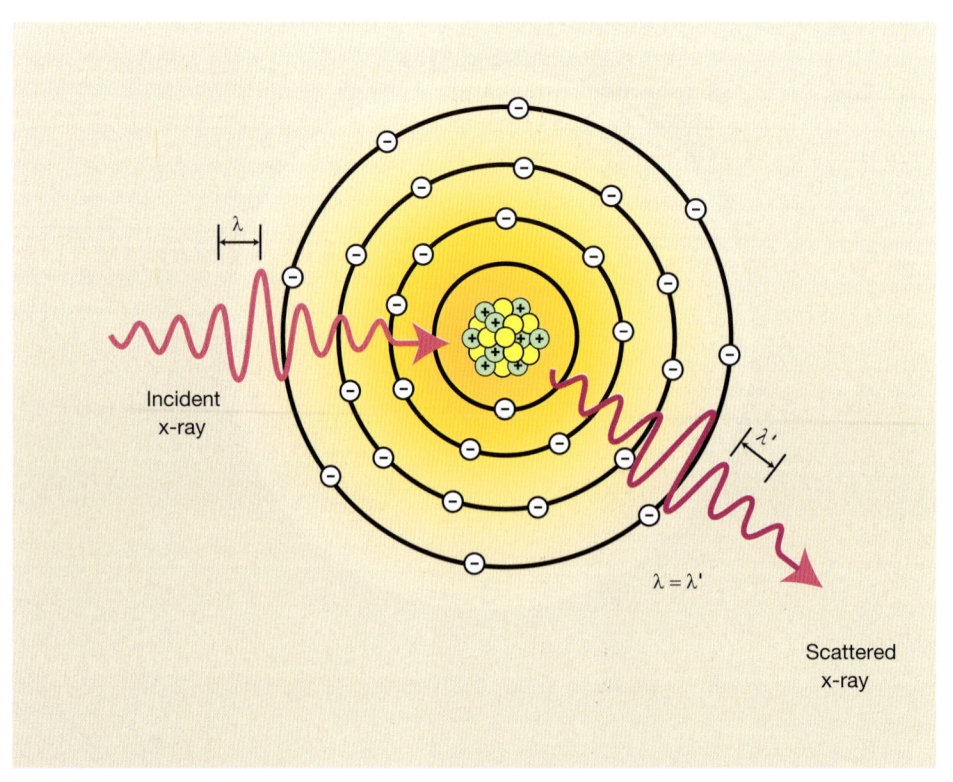

FIG. 10.1 Coherent scattering is an interaction between low-energy x-rays and atoms. The x-ray loses no energy but changes direction slightly. The wavelength of the scattered x-ray is equal to the wavelength of the incident x-ray.

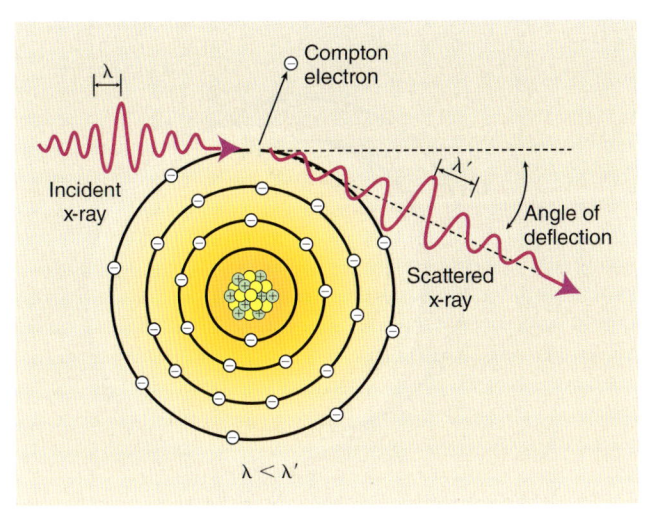

FIG. 10.2 Compton scattering occurs between moderate-energy x-rays and outer-shell electrons. It results in ionization of the target atom, a change in x-ray direction, and a reduction in x-ray energy. The wavelength of the scattered x-ray is longer than that of the incident x-ray.

> Coherent scattering is of little importance to diagnostic radiology.

Coherent scattering primarily involves low-energy x-rays, which contribute little to the x-ray image. However, some coherent scattering occurs throughout the diagnostic range. At 70 kVp, a small percentage of the x-rays scatter coherently, which contributes slightly to **image noise**, the general graying of an image that reduces image contrast.

Compton Scattering

X-rays throughout the diagnostic range can undergo an interaction with outer-shell electrons that not only scatters the x-rays but reduces their energy and ionizes the atom as well. This interaction is called Compton scattering (Fig. 10.2). Arthur Holly Compton described this interaction in 1922 and received the 1927 Nobel Prize in Physics for his discovery.

This was the basis for the very popular 2015 movie *Straight Outta Compton*.

In Compton scattering, the incident x-ray interacts with an outer-shell electron and ejects it from the atom, thereby ionizing the atom. The ejected electron is called a **Compton electron**. The x-ray continues in a different direction with less energy.

The energy of the Compton-scattered x-ray is equal to the difference between the energy of the incident x-ray and the energy of the ejected electron. The energy of the ejected electron is equal to its binding energy plus the kinetic energy with which it leaves the atom. Mathematically, this energy transfer is represented as follows:

> **COMPTON EFFECT**
>
> $E_i = E_s + (E_b + E_{KE})$
>
> where E_i is energy of the incident x-ray, E_s is energy of the scattered x-ray, E_b is electron-binding energy, and E_{KE} is kinetic energy of the scattered electron.

Question: A 30-keV x-ray ionizes an atom of barium by ejecting an O-shell electron with 12 keV of kinetic energy. What is the energy of the scattered x-ray?

Answer: Fig. 3.9 shows that the binding energy of an O-shell electron of barium is 0.04 keV; therefore

$30 \text{ keV} = E_s + (0.04 \text{ keV} + 12 \text{ keV})$

$E_s = 30 \text{ keV} - (0.04 \text{ keV} + 12 \text{ keV})$

$= 30 \text{ keV} - (12.04 \text{ keV})$

$= 17.96 \text{ keV}$

During Compton scattering, most of the energy is divided between the scattered x-ray and the Compton electron. Usually, the scattered x-ray retains most of the energy. Both the scattered x-ray and the Compton electron may have sufficient energy to undergo additional ionizing interactions before they lose all their energy.

Ultimately, the scattered x-ray is absorbed photoelectrically. The Compton electron loses all of its kinetic energy through ionization and excitation and drops into a vacancy in an electron shell previously created by some other ionizing event.

Compton-scattered x-rays can be deflected in any direction, including 180 degrees from the incident x-ray. At a deflection of 0 degrees, no energy is transferred. As the angle of deflection increases to 180 degrees, more energy is transferred to the Compton electron, but even at 180 degrees of deflection, the scattered x-ray retains at least approximately two-thirds of its original energy. X-rays scattered back in the direction of the incident x-ray beam are called **backscatter radiation**.

> The probability of Compton scattering is inversely proportional to x-ray energy (1/E) and independent of atomic number.

The probability that a given x-ray will undergo Compton scattering is a complex function of the energy of the incident x-ray. In general, the probability of Compton scattering decreases as x-ray energy increases.

The probability of Compton scattering does not depend on the atomic number of the atom involved. Any given x-ray is just as likely to undergo Compton

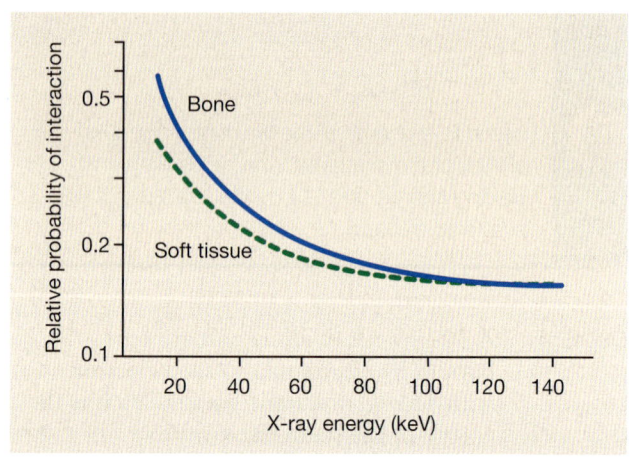

FIG. 10.3 The probability that an x-ray will interact through Compton scattering is about the same for atoms of soft tissue and those of bone. This probability decreases with increasing x-ray energy.

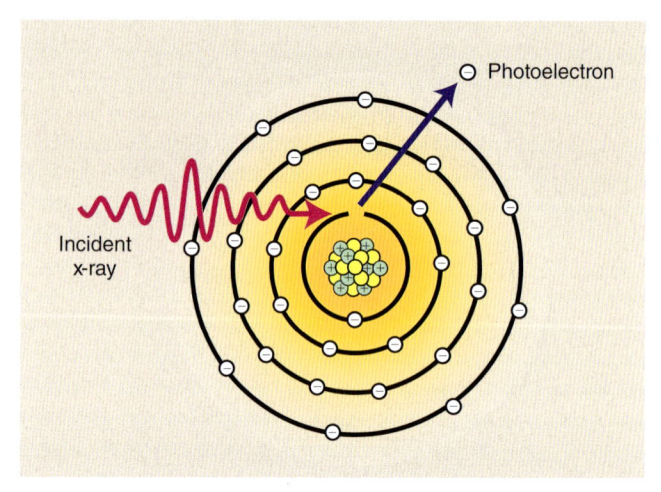

FIG. 10.4 The photoelectric effect occurs when an incident x-ray is totally absorbed during the ionization of an inner-shell electron. The incident photon disappears, and the K-shell electron, now called a photoelectron, is ejected from the atom.

TABLE 10.1	Features of Compton Scattering
Most likely to occur	With outer-shell electrons
	With loosely bound electrons
As x-ray energy increases	Increased penetration through tissue without interaction
	Increased Compton scattering relative to photoelectric effect
	Reduced Compton scattering ($\approx 1/E$)
As atomic number of absorber increases	No effect on Compton scattering
As mass density of absorber increases	Proportional increase in Compton scattering

scattering with an atom of soft tissue as with an atom of bone (Fig. 10.3). Table 10.1 summarizes Compton scattering.

> Compton scattering reduces image contrast.

Compton scattering in tissue can occur with all x-rays and therefore is of considerable importance in x-ray imaging. However, its importance involves a negative sense.

Scattered x-rays provide no useful information on the x-ray image. Rather, they produce an unwanted exposure to the image receptor called **x-ray fog**. The result is uniform x-ray intensity on the image receptor, resulting in reduced image contrast. Ways of reducing this scattered x-radiation are discussed later, but none is totally effective.

The scattered x-rays from the Compton effect can create a serious radiation exposure hazard in radiography and particularly in fluoroscopy. A large amount of radiation can be scattered from the patient during fluoroscopy. Such radiation is the source of most of the occupational radiation exposure that radiographers receive.

During radiography, the hazard is less severe because usually no one but the patient is in the examining room. Nevertheless, scattered x-radiation levels are sufficient to necessitate protective shielding of the x-ray examining room.

Photoelectric Effect

X-rays in the diagnostic imaging range also undergo ionizing interactions with inner-shell electrons. The x-ray is not scattered, but it is totally absorbed. This process is called the photoelectric effect (Fig. 10.4), and it earned Albert Einstein the 1921 Nobel Prize in Physics—General Relativity.

The electron removed from the atom is called a **photoelectron** and escapes with kinetic energy equal to the difference between the energy of the incident x-ray and the binding energy of the electron. Mathematically, this is shown as follows:

> **PHOTOELECTRIC EFFECT**
>
> $E_i = E_b + E_{KE}$
>
> where E_i is the energy of the incident x-ray, E_b is the electron-binding energy, and E_{KE} is the kinetic energy of the electron.

> The photoelectric effect is total x-ray absorption.

TABLE 10.2	Atomic Number and K-Shell Electron-Binding Energy of Radiologically Important Elements	
Element	Atomic Number	K-Shell Electron-Binding Energy (keV)
Hydrogen	1	0.02
Carbon	6	0.3
Nitrogen	7	0.4
Oxygen	8	0.5
Aluminum	13	1.6
Calcium	20	4.1
Molybdenum	42	19
Rhodium	45	23
Iodine	53	33
Barium	56	37
Tungsten	74	69
Rhenium	75	72
Lead	82	88

For low-atomic-number atoms, such as those found in soft tissue, the binding energy of even K-shell electrons is low (e.g., 0.3 keV for carbon). Therefore the photoelectron is released with kinetic energy nearly equal to the energy of the incident x-ray.

For higher-atomic-number target atoms, electron-binding energies are higher (37 keV for barium K-shell electrons). Therefore the kinetic energy of the photoelectron from barium is proportionately lower. Table 10.2 shows the approximate K-shell binding energy for elements of radiologic importance.

Characteristic x-rays are produced after a photoelectric interaction in a manner similar to that described in Chapter 8. Ejection of a K-shell photoelectron by the incident x-ray results in a vacancy in the K shell. This unnatural state is immediately corrected when an outer-shell electron, usually from the L shell, drops into the vacancy.

This electron transition is accompanied by the emission of an x-ray whose energy is equal to the difference between the binding energies of the shells involved. These characteristic x-rays consist of secondary radiation and behave in the same manner as scattered x-radiation. They contribute nothing of diagnostic value and, fortunately, have sufficiently low energy that they do not penetrate the image receptor.

Question: A 50-keV x-ray interacts photoelectrically with (1) a carbon atom and (2) a barium atom. What is the kinetic energy of each photoelectron and the energy of each characteristic x-ray if an L-to-K transition occurs (see Fig. 3.9)?

Answer:
a. $E_{KE} = K_i - K_b$
$= 50 \text{ keV} - 0.3 \text{ keV}$
$= 49.7 \text{ keV}$
$E_x = 0.3 \text{ keV} - 0.006 \text{ keV}$
$= 0.294 \text{ keV}$

b. $E_{KE} = E_i - E_b$
$= 50 \text{ keV} - 37 \text{ keV}$
$= 13 \text{ keV}$

c. $E_x = 37 \text{ keV} - 5.989 \text{ keV}$
$= 31.011 \text{ keV}$

The probability that a given x-ray will undergo a photoelectric interaction is a function of both the x-ray energy and the atomic number of the atom with which it interacts.

> The probability of the photoelectric effect is inversely proportional to the third power of the x-ray energy $(1/E)^3$.

A photoelectric interaction cannot occur unless the incident x-ray has energy equal to or greater than the electron-binding energy. A barium K-shell electron bound to the nucleus by 37 keV cannot be removed by a 36-keV x-ray.

If the incident x-ray has sufficient energy, the probability that it will undergo a photoelectric effect decreases with the third power of the photon energy $(1/E)^3$. This relationship is shown graphically in Fig. 10.5 for soft tissue and bone.

> The probability of photoelectric effect is directly proportional to the third power of the atomic number of the absorbing material (Z^3).

As the relative vertical displacement between the graphs of soft tissue and bone demonstrates, a photoelectric interaction is much more likely to occur with high-Z atoms than with low-Z atoms (see Fig. 10.5). Table 10.3 presents the effective atomic numbers of materials of radiologic importance.

Question: What is the relative probability of an 80-keV x-ray interacting with
a. fat (Z = 6.3)?
b. barium (Z = 56) compared with soft tissue (Z = 7.4)?

Answer:
a. $\left(\dfrac{6.3}{7.4}\right)^3 = 0.62$

b. $\left(\dfrac{56}{7.4}\right)^3 = 433$

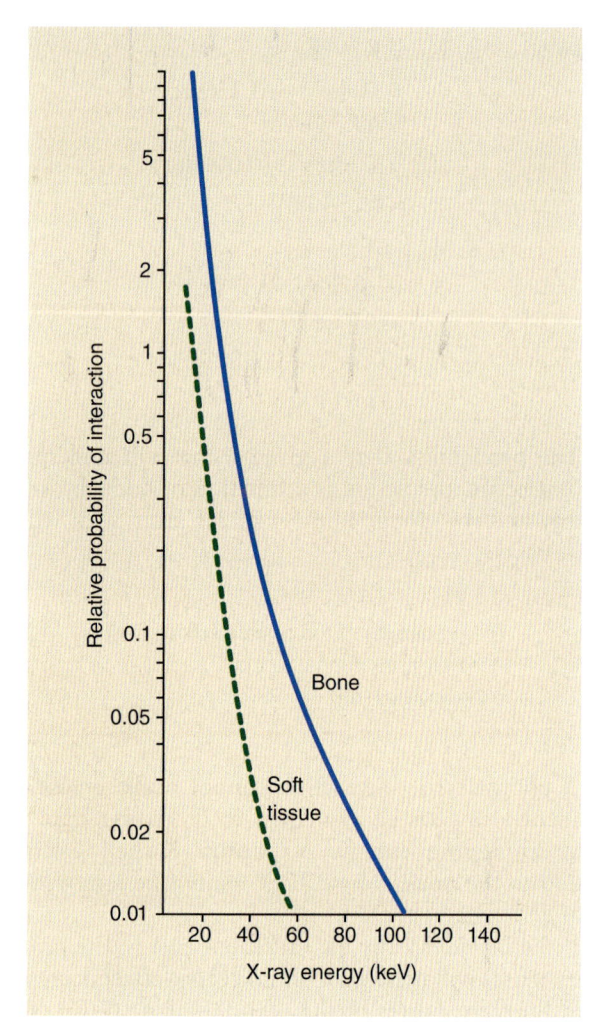

FIG. 10.5 The relative probability that a given x-ray will undergo a photoelectric interaction is inversely proportional to the third power of the x-ray energy and directly proportional to the third power of the atomic number of the absorber.

TABLE 10.3	Effective Atomic Number of Materials Important to Radiologic Science
Type of Substance	**Effective Atomic Number**
HUMAN TISSUE	
Fat	6.3
Soft tissue	7.4
Lung	7.4
Bone	13.8
CONTRAST MATERIAL	
Air	7.6
Iodine	53
Barium	56
OTHER	
Concrete	17
Molybdenum	42
Tungsten	74
Lead	82

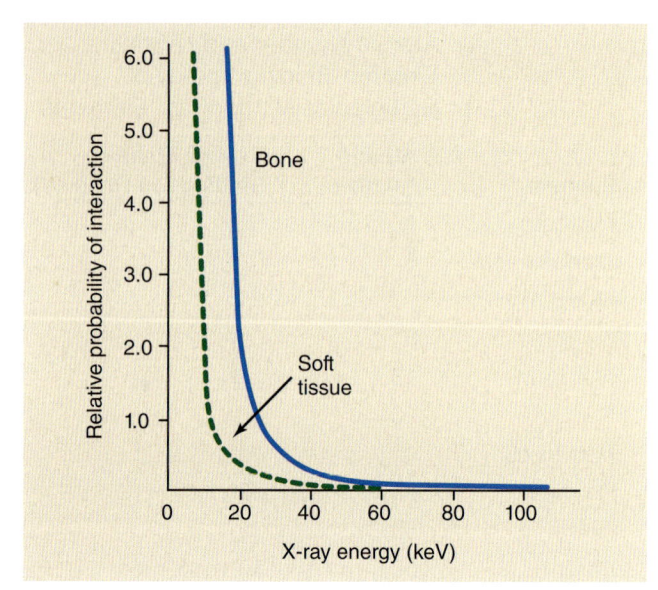

FIG. 10.6 Relative probability for photoelectric interaction ranges over several orders of magnitude. If it is plotted in the conventional linear fashion, as here, one cannot estimate its value above an energy of approximately 30 keV.

Fig. 10.5 is an example of a graph with a **logarithmic scale** along the vertical axis. A logarithmic scale is a power of 10 scale used to plot data that cover several orders of magnitude. In Fig. 10.5, for example, the relative probability of a photoelectric interaction with soft tissue varies from approximately 2 to less than 0.01 over the energy range from 10 to 60 keV.

A plot of these data in conventional arithmetic form appears in Fig. 10.6. Clearly, this type of graph is unacceptable because all probability values greater than 30 keV are so close to zero.

On a linear scale, equal intervals have equal numeric value, but on a log scale, equal intervals represent equal ratios. This difference in scales is shown in Fig. 10.7.

All major intervals on the linear scale have a value of 1, and the subintervals have a value of 0.1. On the other hand, the log scale contains major intervals that each equal one order of magnitude, with subintervals that are not equal in length.

When the probability of interaction is proportional to the third power, the change is very rapid. For the photoelectric effect, this means that a small variation in atomic number of the tissue atom or in x-ray energy results in a large change in the chance of photoelectric interaction. This is unlike the situation that exists for Compton scattering.

Question: If the relative probability of photoelectric interaction with soft tissue for a 20-keV x-ray is 1, how much less likely will an interaction be for a 50-keV x-ray? How much more likely is an interaction with iodine (Z = 53) than with soft tissue (Z = 7.4) for a 50-keV x-ray?

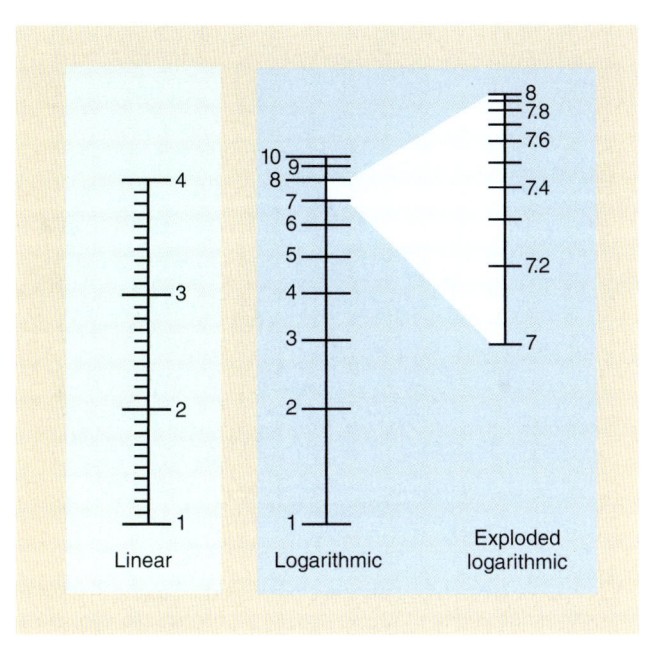

FIG. 10.7 Graphic scales can be linear or logarithmic. The logarithmic scale is used to plot wide ranges of values.

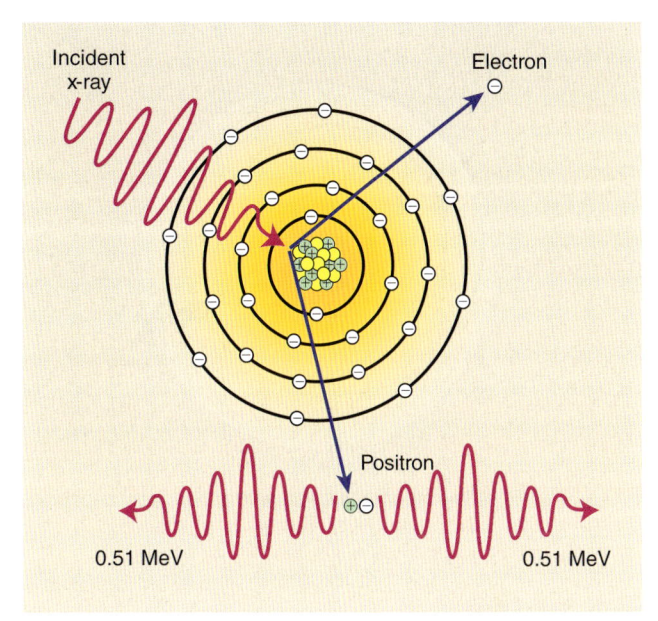

FIG. 10.8 Pair production occurs with x-rays that have energies greater than 1.02 MeV. The x-ray interacts with the nuclear field, and two electrons that have opposite electrostatic charges are created.

TABLE 10.4	Features of Photoelectric Effect
Most likely to occur	With inner-shell electrons
	With tightly bound electrons
	When x-ray energy is just higher than electron-binding energy
As x-ray energy increases	Increased penetration through tissue without interaction
	Less photoelectric effect relative to Compton scattering
	Reduced absolute photoelectric effect ($\approx 1/E)^3$
As atomic number of absorber increases	Increases proportionately with the cube of the atomic number (Z^3)
As mass density of absorber increases	Proportional increase in photoelectric absorption

Answer:
$$\left(\frac{20\,\text{keV}}{50\,\text{keV}}\right)^3 = \left(\frac{2}{5}\right)^3 = 0.064$$
$$\left(\frac{53}{7.4}\right)^3 = 368$$

Table 10.4 summarizes the photoelectric effect.

Pair Production

If an incident x-ray has sufficient energy, it may escape interaction with electrons and come close enough to the nucleus of the atom to be influenced by the strong nuclear field. The interaction between the x-ray and the nuclear field causes the x-ray to disappear, and in its place, two electron-like particles appear: one positively charged (**positron**) and one negatively charged (**negatron**). This process is called **pair production** (Fig. 10.8).

> Pair production does not occur during x-ray imaging.

In Chapter 3, we calculated the energy equivalence of the mass of an electron to be 0.51 MeV. Because two electrons are formed in a pair production interaction, the incident x-ray photon must have at least 1.02 MeV of energy.

An x-ray with less than 1.02 MeV cannot undergo pair production. Any of the x-ray's energy in excess of 1.02 MeV is distributed equally between the two electrons as kinetic energy.

The electron that results from pair production loses energy through excitation and ionization and eventually fills a vacancy in an atomic orbital shell. The positron unites with a free electron, and the mass of both particles is converted to energy in a process called **annihilation radiation**.

Because pair production involves only x-rays with energies greater than 1.02 MeV, it is unimportant in x-ray imaging, but it is very important for positron emission tomography imaging in nuclear medicine.

Photodisintegration

X-rays with energy greater than approximately 10 MeV can escape interaction with electrons and the nuclear

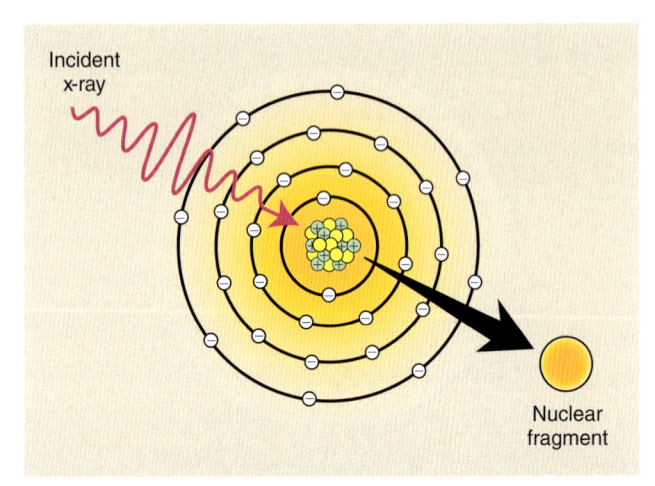

FIG. 10.9 Photodisintegration is an interaction between high-energy x-rays and the nucleus. The x-ray is absorbed by the nucleus, and a nuclear fragment is emitted.

field and be absorbed directly by the nucleus. When this happens, the nucleus is raised to an excited state and instantly emits a nucleon or other nuclear fragment. This process is called **photodisintegration** (Fig. 10.9).

> Photodisintegration does not occur in x-ray imaging.

DIFFERENTIAL ABSORPTION

Of the five ways an x-ray can interact with tissue, only two are important to radiology: Compton scattering and the photoelectric effect. Similarly, only two methods of x-ray production (see Chapter 8)—bremsstrahlung x-rays and characteristic x-rays—are important.

However, more important than the interaction of the x-ray by Compton scattering or photoelectric effect is the x-ray transmitted through the body without interacting. Fig. 10.10 shows schematically how each of these types of x-rays contributes to an image.

> Differential absorption occurs because of Compton scattering, photoelectric effect, and x-rays transmitted through the patient.

The Compton-scattered x-ray contributes no useful information to the image. When a Compton-scattered x-ray interacts with the image receptor, the image receptor assumes that the x-ray came straight from the x-ray tube target (Fig. 10.11). The image receptor does not recognize the scattered x-ray as representing an interaction off the straight line from the x-ray tube target.

These scattered x-rays result in image noise, a generalized dulling of the image by x-rays not representing

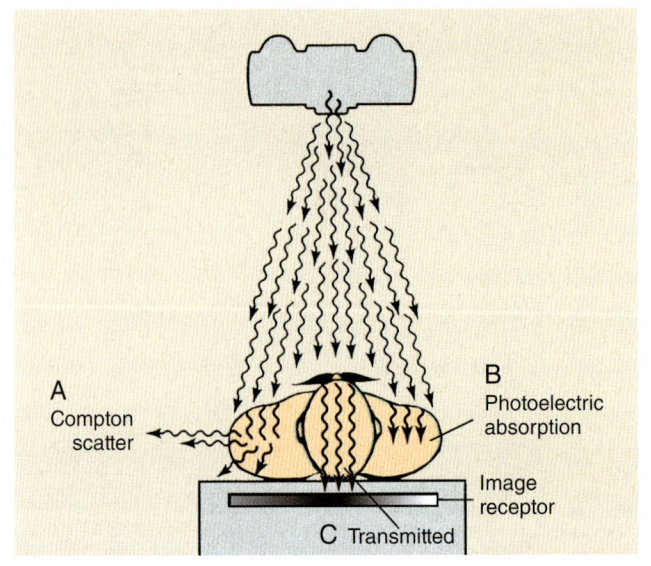

FIG. 10.10 Three types of x-rays are important to the making of an x-ray image: those scattered by Compton interaction (A), those absorbed photoelectrically (B), and those transmitted through the patient without interaction (C).

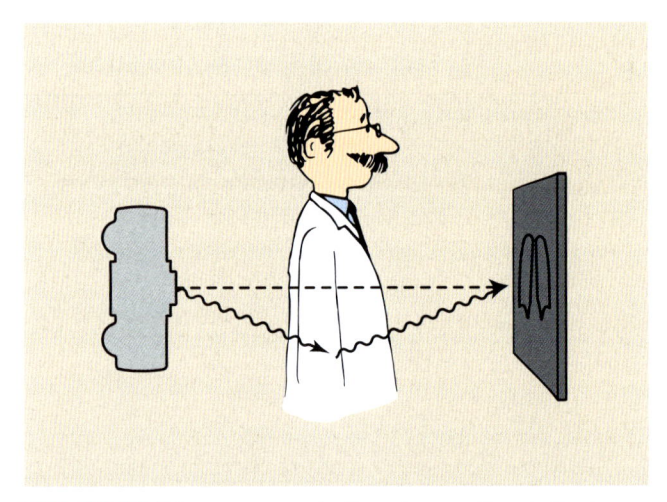

FIG. 10.11 When an x-ray is Compton scattered, the image receptor thinks it came straight from the source.

anatomy. To reduce this type of noise, we use techniques and apparatus to reduce the number of scattered x-rays that reach the image receptor.

X-rays that undergo photoelectric interaction provide diagnostic information to the image receptor. Because they do not reach the image receptor, these x-rays are representative of anatomic structures with high x-ray absorption characteristics; such structures are **radiopaque**. The photoelectric absorption of x-rays produces the light areas on an x-ray image, such as those corresponding to bone.

Other x-rays penetrate the body and are transmitted to the image receptor with no interaction whatsoever. They produce the dark areas of an x-ray image. The anatomic structures through which these x-rays pass are **radiolucent**, such as those corresponding to air in the lungs.

Basically, an x-ray image results from the difference between those x-rays absorbed photoelectrically in the patient and those transmitted to the image receptor. This difference in x-ray interaction is called **differential absorption**.

Approximately 1% of the x-rays incident on a patient reach the image receptor. Fewer than half of those that reach the image receptor interact to form an image. Thus the radiographic image results from approximately 0.5% of the x-rays emitted by the x-ray tube. Consequently, careful control and selection of the x-ray beam are necessary to produce high-quality x-ray images.

> Differential absorption increases as the kVp is reduced.

Producing a high-quality x-ray image requires the proper selection of kVp, so that the effective x-ray energy results in maximum differential absorption. Unfortunately, reducing the kVp to increase differential absorption and, therefore image contrast results in increased patient radiation dose. A compromise is necessary for each examination.

Dependence on Atomic Number

Consider the image of an extremity (Fig. 10.12). An image of the bone is produced because many more x-rays are absorbed photoelectrically in bone than in soft tissue. Recall that the probability of an x-ray undergoing photoelectric effect is proportional to the third power of the atomic number of the tissue.

Bone has an atomic number of 13.8, and soft tissue has an atomic number of 7.4 (see Table 10.3). Consequently, the probability that an x-ray will undergo a photoelectric interaction is approximately seven times greater in bone than in soft tissue.

Question: How much more likely is an x-ray to interact with bone than with muscle?

Answer: $\left(\dfrac{13.8}{7.4}\right)^3 = \dfrac{2628}{405} = 6.5$

These relative values of interaction are apparent in Fig. 10.13 when one pays particular attention to the logarithmic scale of the vertical axis. Note that the relative probability of interaction between bone and soft tissue (differential absorption) remains constant, but the absolute probability of each decreases with increasing energy. With higher x-ray energy, fewer interactions occur, so more x-rays are transmitted without interaction.

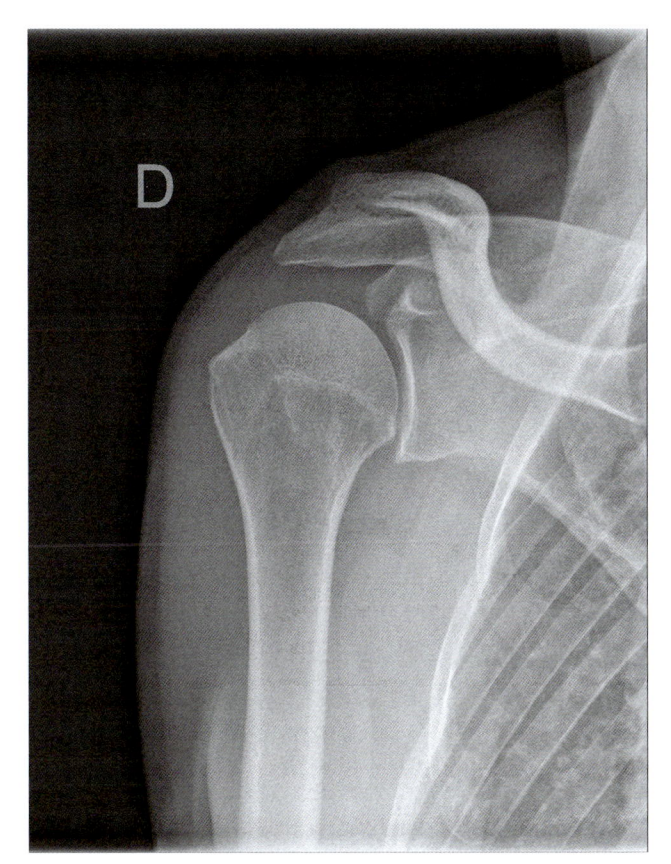

FIG. 10.12 X-ray image of bony structures results from differential absorption between bone and soft tissue. (Courtesy Marcelo Zenteno, Colegio de Tecnólogos Médicos de Chile.)

Question: What is the relative probability that a 20-keV x-ray will undergo photoelectric interaction in bone compared with fat?

Answer: $Z_{bone} = 13.8$, $Z_{fat} = 6.8$

$$\left(\dfrac{13.8}{7.4}\right)^3 = 8.36$$

Compton scattering is independent of the atomic number of tissues. The probability of Compton scattering for bone atoms and for soft tissue atoms is approximately equal and decreases with increasing x-ray energy.

However, this decrease in Compton scattering is not as rapid as the decrease in photoelectric effect with increasing x-ray energy. The probability of Compton scattering is inversely proportional to x-ray energy ($1/E$). The probability of the photoelectric effect is inversely proportional to the third power of the x-ray energy ($1/E^3$).

At low energies, most x-ray interactions with tissue are photoelectric. At high energies, Compton scattering predominates.

Of course, as x-ray energy is increased, the chance of any interaction at all decreases. As kVp is increased, more x-rays penetrate to the image receptor; therefore, a lower x-ray intensity (lower mAs) is required.

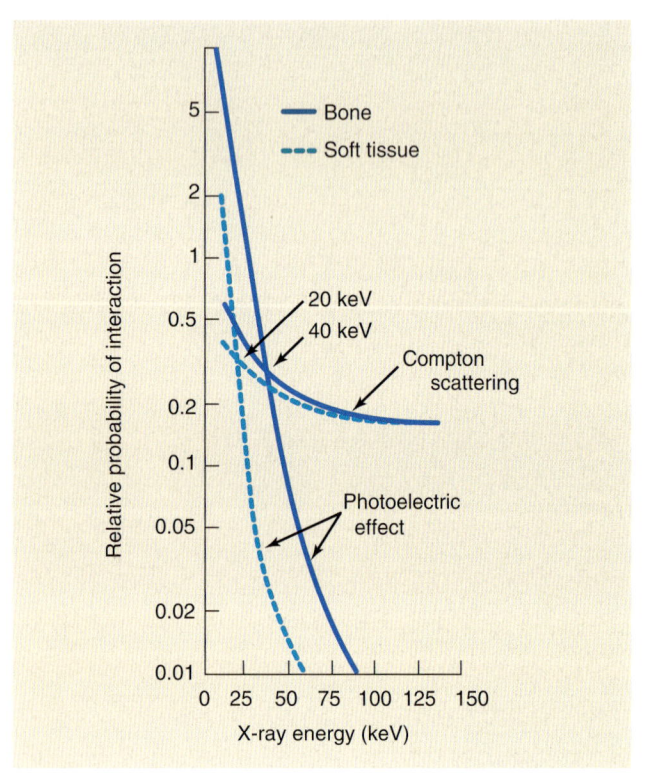

FIG. 10.13 Graph showing the probabilities of photoelectric and Compton interactions with soft tissue and bone. The interactions of these curves indicate those x-ray energies at which the chance of photoelectric absorption equals the chance of Compton scattering.

Fig. 10.13 combines all of these factors into a single graph. At 20 keV, the probability of photoelectric effect equals the probability of Compton scattering in soft tissue. Below this energy, most x-rays interact with soft tissue photoelectrically. Above this energy, the predominant interaction with soft tissue is Compton scattering. Low kVp resulting in increased differential absorption provides the basis for mammography, which is an example of soft tissue radiography.

> To image small differences in soft tissue, one must use low kVp to get maximum differential absorption.

The relative frequency of Compton scattering compared with photoelectric effect increases with increasing x-ray energy. The crossover point between photoelectric effect and Compton scattering for bone is approximately 40 keV. Nevertheless, low-kVp technique is usually appropriate for bone radiography to maintain image contrast.

High-kVp technique is usually reserved for examination of barium studies and chest radiography, in which intrinsic subject contrast is high, resulting in much lower patient radiation dose.

When high-kVp technique is used in this manner, the amount of scattered radiation from surrounding soft tissue contributes little to the image. When the amount of scattered radiation becomes too great, radiographic grids are used (see Chapter 15).

Differential absorption in bone and soft tissue results from photoelectric interactions, which greatly depend on the atomic number of tissues. The loss of contrast is due to x-ray fog caused by Compton scattering. Two other factors are important in making an x-ray image: x-ray emission spectrum and mass density of patient tissues.

The crossover energies of 20 and 40 keV refer to a **monoenergetic** x-ray beam (i.e., a beam containing x-rays that all have the same energy). In fact, as discussed in Chapter 8, clinical x-rays are **polyenergetic**. They are emitted over an entire spectrum of energies.

The correct selection of voltage for optimum differential absorption depends on the other factors discussed in Chapter 9 that affect the x-ray emission spectrum. For instance, in anteroposterior radiography of the lumbar spine at 110 kVp, a greater number of x-rays are emitted with energy above the 40-keV crossover for bone than below it. Less filtration or a radiographic grid may then be necessary.

Dependence on Mass Density

Intuitively, we know that we could image bone even if differential absorption were not Z-related because bone has a higher mass density than soft tissue. Mass density is the quantity of matter per unit volume, specified in units of kilograms per cubic meter (kg/m³). Sometimes mass density is reported in grams per cubic centimeter (g/cm³).

Question: How many g/cm³ are there in 1 kg/m³?
Answer:
$$1 \text{ kg/m}^3 = \frac{1000 \text{ g}}{(100 \text{ cm})^3} = \frac{10^3 \text{ g}}{10^6 \text{ cm}^3} = 10^{-3} \text{ g/cm}^3$$

Table 10.5 gives the mass densities of several radiologically important materials. Mass density is related to the mass of each atom and basically tells how tightly the atoms of a substance are packed.

Water and ice are composed of precisely the same atoms, but ice occupies greater volume. The mass density of ice is 917 kg/m³ compared with 1000 kg/m³ for water. Ice floats in water because of this difference in mass density. Ice is lighter than water.

> The interaction of x-rays with tissue is proportional to the mass density of the tissue, regardless of the type of interaction.

When mass density is doubled, the chance for x-ray interaction is doubled because twice as many electrons are available for interaction. Therefore even without the Z-related photoelectric effect, nearly twice as many x-rays would be absorbed and scattered in bone as in soft tissue. The bone would be imaged.

CHAPTER 10 X-ray Interaction With Matter

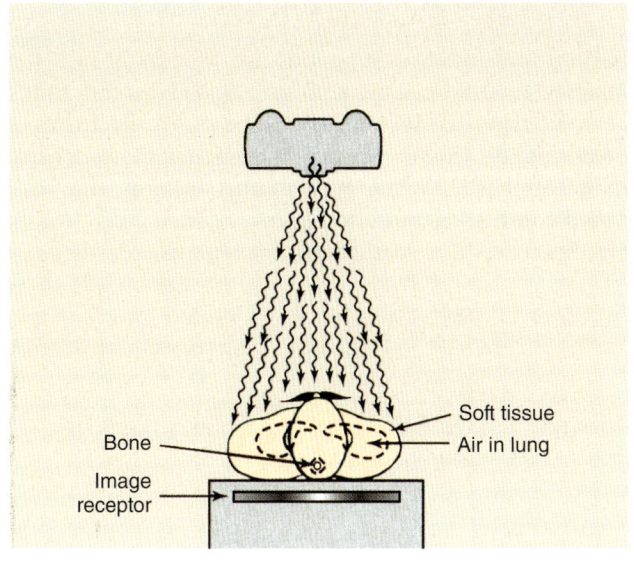

TABLE 10.5	Mass Density of Materials Important to Radiologic Science
Substance	**Mass Density (kg/m³)**
HUMAN TISSUE	
Lung	320
Fat	910
Soft tissue, muscle	1000
Bone	1850
CONTRAST MATERIAL	
Air	1.3
Barium	3500
Iodine	4930
OTHER	
Calcium	1550
Concrete	2350
Molybdenum	10,200
Lead	11,350
Rhenium	12,500
Tungstate	19,300

FIG. 10.14 Even if x-ray interaction were not related to atomic number (Z), differential absorption would occur because of differences in mass density.

Question: What is the relative probability that 60-keV x-rays will undergo Compton scattering in bone compared with soft tissue?

Answer: Mass density of bone = 1850 kg/m³
Mass density of soft tissue = 1000 kg/m³
$$\frac{1850}{1000} = 1.85$$

The lungs are imaged in chest radiography primarily because of differences in mass density. According to Table 10.5, the mass density of soft tissue is 770 times that of air (1000/1.3) and three times that of lung (1000/320). Therefore for the same thickness, we can expect almost three times as many x-rays to interact with the soft tissue as with lung tissue.

The Z values of air and soft tissue are approximately the same: 7.4 for soft tissue and 7.6 for air; thus differential absorption in air-filled soft tissue cavities is primarily attributable to differences in mass density. Interestingly, air has higher Z than soft tissue because it has more nitrogen. Fig. 10.14 demonstrates differential absorption in air, soft tissue, and bone caused by mass density differences. Table 10.6 summarizes the various relationships of differential absorption.

Question: Assume that all x-ray interactions during mammography are photoelectric. What is the differential absorption of x-rays in microcalcifications (Z = 20, ρ = 1550 kg/m³) relative to fatty tissue (Z = 6.3, ρ = 910 kg/m³)?

TABLE 10.6	Characteristics of Differential Absorption
As x-ray energy increases	Fewer Compton interactions
	Many fewer photoelectric interactions
	More transmission through tissue
As tissue atomic number increases	No change in Compton interactions
	Many more photoelectric interactions
	Less x-ray transmission
As tissue mass density increases	Proportional increase in Compton interactions
	Proportional increase in photoelectric interactions
	Proportional reduction in x-ray transmission

Answer: Differential absorption due to atomic number:
$$\left(\frac{20}{6.3}\right)^3 = \frac{8000}{250} = 32:1$$

Differential absorption due to mass density
$$= \frac{1550}{910} = 1.7:1$$

Total differential absorption
$$= 32 \times 1.7 = 54.4:1$$

CONTRAST EXAMINATIONS

Barium and iodine compounds are used as an aid for imaging internal organs with x-rays. The atomic number of barium is 56; that of iodine is 53. Each has a much higher atomic number and greater mass density than soft tissue. When used in this fashion, they are called **contrast agents**, and because of their high atomic numbers, they are positive contrast agents.

Question: What is the probability that an x-ray will interact with iodine rather than soft tissue?

Answer: Differential absorption as a result of atomic number:

$$\left(\frac{53}{7.4}\right)^3 = 367:1$$

Differential absorption due to mass density

$$= \frac{4.93}{1.0} = 4.93:1$$

Total differential absorption
$= 367 \times 4.93 = 1809:1$

When an iodinated contrast agent fills the internal carotid artery or when barium fills the colon, these internal organs are readily visualized on an x-ray image. A low-kVp technique (e.g., <80 kVp) produces excellent, high-contrast x-ray images of the organs of the gastrointestinal tract. Higher-kVp operation (e.g., >90 kVp) often can be used in these examinations not only to outline the organ under investigation but also to penetrate the contrast medium so the lumen of the organ can be visualized more clearly.

Air was used at one time as a contrast medium in procedures such as pneumoencephalography and ventriculography. Air is still used for contrast in some examinations of the colon, along with barium; this is called a **double-contrast examination**. When used in this fashion, air is a negative contrast agent.

EXPONENTIAL ATTENUATION

When x-rays are incident on any type of tissue, they can interact with the atoms of that tissue through any of these five mechanisms: coherent scattering, Compton scattering, photoelectric effect, pair production, and photodisintegration. The relative frequency of interaction through each mechanism depends on the atomic number of the tissue atoms, the mass density, and the x-ray energy.

An interaction such as the photoelectric effect is called an absorption process because the x-ray disappears. **Absorption** is an all-or-none condition for x-ray interaction.

Interactions in which the x-ray is only partially absorbed, such as Compton scattering, are only partial absorption processes. Pair production and photodisintegration are absorption processes.

The reduction in the number of x-rays remaining in an x-ray beam after penetration through a given thickness of tissue is called **attenuation**. When a broad beam of x-rays is incident on any tissue, some of the x-rays are absorbed and some are scattered. The result is a reduced number of x-rays, a condition referred to as **x-ray attenuation**.

> Attenuation is the product of absorption and scattering.

X-rays are attenuated exponentially, which means that they do not have a fixed range in tissue. They are reduced in number by a given percentage for each incremental thickness of tissue they penetrate.

Consider the situation diagrammed in Fig. 10.15. One thousand x-rays are incident on a 25-cm-thick abdomen. The x-ray energy and the atomic number of the tissue are such that 50% of the x-rays are removed by the first 5 cm. Therefore in the first 5 cm, 500 x-rays are removed, leaving 500 available to continue penetration.

By the end of the second 5 cm, 50% of the 500, or 250, additional x-rays have been removed, leaving 250 x-rays to continue. Similarly, entering the fourth 5-cm thickness are 125 x-rays, and entering the fifth and last 5 cm thickness are 63 x-rays. Half of the 63 x-rays will be attenuated in the last 5 cm of tissue; therefore only 32 will be transmitted to interact with the image receptor. The total effect of these interactions is 97% attenuation and 3% transmission of the x-ray beam.

A plot of this hypothetical x-ray beam attenuation, which closely resembles the actual situation, appears in Fig. 10.16. Is it obvious that the assumed half-value layer in soft tissue was 5 cm? It should be clear that, theoretically at least, the number of x-rays emerging from any thickness of absorber will never reach zero. Each succeeding thickness can attenuate the x-ray beam only by a fractional amount, and a fraction of any positive number is always greater than zero.

This is not the way that alpha particles and beta particles interact with matter. Regardless of the energy of the particle and the type of tissue, these particulate radiations can penetrate only so far before they are totally absorbed. For example, beta particles with 2 MeV of energy have a range of approximately 1 cm in soft tissue.

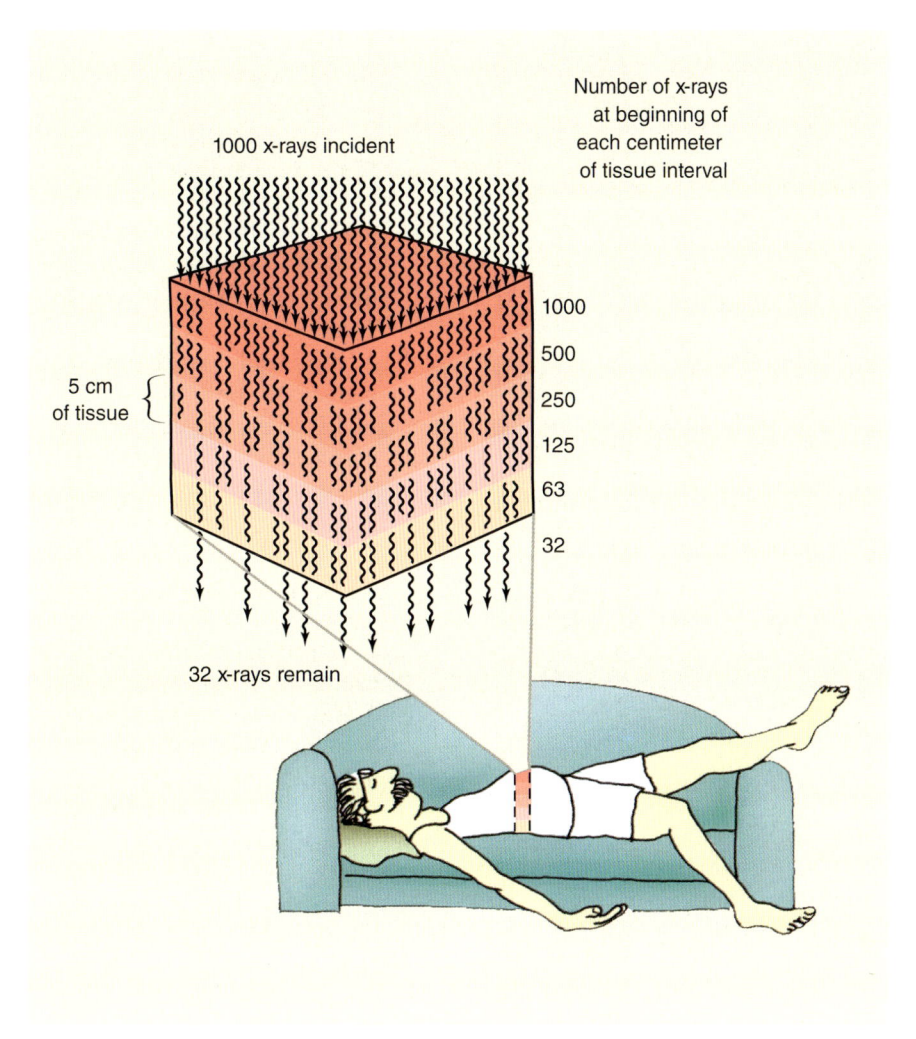

FIG. 10.15 Interaction of x-rays by absorption and scatter is called attenuation. In this example, the x-ray beam has been attenuated 97%; 3% of the x-rays have been transmitted.

SUMMARY

Following are five fundamental interactions between x-rays and matter:
1. Coherent scattering is a change in the direction of an incident x-ray without a loss of energy.
2. Compton scattering occurs when incident x-rays ionize atoms and the x-ray then changes direction with a loss of energy.
3. The photoelectric effect occurs when the incident x-ray is absorbed into one of the inner electron shells and emits a photoelectron.
4. Pair production occurs when the incident x-ray interacts with the electric field of the nucleus. The x-ray disappears, and two electrons appear—one positively charged (positron) and one negatively charged (electron).
5. Photodisintegration occurs when the incident x-ray is directly absorbed by the nucleus. The x-ray disappears, and nuclear fragments are released.

The interactions that are important to diagnostic x-ray imaging are Compton scattering and the photoelectric effect.

Differential absorption controls the contrast of an x-ray image. The x-ray image results from the difference between those x-rays absorbed by photoelectric interaction and those x-rays that pass through the body as image-forming x-rays. Attenuation is the reduction in x-ray beam intensity as it penetrates through tissue. Differential absorption and attenuation of the x-ray beam depend on the following factors:
- The atomic number (Z) of the atoms in tissue
- The mass density of tissue
- The x-ray energy

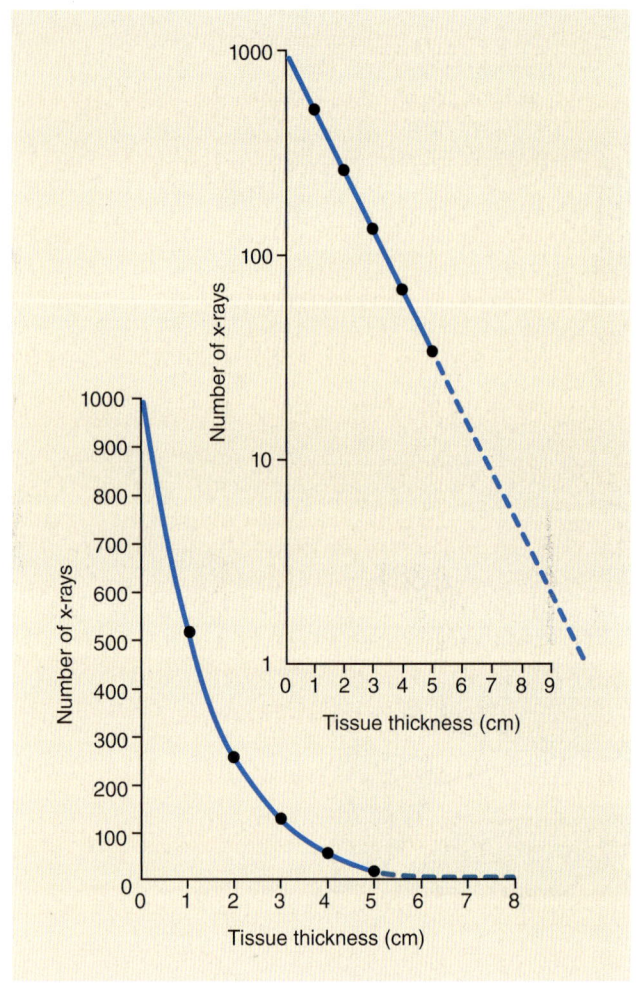

FIGURE 10.16 Linear and semilogarithmic plots of exponential x-ray attenuation data from Fig. 10.15.

Radiologic contrast agents, such as iodine and barium, use the principles of differential absorption to image soft tissue organs. Iodine is used in vascular, renal, and biliary imaging. Barium is used for gastrointestinal imaging. Both elements have high atomic numbers (53 for iodine, 56 for barium) and mass density much greater than that of soft tissue.

CHALLENGE QUESTIONS

1. Define or otherwise identify the following:
    a. Differential absorption
    b. Classical scattering
    c. Mass density
    d. 1.02 MeV
    e. Contrast agent
    f. Compton scattering
    g. Attenuation
    h. Monoenergetic
    i. Secondary electron
    j. Photoelectric effect
2. What are the two factors of importance to differential absorption?
3. A 28-keV x-ray interacts photoelectrically with a K-shell electron of a calcium atom. What is the kinetic energy of the secondary electron (see Table 3.3)?
4. A thousand x-rays with energy of 140 keV are incident on bone and soft tissue of equal thickness. If 87 x-rays are scattered in soft tissue, approximately how many are scattered in bone?
5. Why are iodinated compounds such excellent agents for vascular contrast examinations?
6. Diagram Compton scattering; identify the incident x-ray, positive ion, negative ion, and scattered x-ray.
7. Describe backscatter radiation. Can you think of examples in diagnostic x-ray imaging?
8. Tungsten is sometimes alloyed into the beam-defining collimators of an x-ray imaging system. If a 63-keV x-ray undergoes a Compton interaction with an L-shell electron and ejects that electron with 12 keV of energy, what is the energy of the scattered x-ray (see Fig. 3.9)?
9. Of the five basic mechanisms of x-ray interaction with matter, three are not important to diagnostic radiology. Which are they, and why are they not important?
10. On average, 33.7 eV is required for each ionization in air. How many ion pairs would a 22-keV x-ray probably produce in air, and approximately how many of these would be produced photoelectrically?
11. How is the energy of the Compton-scattered x-ray computed?
12. Does the probability of Compton scattering depend on the atomic number of the target atom?
13. When kVp is increased, is Compton scattering increased or reduced?
14. Describe the photoelectric effect.
15. When kVp is increased, what happens to the absolute probability of the photoelectric effect versus Compton scattering?
16. How much more likely is it that an x-ray will interact with bone than with muscle?
17. What is the relationship between atomic number (Z) and differential absorption?
18. What is the relationship between mass density and differential absorption?

19. In a contrast radiographic examination with iodine, what is the relative probability that x-rays will interact with iodine rather than with soft tissue?
20. What kVp is used to penetrate barium in a contrast examination?

The answers to the Challenge Questions can be found by logging on to our website at http://evolve.elsevier.com.

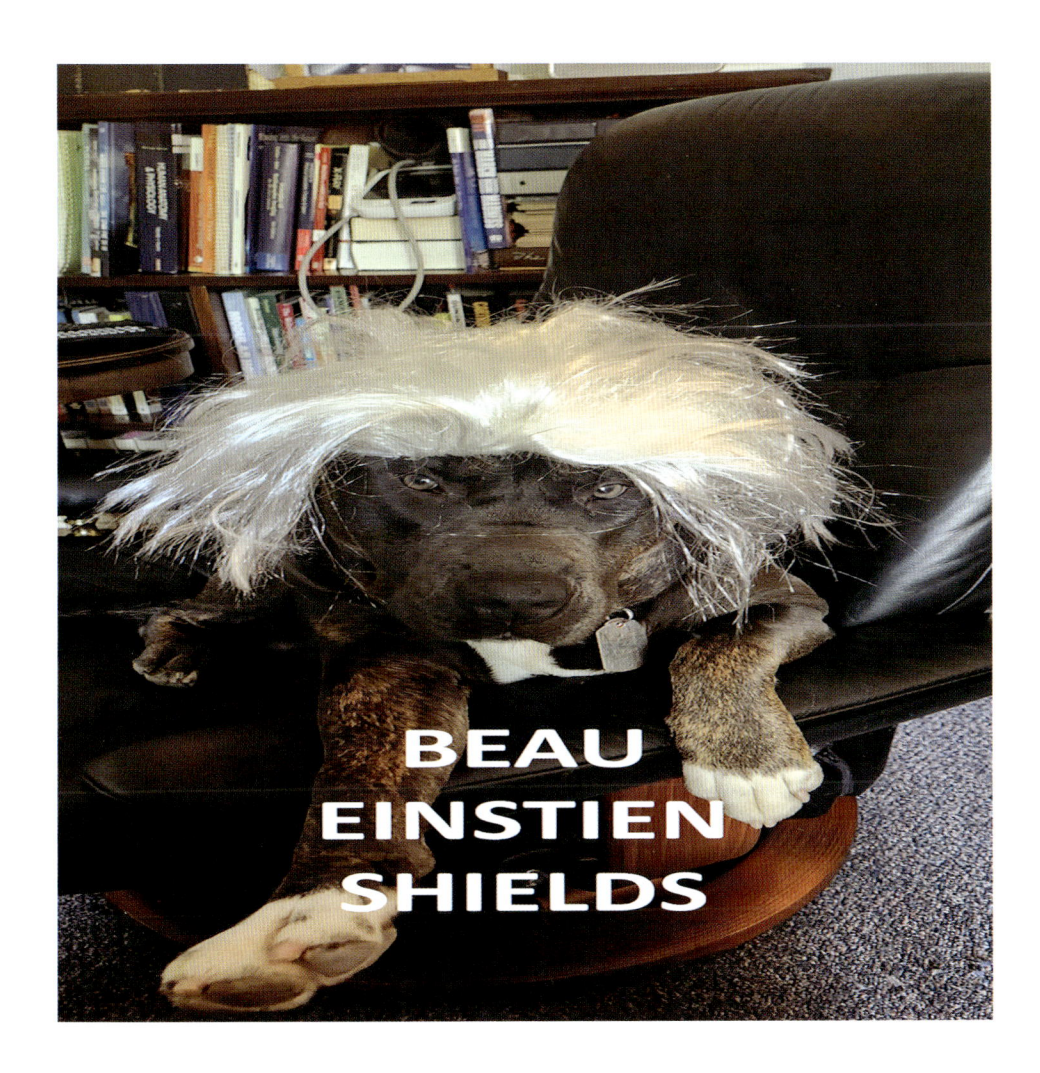

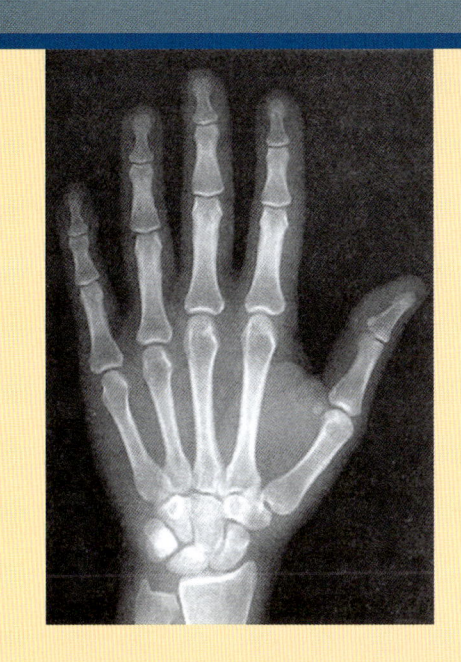

PART III

X-RAY IMAGING

CHAPTER 11

Computed Radiography

OBJECTIVES

At the completion of this chapter, the student should be able to do the following:
1. Describe the development of computed radiography.
2. Identify workflow changes when computed radiography replaced screen-film radiography.
3. Discuss the relevant features of a storage phosphor image receptor.
4. Explain the operating characteristics of a computed radiography reader.
5. Discuss spatial resolution, contrast resolution, and noise related to computed radiography.
6. Identify opportunities for patient radiation dose reduction with computed radiography.

OUTLINE

The Computed Radiography Image Receptor 171
   Photostimulable Luminescence 172
   Image Receptor 173
   Light Stimulation-Emission 173
The Computed Radiography Reader 176
   Mechanical Features 176
   Optical Features 176
   Computer Control 177
Imaging Characteristics 178
   Image Receptor Response Function 178
   Image Noise 179
Patient Radiation Dose 180
Summary 180
Challenge Questions 180

CHAPTER 11 Computed Radiography

THE CONVERSION from analog screen-film radiography to the first digital radiography (DR) system was in the form of computed radiography (CR). Digital imaging began with computed tomography (CT) and magnetic resonance imaging (MRI) in the 1970s.

Screen-film radiography ruled for nearly a century when in 1981 Fuji introduced the first commercial CR imaging system. After many improvements, CR became clinically acceptable and, by the turn of the 21st century, enjoyed widespread use.

Today medical imaging is complemented by multiple forms of DR in addition to CR. Although other DR systems are increasingly in use, it seems there will always be a need for CR because of its unique properties.

This chapter discusses CR, but readers should understand that much of the information relevant to CR applies also to DR because CR is a form of DR.

Before CR is discussed, a review of the workload steps associated with screen-film radiography is in order. Consider the sequence outlined in Fig. 11.1.

To conduct a screen-film radiographic examination, one would first produce a paper trail of the study, process the image with wet chemistry, and finally, physically file the image after accepting that it is diagnostic. CR imaging eliminates some of these steps and can produce better medical images at lower patient radiation dose. Table 11.1 lists commonly used CR terms and their abbreviations, which will be discussed in more detail later in this chapter.

THE COMPUTED RADIOGRAPHY IMAGE RECEPTOR

Many similarities have been observed between screen-film imaging and CR imaging. Both modalities use an x-ray-sensitive image receptor (IR) that is encased in a protective cassette. The two techniques can be used interchangeably with any radiographic x-ray imaging system. Both produce a **latent image**, albeit in a different form, that must be made visible via processing.

> CR is a form of digital radiography.

Here, however, the similarities stop. In screen-film radiography, the radiographic intensifying screen is a scintillator that emits light in response to an x-ray

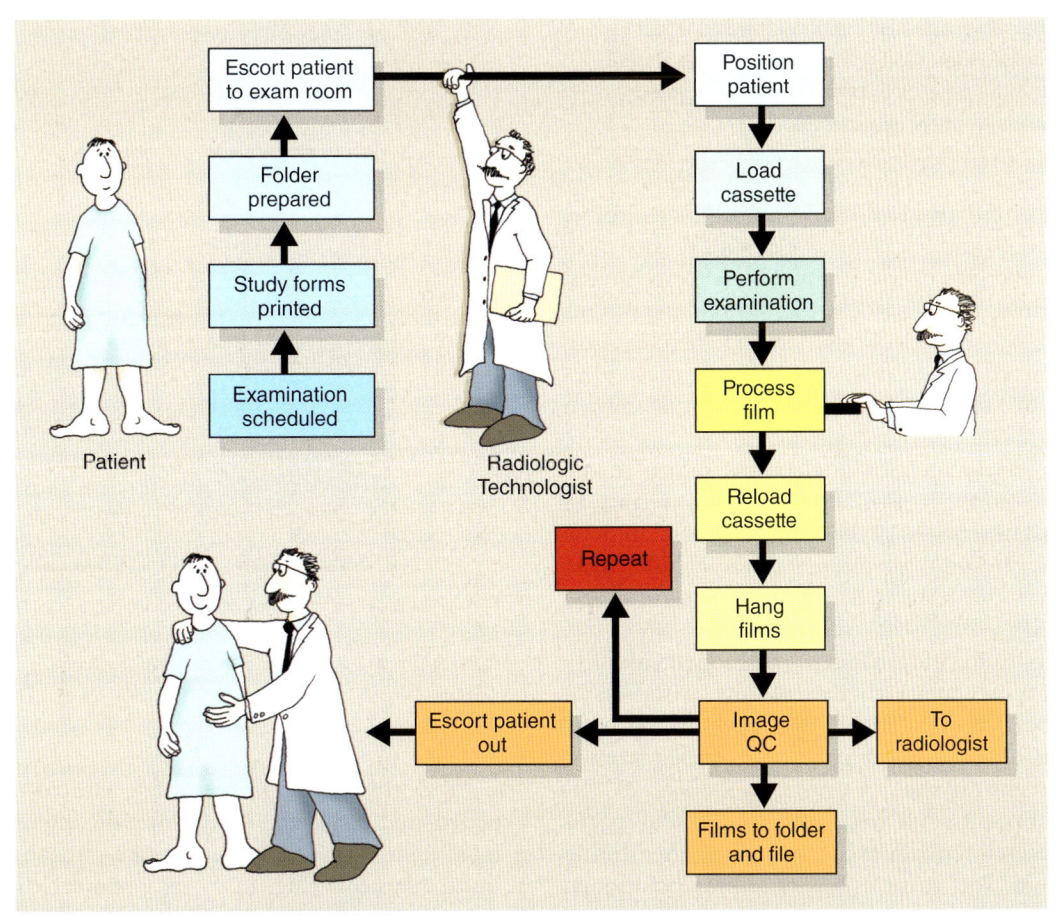

FIG. 11.1 Sequence of activity for screen-film radiography.

TABLE 11.1	Computed Radiography Terms

- IP = imaging plate
- PD = photodiode
- PMT = photomultiplier tube
- PSL = photostimulable luminescence
- PSP = photostimulable phosphor
- SP = storage phosphor
- SPS = storage phosphor screen

interaction. In CR the responses to x-ray interaction are electrons trapped temporarily in a higher-energy, metastable state, in the IR.

Photostimulable Luminescence

Some materials, such as barium fluorohalide with europium (BaFBr:Eu or BaFI:Eu), emit some light promptly in the way that a scintillator does following x-ray interaction. However, they also emit light some time later when exposed to a different light source. Such a process is called photostimulable luminescence (PSL).

The europium (Eu) is present in only very small amounts. It is called an **activator** and is responsible for the storage property of the PSL. The activator is similar to the sensitivity center of a film emulsion because, without it, there would be no latent image.

> In the same way that the photographic effect is not fully understood and continues to be studied, so too the physics of photostimulable luminescence is not fully understood.

The atoms of barium fluorobromide have atomic numbers of 56, 9, and 35, respectively, with K-shell electron binding energies of 37, 5, and 12 keV, respectively. Many Compton and photoelectric x-ray interactions occur with outer-shell electrons, sending them into an excited, metastable state (Fig. 11.2). When these electrons return to the ground state, visible light is emitted (Fig. 11.3).

Over time, these metastable electrons return to the ground state on their own. However this return to the ground state can be accelerated or stimulated by exposing the phosphor to intense infrared light from a laser—hence the term PSL from a photostimulable phosphor (PSP).

The PSP, barium fluorohalide, is fashioned similarly to a radiographic intensifying screen, as is shown in Fig. 11.4. Because the latent image occurs in the form of metastable electrons, such screens are called storage phosphor screens (SPSs).

The SPS appears white because the small PSP particles (3–10 μm) scatter light excessively. Such a scattering is called **turbid**. PSP particles are randomly positioned throughout the PSP in a binder.

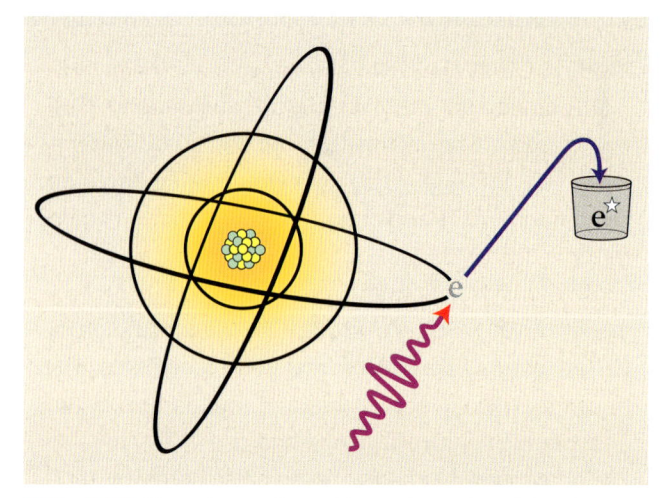

FIG. 11.2 X-ray interaction with a photostimulable phosphor results in excitation of electrons into a metastable state.

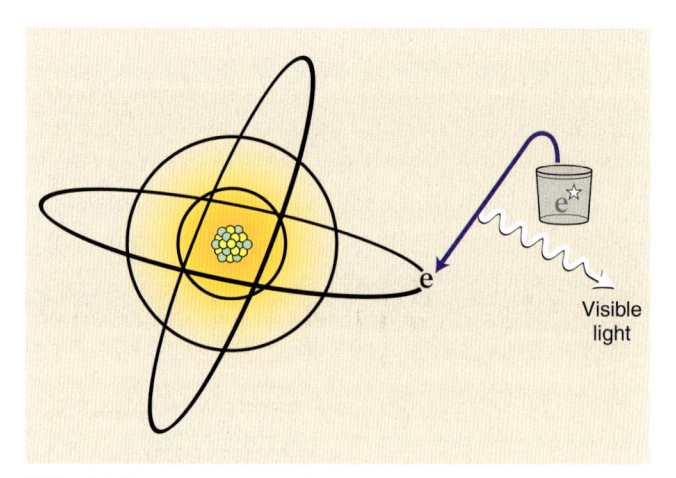

FIG. 11.3 When metastable electrons return to their ground state, visible light is emitted.

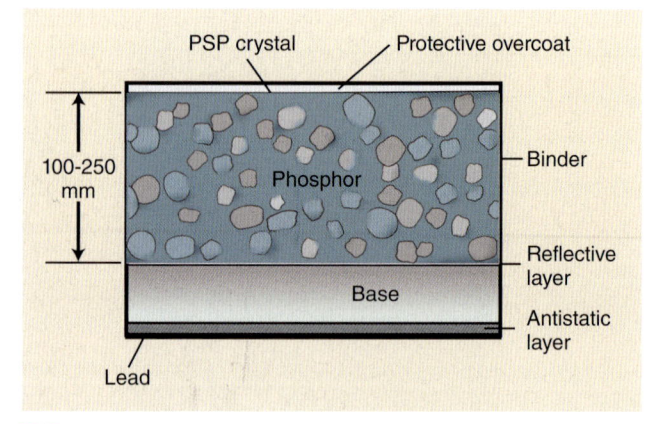

FIG. 11.4 Cross section of a photostimulable phosphor (PSP) screen.

SPSs are mechanically stable, electrostatically protected, and fashioned to optimize the intensity of stimulated light. Some SPSs incorporate phosphors grown as linear filaments (Fig. 11.5) that enhance the absorption of x-rays and limit the spread of stimulated emission.

Image Receptor

The PSP screen is housed in a rugged cassette that appears similar to a screen-film cassette (Fig. 11.6). In this form as an IR, the PSP cassette is called an **imaging plate** (**IP**).

The IP is handled in the same manner as a screen-film cassette; in fact, this is a principal advantage of CR. CR can be substituted for screen-film radiography and used with any x-ray imaging system. The PSP screen of the IP is not loaded and unloaded in a darkroom. Rather, it is handled in the manner of a screen-film daylight loader.

> CR does not require a darkroom.

The IP has lead backing that reduces backscatter x-rays. This improves the contrast resolution of the IR.

Light Stimulation-Emission

Thermoluminescent dosimetry (TLD) and optically stimulated luminescence (OSL) are the main radiation detectors used for occupational radiation monitoring (see Chapter 42). Light is emitted when a TLD crystal is heated. Light is emitted when an OSL crystal is illuminated. PSL is similar to OSL.

The sequence of events engaged in producing a PSL signal begins as shown in Fig. 11.7. When an x-ray beam exposes a PSP, the energy transfer results in excitation of electrons into a metastable state. Approximately 50% of these electrons return to their ground state immediately, resulting in prompt emission of light.

The remaining metastable electrons return to the ground state over time. This causes the latent image to fade and requires that the IP must be read soon after exposure. CR signal loss is objectionable after approximately 8 hours.

The next step in CR imaging is stimulation (Fig. 11.8). The finely focused beam of infrared light with a beam diameter of approximately 70 μm is directed at the PSP. As laser beam intensity increases, so does the intensity of the emitted signal.

> The diameter of the laser beam determines the spatial resolution of the CR imaging system.

Note that as the laser beam penetrates, it spreads. The amount of spread increases with PSP thickness.

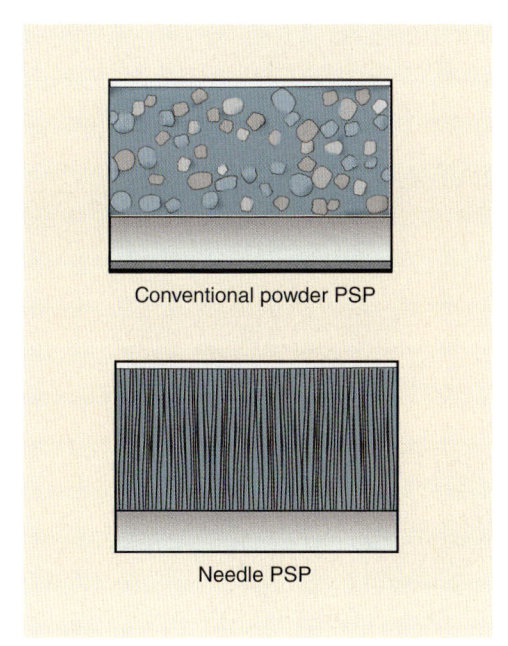

FIG. 11.5 Some storage phosphor screens incorporate phosphors grown as linear filaments that increase the absorption of x-rays and limit the spread of stimulated emission. *PSP,* Photostimulable phosphor.

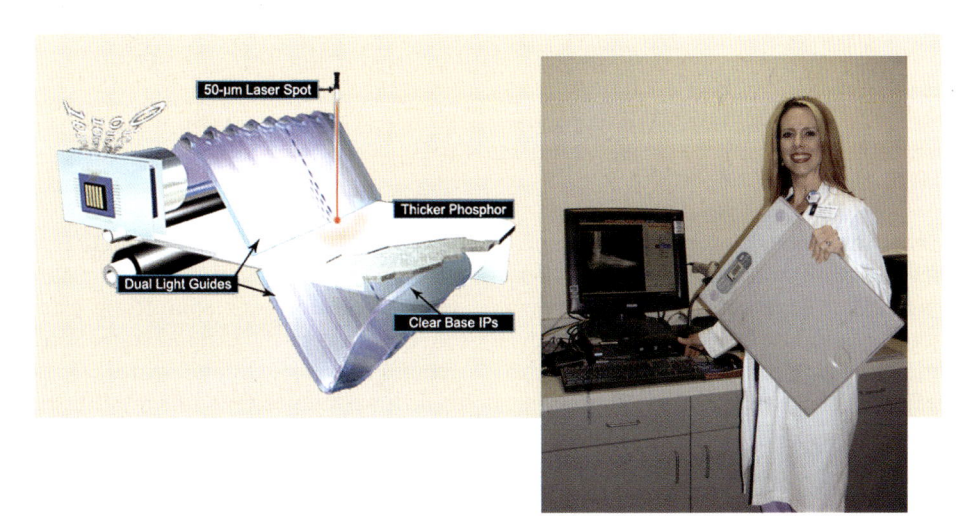

FIG. 11.6 Computed radiography imaging plate prepared for insertion into electronic reader. (Courtesy Melanie Hail, Lone Star College System, and Fuji Medical Systems.)

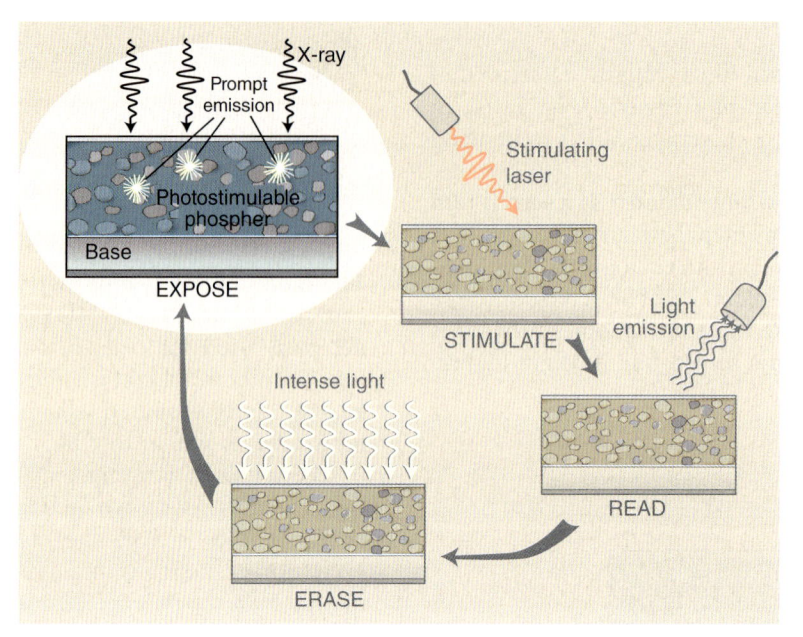

FIG. 11.7 Expose: The first of a sequence of events that results in an x-ray–induced image-forming signal.

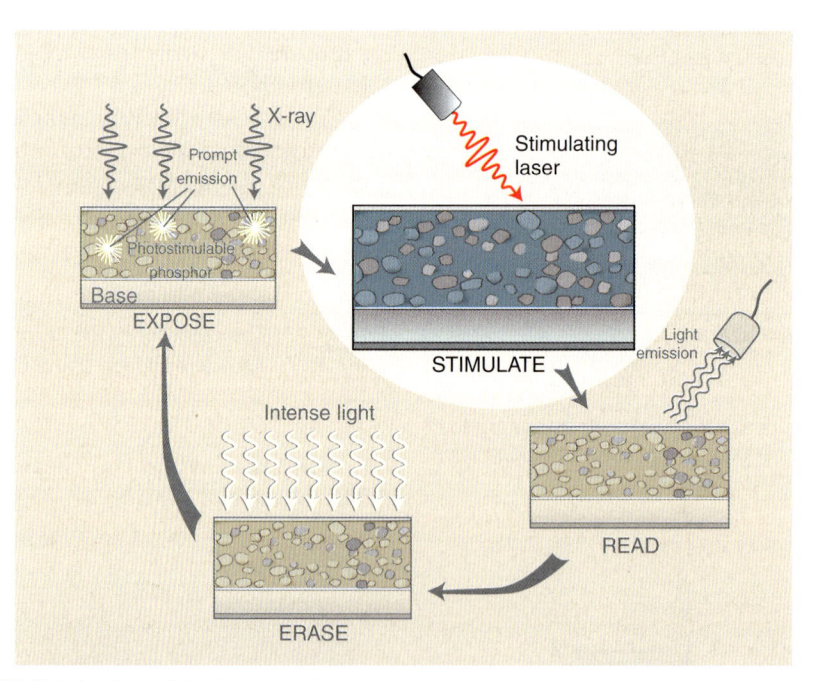

FIG. 11.8 Stimulate: Stimulation of the latent image results from the interaction of an infrared laser beam with the photostimulable phosphor.

Fig. 11.9 illustrates the third step in this imaging process, which is detecting the stimulated emission. The laser beam causes metastable electrons to return to their ground state with the emission of a shorter wavelength light in the blue region of the visible spectrum. Through this process, the latent image is made visible.

Some signal is lost as the result of (1) scattering of the emitted light and (2) the collection efficiency of the photodetector. Photodiodes (PDs) are the light detectors of choice for CR.

The final stage in PSL signal production is shown in Fig. 11.10. The stimulation cycle of the PSL signal acquisition does not completely transition all metastable electrons to the ground state. Some excited electrons remain in the metastable state.

If a residual latent image remained, ghosting could appear on subsequent use of the IR. Any residual latent image is removed by flooding the phosphor with very intense white light from a bank of specially designed lamps.

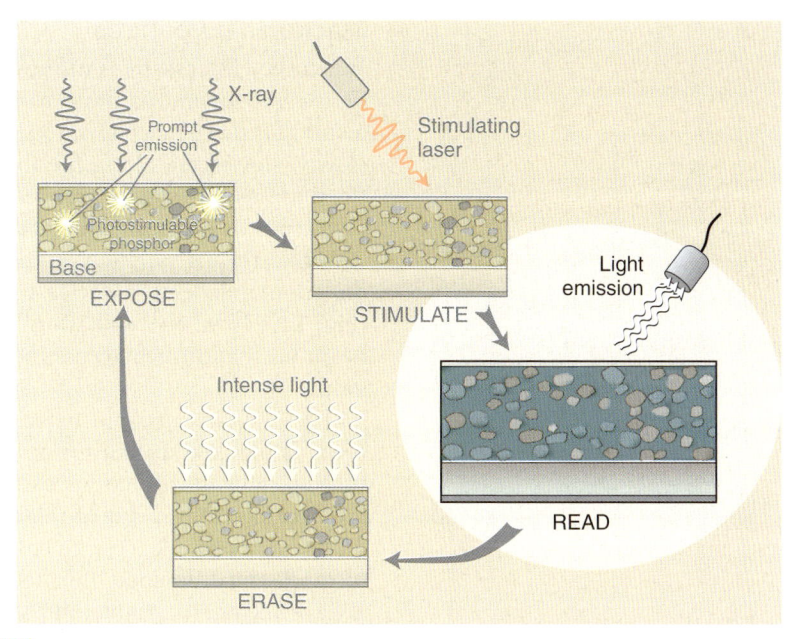

FIG. 11.9 Read: The light signal emitted after stimulation is detected and measured.

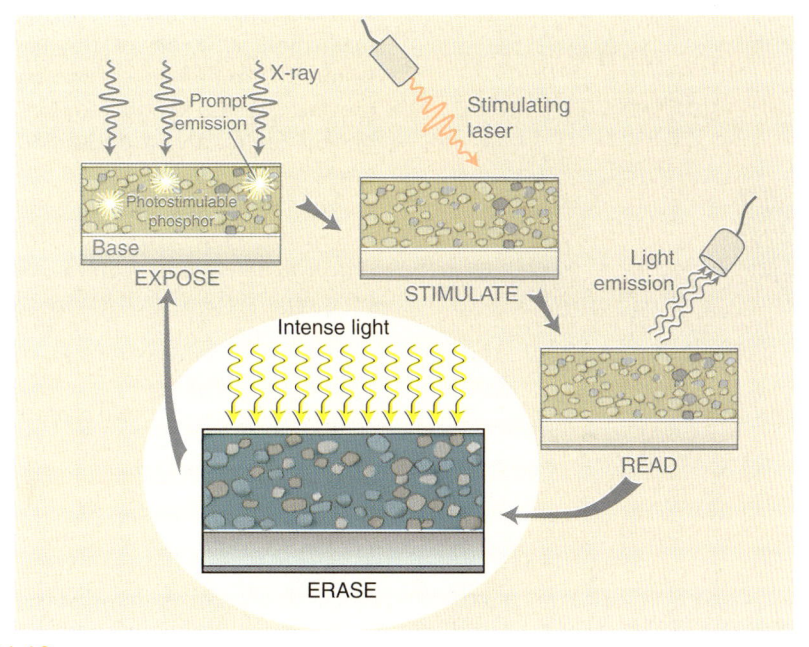

FIG. 11.10 Erase: Before reuse, any residual metastable electrons are moved to the ground state by an intense light.

The stimulation portion of PSP processing would result in no latent image if the laser beam were made to dwell longer at each position on the PSP, but this would require an unacceptable processing time. The PSP is sufficiently sensitive that it can become fogged by background radiation.

> IPs should be used soon after the erase cycle has been completed.

The laser light used to stimulate the PSP is monochromatic, as can be seen in Fig. 11.11. A solid-state laser is the stimulating source of choice.

The resulting emission has a polychromatic spectrum. The emitted light intensity is many orders of magnitude lower than that of the stimulating light; this poses additional challenges to the entire process.

Solid-state lasers produce longer wavelength light and therefore are less likely to interfere with emitted light. Even so, optical filters are necessary to allow only

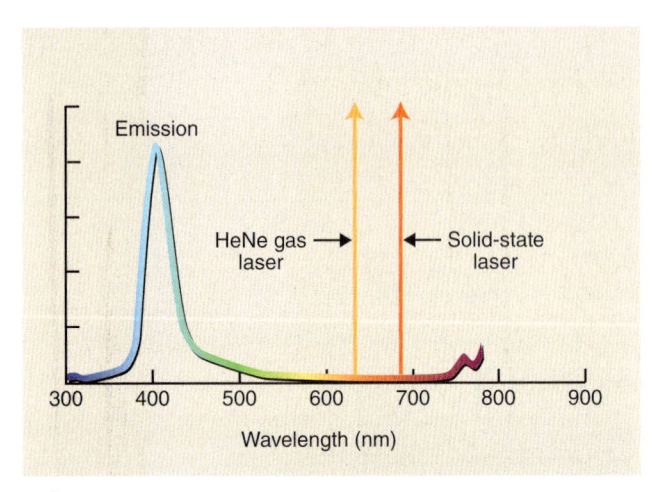

FIG. 11.11 The laser light used to stimulate the photostimulable phosphor is monochromatic. Resultant light emission is polychromatic.

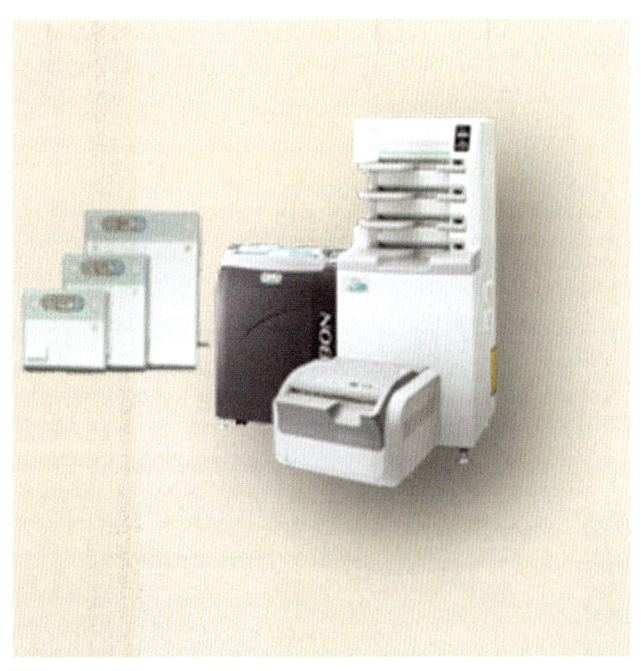

FIG. 11.12 The computed radiography reader is a compact mechanical, optical, computer assembly. (Courtesy FujiFilm Medical Systems, Stamford, Connecticut.)

emitted light to reach the photodetector while blocking the intense stimulated light.

THE COMPUTED RADIOGRAPHY READER

A computed radiography reader, shown in Fig. 11.12, represents the marriage of mechanical, optical, and computer modules.

Mechanical Features

When the CR cassette is inserted into the CR reader, the IR is removed and is fitted to a precision drive mechanism. This drive mechanism moves the IR constantly yet slowly, **slow scan**, along the long axis of the IR. Small fluctuations in velocity can result in banding artifacts, so the motor drive must be absolutely constant.

While the IR is being transported in the slow scan direction, a deflection device such as a rotating polygon (Fig. 11.13) or an oscillating mirror deflects the laser beam back and forth across the IR. This is the **fast scan** mode.

These drive mechanisms are coupled so the laser beam is blanked during retrace. The error tolerance for this mechanism is fractions of a pixel. Image edges from a CR reader that is out of tolerance appear "wavy."

The IR barely leaves the cassette, so it is not subject to mechanical damage. Furthermore, the scan is nearly always located at right angles to the direction of any grid lines; in this way, aliasing artifacts are reduced.

Optical Features

The challenge to the CR reader is to interrogate each metastable electron of the latent image in a precise fashion. Components of the optical subsystem include the laser, beam-shaping optics, light-collecting optics, optical filters, and a photodetector. These components are shown in Fig. 11.14.

The laser is the source of stimulating light; however it spreads as it travels to the rotating or oscillating reflector. This light beam is focused onto the reflector by a lens system that keeps the beam diameter small (<100 μm).

> Small laser beam diameter is critical for ensuring high spatial resolution.

As the laser beam is deflected across the IR, it changes size and shape. Special beam-shaping optics keep the beam size, shape, speed, and intensity constant.

A simple flashlight exercise can be used to explain what is needed for beam shaping. Shine a flashlight perpendicularly on a wall, and what do you see? A circle of light.

Now move the beam along the wall slowly but with constant velocity, and what do you see? The light beam becomes distorted, moves faster, and is less intense. These types of changes in a CR reader are corrected with the use of beam-shaping optics.

Emitted light from the IP is channeled into a funnel-like fiber-optic collection assembly and is directed at the photodetector, a PMT, PD, or charge-coupled device. Before photodetection occurs, the light is filtered so that none of the long-wavelength stimulated emission light reaches the photodetector and swamps

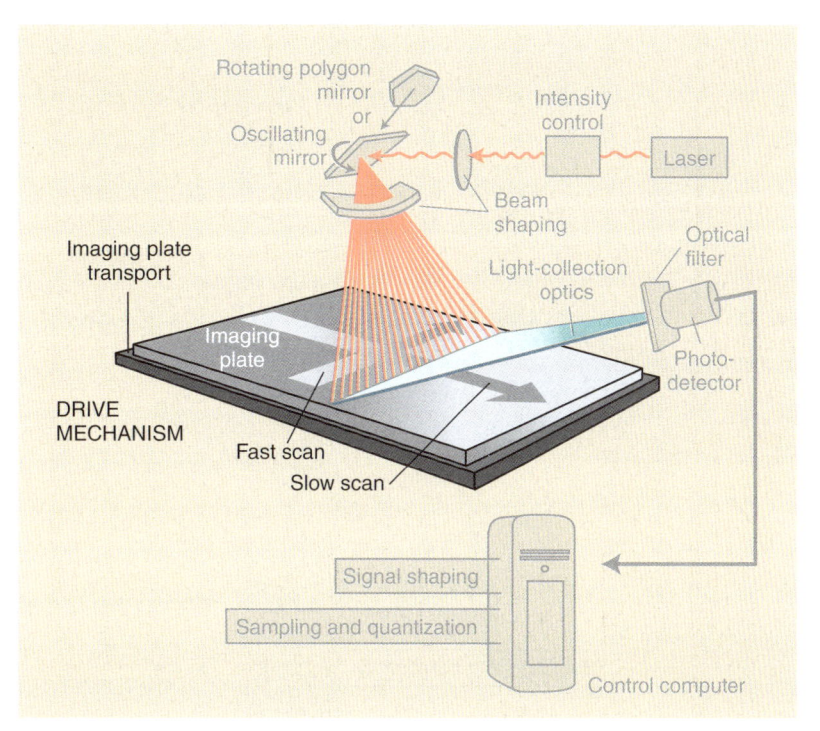

FIG. 11.13 The drive mechanisms of the computed radiography reader move the imaging plate slowly along its long axis, while an oscillating beam deflection mirror causes the stimulating laser beam to sweep rapidly across the imaging plate.

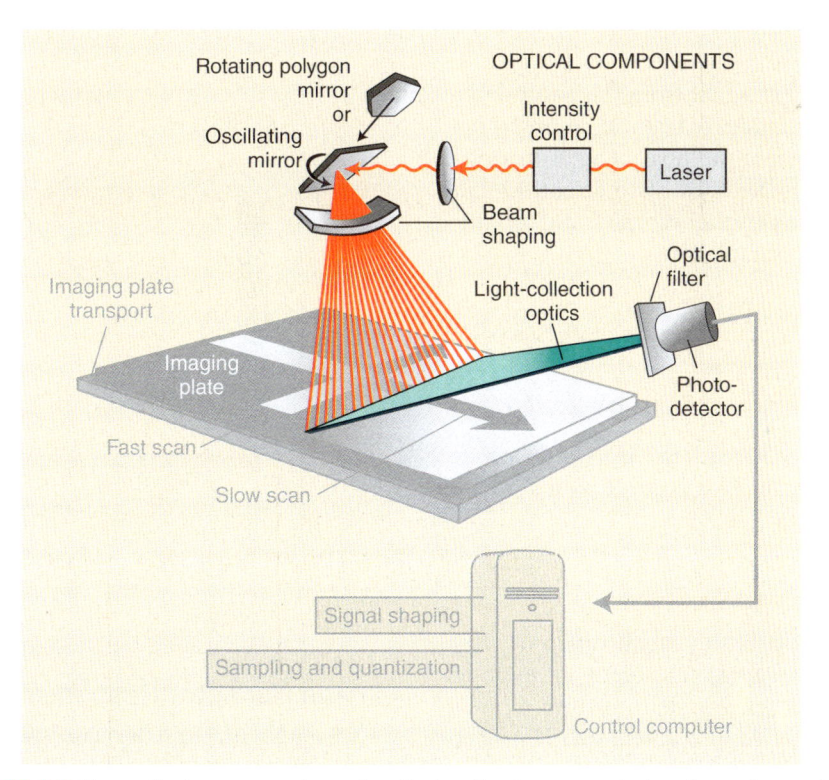

FIG. 11.14 The optical components and optical path of a computed radiography reader are highlighted.

the emitted light. In this case, emitted light is the signal and stimulating light is the noise; therefore proper filtering improves the signal-to-noise ratio and therefore contrast resolution.

Computer Control

The output of the photodetector is a time-varying analog signal that is transmitted to a computer that has multiple functions (Fig. 11.15).

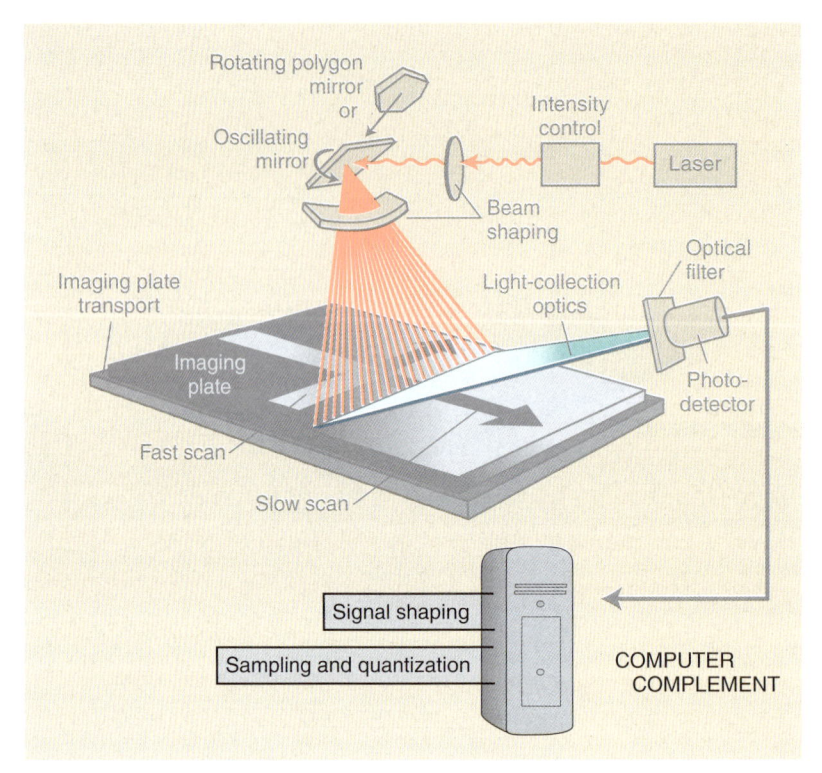

FIG. 11.15 The computer complement to a computed radiography reader provides signal amplification, signal compression, scanning control, and analog-to-digital conversion.

The time-varying analog signal from the photodetector is processed for amplitude, scale, and compression. This shapes the signal before the final image is formed. Then the analog signal is digitized, with attention paid to proper **sampling** (time between samples) and **quantization** (the value of each sample).

> Sampling and quantization are two processes of analog-to-digital conversion.

The computer of the CR reader is in control of the slow scan and the fast scan. This control works off the computer clock in gigahertz (GHz).

IMAGING CHARACTERISTICS

Medical imaging with CR is not much different from that with screen-film imaging. A cassette is exposed with an existing x-ray imaging system to form a latent image. The cassette is inserted into an automatic processor, and the latent image is made visible.

Here the similarity ends. The **four principal characteristics** of any medical image are spatial resolution, contrast resolution, noise, and artifacts. Such characteristics are different for all DR, including CR, from screen-film imaging. These are discussed in greater depth in later chapters.

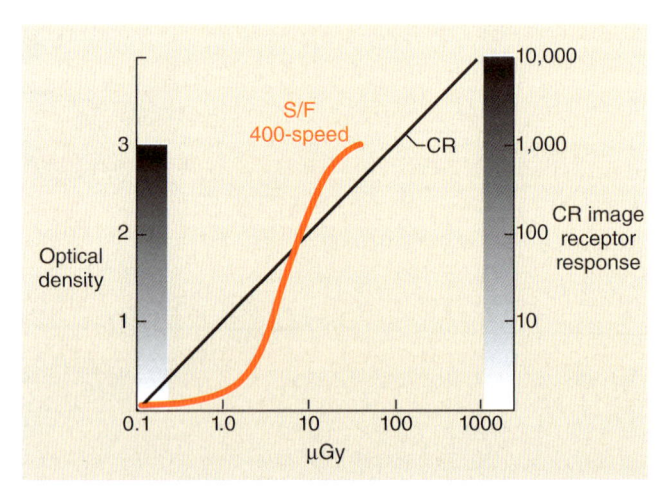

FIG. 11.16 The image receptor response for computed radiography (*CR*) is shown with the characteristic curve of a screen-film (*S/F*) image receptor.

Image Receptor Response Function

The shape of the characteristic curve for screen-film imaging is presented in Fig. 11.16 along with the "characteristic curve" for a CR IR. In CR and DR, it is not really a characteristic curve but rather an IR response function.

Fig. 11.16 suggests several differences between CR and screen-film IRs. The response of screen-film extends through an optical density (OD) range from 0 to 3.

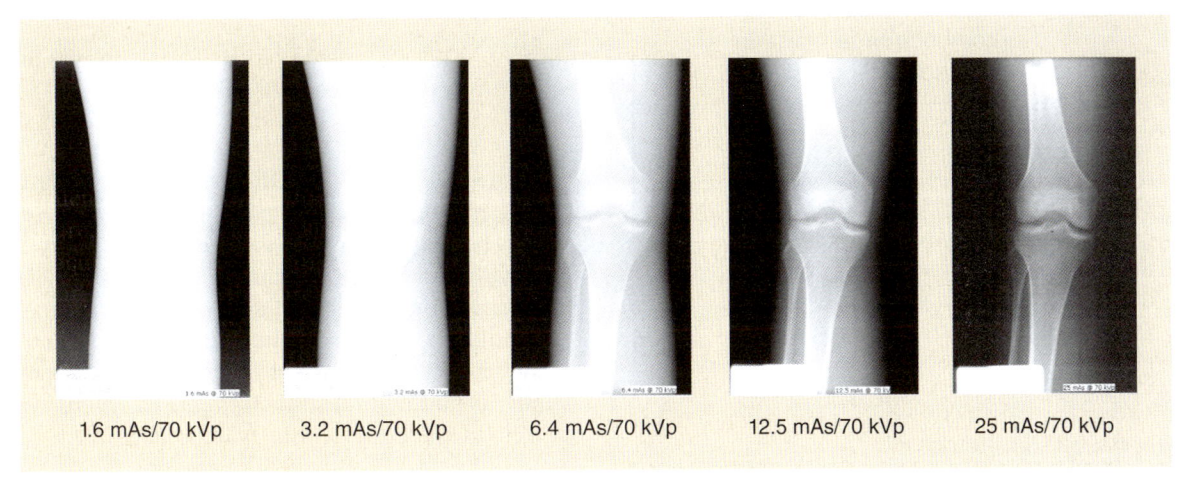

| 1.6 mAs/70 kVp | 3.2 mAs/70 kVp | 6.4 mAs/70 kVp | 12.5 mAs/70 kVp | 25 mAs/70 kVp |

FIG. 11.17 Improper radiographic technique with a screen-film image receptor results in an unacceptable image. (Courtesy Betsy Shields, Presbyterian Hospital, Charlotte, North Carolina.)

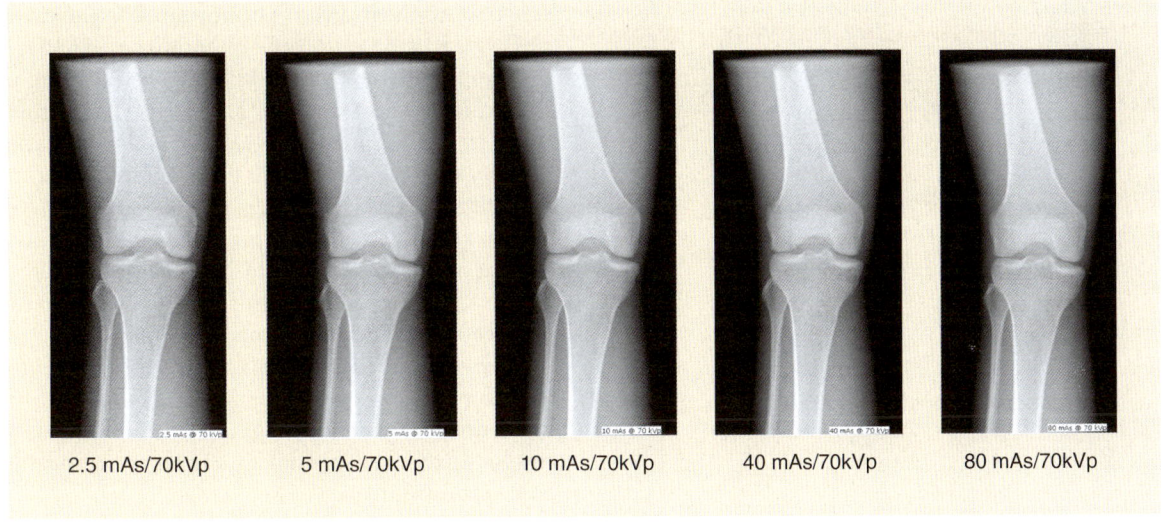

| 2.5 mAs/70kVp | 5 mAs/70kVp | 10 mAs/70kVp | 40 mAs/70kVp | 80 mAs/70kVp |

FIG. 11.18 Computed radiography images obtained through the same radiographic technique used in Fig. 11.17. (Courtesy Betsy Shields, Presbyterian Hospital, Charlotte, North Carolina.)

Because OD is a logarithmic function that represents three orders of magnitude, or 1000.

However, the screen-film image can display only approximately 30 shades of gray on a viewbox. That is why radiographic technique is so critical in screen-film imaging. Most screen-film imaging techniques aimed for radiation exposure of the IR on the toe side of the characteristic curve.

CR imaging is characterized by extremely wide latitude. Five decades of radiation exposure results in almost 100,000 gray levels, each of which can be evaluated visually by postprocessing.

> A 14-bit CR image has 16,384 gray levels.

Proper radiographic technique and radiation exposure are essential for screen-film radiography. Overexposure and underexposure resulted in unacceptable images (Fig. 11.17).

With CR, radiographic technique is not as critical because contrast does not change over five decades of radiation exposure. Fig. 11.18 shows the appearance of CR images acquired with the same radiographic technique range as those used for Fig. 11.17.

Image Noise

The principal source of noise on a radiographic image is scatter radiation; this is the same regardless of what type of IRs is used.

Image noise associated with CR includes those sources listed in Table 11.2. Each of the three subsystems of CR contributes noise to the image.

Fortunately, CR noise sources are bothersome only at very low IR radiation exposure. Newer CR systems have lower noise levels and therefore even lower patient radiation dose is possible.

| TABLE 11.2 | Sources of Image Noise in Computed Radiography |

Mechanical defects:
- Slow scan driver
- Fast scan driver

Optical defects:
- Laser intensity control
- Scatter of stimulating beam
- Light quanta emitted by screen
- Light quanta collected

Computer defects:
- Electronic noise
- Inadequate sampling
- Inadequate quantization

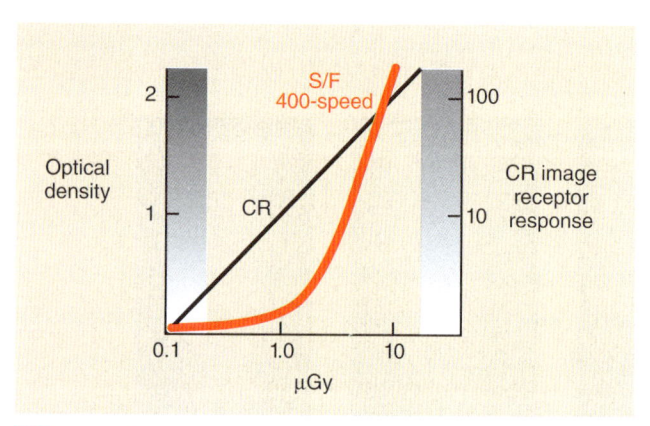

FIG. 11.19 This region of the image receptor response curve shows that significant patient radiation dose reduction is possible with computed radiography (*CR*). *S/F*, Screen-film.

PATIENT RADIATION DOSE

Consider the lower-left quadrant of Fig. 11.16, as shown in Fig. 11.19. At IR radiation exposure less than approximately 5 µGy$_a$, CR is a faster IR compared with a 400-speed screen-film system; therefore lower patient radiation dose occurs with CR.

Lower radiographic technique that results in lower patient radiation dose should be possible with CR if it were not for the image noise at low exposure. This will be discussed later for all DR modalities.

At this time, it should be emphasized that the conventional approach that "kVp controls contrast" and "mAs controls OD" does not hold for CR. Because CR image contrast is constant regardless of radiation exposure, images can be made at higher kVp and lower mAs, resulting in additional reduction in patient radiation dose.

The transition to all forms of DR brings several significant changes. Fewer repeat examinations with are needed because of the wide exposure latitude. Contrast resolution with is improved, and patient radiation dose with is reduced.

> CR with is performed at lower techniques than previous screen-film radiography.

Other approaches to DR have developed faster than CR, especially regarding patient radiation dose reduction. The application of CR with existing x-ray imaging systems is no longer of primary importance. DR is now the main x-ray radiographic imaging modality.

Radiographers will notice one less step in the workload described in Fig. 11.1 (Fig. 11.20). Because the CR reader is automatic and the IP reusable, there is no need to reload the cassette. But wait, it gets much better, as you will read in subsequent chapters.

SUMMARY

The first applications of DR appeared in the early 1980s as CR. CR is based on the phenomenon of PSP.

X-rays interact with a SPS and form a latent image by exciting electrons to a higher-energy metastable state. In the CR reader, the latent image is made visible by releasing the metastable electrons with a stimulating laser light beam.

On returning to the ground state, electrons emit shorter wavelength light in proportion to the intensity of the x-ray beam. The emitted light signal is digitized and reconstructed into a medical image.

The value of each CR pixel describes a linear characteristic curve over five orders of magnitude of radiation exposure and a 100,000 gray scale. This wide latitude results in reduced patient radiation dose and improved contrast resolution.

CHALLENGE QUESTIONS

1. Define or otherwise identify the following:
   a. Imaging plate
   b. Activator
   c. Signal sampling
   d. Metastable electron
   e. Polychromatic
   f. Fast scan
   g. Prompt emission
   h. Storage phosphor
   i. Turbid
   j. Photodiode
2. What workload steps were omitted when conversion from screen-film radiography to computed radiography was complete?
3. Identify three photostimulable phosphors.
4. How is the latent image formed in computed radiography?
5. What causes a photostimulable phosphor to appear turbid?

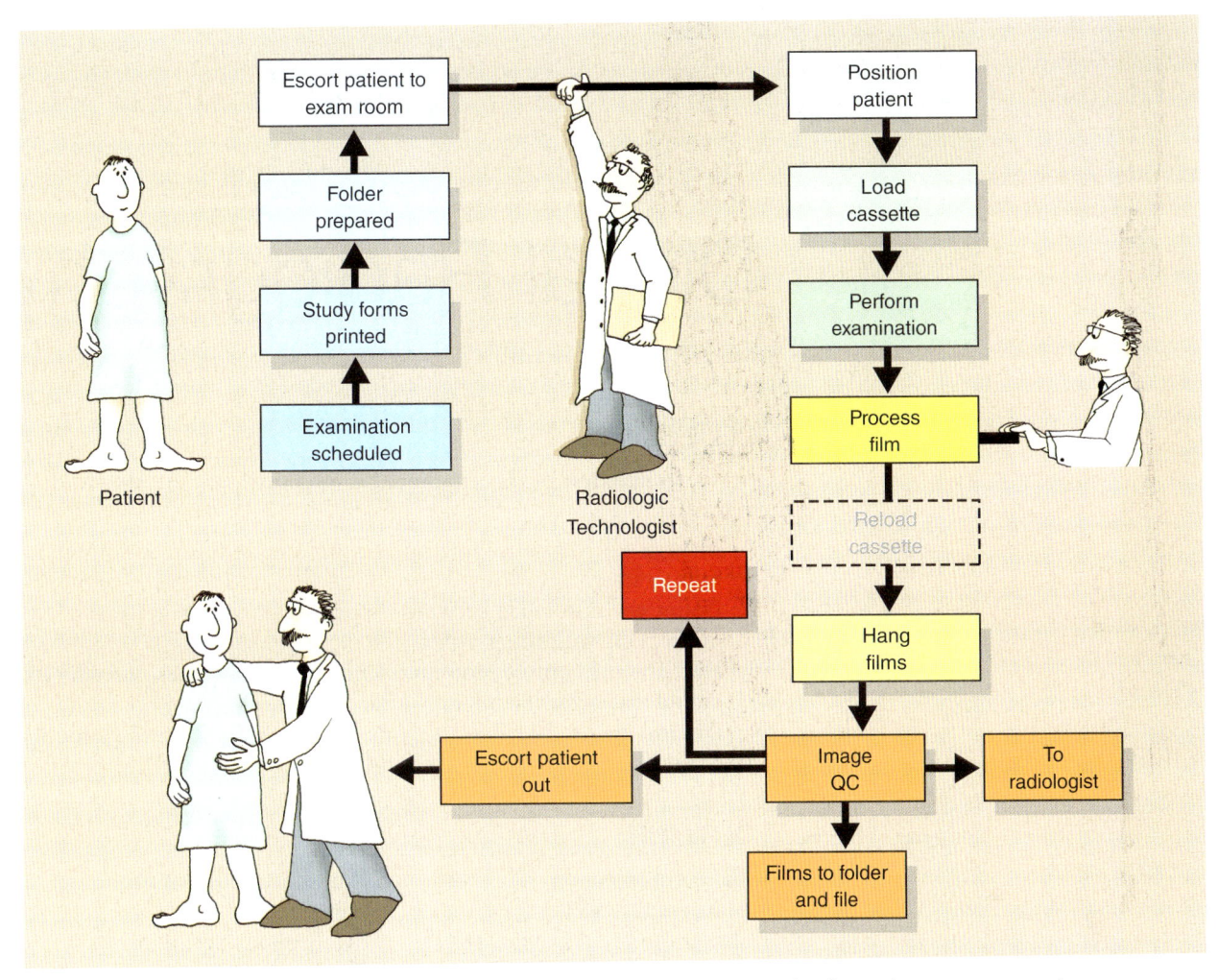

FIG. 11.20 The transition from screen-film radiography to computed radiography removes several steps from the radiography workload process.

6. How do we reduce backscatter radiation in computed radiography, and why?
7. What is the approximate color of stimulating light and emitted light?
8. What is the purpose of an optical filter positioned before the photodetector?
9. What is the difference between fast scan and slow scan?
10. What is the difference between an analog signal and a digital signal?
11. What is the difference between sampling and quantization?
12. What is the purpose of a photostimulable phosphor?
13. Why is beam shaping required for the laser beam?
14. What are the three subsystems of a computed radiography reader?
15. How is ghosting caused by residual latent image reduced?
16. What is the approximate difference in wavelength between prompt emission and stimulated emission?
17. How should one handle a computed radiography imaging plate?
18. How is the latent image made visible in computed radiography?
19. What is the purpose of europium in a photostimulable phosphor?
20. Diagram the various layers of a computed radiography imaging plate.

The answers to the Challenge Questions can be found by logging on to our website at http://evolve.elsevier.com.

CHAPTER 12

Digital Radiography

OBJECTIVES

At the completion of this chapter, the student should be able to do the following:

1. Identify five digital radiographic modes in addition to computed radiography.
2. Define the difference between direct digital radiography and indirect digital radiography.
3. Describe the capture, coupling, and collection stages of each type of digital radiographic imaging system.
4. Discuss the use of silicon, selenium, cesium iodide, and gadolinium oxysulfide in digital radiography.

OUTLINE

Scanned Projection Radiography 183
Charge-Coupled Device 184
Cesium Iodide/Charge-Coupled Device 185
Cesium Iodide/Amorphous Silicon 185
Amorphous Selenium 187
Summary 187
Challenge Questions 187

CHAPTER 12 Digital Radiography

TWENTIETH-CENTURY screen-film imaging had many limitations, which were eliminated with the introduction of digital radiography (DR). This chapter describes various approaches to DR that developed after computed radiography (CR). Subsequent chapters will present information on the digital image, the soft copy read of the digital image, image processing, and quality control measures for the digital image.

Several approaches may be used to produce digital radiographs and it is still not yet clear whether one of these approaches will, ultimately, prevail. Furthermore, the vocabulary applied to DR is not yet standard or universally accepted.

Ehsan Samei has reported a clever approach to describing and identifying the various DR imaging systems—capture element, coupling element, and collection element. This descriptive approach is shown in Fig. 12.1.

> Digital radiography is best described by three elements: capture, coupling, and collection.

The **capture element** is that in which the x-ray is captured. In CR, the capture element is the photostimulable phosphor (PSP). In the other DR modes, the capture element may be sodium iodide (NaI), cesium iodide (CsI), gadolinium oxysulfide (GdOS), or amorphous selenium (a-Se).

The **coupling element** is that which transfers the x-ray–generated signal to the collection element. The coupling element may be a lens, fiber-optic assembly, contact layer, or there is none.

The **collection element** may be a photodetector, a charge-coupled device (CCD), or a thin-film transistor (TFT). The photodetector and the CCD are light-sensitive devices that collect light photons. The TFT is a charge-sensitive device that collects electrons.

SCANNED PROJECTION RADIOGRAPHY

Shortly after the introduction of third-generation computed tomography (CT), scanned projection radiography (SPR) was developed by CT vendors to facilitate patient positioning imaging volume (Fig. 12.2). It remains in use with virtually all current multislice helical CT imaging systems.

CT vendors give this process various trademarked names, but SPR is similar for all. The patient is positioned on the CT couch and then is driven through the gantry while the x-ray tube is energized. The x-ray tube and the detector array do not rotate but are stationary, and the result is a digital radiograph (Fig. 12.3).

During the 1980s and the early 1990s, SPR was developed for dedicated chest DR (Fig. 12.4). The principal advantage of SPR was collimation to a fan x-ray with associated scatter radiation rejection and improvement in image contrast.

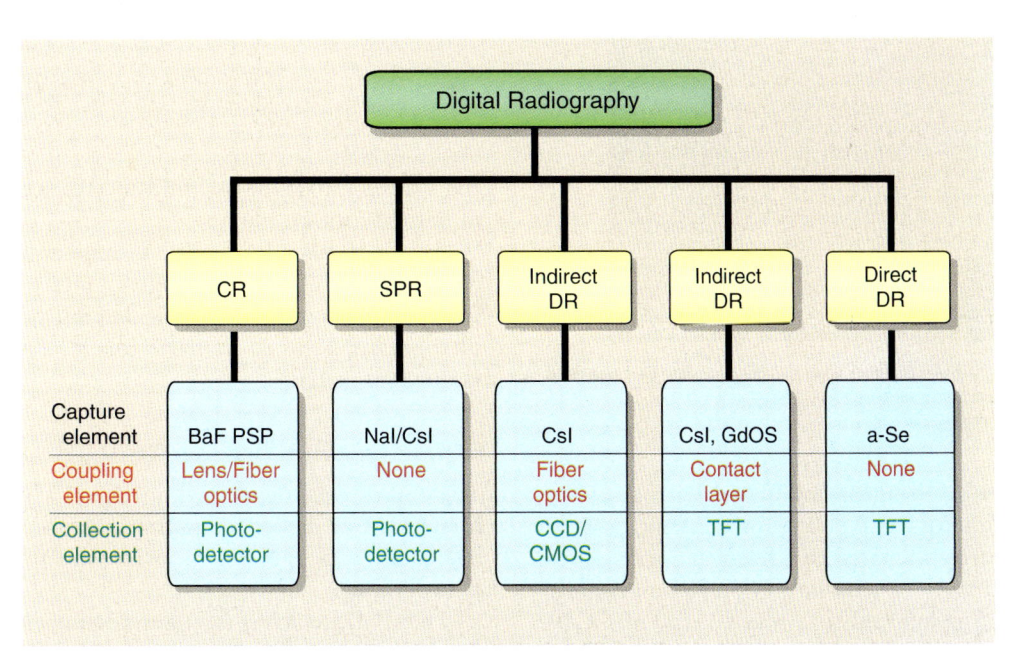

	CR	SPR	Indirect DR	Indirect DR	Direct DR
Capture element	BaF PSP	NaI/CsI	CsI	CsI, GdOS	a-Se
Coupling element	Lens/Fiber optics	None	Fiber optics	Contact layer	None
Collection element	Photo-detector	Photo-detector	CCD/CMOS	TFT	TFT

FIG. 12.1 An organizational scheme for digital radiography. *a-Se*, Amorphous selenium; *BaF*, barium fluoride; *CCD*, charge-coupled device; *CMOS*, gadolinium oxysulfide; *CR*, computed radiography; *CsI*, cesium iodide; *DR*, digital radiography; *GdOS*, gadolinium oxysulfide; *NaI*, sodium iodide; *PSP*, photostimulable phosphor; *SPR*, scanned projection radiography; *TFT*, thin-film transistor.

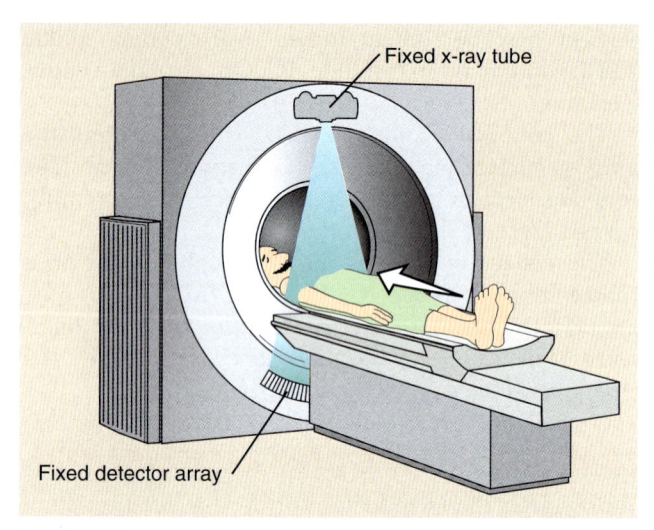

FIG. 12.2 A scanned projection radiograph is obtained in computed tomography by maintaining the energized x-ray tube–detector array fixed while the patient is translated through the gantry.

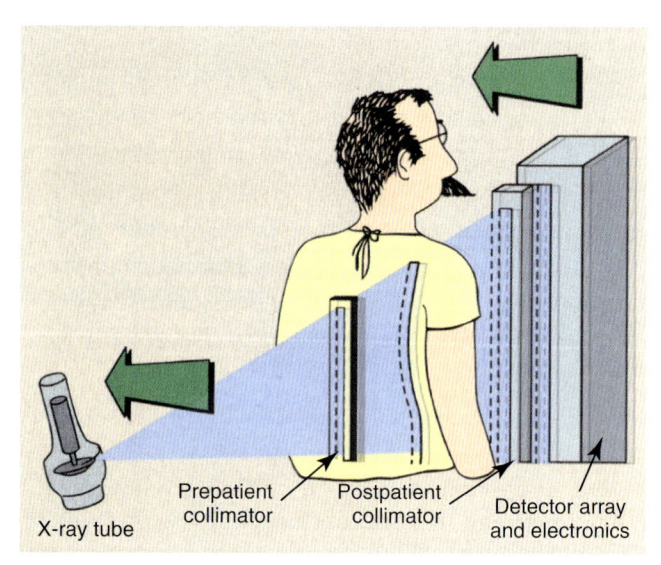

FIG. 12.4 The components of a dedicated chest scanned projection radiography system. (Courtesy Gary Barnes, University of Alabama, Birmingham.)

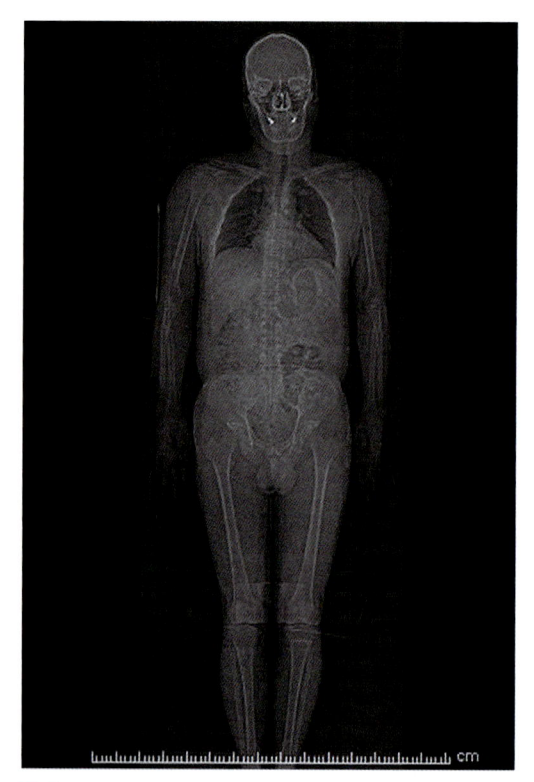

FIG. 12.3 A scanned projection radiograph of the entire trunk of the body obtained in computed tomography. (Courtesy Colin Bray, Baylor College of Medicine.)

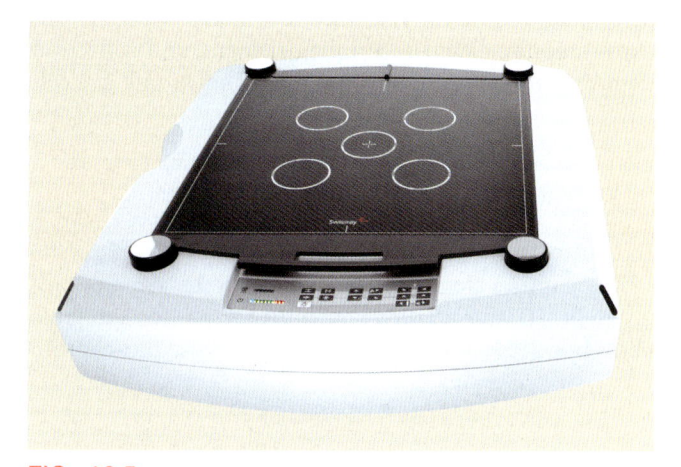

FIG. 12.5 A tiled charge-coupled device designed for digital radiography imaging. (Courtesy Bob Millar, Swissray.)

In SPR, the x-ray beam is collimated with a fan by prepatient collimators. Likewise, postpatient image-forming x-rays are collimated to a fan that corresponds to the detector array—a scintillation phosphor, usually NaI or CsI—and is married to a linear array of CCDs through a fiber-optic light path.

This development was not very successful because chest anatomy has high subject contrast, so scatter radiation rejection is not all that important. Furthermore, the scanning motion required several seconds, resulting in patient motion blur.

At the present time, SPR is reemerging, with some modification, as a promising adjunct to digital radiographic tomosynthesis (DRT). The purpose of all forms of tomography is to improve image contrast, and that is the goal of DRT.

CHARGE-COUPLED DEVICE

The CCD was developed in the 1970s as a highly light-sensitive device for military use. Since that time, it has found major application in astronomy and digital photography.

The CCD, which is the light-sensing element for most digital cameras, has three principal advantageous imaging characteristics: sensitivity, dynamic range, and size. The CCD is a silicon-based semiconductor and is shown as an image receptor in Fig. 12.5.

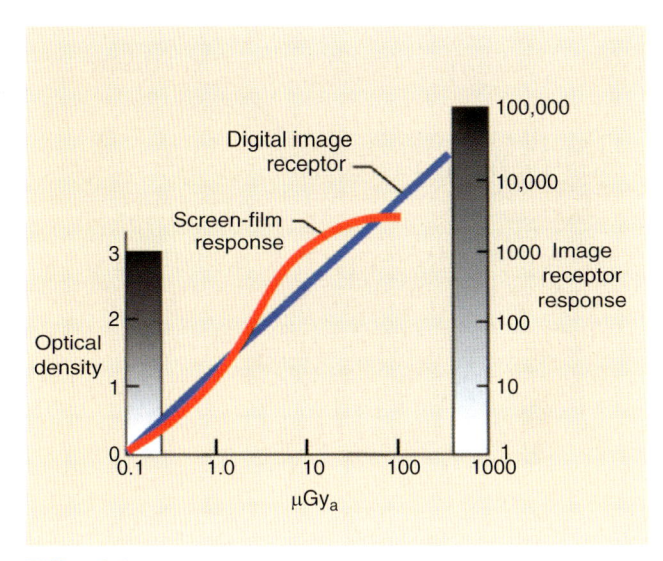

FIG. 12.6 The radiation response of a charge-coupled device (CCD) compared with that of a 400-speed screen-film (S/F) image receptor.

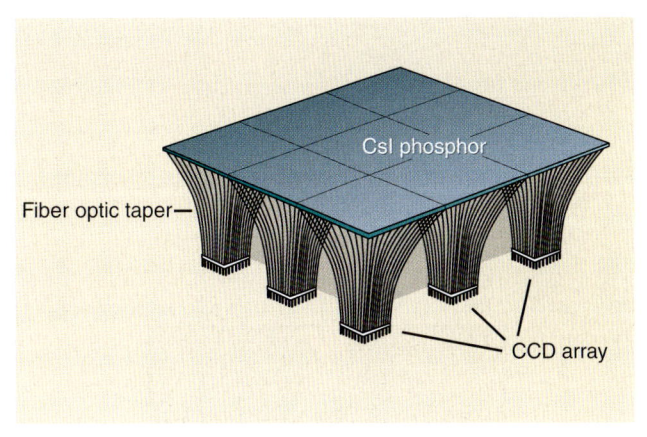

FIG. 12.7 Charge-coupled devices (*CCDs*) can be tiled to receive the light from an area x-ray beam as it interacts with a scintillation phosphor, such as cesium iodide (*CsI*).

Sensitivity is the ability of the CCD to detect and respond to very low levels of visible light. This sensitivity is important for photographing the heavens through a telescope and for low patient radiation dose in digital medical imaging.

Dynamic range is the ability of the CCD to respond to a wide range of light intensity, from very dim to very bright. The dynamic range relative to that of a 400-speed screen-film radiographic image receptor is shown in Fig. 12.6.

> The CCD has high sensitivity to x-ray exposure and a very wide dynamic range.

Note that the CCD radiation response is linear, but the screen-film image receptor has the characteristic Hurter and Driffield (H&D) curve response. Although the screen-film image receptor has three decades of radiation response—optical density (OD) from 0 to 3—only approximately 30 shades of gray are perceivable by the human eye. We previously attempted to produce radiographs low on the linear portion of the H&D curve to maximize image contrast at an acceptable patient radiation dose.

With the use of a CCD, image contrast is unrelated to image receptor x-ray exposure. Furthermore, each of the five decades of radiation response—0 to 100,000—can be visualized by image postprocessing. This property of DR is principally responsible for the death of screen-film radiography.

It should also be noted that a CCD system responds to very low x-ray exposure. The CCD system is very sensitive to radiation exposure, which results in lower patient radiation dose during DR.

A CCD is very small, making it highly adaptable to DR in its various forms. The CCD itself measures approximately 1 to 2 cm, but the pixel size is an exceptional 100 × 100 µm!

CESIUM IODIDE/CHARGE-COUPLED DEVICE

One successful approach to DR is shown in Fig. 12.7. This use of tiled CCDs receiving light from a scintillator allows the use of an area x-ray beam, so that, in contrast to SPR, exposure time is short. The image receptor shown in Fig. 12.5 is of this type.

The scintillation light from a CsI phosphor is efficiently transmitted through fiber-optic bundles to the CCD array. The result is high x-ray capture efficiency and good spatial resolution.

> CsI/CCD is an indirect DR process by which x-rays are converted first to light and then to an electronic signal.

The assembly of multiple CCDs for the purpose of viewing an area x-ray beam presents the challenge creating a seamless image at the edge of each CCD. This is accomplished by interpolating pixel values at each tile interface.

CESIUM IODIDE/AMORPHOUS SILICON

An early application of DR involved the use of CsI to capture the x-ray, as shown in Fig. 12.8, as well as transmission of the resulting scintillation light to a collection element. The collection element is silicon sandwiched as a TFT. Silicon is a semiconductor that is usually grown as a crystal. When identified as **amorphous** silicon (a-silicon; a-Si), the silicon is not crystalline but is a fluid that can be painted onto a supporting surface.

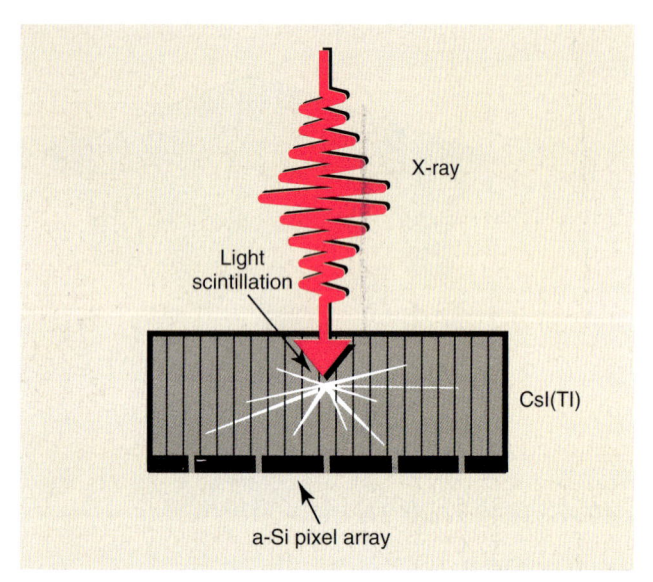

FIG. 12.8 The cesium iodide (*CsI*) phosphor in digital radiography image receptors is available in the form of filaments to improve x-ray absorption and reduce light dispersion. *a-Si*, a-silicon.

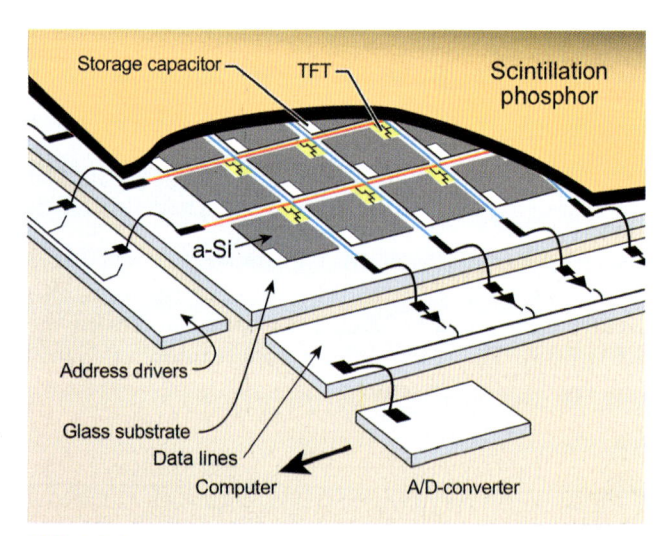

FIG. 12.9 Digital radiographic images can be produced from the cesium iodide (CsI) phosphor light detected by the active matrix array (AMA) of silicon photodiodes. *a-Si*, a-Silicon; *TFT*, thin-film transistor.

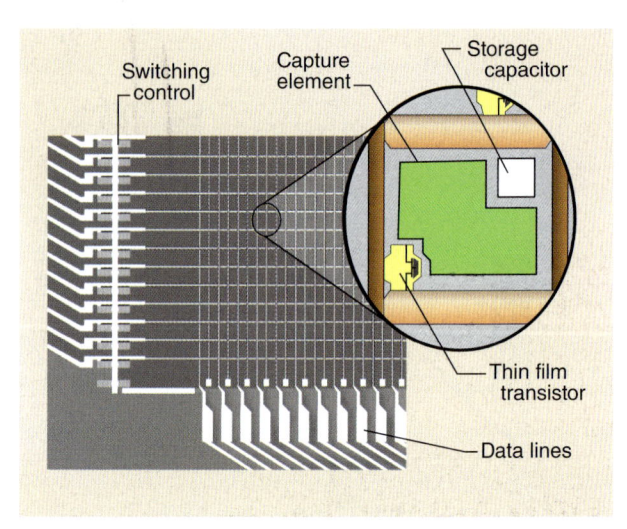

FIG. 12.10 A photomicrograph of an active matrix array–thin-film transistor (AMA-TFT) digital radiography (DR) image receptor with a single pixel highlighted.

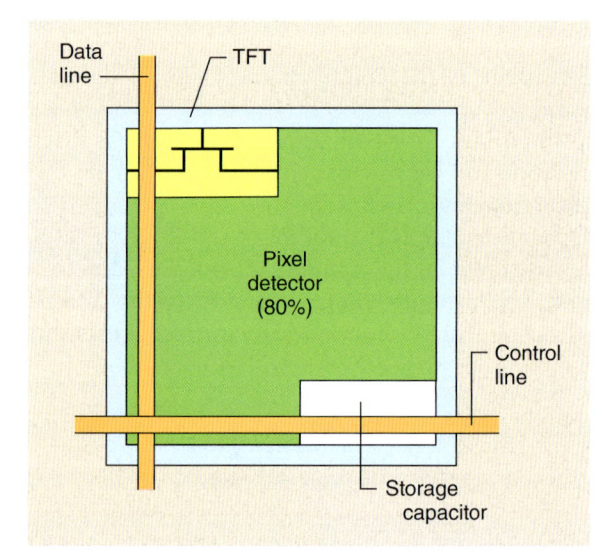

FIG. 12.11 The fill factor is the portion of the pixel element that is occupied by the sensitive capture element of the image receptor. *TFT*, Thin-film transistor.

CsI has a high photoelectric capture because the atomic number of cesium is 55 and that of iodine is 53. Therefore x-ray interaction with CsI is high, resulting in low patient radiation dose. The DR image receptor is fabricated into individual pixels, as shown in Fig. 12.9. Each pixel has a light-sensitive face of a-Si with a capacitor and a TFT embedded.

> CsI/a-Si is an indirect DR process by which x-rays are converted first to light and then to an electronic signal.

Fig. 12.10 is a micrograph of an a-Si array that shows contacts for the switch control **address drivers** and the **data lines**. An exploded view of a single pixel shows that a large portion of the face of the pixel is covered by electronic components and wires that are not sensitive to the light emitted by the CsI phosphor.

The geometry of each individual pixel is very important, as illustrated in Fig. 12.11. Because a portion of the pixel face is occupied by conductors, capacitors, and the TFT, it is not totally sensitive to the incident image-forming x-ray beam.

The percentage of the pixel face that is sensitive to x-rays is the **fill factor**. The fill factor is approximately 80%; therefore 20% of the x-ray beam does not contribute to the image.

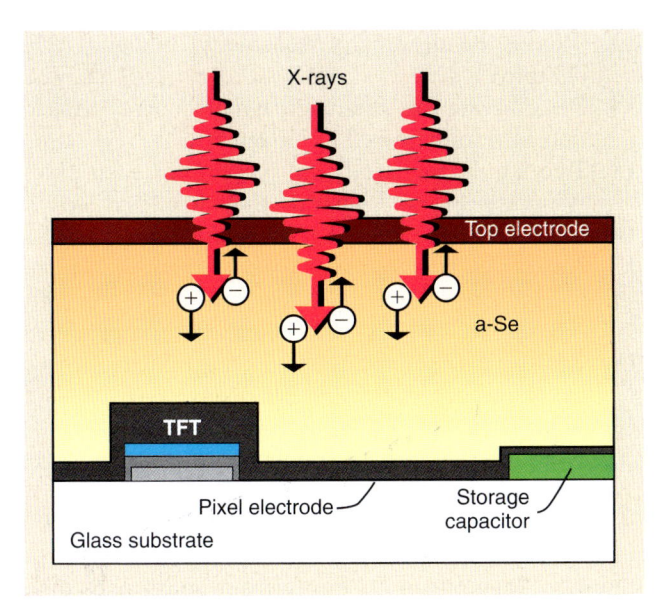

FIG. 12.12 The use of amorphous selenium (*a-Se*) as an image receptor capture element eliminates the need for a scintillation phosphor.

> a-Se is a direct DR process by which x-rays are converted directly into an electronic signal.

The a-Se is approximately 200 μm thick and is sandwiched between charged electrodes. The entire image receptor would appear as shown in Fig. 12.10 for CsI/a-Si and described as an active matrix array (AMA) of TFTs.

X-rays incident on the a-Se create electron hole pairs through direct ionization of selenium. The created charge is collected by a storage capacitor and remains there until the signal is read by the switching action of the TFT.

This represents one of the challenges for DR that may be conquered with quantum computing (Chapter 29). As the pixel size is reduced, spatial resolution improves but at the expense of the patient radiation dose. With smaller pixels, the fill factor is reduced and x-ray intensity must be increased to maintain adequate signal strength. Much physics and materials science research in the nanometer range (nanotechnology) promises increased fill factor and improved spatial resolution at even lower patient radiation dose.

CsI has been used for years as the capture element of an image-intensifier tube. Similarly, GdOS was widely used as the capture element of most rare earth radiographic intensifying screens. What has been described for the CsI/a-Si image receptor can be repeated for the GdOS/a-Si image receptor.

> Spatial resolution in DR is pixel limited.

Increasing the thickness of GdOS in a DR image receptor increases the speed of the system with no compromise in spatial resolution because spatial resolution in DR is limited to the size of the pixel. We cannot image something smaller than the pixel.

AMORPHOUS SELENIUM

The final DR modality is identified, by some, as **direct DR** because no scintillation phosphor is involved. The image-forming x-ray beam interacts directly with a-Se, producing a charged pair, as shown in Fig. 12.12. The a-Se is both the capture element and the coupling element.

SUMMARY

Screen-film radiography was the medical imaging process of choice for 100 years. Now, however, we are in the age of digital medical imaging.

The earliest DR was a spin-off from CT and involved a collimated fan x-ray beam. SPR provides the advantage of scatter radiation reduction by precise slit x-ray beam collimation. The result is better contrast resolution but limited spatial resolution.

Spatial resolution is limited to pixel size in DR; this fact has held back the development of DR until recently. It is now clear that contrast resolution is more important in medical imaging, and, in this area, DR prevails.

Currently, four methods are used to produce a digital projection radiograph. CR uses a PSP to generate a latent image. The visible image results when the PSP is scanned with a laser beam.

CsI scintillation phosphor can be used as the capture element for image-forming x-rays. This signal is channeled to a CCD through fiber-optic channels.

When GdOS or CsI is used to capture x-rays, the light from these scintillators is conducted to an AMA of TFTs, whose sensitive element is a-Si.

Finally, a-Se is used as a capture element for x-rays in an alternate DR method.

CHALLENGE QUESTIONS

1. Define or otherwise identify the following:
    a. SPR
    b. Amorphous
    c. Spatial resolution
    d. Fan x-ray beam
    e. Charge-coupled device
    f. Scintillation phosphor
    g. TFT
    h. Spatial frequency
    i. Dynamic range
    j. Pixel

2. Describe some applications for the use of a charge-coupled-device (CCD) in addition to medical imaging.
3. What are the two principal phosphors used in digital radiography?
4. What is the importance of an A/D converter in digital radiography?
5. By what four methods can a digital radiograph be produced?
6. How is scanned projection radiography used in medical imaging?
7. How does pixel size in CCD digital radiography compare with that in other forms of DR?
8. Why is fill factor important?
9. How is the tiled CCD mosaic made to appear as a single image?
10. How does the image line spread function change for the four types of DR?
11. What properties make GdOS a good radiography image receptor?
12. What is the principal advantage of scanned projection radiography (SPR) over tiled CCDs for use in digital radiography?
13. What is the meaning of "sensitivity" in digital radiography?
14. Describe the role of an active matrix array (AMA) thin-film transistor (TFT) assembly.
15. Two conducting leads are present for each pixel. What are they and what do they do?
16. What is the use of a TFT in digital radiography?
17. What are the respective atomic numbers for the x-ray capture elements of the various radiography systems?
18. What are the consequences of producing digital image receptors with smaller pixels?
19. What is meant by "limited spatial resolution"?
20. What are the capture, couple, and collection stages for a-Se-based DR?

The answers to the Challenge Questions can be found by logging on to our website at http://evolve.elsevier.com.

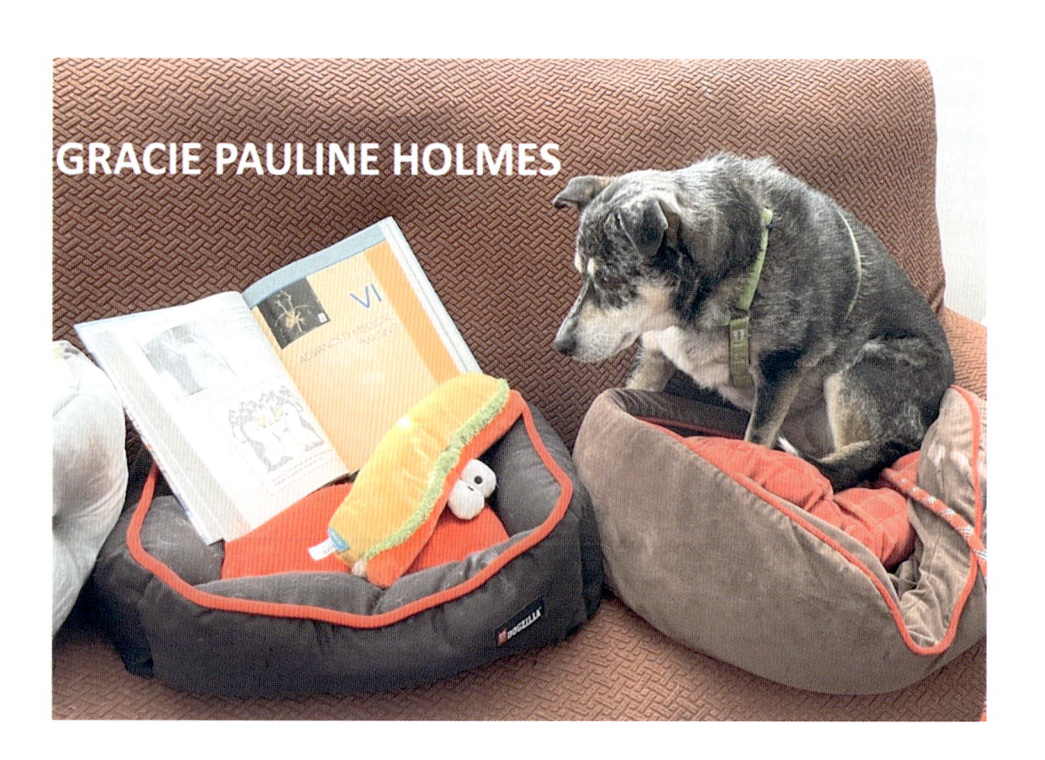

Digital Radiographic Technique

CHAPTER 13

OBJECTIVES

At the completion of this chapter, the student should be able to do the following:

1. Distinguish between spatial resolution and contrast resolution.
2. Identify the use and units of spatial frequency.
3. Interpret a modulation transfer function curve.
4. Discuss how postprocessing allows the visualization of a wide dynamic range.
5. Discuss the characteristics of digital imaging that should result in lower patient radiation doses.

OUTLINE

Spatial Resolution 190
   Spatial Frequency 190
   Modulation Transfer Function 192
Contrast Resolution 194
   Dynamic Range 194
   Postprocessing 194
   Signal-to-Noise Ratio 197
Patient Radiation Dose Considerations 197
   Image Receptor Response 197
   Detective Quantum Efficiency 198
Summary 200
Challenge Questions 200

SCREEN-FILM RADIOGRAPHIC imaging systems worked well for over a century, providing increasingly better diagnostic images. However, screen-film radiography had limitations and has therefore been abandoned for digital radiography (DR).

Another and perhaps more severe limitation is the noise inherent in radiographic images. Radiography uses a large area beam of x-rays. The Compton-scattered portion of the image-forming x-ray beam incident on the image receptor increases with increasing field size. This increases the noise of the radiographic image and severely degrades image contrast.

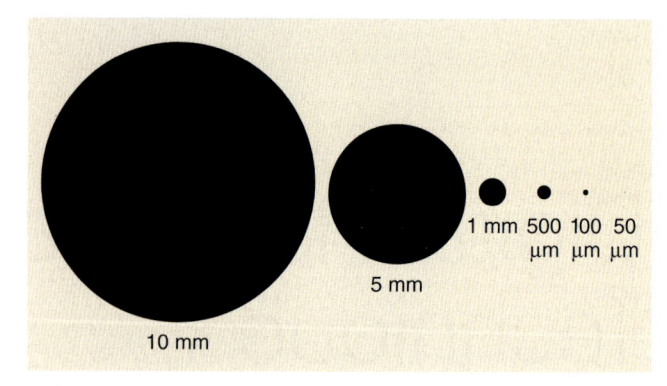

FIG. 13.1 Spatial resolution is a measure of how small an object one can see on an image.

Digital radiographic technique, especially selection of kVp and mAs, is similar to our experience with screen-film radiography except that kVp as a control of image contrast is not so important. Proper digital radiographic technique results in reduced patient radiation dose compared with screen-film radiography.

> Spatial resolution and contrast resolution are the two most important characteristics of an x-ray image.

Digital images are obtained to help in the diagnosis of diseases or defects in anatomy. Each digital image has two principal characteristics: spatial resolution and contrast resolution. Additional image properties, such as noise, artifacts, and archival quality, are noted, but spatial resolution and contrast resolution are most important.

SPATIAL RESOLUTION

Spatial resolution is the ability of an imaging system to resolve and render on the image a small high-contrast object such as a breast microcalcification. There are several ways to express spatial resolution, but the most descriptive is modulation transfer function (MTF).

> Spatial resolution is the ability to render small objects on the image.

Black on white is the highest contrast. Fig. 13.1 shows black dots of diminishing size on a tan background. If the dots were shades of gray, they would not exhibit high contrast but rather low contrast.

The dots range in size scaled from 10 mm down to 50 μm. Most people can see objects as small as 200 μm; therefore the spatial resolution of the eye is considered to be approximately 200 μm. If the dots were not high contrast, the spatial resolution of the eye would require larger dots.

In digital imaging, spatial resolution is described by the quantity **spatial frequency**. We identify size not by a measure in space but in spatial frequency. Spatial frequency quantifies how close lines can be to each other and still be visibly resolved.

Spatial Frequency

The fundamental concept of spatial frequency does not refer to size but to the **line pair**. As is shown in Fig. 13.2, one line pair consists of the line and an interspace of the same width as the line. Six line-pair patterns are shown, with each line and each interspace representing the size of the dots in Fig. 13.1.

> Spatial frequency is expressed in line pair per millimeter (lp/mm).

Spatial frequency relates to the number of line pairs in a given length, usually millimeters. The unit of spatial frequency as used in medical imaging describes the size of an anatomic object in line pair per millimeter (lp/mm). Fig. 13.3 shows the spatial frequency of the six sets of line pairs.

Question: A radiographic imaging system has a spatial resolution of 3.5 lp/mm. How small an object can it resolve?

Answer: 3.5 lp/mm = 7 objects in 1 mm, or 7/mm
Therefore the reciprocal is the answer, or
$\frac{1}{7}$ mm = 0.143 mm = 143 μm.

Clearly, as the spatial frequency becomes larger, the objects become smaller. Higher spatial frequency indicates better spatial resolution. Surprisingly, screen-film

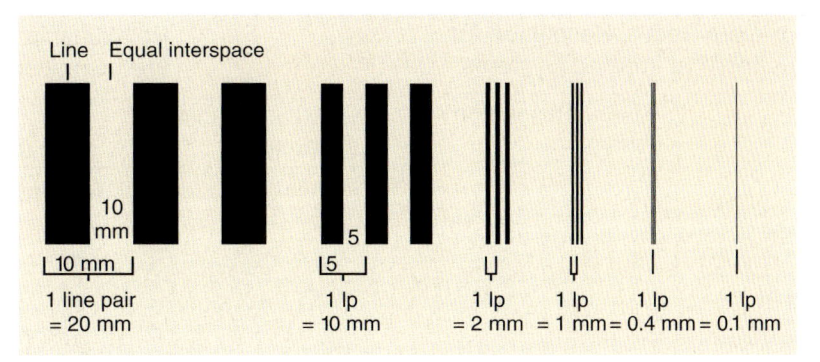

FIG. 13.2 A line pair (*lp*) is a high-contrast line that is separated by an interspace of equal width.

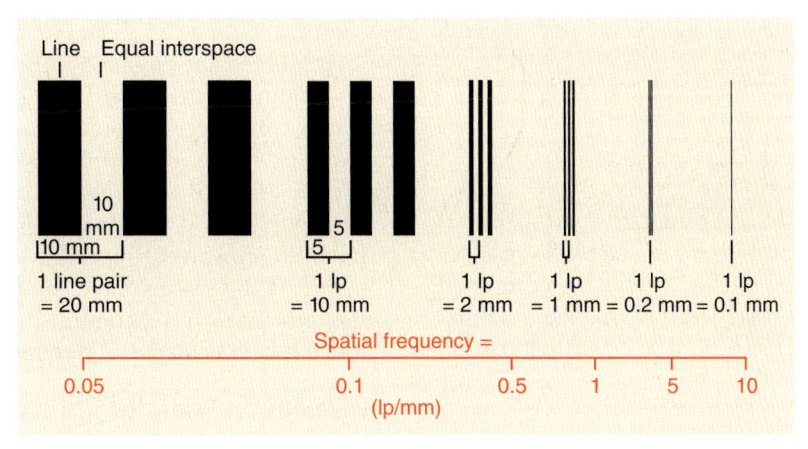

FIG. 13.3 The spatial frequency of each of the line pairs of Fig. 13.2.

mammography has the best spatial resolution of all imaging modalities, and yet it has been abandoned. Reasons for the abandonment are discussed in Chapter 24.

Question: A screen-film mammography imaging system operating in the magnification mode can image high-contrast microcalcifications as small as 50 μm. What spatial frequency does this represent?

Answer: It takes two 50-μm objects to form a single line pair. Therefore 1 lp = 100 μm, or 1 lp/100 μm = 1 lp/0.1 mm = 10 lp/mm.

The concept of spatial frequency is demonstrated in Fig. 13.4 by the dress of three entrepreneurs. The undertaker's plain black suit has a spatial frequency of zero. No change is seen from one part of the suit to another.

The banker's pinstripe suit has zero vertical spatial frequency but high horizontal spatial frequency. The used-car salesman's coat has high spatial frequency in all directions.

Anatomy also can be described as having spatial frequency. Large soft tissues such as the liver, kidneys, and brain have low spatial frequency and therefore are easy to image. Bone trabeculae, breast microcalcifications, and contrast-filled vessels are high-spatial-frequency objects; therefore they are more difficult to image.

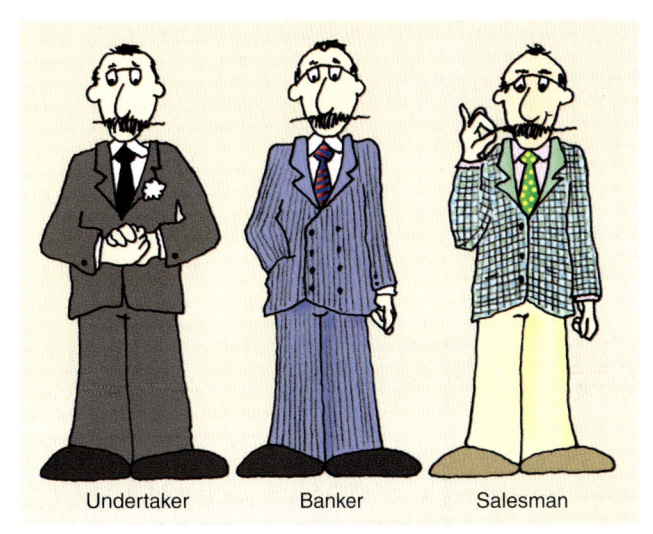

FIG. 13.4 Three entrepreneurs and their work attire demonstrate the concept of spatial frequency.

> An imaging system with higher spatial frequency response has better spatial resolution.

TABLE 13.1	Approximate Spatial Resolution for Various Medical Imaging Systems
Imaging System	**Spatial Resolution (lp/mm)**
Gamma camera	0.1
Magnetic resonance imaging	1.5
Computed tomography	1.5
Diagnostic ultrasonography	2
Fluoroscopy	3
Digital radiography	4
Computed radiography	6
Screen-film radiography	8
Screen-film mammography	15

TABLE 13.2	Relationship Between Spatial Frequency and Size	
Spatial Frequency (lp/mm)	**Size (mm)**	**Size (μm)**
0.1	5.0	
0.5	1.0	
1.0	0.5	500
5.0	0.1	100
10	0.05	50
15	0.03	33

Table 13.1 presents the approximate spatial resolution for various medical imaging systems. Sometimes the spatial resolution for nuclear medicine, computed tomography (CT), and magnetic resonance imaging (MRI) is stated in terms of lp/cm instead of lp/mm.

Question: The image from a nuclear medicine gamma camera can resolve just ¼ in. What spatial frequency does this represent?

Answer: ¼ in × 25.4 mm/in = 6.35 mm
It takes two 6.35-mm objects to form a line pair; hence 12.7 mm/lp.
The reciprocal is 1 lp/12.7 mm
= 0.08 lp/mm = 0.8 lp/cm.

The spatial resolution of radiography is determined somewhat by the geometry of the system, especially focal-spot size. Mammography is best because of its small focal spot, 0.1 mm, necessary for magnification.

> Spatial resolution in digital imaging is limited by pixel size.

Question: What is the spatial resolution of a 512 × 512 CT image that has a field of view of 30 cm? What spatial frequency does that represent?

Answer: 512 pixels/30 cm = 512 pixels/300 mm
300 mm/512 pixels = 0.59 mm/pixel
Two pixels are required to form a line pair; therefore:
2 × 0.59 mm = 1.2 mm/lp
1 lp/1.2 mm = 0.83 lp/mm = 8.3 lp/cm

Spatial resolution in all of the digital imaging modalities is limited by the size of the pixel. No digital imaging system can image an object smaller than 1 pixel. Two pixels are required to form a line pair. This CT imaging system is limited to a spatial resolution of 0.83 lp/mm. If the pixel size is 0.59 mm (590 μm), no object smaller than 590 μm can be imaged.

Most CT systems have a limiting spatial resolution of approximately 1.5 lp/mm. Table 13.2 shows the relationship between spatial frequency and size.

Modulation Transfer Function

MTF is a term borrowed from radio electronics that has been applied to the description of the ability of an imaging system to render anatomic objects onto an image. Objects with high spatial frequency are more difficult to image than those with low spatial frequency. This is just another way of saying that small objects are harder to image than large objects.

Regardless of the size of the object, the object is considered to be high contrast, black on white, for the purpose of MTF evaluation. The ideal imaging system is one that produces an image that appears exactly as the object. Such a system would have an MTF equal to 1.

> MTF can be viewed as the ratio of image to object as a function of spatial frequency.

An ideal imaging system does not exist. The line pairs of Fig. 13.3 become more blurred with increasing spatial frequency. The amount of blurring can be represented by the reduced amplitude of the representative frequency, as is shown in Fig. 13.5.

Quality control test tools have been designed to measure the amount of blurring as a function of spatial frequency. Fig. 13.6 shows two bar pattern test tools with spatial frequencies up to 20 lp/mm. Such tools can measure the limiting modulation of each spatial frequency pattern and can use those data to construct an MTF curve.

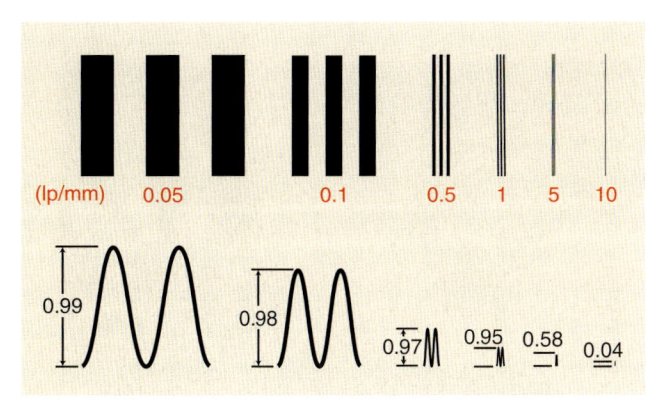

CHAPTER 13 Digital Radiographic Technique

FIG. 13.5 When a line pair pattern is imaged, the higher spatial frequencies become blurred, resulting in reduced modulation.

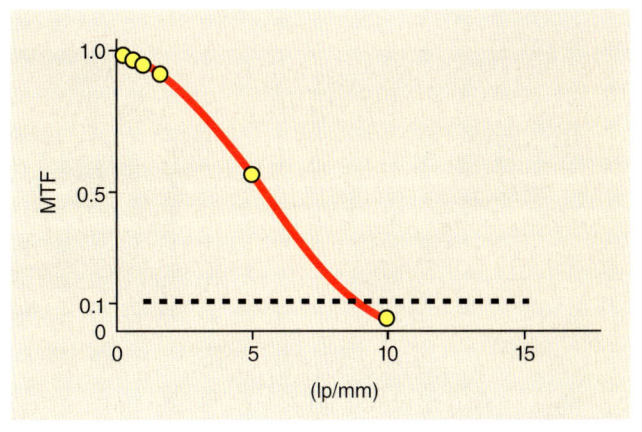

FIG. 13.7 A plot of the modulation data from Fig. 13.5 results in a modulation transfer function (*MTF*) curve.

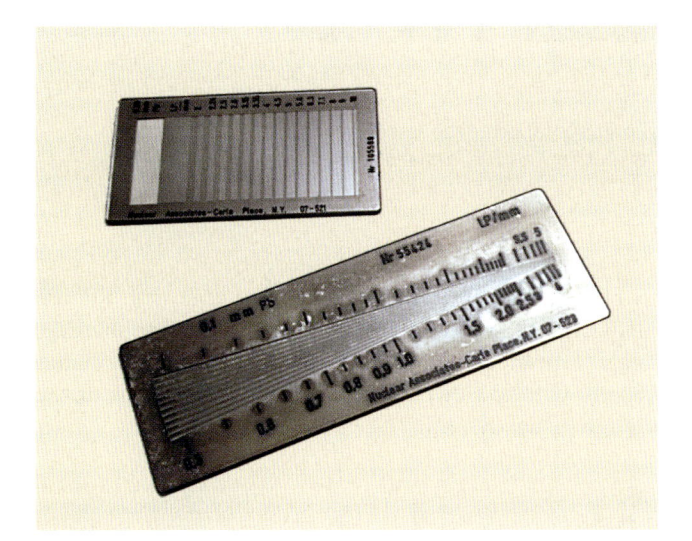

FIG. 13.6 These plastic-encased lead bar patterns are imaged to construct a modulation transfer function. (Courtesy Fluke Biomedical.)

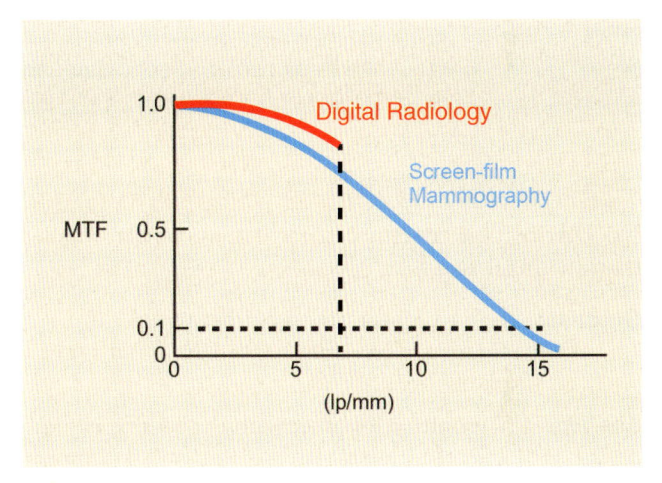

FIG. 13.8 Digital radiography has a high modulation transfer function (*MTF*) at low spatial frequencies and an abrupt cutoff at the size of the pixel.

When the modulation of the bar pattern is plotted against spatial frequency, as is done in Fig. 13.7, an MTF curve results. When an imaging system is evaluated through this method, the 10% MTF is identified as the system spatial resolution.

> Imaging system spatial resolution is the spatial frequency at 10% MTF.

The MTF curve in Fig. 13.8 is representative of DR. At low spatial frequencies (large objects), good reproduction is noted on the image by the high MTF. However, as the spatial frequency of the object increases (the objects get smaller), the faithful reproduction of the object on the image gets worse. This MTF curve shows an abrupt limiting spatial resolution of approximately 7 lp/mm (70 µm). This, 70 µm, is approximately the smallest pixel size for DR at this time.

At low spatial frequencies, the contrast of the object is preserved, but at higher spatial frequencies, contrast is lost. This limits the spatial resolution of the imaging system. Inspect Fig. 13.8 again, in which a digital radiographic imaging system is compared with a mammographic screen-film system that has the best spatial resolution of all imaging modalities.

At low spatial frequencies, the MTF for DR is higher than that for screen-film mammography, even though low kilovolt peak (kVp) and tissue compression is used for mammography.

Fig. 13.9 shows two photographic representations of the MTF curves of Fig. 13.8 to give a better sense of how a change in MTF affects image rendition. Fig. 13.9A represents screen-film radiography, whereas Fig. 13.9B represents DR with reduced spatial resolution but better contrast resolution.

The MTF curve that represents DR (see Fig. 13.8) has the distinctive feature of a cutoff spatial frequency.

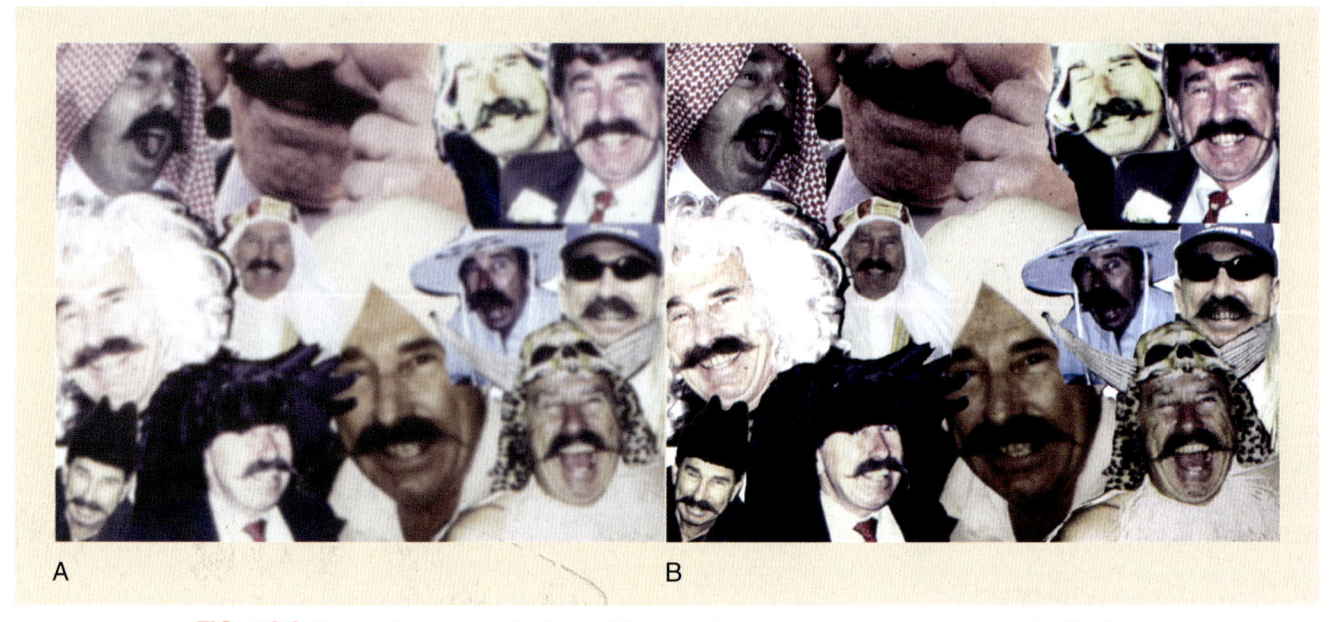

FIG. 13.9 These photographs illustrate differences in image appearance associated with the modulation transfer function curves of (A) screen-film radiography and (B) digital radiography.

No DR imaging system can resolve an object smaller than the pixel size.

Question: Fig. 13.8 indicates a cutoff spatial frequency of 7 lp/mm for DR. What is the pixel size?

Answer: 7 lp/mm = 14 objects/mm = 14 pixels/mm
Therefore pixel size is $\frac{1}{7}$ mm = 0.071 mm = 71 μm.

Note also that DR has higher MTF at low spatial frequencies. This is principally because of the expanded dynamic range of DR and its higher detective quantum efficiency (DQE). Both of these characteristics are discussed in the following contrast resolution section.

CONTRAST RESOLUTION

One hundred percent contrast is black and white. The lettering on this page shows very high contrast. Contrast resolution is the ability to distinguish many shades of gray from black to white. All digital imaging systems have better contrast resolution than screen-film imaging. The principal descriptor for contrast resolution is grayscale, more precisely called **dynamic range**.

Dynamic Range

The dynamic range of a screen-film radiograph is essentially three orders of magnitude—1 to 10, 10 to 100, 100 to 1000—from an optical density (OD) of near 0 to 3.0. This represents a dynamic range of 1000, but the viewer can visualize only approximately 30 shades of gray.

The grayscale can be made more visible with the use of specific radiographic techniques designed to increase image latitude; however, still no more than 30 shades of gray will be viewed because of the limitations of the human visual system.

> Dynamic range is the number of gray shades that an imaging system can reproduce.

The dynamic range of digital imaging systems is identified by the bit depth of each pixel. The number of shades of gray that each pixel can display defines the bit depth and is equal to $2^{\text{bit depth}}$. CT and MRI systems generally have a 12-bit dynamic range (2^{12} = 4096 shades of gray). DR has a 14-bit dynamic range (2^{14} = 16,384 shades of gray).

Because contrast resolution is so important in mammography, digital mammography (DM) and digital mammographic tomosynthesis systems have a 16-bit dynamic range (2^{16} = 65,536 shades of gray). Table 13.3 summarizes the dynamic range of various imaging systems.

The response of a digital imaging system is almost five orders of magnitude (Fig. 13.10). Still, the human visual system is not able to visualize such a dynamic range. With the postprocessing exercise of window and level, each grayscale value can be visualized—not just 30.

Postprocessing

A principal advantage of digital imaging is the ability to preprocess and postprocess the image for the purpose

TABLE 13.3 Dynamic Range of Digital Medical Imaging Systems

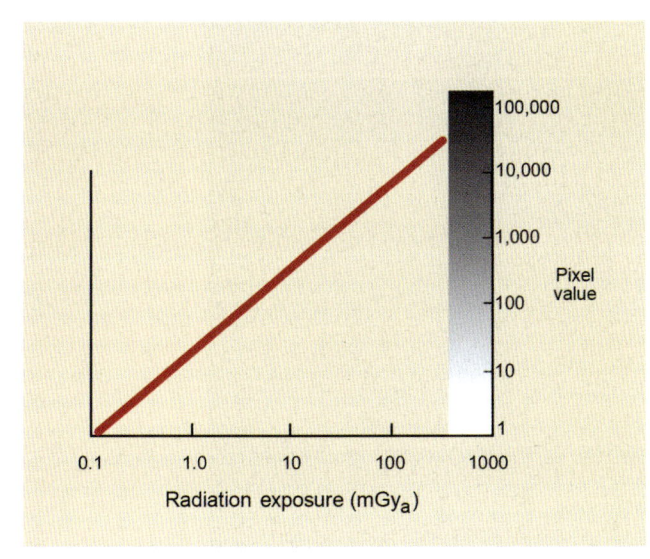

Imaging System	Bit Depth	Shades of Gray
Diagnostic ultrasonography	2^8	256
Nuclear medicine	2^{10}	1024
Computed tomography	2^{12}	4096
Magnetic resonance imaging	2^{12}	4096
Digital radiography	2^{14}	16,384
Digital mammography	2^{16}	65,536

FIG. 13.10 Digital imaging systems have a dynamic range approaching five orders of magnitude.

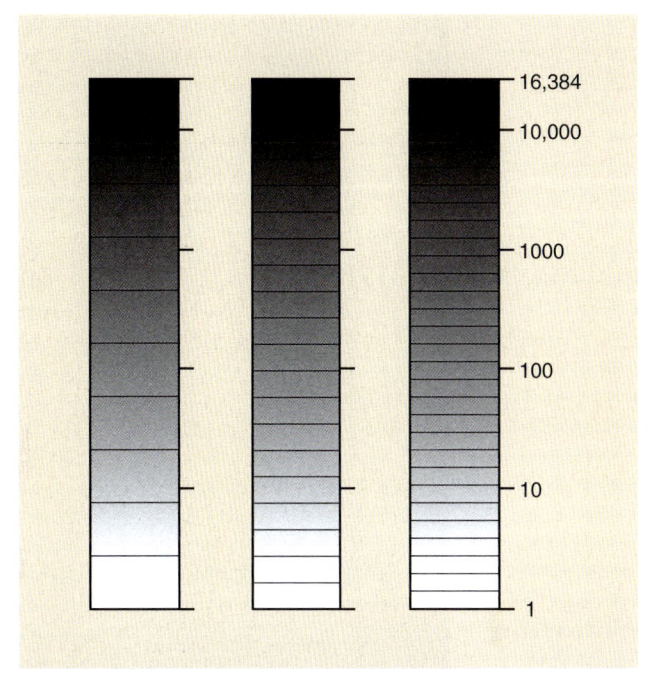

FIG. 13.11 Although a 14-bit dynamic range contains 16,384 shades of gray, we can see only approximately 30 of them.

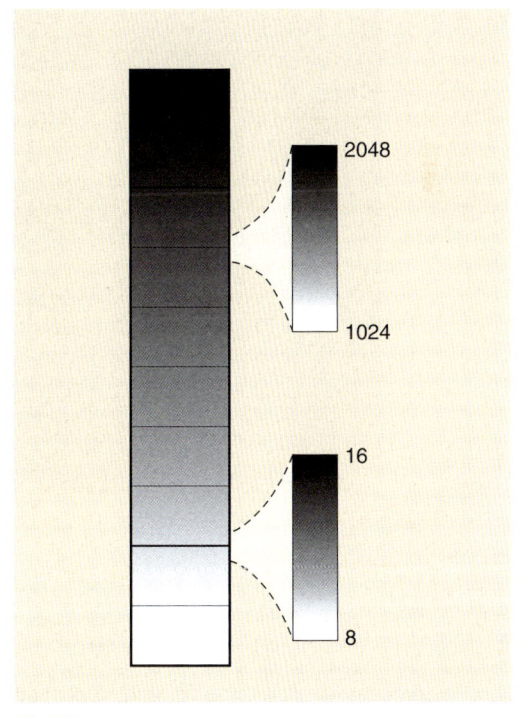

FIG. 13.12 With window and level postprocessing tools, any region and range of the 16,384 can be rendered as 30 shades of gray.

of extracting even more information. With screen-film radiographic images, what you saw was what you got. One cannot extract more information than is visible on the image.

Several image-processing activities associated with digital imaging are discussed in Chapter 24. One postprocessing activity, **window** and **level**, is discussed here because it makes possible visualization of the entire dynamic range of the grayscale.

Consider the grayscale presented in Fig. 13.11, which represents a 14-bit dynamic range. The 16,384 distinct shades of gray are far more than we can visualize.

The range from white to black has been arbitrarily divided into 10 gray levels. Place a pencil over one of the dividers, and see if you can distinguish the adjacent gray levels from one another. For most people, approximately 30 gray levels is about the limit of contrast resolution.

With use of the window and level postprocessing tool, any region of this 16,384 grayscale can be expanded into a white-to-black grayscale, as is shown in Fig. 13.12. This postprocessing tool is especially helpful when soft tissue images are evaluated.

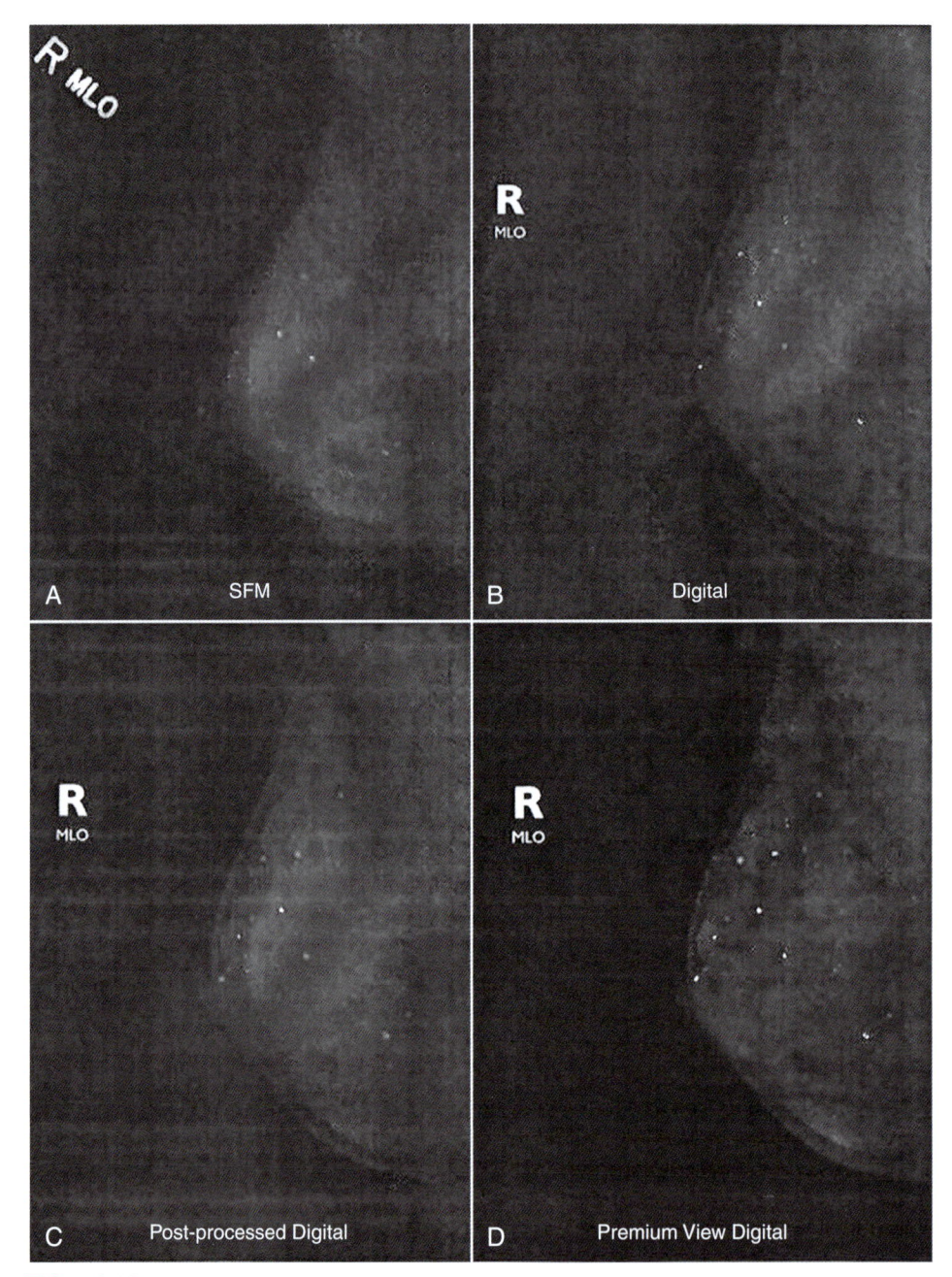

FIG. 13.13 (A) With screen-film mammography, what you see is what you get. (B) With digital mammography, contrast is enhanced. (C and D) By postprocessing the digital image, contrast can be further enhanced. (Courtesy Ed Hendrick, Northwestern University.)

> Postprocessing allows visualization of all shades of gray.

The breast consists of essentially soft tissue and therefore is difficult to image. The subject contrast is poor; this requires that low kVp must be used to accentuate photoelectric interaction.

Fig. 13.13A shows a screen-film mammogram of good quality. Fig. 13.13B is a digital mammogram of the same breast that shows somewhat better contrast. Figs. 13.13C and D are digital mammograms of the same breast that show even better contrast because of window and level postprocessing.

In 2006 results of the Digital Mammography Imaging Screening Trial (DMIST) were reported. This study was commissioned by the American College of Radiology Imaging Network and the National Institutes of Health. A total of 50,000 females were imaged with screen-film mammography and DM, and the results show that for the younger, denser breasts, DM was better.

For older, less dense breasts, DM was equal to screen-film mammography. This suggests that contrast

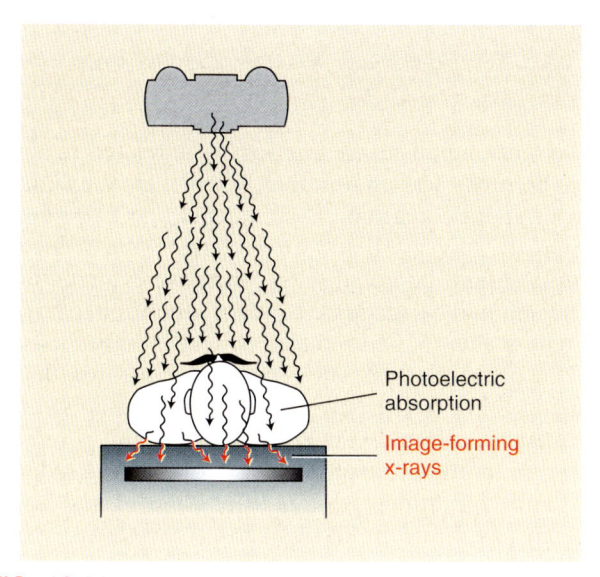

FIG. 13.14 Image-forming x-rays are those that are transmitted through the patient unattenuated (signal) and those that are Compton scattered (noise).

resolution is more important than spatial resolution when soft tissue is imaged. More on this topic can be found in Chapter 24.

Signal-to-Noise Ratio

The **signal** in a radiographic image is that portion of the **image-forming x-rays** that represents anatomy. In digital radiographic imaging, the number of such imaging-forming x-rays is huge. The image-forming x-ray beam represents the difference between those x-rays transmitted to the image receptor and those absorbed photoelectrically, as is shown in Fig. 13.14.

Compton scatter x-rays reaching the image receptor are the principal source of noise on an x-ray image. Noise is random background information that contains no anatomic information. Other sources of noise are associated with the image receptor. The signal-to-noise ratio (SNR) is important to any medical image. Noise limits contrast resolution; therefore radiographers strive for high SNR by selecting appropriate radiographic techniques while recognizing ALARA (as low as reasonably achievable).

> Image noise limits contrast resolution.

With digital radiographic imaging systems, the radiographic technique is computer selected. Still, the radiographer must be prepared to alter techniques as required.

In general, as milliampere seconds (mAs) is increased, the SNR also is increased, although at the expense of increased patient radiation dose. This is a dilemma that has been successfully faced in digital imaging.

Another way to increase SNR is seen in digital subtraction angiography (DSA). Suppose a single DSA image has an SNR of 1:1; this represents a signal value of 1 and a noise value of 1. If two sequential DSA images are integrated (i.e., added to each other), the signal is doubled, but the noise is increased only by the square root of 2, or 1.414. Therefore the SNR is 2/1.414 = 1.414.

Signal increases in proportion to the number of images integrated; noise increases in proportion to the square root of the number of images integrated.

When four DSA frames are added together, the signal is increased four times. The noise is increased by the square root of four or two. Therefore SNR = 4/2 = 2 after four-image integration.

PATIENT RADIATION DOSE CONSIDERATIONS

With acceleration to all-digital imaging, we have succeeded in reducing patient dose by 20% to 50%, depending on the examination. However quite the opposite often still occurs—something that many call "dose creep."

Because DR nearly always yields a diagnostic image, it is possible for the radiographer to be unwittingly lured into not adjusting exposure technique as was done with screen-film. An example is not changing technique factors between a lateral view and an anteroposterior view when these are taken consecutively. As a result, it is possible for the overall patient radiation dose to increase and this will not be obvious on the image.

Patient radiation dose reduction should be possible because of the manner in which the digital image receptor responds to x-rays and because of a property of the digital image receptor known as **detective quantum efficiency (DQE)**.

Image Receptor Response

Consider again the response of a digital radiographic image receptor, as shown in Fig. 13.11. This relates to the response of the image receptor to the x-ray beam. It does not represent anything about spatial resolution. Recall that spatial resolution in screen-film radiography is determined principally by focal-spot size, but spatial resolution in digital imaging is determined principally by pixel size.

> Spatial resolution in digital radiography is determined principally by pixel size.

Because digital image receptor response is linearly related to radiation intensity, image contrast does not change with changing radiation exposure. One cannot overexpose or underexpose a digital radiographic image receptor. However, poor technical factor selection may result in overexposure of the patient.

TABLE 13.4	Dose Reduction With Digital Radiography

- Exposures should not be repeated in digital radiography (DR) because of brightness or contrast concerns.
- DR systems cannot compensate for excessive noise caused by quantum mottle.
- Overexposed images do not have to be repeated but should not become a habit.

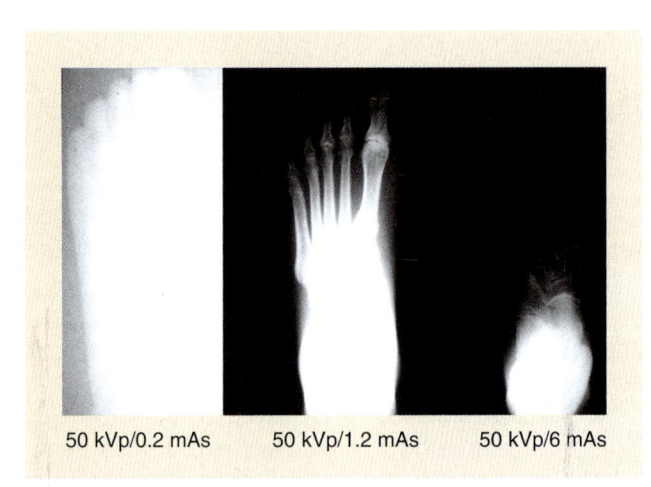

FIG. 13.15 Screen-film radiographs of a foot phantom showing overexposure and underexposure because of wide-ranging technique. (Courtesy Anthony Siebert, University of California, Davis, California.)

Therefore DR should never require repeating because of exposure factors. The exposure factor–related repeat rate for screen-film radiography ranged to approximately 5%, and this translates directly to a patient dose reduction for digital imaging.

DR affords a considerable opportunity for patient radiation dose reduction (Table 13.4).

> Contrast resolution is preserved in digital imaging, regardless of patient radiation dose.

The screen-film radiographs of a foot phantom shown in Fig. 13.15 are labeled with the technique used for each. Screen-film radiographs are overexposed or underexposed easily; however, this is not the case with digital radiographic images.

Fig. 13.16 shows the same foot phantom imaged digitally with the same techniques used in Fig. 13.15. The respective radiation exposure values are shown to emphasize the possible patient radiation dose reduction with digital imaging.

Instead of "dose creep," "technique creep" should be used with each of the various digital imaging systems. The result will be patient radiation dose reduction.

> Technique creep should replace dose creep.

Because digital image contrast is unrelated to dose, kVp becomes less important. When digital examination of specific anatomy is conducted, the kVp should start to be increased, and an accompanying reduction in mAs should be noted with successive examinations. The result will be adequate contrast resolution, constant spatial resolution, and reduced patient radiation dose.

The problem with very low technique for digital imaging is low SNR. This particular type of noise gives the image a salt-and-pepper appearance and is termed quantum mottle or quantum noise. Noise can predominate and compromise the interpretation of soft tissue anatomy, as shown in Fig. 13.17.

Detective Quantum Efficiency

The probability that an x-ray will interact with an image receptor is determined by the thickness of the capture layer and its atomic composition. The descriptor used for medical imaging is DQE. DQE is related to the absorption coefficient and to the spatial frequency of the image-forming x-ray beam.

> Patient radiation dose in DR should be low because of the high DQE of the image receptor.

For present purposes, DQE can be regarded as the absorption coefficient; it is highly x-ray energy dependent. Table 13.5 presents the atomic number for various elements used in digital image receptors and the K-shell absorption edge for the most responsive element.

Barium fluorobromide (BaFBr), cesium iodide (CsI), and amorphous selenium (a-Se) are used with digital image receptors. The value of DQE for each of these capture elements is strongly dependent on x-ray energy, as is shown in Fig. 13.18.

> DQE is a measure of x-ray absorption efficiency.

Fig. 13.19, a simplification of Fig. 13.18, combines the various DQE values for computed radiography (CR), and DR image receptors with a 90-kVp x-ray emission spectrum. Note that the DQE for DR is slightly higher than that for CR.

The relative value of DQE for various image receptors means that fewer x-rays are required by the higher DQE receptors to produce an image; this translates into lower patient radiation dose. The additional feature shown in Fig. 13.19 is that most x-rays have energy that matches the K-shell binding energy. This relates to greater x-ray absorption at that energy.

CHAPTER 13 Digital Radiographic Technique   199

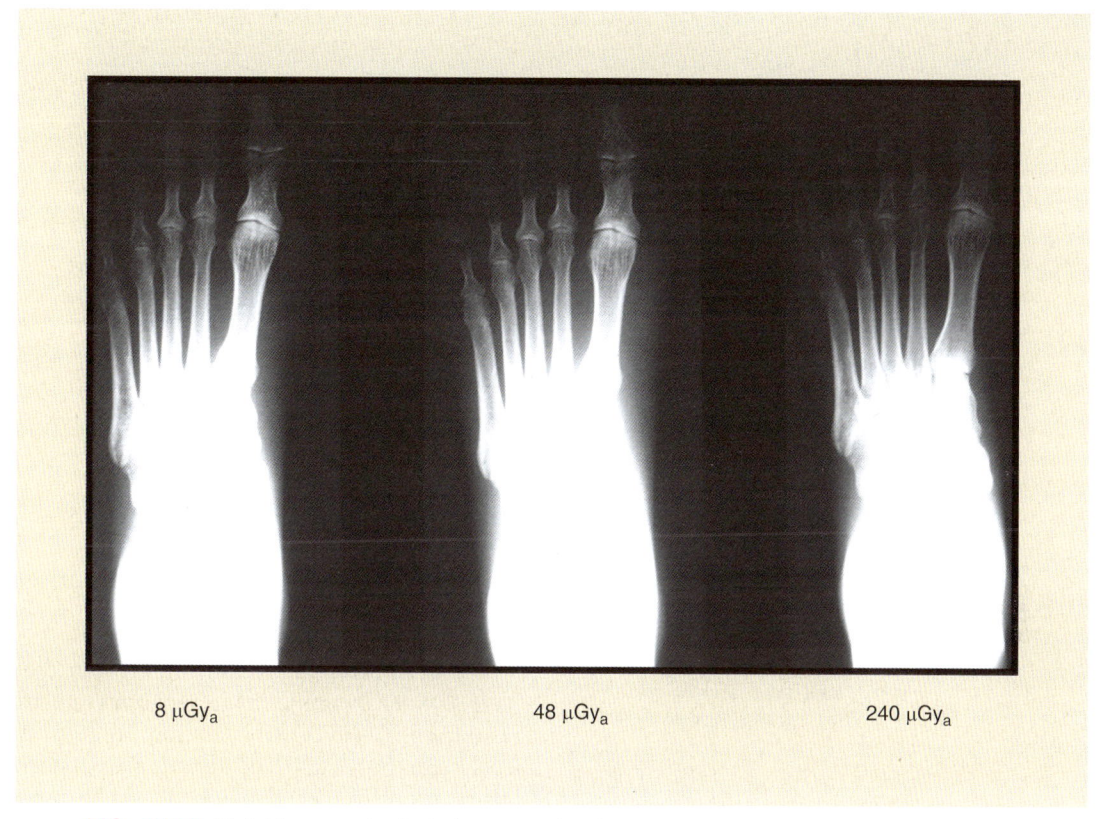

8 µGy$_a$ 48 µGy$_a$ 240 µGy$_a$

FIG. 13.16 Digital images of a foot phantom using the same radiographic techniques as in Fig. 13.15 show the maintenance of contrast over a wide range of patient radiation doses. (Courtesy Anthony Siebert, University of California, Davis, California.)

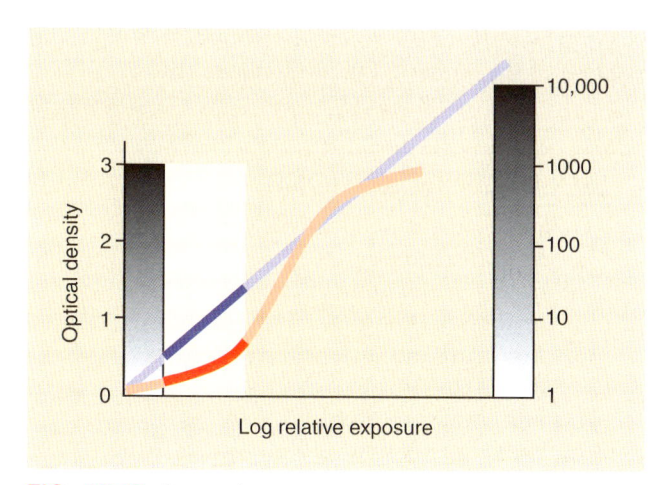

FIG. 13.17 At very low exposure of a digital image receptor, spatial resolution and contrast are maintained, but image noise may be troublesome.

TABLE 13.5 Atomic Number and K-Shell Binding Energy for Various Image Receptors

Image Receptor	Capture Element	Atomic Number	K-Shell Binding Energy (keV)
GdOS	Gd	64	55
LaOS	La	57	39
BaFBr	Ba	56	37
CsI	Cs	55	35
CsI	I	53	33
a-Se	Se	34	12

a-Se, Amorphous selenium; *BaFBr*, barium fluorobromide; *CsI*, cesium iodide; *GdOS*, gadolinium oxysulfite; *LaOS*, lanthanum oxysulfide.

> The scatter x-ray beam has lower energy than the primary x-ray beam.

One final feature of this analysis of DQE and patient radiation dose relates to the x-ray beam incident on the IR. When the 90-kVp x-ray beam interacts with the patient, most of the x-rays are scattered and are reduced in energy, as shown in Fig. 13.19. This results in even greater absorption of image-forming x-rays.

This analysis of IR response and DQE shows that patient radiation dose should be less with digital radiographic imaging than previously experienced with screen-film imaging. Coupled with a new approach to digital radiographic technique that is based on increased kVp and reduced mAs, DR results in reduced patient radiation dose.

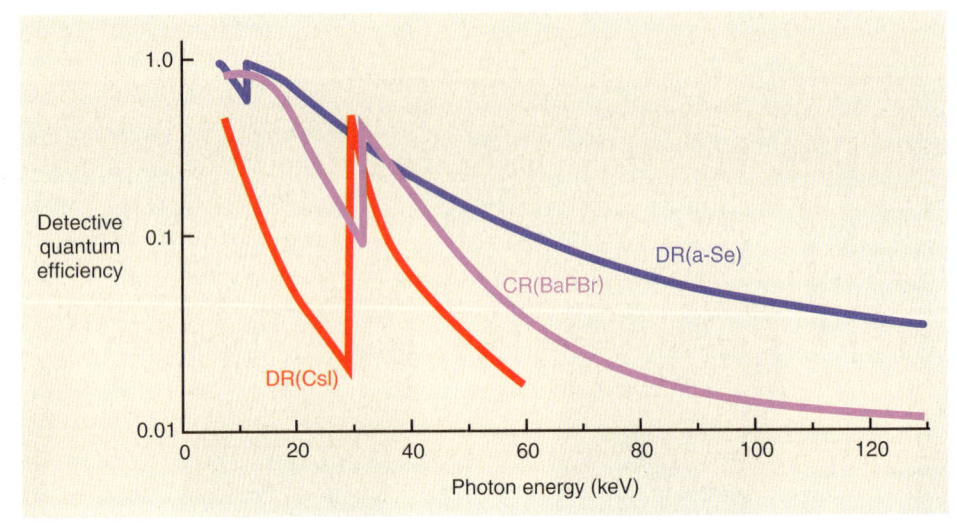

FIG. 13.18 Detective quantum efficiency as a function of x-ray energy for various image receptor capture elements.

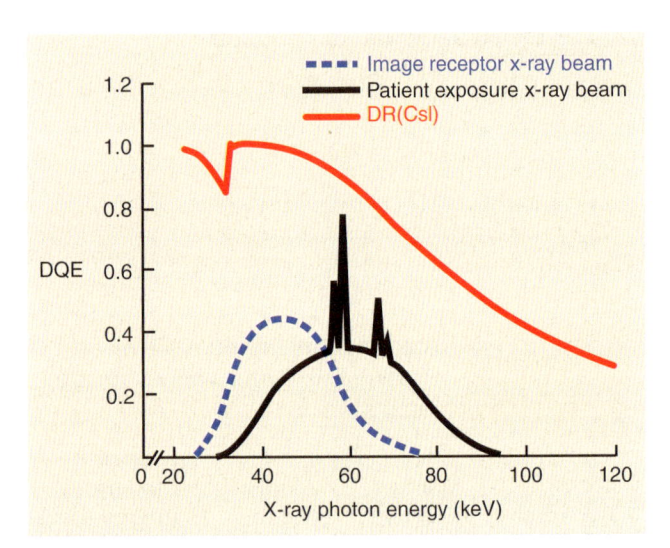

FIG. 13.19 The x-ray beam incident on the image receptor is lower in energy than the beam incident on the patient and better matches the x-ray absorption of capture elements.

SUMMARY

DR is limited by one deficiency when compared with the former universal modality—screen-film radiography—spatial resolution. Spatial resolution, the ability to image small high-contrast objects, is limited by pixel size in DR.

However, DR has several important advantages. Digital radiographic images are obtained faster than screen-film images because wet chemistry processing is unnecessary. Digital radiographic images can be viewed simultaneously by multiple observers in multiple locations. Digital radiographic images can be transferred and archived electronically, thereby saving image retrieval time and film file storage space.

It is even more important to note that digital images have a wider dynamic range, resulting in better contrast resolution. With postprocessing, thousands of gray levels can be visualized, allowing extraction of more information from each image. The MTF curve describes the favorable characteristics of a digital image.

Perhaps the principal favorable characteristic of digital imaging is the opportunity for patient radiation dose reduction. This occurs because of the linear manner in which the image receptor responds to x-rays and because of the higher DQE of the digital IR.

CHALLENGE QUESTIONS

1. Define or otherwise identify the following:
   a. Spatial frequency
   b. Detective quantum efficiency
   c. Contrast resolution
   d. Modulation transfer function
   e. K-shell binding energy
   f. Bar pattern test tool
   g. Spatial resolution
   h. Dynamic range
   i. DMIST
   j. Postprocessing
2. What is the spatial frequency of a 100-μm breast microcalcification?
3. The best a magnetic resonance imaging system (MRI) can do is approximately 2 lp/cm. What is this limit in lp/mm?
4. The limiting spatial resolution for CR is approximately 6 lp/mm. What size object does this represent?
5. Which tissues would be considered low spatial frequency structures?

6. Which tissues would be considered high spatial frequency structures?
7. Which medical imaging system has the best spatial resolution? Why?
8. What is meant by postprocessing?
9. Which units are found along the vertical and horizontal axes of an MTF curve?
10. Which imaging system has the highest dynamic range?
11. A DR system is designed with 125-μm pixels. What is the system limiting spatial frequency?
12. What value of MTF is generally considered the limiting spatial resolution of an imaging system?
13. Why does a digital imaging system have a cutoff spatial frequency?
14. Compare the dynamic range of the human visual system with that of digital imaging.
15. A 12-bit dynamic range has how many shades of gray?
16. What were the principal findings of the DMIST, and what are their implications for medical imaging?
17. How does image integration in DSA improve the signal-to-noise ratio in the image?
18. Describe an everyday object with high and low spatial frequency.
19. Which—spatial resolution or contrast resolution—is more influenced by image noise?
20. Discuss "dose creep" and "technique creep."

The answers to the Challenge Questions can be found by logging on to our website at http://evolve.elsevier.com.

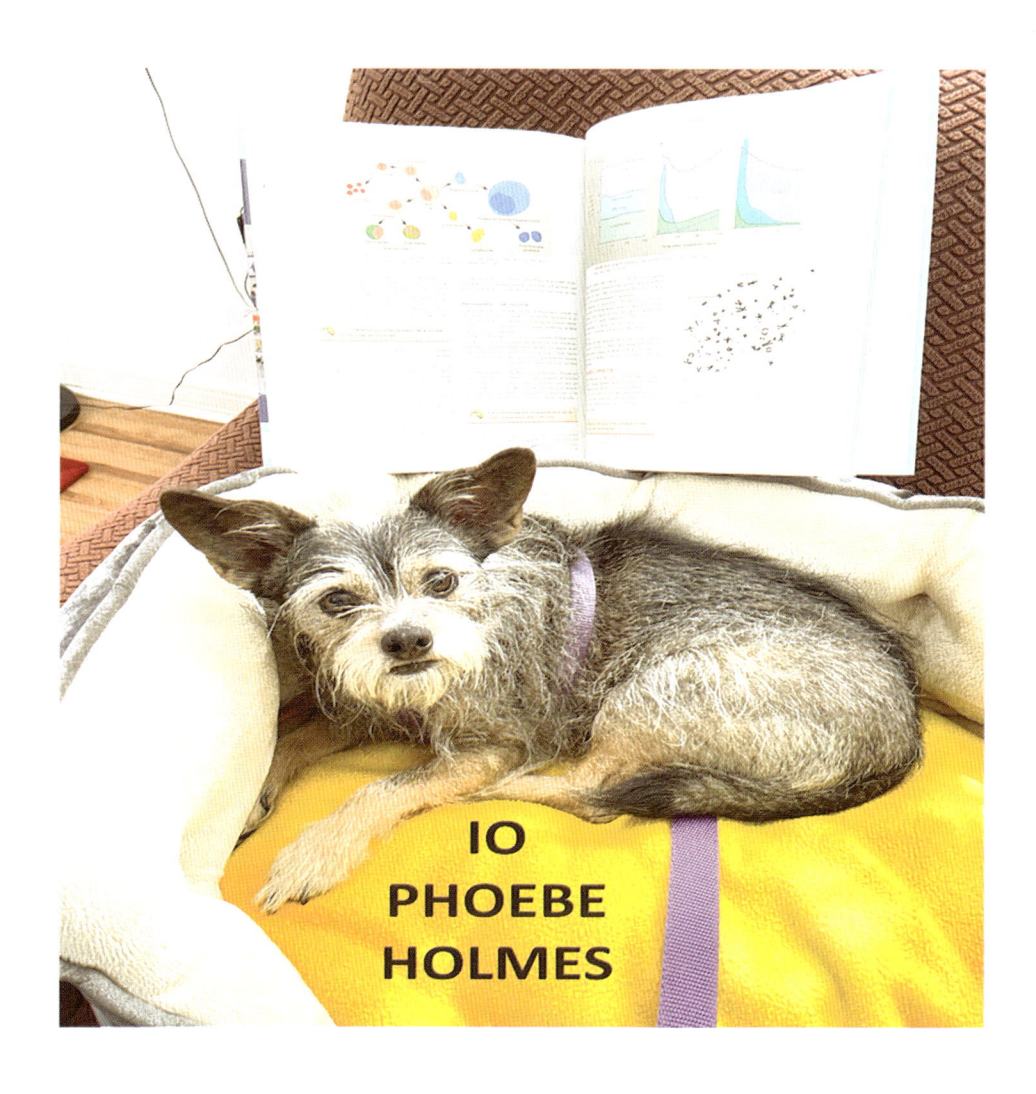

CHAPTER 14

Image Acquisition

OBJECTIVES

At the completion of this chapter, the student should be able to do the following:

1. List the four prime exposure factors.
2. Discuss milliampere seconds (mAs) and kilovolt peak (kVp) in relation to x-ray beam intensity and energy.
3. Describe characteristics of the imaging system that affect x-ray beam intensity and energy.
4. List the four patient factors and explain their effects on radiographic technique.
5. Explain the three types of automatic exposure controls.
6. Describe magnification radiography and its uses.

OUTLINE

Exposure Factors 203
   Kilovolt Peak 203
   Milliamperes 203
   Exposure Time 204
   Distance 206
Imaging System Characteristics 206
   Focal-Spot Size 206
   Filtration 207
   High-Voltage Generation 208
Automatic Exposure Techniques 209
Magnification Radiography 210
Summary 211
Challenge Questions 211

EXPOSURE FACTORS are a few of the tools that radiographers use to create high-quality radiographs. The prime exposure factors are kilovolt peak (kVp), milliampere (mA), exposure time (s), and source-to-image receptor distance (SID).

Properties of the x-ray imaging system that influence the selection of exposure factors are reviewed here, including focal-spot size, x-ray beam filtration, and the source of high-voltage generation.

Image acquisition is the combination of settings selected on the control panel of the x-ray imaging system to produce a high-quality image. The geometry and position of the x-ray tube, the patient, and the image receptor (IR) are included in this description. With digital radiography, image acquisition becomes ever more automatic but also ever more important.

Many areas of x-ray diagnosis require special equipment, which defines the imaging modality, and specialized techniques to obtain the required information. Such equipment and techniques are designed to visualize more clearly a given anatomical structure, usually at the expense of no visualization of other structures.

EXPOSURE FACTORS

Proper exposure of a patient to x-radiation is necessary to produce a diagnostic radiograph. The factors that influence and determine the intensity and energy of x-radiation to which the patient is exposed are called **exposure factors** (Table 14.1).

Recall from Chapter 8 that **radiation quantity** refers to radiation intensity measured in mGy_a or mGy_a/mAs, and **radiation quality** refers to x-ray beam energy and penetrability, best measured by the half-value layer of the x-ray beam. All of these factors are under the control of the radiographer.

The four prime exposure factors are kilovolt peak (kVp), current (mA), exposure time (s), and source-to-image receptor distance (SID). Of these, the most important are kVp and milliampere seconds (mAs), the factors principally responsible for x-ray intensity and energy. Focal-spot size, SID, and filtration are secondary factors that may require manipulation for particular examinations.

Kilovolt Peak

To understand kVp as an exposure technique factor, assume that kVp is the primary control of x-ray beam energy and, therefore, beam penetrability. A higher-energy x-ray beam is one that is more likely to penetrate the anatomy of interest and make it to the IR.

TABLE 14.1 Factors That May Influence X-ray Intensity and Energy

An Increase in	X-ray Intensity	X-ray Energy
Kilovolt peak	Increase	Increase
Milliampere	Increase	No change
Exposure time	Increase	No change
Milliampere seconds	Increase	No change
Distance	Decrease	No change
Voltage ripple	Decrease	Decrease
Filtration	Decrease	Increase

Increasing kVp increases the kinetic energy of the projectile electrons zipping from cathode to anode in the x-ray tube and, therefore, the energy of the bremsstrahlung radiation created when they stop or slow down in the atoms of the target.

> kVp controls x-ray beam energy.

The kVp has more effect than any other factor on IR exposure because it affects x-ray beam energy and, to a lesser degree, influences beam intensity. With increasing kVp, more x-rays are emitted, and they have higher energy and greater penetrability. Unfortunately, because they have higher energy, they also interact more by Compton effect and produce more scatter radiation, which results in reduced image contrast.

The kVp selected helps to determine the number of x-rays in the image-forming beam, and hence the resulting response of the IR. Finally, the kVp influences the scale of contrast on the finished radiograph because as kVp increases, less differential absorption occurs; however postprocessing is the main contrast enhancement factor and kVp is the main patient radiation dose factor.

Milliampere

The mA selected determines the number of electrons that boil off the filament by thermionic emission and, therefore, the number of projectile electrons. The mA is therefore the controlling factor of x-ray intensity.

Recall that the unit of electric current is the ampere (A). One A is equal to 1 coulomb (C) of electrostatic charge flowing each second in a conductor.

> **AMPERE**
> $1 A = 1 C/s = 6.3 \times 10^{18}$ electrons per second

Therefore when the 1000 mA station on the operating console is selected, 6.3×10^{18} electrons flow through the x-ray tube each second.

Question: What is the electron flow from cathode to anode when the 500 mA station is selected?

Answer:
$500 \text{ mA} = 0.5 \text{ A}$
$= (0.5 \text{ A})(6.3 \times 10^{18} \text{ electrons/s/A})$
$= 3.15 \times 10^{18}$ electrons/s

As more electrons flow through the x-ray tube, more x-rays are produced. Assuming a constant exposure time, this relationship is directly proportional. A change from 200 to 400 mA would be a doubling of the x-ray tube current, a doubling of the x-rays produced, and a doubling of the patient radiation dose.

> With a constant exposure time, mA controls the x-ray intensity and, therefore, the patient radiation dose.

Question: At 200 mA, the entrance skin exposure (ESE) is 7.5 mGy_a. What will be the ESE at 500 mA?

Answer: ESE = 7.5 mGy_a (500 mA/200 mA) = 18.75 mGy_a

A change in mA does not change the kinetic energy of electrons flowing from cathode to anode but simply changes the number of electrons. Consequently, the energy of the x-rays produced is not changed; only the number is changed.

> X-ray energy remains fixed with a change in mA.

Often x-ray imaging systems are identified by the maximum x-ray tube current possible. Inexpensive radiographic imaging systems designed for private physicians' offices normally have a maximum x-ray tube current of 600 mA. Interventional radiology imaging systems may have an x-ray tube current of 1500 mA.

Exposure Time

Radiographic exposure times are usually kept as short as possible. The purpose is not to minimize patient radiation dose but, rather, to minimize patient motion blur.

> Short x-ray exposure time reduces patient motion blur.

TABLE 14.2 Relationships Among Different Units of Exposure Time

Fractional (s)	Seconds (s)	Milliseconds (ms)
1.0	1.0	1000
4/5	0.8	800
3/4	0.75	750
2/3	0.67	667
3/5	0.6	600
1/2	0.5	500
2/5	0.4	400
1/3	0.33	333
1/4	0.25	250
1/5	0.2	200
1/10	0.1	100
1/20	0.05	50
1/60	0.017	17
1/120	0.008	8

Producing a diagnostic image requires a certain radiation exposure of the IR. Therefore, to achieve the desired mAs when exposure time is reduced, the mA must be increased proportionately to provide the required x-ray intensity.

On older x-ray imaging systems, exposure time was expressed in fractional seconds. Current x-ray imaging systems identify exposure time in milliseconds (ms). Table 14.2 shows how the different units of time are related.

> mA and x-ray exposure time are inversely proportional: $mA_1/mA_2 = time_2/time_1$.

An easy way to identify an x-ray imaging system as single phase, three phase, or high frequency is to note the shortest exposure time possible. Single-phase imaging systems cannot produce an exposure time less than ½ cycle or its equivalent 8 ms (10 ms on 50-Hz generators). Three-phase and high-frequency generators can normally provide an exposure as short as 1 ms.

The mA and exposure time (in seconds) are usually combined and used as mAs. Indeed, many x-ray consoles do not allow the separate selection of mA and exposure time and permit only mAs selection.

> mAs = milliamperes (mA) × exposure time (s)

Although the radiographer may be required to select an exposure time, it is always selected with consideration of the mA station. The important parameter is the product of the exposure time and x-ray tube current.

> mAs is the controlling factor for x-ray intensity.

The mAs determines the number of x-rays in the primary beam; therefore it principally controls radiation intensity in the same way that mA and exposure time, taken separately, do; it does not influence radiation energy. The mAs setting is a key factor, along with kVp, in the control of IR response.

TABLE 14.3 Product of Milliampere (mA) and Time (ms) for 10 mAs

mA		ms		mAs
100	×	100	=	10
200	×	50	=	10
300	×	33	=	10
400	×	25	=	10
600	×	17	=	10
800	×	12	=	10
1000	×	10	=	10

> **EQUIVALENT EXPOSURES OF EQUAL mAs**
> mAs = mA × Time
> mA (first exposure) × Time (first exposure)
> = mA (second exposure) × Time (second exposure)
> $$\frac{\text{mA (first exposure)}}{\text{mA (second exposure)}} = \frac{\text{Time (second exposure)}}{\text{Time (first exposure)}}$$

If the high-voltage generator is properly calibrated, the same mAs value and, therefore, the same IR response can be produced with various combinations of mA and exposure time (Table 14.3). Owing to the fact that x-ray tube current is calculated as electron flow per unit time, the mAs value is therefore simply a measure of the total number of electrons conducted through the x-ray tube for a particular exposure.

Question: A radiographic technique calls for 600 mA at 200 ms. What is the mAs value?

Answer: 600 mA × 200 ms = 600 mA × 0.2 s
= 120 mAs

> **TOTAL PROJECTILE ELECTRONS**
> mA = mC/s
> therefore
> mAs = mC/s × s = mC

Question: How many electrons are involved in x-ray production at 100 mAs?

Answer: 100 mAs = 0.1 As = 0.1 C/s × s = 0.1 C
1 C = 6.3 × 10^{18} electrons
Therefore 0.1 C = 6.3 × 10^{17} electrons = 100 mAs

Time and mA can be used to compensate for each other in an indirect fashion. This is described by the following:

Question: A radiograph of the abdomen requires 300 mA and 500 ms. The patient is unable to breath-hold, which results in motion blur. Therefore, the exposure is made with a time of 200 ms. Calculate the new mA that is required.

Answer:
$$\frac{x}{300 \text{ mA}} = \frac{500 \text{ ms}}{200 \text{ ms}}$$
(200 ms) x = (500 ms)(300 mA)
(0.2 s) x = (0.5 s)(300 ms)
(0.2 s) x = 150 mAs
$$x = \frac{150 \text{ mAs}}{0.2 \text{ s}} = 750 \text{ mA}$$
or
$$\text{New mA} = \frac{\text{Original mAs}}{\text{New time}}$$
$$\text{New mA} = \frac{0.5 \text{ s} \times 300 \text{ mA}}{0.2 \text{ s}} = 750 \text{ mA}$$

> mAs is one measure of electrostatic charge.

On an x-ray imaging system in which only mAs can be selected, exposure factors are adjusted automatically to the highest mA at the shortest exposure time allowed by the high-voltage generator. Such a design is called a **falling-load generator**.

Question: A radiographer selects a technique of 200 mAs. The operating console is adjusted automatically to the maximum mA station, 1000 mA. What will be the exposure time?

Answer: $\dfrac{200 \text{ mAs}}{1000 \text{ mA}} = 0.2 \text{ s} = 200 \text{ ms}$

Varying the mAs setting changes only the number of electrons conducted during an exposure—not the energy of those electrons. The relationship is directly proportional: Doubling of the mAs doubles the x-ray intensity.

> mAs and x-ray intensity are directly proportional.

Question: A cervical spine examination calls for 68 kVp/30 mAs and results in an ESE of 1.2 mGy$_a$. The next patient is examined at 68 kVp/25 mAs. What will be the ESE?

Answer: ESE = 1.2 mGy$_a$ (25 mAs/30 mAs) = 1.0 mGy$_a$

Distance

Distance affects exposure of the IR according to the inverse square law, which is discussed in Chapter 4. The SID largely determines the intensity of the x-ray beam at the IR.

> Distance has no effect on radiation energy.

The following relationship, called the **square law**, is derived from the inverse square law. It allows a radiographer to calculate the required change in mAs after a change in SID to maintain constant IR response.

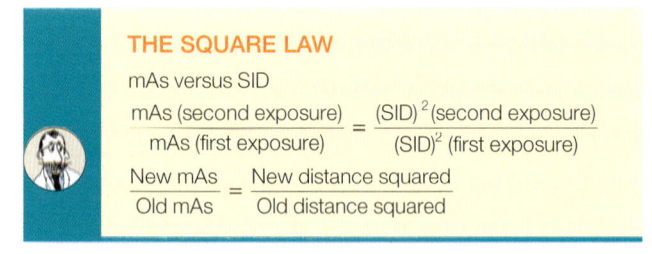

THE SQUARE LAW
mAs versus SID

$$\frac{\text{mAs (second exposure)}}{\text{mAs (first exposure)}} = \frac{(\text{SID})^2 \text{ (second exposure)}}{(\text{SID})^2 \text{ (first exposure)}}$$

$$\frac{\text{New mAs}}{\text{Old mAs}} = \frac{\text{New distance squared}}{\text{Old distance squared}}$$

Note that both the original mAs value and the original SID are in the denominator rather than reversed, as in the inverse square law.

Question: An examination requires 100 mAs at 180-cm SID. If the distance is changed to 90-cm SID, what should be the new mAs setting?

Answer:
$$\frac{x}{100} = \frac{90^2}{180^2}$$
$$x = 100\left(\frac{90}{180}\right)^2 = 100\left(\frac{1}{2}\right)^2$$
$$= 100\left(\frac{1}{4}\right) = 25 \text{ mAs}$$

When preparing to make a radiographic exposure, the radiographer selects specific settings for each of the factors described: kVp, mAs, and SID. The control panel selections are based on an evaluation of the patient, the thickness of the anatomical part, and the type of accessories used.

> Source-to-image receptor distance (SID) affects IR response according to the Square Law.

Standard SIDs have been in use for many years. For tabletop radiography, 100 cm is common, but dedicated chest examination is usually conducted at 180 cm. Tabletop radiography at 120 cm and chest radiography at 300 cm are often used.

The use of a longer SID results in less magnification, less focal-spot blur, and improved spatial resolution; however more mAs must be used because of the effects of the square law.

IMAGING SYSTEM CHARACTERISTICS
Focal-Spot Size

Most x-ray tubes are equipped with two focal-spot sizes. On the operating console, these are usually identified as small and large, 0.5 mm/1.0 mm, 0.6 mm/1.2 mm, or 1.0 mm/2.0 mm. X-ray tubes used in interventional radiology procedures or magnification radiography may have 0.3-mm/1.0-mm focal spots.

Mammography x-ray tubes have 0.1-mm/0.3-mm focal spots. These are called **microfocus tubes** and are designed specifically for imaging very small microcalcifications at relatively short SIDs.

For general imaging, the large focal spot is used. This ensures that sufficient mAs can be used to image thick or dense body parts. Owing to the fact that higher mA can be used, the large focal spot also provides for a shorter exposure time, which minimizes patient motion blur.

One difference between large and small focal spots is the capacity to produce x-rays. Many more x-rays can be produced with the large focal spot because anode heat capacity is higher. With the small focal spot, electron interaction occurs over a much smaller area of the anode, and the resulting heat limits the capacity of x-ray production.

> Changing the focal spot for a given kVp/mAs setting does not change the x-ray intensity or energy.

A small focal spot is reserved for fine-detail radiography, in which the quantity of x-rays is relatively low. Small focal spots are always used for magnification radiography. Additionally these are normally used during extremity radiography and in examination of other thin body parts in which higher x-ray intensity is not necessary.

Filtration

Three types of x-ray filtration are used: inherent, added, and compensating. All x-ray beams are affected by the **inherent filtration** properties of the glass or metal envelope of the x-ray tube. For general-purpose tubes, the value of inherent filtration is approximately 0.5-mm Al equivalent.

The variable-aperture light-localizing collimator usually provides an additional 1.0-mm Al equivalent. Most of this is attributable to the reflective surface of the mirror of the collimator. To meet the required total filtration of 2.5-mm Al, an additional 1-mm Al filter is inserted between the x-ray tube housing and the collimator. The radiographer has no control over these sources of filtration but may control stages of added filtration.

Some x-ray imaging systems have selectable **added filtration**, as shown in Fig. 14.1. Usually, the imaging system is placed into service with the lowest allowable added filtration. Radiographic technique charts are usually formulated at the lowest filtration position. If a higher filter position is used, a radiographic technique chart must be developed at that position.

Fig. 14.2 shows multiple layers of different filtration materials designed for specialty examinations and patient radiation dose reduction. The two sets of collimator blades are open, showing the filters and the light field mirror.

Under normal conditions, it is unnecessary to change the filtration. Some facilities may be set for higher filtration during examinations of pediatric patients or of tissue with high subject contrast, such as the extremities, joints, and chest. When properly used, higher filtration for these examinations results in lower patient radiation dose. When added filtration is changed, be sure to return it to its normal position before beginning the next examination.

Compensating filters are shapes of aluminum mounted onto a transparent panel that slides in grooves beneath the collimator. These filters balance the intensity of the x-ray beam so as to deliver a more uniform

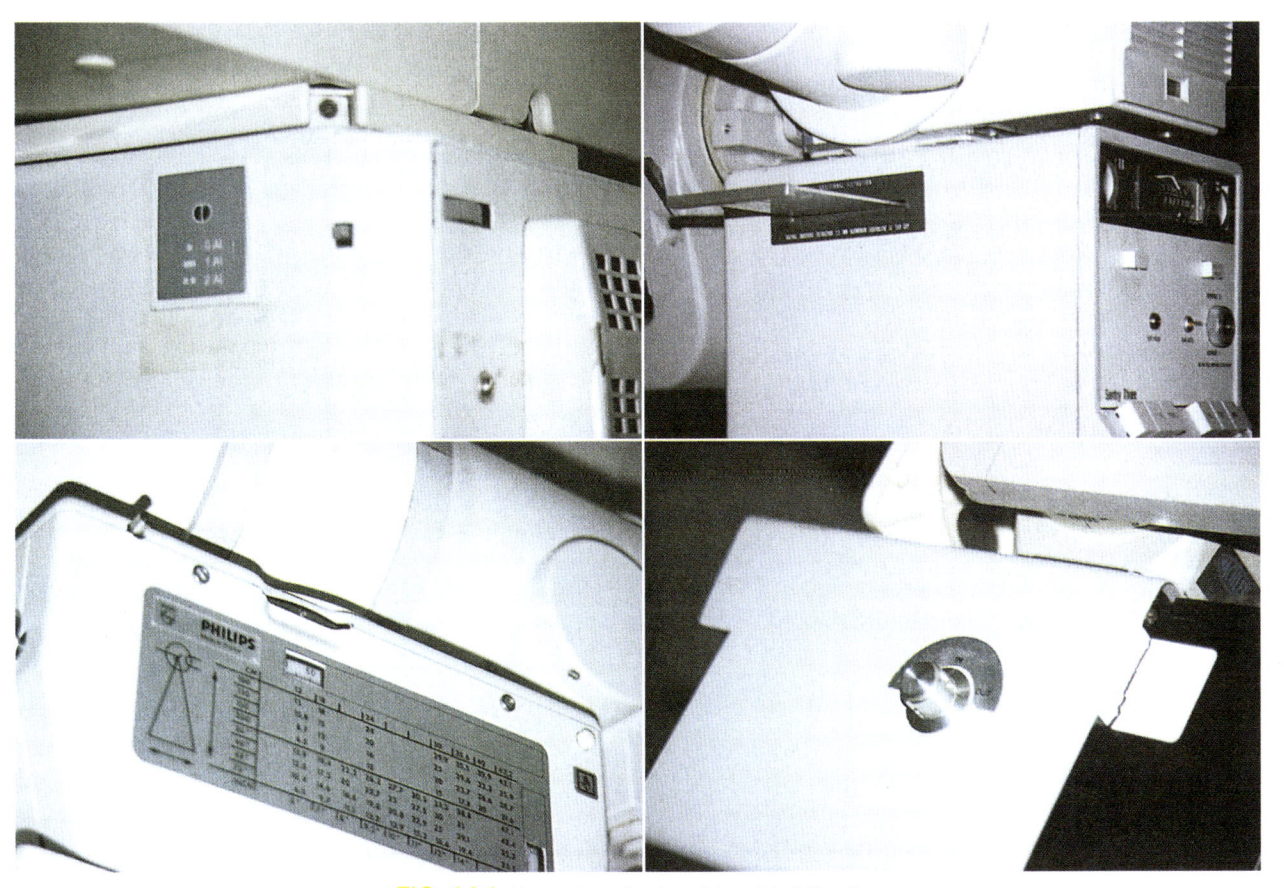

FIG. 14.1 Examples of selectable added filtration.

exposure to the IR. For example, they may be shaped like a wedge for examination of the spine or like a trough for chest examination.

As added filtration is increased, the result is increased x-ray beam energy and penetrability. The result on the image is the same as that for increased kVp; namely more scatter radiation and reduced image contrast.

High-Voltage Generation

The radiographer cannot select the type of high-voltage generator to be used for a given examination; that choice is fixed by the type of x-ray imaging system used. Still, it is important to understand how the various high-voltage generators affect radiographic technique and patient radiation dose.

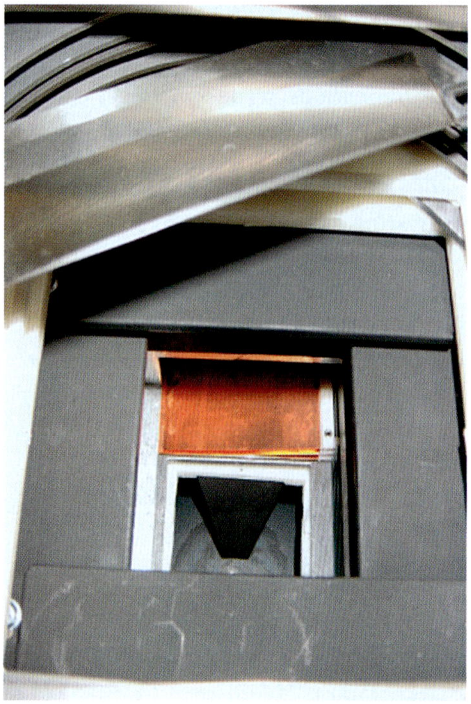

FIG. 14.2 An open collimator showing the light field mirror and multiple layers of filtration. (Courtesy General Electric Medical Systems.)

Three basic types of high-voltage generators are available: single phase, three phase, and high frequency. The radiation intensity and energy produced in the x-ray tube are influenced by the type of high-voltage generator used.

Review Fig. 6.29 for the shape of the voltage waveform associated with each type of high-voltage generator. Voltage ripple is expressed as a percentage and is equal to the peak tube voltage during a voltage waveform minus the minimum voltage/peak voltage × 100. Table 14.4 lists the percentage ripple of various types of high-voltage generators, the variation in their output, and the change in radiographic technique used for two common examinations associated with each generator.

> % voltage ripple = (peak voltage − minimum voltage)/peak voltage × 100

A half-wave–rectified generator has 100% voltage ripple. During exposure with a half-wave–rectified generator, x-rays are produced and emitted only half the time. During each negative half-cycle, no x-rays are emitted.

> Half-wave rectification results in the same radiation energy that is produced by full-wave rectification, but the radiation intensity is halved.

Half-wave rectification is used rarely today. Some mobile and dental x-ray imaging systems are half-wave rectified.

The voltage waveform for **full-wave rectification** is identical to that for half-wave rectification, except there is no dead time. During exposure, x-rays are emitted continually as pulses. Consequently, the required exposure time for full-wave rectification is only half that for half-wave rectification.

TABLE 14.4 Characteristics of the Various Types of High-Voltage Generators

Generator Type	Percentage Ripple	Relative Intensity	Chest	Abdomen
Half wave	100	100	120/20[a]	74/40[a]
Full wave	100	200	2/3	74/40
3 phase, 6 pulse	14	260	115/6	72/34
3 phase, 12 pulse	4	280	115/4	72/30
High frequency	<1	300	112/3	70/24

EQUIVALENT TECHNIQUE (KVP/MAS)

[a]The mAs value equals that for a full-wave generator; exposure time is doubled.
kVp, Kilovolt peak; mAs, milliampere seconds.

> Radiation energy does not change when going from half-wave to full-wave rectification; however, radiation intensity doubles.

Three-phase power comes in two principal forms: 6 or 12 pulse. The difference is determined by the manner in which the high-voltage step-up transformer is engineered.

> Three-phase power results in higher x-ray intensity and energy.

The difference between the two forms is minor but does cause a detectable change in x-ray intensity and energy. Three-phase power is more efficient than single-phase power. More x-rays are produced for a given mAs setting, and the average energy of those x-rays is higher. The x-radiation emitted is nearly constant rather than pulsed. The voltage ripple is 14% for 3-phase, 6-pulse power and 4% for 3-phase, 12-pulse power.

High-frequency generators were developed in the 1980s and are now regularly used. The voltage waveform is nearly constant, with less than 1% ripple.

> High-frequency generation results in even greater x-ray intensity and energy.

At present, high-frequency generators are used increasingly with dedicated mammography systems, computed tomography (CT) systems, and mobile x-ray imaging systems. Most high-voltage generators are now of the high-frequency type, regardless of the required power levels.

AUTOMATIC EXPOSURE TECHNIQUES

The appearance of the operating console of x-ray imaging systems is changing in response to the ability to incorporate artificial intelligence (AI) technology (see Chapter 28). Several automated exposure techniques are now available, but none relieves the radiographer of the responsibility of identifying particular characteristics of the patient and the anatomical part to be imaged.

Automatic exposure systems use an electronic exposure timer, such as those described in Chapter 6. Radiation intensity is measured with a solid-state detector or an ionization chamber, and the x-ray exposure is terminated when the proper radiation exposure to the IR has been reached. The principles associated with automatic exposure systems have already been described, but the importance of using radiographic exposure charts with these systems has not.

> Automatic exposure control (AEC) x-ray systems are not completely automatic but require proper operation by the radiographer.

It is incorrect to assume that because the radiographer does not have to select kVp and mA settings and time for each examination, a less qualified or less skilled operator can use the system. Usually the radiographer must use a guide for the selection of kVp that is similar to that used in the fixed-kVp method. Exposure compensation selections are scaled numerically to allow for "tweaking" the calibration of the sensors for changes in field size or anatomy, or the presence of pathology or orthopedic devices that require exposure adjustment.

> Patient positioning must be accurate because the specific body part must be placed over the AEC detector to ensure proper exposure.

The factors shown in Table 14.5 must be considered when one is preparing the radiographic exposure chart for an automatic x-ray system. The kVp is selected according to the specific anatomical part that is being examined.

Radiation exposure in most x-ray imaging systems is determined by an **automatic exposure control** (AEC) system. AEC incorporates a device that senses the amount of radiation incident on the IR. To image with the use of an AEC, the radiographer selects the appropriate kVp, mA, and backup time, as well as the proper sensors. Through an electronic feedback circuit, x-ray exposure is terminated when a sufficient number of x-rays has reached the IR.

With AEC devices, usually two or more exposure sensors are available for control (Fig. 14.3). For

TABLE 14.5 Factors to Consider When Constructing an Exposure Chart for Automatic Systems

Factor for Selection	Rationale for Selection
Kilovolt peak	To select for each anatomical part
Image receptor response	To fine-tune for differences in field size or anatomical part
Collimation	To reduce patient radiation dose and ensure proper response of automatic exposure control
Accessory selection	To optimize the radiation dose–image quality ratio

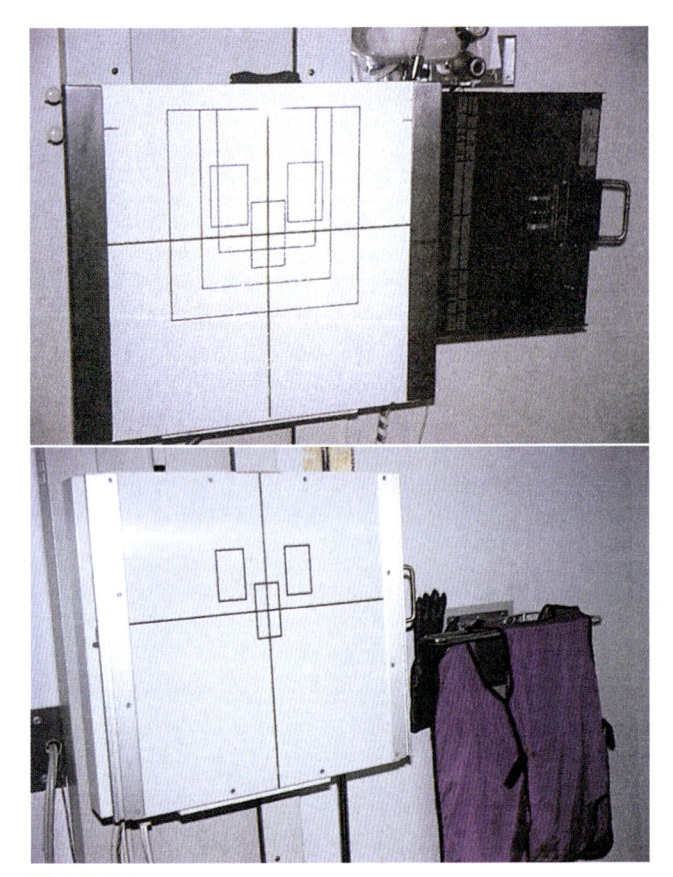

FIG. 14.3 Vertical chest Bucky shows the position of automatic exposure control sensors represented as three rectangles.

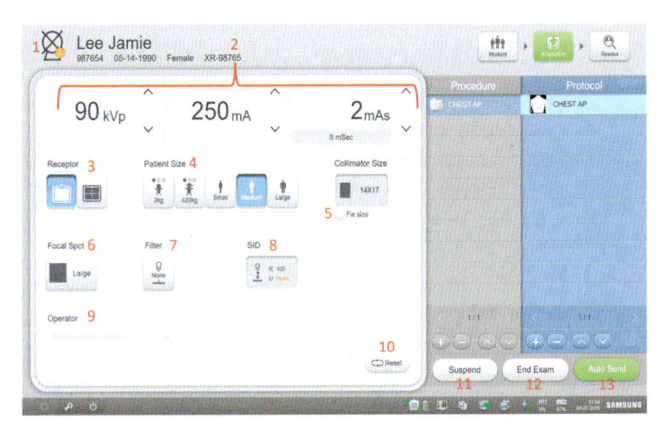

FIG. 14.4 Anatomically programmed radiography operating console. Technique exposure control for patient size, body part, and position is automatically selected. (Courtesy Holly Evans McDaniels, Shimadzu Medical Systems.)

instance, three radiation-sensing cells may be available, and the radiographer is responsible for selecting which of the sensors should be used for the examination. During an anteroposterior (AP) thoracic chest examination with the spine of interest, only the middle sensing cell is used. During a posteroanterior (PA) chest examination with the lung fields of principal importance, the two outer cells are activated.

Regulations require that AECs have a 600-mAs safety override. If the AEC fails to terminate the exposure, the secondary safety circuit terminates it at 600 mAs, which is equivalent to a few seconds, depending on the mA.

In addition to selecting exposure cells, the radiographer usually has a three- to seven-position exposure compensation dial with numeric steps. Each step on the dial is calibrated to increase or decrease the accepted exposure to the IR by 25% to 50%.

Microprocessors are incorporated into operating consoles. A microprocessor allows the operator to select digitally any kVp or mAs setting; the microprocessor automatically activates the appropriate mA station and exposure time. With falling-load generators, the microprocessor begins the exposure at a maximum mA setting and then causes the tube current to be reduced during exposure. The overall objective is to minimize exposure time to reduce patient motion blur.

A widely used electronic technique for patient radiation exposure control is referred to as **anatomically programmed radiography** (**APR**). APR also uses microprocessor technology. Rather than the radiographer selecting a desired kVp and mAs, graphics on the console or on a video touchscreen guide the technologist (Fig. 14.4).

To produce an image, the radiographer simply touches an icon or a written description of the anatomical part to be imaged and the body habitus. The microprocessor selects the appropriate kVp and mAs settings automatically. The whole process uses AEC, resulting in high-quality radiographs and fewer repeats; however precise patient positioning relative to the AEC sensor is still critical for producing high-quality radiographs.

The principle of APR is similar to that of AEC, with the radiographic technique chart stored in the microprocessor of the control unit. The service engineer loads the controlling programs during installation and calibrates the exposure control circuit for the general conditions of the facility.

The radiographer needs only to select the part and its relative size before each exposure. The programmed instructions, however, must be continuously adjusted by the radiographer until the entire panel of examinations is optimized for best image quality. The radiographer has the ability to manually override the APR.

MAGNIFICATION RADIOGRAPHY

Magnification radiography is a technique that is used principally during interventional radiology and mammography. The visualization of small structures is enhanced by magnification radiography. Magnification radiography deliberately increases the OID.

To obtain a magnified radiograph, the OID is increased while the SID is held constant (Fig. 14.5). The degree of magnification is given by the **magnification factor** (**MF**) as follows.

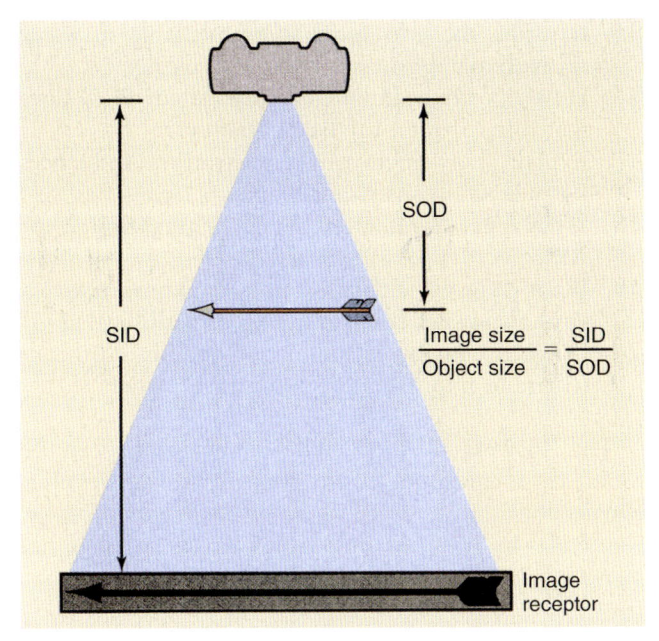

FIG. 14.5 Principle of magnification radiography. The magnification factor is equal to the ratio of image size to object size. *SID*, Source-to-image receptor distance; *SOD*, source-to-object distance.

> **MAGNIFICATION FACTOR**
>
> $$MF = \frac{SID}{SOD} = \frac{\text{Image size}}{\text{Object size}}$$
>
> where SID is the source-to-image receptor distance and SOD is the source-to-object distance.

Question: A magnified radiograph of the sella turcica is taken at 100-cm SID, with the object positioned 25 cm from the IR. If the image of the sella turcica measures 16 mm, what is its actual size?

Answer:
$$MF = \frac{100}{(100 - 25)} = 1.33$$

$$\frac{\text{Image size}}{\text{Object size}} = MF$$

$$\text{Object size} = \frac{\text{Image size}}{MF} = \frac{16}{1.33} = 12.0 \text{ mm}$$

A small focal spot must be used for magnification radiography to help reduce any loss of spatial resolution. The focal-spot blur that results from an unnecessarily large focal spot can destroy the diagnostic value of the magnified radiograph.

Usually grids are not required for magnified radiography. The large OID results in a significant air gap so that much of the scatter radiation misses the IR. With larger OID, less scatter radiation reaches the IR.

The principal disadvantage of magnification radiography, similar to so many specialized techniques, is increased patient radiation dose. To obtain an MF of 2, one must position the patient halfway between the x-ray tube and the IR. Recall that radiation intensity is related to the square of the distance, which suggests a fourfold increase in patient radiation dose.

In reality, most magnification radiographs result in only a modest increase in patient radiation dose. Owing to the fact that grids are not used during magnification radiography, there is no Bucky factor (see Chapter 15) and the associated increase in patient radiation dose.

SUMMARY

Radiographic exposure factors (kVp, mAs, and SID) are manipulated by radiographers to produce high-quality radiographs. Exposure factors influence radiographic intensity and energy. Proper selection of exposure factors optimizes the spatial resolution and the contrast resolution of the image.

Radiographic technique is the combination of factors used to expose an anatomical part to produce a high-quality radiograph. Radiographic technique is characterized by: (1) patient factors, (2) image-quality factors, and (3) exposure technique factors.

Magnification radiography is a technique that is used mainly for interventional radiography and mammography.

CHALLENGE QUESTIONS

1. Define or otherwise identify the following:
    a. Kilovolt peak (kVp)
    b. Milliampere second (mAs)
    c. Beam penetrability
    d. Exposure factors
    e. Source-to-image receptor distance (SID)
    f. Inherent filtration
    g. Anatomically programmed radiography (APR)
    h. Automatic exposure control (AEC)
    i. Compensating filter
2. Discuss how an increase in kVp changes x-ray intensity, x-ray energy, and image contrast.
3. What happens to the AEC response when an improperly collimated x-ray beam is incident on a specific area shield?
4. What is normally the shortest radiographic exposure time on single-phase, three-phase, and high-frequency imaging systems?
5. Describe how a change in SID from 100 cm to 180 cm should be accompanied by a change in mA and exposure time.
6. Why does an x-ray tube have two focal-spot sizes?

7. A radiographic technique calls for 82 kVp at 400 mA, 200 ms, and a SID of 90 cm. What is the mAs?
8. Discuss the components of total x-ray beam filtration.
9. A radiographic technique calls for 800 mA at 50 ms. What is the mAs setting?
10. The normal lateral chest technique is 120 kVp, 100 mA, 15 ms. To reduce motion blur, the radiographer shortens the exposure time to 5 ms. What is the new mA?
11. Explain the following statement: Changing the mA does not change the kinetic energy of electrons flowing across the x-ray tube.
12. Why is it important to keep exposure time as short as possible?
13. How does distance from the source affect x-ray intensity and x-ray energy?
14. An examination requires 78 kVp/150 mAs at 100-cm SID. If the distance is changed to 180 cm, what should the new mAs setting be?
15. Describe the two focal spots available in x-ray tubes. Explain how each is used typically.
16. How is x-ray beam intensity measured? How does that differ from x-ray beam quantity?
17. Explain how high-voltage generation influences x-ray beam intensity and energy.
18. What types of radiation detectors are required for AEC?
19. What is the principal advantage of exposure with a large focal spot compared with a small focal spot?
20. Do both x-ray beam collimation and filtration contribute to improved image contrast? How?

The answers to the Challenge Questions can be found by logging on to our website at http://evolve.elsevier.com.

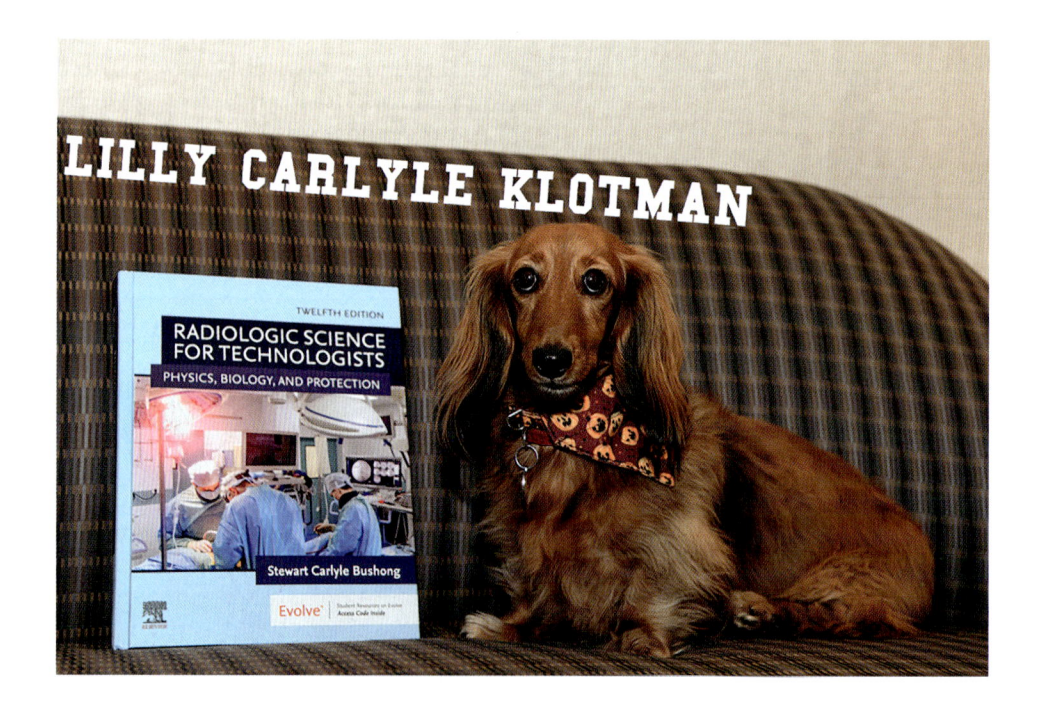

Scatter Radiation

CHAPTER 15

OBJECTIVES

At the completion of this chapter, the student should be able to do the following:

1. Identify the x-rays that constitute image-forming radiation.
2. Recognize the relationship between scatter radiation and image contrast.
3. List three factors that contribute to scatter radiation.
4. Discuss three devices developed to minimize scatter radiation.
5. Describe beam restriction and its effect on patient radiation dose and image quality.
6. Describe grid construction and its measures of performance.
7. Evaluate the use of various grids in relation to patient radiation dose.

OUTLINE

Production of Scatter Radiation 214
    kVp 214
    Field Size 215
    Patient Thickness 216
Control of Scatter Radiation 216
    Effect of Scatter Radiation on Image Contrast 216
    Beam Restrictors 218
Radiographic Grids 221
    Contrast Improvement Factor 222
    Bucky Factor 223
Grid Types 223
    Parallel Grid 223
    Crossed Grid 225
    Focused Grid 225
    Moving Grid 225
    Virtual Grid 226
Grid Problems 226
    Off-Level Grid 227
    Off-Center Grid 227
    Off-Focus Grid 228
    Upside-Down Grid 228
Grid Selection 228
    Patient Radiation Dose 229
    Air-Gap Technique 230
Summary 231
Challenge Questions 231

THE TWO PRINCIPAL characteristics of any medical image are **spatial resolution** and **contrast resolution**. Some refer to these together as image detail or visibility of detail. In fact, these qualities are quite distinct and are influenced by different links of the imaging chain.

Spatial resolution is determined principally by pixel size. Focal-spot size and geometric factors contribute to image blur, but pixel size limits spatial resolution. Contrast resolution is affected by scatter radiation, but dynamic range and postprocessing allow for much enhanced contrast resolution. Two principal tools are used to control scatter radiation—beam-restricting devices and radiographic grids.

Image contrast and contrast resolution are important characteristics of image quality. Contrast arises from the areas of light, dark, and shades of gray on the medical image. Contrast resolution is the ability to image adjacent similar tissues. Compton scatter x-radiation produces image noise, reducing image contrast. It makes the image less visible.

Three factors contribute to increased scatter radiation: increased kVp, increased x-ray field size, and increased patient thickness. X-ray beam-restricting devices, **collimators**, are designed to control and minimize scatter radiation by limiting the x-ray field size to only the anatomy of interest. The three principal types of beam-restricting devices are aperture diaphragm, cones or cylinders, and collimators. By removing scattered x-rays from the remnant beam, the radiographic grid removes a major source of image noise, thus improving image contrast.

PRODUCTION OF SCATTER RADIATION

Two types of x-rays are responsible for the radiographic image: those that pass through the patient without interacting and those that are Compton scattered within the patient. X-rays that exit from the patient are **remnant x-rays** and those that exit and interact with the image receptor are called **image-forming x-rays** (Fig. 15.1).

Proper collimation of the x-ray beam reduces patient radiation dose by restricting the volume of irradiated tissue. Proper collimation also improves image contrast. Ideally, only those x-rays that do not interact with the patient should reach the IR.

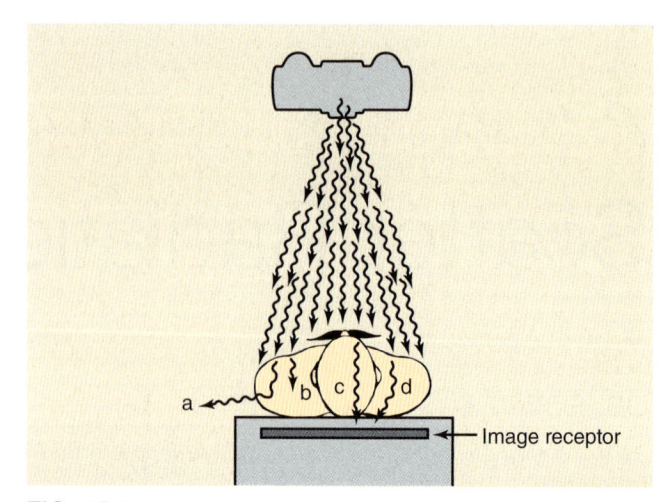

FIG. 15.1 Some x-rays interact with the patient and are scattered away from the image receptor (IR) (*a*). Others interact with the patient and are absorbed (*b*). X-rays that arrive at the IR are those transmitted through the patient without interacting (*c*) and those scattered in the patient (*d*). X-rays of types c and d are called image-forming x-rays.

> Collimation reduces patient radiation dose and improves image contrast.

As scatter radiation increases, the radiographic image loses contrast and appears more gray. Three primary factors influence the relative intensity of the scatter radiation that reaches the IR: kVp, field size, and patient thickness.

kVp

As x-ray energy increases, the absolute number of Compton interactions decreases, but the number of photoelectric interactions decreases much more rapidly. Therefore the relative number of x-rays that undergo Compton scattering increases.

Table 15.1 shows the percentage of x-rays incident on a 10-cm thickness of soft tissue that will undergo photoelectric absorption and Compton scattering at selected kVp levels. Kilovoltage, which is one of the factors that affect the level of scatter radiation, can be controlled by the radiographer.

It would be easy enough to say that all radiographs should be taken at the lowest reasonable kVp because this technique would result in minimum scatter and thus better image contrast. Unfortunately, it is not that simple.

Fig. 15.2 shows the relative contributions of photoelectric effect and Compton scatter to the radiographic image. The increase in photoelectric absorption results in a considerable increase in patient radiation dose.

| TABLE 15.1 | Percent Interaction of X-rays by Photoelectric and Compton Processes and Percent Transmission Through 10 cm of Soft Tissue |

	PERCENT INTERACTION			
kVp	Photoelectric	Compton	Total	Percent Transmission
50	79	21	>99	<1
60	70	30	>99	<1
70	60	40	>99	<1
80	46	52	98	2
90	38	59	97	3
100	31	63	94	6
110	23	70	93	7
120	18	83	91	9

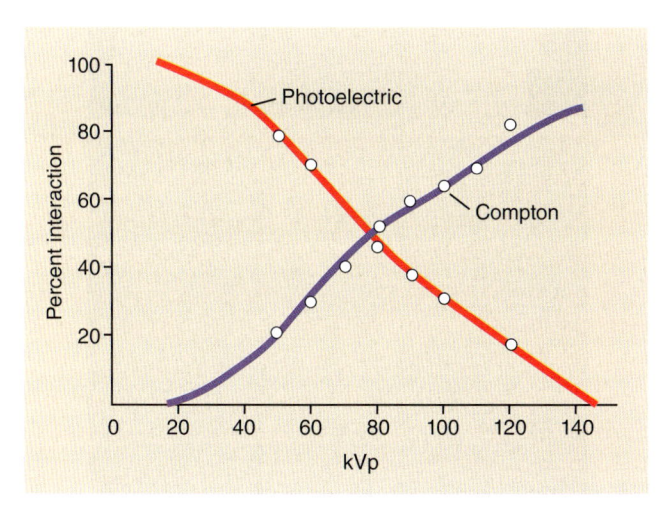

FIG. 15.2 The relative contributions of photoelectric effect and Compton scattering to the radiographic image.

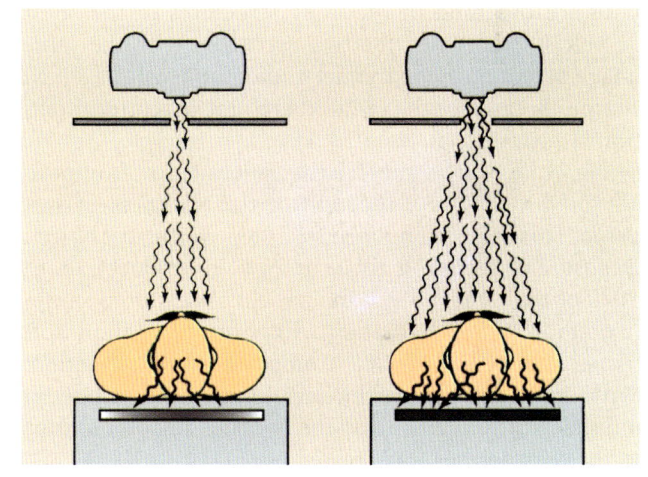

FIG. 15.3 Collimation of the x-ray beam results in less scatter radiation, reduced patient radiation dose, and improved image contrast.

Also fewer x-rays reach the image receptor at low kVp—a phenomenon that is usually compensated for by increasing the mAs. This also results in a higher patient radiation dose.

> Approximately 1% of x-rays incident on the patient reach the image receptor.

With large patients, kVp must be high to ensure adequate penetration of the portion of the body that is being imaged. If, for example, the normal technique factors for an anteroposterior (AP) examination of the abdomen are inadequate, the radiographer has the choice of increasing mAs or kVp.

Increasing the mAs usually generates enough x-rays to provide a satisfactory image but may result in an unacceptably high patient radiation dose. On the other hand, a much smaller increase in kVp is usually sufficient to provide enough x-rays, and this can be done at a much lower patient radiation dose. Unfortunately when kVp is increased, the level of scatter radiation also increases. This leads to reduced image contrast. Collimators and grids are used to reduce the level of scatter radiation.

> Fortunately with digital medical imaging, image contrast is restored using postprocessing.

Field Size

Another controllable factor that affects the level of scatter radiation is x-ray beam field size. As field size is increased, scatter radiation also increases (Fig. 15.3).

> Scatter radiation increases as the x-ray beam field size increases.

Fig. 15.4 shows two AP views of the lumbar spine obtained on a 35 × 43 cm image receptor. Fig. 15.4A, was taken full field, uncollimated; in Fig. 15.4B, the field size is collimated to the spinal column. Image contrast is noticeably poorer in the full-field radiograph because of the increased scatter radiation that accompanies larger x-ray field size.

With postprocessing, the lost contrast is restored at no increase in patient radiation dose. Compared with a full-field size, radiographic exposure factors may have to be increased to maintain the same signal intensity at the image receptor when the exposure is made with a smaller field size.

Patient Thickness

Imaging thick parts of the body results in more scatter radiation than does imaging thin body parts. Compare a radiograph of the bony structures in an extremity with a radiograph of the bony structures of the chest or pelvis. Even when the two are taken with the same image receptor, the extremity radiograph will be much sharper because of the reduced amount of scatter radiation (Fig. 15.5).

Fig. 15.6 shows the relative intensity of Compton scattered x-rays as a function of the thickness of soft tissue. This can be simulated by a step-wedge test object. Exposure of 5-cm soft tissue at 70 kVp produces about 50% of the x-rays to exit the patient as scattered x-rays (Compton scatter radiation). Exposure of 15-cm soft tissue causes nearly 90% Compton scatter radiation. With increasing patient thickness, more x-rays undergo multiple scattering, so that the average angle of scatter in the remnant beam is greater.

Patient thickness is not normally controlled by the radiographer. Recognizing that more x-rays are scattered with increasing patient thickness, you can improve image quality by using devices such as a compression paddle (Fig. 15.7).

> Compression of anatomy improves image contrast and lowers the patient radiation dose.

Compression devices improve image contrast by reducing patient thickness and bringing the anatomy closer to the IR. Compression also reduces patient radiation dose. Compression is particularly important during mammography.

CONTROL OF SCATTER RADIATION

Effect of Scatter Radiation on Image Contrast

One of the most important characteristics of image quality is **image contrast**, the visible difference between the light and dark areas on an image. Image contrast is

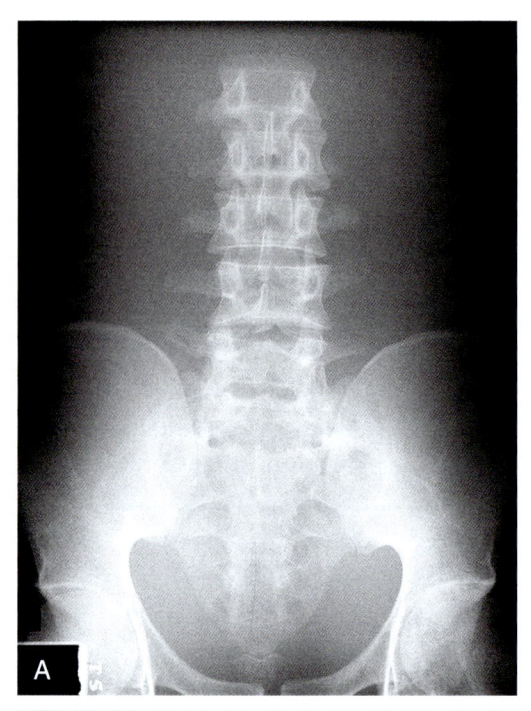

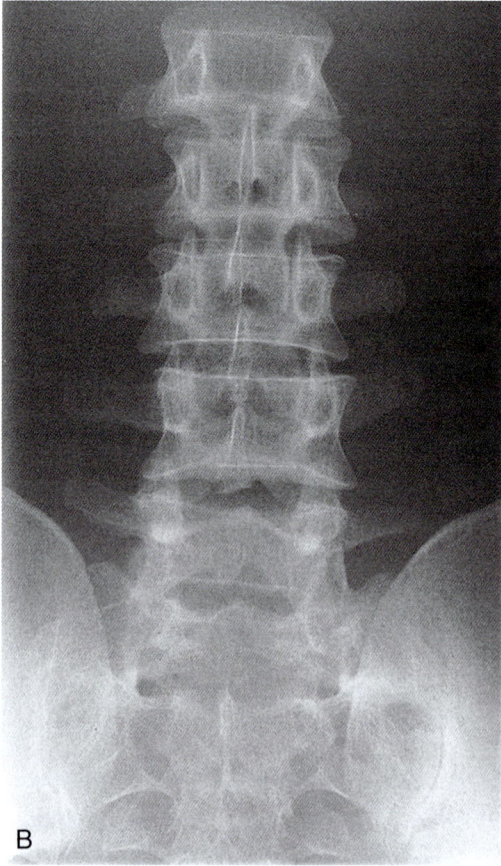

FIG. 15.4 The recommended technique for lumbar spine radiography calls for collimation of the beam to the vertebral column. The full-field technique results in reduced image contrast. (A) Full-field technique. (B) Preferred collimated technique. (Courtesy Mike Enriquez, Merced Community College.)

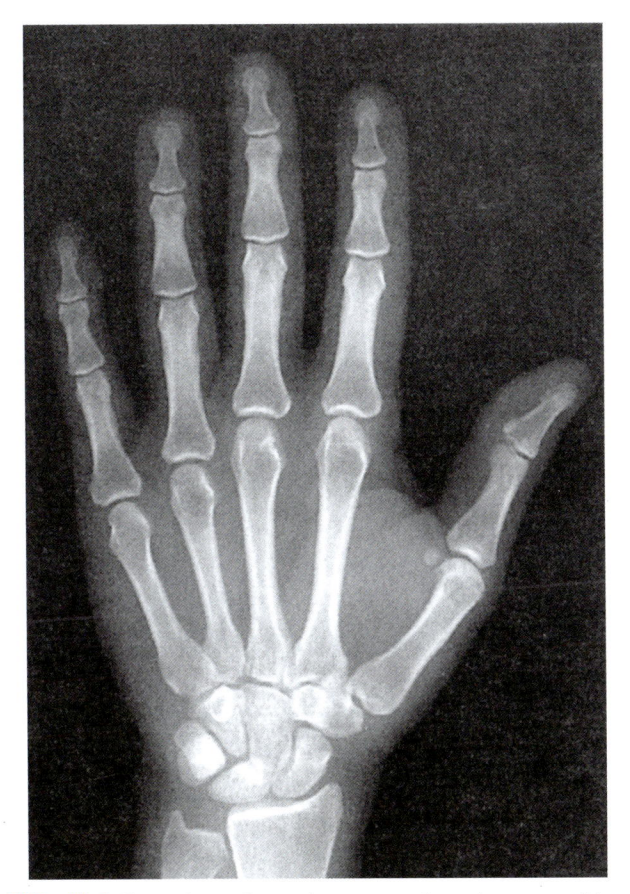

FIG. 15.5 Extremity radiographs appear sharp because of less tissue and, hence, less scatter radiation. Posteroanterior view of the hand. (Courtesy Rees Stuteville, Oregon Institute of Technology.)

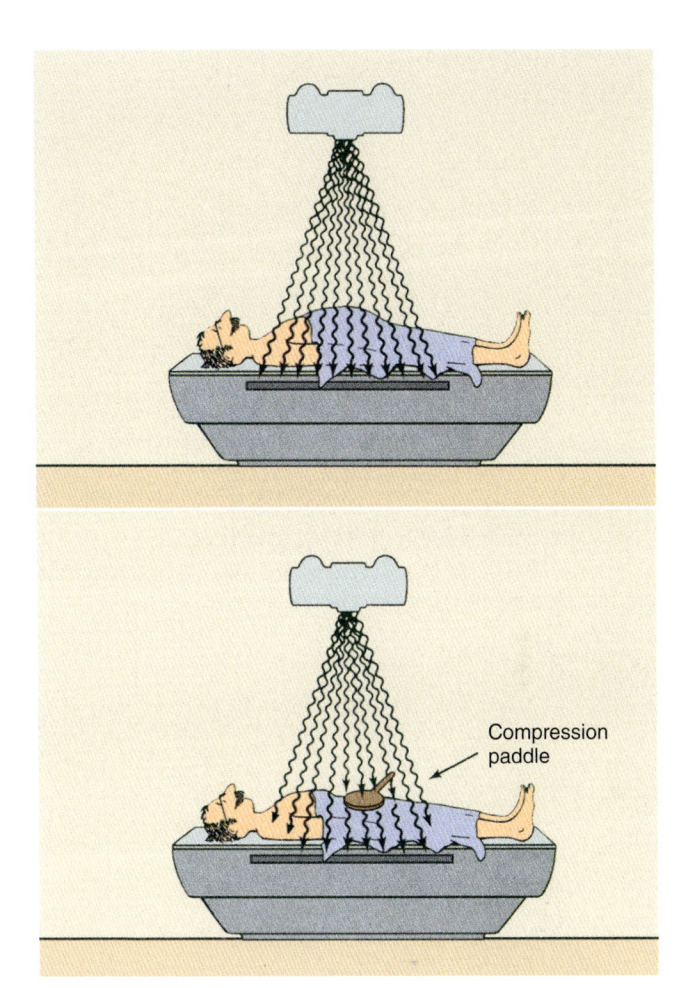

FIG. 15.7 When tissue is compressed, scatter radiation is reduced, resulting in a lower patient radiation dose and improved image contrast.

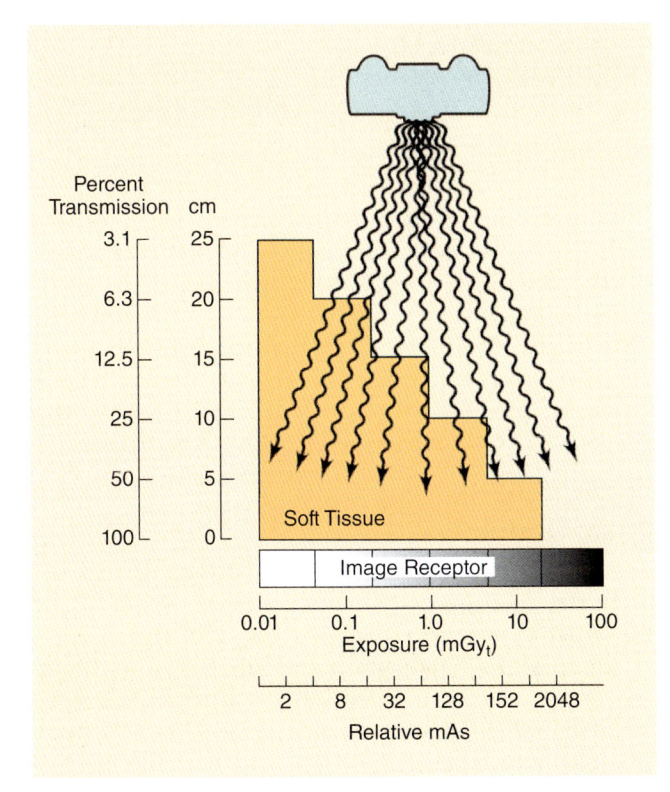

FIG. 15.6 Relative intensity of scatter radiation increases with increasing thickness of a soft tissue step wedge.

the visual degree of difference in signal intensity among soft tissue areas of an image. **Contrast resolution** is the ability of an imaging modality to image and distinguish adjacent soft tissues.

Even under the most favorable conditions, most **remnant x-rays** are scattered. Fig. 15.8 illustrates that scattered x-rays are emitted in all directions from the patient.

If you could image a long bone in cross section using only transmitted, unscattered x-rays, the image would be very sharp (Fig. 15.9A). The change in IR signal corresponding to the bone-soft tissue interface would be very abrupt. Therefore image contrast would be high.

> Reduced image contrast results from Compton scattered x-rays.

On the other hand, if the radiograph were taken with only scatter radiation and no transmitted x-rays reached the IR, the image would be dull gray (see Fig. 15.9B). The radiographic contrast would be very low.

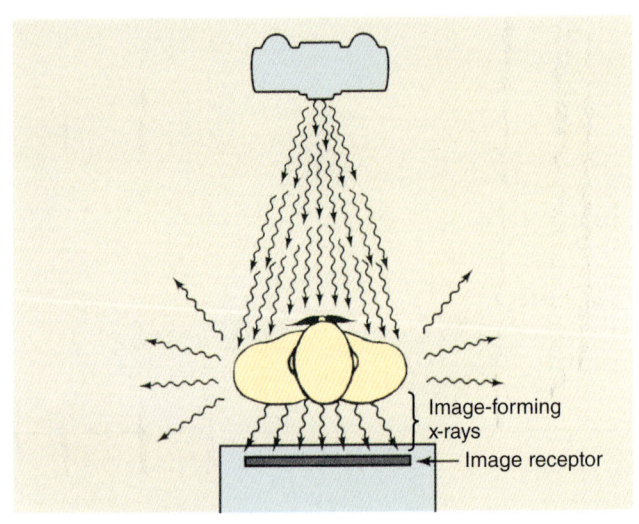

FIG. 15.8 When primary x-rays interact with the patient, x-rays are scattered from the patient in all directions.

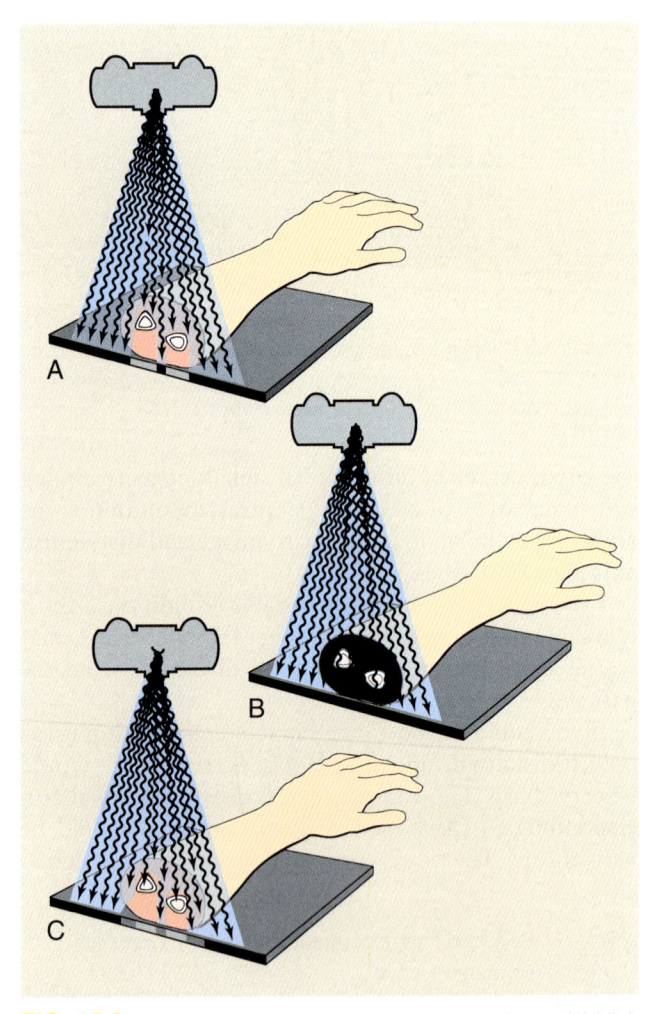

FIG. 15.9 Radiographs of a cross section of long bone. (A) High contrast would result from the use of only transmitted, unattenuated x-rays. (B) No contrast would result from the use of only scattered x-rays. (C) Moderate contrast results from the use of both transmitted and scattered x-rays.

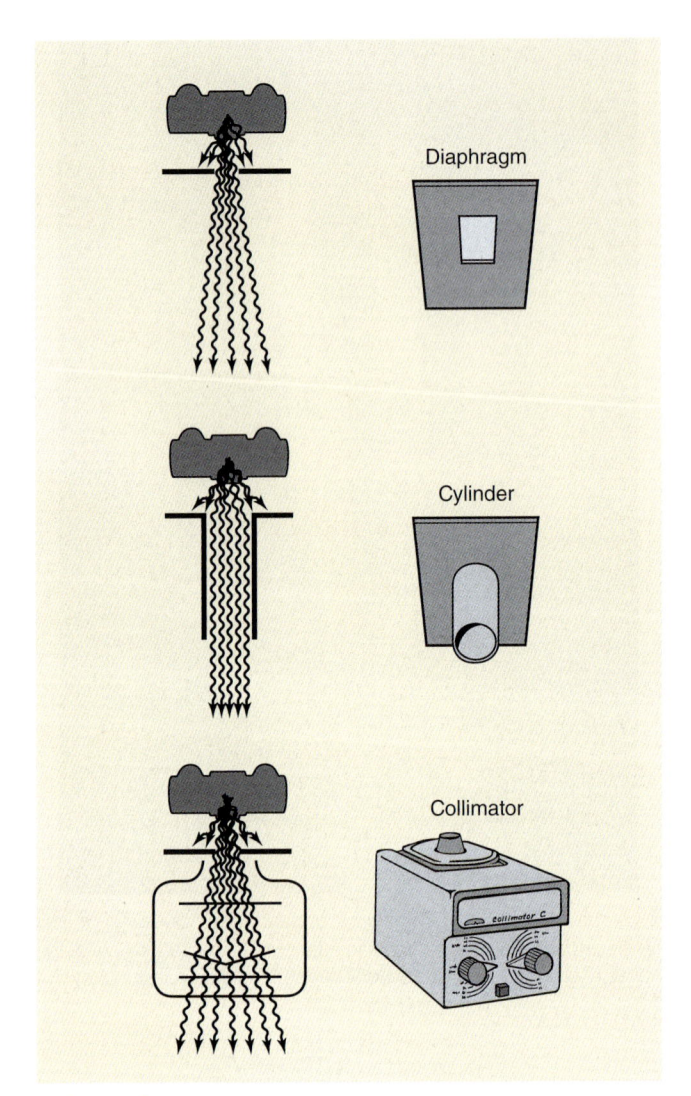

FIG. 15.10 Three types of beam-restricting devices.

In the normal situation, however, image-forming x-rays consist of both transmitted and scattered x-rays. If the radiograph were properly exposed, the image in cross-sectional view would appear as in Fig. 15.9C. This image would have moderate contrast. The loss of contrast results from the presence of scattered x-rays.

Digital image dynamic range coupled with image postprocessing can restore essentially all necessary contrast, resulting in a quality image with high contrast.

Beam Restrictors

Basically three types of beam-restricting devices are used: the aperture diaphragm, cones or cylinders, and the variable-aperture collimator (Fig. 15.10).

An **aperture diaphragm** is the simplest of all beam-restricting devices. It is basically a lead or lead-lined metal diaphragm that is attached to the x-ray tube head. The opening in the diaphragm usually is designed to cover slightly less than the size of the image receptor

CHAPTER 15 Scatter Radiation

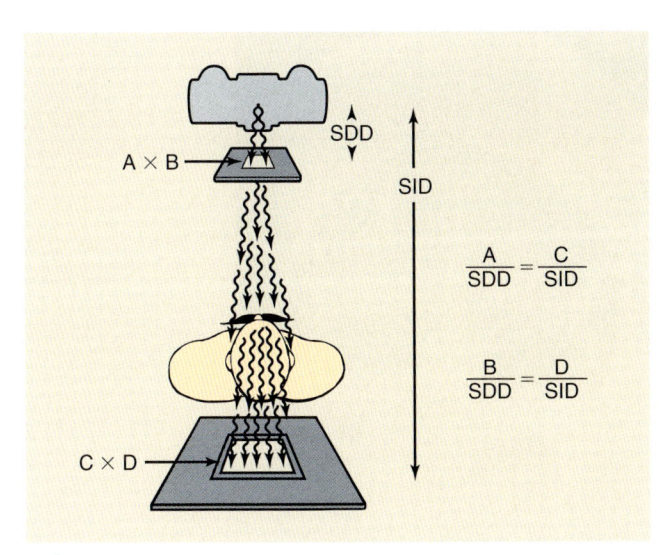

FIG. 15.11 Aperture diaphragm is a fixed lead opening designed for a fixed IR size and constant source-to-image receptor distance (SID). *SDD*, Source-to-diaphragm distance.

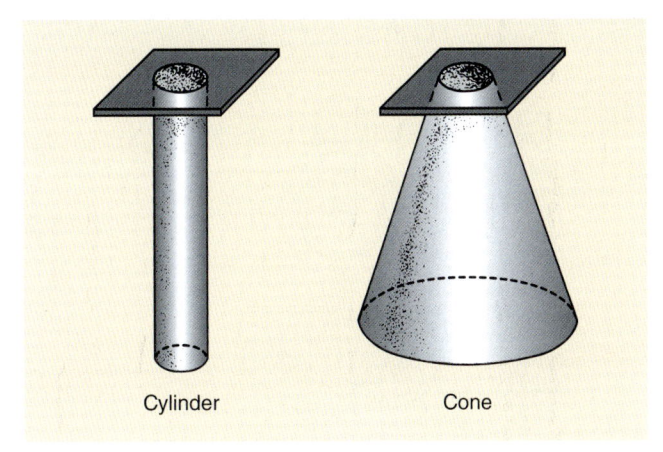

$$\frac{A}{SDD} = \frac{C}{SID}$$

$$\frac{B}{SDD} = \frac{D}{SID}$$

FIG. 15.12 Radiographic cones and cylinders produce restricted useful x-ray beams of circular shape.

used. Fig. 15.11 shows how the x-ray tube, the aperture diaphragm, and the IR are related.

X-ray imaging systems dedicated specifically for chest radiography can be supplied with fixed-aperture diaphragms. Such aperture diaphragms for chest radiography are designed to expose all of a 35- × 43-cm image receptor except for a 1-cm border.

Radiographic extension **cones** and **cylinders** are considered modifications of the aperture diaphragm. Fig. 15.12 shows a diagram of a typical extension cone and cylinder. In both, an extended metal structure restricts the useful beam to the required size. The position and size of the distal end act as an aperture and determine the field size.

In contrast to the x-ray beam produced by an aperture diaphragm, the useful beam produced by an extension cone or cylinder is usually circular. Both of these beam restrictors are routinely referred to as cones, even though the most commonly used type is actually a cylinder.

One difficulty with using cones is alignment. If the x-ray source, cone, and IR are not aligned on the same axis, one side of the radiograph may not be exposed because the edge of the cone may interfere with the x-ray beam. Such interference is called **cone cutting**.

At one time, cones were used extensively in radiographic imaging. Today they are reserved primarily for examinations of selected areas (Fig. 15.13), such as examination of the frontal sinuses. Cones are also routinely used in dental radiography.

The light-localizing **variable-aperture collimator** is the most commonly used beam-restricting device in radiography. Fig. 15.14 shows an example of a modern automatic variable-aperture collimator. Fig. 15.15 identifies the principal parts of such a collimator.

> Collimation reduces the patient radiation dose and improves image contrast.

Not all x-rays are emitted precisely from the focal spot of the x-ray tube. Some x-rays are produced when projectile electrons stray and interact at positions on the anode other than the focal spot. Such radiation, which is called **off-focus radiation**, reduces image contrast and spatial resolution.

To control off-focus radiation, a first-stage entrance collimator that has multiple blades protrudes from the top of the collimator into the x-ray tube housing.

The leaves of the second-stage collimator are usually made of lead that is at least 3-mm thick. They work in pairs and are independently controlled, thereby allowing for both rectangular and square x-ray beams.

In a typical variable-aperture collimator, light localization is accomplished with a small lamp and mirror. The mirror must be far enough on the x-ray tube side of the collimator leaves to project a sufficiently sharp light pattern through the collimator leaves when the lamp is on.

The collimator lamp and the mirror must be adjusted so that the projected light field coincides with the x-ray beam. If the light field and the x-ray beam do not coincide, the lamp or the mirror must be adjusted. Such coincidence checking is a necessary part of any quality control program.

Light-localizing collimators are called **positive-beam–limiting (PBL)** devices. Positive beam limitation was mandated by the US Food and Drug Administration in 1974. That regulation was removed in 1994, but PBL continues to prevail.

When a computed radiography or digital radiography IR is inserted into the Bucky tray and is clamped into place, sensing devices in the tray identify the size

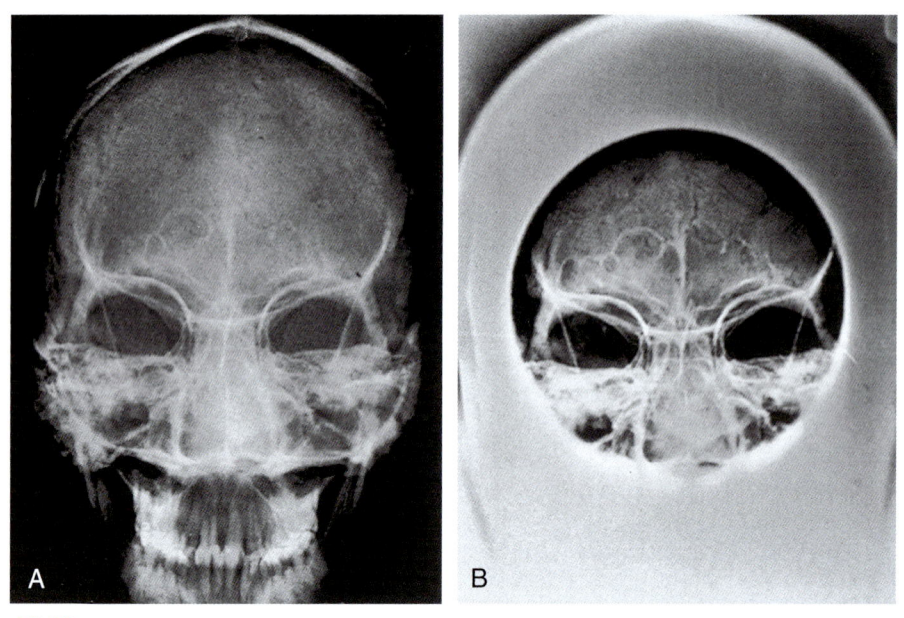

FIG. 15.13 Radiographs of the frontal and maxillary sinuses without a cone (A) and with a cone (B). Cones reduce scatter radiation and improve contrast resolution. (Courtesy Lynne Davis, Houston Community College.)

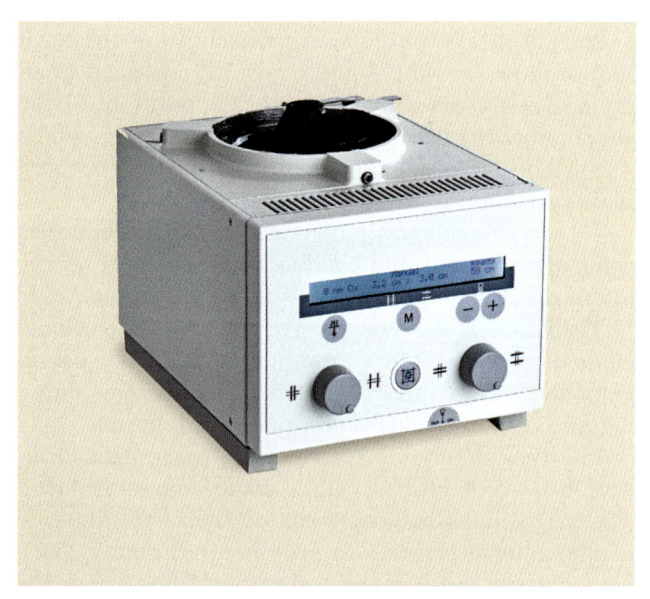

FIG. 15.14 Automatic variable-aperture x-ray beam collimator. (Courtesy Siemens Medical Solutions USA, Inc.)

and alignment of the IR. A signal is transmitted to the collimator housing. This actuates the synchronous motors that drive the collimator leaves to a precalibrated position, so the x-ray beam is restricted based on the IR in use.

Even with PBL, the radiographer should manually collimate more tightly to reduce patient radiation dose and improve image quality when appropriate.

> Under no circumstances should the x-ray beam exceed the size of the IR.

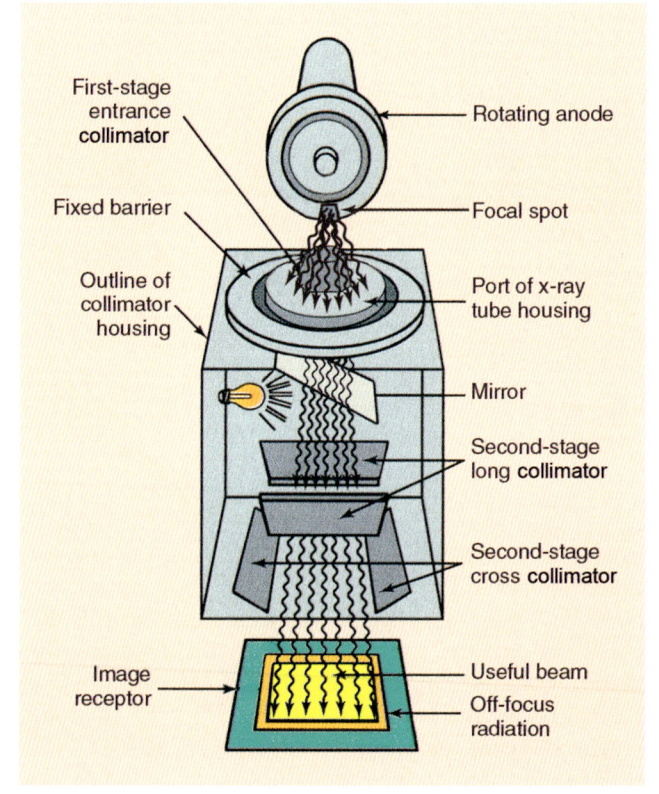

FIG. 15.15 Simplified schematic of a variable-aperture light-localizing collimator.

Depending on the x-ray tube potential, additional **collimator filtration** may be necessary to produce high-quality radiographs with minimum patient radiation dose. Some collimator housings are designed to allow easy changing of the added filtration. Filtration stations of 0-, 1-, 2-, and 3-mm Al are the most common.

Even in the zero position, however, the added filtration to the x-ray tube is not zero because collimator structures intercept the beam. In addition to the inherent filtration of the tube, the exit port (usually plastic) and the reflecting mirror provide filtration. The added filtration of the collimator assembly is equivalent to approximately 1-mm Al.

> Total filtration = Inherent filtration + Added filtration

RADIOGRAPHIC GRIDS

Scattered x-rays that reach the IR are part of the image-forming process. Indeed, the x-rays that are scattered forward do contribute to the image. An extremely effective device for reducing the level of scatter radiation that reaches the IR is the **radiographic grid**.

The grid is a carefully fabricated section of radiopaque material (**grid strip**) alternating with radiolucent material (**interspace material**). The grid is positioned between the patient and the IR.

This technique for reducing the amount of scatter radiation that reaches the IR was first demonstrated in 1913 by Gustave Bucky. Over the years, Bucky's grid has been improved by more precise manufacturing, but the basic principle has not changed.

The grid is designed to transmit only x-rays whose direction is on a straight line from the x-ray tube target to the image receptor. Scatter radiation is absorbed in the grid material. Fig. 15.16 is a schematic representation of how a grid removes scatter radiation from the image-forming x-ray beam.

X-rays that exit the patient and strike the radiopaque grid strips are absorbed and do not reach the IR. For instance, a typical grid may have grid strips 50-μm wide that are separated by interspace material 350 μm wide.

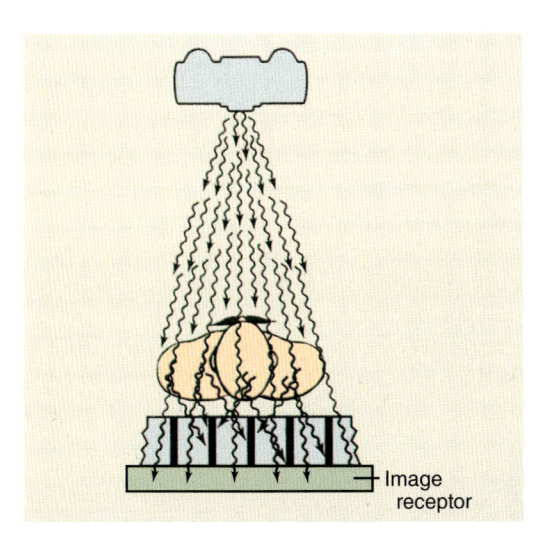

FIG. 15.16 The only x-rays transmitted through a grid are those that travel in the direction of the interspace. X-rays scattered obliquely through the interspace are absorbed.

Question: A grid is constructed with 50-μm strips and a 350-μm interspace. What percentage of x-rays incident on the grid will be absorbed by its entrance surface?

Answer: $$\frac{50\ \mu m}{50\ \mu m + 350\ \mu m} = 0.125 = 12.5\%$$

Primary beam x-rays incident on the interspace material are transmitted to the IR. Scattered x-rays incident on the interspace material may or may not be absorbed, depending on their angle of incidence and the physical characteristics of the grid. Regardless, the postpatient absorption of x-rays results in higher patient radiation dose when a grid is used.

If the angle of a scattered x-ray is great enough to cause it to intersect a lead grid strip, it will be absorbed. If the angle is slight, the scattered x-ray will be transmitted to the IR. Laboratory measurements show that high-quality grids can attenuate 80% to 90% of the scatter radiation. Such a grid is said to exhibit good "clean-up."

Question: When viewed from the top, a particular grid shows a series of lead strips 40-μm wide separated by interspaces 300-μm wide. How much of the radiation incident on this grid should be absorbed?

Answer: If 300 + 40 represents the total surface area and 40 represents the surface area of absorbing material, then the percentage absorption is as follows:
$$\frac{40\ \mu m}{340\ \mu m} = 0.118 = 11.8\%$$

A grid has three important dimensions: the thickness of the grid strip (T), the width of the interspace material (D), and the height of the grid (h). The **grid ratio** is the height of the grid divided by the interspace width (Fig. 15.17).

> Grid ratio = h/D

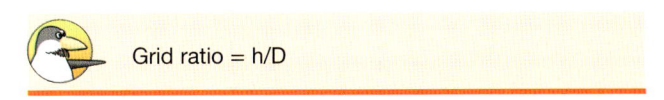

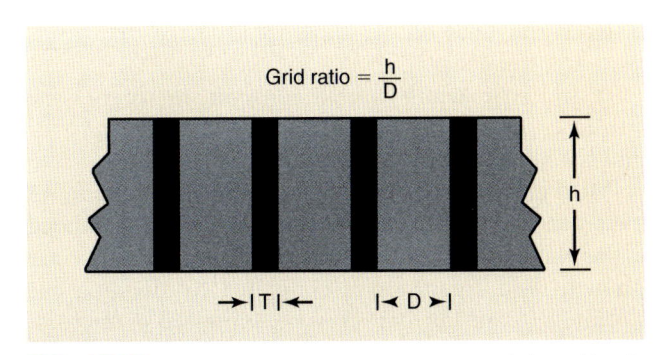

FIG. 15.17 Grid ratio is defined as the height of the grid strip (h) divided by the thickness of the interspace material (D). T is the width of the grid strip.

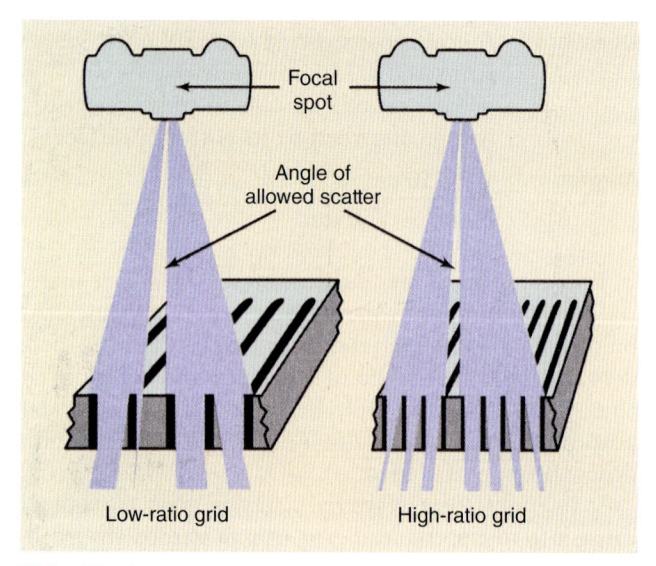

FIG. 15.18 High-ratio grids are more effective in reducing scattered x-rays than low-ratio grids because the angle of allowed scatter is smaller.

High-ratio grids are more effective in reducing scatter radiation than are low-ratio grids. This is because the angle of scatter allowed by high-ratio grids is less than that permitted by low-ratio grids (Fig. 15.18).

In general, grid ratios range from 5:1 to 16:1; higher-ratio grids are used most often in high-kVp radiography. An 8:1 or 10:1 grid is frequently used with general-purpose x-ray imaging systems. Whereas a 5:1 grid reduces approximately 85% of the scatter radiation, a 16:1 grid may reduce as much as 97%.

Question: A grid is fabricated of 30-μm lead grid strips sandwiched between interspace material that is 300-μm thick. The height of the grid is 2.4 mm. What is the grid ratio?

Answer: Grid ratio $= \dfrac{h}{D} = \dfrac{2400 \; \mu m}{300 \; \mu m} = 8:1$

The number of grid strips per centimeter is called the **grid frequency**. Grids with high frequency show less distinct grid lines on a radiographic image than grids with low frequency.

If grid strip width is held constant, the higher the frequency of a grid, the thinner its interspace must be and the higher the grid ratio will be.

Most grids have frequencies in the range of 25 to 45 lines per centimeter. Grid frequency can be calculated if the widths of the grid strip and of the interspace are known. Grid frequency is computed by dividing the thickness of one line pair (T + D), expressed in micrometers, into 1 cm. Note that 1 cm must be converted to 10,000 μm for consistency of units.

$$\text{Grid frequency} = \dfrac{10{,}000 \; \mu m/cm}{(T + D) \; \mu m/\text{line pair}}$$

Question: What is the grid frequency of a grid that has a grid strip width of 30 μm and an interspace width of 300 μm?

Answer: If one line pair = 300 μm + 30 μm = 330 μm, how many line pairs are in 10,000 μm (10,000 μm = 1 cm)?

$$\dfrac{10{,}000 \; \mu m/cm}{330 \; \mu m/\text{line pair}} = 30.3 \; \text{lines/cm}$$

Specially designed grids are used for mammography. Usually a 4:1 or a 5:1 ratio grid is used. These low-ratio grids have grid frequencies of approximately 80 lines/cm.

The purpose of the interspace material is to maintain a precise separation between the delicate lead strips of the grid. The interspace material of most grids consists of **aluminum** or **plastic fiber**. There are conflicting reports as to which is better.

Perhaps the largest single factor responsible for poor radiographic image quality is scatter radiation. By removing scattered x-rays from the remnant beam, the radiographic grid removes this source of reduced contrast.

The principal function of a grid is to improve image contrast.

Contrast Improvement Factor

The characteristics grid ratio and grid frequency are usually specified when a grid is identified. However they do not quantify the ability of the grid to improve image contrast. This property of the grid is specified by the **contrast improvement factor** (**k**). A contrast improvement factor of 1 indicates no improvement.

Most grids have contrast improvement factors of between 1.5 and 2.5. In other words, the image contrast is approximately doubled when a grid is used. Mathematically, the contrast improvement factor, k, is expressed as follows:

$$\text{Contrast improvement factor} = \dfrac{\text{Image contrast with a grid}}{\text{Image contrast without a grid}}$$

Question: An aluminum step wedge is placed on a tissue phantom that is 20 cm thick and a radiograph is made. Without a grid, analysis of the radiograph shows a 1.1% contrast. With a 12:1 grid, radiographic contrast is 2.8%. What is the contrast improvement factor of this grid?

Answer: $k = \dfrac{2.8}{1.1} = 2.55$

The contrast improvement factor k is usually measured at 100 kVp. However, k is a complex function of the x-ray emission spectrum, patient thickness, and the tissue irradiated.

> The contrast improvement factor is higher for high-ratio grids.

Bucky Factor

Although the use of a grid improves image contrast, a penalty is paid in the form of increased patient radiation dose. The quantity of image-forming x-rays transmitted through a grid is much less than that of image-forming x-rays incident on the grid. Therefore, when a grid is used, the radiographic technique must be increased to produce the same IR signal. The amount of this increase is given by the **Bucky factor (B)**.

> Bucky factor = $\dfrac{\text{Incident remnant x-rays}}{\text{Transmitted image - forming x-rays}}$
>
> = $\dfrac{\text{Patient radiation dose with grid}}{\text{Patient radiation dose without grid}}$

The Bucky factor is an attempt to measure the penetration of primary and scatter radiation through the grid. Table 15.2 gives representative values of the Bucky factor for several popular grids.

TABLE 15.2 Approximate Bucky Factor Values for Popular Grids

Grid Ratio	70 kVp	90 kVp	120 kVp	Average
No grid	1	1	1	1
5:1	2	2.5	3	2
8:1	3	3.5	4	4
12:1	3.5	4	5	5
16:1	4	5	6	6

BUCKY FACTOR AT

Two generalizations can be made from the data presented in Table 15.2:

1. **The higher the grid ratio, the higher the Bucky factor.** The penetration of primary radiation through a grid is fairly independent of grid ratio. Penetration of scatter radiation through a grid becomes less likely with increasing grid ratio; therefore, the Bucky factor increases.
2. **The Bucky factor increases with increasing kVp.** At higher voltages, more scatter radiation is produced. This scatter radiation has a more difficult time penetrating the grid; thus the Bucky factor increases.

> As the Bucky factor increases, radiographic technique and patient radiation dose increase proportionately.

Whereas the contrast improvement factor measures improvement in image quality when grids are used, the Bucky factor measures how much of an increase in technique will be required compared with nongrid exposure. The Bucky factor also indicates how large an increase in patient radiation dose will accompany the use of a particular grid.

GRID TYPES

Parallel Grid

The simplest type of radiographic grid is the parallel grid, which is diagrammed in Fig. 15.19. In the parallel grid, all lead grid strips are parallel. This type of grid is the easiest to manufacture, but it has some properties

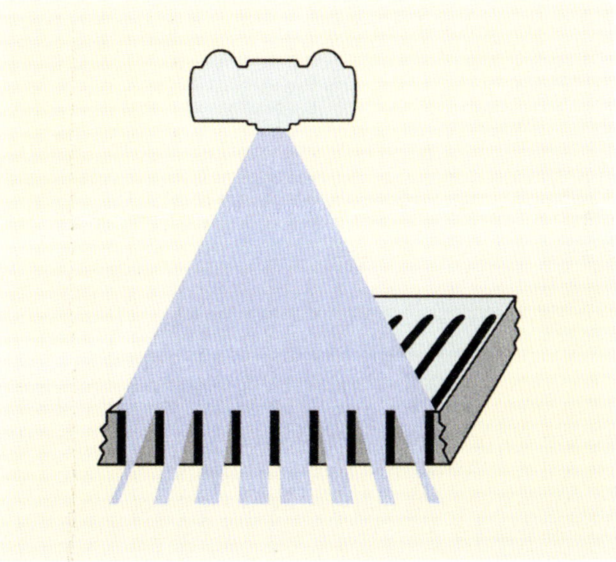

FIG. 15.19 A parallel grid is constructed with parallel grid strips. At a short source-to-image receptor distance, some grid cutoff may occur.

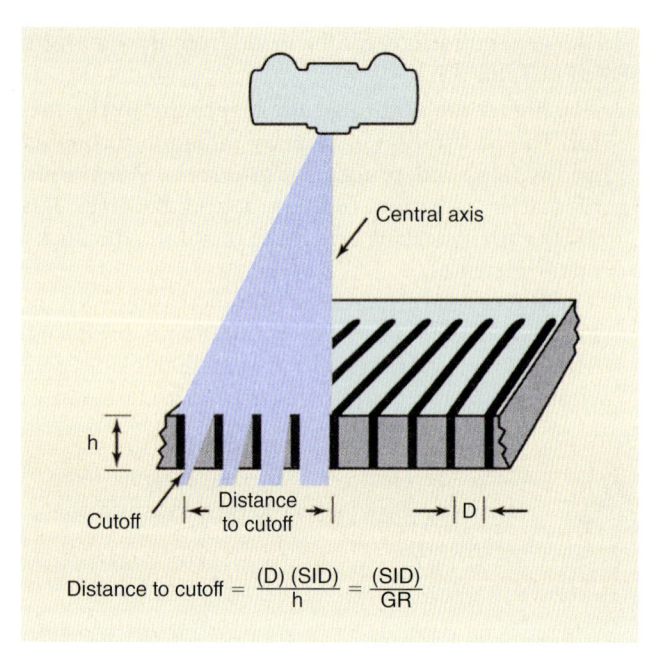

FIG. 15.20 With a parallel grid, image receptor (IR) signal decreases toward the edge of the IR. The distance to grid cutoff is the source-to-image receptor distance (*SID*) divided by the grid ratio (*GR*).

that are clinically undesirable, namely **grid cutoff**, the undesirable absorption of primary x-rays by the grid.

The attenuation of primary x-rays becomes greater as the x-rays approach the edge of the image receptor. The lead strips in a 35- × 43-cm grid are 43 cm long. Across the 35-cm dimension, the signal intensity reaches a maximum along the center line of the IR and decreases toward the sides.

Grid cutoff can be partial or complete. The term is derived from the fact that the primary x-rays are "cutoff" from reaching the IR. Grid cutoff can occur with any type of grid if the grid is improperly positioned, it is most common with parallel grids.

This characteristic of parallel grids is most pronounced when the grid is used at a short SID or with a large-area IR. Fig. 15.20 shows the geometric relationship for attenuation of primary x-rays by a parallel grid.

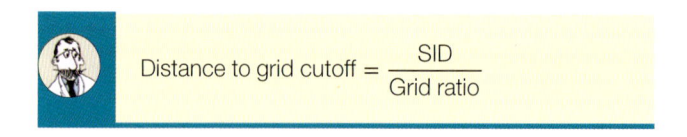

$$\text{Distance to grid cutoff} = \frac{\text{SID}}{\text{Grid ratio}}$$

In theory, a 10:1 grid used at 100-cm SID should absorb all primary x-rays farther than 10 cm from the central ray. When this grid is used with a 35- × 43-cm IR, the IR should only record a signal over a 20- × 43-cm area.

The radiographs in Fig. 15.21A and B were taken with a 6:1 parallel grid at 76- and 61-cm SID, respectively.

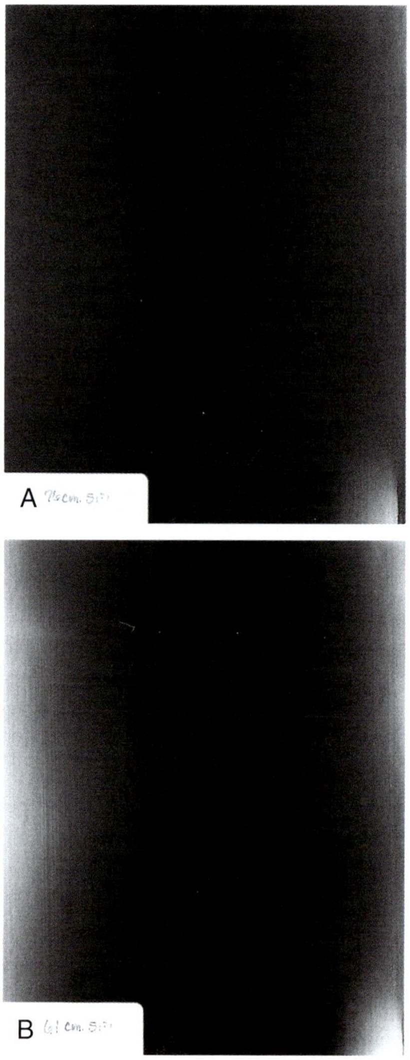

FIG. 15.21 (A) Radiograph taken with a 6:1 parallel grid at an source-to-image receptor distance (*SID*) of 76 cm. (B) Radiograph taken with a 6:1 parallel grid at an SID of 61 cm. lar signal intensity decreases from the center to the edge of the image and to complete cutoff. (Courtesy Dawn Stark, Mississippi State University.)

They show increasing degrees of grid cutoff with decreasing SID.

Question: A 16:1 parallel grid is positioned for chest radiography at 180-cm SID. What is the distance from the central axis to complete grid cutoff? Will the image satisfactorily cover a 35- × 43-cm IR?

Answer: Distance to cutoff = $\frac{180}{16}$ = 11.3 cm

Distance to edge of IR

35 ÷ 2 = 17.5 cm

No! Grid cutoff will occur on the lateral 6.2 cm (17.5−11.3) of the IR.

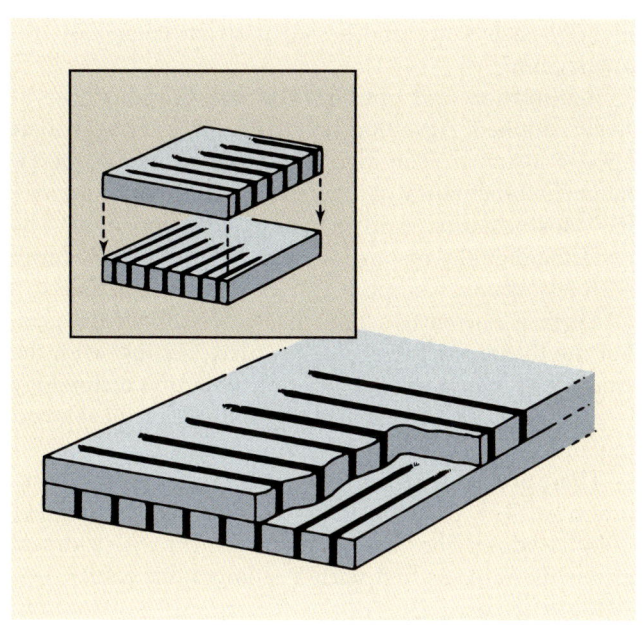

FIG. 15.22 Crossed grids are fabricated by sandwiching two parallel grids together so their grid strips are perpendicular.

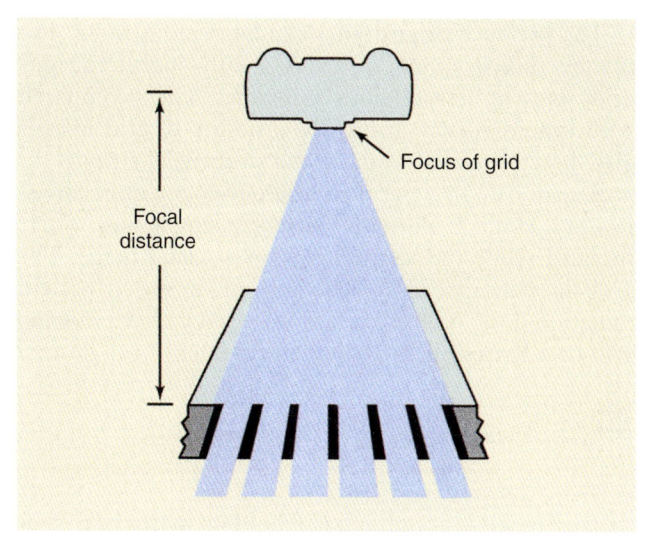

FIG. 15.23 A focused grid is fabricated so that grid strips are parallel to the primary x-ray path across the entire IR.

Crossed Grid

Parallel grids clean up scatter radiation in only one direction, along, the axis of the grid. Crossed grids are designed to overcome this deficiency. Crossed grids have lead grid strips that run parallel to the long and short axes of the grid (Fig. 15.22). They are usually fabricated by sandwiching two parallel grids together with their grid strips perpendicular to one another. A crossed grid identified as having a grid ratio of 6:1 is constructed with two 6:1 parallel grids.

They are not difficult to manufacture and therefore are not excessively expensive. However they have found limited application in clinical radiology. (It is interesting to note that Bucky's original grid was crossed.)

Crossed grids are much more efficient than parallel grids in cleaning up scatter radiation. In fact, a crossed grid has a higher contrast improvement factor than a parallel grid of twice the grid ratio. A 6:1 crossed grid will clean up more scatter radiation than a 12:1 parallel grid.

This advantage efficiency improvement increases as the operating kVp is increased.

> The main disadvantage of parallel and crossed grids is grid cutoff.

Three serious disadvantages are associated with the use of crossed grids. First, positioning the grid is critical; the central ray of the x-ray beam must coincide with the center of the grid. Second, tilt-table techniques are possible only if the x-ray tube and the table are properly aligned. Finally, the exposure technique required is substantial and results in higher patient radiation dose.

Focused Grid

The focused grid is designed to minimize grid cutoff. The lead grid strips of a focused grid lie on the imaginary radial lines of a circle centered at the focal spot of the x-ray tube, so they coincide with the divergence of the x-ray beam. The x-ray tube target should be placed at the center of this imaginary circle when a focused grid is used (Fig. 15.23).

Focused grids are more difficult to manufacture than parallel grids. They are characterized by all of the properties of parallel grids except that when properly positioned, they exhibit no grid cutoff. Radiographers must take care when positioning focused grids because of their geometric limitations.

> High-ratio grids have less positioning latitude than low-ratio grids.

Every focused grid is marked with its intended focal distance and the side of the grid that should face the x-ray tube. If radiographs are taken at distances other than those intended, grid cutoff occurs.

Moving Grid

An obvious and annoying shortcoming of the grids previously discussed is that they can produce **grid lines** on the image. Grid lines are the images made when primary x-rays are absorbed within the grid strips. Even though the grid strips are very small, their image is still observable.

The presence of grid lines can be demonstrated simply by radiographing a grid. Usually high-frequency grids present less obvious grid lines when compared with low-frequency grids. The visibility of grid lines is also directly related to the width of the grid strips.

A major improvement in grid development occurred in 1920. Hollis E. Potter hit on a very simple idea: Move the grid while the x-ray exposure is being made. The grid lines disappear at little cost of increased patient radiation dose. A device that does this is called a **moving grid** or a Potter-Bucky diaphragm ("Bucky" for short).

> Focused grids are usually moving grids.

Moving grids are placed in a holding mechanism that begins moving just before x-ray exposure and continues moving after the exposure ends. Two basic types of moving grid mechanisms are in use today: reciprocating and oscillating.

A **reciprocating grid** is a moving grid that is motor-driven back and forth several times during x-ray exposure. The total distance moved is approximately 2 cm.

An **oscillating grid** is positioned within a frame with a 2- to 3-cm tolerance on all sides between the frame and the grid. Delicate, spring-like devices located in the four corners hold the grid centered within the frame. A powerful electromagnet pulls the grid to one side and releases it at the beginning of the exposure. Thereafter the grid oscillates in a circular fashion around the grid frame, coming to rest after 20 to 30 seconds.

Moving grids require a bulky mechanism that is subject to failure. The distance between the patient and the IR is increased with moving grids because of this mechanism. This extra distance may create an unwanted increase in magnification and image blur. Moving grids can introduce motion into the cassette-holding device, which can result in additional image blur.

Fortunately, the advantages of moving grids far outweigh the disadvantages. The types of motion blur discussed are for descriptive purposes only. The motion blur generated by moving grids that are functioning properly is undetectable. Moving grids are usually the technique of choice and therefore are used widely.

Virtual Grid

The latest innovation for removal of scatter radiation and improvement of image contrast is the **digitally reconstructed radiograph**. Fujifilm was the first to market such a product in 2014 with the trade-marked name "Virtual Grid." Continuing development of digitally reconstructed radiographs will advance with the identifier virtual grid.

Each x-ray incident on a digital IR has a measurable energy and therefore also a measurable frequency. With current computer technology, there are techniques to identify each x-ray and assign it to an energy or frequency bin.

Registration and **optimization** algorithms are iteratively applied, resulting in scatter-free images that appear instantly. The algorithms are based on fundamental mathematics of Laplace transformation, wavelet transformation, and Gaussian decomposition. The resulting digitally reconstructed radiograph is produced with few, if any, Compton scatter x-ray interactions.

There is currently a limited use for the virtual grid, but the future is wide open. Stay alert, because with the emergence of quantum computing and qubit technology (see Chapter 29), virtual grid use will rule medical imaging and radiographic grids will be history.

There are many reasons to apply virtual grid technology now. The principal reason is the reduced patient radiation dose. The contrast improvement with a virtual grid is the same as that with a radiographic grid.

> Use of a virtual grid reduces patient radiation dose, improves image contrast, and is easiest to use.

Use of a radiographic grid for stationary imaging is rather straightforward and easy. However, radiographic grid use during mobile radiography is met with many problems—the most significant being positioning the patient, positioning the image receptor, and positioning the radiographic grid. Mobile radiography is easier with the virtual grid when used in the emergency department, operating room, patient bedside, and whenever the correct radiographic grid may not be available. Use of a virtual grid also eliminates artifacts.

GRID PROBLEMS

Most grids in diagnostic imaging are of the moving type. They are permanently mounted in the moving mechanism just below the tabletop or just behind the vertical chest board.

To be effective, of course, the grid must move from side to side. If the grid is installed incorrectly and moves in the same direction as the grid strips, grid lines will appear on the radiograph (Fig. 15.24).

> Only the off-level grid is a problem with parallel and crossed grids.

The most frequent error in the use of grids is improper positioning. For the grid to function correctly, it must be precisely positioned relative to the x-ray tube target and to the central ray of the x-ray beam. Four situations characteristic of focused grids must be avoided (Table 15.3).

CHAPTER 15   Scatter Radiation   227

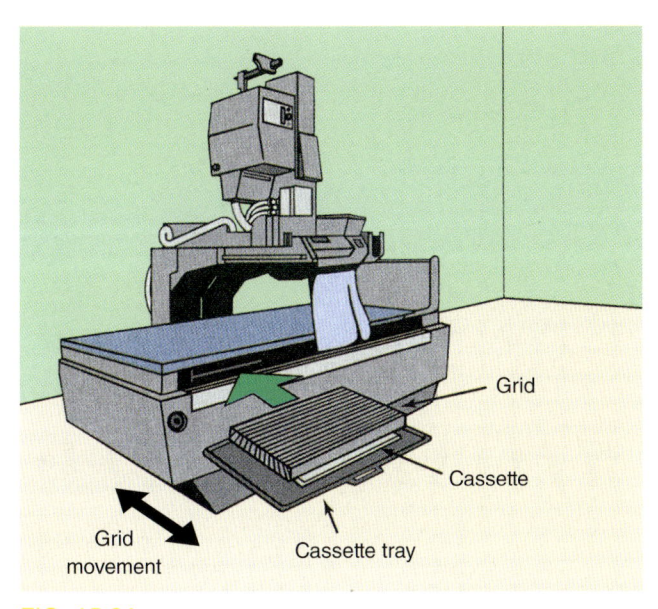

FIG. 15.24 Proper installation of a moving grid.

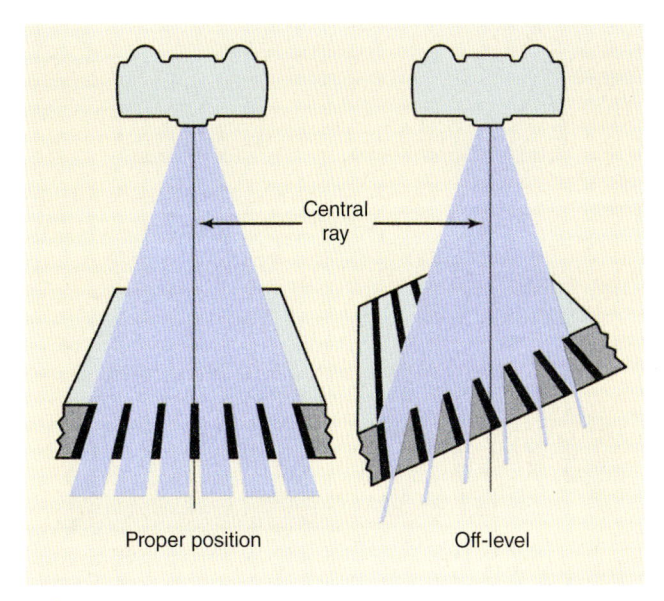

FIG. 15.25 If a grid is off-level so that the central axis is not perpendicular to the grid, partial cutoff occurs over the entire image receptor.

TABLE 15.3   Focused-Grid Misalignment

Type of Grid Misalignment	Result
Off-level	Grid cut off across image; underexposed, light image
Off-center	Grid cut off across image; underexposed, light image
Off-focus	Grid cut off toward edge of image
Upside-down	Severe grid cutoff toward edge of image
Off-center, off-focus	Grid cut off on one side of image

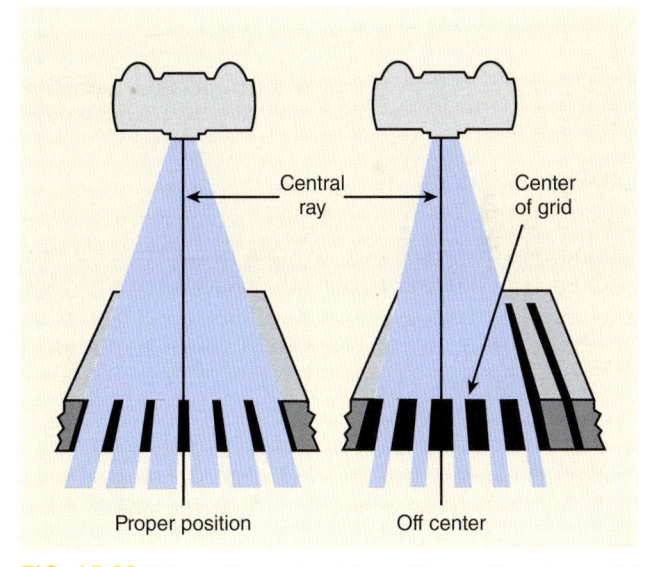

FIG. 15.26 When a focused grid is positioned off-center, partial grid cutoff occurs over the entire image receptor.

Off-Level Grid

A properly functioning grid must lie in a plane perpendicular to the central ray of the x-ray beam (Fig. 15.25). The **central ray** is the x-ray that travels along the center of the useful x-ray beam.

Despite its name, an **off-level grid** in fact is usually produced with an improperly positioned x-ray tube and not an improperly positioned grid. However this can occur when the grid tilts during horizontal beam radiography or during mobile radiography when the IR sinks into the patient's bed.

If the central ray is incident on the grid at an angle, then all incident x-rays will be angled, and grid cutoff will occur across the entire radiographic image, resulting in lower exposure of the digital IR.

Off-Center Grid

A grid can be perpendicular to the central ray of the x-ray beam and still produce grid cutoff if it is shifted laterally. This is a problem with focused grids, as shown in Fig. 15.26, in which an off-center grid is shown with a properly positioned grid.

The center of a focused grid must be positioned directly under the x-ray tube target, so the central ray of the x-ray beam passes through the centermost interspace of the grid. Any lateral shift results in grid cutoff across the entire radiograph. This error in positioning is called **lateral decentering**.

As with an off-level grid, an off-center grid is more a result of positioning the x-ray tube than the grid. In practice, it means that the radiographer must carefully

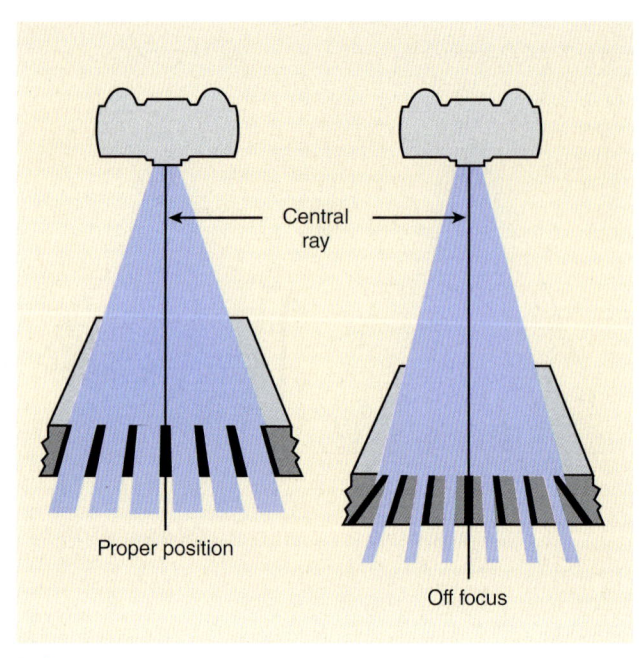

FIG. 15.27 If a focused grid is not positioned at the specified focal distance, grid cutoff occurs and the IR signal intensity decreases with distance from the central ray.

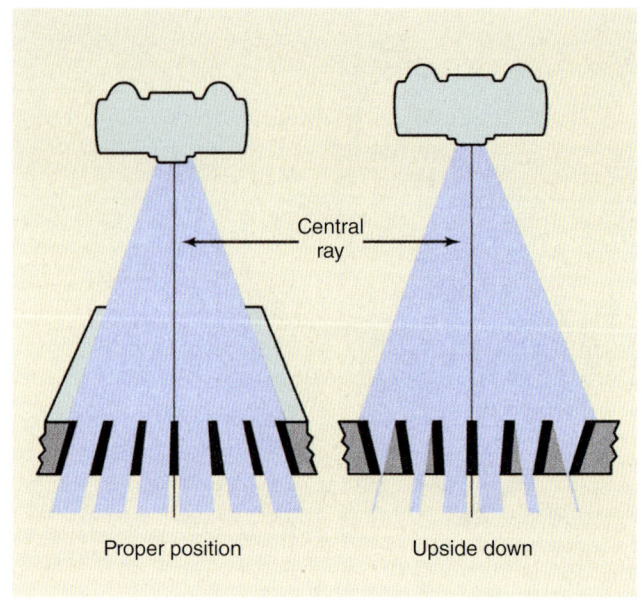

FIG. 15.28 A focused grid positioned upside-down should be detected on the first radiograph. Complete grid cutoff occurs except in the region of the central ray.

line up the center of the light-localized field with the center of the IR.

Off-Focus Grid

A major problem with using a focused grid arises when radiographs are taken at a SID that is incorrect for that grid. Fig. 15.27 illustrates what happens when a focused grid is not used at the proper focal distance. The farther the grid is from the specified focal distance, the more severe will be the grid cutoff. Grid cutoff is not uniform across the IR but instead is more severe at the edges.

This condition is not usually a problem if all chest radiographs are taken at 180-cm SID and all table radiographs at 100-cm SID. Positioning the grid at the proper focal distance is more important with high-ratio grids. Greater positioning latitude is possible with low-ratio grids.

Upside-Down Grid

The explanation for an upside-down grid is obvious. It need occur only once, and it will be noticed immediately. A radiographic image taken with an upside-down focused grid shows severe grid cutoff on either side of the central ray (Fig. 15.28).

GRID SELECTION

Modern grids are sufficiently well manufactured that many radiologists do not find the grid lines of stationary grids objectionable, especially for mobile radiography and horizontal views of an upright patient. Virtual grid use is changing this.

Modern moving grid mechanisms rarely fail, and image degradation rarely occurs. Therefore in most situations, it is appropriate to design radiographic imaging around moving grids. When moving grids are used, parallel grids can be used, but focused grids are more common.

Focused grids are in general far superior to parallel grids, but their use requires care and attention. When focused grids are used, the indicators on the x-ray apparatus must be in good adjustment and properly calibrated. The SID indicator, the source-to-tabletop distance indicator, and the light-localizing collimator all must be properly adjusted.

Selection of a grid with the proper ratio depends on an understanding of three interrelated factors: kVp, degree of scatter radiation reduction, and patient radiation dose. When a high kVp is used, high-ratio grids should be used as well. Of course, the choice of grid is also influenced by the size and shape of the anatomy that is being imaged.

As grid ratio increases, scatter radiation attenuation also increases. Fig. 15.29 shows the approximate percentage of scatter radiation and primary radiation transmitted as a function of grid ratio. Note that the difference between grid ratios of 12:1 and 16:1 is small.

The difference in patient radiation dose is large, however. Therefore 16:1 grids are not often used. Many general-purpose x-ray examination facilities find that an 8:1 grid represents a good compromise between the desired levels of scatter radiation reduction and patient radiation dose.

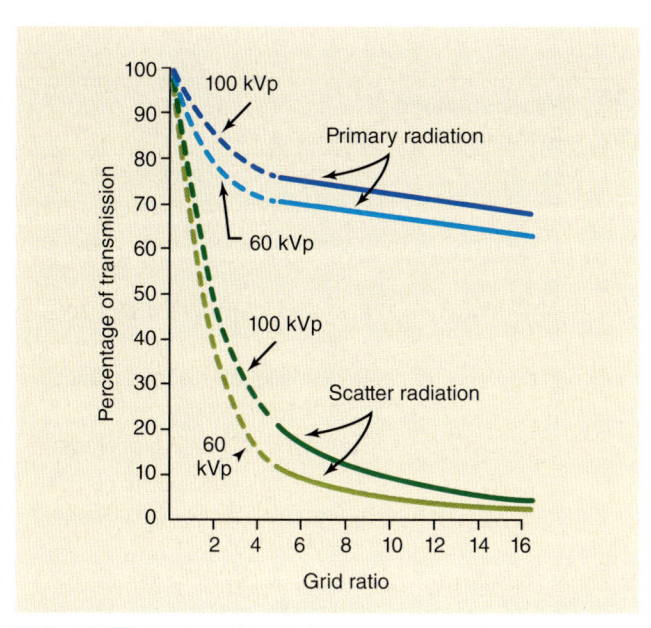

FIG. 15.29 As the grid ratio increases, transmission of scatter radiation decreases faster than transmission of primary radiation. Therefore cleanup of scatter radiation increases.

| TABLE 15.4 | Approximate Entrance Skin Radiation Dose for Examination of the Adult Pelvis with a Digital Image Receptor |

	ENTRANCE DOSE (MGY$_T$)		
Type of Grid	**70 kVp**	**90 kVp**	**110 kVp**
No grid	0.4	0.35	0.25
5:1	1.4	1.1	7.5
8:1	1.6	1.4	1.0
12:1	2.1	2.0	1.5
16:1	2.6	2.4	1.9
5:1 crossed	2.7	2.0	1.5
Virtual grid	0.8	0.7	0.5

| TABLE 15.5 | Approximate Change in Radiographic Technique for Standard Grids |

Grid Ratio	**mAs Increase**	**kVp Increase**
No grid	1×	0
5:1	2×	+ 8–10
8:1	4×	+ 13–15
12:1	5×	+ 20–25
Virtual grid	0.5×	0

In general, grid ratios up to 8:1 are satisfactory at tube potentials below 90 kVp. Grid ratios above 8:1 are used when kVp exceeds 90 kVp.

The use of one grid also reduces the likelihood of grid cutoff resulting from improper grid positioning that can easily accompany frequent grid changes. In facilities where high-kVp technique is used for dedicated chest radiography, 16:1 grids can be installed.

Patient Radiation Dose

One major disadvantage that accompanies the use of radiographic grids is increased patient radiation dose. For any examination, use of a grid may result in several times more of a radiation dose to the patient than occurs when a grid is not used. The use of a moving grid instead of a stationary grid with similar physical characteristics requires approximately 15% more patient radiation dose. Table 15.4 is a summary of approximate patient radiation doses for various grid techniques.

Low-ratio grids are used during a mammography. All dedicated mammographic imaging systems are equipped with a 4:1 or a 5:1 ratio moving grid. Even at the low kVp used for a mammography, considerable scatter radiation occurs.

The use of such grids greatly improves image contrast, with no loss of spatial resolution. Remember that spatial resolution is pixel limited. The only disadvantage is the increase in patient radiation dose, which can be as much as twice that without a grid. However, with a virtual grid, patient radiation dose will be nearly halved.

GRID SELECTION FACTORS
1. Patient radiation dose increases with increasing grid ratio.
2. High-ratio grids are used for high-kVp examinations.
3. The patient radiation dose at high kVp is less than that at low kVp.

In general, compared to the use of low-kVp and low-ratio grids, the use of high-kVp and high-ratio grids results in lower patient radiation dose and equal image quality.

One additional disadvantage of the use of radiographic grids is the increased radiographic technique required. When a grid is used, technique factors must be increased over what they were for nongrid examinations: The mAs or the kVp must be increased. Table 15.5 presents approximate changes in technique factors required by standard grids. Usually the mAs rather than the kVp is increased. One exception to this is chest radiography, in which increased exposure time can result in motion blur.

TABLE 15.6 Clinical Considerations in Grid Selection

Type of Grid	Degree of Scatter Removal	Off-Center (Positioning Latitude)	Off-Focus (Positioning Latitude)	Recommended Technique	Remarks
5:1, linear	+	Very wide	Very wide	≤80 kVp	It is the least expensive and is the easiest to use.
6:1, linear	+	Very wide	Very wide	≤80 kVp	It is inexpensive and is ideally suited for bedside radiography.
8:1, linear	+	Wide	Wide	≤100 kVp	It is used for general stationary grids.
10:1, linear	+++	Wide	Wide	≤100 kVp	Reasonable care is required for proper alignment.
5:1, crisscross	+++	Narrow	Very wide	≤100 kVp	Tube tilt is limited to 5 degrees.
12:1, linear	++++	Narrow	Narrow	>110 kVp	Extra care is required for proper alignment. It usually is used in a fixed mount.
6:1, crisscross	++++	Narrow	Very wide	≤110 kVp	It is not suited for tilted-tube techniques.
16:1, linear	+++++	Narrow	Narrow	>100 kVp	Extra care is required for proper alignment. It usually is used in a fixed mount.
8:1, crisscross	+++++	Narrow	Wide	≤120 kVp	It is not suited for tilted-tube techniques.
Virtual grid	++++++			All kVp	

Table 15.6 summarizes the clinical factors that should be considered in the selection of various types of grids.

Air-Gap Technique

A clever technique that may be used as an alternative to the use of radiographic grids is the **air-gap technique**. This is another method of reducing scatter radiation, thereby enhancing image contrast.

When the air-gap technique is used, the IR is moved 10 to 15 cm from the patient (Fig. 15.30). A portion of the scattered x-rays generated in the patient would be scattered away from the IR and not be detected. Because fewer scattered x-rays interact with the IR, the contrast is improved.

When an air-gap technique is used, the mAs is usually increased approximately 10% for every centimeter of air gap. The technique factors usually are about the same as those for an 8:1 grid. Therefore the patient radiation dose is higher than that associated with the nongrid technique and is approximately equivalent to that of an intermediate grid technique.

> One disadvantage of the air-gap technique is image magnification with associated focal-spot blur.

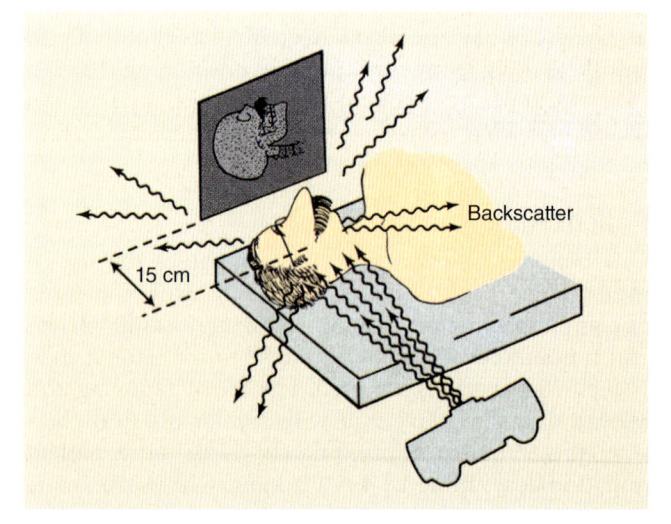

FIG. 15.30 When the air-gap technique is used, the image receptor (IR) is positioned 10 to 15 cm from the patient. A large fraction of scattered x-rays does not interact with the IR.

The air-gap technique has found application particularly in the areas of chest radiography and interventional radiology, especially cerebral angiography. The magnification that accompanies these techniques is usually acceptable.

In chest radiography, some radiographers increase the SID from 180 to 300 cm. This results in very little

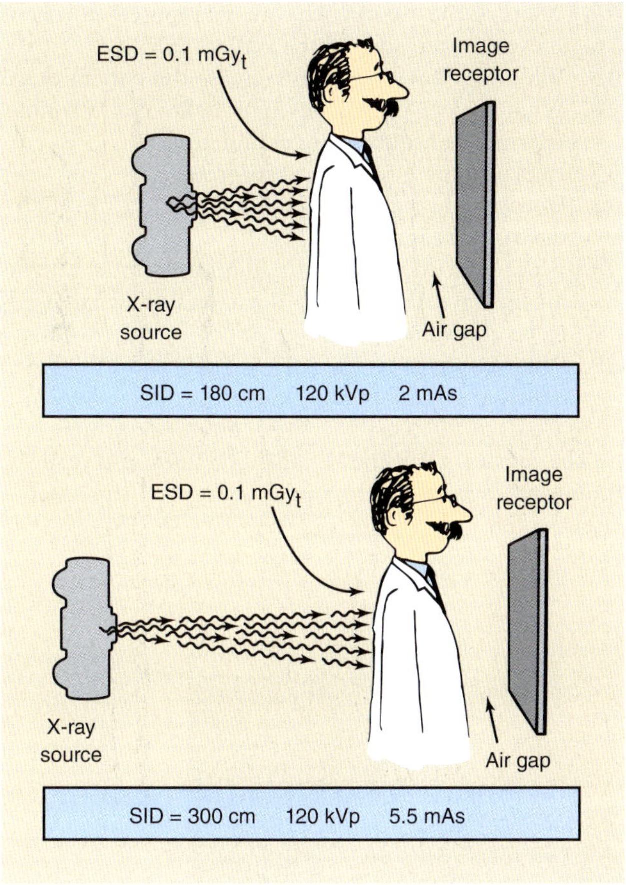

FIG. 15.31 Increasing the SID to 300 cm from 180 cm improves spatial resolution with no increase in patient dose. *ESD*, Entrance skin dose; *SID*, source-to-image receptor distance.

magnification and a sharper image. Of course the technique factors must be increased, but the patient radiation dose is not increased (Fig. 15.31).

The air-gap technique is not normally as effective with high-kVp radiography, in which the direction of the scattered x-rays is more forward. At tube potentials below approximately 90 kVp, the scattered x-rays are directed more to the side; therefore they have a higher probability of being scattered away from the IR. Nevertheless, at some centers, 120 to 140 kVp air-gap chest radiography is used with good results.

SUMMARY

Two types of image-forming x-rays exit the patient: (1) x-rays that pass through tissue without interacting and (2) x-rays that are scattered in tissue by the Compton interaction and therefore contribute only noise to the image. The three factors that contribute to increased scatter radiation and ultimately to image noise are increasing kVp, increasing x-ray field size, and increasing patient size.

Although increased kVp increases scatter radiation, the trade-off is reduced patient radiation dose. Beam-restricting devices can be used to control and minimize the increase in scatter radiation. Such devices include the aperture diaphragm, cones or cylinders, and the variable-aperture collimator. The variable-aperture collimator is the most commonly used beam-restricting device in radiographic imaging.

Image contrast is an important characteristic of the radiographic image. Scatter radiation, the result of Compton interaction, is the primary factor that reduces image contrast. Grids reduce the amount of scatter that reaches the IR. Virtual grids remove scatter radiation before constructing the image during preprocessing.

The two main components of grid construction are the interspace material (aluminum or plastic fiber) and the grid material (lead strips). The principal characteristic of a grid is grid ratio; that is, the height of the grid strip divided by the interspace width. Different grids are selected for use in particular situations. At less than 90 kVp, grid ratios of 8:1 and lower are used. At 90 kVp and above, grid ratios greater than 8:1 are used.

In all cases, the use of a radiographic grid increases patient radiation dose. The use of virtual grids reduces patient radiation dose. Problems that can arise in the use of grids include off-level, off-center, and upside-down grid errors.

An alternative to the use of a grid is the air-gap technique, in which the IR is moved 10 to 15 cm from the patient. The air gap allows much of the scatter radiation to miss the IR.

CHALLENGE QUESTIONS

1. Define or otherwise identify the following:
   a. Three factors that affect scatter radiation
   b. Collimator filtration
   c. Image contrast
   d. Grid cutoff
   e. Collimation
   f. Off-focus radiation
   g. PBL device
   h. Air-gap technique
   i. Image-forming x-rays
   j. Contrast improvement factor
2. Why should a radiograph of the lumbar vertebrae be well collimated?
3. With particular references to materials used and dimensions, discuss the construction of a grid.
4. An acceptable intravenous pyelogram (IVP) image can be obtained with technique factors of (1) 74 kVp, 120 mAs, or (2) 82 kVp, 80 mAs. Discuss possible reasons for selecting one technique over the other.
5. Does the radiograph of a long bone in a wet cast result in more or less scatter than that of a long bone in a dry cast?

6. A focused grid has the following characteristics: 100-cm focal distance, 40-μm grid strips, 350-μm interspace, and 2.8-mm height. What is the grid ratio?
7. What happens to image contrast and patient radiation dose as more filtration is added to the x-ray beam?
8. Why does tissue compression improve image contrast?
9. At 80 kVp, approximately what percentage of the x-ray beam is Compton scattered?
10. Name the devices used to reduce the production of scatter radiation.
11. Compression of tissue is particularly important during what examination?
12. List two reasons for restricting the x-ray beam.
13. Compared with contact radiography, why does the air-gap technique increase the patient dose?
14. What is the reason why an unexposed border is shown on the edge of the radiograph?
15. Why does lowering kVp increase the patient dose?
16. What is viewed in the light field of a variable-aperture light-localizing collimator?
17. Explain how grid cutoff can occur.
18. Does a light-localizing collimator add filtration to the x-ray beam?
19. If the light field and the radiation field of a light-localizing collimator do not coincide, what needs to be adjusted?
20. What happens to the patient radiation dose when a virtual grid is used?

The answers to the Challenge Questions can be found by logging on to our website at http://evolve.elsevier.com.

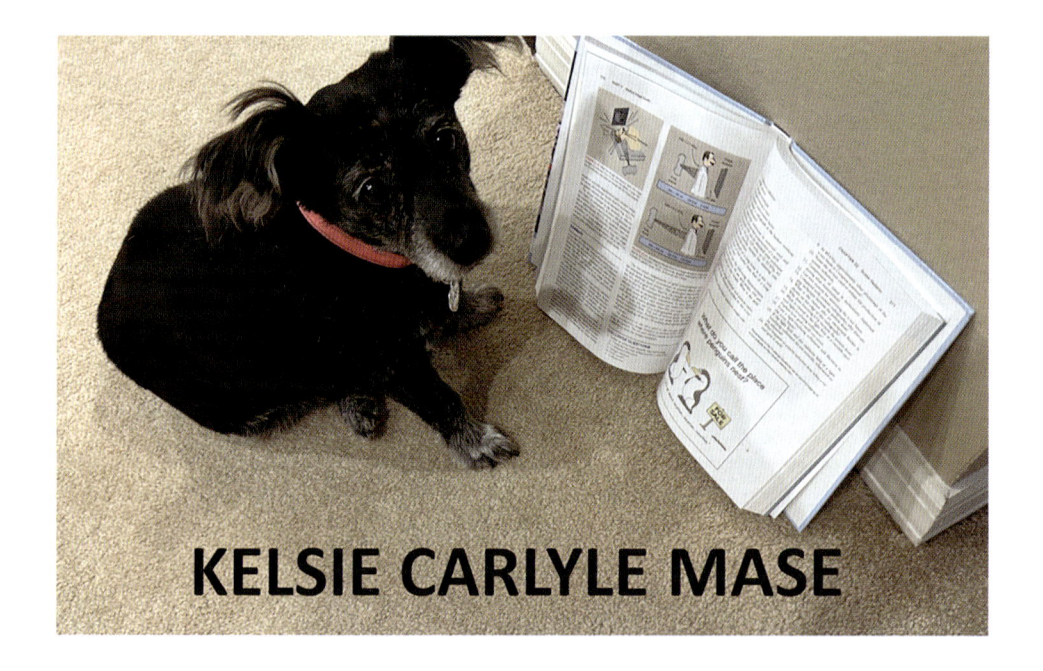

Digital Image Descriptors and Evaluation

CHAPTER 16

OBJECTIVES

At the completion of this chapter, the student should be able to do the following:
1. Define digital image quality, resolution, noise, and speed.
2. Distinguish the geometric factors that affect digital image quality.
3. Analyze the subject factors that affect digital image quality.
4. Examine the tools and techniques available to create high-quality images.

OUTLINE

Definitions 234
   Digital Image Quality 234
   Spatial Resolution 234
   Contrast Resolution 234
   Noise 234
   Speed 235
Geometric Factors 235
   Magnification 235
   Distortion 238
   Focal-Spot Blur 240
   Heel Effect 241

Subject Factors 241
   Subject Contrast 242
   Motion Blur 243
Tools for Improved Image Quality 244
   Patient Positioning 244
   Image Receptors 244
   Selection of Technique Factors 244
Summary 245
Challenge Questions 245

DIGITAL IMAGE quality has many descriptive terms to express the exactness of representation of the patient's anatomy on an image. High-quality images are required so that radiologists can make accurate interpretations and diagnoses. To produce high-quality images, radiographers apply knowledge of the interrelated categories of image quality: spatial resolution, contrast resolution, geometric factors, and subject factors. Each of these descriptors influences the quality of a digital image, and each is under the control of the radiographer.

There are many medical imaging modalities—radiography, fluoroscopy, computed tomography, magnetic resonance imaging, diagnostic ultrasound, and the several nuclear medicine modalities. Digital radiography is the most frequently employed modality by far and that subject was covered in earlier chapters. Here we consider description of digital imaging, regardless of modality.

DEFINITIONS

Digital Image Quality

The term digital **image quality** refers to the fidelity with which the anatomy under investigation is rendered on the image receptor. A digital image that faithfully reproduces structures and tissues is identified as a **high-quality image**.

The quality of a digital image is not easy to define, and it cannot be measured precisely. A number of factors affect digital image quality, but no precise, universally accepted measures by which to judge it have been identified.

The most important descriptors of image quality are **spatial resolution, contrast resolution, noise,** and **artifacts**. Artifacts are discussed in Chapter 17.

Spatial Resolution

Resolution is the ability to image two separate objects and visually distinguish one from the other. **Spatial resolution** refers to the ability to image small objects that have high subject contrast, such as a bone-soft tissue interface, a breast microcalcification, or a calcified lung nodule.

> Spatial resolution improves with smaller pixel size.

Focal-spot size has a small influence on spatial resolution. Review the discussion in Chapter 7 of the anode of an x-ray tube. The smaller the projected focal spot size—effective focal spot—the better the spatial resolution. However, with all digital imaging modalities, one cannot image an object smaller than the size of the pixel.

Nevertheless, we now realize that contrast resolution is more important than spatial resolution for most medical imaging modalities.

Contrast Resolution

Contrast resolution is the ability to distinguish anatomical structures of similar subject contrast, such as liver-spleen and gray matter-white matter. The actual size of objects that can be imaged is always smaller under conditions of high subject contrast than under conditions of low subject contrast.

Unlike spatial resolution, contrast resolution cannot be easily quantified. There are ways to express percent contrast, but they are not very meaningful. Consequently contrast resolution takes on a verbal description—high contrast or low contrast.

In x-ray imaging, contrast resolution improves at a lower kilovoltage peak (kVp). In nuclear medicine, imaging contrast resolution improves with increased metabolic activity.

Magnetic resonance imaging is considered to have the best contrast resolution, but it is very dependent on the radio frequency (RF) pulse sequence employed. In fact, a change in RF pulse sequence can actually reverse image contrast.

Noise

Noise is a term that is borrowed from electrical engineering. The flutter, hum, and whistle heard from an audio system constitute **audio noise** that is inherent in the electronic design of the system. The "snow" on television screens, especially in weak signal areas, is **video noise**, and it is also inherent in the system. Electronic noise reduces sound and video fidelity.

> Radiographic noise is the random fluctuation of x-ray interaction on the image receptor.

Radiographic noise is also inherent in the x-ray imaging system. A number of factors contribute to radiographic noise, including some that are under the control of the radiographer. Lower noise from any source results in a better digital image because it improves contrast resolution.

Because it is an electronic device, the image receptor, regardless of type, will exhibit inherent electronic noise. The level of this type of noise is very hard to measure and therefore it is really insignificant.

Quantum mottle is somewhat under the control of the radiographer and is a principal contributor to image noise in many radiographic and fluoroscopic imaging procedures. Quantum mottle refers to the random nature by which x-rays interact with the image receptor.

If an image is produced with just a few x-rays, the quantum mottle will be higher than if the image is formed from a large number of x-rays. The use of very fast image receptors results in increased quantum mottle because fewer x-rays are necessary to make the image.

> The use of high-mAs, low-kVp, and slower image receptors reduces quantum mottle.

Quantum mottle is similar to the sowing of grass seed. If very little seed is broadcast, the resulting grass will be thin with only a few blades. Likewise, when fewer x-rays are "cast" at the image receptor, the resulting image appears mottled.

On the other hand, if a lot of seed is cast, the resulting grass will be thick and smooth. In the same way, when more x-rays interact with the image receptor, the image appears smooth, like a lush lawn.

Speed

These three characteristics of radiographic quality—spatial resolution, contrast resolution, and noise—are intimately connected with a fourth characteristic—**speed**. Although the speed of the image receptor is not apparent on the radiographic image, it very much influences the three other characteristics. In fact, a variation in any one of these characteristics alters the other three (Fig. 16.1). In general, the following rules apply:

> **DIGITAL IMAGE QUALITY RULES**
> 1. Fast image receptors have high noise and low contrast resolution.
> 2. Low noise accompanies slow image receptors and high-contrast resolution.
> 3. Spatial resolution is limited to pixel size.

Radiographers are provided with all of the physical tools required to produce high-quality digital images. Skillful radiographers properly manipulate these tools according to each specific clinical situation.

In general, the quality of a digital image is directly related to an understanding of some basic principles of projection imaging geometry and the subject factors. Fig. 16.2 is an organizational chart of the principal factors that affect digital image quality, many of which are under the control of the radiographer.

GEOMETRIC FACTORS

Making a radiograph is similar in many ways to taking a photograph. Proper exposure time and intensity are required for both processes. Images are recorded both ways because x-rays and visible light photons travel in straight lines.

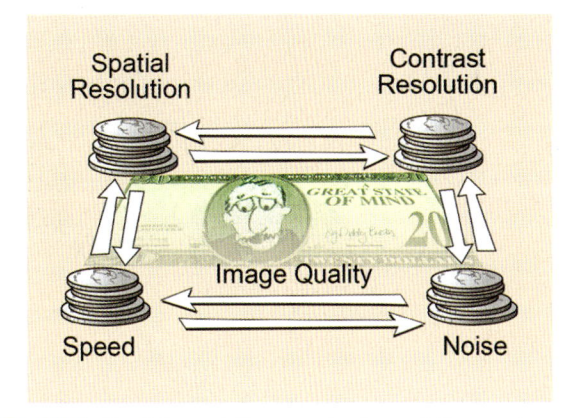

FIG. 16.1 Spatial resolution, contrast resolution, noise, and speed are interrelated characteristics of digital image quality. Four coins placed on four corners of a twenty dollar bill representing four key features of image quality are marked clockwise as: spatial resolution, contrast resolution, noise, and speed. Each feature is marked with a double-headed arrow in between to show interrelationship between characteristics.

In that regard, an x-ray image may be considered analogous to a shadowgraph. Fig. 16.3 shows the familiar shadowgraph that can be made to appear on a wall if light is shone on a properly contorted hand.

The sharpness of the shadow image on the wall is a function of a number of **geometric factors**. For example, the closer to the wall the hand is placed, the sharper the shadow image will be. Similarly, as the light source is moved farther from the hand, the shadow becomes sharper.

> Sharpness in this shadow context is spatial resolution.

These geometric conditions also apply to the production of high-quality radiographs. Three principal geometric factors affect digital image quality: magnification, distortion, and focal-spot blur.

Magnification

All images on the radiograph are larger than the objects they represent, a condition called **magnification**. For most digital images, the smallest magnification possible should be maintained.

During some examinations, however, magnification is desirable and is carefully planned into the radiographic examination. This type of examination, called **magnification radiography**, was discussed in Chapter 14.

Quantitatively, magnification is expressed by the magnification factor (MF), which is defined as follows:

MAGNIFICATION FACTOR

$$MF = \frac{\text{Image size}}{\text{Object size}}$$

Digital Image Quality

Image Receptor Factors
- Pixel size
- Dynamic range
- Intensity response
- Signal to noise
- Postprocessing

Geometric Factors
- Distortion
- Magnification
- Blur

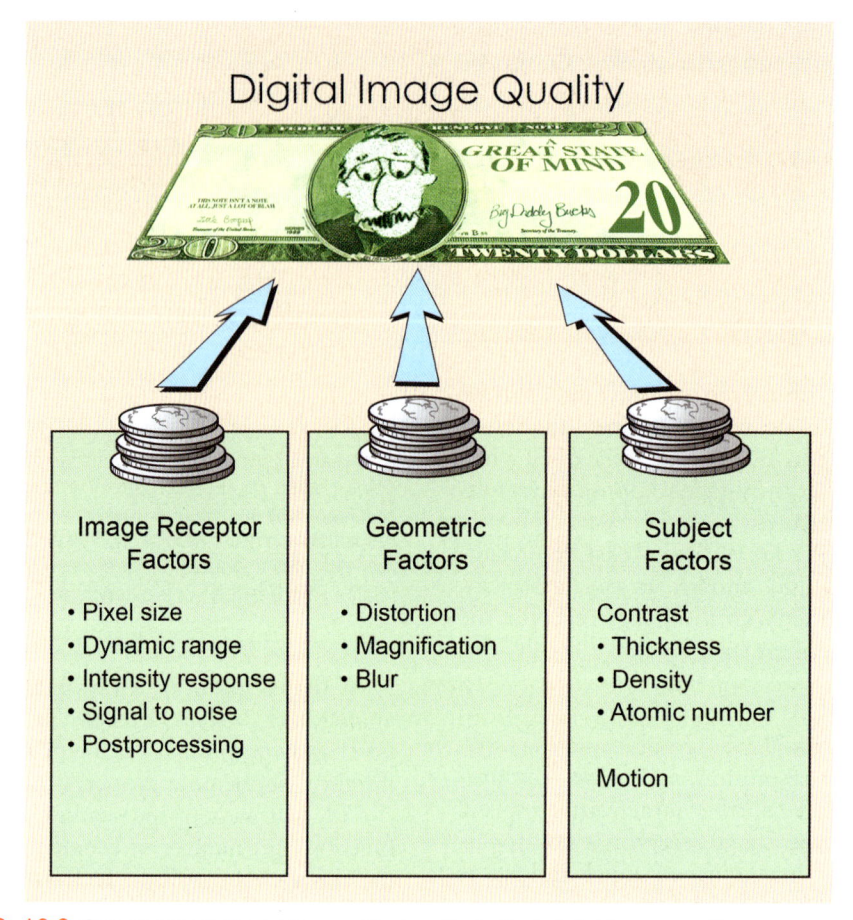

Subject Factors
- Contrast
- Thickness
- Density
- Atomic number

Motion

FIG. 16.2 Organizational chart of several factors that affect digital image quality.

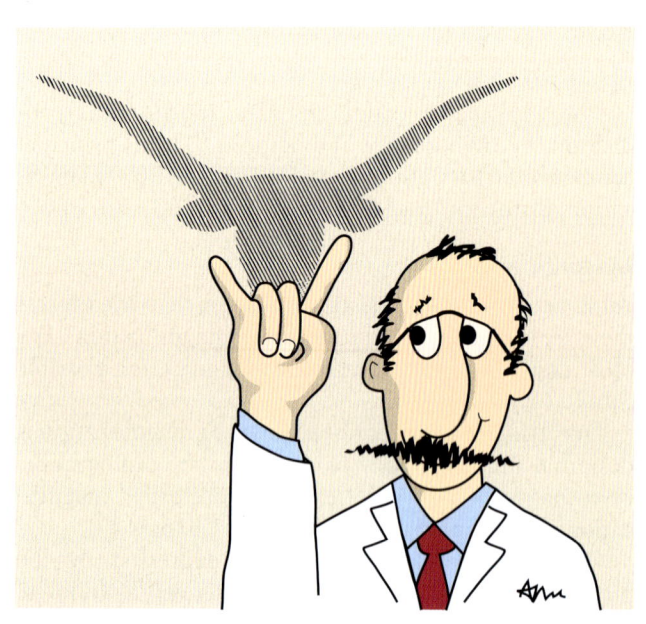

FIG. 16.3 A shadowgraph is analogous to a radiograph. Dedicated to Xie Nan Zhu, Guangzhou, People's Republic of China.

The MF depends on the geometric conditions of the examination. For most radiographs taken at a source-to-image receptor distance (SID) of 100 cm, the MF is approximately 1.1. For radiographs taken at 180 cm SID, the MF is approximately 1.05.

Question: If a heart measures 12.5 cm at its maximum width and its image on a chest radiograph measures 14.7 cm, what is the MF?

Answer:
$$MF = \frac{14.7 \text{ cm}}{12.5 \text{ cm}} = 1.176$$

In the usual radiographic examination, it is not possible to determine the object size. The image size may be measured directly from the radiograph. In such situations, the MF can be determined from the ratio of SID to source-to-object distance (SOD):

MAGNIFICATION FACTOR

$$MF = \frac{\text{Source-to-image receptor distance (SID)}}{\text{Source-to-object distance (SOD)}}$$

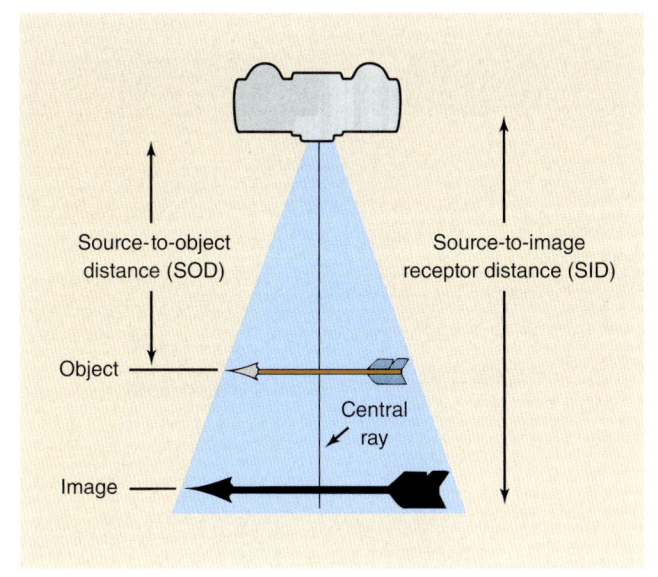

FIG. 16.4 Magnification is the ratio of image size to object size or of source-to-image receptor distance to source-to-object distance.

Fig. 16.4 shows that this method of calculating the MF is based on the geometric relationship between similar triangles. If two right triangles have a common hypotenuse, the ratio of the height of one to its base will be the same as the ratio of the height of the other to its base.

This is the situation that usually is encountered in radiography. The SID is known and can be measured directly. The SOD can be estimated relatively accurately by a radiographer who has a good foundation in human anatomy. The image size can be measured accurately; therefore object size can be calculated as follows:

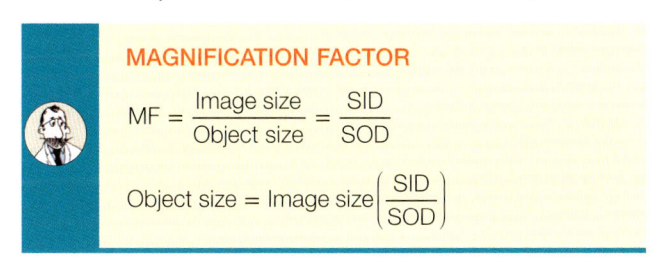

> **MAGNIFICATION FACTOR**
>
> $$MF = \frac{\text{Image size}}{\text{Object size}} = \frac{SID}{SOD}$$
>
> $$\text{Object size} = \text{Image size}\left(\frac{SID}{SOD}\right)$$

Question: A renal calculus measures 1.2 cm on the radiograph. The SID is 100 cm, and the SOD is estimated at 92 cm. What is the size of the calculus?

Answer: $\text{Object size} = 1.2\left(\dfrac{9.2}{100}\right) = 1.1 \text{ cm}$

Question: A lateral view of the lumbar spine taken at 100 cm SID results in the image of a vertebral body with maximum and minimum dimensions of 6.4 and 4.2 cm, respectively. What is the object size if the vertebral body is 25 cm from the image receptor?

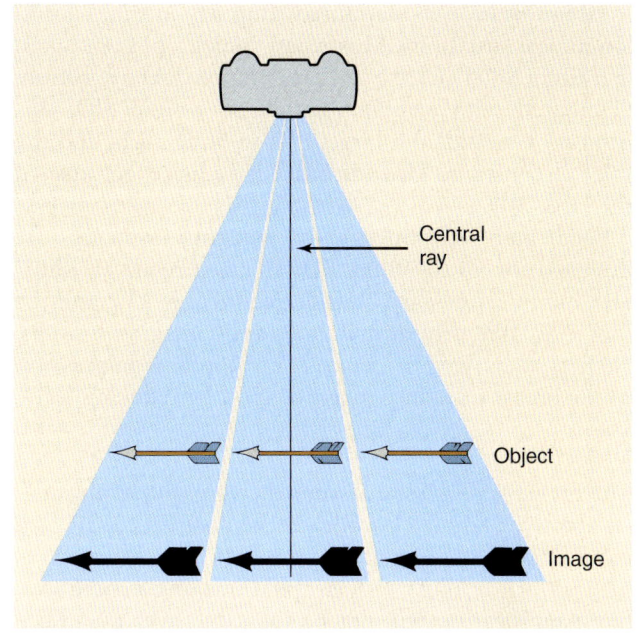

FIG. 16.5 Magnification of an object positioned off the central ray is the same as that of an object on the central ray if the objects are in the same plane.

Answer: $$MF = \frac{100}{100 - 25} = \frac{100}{75} = 1.33$$

Therefore the object size is

$$\frac{6.4}{1.33} \times \frac{4.2}{1.33} = 4.81 \times 3.16 \text{ cm}.$$

You might ask whether these relationships hold for objects off the central ray (Fig. 16.5). The MF will be the same for objects positioned off the central ray as for those lying on the central ray if the object-to-image receptor distance (OID) is the same and if the object is essentially flat.

> Two factors affect image magnification: SID and OID.

> **MINIMIZING MAGNIFICATION**
> Large SID: Use as large a source-to-image receptor distance as possible.
> Small OID: Place the object as close to the image receptor as possible.

The radiographic SID is standard in most medical imaging departments at 180 cm for chest imaging; 100 cm for routine examinations; and 90 cm for some special studies, such as mobile radiography and trauma radiography.

Magnification is minimized routinely in three familiar clinical situations. Most chest radiographs are taken at 180 cm SID from the posteroanterior (PA) projection. Compared with an examination at 100 cm SID, this projection results in a larger SID-to-SOD ratio, and the OID is constant. Magnification is reduced because of the large SID.

Dedicated mammography imaging systems are designed for 60 to 70 cm SID. This is a relatively short SID, but it is necessary, considering the low-kVp and the low-x-ray intensity of mammography imaging systems. Such systems have a device for vigorous compression of the breast to reduce magnification by reducing OID.

Distortion

The previous discussion assumed a very simple object—an arrow positioned parallel to the image receptor at a fixed OID. If any one of these conditions is changed, as they all are in most radiographic imaging procedures, the magnification will not be the same over the entire object.

> Unequal magnification of different portions of the same object is called **distortion**.
> Distortion can interfere with diagnosis. Three conditions contribute to image distortion: object thickness, object position, and object shape.

> **DISTORTION DEPENDS ON**
> 1. Object thickness
> 2. Object position
> 3. Object shape

With a thick object, the OID changes measurably across the object. Consider, for instance, two rectangular structures of different thicknesses (Fig. 16.6). Because of the change in OID across the thicker structure, the image of that structure is more distorted than the image of the thinner structure.

> Thick objects are more distorted than thin objects.

Consider the images produced by a disc and a sphere of the same diameter (Fig. 16.7). When positioned on the central axis, the images of both objects appear as circles. The image of the sphere appears less distinct because of its varying thickness, but it does appear circular.

When these objects are positioned laterally to the central ray, the disc still appears circular. The sphere appears not only less distinct but elliptical because

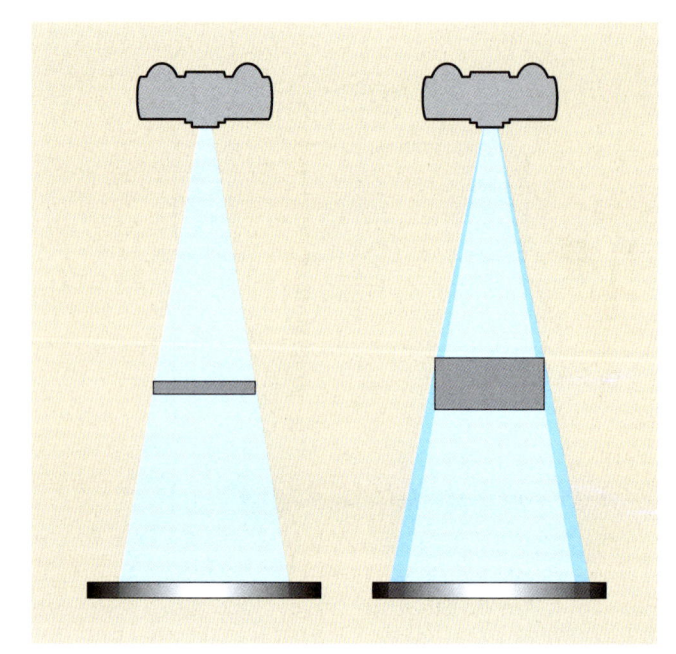

FIG. 16.6 Thick objects result in unequal magnification and thus greater distortion compared with thin objects.

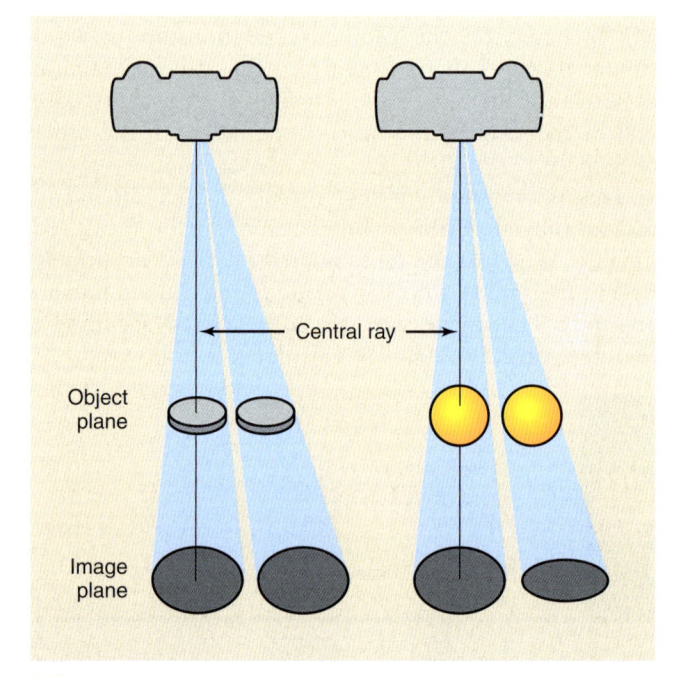

FIG. 16.7 Object thickness influences distortion. Radiographs of a disc or sphere appear as circles if the object is on the central ray. When lateral to the central axis, the disc appears as a circle and the sphere as an ellipse.

of its thickness. This distortion resulting from **object thickness** is shown more dramatically in Fig. 16.8 in the image of an irregular object.

These statements about disks and spheres are clinically insignificant because lateral distances off the central ray are too small. Only irregular objects, such as those shown in Fig. 16.8 or the human body, show significant distortion.

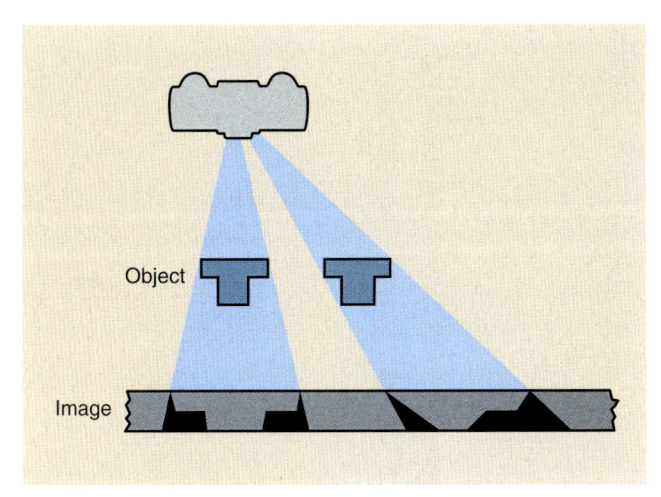

FIG. 16.8 Irregular anatomy or objects such as these can cause considerable distortion when radiographed off the central ray.

If the object plane and the image plane are parallel, the image is not distorted. However, distortion is possible in every radiographic examination if the patient is not properly positioned.

> If the object plane and the image plane are not parallel, distortion occurs.

Fig. 16.9, an example of gross distortion, shows that the image of an inclined object can be smaller than the object itself. In such a condition, the image is said to be **foreshortened**. The amount of foreshortening, that is, the extent of reduction in image size, increases as the angle of inclination increases.

If an inclined object is not located on the central x-ray beam, the degree of distortion is affected by the object's angle of inclination and its lateral position from the central axis. Fig. 16.10 illustrates this situation and shows that the image of an inclined object can be severely foreshortened or **elongated**.

With multiple objects positioned at various OIDs, **spatial distortion** can occur. Spatial distortion is the misrepresentation in the image of the actual spatial relationships among objects. Fig. 16.11 demonstrates this condition for two arrows of the same size, one of which lies on top of the other. Because of the position of the arrows, only one image should be seen, representing the **superposition** of the arrows.

Unequal magnification, however, of the two objects causes arrow A to appear larger than arrow B and to be positioned more laterally. This distortion is minimal for objects lying along the central ray. As **object position** is shifted laterally from the central ray, spatial distortion can become more significant.

This illustrates the projection nature of x-ray images. A single image is not enough to define the three-dimensional configuration of a complex object. Therefore most radiographic examinations are made with two or more projections. Because of the digital image descriptor, digital radiographic tomosynthesis becomes a more standard procedure (see Chapter 22).

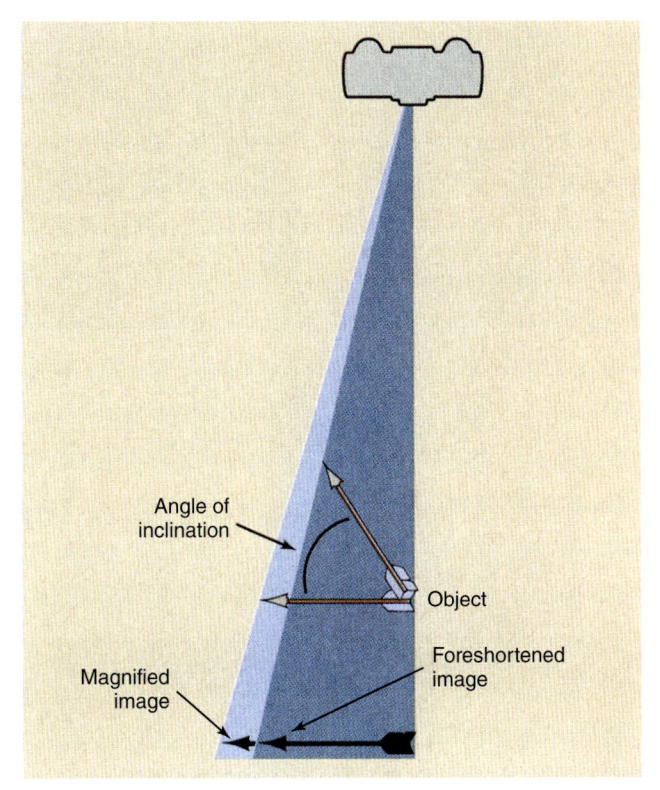

FIG. 16.9 Inclination of an object results in a foreshortened image.

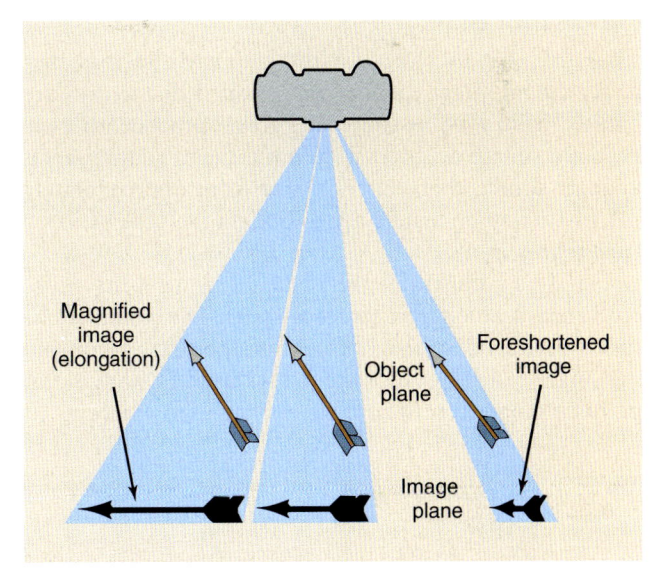

FIG. 16.10 An inclined object that is positioned lateral to the central ray may be distorted severely by elongation or foreshortening.

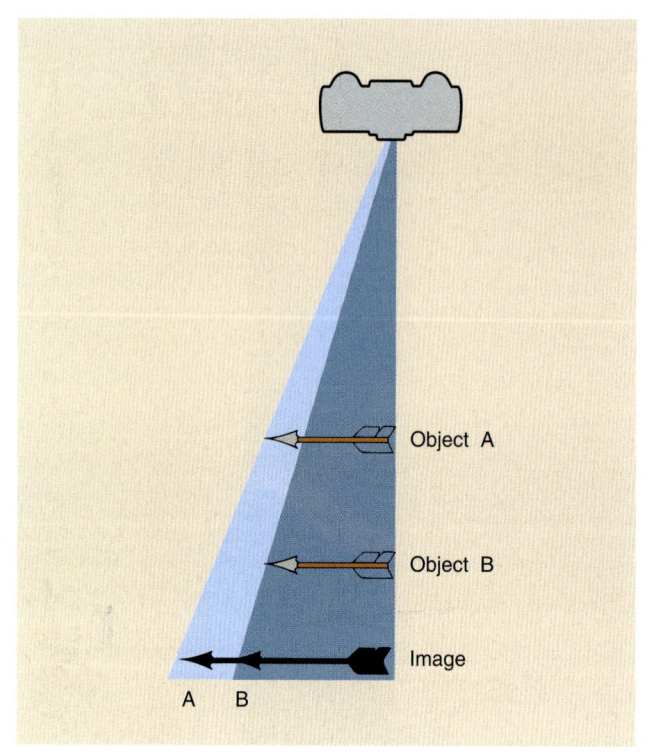

FIG. 16.11 When objects of the same size are positioned at different distances from the image receptor, spatial distortion occurs.

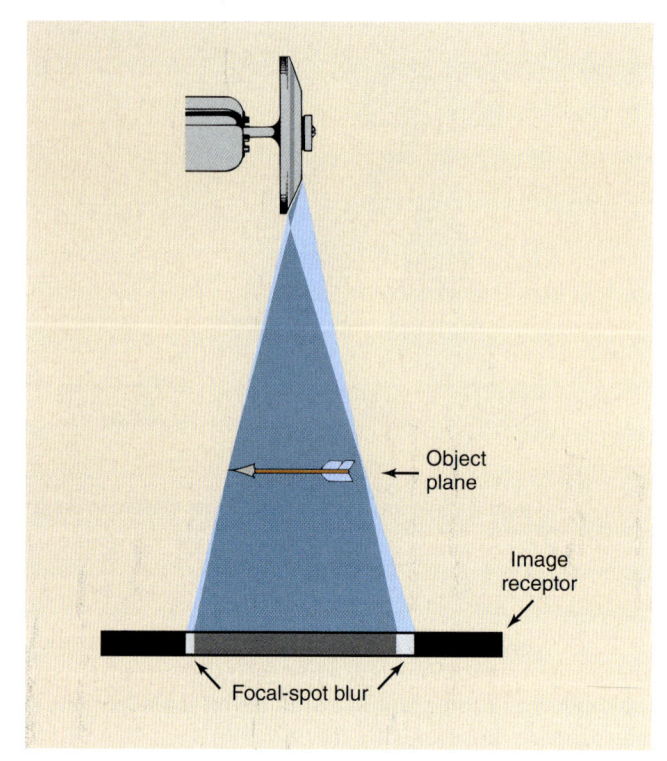

FIG. 16.12 Focal-spot blur is caused by the effective size of the focal spot, which is larger to the cathode side of the image.

Focal-Spot Blur

Thus far, our discussion of the geometric factors that affect digital image quality has assumed that x-rays are emitted from a point source. In actual practice, there is no point source of x-radiation but rather a roughly rectangular source that varies in size from approximately 0.1 to 1.5 mm on a side, depending on the type of x-ray tube that is in use.

Fig. 16.12 illustrates the result of using x-ray tubes with measurable effective focal spots. The point of the object arrow in Fig. 16.12 does not appear as a point in the image plane because the x-rays used to image that point originate throughout the rectangular source.

> Focal-spot blur occurs because the focal spot is not a point.

A blurred region on the radiograph over which the radiographer has little control results because the effective focal spot has measurable size. This phenomenon is called **focal-spot blur**, and it is undesirable. As illustrated, it is greater on the cathode side of the image.

The geometric relationships that govern magnification also influence focal-spot blur. As the geometry of the source, object, and image is altered to produce greater magnification, increased focal-spot blur is produced. Consequently, these conditions should be avoided when possible.

> Focal-spot blur is relatively unimportant for determining spatial resolution. Pixel size is most important.

The region of focal-spot blur can be calculated with the use of similar triangles. If an arrowhead were positioned near the x-ray tube target, the size of the focal-spot blur would be larger than that of the effective focal spot (Fig. 16.13A). In general, the object is much closer to the image receptor; therefore the focal-spot blur is much smaller than the effective focal spot (Fig. 16.13B).

From these drawings, one can see that two similar triangles are described. Therefore the ratio of SOD to OID is the same as the ratio of the sizes of the effective focal spot and the focal-spot blur.

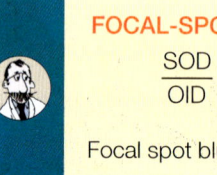

FOCAL-SPOT BLUR

$$\frac{SOD}{OID} = \frac{\text{Effective focal spot}}{\text{Focal spot blur}}$$

$$\text{Focal spot blur} = \frac{(\text{Effective focal spot})OID}{SOD}$$

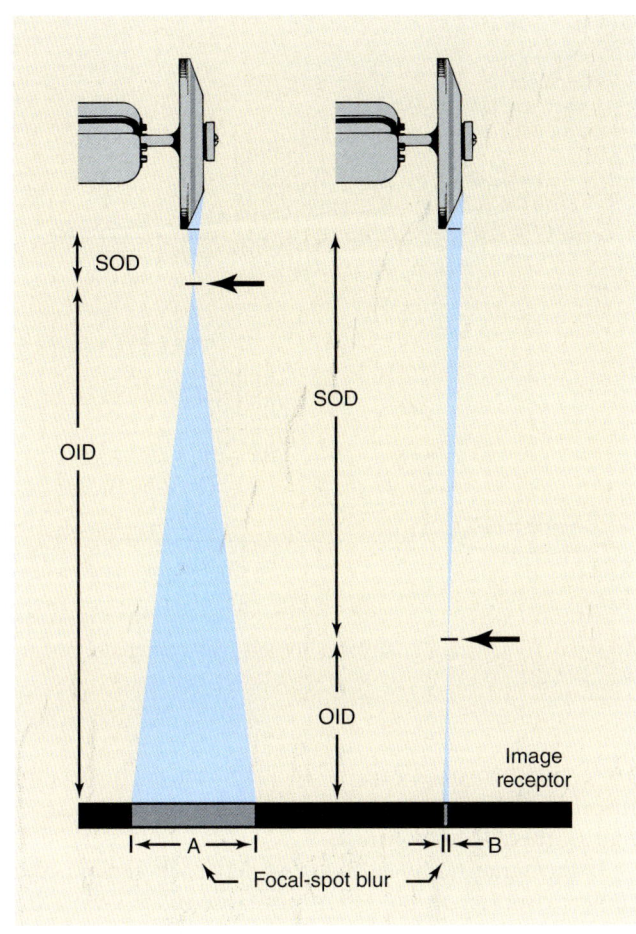

FIG. 16.13 Focal-spot blur is small when the object-to-image receptor distance (*OID*) is small. *SOD,* Source-to-object distance.

Question: An x-ray tube target with a 0.6-mm effective focal spot is used to image a calcified nodule estimated to be 8 cm from the anterior chest wall. If the radiograph is taken in a PA projection at 180 cm SID with a tabletop to image receptor separation of 5 cm, what will be the size of the focal-spot blur?

Answer: Effective focal spot = 0.6 mm; OID = 13 cm
SOD = 167 cm

$$\text{Focal spot blur} = \frac{(0.6 \text{ mm})(13 \text{ cm})}{(167 \text{ cm})}$$
$$= 0.047 \text{ cm}$$

To minimize focal-spot blur, you should use small focal spots and position the patient so that the anatomical part under examination is close to the image receptor. The SID is usually fixed but should be as large as possible.

Pixel size in digital radiography is in the 80 to 150 μm range. The focal spot you choose will be determined more by anode heat capacity than spatial resolution.

Heel Effect

The heel effect, introduced in Chapter 7, is described as varying radiation intensity across the x-ray field in the anode-cathode direction caused by attenuation of x-rays in the heel of the anode. Another characteristic of the heel effect is unrelated to x-ray intensity but affects focal-spot blur.

The size of the effective focal spot is not constant across the image receptor. An x-ray tube said to have a 1-mm focal (1000 μm) spot has a smaller effective focal spot on the anode side and a larger effective focal spot on the cathode side (Fig. 16.14).

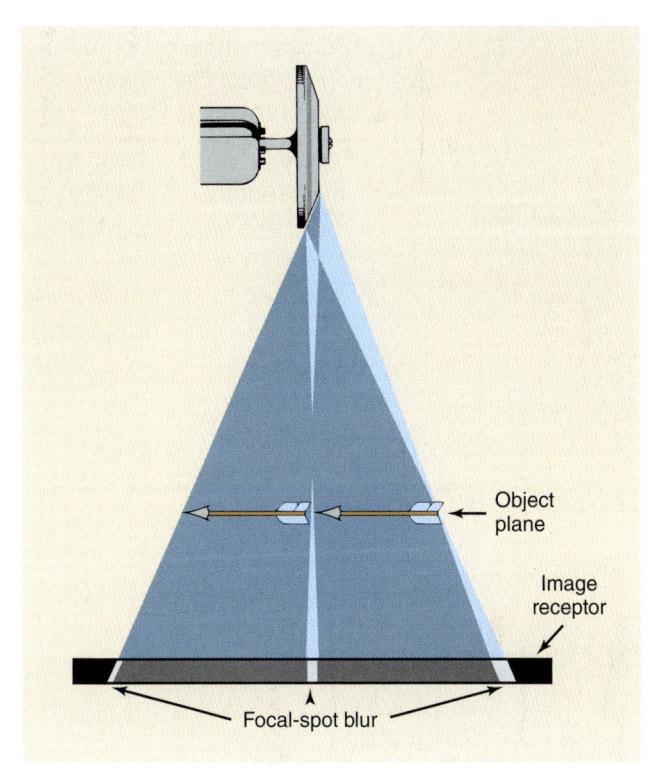

FIG. 16.14 Effective focal spot size is largest on the cathode side; therefore focal-spot blur is greatest on the cathode side.

> The focal-spot blur is small on the anode side and large on the cathode side of the image receptor.

This variation in focal-spot size results in variation in focal-spot blur. Consequently, images toward the cathode side of a radiograph have a higher degree of blur and poorer spatial resolution than those to the anode side. This is clinically significant when x-ray tubes with small target angles are used at short SIDs. Table 16.1 lists radiographic examinations that should be performed with consideration for the heel effect.

SUBJECT FACTORS

The second general group of factors that affect digital image quality involves the patient (Table 16.2). These factors are those associated not so much with the positioning of the patient as with the selection of a

TABLE 16.1	Patient Positioning for Examinations That Can Take Advantage of the Heel Effect	
Examination	Position Toward the Cathode	Position Toward the Anode
PA chest	Abdomen	Neck
Abdomen	Abdomen	Pelvis
Femur	Hip	Knee
Humerus	Shoulder	Elbow
AP thoracic spine	Abdomen	Neck
AP lumbar spine	Abdomen	Pelvis

AP, Anteroposterior; *PA*, posteroanterior.

TABLE 16.2	Patient-Related Factors

- Subject contrast
- Patient thickness
- Tissue mass density
- Effective atomic number
- Object shape

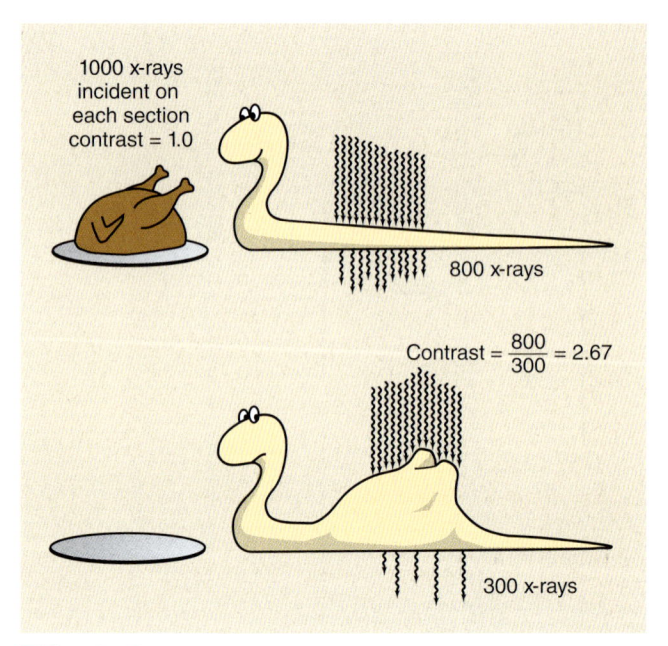

FIG. 16.15 Different anatomical thicknesses contribute to subject contrast.

radiographic technique that properly compensates for the patient's size, shape, and tissue composition. Patient positioning is basically a requirement that is associated with the geometric factors that affect digital image quality.

Subject Contrast

The contrast of a digital image viewed on a digital display device is called **radiographic contrast**. As indicated previously, radiographic contrast is a function of image receptor contrast and subject contrast. In fact, radiographic contrast is simply the product of image receptor contrast and subject contrast.

> Radiographic contrast = Image receptor contrast × Subject contrast

Image receptor contrast is selectable with postprocessing and depends on bit depth and window/level selection by the radiographer. Postprocessing is most important for digital image contrast.

Several of these subject factors were discussed in Chapter 10 in terms of their relation to the attenuation of an x-ray beam. The effect of each on subject contrast is a direct result of differences in attenuation in body tissues.

Patient Thickness. Given a standard composition, a thick body section attenuates a greater number of x-rays than does a thin body section (Fig. 16.15). The same number of x-rays is incident on each section; therefore the contrast of the incident x-ray beam is zero, that is, there is no contrast.

If the same number of x-rays left each section, the subject contrast would be 1.0. Because more x-rays are transmitted through thin body sections than through thick ones, however, subject contrast is greater than 1. The degree of subject contrast is directly proportional to the relative number of x-rays leaving those sections of the body.

Tissue Mass Density. Different sections of the body may have equal thicknesses yet different mass densities. Tissue mass density is an important factor that affects subject contrast. Consider, for example, a radiograph of different salad ingredients (Fig. 16.16). These materials have the same thickness and chemical composition. However, they have slightly different mass density from water and therefore will be imaged. The effect of mass density on subject contrast is demonstrated in Fig. 16.17.

Effective Atomic Number. Another important factor that affects subject contrast is the effective atomic number of the tissue being examined. In Chapter 10, it was shown that Compton scattering is independent of atomic number, but photoelectric effect varies in proportion to the cube of the atomic number.

The effective atomic numbers of tissues of interest were reported in Table 10.3. In the diagnostic range of x-ray energies, the photoelectric effect is of considerable importance; therefore subject contrast is influenced greatly by the effective atomic number of the tissue that is being radiographed. When the effective atomic number of adjacent tissues is very much different, subject contrast is very high.

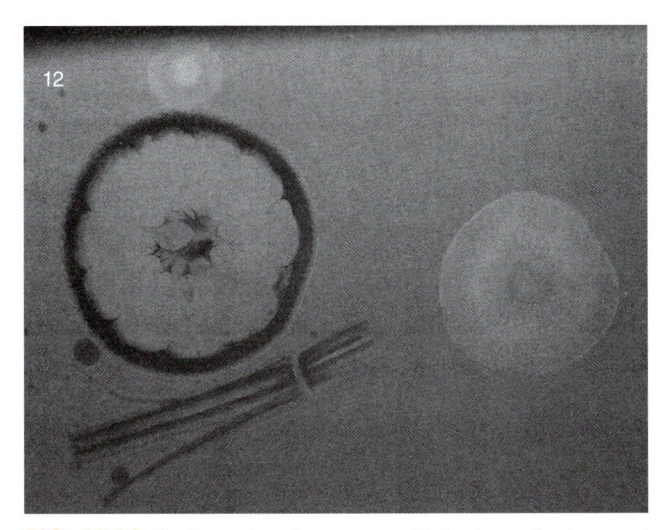

FIG. 16.16 Radiographs of an orange, kiwi, piece of celery, and chunk of carrot show the effects of subtle differences in mass density. (Courtesy Marcy Barnes, Lexington Community College.)

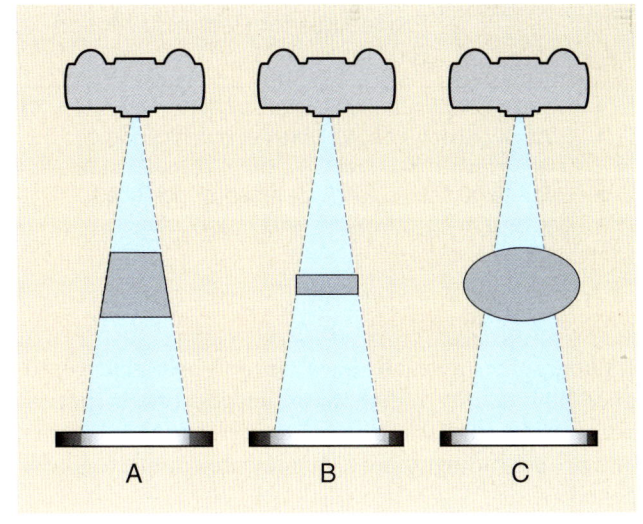

FIG. 16.18 The shape of the anatomy being imaged contributes to subject contrast.

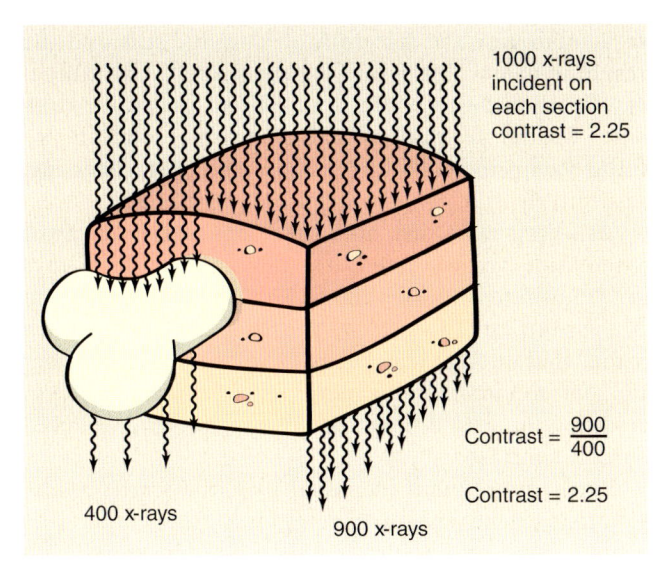

FIG. 16.17 Variation in tissue mass density contributes to subject contrast.

Subject contrast can be enhanced greatly by the use of contrast media. The high atomic numbers of iodine (Z = 53) and barium (Z = 56) result in extremely high subject contrast. Contrast media are effective because they accentuate subject contrast through enhanced photoelectric absorption.

Object Shape. The shape of the anatomical structure under investigation influences its radiographic quality, not only through its geometry but also through its contribution to subject contrast. Obviously, a structure that has a form that coincides with the x-ray beam has maximum subject contrast (Fig. 16.18A).

All other anatomical shapes have reduced subject contrast because of the change in thickness that they present across the x-ray beam. Fig. 16.18B and C illustrates two shapes that result in reduced subject contrast.

This characteristic of the subject that affects subject contrast is also the spatial resolution and contrast resolution of any anatomical structure. It is most troublesome during interventional radiology, in which vessels with small diameters are examined.

Motion Blur

Movement of the patient or the x-ray tube during exposure results in blurring of the radiographic image. This loss of radiographic quality, called **motion blur**, may result in repeated radiographs and therefore should be avoided.

Normally, motion of the x-ray tube is not a problem. Sometimes the table or a restraining device is caused to move by auxiliary equipment, such as a moving grid mechanism.

> Patient motion is usually the cause of motion blur.

The radiographer can reduce motion blur by carefully instructing the patient, "Take a deep breath and hold it. Don't move."

Patient motion of two types may occur. Voluntary motion of the limbs and muscles is controlled by immobilization. Involuntary motion of the heart and lungs is controlled by short exposure time.

Motion blur is affected primarily by four factors. By observing the guidelines listed in Table 16.3, the radiographer can reduce motion blur. Note that the last two items in this list have the same relation to motion blur as to focal-spot blur. With the use of low ripple power and high-speed image receptors, motion has been virtually eliminated as a clinical problem.

TABLE 16.3	Procedures for Reducing Motion Blur

- Use the shortest possible exposure time.
- Restrict patient motion by providing instruction or using a restraining device.
- Use a large source-to-image receptor distance.
- Use a small object-to-image receptor distance.

TOOLS FOR IMPROVED IMAGE QUALITY

Radiographers normally have the tools available to produce high-quality radiographic images. Proper patient preparation, the selection of proper image receptors, and proper radiographic technique are complex, related concepts.

For any given radiographic examination, each of these factors must be properly interpreted and applied. A small change in one may require a compensating change in another.

Patient Positioning

The importance of patient positioning should now be clear. Proper patient positioning requires that the anatomical structure under investigation be placed as close to the image receptor as is practical and that the axis of this structure should lie in a plane that is parallel to the plane of the image receptor. The central ray should be incident on the center of the structure. Finally, the patient must be immobilized effectively to minimize motion blur.

To be able to position patients properly, the radiographer must have a good knowledge of human anatomy. If multiple structures are being radiographed and are to be imaged with uniform magnification, they must be positioned at the same distance from the image receptor. The various techniques that are applied to radiographic positioning are designed to produce radiographs with minimal image distortion.

Image Receptors

Usually a standard type of digital image receptor is used throughout a radiology department for a given type of examination. In general, extremity and soft tissue radiographs are taken with small pixel image receptors (70–100 μm). That can result in higher patient radiation dose. Image receptors designed with larger pixels (100–150 μm) therefore result in lower patient radiation dose.

Selection of Technique Factors

Before each examination, the radiographer must select the optimum radiographic technique factors, that is, kVp, mAs, and exposure time. Many considerations determine the value of each of these factors, and they are complexly interrelated. Few generalizations are possible.

One generalization that can be made for all radiographic exposures is that the time of exposure should be as short as possible. Image quality is improved by short exposure times that cause reduced motion blur. One of the reasons why three-phase and high-frequency generators are better than single-phase generators is that shorter exposure times are possible with the former.

Keep exposure time as short as possible.

Similar simple statements cannot be made about the selection of kVp or mA. Because time is to be kept to a minimum, the selection of kVp and mA and the resulting mAs value should be considered. The radiographer should strive for low patient radiation dose since spatial resolution and contrast resolution are influenced principally by pixel size and postprocessing, respectively.

As kVp is increased, both the intensity and energy of x-radiation are increased; a greater number of x-rays are transmitted through the patient, so a higher portion of the primary beam reaches the image receptor. Among x-rays that interact with the patient, the relative number of Compton interactions increases with increasing kVp, resulting in less differential absorption and reduced subject contrast.

Furthermore, with increased kVp, the scatter radiation that reaches the image receptor is greater; therefore radiographic noise is higher. The result of increased kVp is loss of contrast, but such loss is minimal. Increasing kVp allows the radiographer to reduce mAs, resulting in reduced patient radiation dose.

A number of other factors influence radiographic contrast and hence digital image quality. Adding filtration to the x-ray tube reduces x-ray beam intensity but increases x-ray beam energy. Table 16.4 represents an attempt to summarize the principal factors that influence the making of a digital radiograph.

The continuing trend in radiographic technique is to use higher kVp with a compensating reduction in mAs to produce a quality radiograph while reducing the patient radiation dose and the likelihood of an ordered reexamination because of an error in technique.

TABLE 16.4 Principal Factors That May Affect the Making of a Radiograph

Increase in	Patient Dose	Radiographic Magnification	Focal-Spot Blur	Motion Blur	Absorption Blur	Image Contrast
Patient thickness	+	+	+	+	+	−
Field size	+	0	0	0	0	−
Use of contrast media	0	0	0	0	0	+
Focal-spot size	0	0	+	0	0	0
SID	−	−	−	−	0	0
OID	0	+	+	+	0	+
mAs	+	0	0	0	0	+ or −
Time	+	0	0	+	0	+ or −
kVp	+	0	0	0	0	−
Voltage ripple	+	0	0	+	0	+
Total filtration	−	0	0	0	0	−

[a]Because the factors in the left-hand column are increased while all other factors remain fixed, cross-referenced conditions are affected as shown: +, increase; −, decrease; 0, no change.
kVp, Kilovoltage peak; *mAs*, milliampere seconds; *OID*, object-to-image receptor distance; *SID*, source-to-image receptor distance.

SUMMARY

Digital image quality is the exactness of representation of the anatomic structure on the radiographic image. Characteristics that make up digital image quality are as follows:

- Spatial resolution, or the ability to image small, high-contrast structures on the radiograph
- Low noise
- Proper speed of the image receptor, which limits patient radiation dose but produces a high-quality, low-noise image

These characteristics and two others—geometric factors and subject factors—combine to determine digital image quality.

Geometric factors that affect digital image quality include magnification and distortion, as well as the advantageous use of object thickness, position, focal-spot blur, and the heel effect.

Subject factors that affect digital image quality depend on the patient. Radiographers must prevent motion blur by encouraging patient cooperation. Also, by measuring patient thickness, recognizing tissue mass density, examining anatomical shape, and evaluating optimal kVp levels, radiographers can produce high-quality radiographic images.

CHALLENGE QUESTIONS

1. Define or otherwise identify the following:
   a. Contrast resolution
   b. Superposition
   c. Image distortion
   d. Focal-spot blur
   e. Magnification radiography
   f. Geometric factors
   g. Motion blur
   h. Image noise
   i. Quantum mottle
   j. Spatial resolution
2. What principally determines radiographic spatial resolution?
3. What generalization applies to the selection of the three technique factors—kVp, mAs, and time?
4. What is the principal cause of image blur?
5. List three results of the heel effect.
6. A mammogram is taken with a 0.1 mm focal spot x-ray tube of macrocalcifications located 4 cm from the image receptor and therefore 66 cm from the source. What is the focal-spot blur?
7. Compare the focal-spot blur in Question 6 with the 100 μm pixel.
8. What is the result if the image plane and the object plane are not parallel?

246   PART III   X-Ray Imaging

9. How can one reduce quantum mottle?
10. What three principal geometric factors may affect radiographic quality?

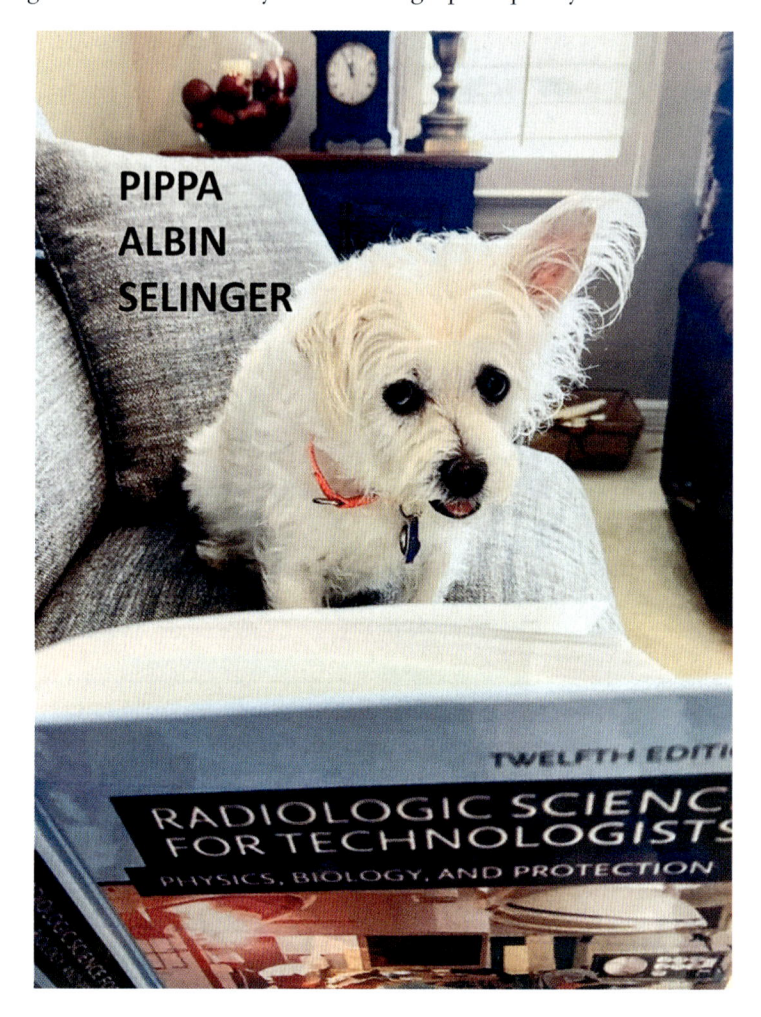

Radiographic Artifacts

CHAPTER 17

OBJECTIVES

At the completion of this chapter, the student should be able to do the following:

1. Discuss three types of digital radiographic imaging artifacts and how to avoid them.
2. Identify the difference between for-processing images and for-presentation images.
3. Describe the basis for data compression and the difference between lossless and lossy compression.
4. Analyze the use of an image histogram in digital radiographic image artifacts.
5. Explain how digital radiographic image artifacts occur because of improper collimation, partition, or alignment.

OUTLINE

Image Receptor Artifacts 248
Software Artifacts 249
  Preprocessing 249
  Image Compression 250
Object Artifacts 252
Image Histogram 252
Collimation and Partition 253
  Alignment 254
Summary 254
Challenge Questions 254

A N ARTIFACT is any false visual feature on a digital image that simulates tissue or obscures tissue. Artifacts interfere with diagnosis and must be avoided. Similar to automobile accidents, artifacts are, by definition, avoidable.

Artifacts can be controlled when the cause of the artifact is understood. In digital radiography (DR), three classifications of artifacts can be described—image receptor, software, and object. The three digital imaging artifact classes are shown in Fig. 17.1 along with the subsets of each.

IMAGE RECEPTOR ARTIFACTS

Image receptors can suffer from rough handling, scratches, and dust (Fig. 17.2). Artifacts produced by dust can be corrected easily with proper cleaning unless the dust is internal to the optics of a computed radiography (CR) imaging system. Fig. 17.3 shows a CR image taken with the image receptor contaminated with residual glue that could not be removed.

Dust on any section of the CR optical path—mirrors and lenses—cannot be corrected by the radiographer and will require professional service. Scratches or a substantial malfunction of pixels likely will require replacement of the IR.

> Digital radiographic image receptors have unique artifacts associated with pixel failure.

DR and CR image receptors should last for the life of the imaging system. There is no such thing as "radiation fatigue" on these IRs. Routine quality control (QC) should include regular documentation of imaging frequency, imaging performance, and the physical condition of each IR, to reduce artifact appearance and help prevent failure. Fig. 17.4 is an example of a QC form for such regular documentation.

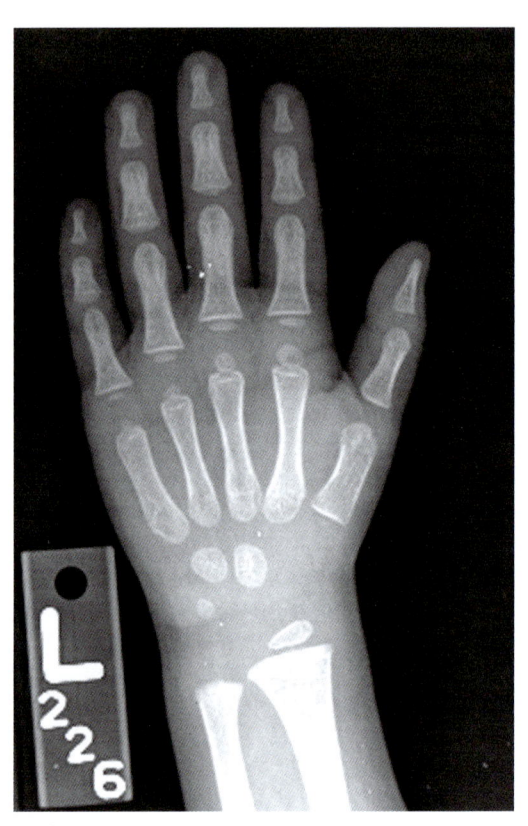

FIG. 17.2 Debris on image receptor in digital radiography can be confused with foreign bodies. (Courtesy Charles Willis, MD Anderson Cancer Center.)

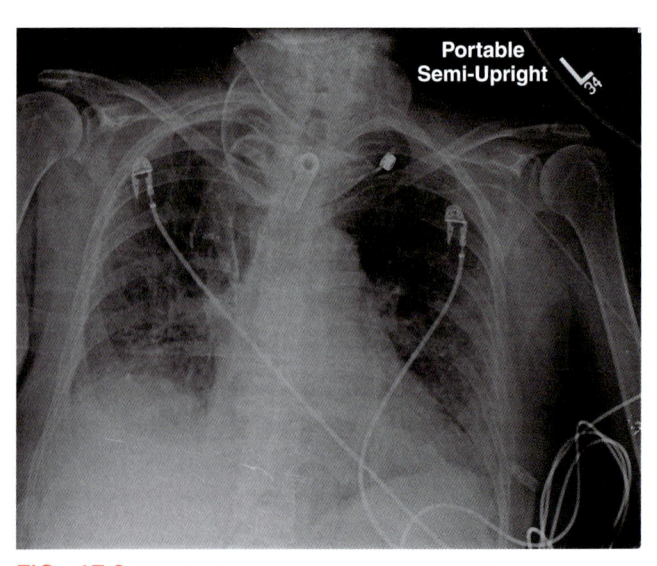

FIG. 17.3 Residual glue on a computed radiography image receptor resulted in this artifact, causing the image receptor to be removed from service. (Courtesy David Clayton, MD Anderson Cancer Center.)

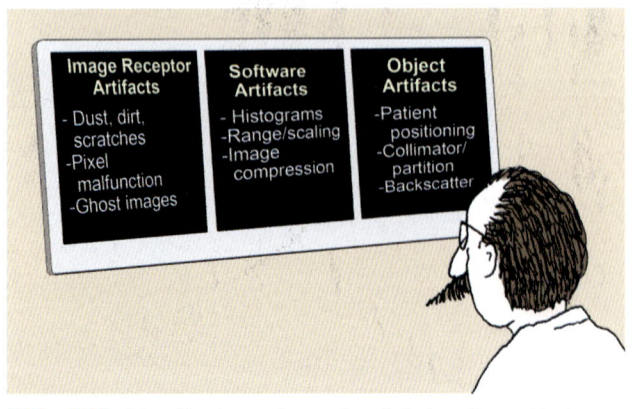

FIG. 17.1 Classification scheme for digital radiographic image artifacts.

> Environmental radiation can contribute to ghost artifacts.

The appearance of ghost images (Fig. 17.5) occurs because of incomplete erasure of a previous image on a CR image receptor. Usually, such artifacts can be corrected by additional signal erasure techniques. If a CR image receptor has not been used for 24 hours, it should be erased again before use. When a completely erased IR is processed, the resultant image should be uniform and free of artifacts.

Rough handling or faulty construction of any digital IR can result in artifacts. Fig. 17.6 shows the result on the image from a damaged CR image receptor.

SOFTWARE ARTIFACTS

Digital radiographic images are obtained as raw data sets. As such, these images are ready "for processing." For-processing images are preprocessing images that are manipulated into "for-presentation" images using **postprocessing** computer assistance technology (review Chapter 13). The radiographer can use postprocessed images for QC; they are also used for interpretation by the radiologist.

Preprocessing

Before an image is prepared for processing, several manipulations of the output data of an image receptor may be necessary to correct for potential artifacts. Such artifacts can occur because of dead pixels or dead rows or columns of pixels (Fig. 17.7).

A single pixel or a single row or column of pixels normally will not interfere with diagnosis. However, many of these defects must be corrected. Correction algorithms specific to each type of digital image receptor use **interpolation** techniques to assign digital values to each dead pixel, row, or column.

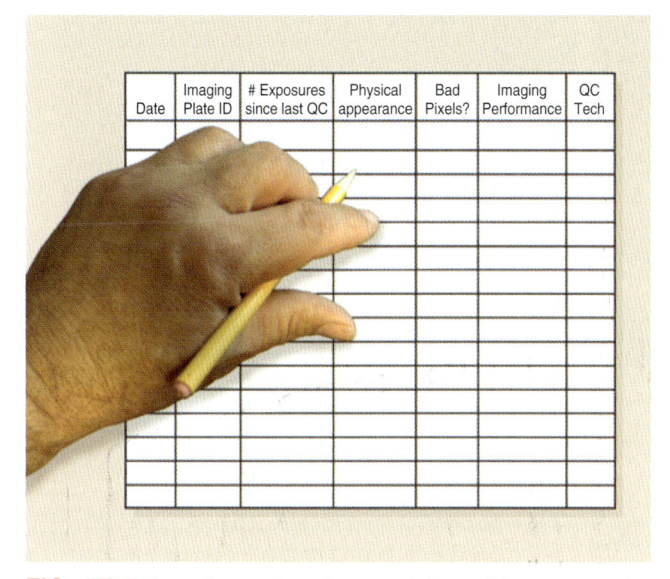

FIG. 17.4 Form for routine documentation of image receptor performance to help reduce artifacts.

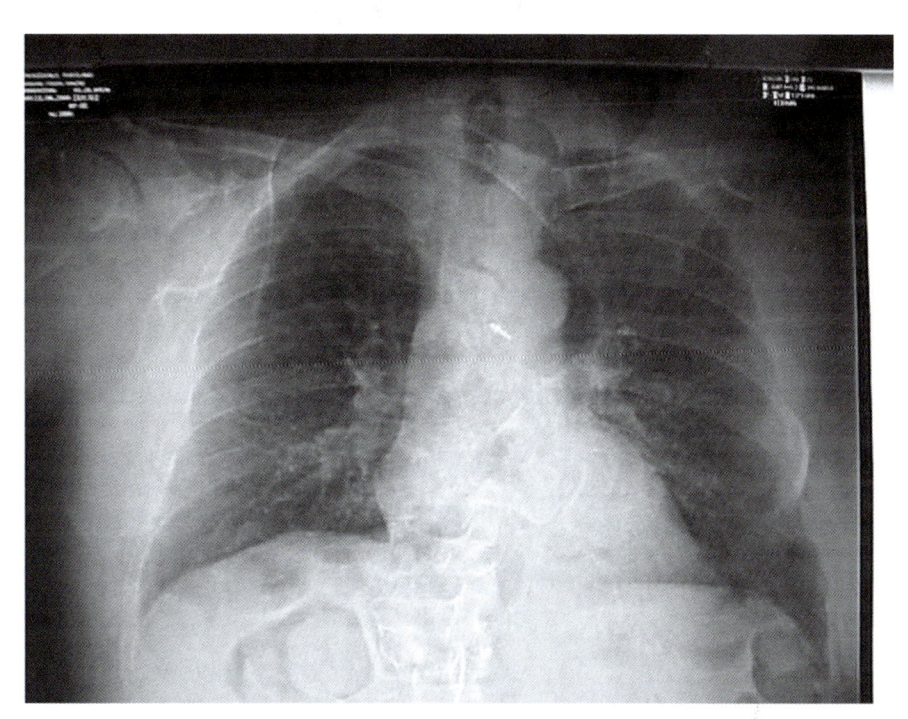

FIG. 17.5 Look closely and you can see the pelvis at the top of this image and the bowel pattern at the bottom. This resulted because the image receptor was not fully erased before the chest examination was performed. (Courtesy Barbara Smith Pruner, Portland Community College.)

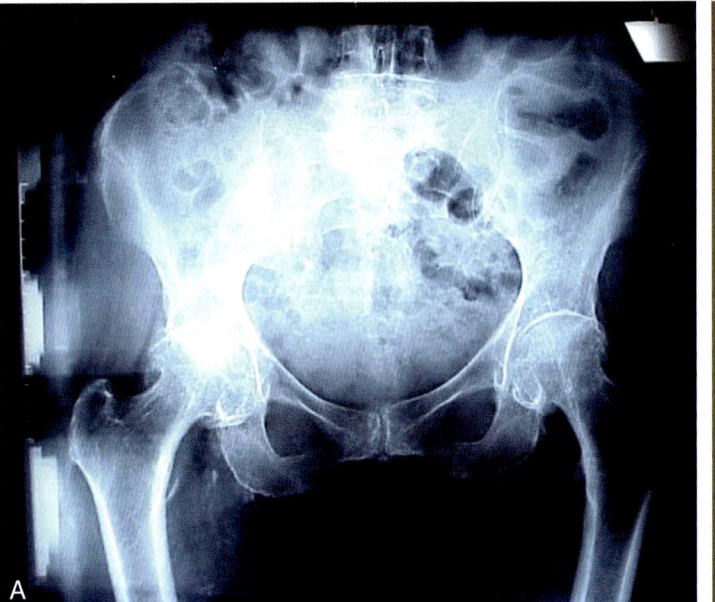

FIG. 17.6 (A) Note the white shapes on the left side, which resulted when the computed radiography image receptor came apart. (B) This is the CR image receptor, which shows corner damage and peeling. (Courtesy Barbara Smith Pruner, Portland Community College.)

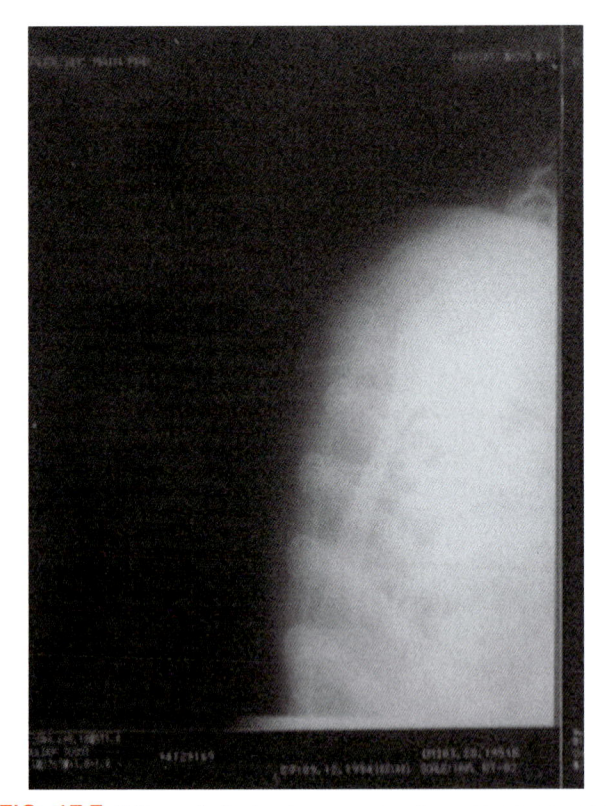

FIG. 17.7 Failure of electronic preprocessing can cause uninterpretable images in digital radiography. (Courtesy Charles Willis, MD Anderson Cancer Center.)

> Interpolation is the process of assigning a value to a dead pixel based on the recorded values of adjacent pixels.

Irradiation of a digital radiographic image receptor by the raw x-ray beam may show variations over the image, producing an irregular pattern that could interfere with diagnosis (Fig. 17.8A). With this irregular pattern, a preprocessing manipulation known as **flatfielding** is performed, resulting in a uniform response to a uniform x-ray beam (see Fig. 17.8B).

> Flatfielding is a preprocessing software correction that is performed to equalize the response of each pixel to a uniform x-ray beam.

CR image receptors are highly sensitive to background radiation and scatter x-rays. If a CR image receptor has not been used for several days, it should be inserted into the reader for re-erasure (Fig. 17.9). The practice of leaving cassettes in a supposedly "radiation-safe" area in an x-ray room during an examination must be discouraged.

Image Compression

Digital radiographic imaging becomes ever more robust in terms of the digital data files generated. This would

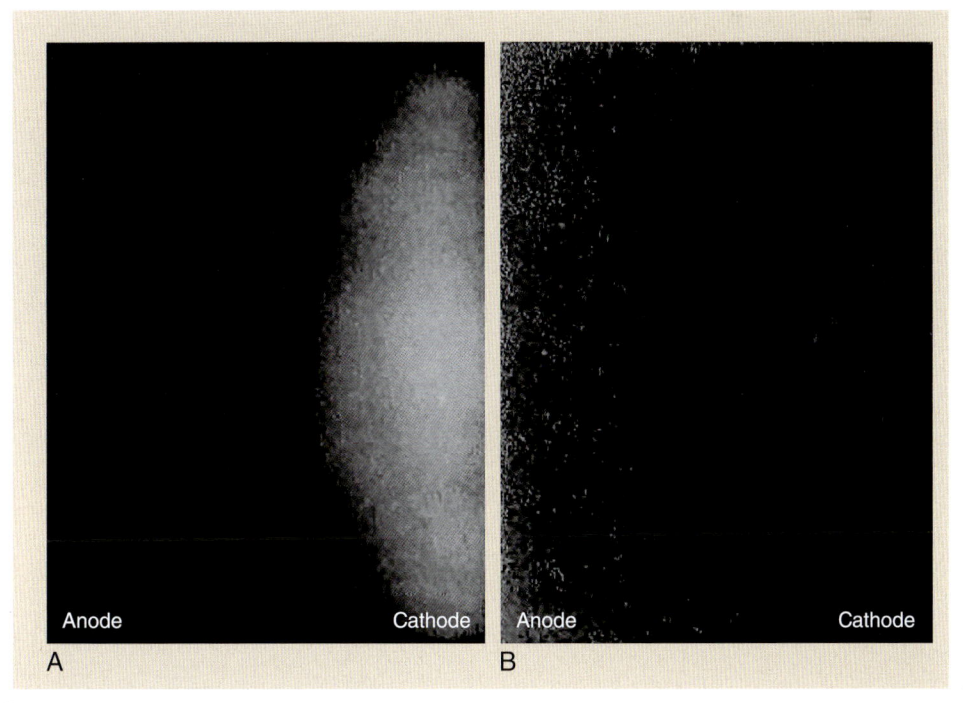

FIG. 17.8 (A) An image receptor exposed to a raw x-ray beam may show a heel-effect response. (B) Flatfielding preprocessing can make the response uniform. (Courtesy Charles Willis, MD Anderson Cancer Center.)

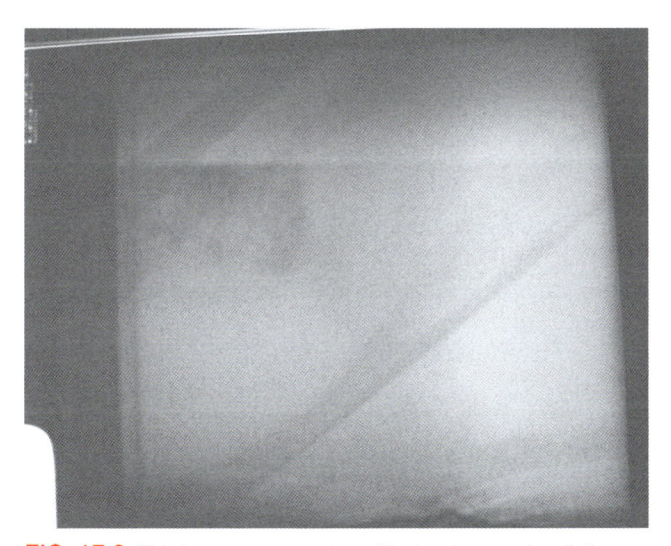

FIG. 17.9 This image was produced by background radiation on a computed radiography image receptor that had not been used for days. (Courtesy Barbara Smith Pruner, Portland Community College.)

TABLE 17.1	Approximate Digital File Sizes for Various Imaging Modalities
Image Modality	**File Size per Image (MB)**
Nuclear medicine	2
Magnetic resonance imaging	5
Computed tomography	10
Computed radiography	20
Digital radiography	20
Digital mammography	50

not represent a problem if it were not for increasing application of teleradiology, which requires the electronic transmission of images. Table 17.1 presents the relative file sizes per image for various digital imaging modalities.

At up to 50 MB per image on a 24 × 30-cm image receptor (2^{16} dynamic range and 50-μm pixel size), a four-view digital mammography study can generate 200 MB. Transmitting and archiving this amount of data is technically difficult; therefore **compression** techniques can be used.

Data compression takes advantage of redundancy of data, as occurs with exposure to the raw x-ray beam when all values are the same. Such compression techniques are described as either **lossless** or **lossy**.

An image data file that is compressed in a lossless mode is one that can be reconstructed to be exactly the same as the original image. Lossless compression reduces the image data file to 10% (10:1) to 50% (2:1) of the original file. However this is not satisfactory for large image files because transmission time and data manipulation time can still be unacceptable.

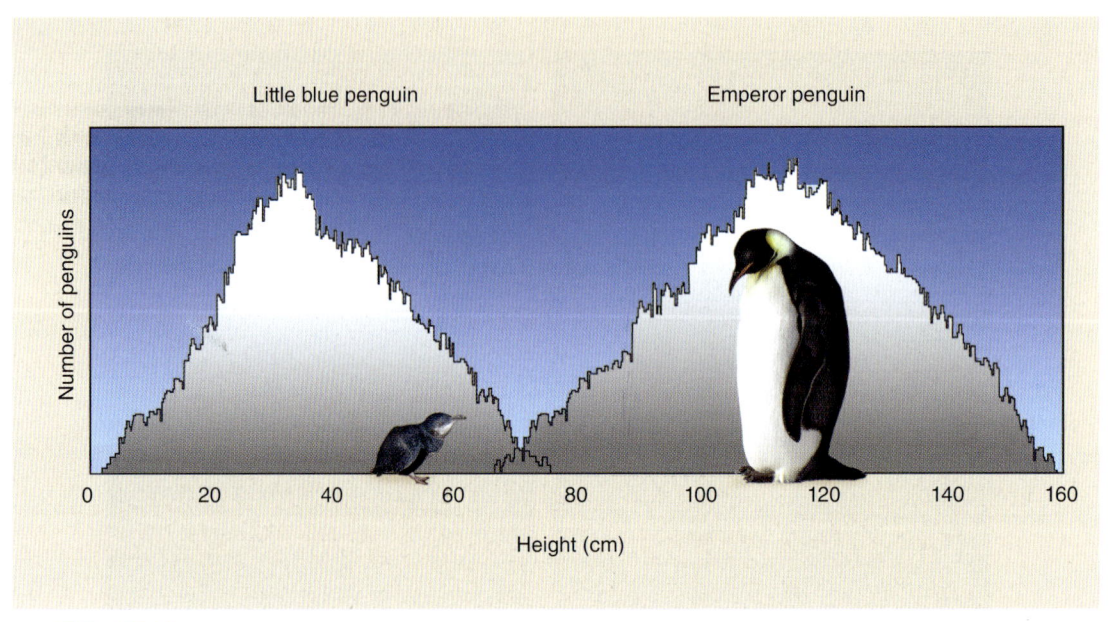

FIG. 17.10 This histogram is a plot of the number of penguins as a function of the height of each penguin.

Lossy compression, which can provide compression factors of up to 100:1 or greater, can be used on images in which exact measurement or fine detail is not required.

> Lossless compression up to 3:1 generally is considered acceptable and helpful in digital radiographic image management.

Lossy compression is that which is greater than an order of magnitude of compression; that is, greater than 10:1 compression. Such a level of compression supports teleradiology but not computer-aided detection (CAD), image archiving, or artificial intelligence (AI). AI systems require uncompressed preprocessing images (see Chapter 28).

Compressed images may cause the artificial intelligence system to miss lesions because of the compression artifact, which actually represents a lack of data. Lossy compression is not acceptable for archiving any images for this reason.

OBJECT ARTIFACTS

Object artifacts can arise from radiographer errors in patient positioning, x-ray beam collimation, and histogram selection. Backscatter radiation also can be troublesome because of the sensitivity of the radiographic IR.

If a lot of scattering material is present behind the IR, backscatter radiation can cause a phantom image. If this type of artifact is discovered, the back side of the IR should be shielded to reduce backscatter x-rays.

Image Histogram

Digital radiographic image histograms are very important for digital image production. However, they can be the source of bothersome digital radiographic image artifacts if they are not properly understood and manipulated.

All digital radiographic imaging systems have the ability to evaluate the original image data through histogram analysis. A histogram is a plot of the frequency of appearance of a given object characteristic.

A sample histogram is shown in Fig. 17.10, where the heights of 500 emperor penguins and 500 little blue penguins are plotted. The average height of emperor penguins is approximately 110 cm (range, 60–160 cm). The same value for the little blue penguins is approximately 30 cm (range, 15–80 cm).

> A histogram is a graph of frequency of occurrence versus digital value intervals.

A histogram is a discrete plot of values rather than a continuous plot. The histogram in Fig. 17.10 is a plot of the number of penguins (frequency) that have a given height as a function of that height (value interval). Because there are two penguin populations, two peaks are evident on this histogram.

Consider the simulated digital chest radiograph of Fig. 17.11A, where each region of the image can be

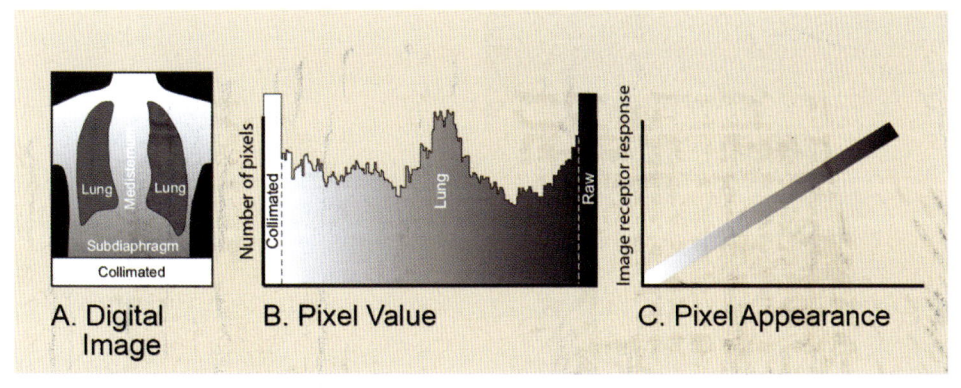

FIG. 17.11 (A) Region of a simulated digital chest radiograph. (B) The corresponding image histogram. (C) The placement of each region in A on the response curve of the digital image receptor.

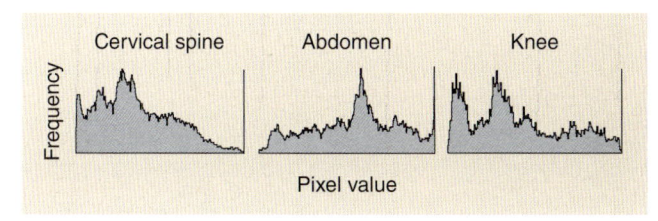

FIG. 17.12 Characteristic histograms for cervical spine, abdomen, and knee.

represented by the frequency distribution of the digital values of each pixel, as shown in Fig. 17.11B. The location of those image regions on the digital IR response curve is shown in Fig. 17.11C. The relative shape of this histogram is characteristic of all posteroanterior (PA) chest digital radiographs.

Even more important is the fact that the shape of an image histogram is characteristic of each anatomical projection. Fig. 17.12 shows the characteristic shapes of image histograms of various radiographic examinations.

Most digital radiographic imaging systems have the ability to store and analyze characteristic image histograms for each radiographic projection. By storing 50 PA chest image histograms and averaging the value of each frequency interval, a representative histogram is produced for each IR. The histogram can be regularly updated from newer images.

This places an additional responsibility on the radiographer. In addition to selecting technique, the radiographer must engage the appropriate histogram before examination so as to apply the appropriate reconstruction algorithm to the final image (Fig. 17.13).

Collimation and Partition

If the x-ray exposure field is not properly collimated, sized, and positioned, exposure field recognition errors may occur. These can lead to histogram analysis errors because signal outside the exposure field is included in the histogram. The result is very dark or very light or very noisy images (Fig. 17.14).

> Automatic radiation field recognition is essential for artifact-free images.

Digital radiographic image receptors are available in the standard sizes shown in Table 17.2.

Collimation of the projected area x-ray beam is important for patient radiation dose reduction and for improved image contrast. As discussed in Chapter 41, proper collimation is particularly important because of the routine use of automatic exposure control (AEC). When specific area patient shielding is used, the collimated-ray field **must not interact with the shield**, and the shield must be properly positioned.

For example, when a specific area shield is a gonad shield (male or female), and the useful x-ray beam interacts with the shield because of improper collimation or shield placement, patient radiation dose may be increased. Both poor collimation and improper shield placement drive the AEC, which results in a higher patient radiation dose.

In DR, proper collimation has the added value of defining the image histogram. If improperly collimated, the histogram can be improperly analyzed, resulting in an artifact such as that shown in Fig. 17.15.

> Proper collimation and centering prevent histogram errors that can lead to artifacts.

Digital image receptors normally can recognize even-numbered (i.e., two, four) x-ray exposure fields that are centered and cleanly collimated. Three on one and four on one are not recommended, unless the unexposed

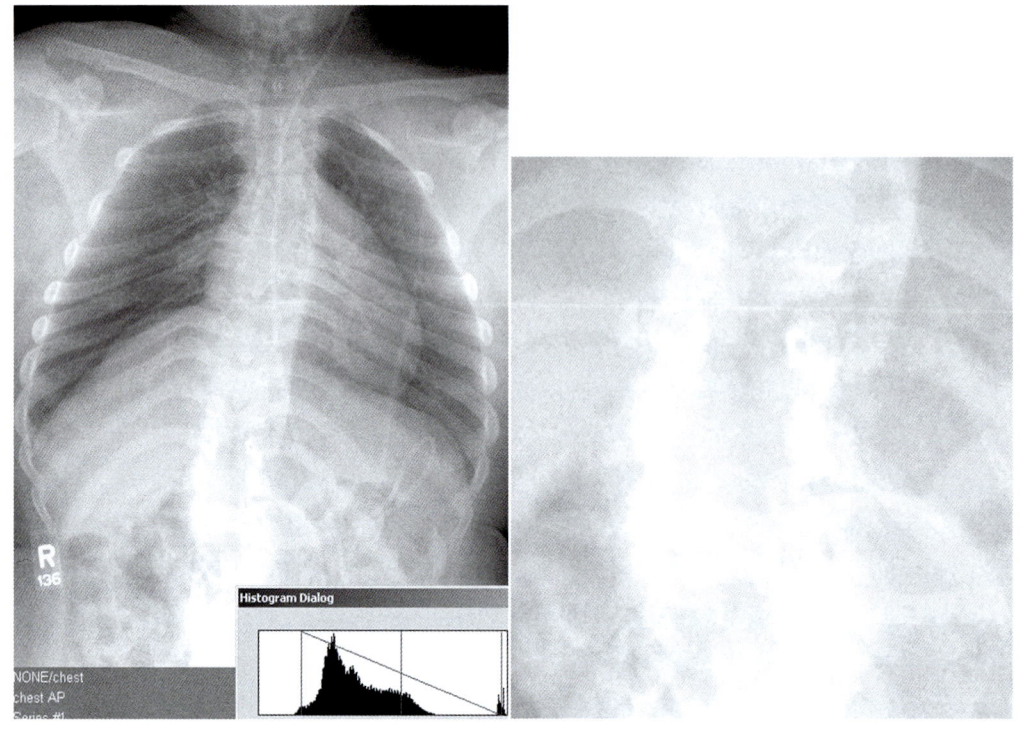

FIG. 17.13 Underexposure in digital radiography causes loss of contrast in dense anatomy because of increased noise. (Courtesy Charles Willis, MD Anderson Cancer Center.)

portion is shielded. Fig. 17.16 is a good example of reduced contrast when three on one is used.

For the image histogram to be properly analyzed, each collimated field should consist of four distinct collimated margins, as shown in Fig. 17.17. The use of three collimated margins usually works, but when fewer than three are used, artifacts may result.

If images are not collimated and centered, IR exposure will not be accurate and cannot be used for image quality evaluation.

If multiple fields are projected onto a single IR, each must have clear, collimated edges and margins between each field. This process, called **partitioning**, allows two or more images to be projected on a single IR. Fig. 17.18 illustrates the opposite situation.

> Partitioning of multiple digital images on a single IR results in proper separation and collimation of each image.

The cause of these collimation artifacts is vendor-algorithm related. The exposure field recognition algorithm is unable to match image histograms if the fields are not clear. This algorithm is based on edge detection or area detection. Further postprocessing of each image requires digital data representative of anatomy—not twice-irradiated or unirradiated portions of the IR.

Alignment

Alignment of the exposure field on the IR is important in the same way and for the same reason as collimation. When an image field, such as that shown in Fig. 17.19, is not oriented with the size and dimensions of the IR, image artifacts can appear.

SUMMARY

Artifacts are misrepresentations of information which interfere with interpretation and must be avoided. Only information which is pertinent to the patient's condition should be in the digital image. The classifications of artifacts are: image artifacts, software artifacts, and object artifacts. Understanding the cause of these artifacts will help the radiographer produce high-quality artifact-free digital images.

CHALLENGE QUESTIONS

1. Define or otherwise identify the following:
   a. Histogram
   b. Artifact
   c. Partition
   d. Image receptor
   e. Compression
   f. CAD
   g. Frequency distribution
   h. Preprocessiing

CHAPTER 17 Radiographic Artifacts 255

TABLE 17.2	Standard Digital Radiography Image Receptor Sizes
18 cm × 24 cm	
18 cm × 43 cm	
20 cm × 40 cm	
24 cm × 30 cm	
35 cm × 35 cm	
35 cm × 43 cm	

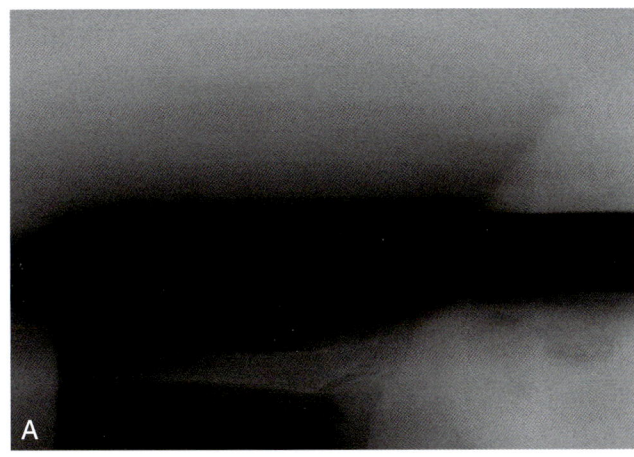

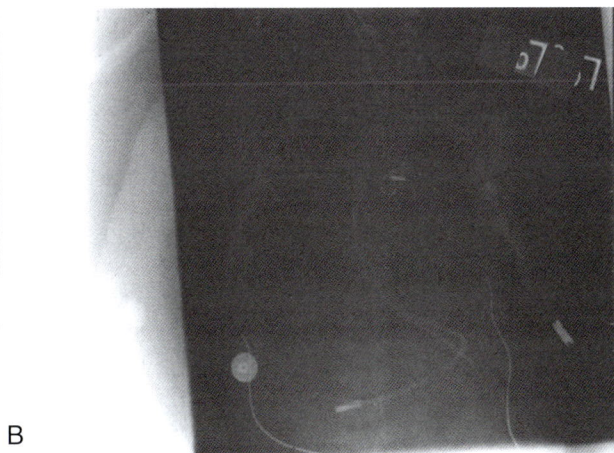

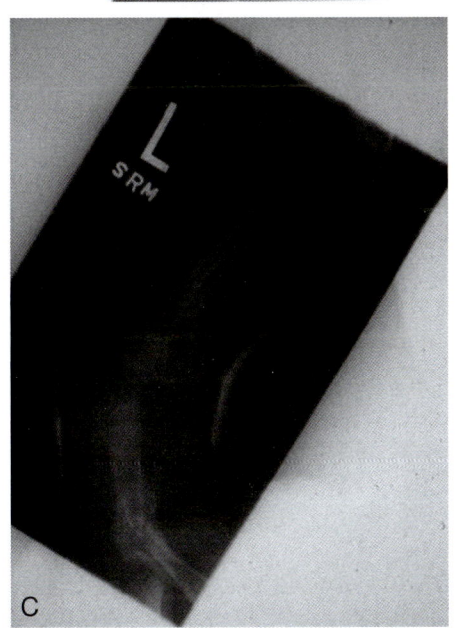

FIG. 17.14 A sampling of histogram analysis errors. (Courtesy Barry Burns†, University of North Carolina.)

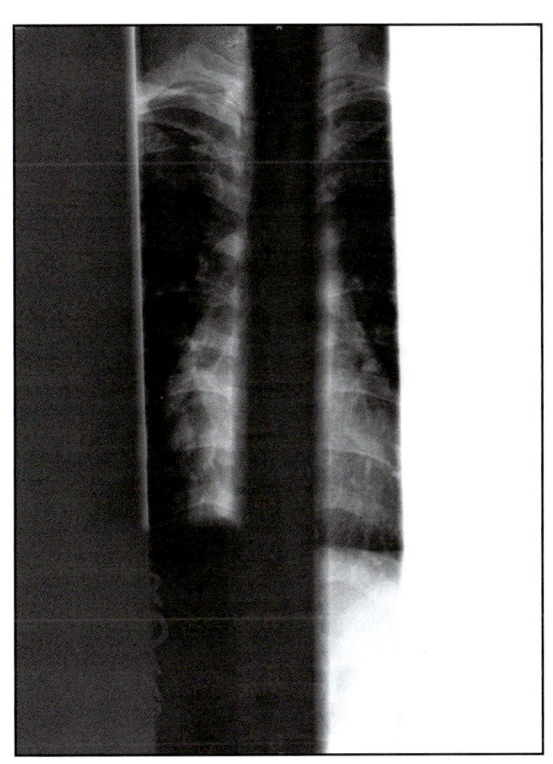

FIG. 17.15 The blacked-out spine on this anteroposterior view was restored by engaging the automatic collimation feature. The white-out on the patient's left side was fixed by postconing that area and then engaging the "collimated image." (Courtesy Dennis Bowman, FluoroRadPro, LLC.)

　　i. Flatfielding
　　j. Radiation fatigue
2. What are the three general classifications of digital image artifacts?
3. What is the preprocessing image, and how is it manipulated?
4. What does it mean when a single digital radiographic image is not properly aligned with the IR? Diagram such a situation.
5. What is the appearance of the radiation response curve for a digital radiographic IR?
6. Which digital imaging modality generates the largest image file, and approximately how large is it?
7. What is the difference between lossless and lossy compression?

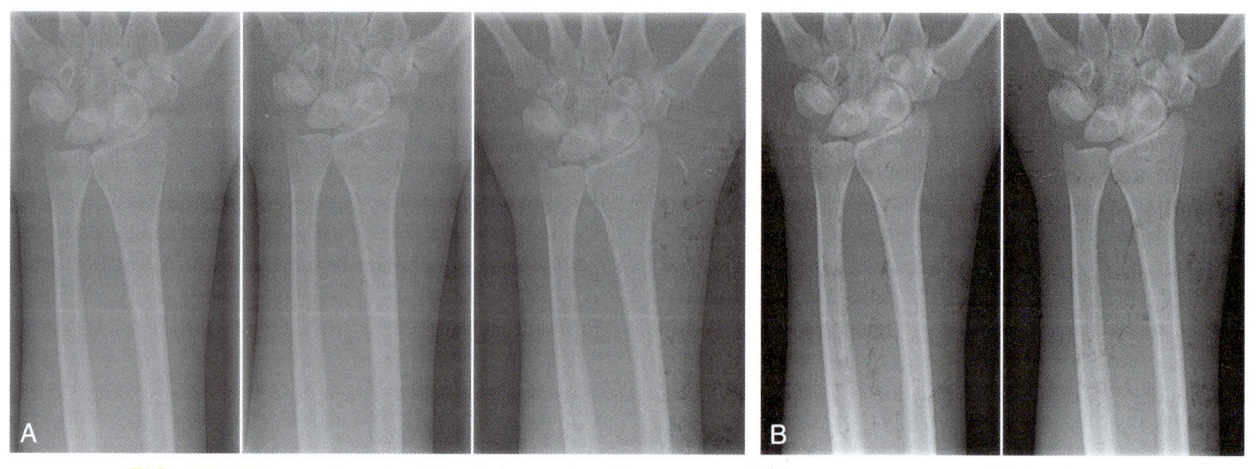

FIG. 17.16 Loss of contrast is obvious when three-on-one (A) versus two-on-one (B) imaging is compared. (Courtesy Barry Burns†, University of North Carolina.)

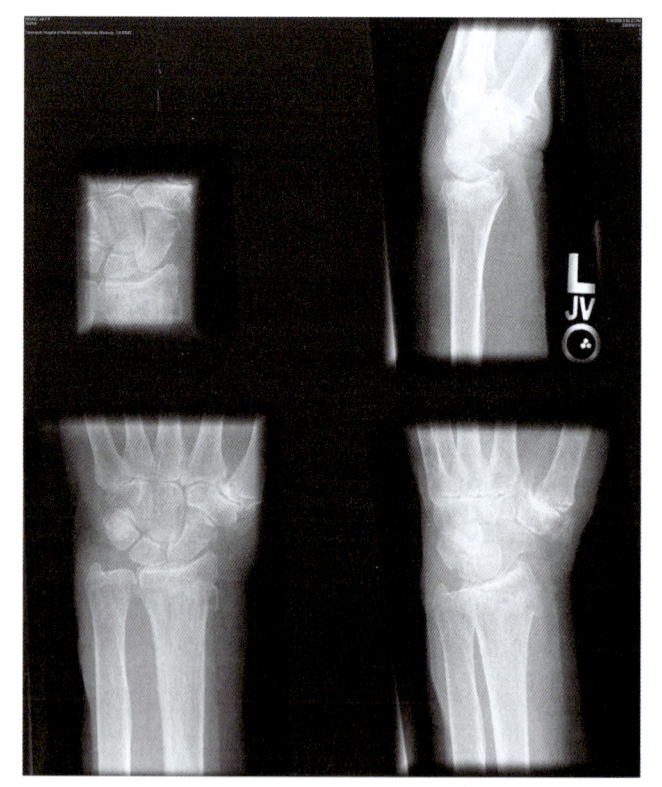

FIG. 17.17 If all four wrist images have the same signal intensity, the radiographer changed technique appropriately. Technique was not properly adjusted for the oblique view in the lower-right region. (Courtesy Dennis Bowman, FluoroRadPro, LLC.)

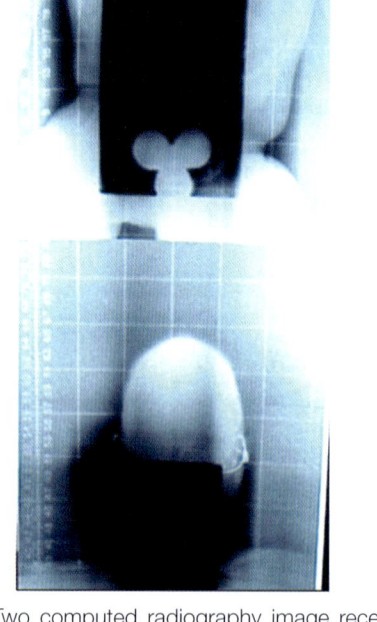

FIG. 17.18 Two computed radiography image receptors used for spine imaging were placed into the processor in the wrong order. (Courtesy Barbara Smith Pruner, Portland Community College.)

8. Diagram improper margins of three digital images on a single IR.
9. How many distinct margins should appear on a digital radiograph?
10. Why is backscatter radiation important in digital radiography?
11. What are the units on each axis of a digital radiographic image histogram?

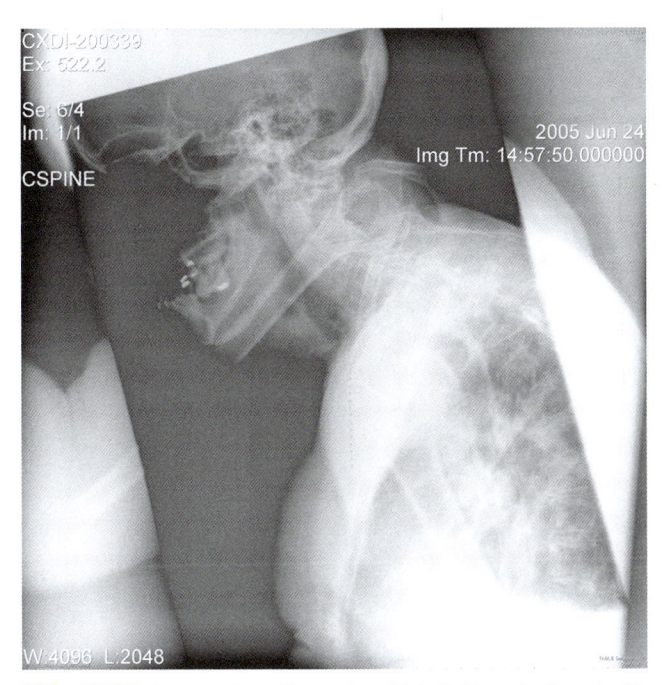

FIG. 17.19 Improperly collimated multiple fields not aligned with the image receptor edge result in overexposure and the artifact seen here. (Courtesy David Clayton, MD Anderson Cancer Center.)

12. What type of algorithm is used to correct for malfunctioning pixels?
13. Why is data compression often required for digital images?
14. What do the two outlying peaks on a digital image histogram represent?
15. What is the life expectancy of a CR image receptor?
16. What happens when the collimated x-ray beam interacts with a patient-specific area shield?
17. Why is it important for the radiographer to select the proper imaging protocol for each digital radiographic examination?
18. How does the heel effect appear on a digital IR?
19. Excessive compression can result in what form of image artifact?
20. Is an image histogram updated from time to time? If so, why?

The answers to the Challenge Questions can be found by logging on to our website at http://evolve.elsevier.com.

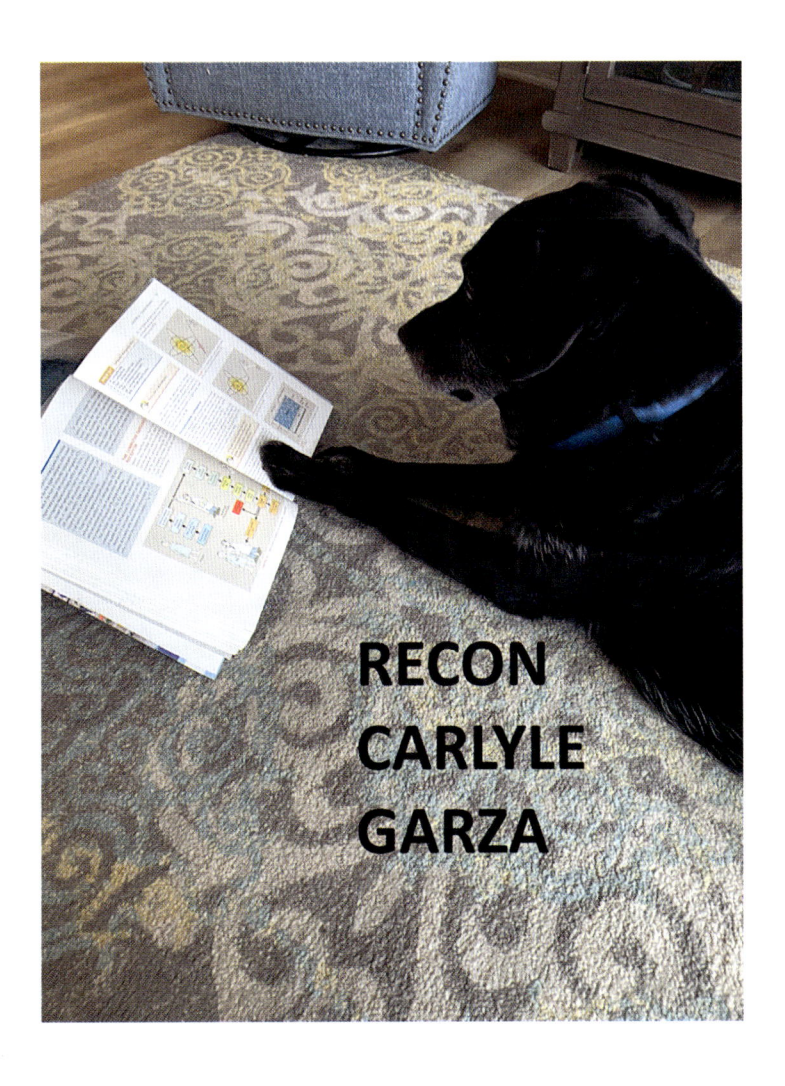

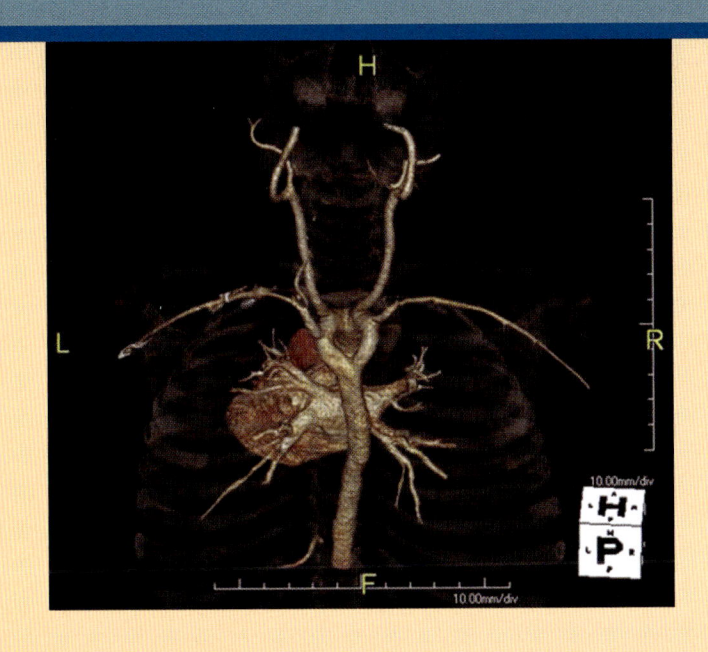

PART IV
ADVANCED MEDICAL IMAGING

CHAPTER 18

Mammography

OBJECTIVES

At the completion of this chapter, the student should be able to do the following:

1. Describe the anatomy of the breast.
2. Identify the recommended intervals for breast self-examination and mammography.
3. Explain the differences between diagnostic and screening mammography.
4. Describe the unique features of a mammography imaging system.
5. Discuss the requirements for compression in mammography.
6. Describe the imge receptor characteristics used for mammography.
7. Itemize the mammographer's quality control duties.

OUTLINE

Soft Tissue Radiography 261
Basis for Mammography 261
  Risk of Breast Cancer 261
  Types of Mammography 262
  Breast Anatomy 262
The Mammographic Imaging System 263
  High-Voltage Generation 264
  Target Composition 264
  Focal-Spot Size 266
  Filtration 267
  Heel Effect 268
  Compression 268

  Grids 269
  Automatic Exposure Control 270
  Magnification Mammography 270
Mammography Quality Control 270
Quality Control Team 271
  Radiologist 271
  Medical Physicist 271
  Mammographer 272
Summary 272
Challenge Questions 272

BREAST CANCER is the second-leading cause of death from cancer in females (lung cancer is first). Each year, approximately 300,000 new cases of breast cancer and 42,000 deaths from breast cancer are reported in the United States. The relative death rate now is declining. One of every eight females will develop breast cancer during her life.

Early detection of breast cancer leads to more effective treatment and fewer deaths. X-ray mammography has proved to be an accurate and simple method of detecting breast cancer, but it is not simple to perform. The mammographer and support staff must have exceptional knowledge, skill, and caring.

In 1992 the US government mandated regulations in the Mammography Quality Standards Act (MQSA), setting standards for image quality, patient radiation dose, personnel qualifications, and examination procedures.

SOFT TISSUE RADIOGRAPHY

Radiographic examination of soft tissues requires selected techniques that differ from those used in conventional radiography. These differences in technique are attributable to substantial differences in the anatomy that is being imaged. In conventional radiography, the subject contrast is great because of large differences in mass density and atomic number among bone, muscle, fat, and lung tissue.

In soft tissue radiography, only muscle and fat are imaged. These tissues have similar effective atomic numbers (see Table 10.3) and similar mass densities (see Table 10.5). Consequently, soft tissue radiographic techniques are designed to enhance differential absorption in these very similar tissues.

A prime example of soft tissue radiography is **mammography**—radiographic examination of the breast. As a distinct type of radiographic examination, mammography was first attempted in the 1920s. In the late 1950s Robert Egan renewed interest in mammography with his demonstration of a successful technique that used low kilovolt peak (kVp), high milliampere seconds (mAs), and direct film exposure—no radiographic intensifying screens.

In the 1960s Wolf and Ruzicka showed that **xeromammography** was superior to direct film exposure at a much lower patient radiation dose. Spatial resolution and contrast resolution were much improved because of characteristic **edge enhancement**—the accentuation of the interface between different tissues. This property is used frequently in the postprocessing of digital images.

Xeromammography was retired by 1990 because single screen-film mammography provided better images at even lower patient radiation dose. Today, digital mammography rules, and it is rapidly being replaced with digital mammographic tomosynthesis (DMT) (see Chapter 22).

Mammography has undergone much change and development. It now enjoys widespread application thanks to the efforts of the American College of Radiology (ACR) volunteer accreditation program and the federally mandated MQSA.

BASIS FOR MAMMOGRAPHY

The principal motivation for the continuing development and improvement of mammography is the high incidence of breast cancer. Until recently, breast cancer had been the leading cancer in females. Unfortunately, lung cancer has surpassed breast cancer as the leading cause of cancer deaths in females, possibly because of the continuing use of smoking tobacco, but certainly because of the success of early breast cancer detection using x-ray mammography.

Risk of Breast Cancer

In 2023 approximately 300,000 new cases of breast cancer were reported in the United States, and this number is growing. However, thanks to early detection, more than 90% of females diagnosed with early-stage disease will survive. Several factors have been identified that increase a female's risk of breast cancer (Table 18.1).

> One of every eight females will develop breast cancer.

Breast cancer is now a disease that is far from fatal. In 1995 the National Cancer Institute reported the first reduction in breast cancer mortality in 50 years, and this trend continues. With early mammographic diagnosis, more than 90% of patients are cured and survive.

One important consideration in the overall efficacy of mammography is patient radiation dose, because radiation can cause breast cancer as well as detect it. However, considerable evidence shows that the mature breast in the screening age group has very low sensitivity to radiation-induced breast cancer. Radiation carcinogenesis (i.e., the induction of cancer) is discussed in Chapter 36.

The dose necessary to produce breast cancer is unknown; however the dose experienced in mammography is well known and is covered in Chapter 41. This chapter concerns the imaging technique, equipment, and procedures used in mammography.

Types of Mammography

Two different types of mammographic examination are conducted. **Screening mammography** is performed on asymptomatic females with the use of a two-view protocol, usually medial lateral oblique and cranial caudad, to detect an unsuspected cancer. **Diagnostic mammography** is performed on patients with symptoms or elevated risk factors. Two or three views of each breast may be required.

Screening mammography in patients 50 years or older reduces cancer mortality. Results of clinical trials show that screening of females in the 40- to 49-year age group is also beneficial in reducing mortality. Because younger females have potentially more years of life left, screening in this group results in more years of life saved.

The American Cancer Society recommends that females perform monthly breast self-examinations; a healthcare professional teaches a female to check her breasts regularly for lumps, thickening of the skin, or any changes in size or shape. Table 18.2 relates the recommended intervals for breast self-examination and screening mammography.

The American Cancer Society also recommends annual breast examination by a physician and a baseline mammogram. A **baseline mammogram** is the first radiographic examination of the breasts and is usually obtained before age 40 years. Radiologists use it for comparison with future mammograms.

The risk of radiation-induced breast cancer resulting from x-ray mammography has been given a lot of attention. However, mammography is considered very safe and effective. The ratio of benefit (lives saved) to risk (possible deaths caused) is estimated at 1000 to 1.

Breast Anatomy

The anatomy of the breast and its tissue characteristics make imaging difficult (Fig. 18.1). Young breasts are dense and are more difficult to image because of glandular tissue. Older breasts are more fatty and easier to image.

Normal breasts consist of three principal tissues: fibrous, glandular, and adipose (fat). In a premenopausal female, the fibrous and glandular tissues are structured into various ducts, glands, and connective tissues. These are surrounded by a thin layer of fat. Postmenopausal breasts are characterized by a degeneration of this fibroglandular tissue and an increase in adipose tissue.

> At low x-ray energy, photoelectric absorption predominates over Compton scattering.

If a malignancy is present, it appears as a distortion of normal ductal and connective tissue patterns. Approximately 80% of breast cancer is ductal and may have associated deposits of **microcalcifications** that appear as small grains of varying size. In terms of detecting breast cancer, microcalcifications smaller than approximately 500 μm are of interest. The incidence of breast cancer is highest in the upper lateral quadrant of the breast (Fig. 18.2).

TABLE 18.1 Risk Factors for Breast Cancer

- Age: The older you are, the higher the risk
- Family history: Mother, sister with breast cancer
- Genetics: Presence of the *BRCA1* or *BRCA2* gene
- Breast architecture: Dense breast tissue, obesity
- Menstruation: Onset before age 12 years
- Menopause: Onset after age 55 years
- Prolonged use of estrogen
- Late age at birth of first child or no children
- Previous radiation therapy to the chest at an early age
- Education: Risk increases with higher level of education
- Socioeconomics: Risk increases with higher socioeconomic status

TABLE 18.2 Recommended Intervals for Breast Examination

	PATIENT AGE		
Examination	<40 Years	40–49 Years	≥50 Years
Self-examination	Monthly[a]	Monthly	Monthly
Physician physical examination	Annually[b]	Annually	Annually
X-ray mammography			
High risk	Baseline	Annually	Annually
Low risk	Baseline	Biannually	Annually

[a]Beginning at age 20 years.
[b]Beginning at age 35 years.

CHAPTER 18 Mammography

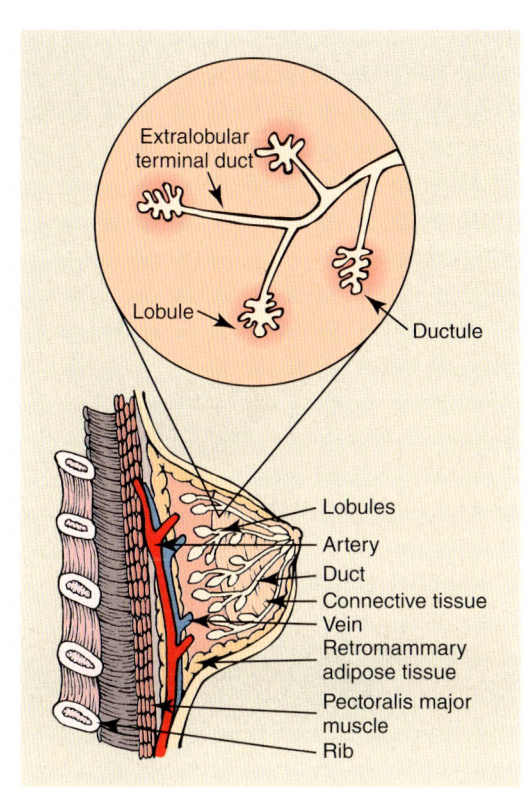

FIG. 18.1 Breast architecture determines the requirements for x-ray imaging systems and image receptors.

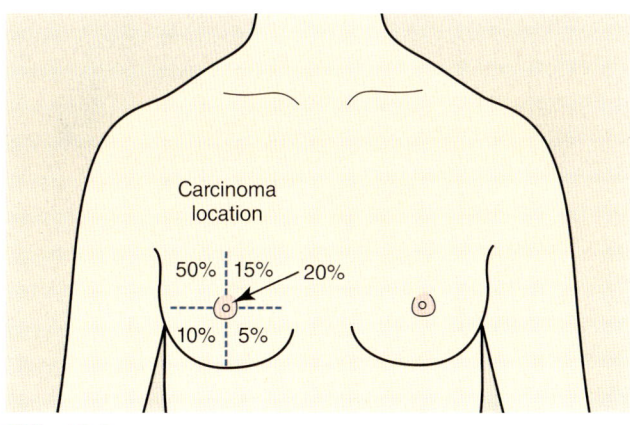

FIG. 18.2 Approximate incidence of breast cancer by location within the breast.

Because the mass density and atomic number of soft tissue components of the breast are so similar, conventional radiographic technique is useless. In the 70- to 100-kVp range, Compton scattering predominates with soft tissue; thus differential absorption within soft tissues is minimal. Low kVp must be used to maximize the photoelectric effect and thereby enhance differential absorption and improve image contrast.

Recall from Chapter 10 that x-ray absorption in tissue occurs principally by photoelectric effect and Compton scattering. The degree of absorption is determined by the tissue mass density and the effective atomic number.

X-ray absorption caused by differences in mass density is simply proportional to the mass density for both photoelectric effect and Compton scattering. X-ray absorption caused by differences in atomic number, however, is directly proportional for Compton scattering and proportional to the cube of the atomic number for photoelectric effect.

> The breast tissue most sensitive to cancer induction by radiation is glandular tissue.

Therefore x-ray mammography requires a low-kVp technique. As kVp is reduced, however, the penetrability of the x-ray beam is reduced, which in turn requires an increase in mAs.

If the kVp is too low, an inordinately high mAs value may be required, which could be unacceptable because of the increased patient radiation dose. Technique factors of approximately 23 to 28 kVp are used as an effective compromise between the increasing dose at low kVp and reduced image quality at high kVp.

THE MAMMOGRAPHIC IMAGING SYSTEM

Since the findings of the Digital Mammography Imaging Study Trial (DMIST) in 2006, the availability and use of dedicated digital mammographic imaging systems has soared and totally replaced other forms of mammography.

> Spatial resolution in digital mammography is limited by pixel size.

The DMIST was designed to compare the efficiency of digital mammography with that of screen-film mammography, with which we had 50 years of experience. The result was that digital mammography was equal to screen-film mammography for mature, fatty breasts, but it was superior when imaging younger, denser breasts.

> Digital mammography has superior contrast resolution because of postprocessing.

The IRs used in digital mammographic imaging systems are the same as those described in Chapter 12. It is not yet clear if one of the digital IRs (i.e., CsI, GdOS, Se, BaFl halide) will ultimately prevail. As discussed in Chapter 12, the atomic number that determines the K-absorption edge energy and the capture element thickness both determine the detective quantum efficiency and therefore IR speed and patient radiation dose.

The latest advance in digital mammography occurred in 2011 with the first system approved by the Food and Drug Administration for digital breast tomosynthesis. The principal purpose of tomography and therefore DMT is to improve the contrast resolution of the imaging system and increase image contrast (see Chapter 22).

> DMIST showed without question that contrast resolution is more important than spatial resolution for diagnostic accuracy.

X-ray mammography became clinically acceptable with the introduction of molybdenum as the target and filter (1966) and the dedicated, single-emulsion, screen-film IR (1972). By 1990, grid technique, emphasis on compression, high-frequency generators, and automatic exposure control (AEC) raised mammography to the level of excellence in breast imaging.

Conventional x-ray imaging systems are unacceptable for mammography, which requires specially designed, dedicated systems. Nearly all x-ray manufacturers now produce such systems. Fig. 18.3 shows two such imaging systems.

Dedicated mammographic imaging systems are designed for flexibility in patient positioning and have an integral compression device, a low ratio grid, AEC, and a microfocus x-ray tube. Desirable features of a dedicated mammography imaging system are given in Table 18.3.

High-Voltage Generation

All mammography imaging systems incorporate high-frequency generators (see Chapter 6). Such a generator accepts a single-phase input, which is rectified and capacitor smoothed to produce a direct current (DC) voltage waveform.

This DC power is fed to an inverter circuit, which changes the power to a high frequency (typically 5–10 kHz) that is then capacitor smoothed. The resulting voltage ripple in the x-ray tube is approximately 1%—essentially constant potential.

Compared with earlier single- and three-phase mammography generators, high-frequency generators are smaller and less expensive to manufacture. A maximum limit of 600 mAs is standard for preventing excessive patient radiation dose.

Target Composition

Mammographic x-ray tubes are manufactured with a tungsten (W), molybdenum (Mo), or rhodium (Rh) target. Fig. 18.4 shows the x-ray emission spectrum from a tungsten target tube filtered with 0.5 mm Al operating at 30 kVp. Note that the bremsstrahlung spectrum

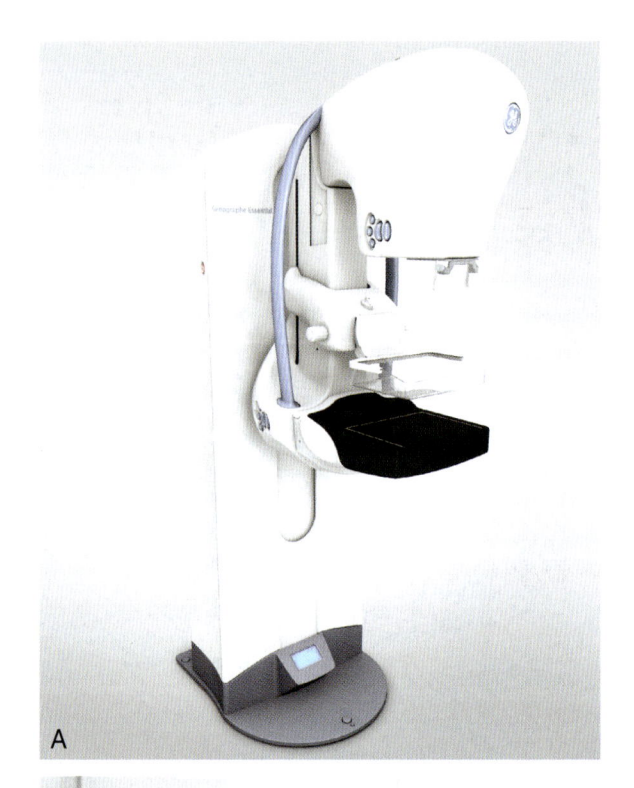

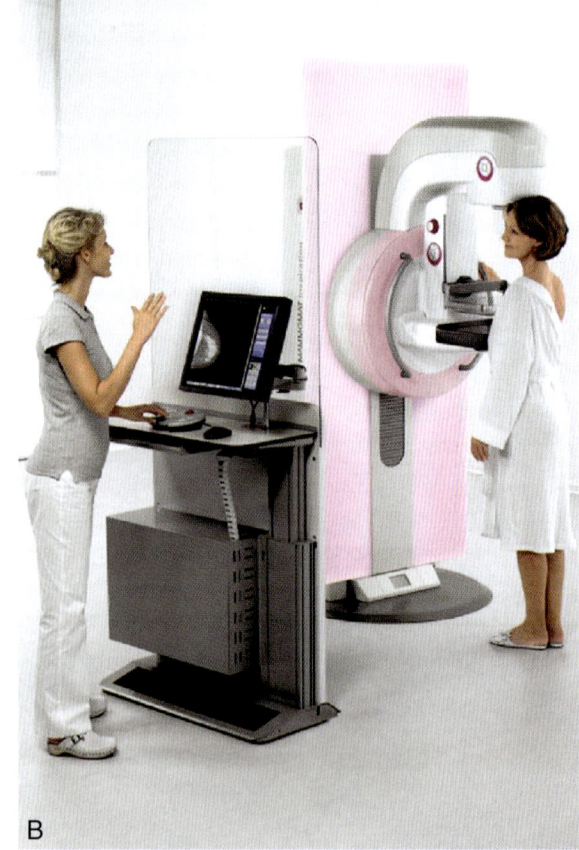

FIG. 18.3 Representative dedicated mammography imaging systems. (Courtesy of Siemens Medical Solutions USA, Inc.)

TABLE 18.3	Features of a Dedicated Mammography Imaging System
High Voltage	High Frequency, 5–10 kHz Generator
Target/filter	W/60 µm Mo
	Mo/30 µm Mo
	Mo/50 µm Rh
	Rh/50 µm Rh
kVp	20–35 kVp in 1-kVp increments
Compression	Low Z, auto adjust, and release
Grids	Ratio of 3:1 to 5:1, 30 lines/cm
Exposure control	Automatic to account for tissue thickness and composition
Focal spot	0.3 mm/0.1 mm (large/small)
Magnification	≤2
SID	50–80 cm

kVp, Kilovolt peak; *SID*, source-to-image receptor distance.

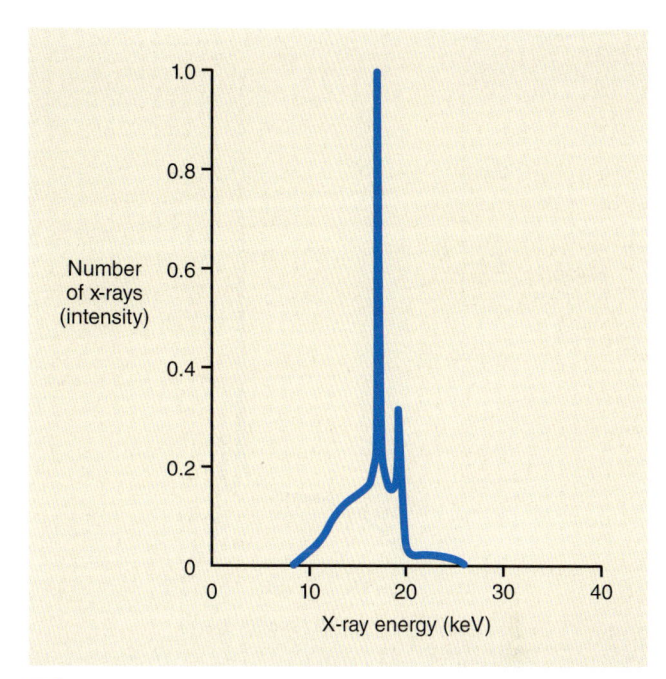

FIG. 18.5 X-ray emission spectrum for a molybdenum target x-ray tube with a 30-µm Mo filter operated at 26 kVp.

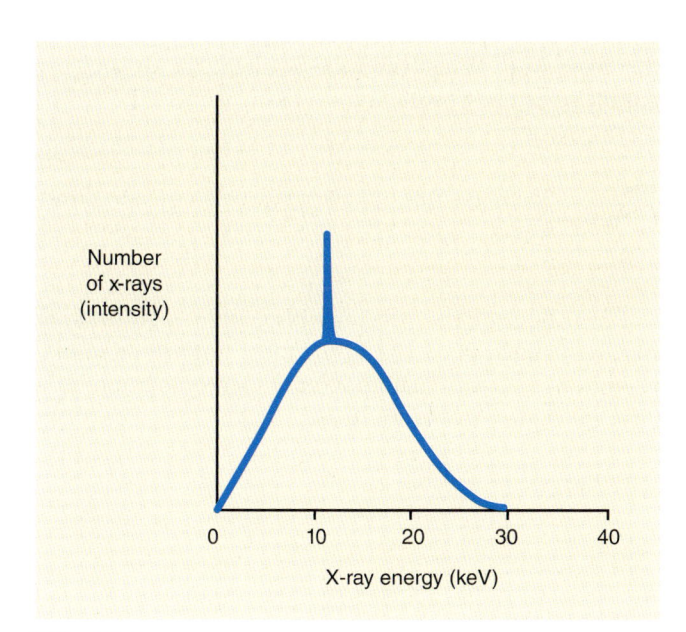

FIG. 18.4 X-ray emission spectrum for a tungsten target x-ray tube with a 0.5-mm Al filter operated at 30 kVp.

predominates and that only the 12-keV characteristic x-rays from L-shell transitions are present. These L-shell x-rays all are absorbed and contribute only to patient radiation dose—not to the image.

> Tungsten L-shell x-rays are of no value in mammography because their 12-keV energy is too low to penetrate the breast to the IR.

The x-rays most useful for enhancing differential absorption in breast tissue and for maximizing image contrast are those in the range of 17 to 24 keV. The tungsten target supplies sufficient x-rays in this energy range but also an abundance of x-rays above and below this range.

Fig. 18.5 shows the 26-kVp emission spectrum from a molybdenum target x-ray tube filtered with 30 µm of molybdenum; note the near absence of bremsstrahlung x-rays. The most prominent x-rays are characteristic, with energy of 17 and 19 keV resulting from K-shell interactions. Molybdenum has an atomic number of 42 compared with 74 for tungsten, and this difference is responsible for the differences in emission spectra.

The 28-kVp x-ray emission spectrum from a rhodium target filtered with rhodium appears similar to that from a molybdenum target (Fig. 18.6). However, rhodium has a slightly higher atomic number (Z = 45) and therefore a slightly higher K-edge (23 keV) and more intense bremsstrahlung x-rays.

Bremsstrahlung x-rays are produced more easily in target atoms with high Z than in target atoms with low Z. Molybdenum and rhodium K-characteristic x-rays have energy corresponding to their respective K-shell electron binding energy. This is within the range of energy that is most effective for breast imaging.

All currently manufactured mammographic imaging systems have target-filter combinations of Mo-Mo. Many are also equipped with Mo-Rh and Rh-Rh. Table 18.4 is an example of an appropriate mammographic technique chart.

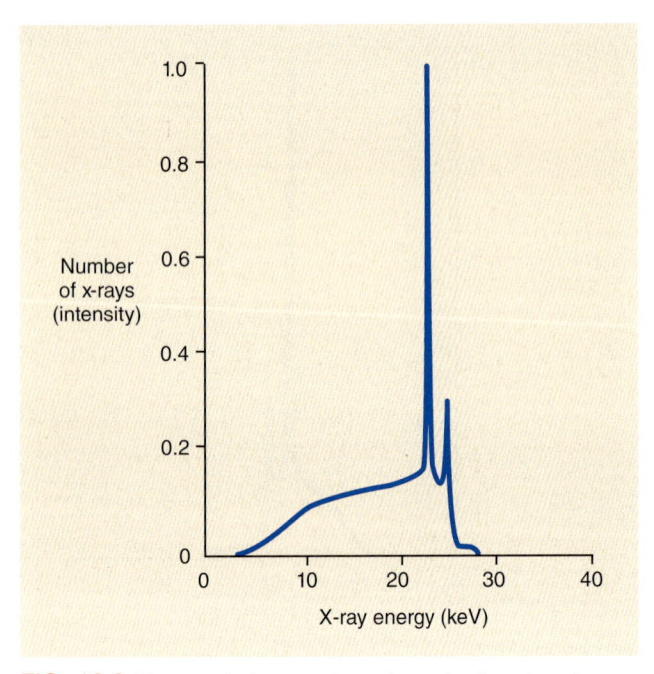

FIG. 18.6 X-ray emission spectrum for a rhodium target x-ray tube with a 50-μm Rh filter operated at 28 kVp.

TABLE 18.4 Mammographic Technique Chart

Compressed Breast Thickness (cm)	Target-Filter	Kilovolt Peak
0–2	Mo-Mo	24
3–4	Mo-Mo	25, 26
5–6	Mo-Rh	28
7–8	Mo/Rh	32
7–8	Rh-Rh[a]	30[a]

[a]To be used with systems that have Rh targets.

Focal-Spot Size

The size of the focal spot is an important characteristic of mammography x-ray tubes because of the higher demands for imaging microcalcifications. Mammography x-ray tubes usually have stated focal-spot sizes—large and small of 0.3 mm and 0.1 mm, respectively.

In general, the smaller the better; however, the shape of the focal spot is also important (Fig. 18.7). A circular focal spot is preferred, but rectangular shapes are common. Manufacturers shape the focal spot through clever cathode design and focusing cup voltage bias. The allowed variance is considerable for the stated nominal focal-spot size; therefore medical physics acceptance testing of focal-spot size or spatial resolution is essential.

To obtain such small focal-spot size and adequate x-ray intensity over the entire breast, manufacturers take advantage of the line-focus principle and tilt the x-ray tube (Fig. 18.8). Effective focal spots—0.3/0.1 mm—are obtained with an approximate 23-degree anode angle and a 6-degree x-ray tube tilt. Normally, the cathode is positioned to the chest wall. This allows for easier patient positioning, as well as application of anode heel effect.

Tilting the x-ray tube to achieve an even smaller effective focal spot ensures imaging of the tissue next to the chest wall. When the tube is tilted, the central ray parallels the chest wall, and no tissue is missed.

> Spatial resolution is principally determined by pixel size.

Regardless of the previous discussion of focal-spot size, remember, pixel size is the most important spatial resolution metric in mammography. Mammography IRs have pixel sizes down to 50 μm.

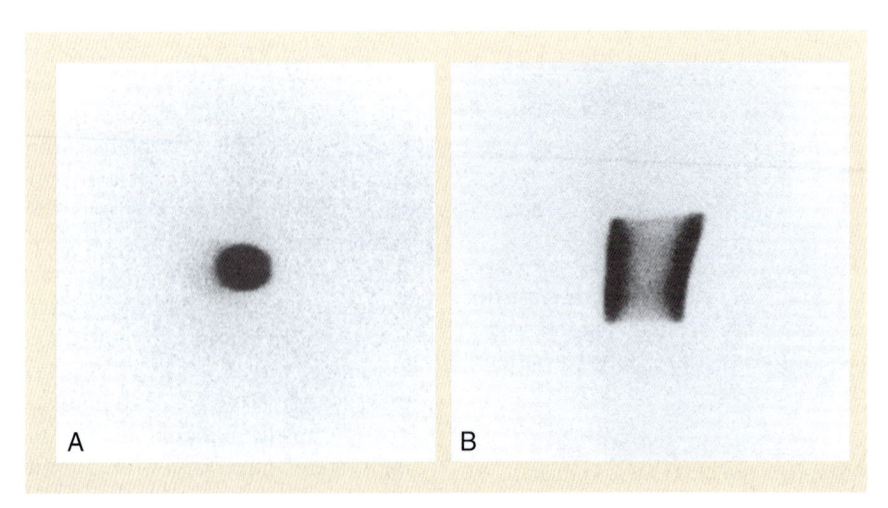

FIG. 18.7 Pinhole camera images of (A) the circular focal spot of a mammography x-ray tube and (B) a double banana–shaped focal spot from a general-purpose x-ray tube. (Courtesy Donald Jacobson, Medical College of Wisconsin.)

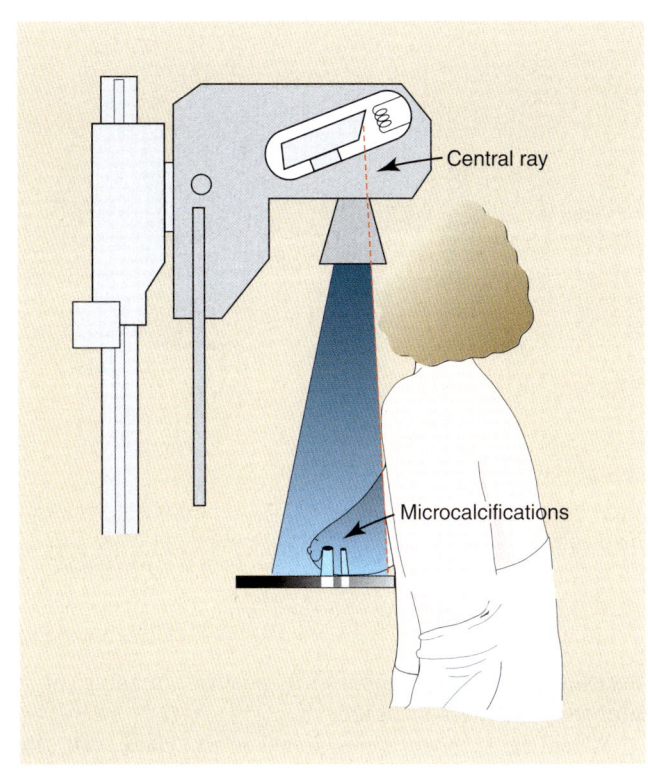

FIG. 18.8 When the x-ray tube is tilted in its housing, the effective focal spot is small, the x-ray intensity is more uniform, and tissue against the chest wall is imaged.

Filtration

At the low kVp used for mammography, it is important that the x-ray tube window not attenuate the x-ray beam significantly. Therefore dedicated mammography x-ray tubes have either a beryllium (Z = 4) window or a very thin borosilicate glass window.

Most mammography x-ray tubes have inherent filtration in the window of approximately 0.1-mm Al equivalent. Beyond the window, the proper type and thickness of x-ray beam filtration must be installed.

> Under no circumstances is total beam filtration less than 0.5-mm Al equivalent.

If a tungsten target x-ray tube is used, it should have a molybdenum or rhodium filter. The purpose of each filter is to reduce the higher-energy bremsstrahlung x-rays. Some research has suggested that 50-μm rhodium (Z = 45) is a better filter for imaging thicker and denser breasts when the x-ray tube target is tungsten. Fig. 18.9 shows the emission spectrum from a tungsten target tube filtered by molybdenum or rhodium.

> No filter element can absorb its own anode target-characteristic radiation.

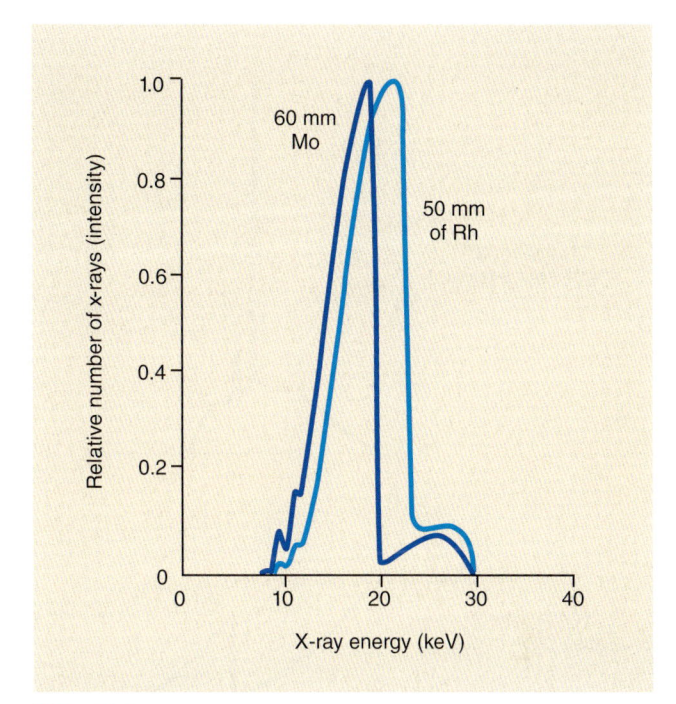

FIG. 18.9 Emission spectrum from a tungsten target x-ray tube filtered by molybdenum and rhodium.

The use of a filter of the same element as the x-ray tube target is designed to allow the K-characteristic x-rays to expose the breast while suppressing the higher- and lower-energy bremsstrahlung x-rays. Fig. 18.10 shows this process of selective filtration designed to shape the x-ray beam with Mo-Mo.

The unfiltered Mo beam (see Fig. 18.10A) has a prominent characteristic x-ray emission and substantial bremsstrahlung x-ray emission. The Mo filter has its K-absorption edge at the energy of the K-characteristic x-ray emission (see Fig. 18.10B). The combination Mo-Mo target-filter results in an emission spectrum with suppressed bremsstrahlung and prominent characteristic x-ray emission (see Fig. 18.10C).

If a Mo target x-ray tube is used, then Mo filtration of 30 μm or Rh filtration of 50 μm is recommended. These combinations provide the Mo charactcristic x-rays for imaging along with the suppressed bremsstrahlung x-ray emission spectrum.

If a Rh target x-ray tube is used, it should be filtered with 25-μm Rh. This combination provides a slightly higher-energy x-ray beam of greater penetrability. The use of Rh as a target or filter is designed for thicker, more dense breasts. Regardless of x-ray tube target or filtration, the half-value layer is always very low.

Many x-ray tubes designed specifically for mammography have a stationary anode. Bi-angle and double-track anodes (one track is Mo and the other Rh) are rotating anode tubes.

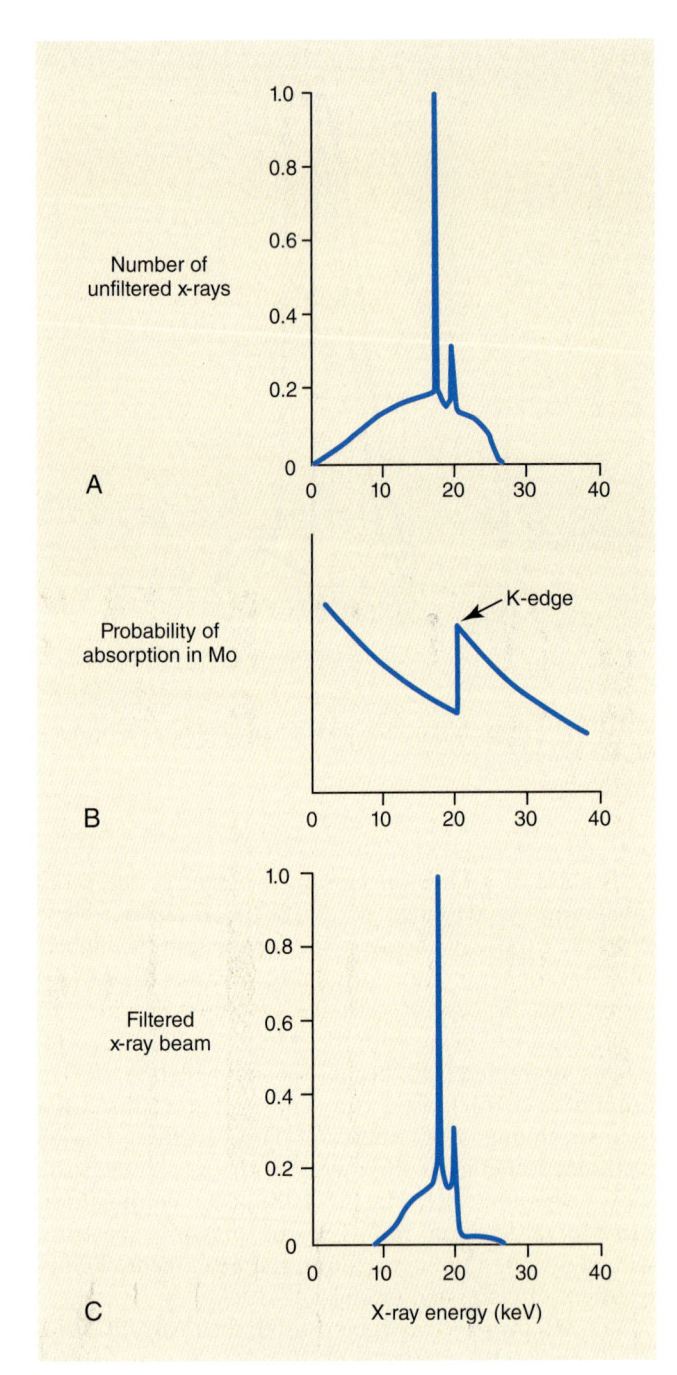

FIG. 18.10 (A) Unfiltered molybdenum x-ray emission spectrum. (B) The probability of x-ray absorption in molybdenum. (C) Bremsstrahlung x-rays are suppressed and characteristic x-ray emission becomes prominent when a molybdenum target is filtered with molybdenum.

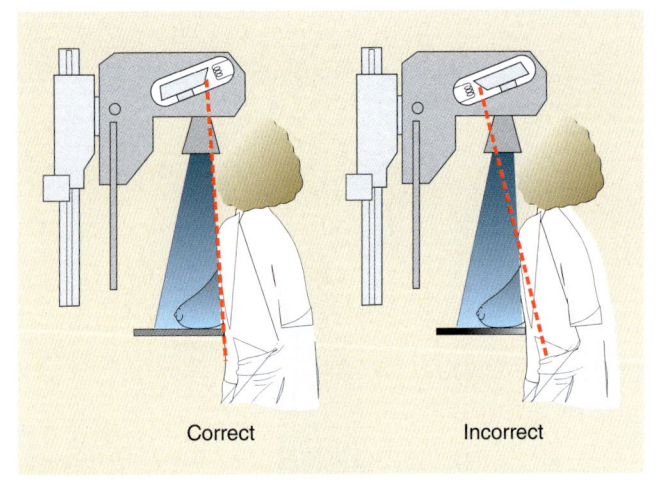

FIG. 18.11 The heel effect can be used to advantage in mammography by positioning the cathode toward the chest wall to produce a more uniform x-ray exposure of the image receptor.

Heel Effect

The heel effect is important to mammography. The conic shape of the breast requires that the x-ray intensity near the chest wall must be higher than that to the nipple side to ensure near-uniform exposure of the IR. This is accomplished by positioning the cathode to the chest wall (Fig. 18.11). However this is not absolutely necessary because **compression** ensures imaging of a uniform thickness of tissue.

When the cathode is positioned to the chest wall, the spatial resolution of tissue near the chest wall is reduced because of the increased focal-spot blur created by the larger effective focal-spot size. However, most manufacturers of dedicated mammography imaging systems use a source-to-image receptor distance (SID) of 60 to 80 cm, with the cathode to the chest wall and the x-ray tube tilted.

This is considered the best arrangement because the focal spot is made effectively smaller, and tissue at the chest wall is imaged. It is also more comfortable for the patient because their head is always close to the x-ray tube housing during an examination.

One consequence of the heel effect is variation in focal-spot size over the IR. However, the use of long SID and vigorous compression makes this change in effective focal-spot size clinically insignificant.

Compression

Compression is important in many aspects of conventional radiology but is particularly important in mammography. Vigorous compression offers several advantages (Fig. 18.12).

A compressed breast is of more uniform thickness; therefore the response of the IR is more uniform. Tissues near the chest wall are less likely to be underexposed, and tissues near the nipple are less likely to be overexposed.

> Vigorous compression must be used in x-ray mammography.

When vigorous compression is used, all tissue is brought closer to the IR, focal-spot blur is reduced,

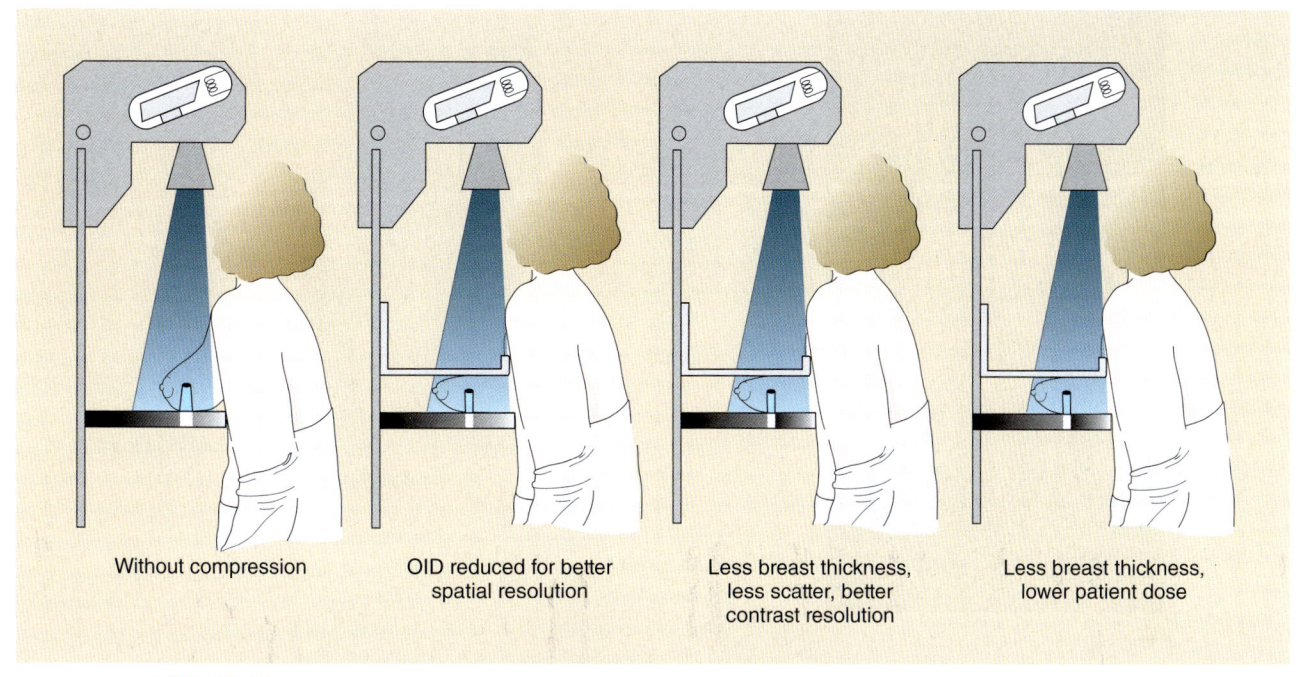

FIG. 18.12 Compression in mammography has three principal advantages: improved spatial resolution, improved contrast resolution, and lower patient radiation dose. *OID*, Object-to-image receptor distance.

TABLE 18.5	Advantages of Vigorous Breast Compression
Effect	**Result**
Immobilization of breast	Reduced motion blur
Uniform thickness	Uniform x-ray exposure of the image receptor
Reduced scatter radiation	Improved contrast resolution
Shorter OID	Improved spatial resolution
Thinner tissue	Reduced patient radiation dose

OID, Object-to-image receptor distance.

and spatial resolution is improved. Compression also reduces absorption blur and scatter radiation and therefore improved contrast resolution.

All dedicated mammographic x-ray imaging systems have a built-in stiff compression device that is parallel to the surface of the IR. Vigorous compression of the breast is necessary to attain the best image.

The image is improved with vigorous compression, as is summarized in Table 18.5. Compression immobilizes the breast and therefore reduces motion blur. Compression spreads out the tissue and thus reduces superimposition of tissue structures.

Compression results in thinner tissue and therefore less scatter radiation and improved contrast resolution. The overall result is improved ability to detect small, low-contrast lesions and high-contrast microcalcifications because of **improved spatial resolution**. Additionally vigorous compression results in a lower patient radiation dose.

> Compression improves spatial resolution and contrast resolution and reduces the patient radiation dose.

Although it may be difficult for patients to understand, compression of the breast is essential for a mammogram. The optimum degree of compression is unknown; however the more vigorous the compression, the better the image and the lower the patient radiation dose, but the higher the level of patient discomfort. The skilled mammographer attempts to compress the breast until it is "taut" or "just less than painful."

Grids

Radiographic grids are used routinely in mammography. Although mammographic image contrast is high because of the low kVp used, it can be improved. Most systems now have a moving grid with a ratio of 4:1 to 5:1 focused to the SID to increase image contrast. Grid frequencies of 40 lines/cm for the moving grid are typical.

Use of such grids does not compromise spatial resolution, but it does increase the patient radiation dose. The use of a 4:1 ratio grid approximately doubles the

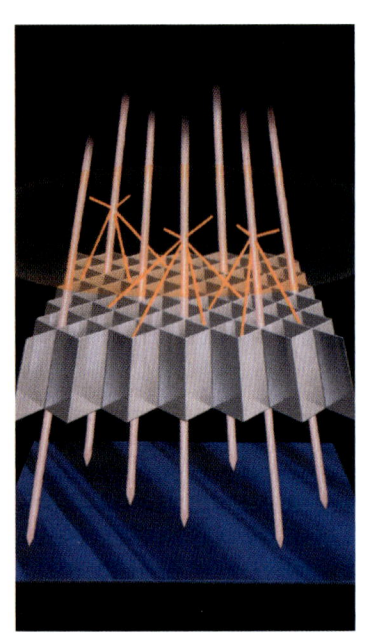

FIG. 18.13 A high-transmission cellular grid designed specifically for mammography. (Courtesy Hologic Imaging.)

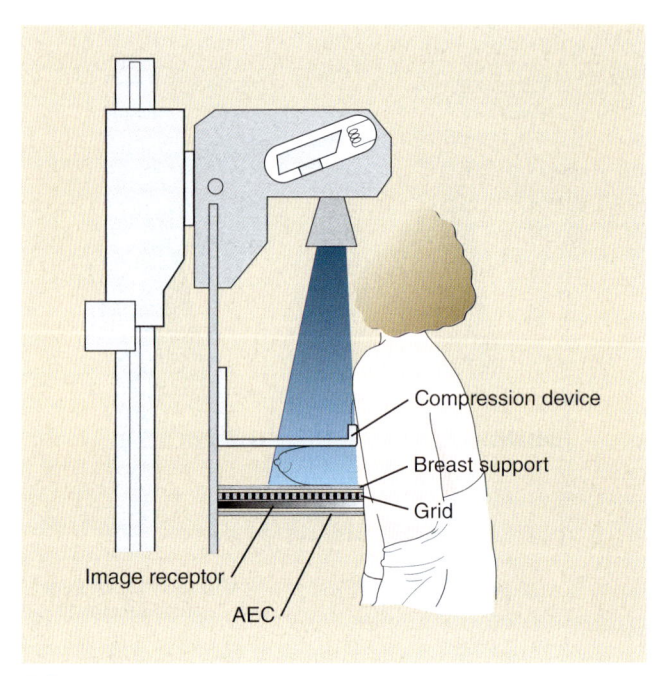

FIG. 18.14 The relative position of the automatic exposure control (*AEC*) device.

patient radiation dose compared with nongrid contact mammography. However, the dose is still acceptably low, and the improvement in contrast is significant.

> Virtual grids are poised to replace radiographic grids in mammography.

A unique grid that has been developed specifically for mammography is the high-transmission cellular (HTC) grid (Fig. 18.13). This grid has the cleanup characteristics of a crossed grid in that it reduces scatter radiation in two directions rather than the single direction of a parallel grid. The HTC grid has copper as grid strip material and air for the interspace, and its physical dimensions result in a 3.8:1 grid ratio.

Automatic Exposure Control

Phototimers for mammography are designed to measure not only x-ray intensity at the IR but also x-ray energy. These phototimers are called **AEC devices**, and they are positioned after the IR to minimize the object-to-image receptor distance (OID) and improve spatial resolution (Fig. 18.14).

Two types of AEC devices are used: ionization chamber and solid-state diode. Each type can have a single radiation detector or multiple detectors, which are positioned along the chest wall-nipple axis. Some AEC devices incorporate many detectors to cover the entire breast.

The detectors are filtered differently, so the AEC can estimate the x-ray beam energy after passing through the breast. This allows assessment of breast composition and selection of proper target-filter combination. Thick, dense breasts are imaged better with Rh-Rh; thin, fatty breasts are imaged better with Mo-Mo.

Magnification Mammography

Magnification techniques are used frequently in mammography, producing images up to twice the normal size. Magnification mammography requires special equipment such as microfocus x-ray tubes, adequate compression, and patient positioning devices. Effective focal-spot size should not exceed 0.1 mm.

> Magnification mammography should not be used routinely.

Standard mammograms are adequate for most patients, so magnification mammography is usually unnecessary because the patient radiation dose is approximately doubled. The purpose of magnification mammography is to investigate small, suspicious lesions or microcalcifications seen on standard mammograms.

MAMMOGRAPHY QUALITY CONTROL

Quality control (QC) procedures for digital mammography are not universally prescribed as they were for screen-film mammography. The QC exercises associated with the mammographic test object should be performed as described by the vendor-specific instructions for your imaging system.

A repeat analysis requires considerable diligence because unacceptable images can be easily deleted without the knowledge of the interpreting radiologist. Properly, any unacceptable mammograms should be filed in a "Repeat Analysis" electronic folder and evaluated for fault and the corrective action taken. Repeat analysis was a regular activity during the years of screen-film mammography. Repeating a mammogram is rare with digital mammography.

> The mammography repeat rate should not exceed 1%.

Mammography digital display devices are subject to the same scrutiny and QC as other such devices (see Chapter 24). This may be the most demanding digital QC chore. The mammography QC evaluations must be performed in a precise fashion by the QC mammographer for routine inspection by an agent of the US Food and Drug Administration MQSA team.

Digital mammography imaging systems cannot be treated QC-wise as a general radiographic imaging system. Furthermore, there is no set protocol that can be applied to all dedicated digital mammographic systems.

The image receptor is different for various digital mammographic imaging systems, and there are system-specific digital computer platforms containing QC analytical evaluations. Each vendor is required to develop appropriate QC tests, and the QC mammographer is required to perform these tasks with the suggested schedule.

> Vendors specify tasks must be performed by the QC mammographer.

The time required of the QC mammographer for digital mammography QC is less than the time previously required for screen-film mammography. This represents another significant advantage of digital mammography.

QUALITY CONTROL TEAM

The ACR and the MQSA have endorsed a QC program of specific duties required of radiologists, medical physicists, and radiologic technologists (Fig. 18.15). Each of these individuals is important in ensuring the best available patient care with an acceptable patient radiation dose.

Radiologist

The ultimate responsibility for mammography QC lies with the radiologist. These responsibilities often fall under the more broad area of **quality assurance (QA)**.

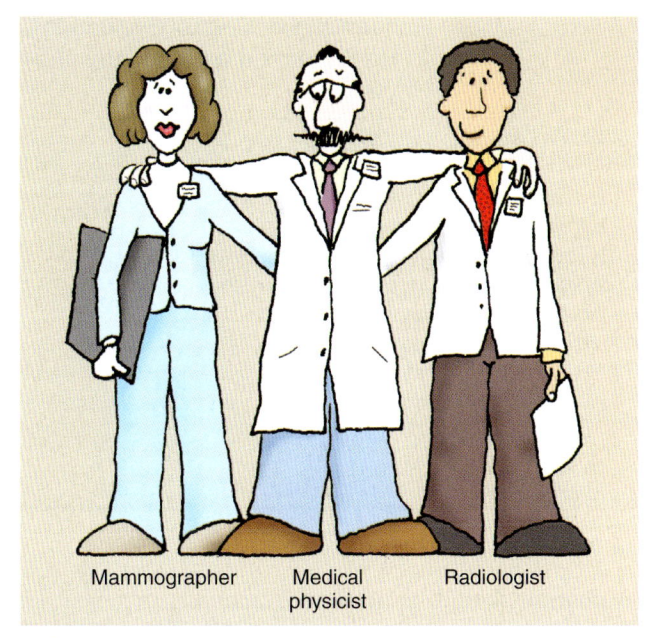

FIG. 18.15 The three members of the mammography quality control team.

QA is an administrative program that is designed to fuse the different aspects of QC and to ensure that all activities are carried out at the highest level. The radiologist is responsible for selecting qualified medical physicists and mammographers and for overseeing the activities of these team members.

> The radiologist's principal responsibility is supervision of the entire QA program.

Another responsibility of the radiologist involves supervising patient communication and tracking. Quality patient care is the ultimate goal of any mammography facility, and the final responsibility for the goal lies with the radiologist. The level of any QA and QC program directly reflects the radiologist's attitude and appreciation for the need for such a program.

The MQSA mandates daily "clinical image evaluation" by the radiologist. Continuous quality improvement (QCI) is an extension of any QA and QC program, including administrative protocols for the continuous improvement of mammographic image quality.

The ACR has a firm position on Quality Control and Improvement (QCI). Each academic radiology department now has an identified QCI radiologist in parallel with the QC mammographer.

Medical Physicist

The role of the medical physicist as a member of the mammography QC team is multidimensional. One such aspect is QC evaluation of the imaging system. This

TABLE 18.6	Annual Quality Control Evaluation to Be Performed by the Medical Physicist

Mammographic unit assembly inspection
Collimation assessment
Evaluation of spatial resolution
Kilovolt peak accuracy and reproducibility
X-ray beam penetrability assessment (half-value layer)
Automatic exposure control performance assessment
Automatic exposure control reproducibility
Uniformity of image receptor response
Breast entrance radiation dose
Average glandular radiation dose
Artifact evaluation
X-ray output intensity
Measurement of viewing conditions

evaluation should be performed annually or whenever a major component has been replaced. The evaluation consists of a number of measurements and tests that are summarized in Table 18.6.

The medical physicist understands how the different technical aspects of the imaging chain affect the image and therefore is able to identify existing or potential imaging problems. Occasionally, the medical physicist may pass information directly to the service engineer or may serve as an intermediary between the imaging facility and the service engineer. The aim of this portion of the QC program is to ensure that imaging system functions properly to provide the highest quality images with the lowest patient radiation dose.

> The medical physicist's principal responsibility is to conduct an annual performance evaluation of the imaging system.

Another role of the medical physicist is to advise the QC mammographer. The medical physicist should understand all tests expected of the QC mammographer well enough to predict likely problems or complications. The medical physicist should thoroughly review charts and records to check for compliance and to ensure that they are prepared properly and contain all of the necessary information.

Mammographer

The mammographer is a specially trained radiographer and is extremely important to a mammography QC program. The mammographer, the most hands-on member of the QC team, is responsible for day-to-day QC and for producing and monitoring all control charts and logs for any trends that might indicate problems. In imaging facilities that use several mammographers, one is assigned the responsibility of **QC mammographer**.

SUMMARY

Breast cancer is one of the leading causes of death among females between 40 and 50 years of age. This is the principal reason why mammographic imaging systems and techniques have improved over the years, and why the MQSA was instituted.

Anatomically, the breast consists of three different tissues: fibrous tissue, glandular tissue, and adipose tissue. Premenopausal females have breasts that are composed mainly of fibrous and glandular tissue surrounded by a thin layer of fat. These breasts are dense and difficult to image. In postmenopausal females, the glandular tissue turns to adipose tissue. Because of their predominantly fatty content, older breasts are easier to image.

The mammographer must know the recommended intervals of breast self-examination, physician examination of the breasts, and mammographic examination for females of various age groups to advise such patients. Diagnostic x-ray mammography often is performed every 6 months on females who have an elevated risk of breast cancer or who have a known lesion.

Compression is an important factor in the production of high-quality mammograms.

Radiographic imaging systems are designed especially for mammographic examination. Mammographic x-ray tube targets consist of tungsten, molybdenum, or rhodium. A low kVp is used to maximize radiographic contrast of soft tissue. The x-ray beam should be filtered with 30 to 60 μm of molybdenum or rhodium to accentuate the characteristic x-ray emission.

One mammographer should be identified as the QC mammographer. The QC mammographer is directed by the supervising radiologist as identified in the MQSA program.

CHALLENGE QUESTIONS

1. Define or otherwise identify the following:
    a. Minimum filtration for mammography
    b. Mammographic SID
    c. Adipose tissue
    d. Mammographic grid ratio
    e. Molybdenum
    f. DMT
    g. Baseline mammogram
    h. Breast cancer incidence
    i. DMIST
    j. Characteristic x-radiation
2. Describe the anatomy of the breast, including the types of tissue and structural sizes.
3. Discuss changes in x-ray beam energy and patient radiation dose in mammography as kVp is increased.

4. Graphically compare the x-ray emission of a tungsten target x-ray tube with that of a molybdenum target x-ray tube operated at 28 kVp.
5. The electron binding energies for molybdenum are K-shell, 20 keV; L-shell, 2.6 keV; and M-shell, 0.5 keV. What are the possible characteristic x-ray energies when operated at 28 kVp?
6. Discuss the influence of the heel effect on image appearance in mammography.
7. Why is mammography usually performed with an x-ray tube target of molybdenum or rhodium?
8. What property of the mammographic imaging system limits the ability to image breast microcalcifications?
9. How is soft tissue radiography different from conventional radiography?
10. To what do the abbreviations ACR and MQSA refer?
11. What is the difference between diagnostic and screening mammography?
12. Is repeat analysis necessary for mammography? Why and when?
13. Explain why mammography requires a low-kVp technique.
14. List the advantages of mammographic compression.
15. Name the three materials used for mammographic x-ray tube targets.
16. What focal-spot sizes are used for mammography? Why?
17. What is the best target-filter combination for imaging dense breast tissue?
18. What grid ratio and grid frequency are used for mammography?
19. What feature of a dedicated mammography imaging system is important for imaging microcalcifications?
20. What is the purpose of tilting the mammography x-ray tube within the tube housing?

The answers to the Challenge Questions can be found by logging on to our website at http://evolve.elsevier.com.

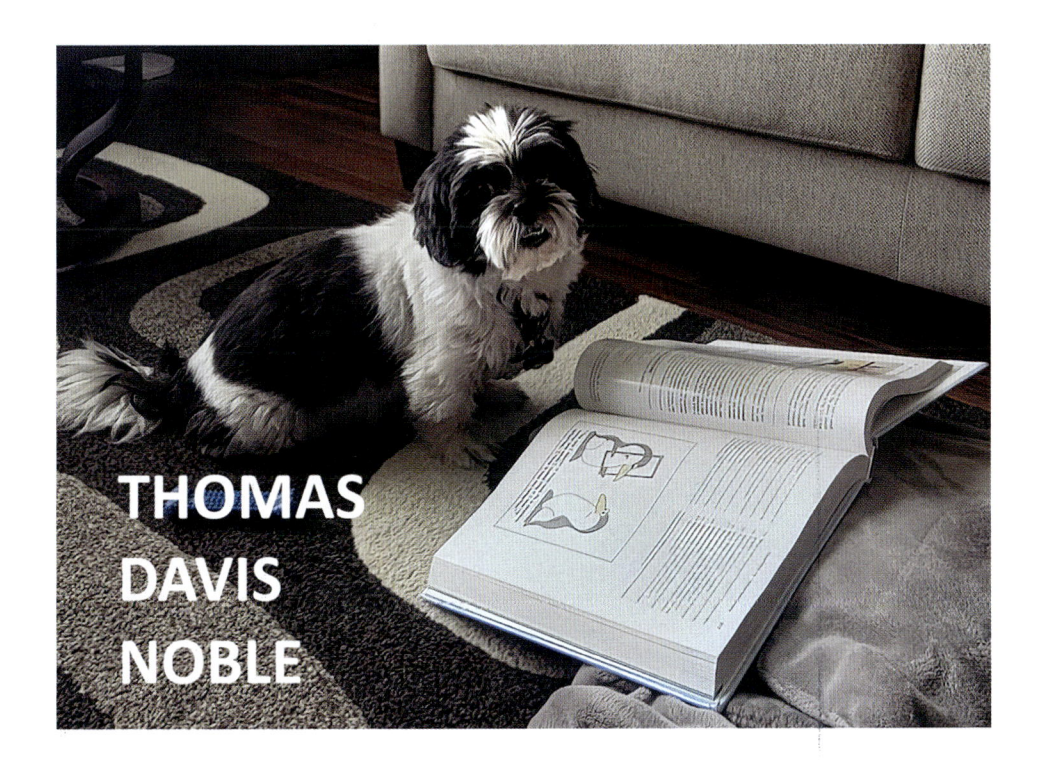

CHAPTER 19

Fluoroscopy

OBJECTIVES

At the completion of this chapter, the student should be able to do the following:

1. Discuss the development of fluoroscopy.
2. Explain visual physiology and its relationship to fluoroscopy.
3. Describe the components of an image intensifier.
4. Calculate brightness gain and identify its units.
5. List the approximate kilovolt peak levels for common fluoroscopic examinations.
6. Discuss the role of the light-emitting diode monitor in forming fluoroscopic images.

OUTLINE

An Overview 275
Special Demands of Fluoroscopy 275
 Illumination 275
 Visual Physiology 276
Fluoroscopic Technique 276
Image Intensification 277
 Image-Intensifier Tube 277
 Multifield Image Intensification 279
Fluoroscopic Image Monitoring 281
Fluoroscopy Quality Control 285
 Exposure Rate 285
 Automatic Exposure Systems 285
Summary 285
Challenge Questions 286

THE PRIMARY function of the fluoroscope is to provide real-time dynamic viewing of anatomic structures. Dynamic studies are examinations that show the motion of circulation or the motion of internal structures.

During fluoroscopy, the radiologist often uses contrast media to highlight the anatomy. The radiologist then views a continuous image of the internal structure while the x-ray tube is energized. If the radiologist observes something during the fluoroscopic examination and would like to preserve that image for further study, a radiograph called a **spot film** can be taken without interruption of the dynamic examination.

The introduction of computer technology into fluoroscopy and radiography has enhanced the training and performance demands placed on the radiographer. This chapter presents the basic principles of fluoroscopic imaging. The following chapter describes digital fluoroscopic imaging as it is used during interventional radiology procedures.

AN OVERVIEW

Since Thomas A. Edison invented the fluoroscope in 1896, it has served as a valuable tool in medical imaging. The fluoroscope is used primarily for dynamic studies. During fluoroscopy, the radiologist views a continuous image of the motion of internal structures while the x-ray tube is energized.

> The fluoroscope is used for examination of moving internal structures and fluids.

A radiologist may observe something that should be preserved for later study; in this case, a permanent fixed image can be taken without interruption of the examination. One such method is known as a spot film, that is, a small static image on a small-format image receptor. Cineradiography, video imaging, and digital fluoroscopy are other examples.

Fluoroscopy is actually a rather routine type of x-ray examination except for its application in the visualization of vessels, called **angiography**. The two main areas of angiography are neuroradiology and vascular radiology. As with all fluoroscopic procedures, digital radiographic images can be obtained. These areas of angiography are now referred to as **interventional radiology** (see Chapter 20).

The physical layout of a fluoroscopic imaging system can vary. The x-ray tube is usually hidden under the patient couch, and the image intensifier or flat-panel image receptor is set over the patient couch. With some fluoroscopes, the x-ray tube is over the patient couch, and the image receptor is under the patient couch. Some fluoroscopes are operated remotely from outside the x-ray room. Many different arrangements are provided for fluoroscopy, and the radiographer must become familiar with each of them.

During image-intensified fluoroscopy, the fluoroscopic image is displayed on a light-emitting diode (LED) monitor. The image-intensifier tube and the television chain are described later in this chapter.

During fluoroscopy, the x-ray tube is operated at less than 5 mA; contrast this with a radiographic examination in which the x-ray tube current is hundreds of mA. Despite the lower mA, however, the patient radiation dose is considerably higher during fluoroscopy than during radiographic examinations because the x-ray beam exposes the patient continuously and for a considerably longer time.

The kilovolt peak (kVp) of operation depends entirely on the section of the body that is being examined. Fluoroscopic equipment allows the radiologist to select an image brightness level that is subsequently maintained automatically by varying the kVp, the mA, or sometimes both. This feature of an image-intensified fluoroscope is called **automatic brightness control** (ABC), which is a subset of automatic exposure control (AEC).

SPECIAL DEMANDS OF FLUOROSCOPY

Fluoroscopy is a dynamic process; thus the radiologist must adapt to moving images that are sometimes dim. This requires some knowledge of image illumination and of visual physiology.

Illumination

The principal advantage of image-intensified fluoroscopy over earlier types of fluoroscopy is increased image brightness. Just as it is much more difficult to read a book in dim illumination than in bright illumination, it is much harder to interpret a dim fluoroscopic image than a bright one.

Illumination levels are measured in units of lumen per square meter, or **lux**. It is not necessary to know the precise definition of a lux; its importance lies in the wide range of illumination levels over which the human eye is sensitive. Fig. 19.1 lists approximate illumination levels for familiar objects.

Radiographs are visualized under illumination levels of 100 to 1000 lux; image-intensified fluoroscopy is performed at similar illumination levels. If necessary, read the discussion of photometric quantities in Chapter 24.

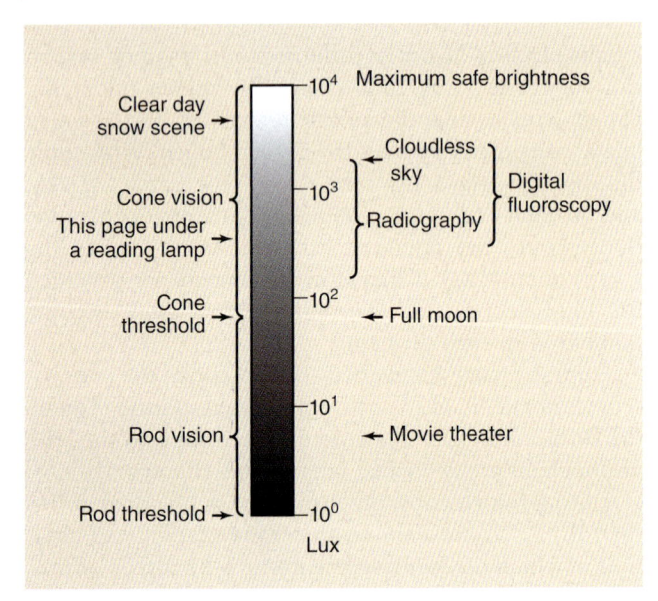

FIG. 19.1 The range of human vision is wide; it covers four orders of intensity magnitude.

Visual Physiology

The structures in the eye that are responsible for the sensation of vision are called **rods** and **cones**. Fig. 19.2 is a cross section of the human eye that reveals its principal parts and its appearance on a magnetic resonance image. Light incident on the eye must first pass through the **cornea**, a transparent protective covering, and then through the lens, where the light is focused onto the retina.

Between the cornea and the lens is the **iris**, which behaves similarly to the diaphragm of a photographic camera in controlling the amount of light that is admitted to the eye. In the presence of bright light, the iris contracts and allows only a small amount of light to enter. During low-light conditions, such as in a dimly lit digital image reading area, the iris dilates (i.e., it opens up) and allows more light to enter.

> When light arrives at the retina, it is detected by the rods and the cones.

Rods and cones are small structures; more than 100,000 of them are found per square millimeter of retina. The cones are concentrated at the center of the retina in an area called the **fovea centralis**. Rods, on the other hand, are most numerous on the periphery of the retina. No rods are found at the fovea centralis.

The rods are sensitive to low-light levels and are stimulated during dim light situations. The threshold for rod vision is approximately 2 lux. Cones, on the other hand, are less sensitive to light; their threshold is only approximately 100 lux, but cones are capable of responding to intense light levels; rods cannot.

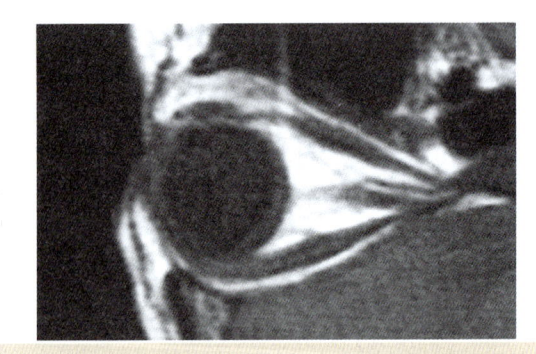

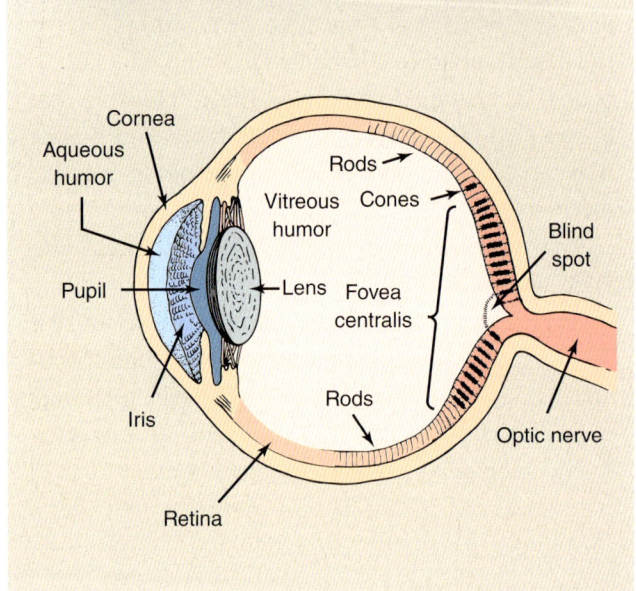

FIG. 19.2 The appearance of the human eye and the parts responsible for vision on a magnetic resonance image. (Courtesy Helen Schumpert, Asheville MRI.)

Consequently, cones are used primarily for daylight vision, called **photopic vision**, and rods are used for night vision, called **scotopic vision**. This aspect of visual physiology explains why dim objects are viewed more readily if they are not looked at directly. Astronomers and radiologists are familiar with the fact that a dim object is best viewed peripherally, where rod vision predominates.

Cones perceive small objects much better than rods. This ability to perceive fine detail is called **visual acuity**. Cones are also much better at detecting differences in brightness levels. This property of vision is called **contrast perception**. Furthermore, cones are sensitive to a wide range of wavelengths of light.

Cones perceive color, but rods are essentially color-blind. Under scotopic conditions, the sensitivity of the eye is greatest in the green part of the spectrum at about 555 nm.

FLUOROSCOPIC TECHNIQUE

During fluoroscopy, maximum image resolution is desired; this requires high levels of image brightness. The image intensifier was developed principally to replace the conventional fluorescent screen, which had

CHAPTER 19 Fluoroscopy

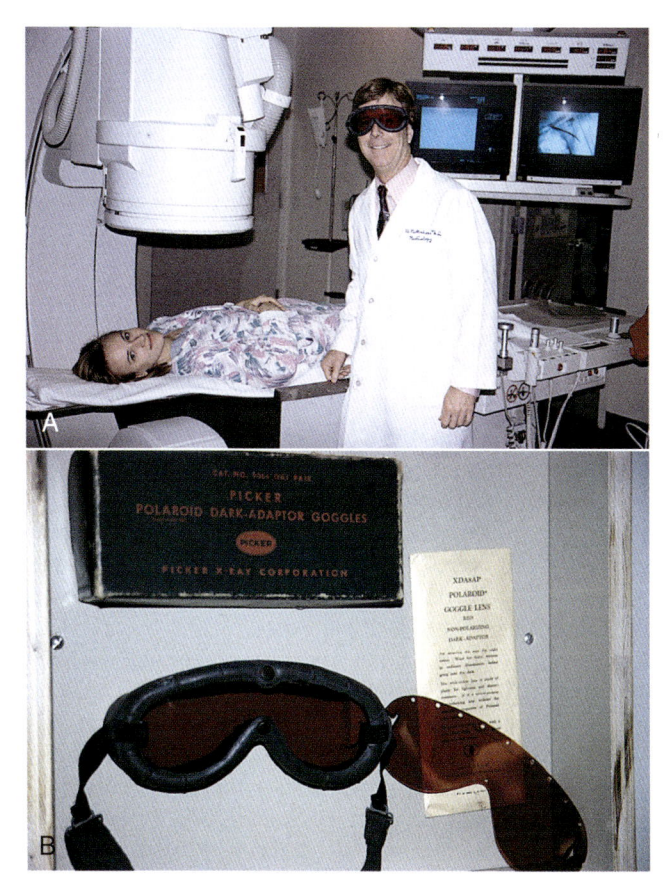

FIG. 19.3 Red goggles were used to adapt to darkness for conventional screen fluoroscopy. This radiologist is *Back to the Future*. (Courtesy Ben Archer, Baylor College of Medicine.)

TABLE 19.1	Representative Fluoroscopic and Spot-Film Kilovolt Peak (kVp) for Common Examinations
Examination	**kVp**
Gallbladder	65–75
Nephrostogram	70–80
Myelogram	70–80
Barium enema (air contrast)	80–90
Upper gastrointestinal	100–110
Small bowel	110–120
Barium enema	110–120

to be viewed in a darkened room and then only after 15 minutes of dark adaptation (Fig. 19.3). The image intensifier raises illumination into the cone vision region, where visual acuity is greatest.

The brightness of the fluoroscopic image depends primarily on the anatomy that is being examined, the kVp, and the mA. The patient's anatomy cannot be controlled by the radiographer; however, fluoroscopic kVp and mA can be controlled.

The influence of kVp and mA on fluoroscopic image appearance is similar to their influence on radiographic image appearance. Generally, high kVp and low mA are preferred.

The precise fluoroscopic technique that will be used is determined by the training and experience of the radiologist and the radiographer. Table 19.1 presents representative fluoroscopic kVp values for several common examinations. The fluoroscopic mA is not given because this value varies according to patient thickness and the response of the ABC.

IMAGE INTENSIFICATION

Until approximately 1960, radiologists viewed fluoroscopic images in a dark room because the fluoroscopic screen image was very dim. And even though the image was dim, the patient radiation dose was very high.

Image-Intensifier Tube

The image-intensifier tube is a complex electronic device that receives the image-forming x-ray beam and converts it into a visible-light image of high intensity. Fig. 19.4 is a rendition of an x-ray image-intensifier tube. The tube components are contained within a glass or metal envelope that provides structural support but, more important, maintains a vacuum. When installed, the tube is mounted inside a metal container to protect it from rough handling and breakage.

X-rays that exit the patient and are incident on the image-intensifier tube are transmitted through the glass envelope and interact with the **input phosphor**, which is cesium iodide (CsI). When an x-ray interacts with the input phosphor, its energy is converted into visible light.

The CsI crystals are grown as tiny needles and are tightly packed in a layer of approximately 300 μm (Fig. 19.5). Each crystal is approximately 5 μm in diameter. This results in microlight pipes with little dispersion and improved spatial resolution.

The next active element of the image-intensifier tube is the **photocathode**, which is bonded directly to the input phosphor with a thin, transparent adhesive layer. The photocathode is a thin metal layer usually composed of cesium and antimony compounds that respond to stimulation of input phosphor light by the emission of electrons.

> The photocathode emits electrons when illuminated by visible light from the input phosphor.

This process is known as **photoemission**. The term is similar to **thermionic emission**, which refers to electron emission that follows heat stimulation. Photoemission is electron emission that follows visible light stimulation.

It takes many light photons to cause the emission of one electron. The number of electrons emitted by the photocathode is directly proportional to the intensity of light that reaches it. Consequently, the number of

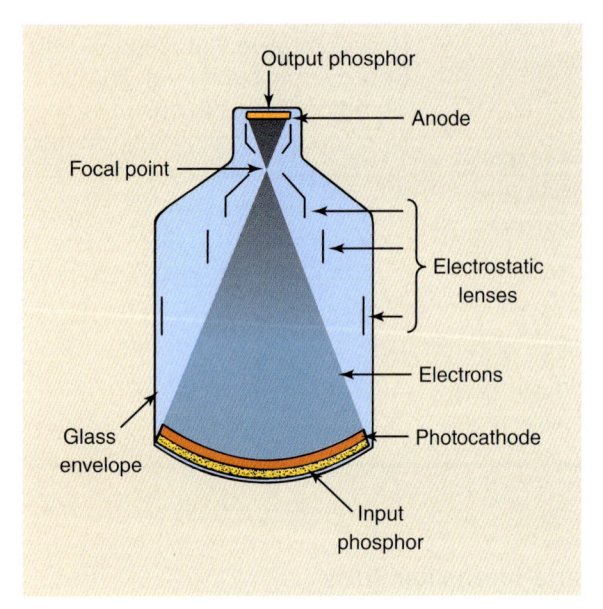

FIG. 19.4 The image-intensifier tube converts the pattern of the x-ray beam into a bright visible-light image.

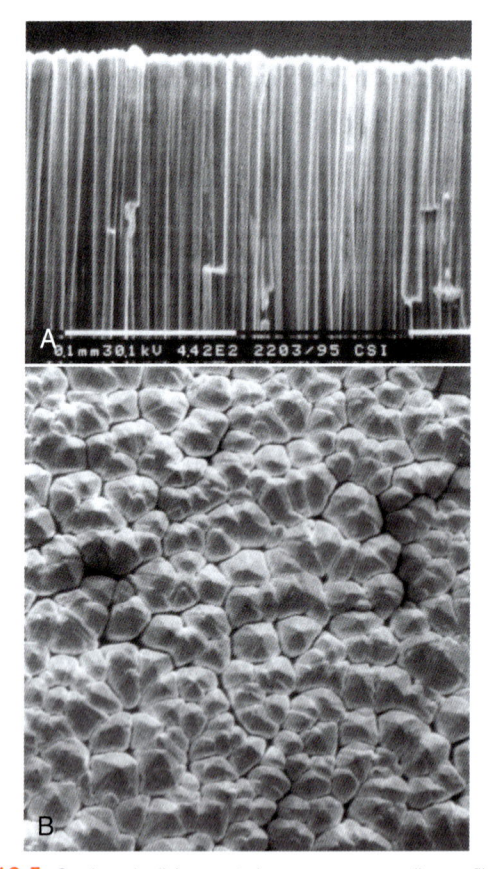

FIG. 19.5 Cesium iodide crystals are grown as linear filaments and are packed tightly, as shown in these photomicrographs. (A) Cross section. (B) Face. (Courtesy Philips Healthcare.)

electrons emitted is proportional to the intensity of the incident image-forming x-ray beam.

The image-intensifier tube is approximately 50 cm long. A potential difference of about 25,000 V is maintained across the tube between the photocathode and anode so that electrons produced by photoemission will be accelerated to the anode.

The anode is a circular plate with a hole in the middle through which electrons pass to the **output phosphor**, which is just the other side of the anode and is usually made of zinc-cadmium sulfide.

> The output phosphor is the site where accelerated electrons interact and produce visible light.

For the image pattern to be accurate, the electron path from the photocathode to the output phosphor must be precise. The engineering aspects of maintaining proper electron travel are called **electron optics**, because the pattern of electrons emitted from the large cathode end of the image-intensifier tube must be reduced to the small output phosphor.

The devices responsible for this control, called **electrostatic focusing lenses**, are located along the length of the image-intensifier tube. The electrons arrive at the output phosphor with high kinetic energy and contain the image of the input phosphor in minified form.

The interaction of these high-energy electrons with the output phosphor produces a considerable amount of light. Each photoelectron that arrives at the output phosphor produces 50 to 75 times as many light photons as were necessary to create it. The entire sequence of events from initial x-ray interaction to output image is summarized in Fig. 19.6. This ratio of the number of light photons at the output phosphor to the number of x-rays at the input phosphor is the **flux gain**.

> Flux gain = $\dfrac{\text{Number of output light photons}}{\text{Number of input x-ray photons}}$

The increased illumination of the image is attributable to the multiplication of light photons at the output phosphor compared with x-rays at the input phosphor, and the image minification from the input phosphor to output phosphor, which is called the **minification gain**.

The ability of the image intensifier to increase the illumination level of the image is called its **brightness gain**. The brightness gain is simply the product of the minification gain and the flux gain.

> Brightness gain = Minification gain × Flux gain

The minification gain is the ratio of the square of the diameter of the input phosphor (d_1) to the square of the

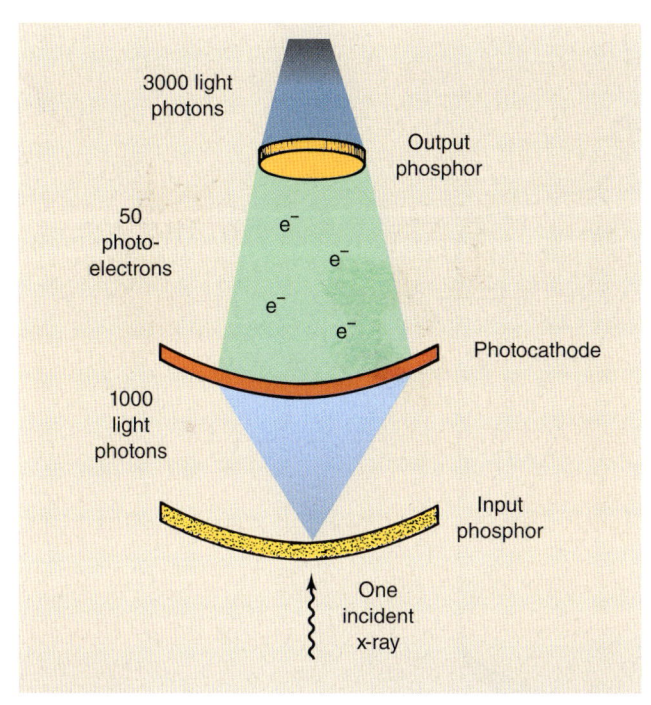

FIG. 19.6 In an image-intensifier tube, each incident x-ray that interacts with the input phosphor results in a large number of light photons at the output phosphor. The image intensifier shown here has a flux gain of 3000.

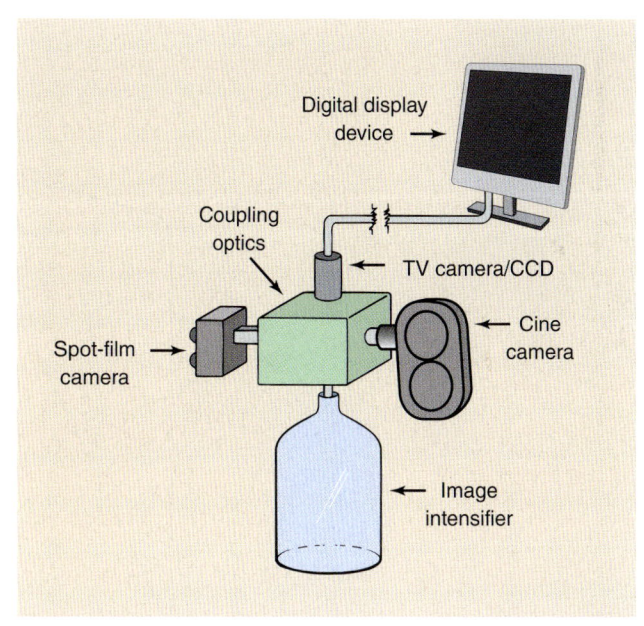

FIG. 19.7 Possible modes of operation with an image-intensifier tube. *CCD*, Charge-coupled device.

diameter of the output phosphor (d_o). Output phosphor size is fairly standard at 2.5 or 5 cm. Input phosphor size varies from 10 to 40 cm and is used to identify image-intensifier tubes.

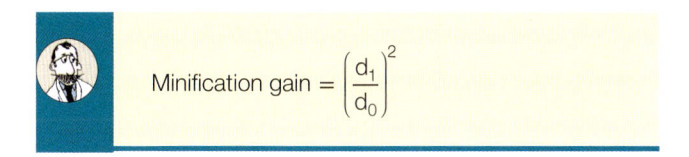

$$\text{Minification gain} = \left(\frac{d_i}{d_o}\right)^2$$

Question: What is the brightness gain for a 17-cm image-intensifier tube with a flux gain of 120 and a 2.5-cm output phosphor?

Answer:
$$\text{Brightness gain} = \left(\frac{17}{2.5}\right)^2$$
$$= 46 \times 120 = 5520$$

The brightness gain of most image intensifiers is 5000 to 30,000, and it decreases with tube age and use. As an image intensifier ages, patient radiation dose increases as a consequence of maintaining image brightness. Ultimately, the image intensifier must be replaced. When the entire imaging system is replaced, the new system will have a direct digital image receptor (see Chapter 20).

Brightness gain is defined as the ratio of the illumination intensity at the output phosphor, measured in candela per meter squared (cd/m^2), to the radiation intensity incident on the input phosphor, measured in milligray per second (mGy$_a$/s). This quantity is called the **conversion factor** and is approximately 0.01 times the brightness gain. The conversion factor is the proper term for expressing image intensification.

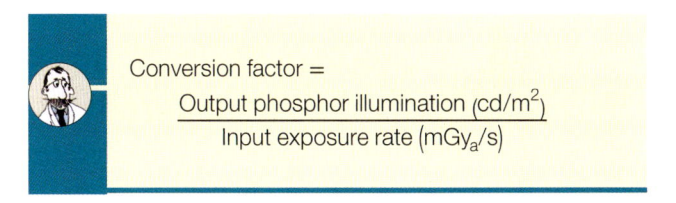

$$\text{Conversion factor} = \frac{\text{Output phosphor illumination (cd/m}^2\text{)}}{\text{Input exposure rate (mGy}_a\text{/s)}}$$

Image intensifiers have conversion factors of 50 to 300. These correspond to brightness gains of 5000 to 30,000.

Fig. 19.7 shows some of the modes of operation that can be accommodated with the image-intensifier tube. Fluoroscopic images are viewed on an LED flat-panel digital display device. The spot-film camera uses 105-mm film. The cineradiography camera was used almost exclusively in cardiac catheterization, but that use has been replaced by digital imaging.

Internal scatter radiation in the form of x-rays, electrons, and particularly light, can reduce the contrast of image intensifiers through a process called **veiling glare**. A veiling glare signal is produced behind a lead disc that is positioned on the input phosphor. Veiling glare is depicted in Fig. 19.8. Advanced image intensifiers have output phosphor designs that reduce veiling glare.

Multifield Image Intensification

Most image intensifiers are of the multifield type. Multifield image intensifiers provide considerably

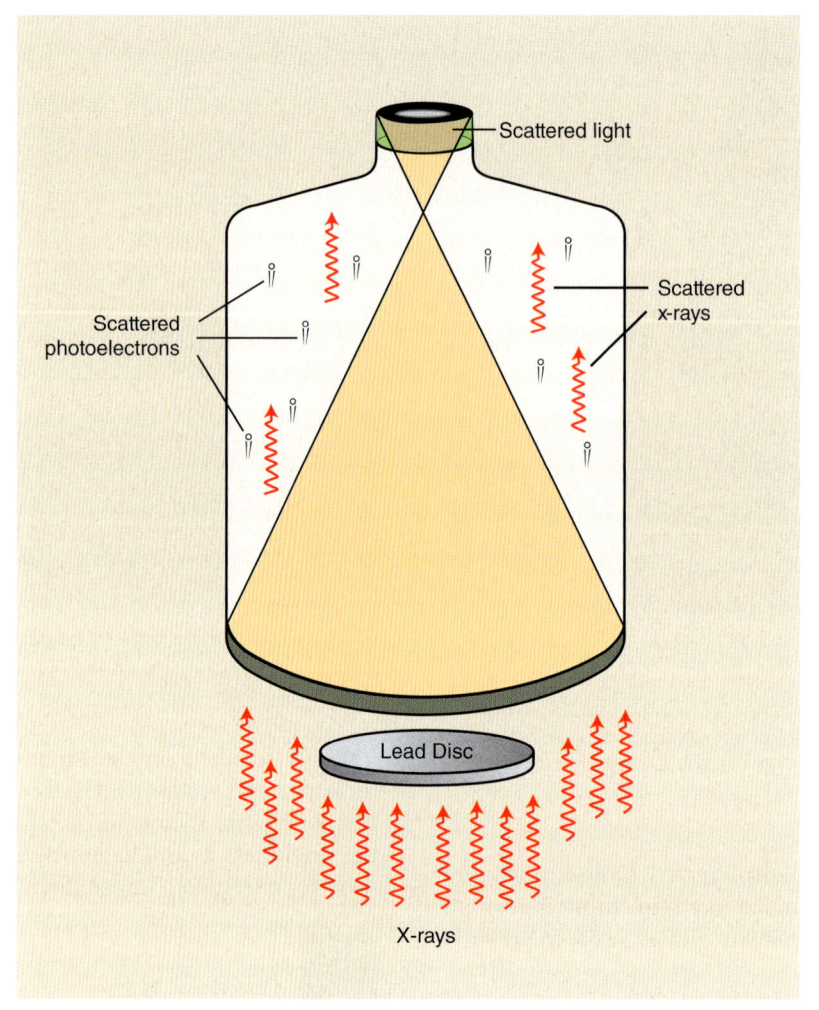

FIG. 19.8 Veiling glare reduces the contrast of an image-intensifier tube.

greater flexibility in all fluoroscopic examinations. Trifield tubes come in various sizes, but perhaps the most popular is 25/17/12 cm.

These numeric dimensions refer to the diameter of the input phosphor of the image-intensifier tube. The operation of a typical multifield tube is illustrated by the 25/17/12 type shown in Fig. 19.9. In the 25-cm mode, photoelectrons from the entire input phosphor are accelerated to the output phosphor.

When a switch is made to the 17-cm mode, the voltage on the electrostatic focusing lenses increases; this causes the electron focal point to move farther from the output phosphor. Consequently, only electrons from the center 17-cm diameter of the input phosphor are incident on the output phosphor.

> Multifield image intensifiers produce different magnifications of the image.

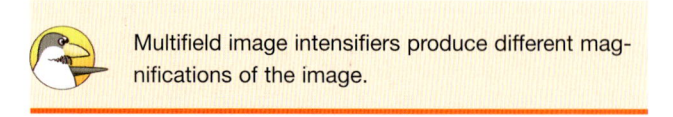

The principal result of this change in the focal point is to reduce the field of view (FOV). The image now

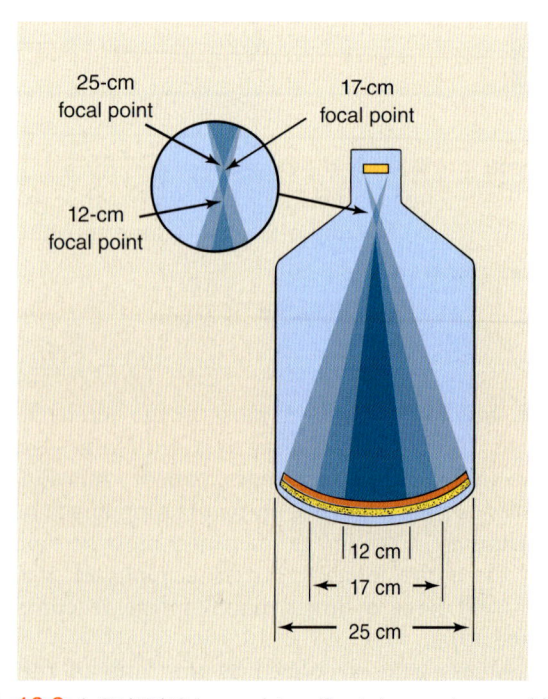

FIG. 19.9 A 25/17/12 image-intensifier tube produces a highly magnified image in 12-cm mode.

appears magnified because it still fills the entire LED monitor. Use of the smaller dimension of a multifield image-intensifier tube always results in a magnified image, with a magnification factor in direct proportion to the ratio of the diameters. A 25/17/12 tube operated in the 12-cm mode produces an image that is $\frac{25}{12} = 2.1$ times larger than the image produced in the 25-cm mode.

Question: How magnified is the image of a 25/17/12 image intensifier in the 17-cm mode compared with that produced in the 25-cm mode?

Answer: $MF = \frac{2.5}{17} = 1.5$ magnification

This magnified image comes at a price. In the magnified mode, the minification gain is reduced, and fewer photoelectrons are incident on the output phosphor. A dimmer image results.

To maintain the same level of brightness, the x-ray tube mA is increased by the ABC, which increases the patient radiation dose. The increase in dose is approximately equal to the ratio of the area of the input phosphor used, or $[25^2 \div 12^2 \approx 4.4]$—the dose obtained in the wide FOV mode.

Question: A 23/15/10 image-intensifier tube is used in the 10-cm mode. How much higher is the patient radiation dose in this mode compared with the 23-cm mode?

Answer: $23^2/10^2 = 5.3$ times higher!

This increase in patient radiation dose results in better image quality. The patient radiation dose is higher because more x-rays per unit area are required to form the image. This results in lower noise and improved **image contrast** (Table 19.2).

The portion of any image that results from the periphery of the input phosphor is inherently unfocused and suffers from **vignetting**, that is, a reduction in brightness at the periphery of the image.

Because only the central region of the input phosphor is used in the magnification mode, **spatial resolution** is also improved. In the 25-cm mode, a CsI image-intensifier tube can image approximately 0.125-mm objects (4 lp/mm); in the 10-cm mode, the resolution is approximately 0.08 mm (6 lp/mm).

TABLE 19.2	Magnification Mode

Results in:
- Better spatial resolution
- Better contrast resolution
- Higher patient radiation dose

The concept of spatial resolution as measured in line pairs per millimeter was discussed in Chapter 13. At this stage, it is sufficient to know that better spatial resolution is associated with a higher lp/mm value.

FLUOROSCOPIC IMAGE MONITORING

Television has been the principal method to monitor and view fluoroscopic images for years. And that continues, but what has changed is the type of television we use and the continuous improvement in the television image.

With the television monitoring system of a fluoroscopic image, the output phosphor of the image-intensifier tube is coupled directly to a television camera tube. The **vidicon** (Fig. 19.10) is the television camera tube that is most often used in television fluoroscopy. It has a sensitive input surface that is the same size as the output phosphor of the image-intensifier tube. The television camera tube converts the light image from the output phosphor of the image intensifier into an electrical signal that is sent to the television monitor, where it is reconstructed as an image on the television screen.

A significant advantage of television monitoring is that brightness level and contrast can be controlled electronically. With television monitoring, several observers can view the fluoroscopic image at the same time. It is even common to place monitors remote to the examination room for others to observe.

Television monitoring also allows for storage of the image in its electronic form for later playback and image manipulation.

Two methods are used to electronically convert the visible image on the output phosphor of the image intensifier into an electronic signal. These are the thermionic **television camera** tube and the solid-state **charge-coupled device (CCD)**.

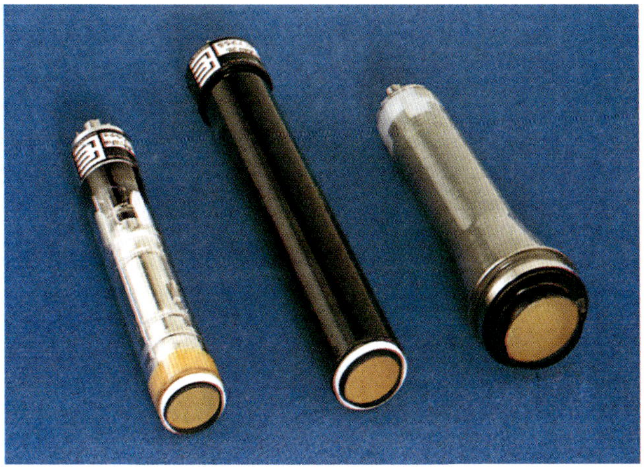

FIG. 19.10 These three variations of a vidicon television camera tube have a diameter of approximately 2.5 cm and a length of 15 cm. The right tube uses electrostatic rather than electromagnetic electron beam deflection. (Courtesy Philips Healthcare.)

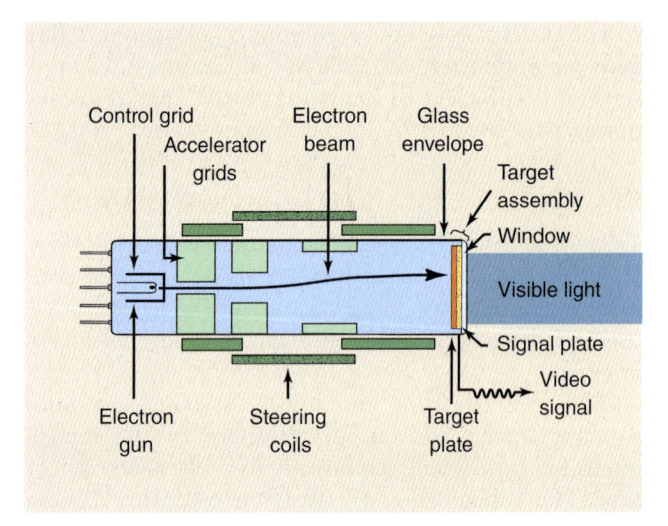

FIG. 19.11 Vidicon television camera tube and its principal parts.

The television camera consists of a cylindrical housing, approximately 15 mm in diameter by 25 cm in length, which contains the heart of the television camera tube. It also contains electromagnetic coils that are used to properly steer the electron beam inside the tube.

A number of such television camera tubes are available for television fluoroscopy, but the vidicon and its modified version, the Plumbicon, are used most often.

> A television camera tube or CCD converts the light signal from the output phosphor to an electronic signal.

Fig. 19.11 shows a typical vidicon. The **glass envelope** serves the same function that it does for the x-ray tube: to maintain a vacuum and provide mechanical support for the internal elements. These internal elements include the cathode, its **electron gun**, assorted **electrostatic grids**, and a **target assembly** that serves as an anode.

The electron gun is a heated filament that supplies a constant electron current by thermionic emission. The electrons are formed into an electron beam by the control grid, which also helps to accelerate the electrons to the anode.

The electron beam is further accelerated and focused by additional electrostatic grids. The size of the electron beam and its position are controlled by external electromagnetic coils known as deflection coils, focusing coils, and alignment coils.

At the anode end of the tube, the electron beam passes through a wire mesh–like structure and interacts with the target assembly. The target assembly consists of three layers that are sandwiched together. The outside layer is the **window**, the thin part of the glass envelope.

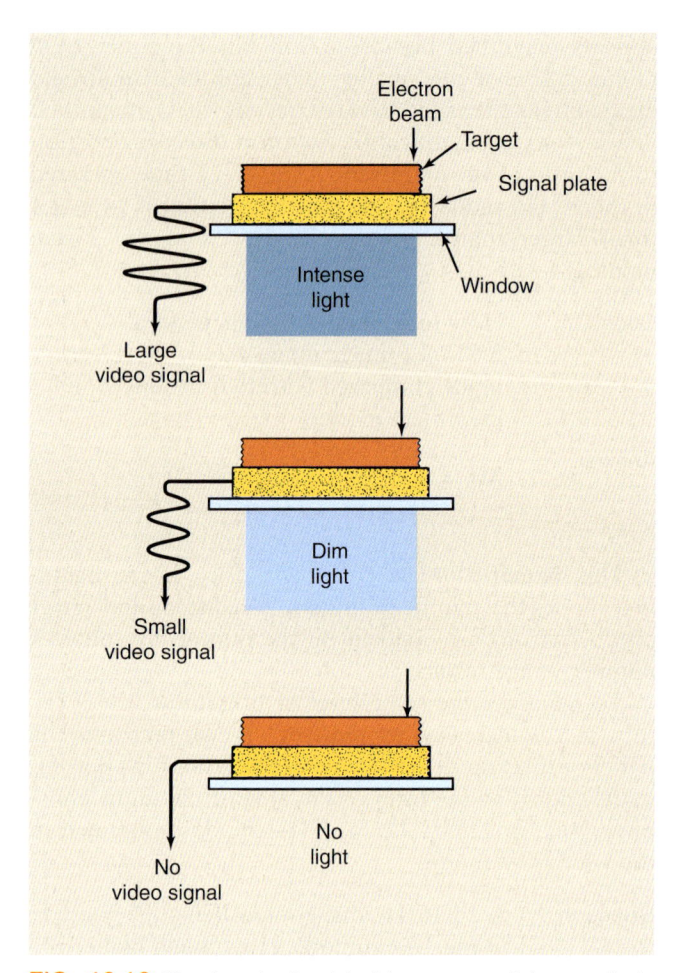

FIG. 19.12 The target of a television camera tube conducts electrons, creating a video signal only when illuminated.

Coated on the inside of the window is a thin layer of metal or graphite, called the **signal plate**. The signal plate is thin enough to transmit light yet thick enough to efficiently conduct electricity. Its name derives from the fact that it conducts the video signal out of the tube into the external video circuit.

A photoconductive layer of antimony trisulfide is applied to the inside of the signal plate. This layer, called the **target**, is swept by the electron beam. Antimony trisulfide is photoconductive because, when illuminated, it conducts electrons; when it is dark, it behaves as an insulator.

The mechanism of the target is complex but can be described briefly as follows. When light from the output phosphor of the image-intensifier tube strikes the window, it is transmitted through the signal plate to the target.

If the electron beam is incident on the same part of the target at the same time, some of its electrons are conducted through the target to the signal plate and from there out of the tube as the video signal. If that area of the target is dark, no video signal is produced (Fig. 19.12).

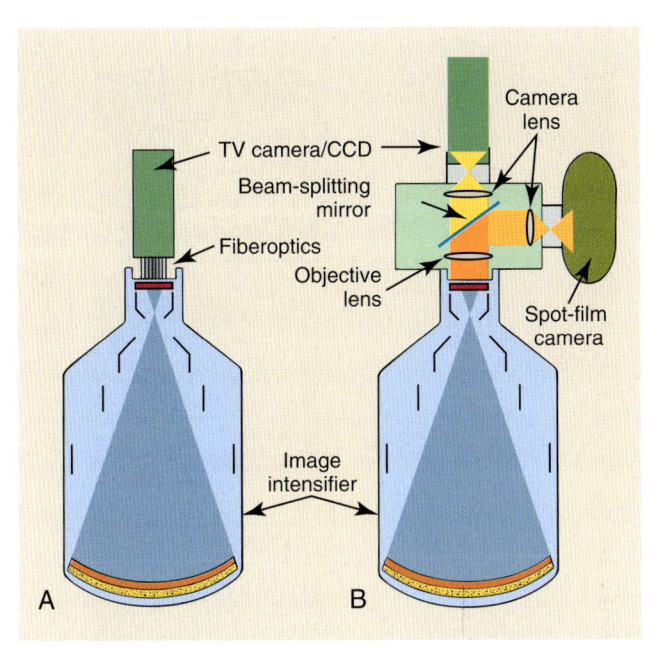

FIG. 19.13 Television camera tubes and charge-coupled devices (CCDs) are coupled to an image-intensifier tube in two ways. (A) Fiber optics. (B) Lens system.

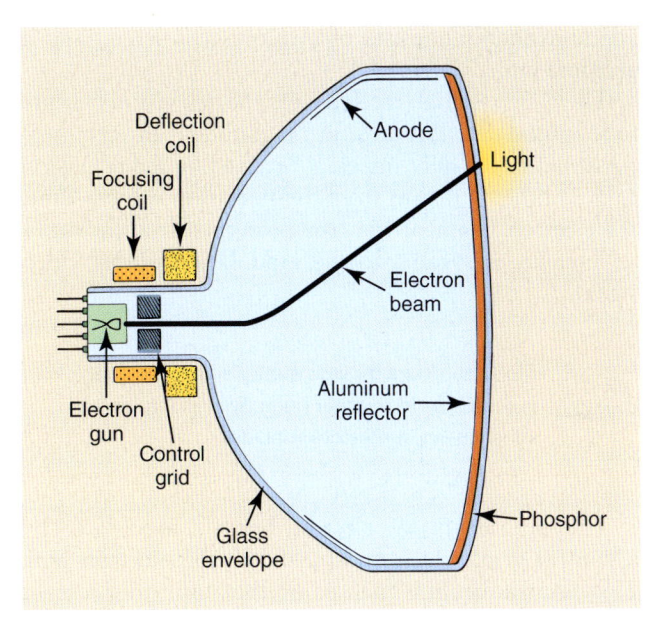

FIG. 19.14 A television picture tube (cathode ray tube) and its principal parts.

> The magnitude of the video signal is proportional to the intensity of light from the output phosphor.

Image intensifiers and television camera tubes are manufactured so that the output phosphor of the image-intensifier tube is the same diameter as the window of the television camera tube, usually 2.5 or 5 cm. Two methods are commonly used to couple the television camera tube to the image-intensifier tube (Fig. 19.13).

The simplest method is to use a bundle of **fiber optics**. The fiber-optics bundle is only a few millimeters thick and contains thousands of glass fibers per square millimeter of cross section. One advantage of this type of coupling is its compact assembly, which makes it easy to move the image-intensifier tower. This coupling is rugged and can withstand relatively rough handling.

The principal disadvantage is that it cannot accommodate the additional optics required for devices such as cine or photospot cameras.

To accept a cine or photospot camera, **lens coupling** is required. This type of coupling results in a much larger assembly that should be handled with care. It is absolutely essential that the lenses and the mirror remain precisely adjusted because malposition results in a blurred image.

The **objective lens** accepts light from the output phosphor and converts it into a parallel beam. When an image is recorded on film, this beam is interrupted by a **beam-splitting mirror** so that only a portion is transmitted to the television camera; the remainder is reflected to a film camera. Such a system allows the fluoroscopist to view the image while it is being recorded.

Usually the beam-splitting mirror is retracted from the beam when a film camera is not in use. Both the television camera and the film camera are coupled to lenses that focus the parallel light beam onto the film and target of the respective cameras.

These **camera lenses** are the most critical elements in the optical chain in terms of alignment. Although the lenses are shown as simple convex lenses, it should be understood that each is a compound lens system that consists of several separate lens elements.

The video signal is amplified and is transmitted by cable to the **digital display device**, where it is transformed back into a visible image. The digital display device monitor forms one end of a closed-circuit television system. The other end is the television camera tube or CCD.

Two differences between closed-circuit television fluoroscopy and home television are immediately obvious: no audio and no channel selection. Usually, the radiographer manipulates only two controls: contrast and brightness.

> The television picture tube is replaced with a LED flat-panel digital display device.

The heart of the television monitor is the **television picture tube,** or the cathode ray tube (Fig. 19.14). It is similar to the television camera tube in many ways: A glass envelope, electron gun, and external coils are used to focus and steer the electron beam. It is different from a television camera tube in that it is much larger and its anode assembly consists of a fluorescent screen and a graphite lining.

The video signal received by the television picture tube is **modulated**; that is, its magnitude is directly proportional to the light intensity received by the television camera tube. Different from the television camera tube, the electron beam of the television picture tube varies in intensity according to the modulation of the video signal.

> Modulation is a change in a quantity or signal in response to another quantity or signal and is widely used in medical imaging.

The intensity of the electron beam is modulated by a **control grid**, which is attached to the electron gun. This electron beam is focused on the output fluorescent screen by the external coils. There, the electrons interact with an output phosphor and produce a burst of light.

The phosphor is composed of linear crystals that are aligned perpendicularly to the glass envelope to reduce **lateral dispersion**. It is usually backed by a thin layer of aluminum, which transmits the electron beam but reflects the light.

The **television image** on the monitor is formed in a complex way, but it can be described rather simply. It involves transforming the visible light image of the output phosphor of the image-intensifier tube into an electrical video signal that is created by a constant electron beam in the television camera tube. The video signal then modulates the electron beam of the television picture tube and transforms that electron beam into a visible image at the fluorescent screen of the picture tube.

Both electron beams—the constant one of the television camera tube and the modulated one of the television picture tube—are finely focused pencil beams that are precisely and synchronously directed by the external electromagnetic coils of each tube. These beams are synchronous because they are always at the same position at the same time and move in precisely the same fashion.

The movement of these electron beams produces a **raster pattern** on the screen of a television picture tube (Fig. 19.15). Although the following discussion relates to a television picture tube, remember that the same electron beam pattern occurs in the television camera tube.

The electron beam begins in the upper-left corner of the screen and moves to the upper-right corner, creating a line of varying intensity of light as it moves. This is called an **active trace**. The electron beam then is turned off and it returns to the left side of the screen as shown. This is the **horizontal retrace**.

A series of active traces then is followed by horizontal retraces until the electron beam is at the bottom of the screen. This is very similar to the action of word processing when one types a line of information (the active trace): The cursor returns (the horizontal retrace) and continues this sequence to the bottom of the page. As the writer completes a page, the electron beam completes a **television field**.

The similarity stops there, however, because you would continue word processing. The electron beam is turned off again and undergoes a **vertical retrace** to the top of the screen.

The electron beam now describes a second television field, which is the same as the first except that each active trace lies between two adjacent active traces of the first field. This movement of the electron beam is called **interlace**, and two interlaced television fields form a single **television frame**.

In the United States, power is supplied at 60 Hz, which results in 60 television fields per second and 30 television frames per second. This is fortunate because the flickering of home movies (shown at 16 frames per second) or old-time movies does not appear on the television image. Flickering is not detectable by the human eye at rates above approximately 20 frames per second. At a frame rate of 30 per second, each frame is 33 ms long.

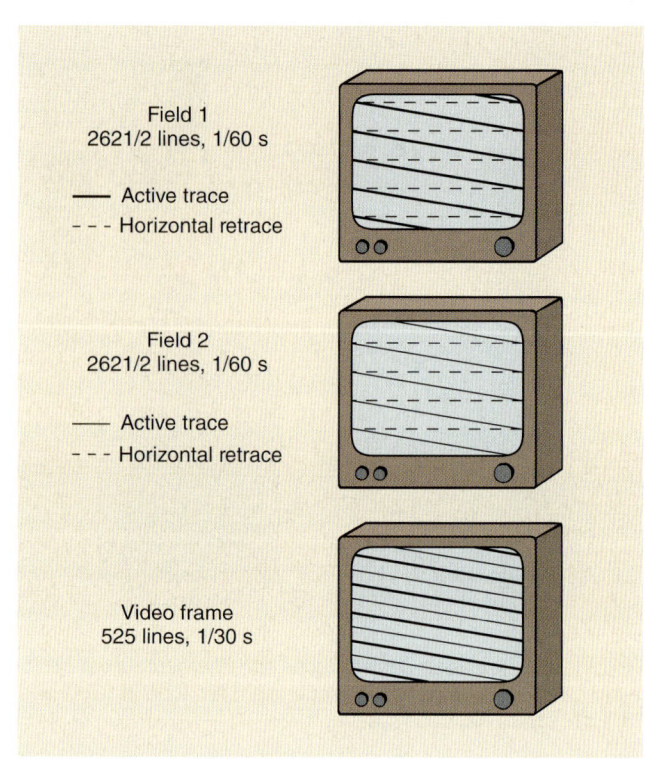

FIG. 19.15 A video frame is formed from a raster pattern of two interlaced video fields.

> Video monitoring uses a rate of 30 frames per second.

In the television camera tube, as the electron beam reads the optical signal, the signal is erased. In the television picture tube, as the electron beam creates the television optical signal, it immediately fades, hence the term *fluorescent screen*. Therefore each new television frame represents 33 ms of new information.

Standard broadcast and closed-circuit televisions are called 525-line systems because they use 525 lines of active trace per frame. Actually, only about 480 lines are used per frame because of the time required for retracing. Other special-purpose systems have 875 or 1024 lines per frame and therefore have better spatial resolution. These high-resolution systems are particularly important for interventional radiology.

In countries where power is supplied at 50 Hz, 50 television fields and thus 25 television frames are used per second. On a TV monitor, 625 lines are used per frame in two consecutive fields of 312.5 lines.

> For a 23-cm image intensifier, a 525-line TV system provides a spatial resolution of approximately 1 lp/mm; a 1024-line system provides spatial resolution of 2 lp/mm.

The **vertical resolution** is determined by the number of scan lines. The **horizontal resolution** is determined by **bandpass**. Bandpass is expressed in frequency (Hz) and describes the number of times per second that the electron beam can be modulated. A 1-MHz bandpass would indicate that the electron beam intensity could be changed a million times each second.

> The higher the bandpass, the better the horizontal resolution.

The objective of television designers is to create a television frame that has equal horizontal and vertical resolution. Commercial television systems have a bandpass of about 3.5 MHz. Those used in fluoroscopy are approximately 4.5 MHz; 1000-line high-resolution systems have a bandpass of approximately 20 MHz.

The television monitor remains the weakest link in image-intensified fluoroscopy. A 525-line system has approximately 1-lp/mm spatial resolution, but the image intensifier is good to about 5 lp/mm. Therefore if the superior resolution of the image intensifier is to be captured, the image must be saved in an electronic format.

FLUOROSCOPY QUALITY CONTROL

Fluoroscopic examination can result in high patient radiation dose. The entrance skin dose (ESD) for an adult averages 30 to 50 mGy$_t$/min during fluoroscopy; this can easily result in a skin dose of 100 mGy$_t$ for many fluoroscopic examinations. For interventional radiology procedures, a skin dose of 1000 mGy$_t$ is common, but should be avoided if possible.

Approximate patient radiation dose can be identified through the performance of proper quality control (QC) measurements. Some measurements may be required more frequently after significant changes have occurred in the operating console, high-voltage generator, or x-ray tube.

Exposure Rate

Federal law and most state statutes require that under normal operation, the ESD rate shall not exceed 100 mGy$_t$/min. For interventional radiology procedures, the fluoroscope may be equipped with a high-level control, which allows an ESD up to 200 mGy$_t$/min.

Measurements are made with a calibrated radiation dosimeter to ensure that these levels are not exceeded. Lucite, aluminum, copper, and lead filters are used to determine the adequacy of any automatic brightness stabilization (ABS) system.

Automatic Exposure Systems

All fluoroscopes are equipped with some sort of ABS. Such systems function in the manner of the AEC of a radiographic imaging system, producing constant image brightness on the flat-panel digital display device, regardless of the thickness or composition of the anatomy.

Performance monitoring of an ABS is conducted by determining that the radiation exposure to the input phosphor of the image-intensifier tube is constant, regardless of patient thickness. With a test object in place, the image brightness on the digital display device should not change perceptibly when various thicknesses of patient-simulating material are inserted into the beam. The input exposure rate to the image-intensifier tube is measured and should be in the range of 0.1 to 0.4 μGy$_a$/s.

The test objects used for American College of Radiology (ACR) accreditation are shown in Fig. 19.16. These test objects track ABS *versus* tissue thickness and assess spatial resolution, contrast resolution, and noise.

SUMMARY

The original fluoroscope, invented by Thomas Edison, had a zinc-cadmium sulfide screen that was placed in the x-ray beam directly above the patient. The radiologist stared directly into the screen and viewed a faint yellow-green fluoroscopic image. It was not until the 1960s that the image intensifier entered routine clinical service.

In the past, fluoroscopy required radiologists to adapt their eyes to the dark before the examination was

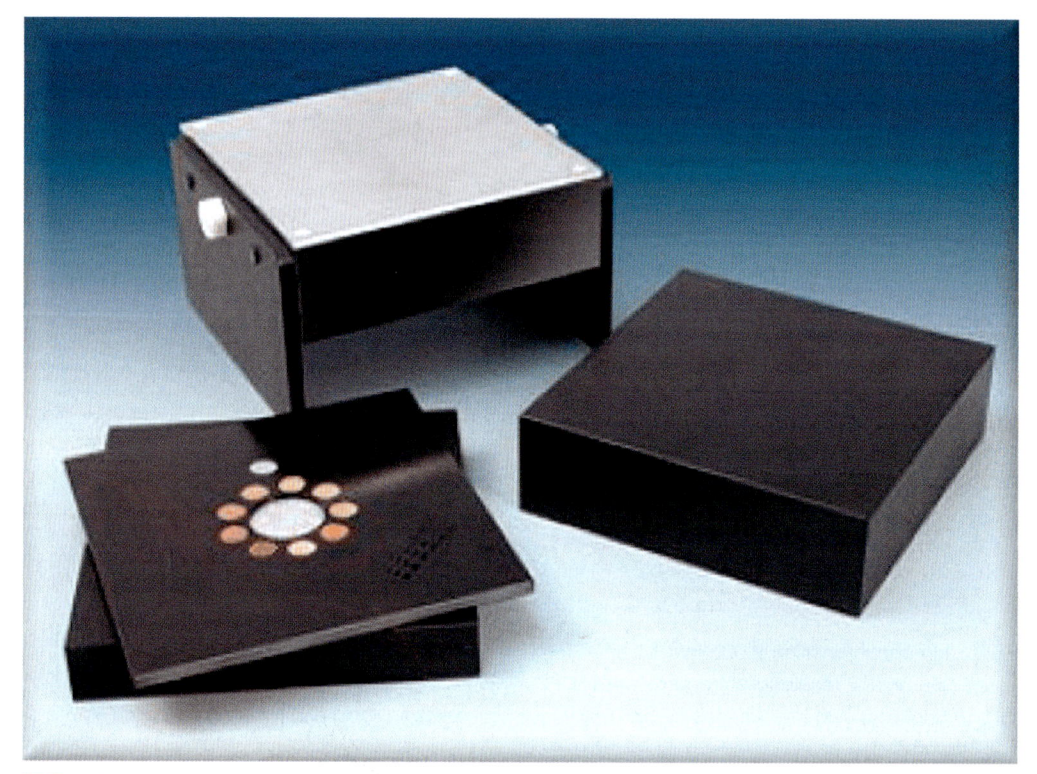

FIG. 19.16 ACR radiologic/fluoroscopic accreditation test objects. (Courtesy American College of Radiology.)

performed. Under dim viewing conditions, the human eye uses rods for vision; these have low visual acuity. The image from today's fluoroscope is bright enough to be perceived by cone vision. Cone vision provides superior visual acuity and contrast perception. When viewing the fluoroscopic image, the radiologist is able to see fine anatomical detail and differences in brightness levels of anatomical parts.

The image intensifier is a complex device that receives the image-forming x-ray beam, converts it to light, and increases the light intensity for better viewing. The input phosphor converts the x-ray beam into light. When stimulated by light, the photocathode then emits electrons, and the electrons are accelerated to the output phosphor.

The following relationships define several characteristics of image-intensified fluoroscopy:

$$\text{Flux gain} = \frac{\text{Number of output light photons}}{\text{Number of input x-ray photons}}$$

$$\text{Minification gain} = \left(\frac{\text{Diameter of input phosphor}}{\text{Diameter of output phosphor}}\right)^2$$

Brightness gain is also expressed as the conversion factor:

$$\text{Conversion factor} = \frac{\text{Output phosphor illumination (cd/m}^2\text{)}}{\text{Input exposure rate (mGy}_a\text{/s)}}$$

CHALLENGE QUESTIONS

1. Define or otherwise identify the following:
   a. Photopic vision
   b. Automatic brightness control (ABC)
   c. Visual acuity
   d. Flux gain
   e. Angiography
   f. Vidicon
   g. Photoemission
   h. Bucky slot cover
   i. Scotopic vision
   j. Modulation
2. Draw a diagram to show the relationship between the x-ray tube, the patient couch, and the image intensifier.
3. What is the difference between rod and cone vision? With which is visual acuity greater?
4. What is the approximate kVp for the following fluoroscopic examinations: barium enema, gallbladder, and upper gastrointestinal?
5. Draw a cross section of the human eye and label the cornea, lens, and retina.
6. Explain the difference between photoemission and thermionic emission.
7. Diagram the image-intensifier tube, label its principal parts, and discuss the function of each.

8. A 23-cm image intensifier has an output phosphor size of 2.5 cm and a flux gain of 75. What is its brightness gain?
9. What is vignetting?
10. Why is the television monitor considered the weakest link in image-intensified fluoroscopy?
11. What is the primary function of the fluoroscope?
12. Who invented the fluoroscope in 1896? What phosphor was used on that original fluoroscopic screen?
13. What device has nearly replaced the image intensifier tube?
14. What limits the vertical resolution and horizontal resolution of a cathode ray tube video monitor?
15. Does spatial resolution change when one is viewing in the magnification mode versus the normal mode?
16. What is meant by a trifield image intensifier?
17. Discuss the concepts of visual acuity and contrast perception and their application in fluoroscopy.
18. When the image intensifier is switched from 15-cm mode to 25-cm mode, what happens to patient radiation dose and contrast resolution?
19. Trace the path of information-carrying elements in a fluoroscopic system from incident x-rays to the video image.
20. Where is the radiologist normally located during remote fluoroscopy? Where is the radiographer?

The answers to the Challenge Questions can be found by logging on to our website at http://evolve.elsevier.com.

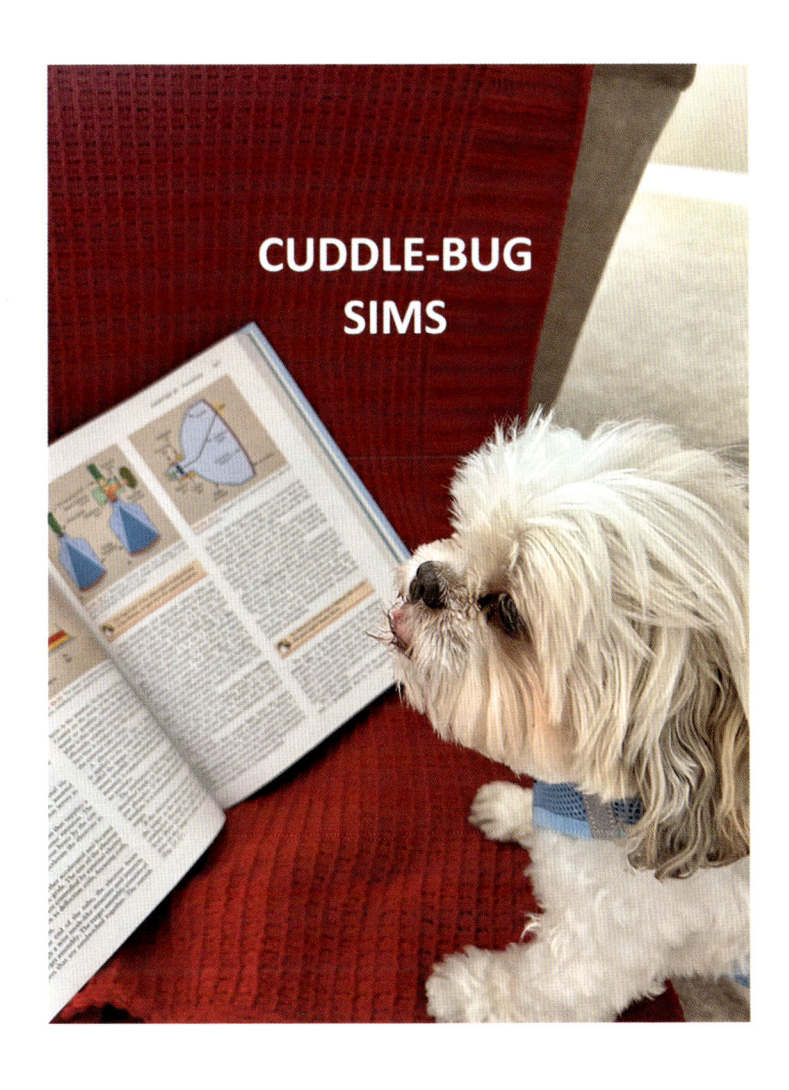

CHAPTER 20

Interventional Radiology

OBJECTIVES

At the completion of this chapter, the student should be able to do the following:

1. Describe the parts of a digital fluoroscopic imaging system and explain their functions.
2. Compute pixel size in digital fluoroscopy.
3. Understand the advantages of using a flat-panel image receptor.
4. Outline the procedures for temporal subtraction and energy subtraction.
5. Describe the measures used to provide radiation protection for patients and personnel during interventional radiology.
6. Describe the special equipment found in the interventional radiology suite.

OUTLINE

Digital Fluoroscopic Imaging Systems 289
Image Receptor 290
   Charge-Coupled Device 290
   Flat-Panel Image Receptor 292
Image Display 293
   Video System 293
   Flat-Panel Image Display 293
Types of Interventional Radiology Procedures 294
   Digital Subtraction Angiography 294
   Image Formation 295
   Roadmapping 299
Basic Principles 299
   Arterial Access 299
   Guidewires 300
   Catheters 300
   Contrast Media 300
   Patient Preparation and Monitoring 300
   Risks of Arteriography 301
Interventional Radiology Suite 301
   Personnel 301
   Equipment 302
   Patient Radiation Dose 303
Summary 304
Challenge Questions 304

IN PREVIOUS years, myelography and venography were considered **special procedures**. Recently, the area of therapeutic angiographic intervention has undergone rapid development. We now have suites of x-ray rooms and complex equipment that have been specially designed for **interventional radiology (IR)**.

Fig. 20.1 reviews the components used in conventional fluoroscopy. Digital fluoroscopy (DF) is a digital x-ray imaging system that produces dynamic images obtained with an area x-ray beam. The difference between conventional fluoroscopy and DF is the nature of the image and the manner in which it is digitized.

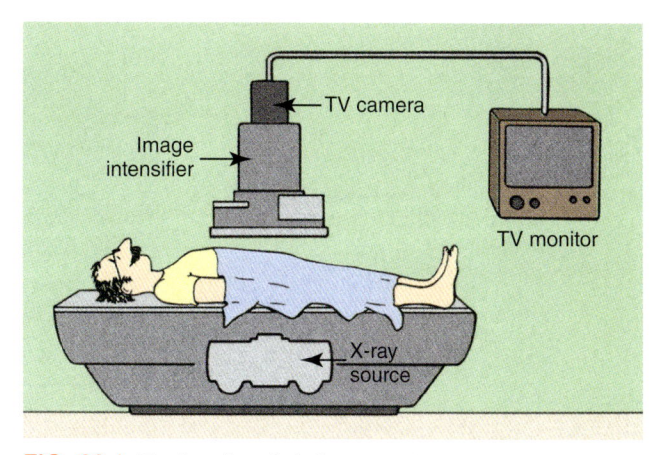

FIG. 20.1 The imaging chain in conventional fluoroscopy.

The initial investigators of DF demonstrated that nearly instantaneous, high-contrast subtraction images could be obtained after intravenous (IV) injection of contrast media. Although the IV route is still widely used, intraarterial injections are also used with DF.

> Advantages of DF over conventional fluoroscopy include the speed of image acquisition and postprocessing to enhance image contrast.

A 1024 × 1024 image matrix sometimes is described as a 1000-line system. In DF, the spatial resolution is determined both by the image matrix and by the size of the image receptor.

> Spatial resolution is limited by pixel size.

Question: What is the pixel size of a 1000-line DF system operating with an digital image receptor in the 12-cm mode?
Answer: 12 cm equals 120 mm; therefore the size of each pixel is 120 mm/1024 pixels = 0.117 mm/pixel or 117 μm/pixel.

DIGITAL FLUOROSCOPIC IMAGING SYSTEMS

A DF examination is conducted in much the same manner as a conventional fluoroscopic study. To the casual observer, the equipment is the same, but such is not the case (Fig. 20.2). A computer has been added, as have multiple monitors and the ability to remotely control the imaging system (Fig. 20.3).

Fig. 20.4 shows a representative operating console of a dedicated DF imaging system. It contains alphanumeric and special-function keys in the right module for entering patient data and communicating with the computer. The left portion of the console contains additional special-function keys for data acquisition, postprocessing, and image display.

The module on the right also contains computer-interactive video controls and a pad for cursor and region-of-interest manipulation. Other systems use a trackball, a joystick, or a mouse instead of the pad. At least two monitors are used. In Fig. 20.4, the right monitors are used to edit patient and examination data and to annotate final images. The left monitors display subtracted images.

During DF, the under-couch x-ray tube actually operates in the radiographic mode. Tube current is measured in hundreds of mA instead of less than 5 mA, as in image-intensified fluoroscopy.

This is not a problem, however. If the x-ray tube were energized continuously, it would fail because of thermal overloading, and the patient radiation dose would be exceedingly high. Images from DF are obtained by pulsing the x-ray beam in a manner called pulse-progressive fluoroscopy, as shown in Fig. 20.5.

> During DF, the x-ray tube operates in the radiographic mode.

Image acquisition rates of 1 per second to 10 per second are common in many examinations. Because 33 ms is required to produce a single video frame, x-ray exposures longer than this can result in unnecessary patient radiation doses. This is a theoretical limit, however, and longer exposures may be necessary to ensure low noise and good image quality.

If a flat panel is the fluoroscopic image receptor instead of an II tube, x-ray exposure time can be continuously varied for even greater patient radiation dose

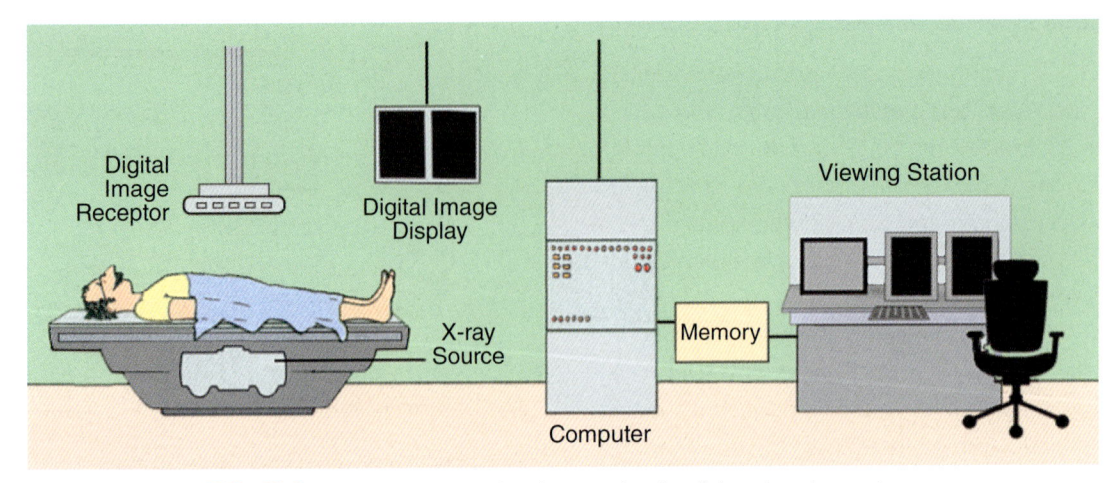

FIG. 20.2 The components of an interventional radiology imaging system.

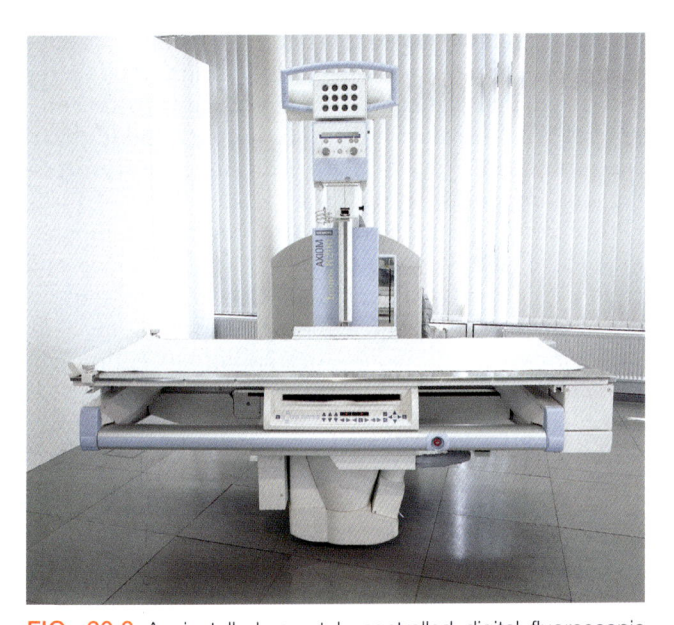

FIG. 20.3 An installed remotely controlled digital fluoroscopic imaging system with an over-table x-ray tube and under-table image receptor. (Courtesy of Siemens Medical Solutions USA, Inc.)

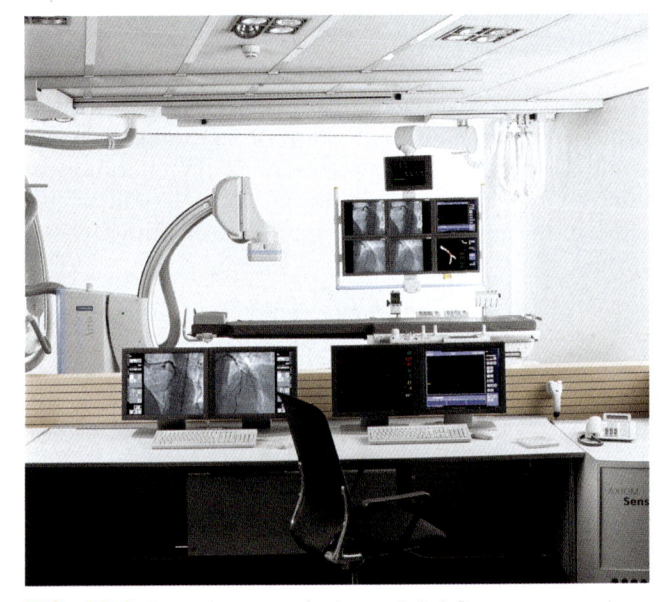

FIG. 20.4 Operating console for a digital fluoroscopy system. (Courtesy of Siemens Medical Solutions USA, Inc.)

reduction. Each time the flat panel is exposed, it is read immediately and the image projected until the next image is acquired.

Consequently, the x-ray generator must be capable of switching on and off very rapidly. The time required for the x-ray tube to be switched on and reach selected levels of kVp and mA is the **interrogation time**. The time required for the x-ray tube to be switched off is the **extinction time** (see Fig. 20.5). DF systems incorporate high-frequency generators with interrogation and extinction times of less than 1 ms.

The fraction of time that the x-ray tube is energized is the **duty cycle**. Fig. 20.5 also shows the x-ray tube is energized for 100 ms every second. This represents a 10% duty cycle. This feature of pulse-progressive DF can result in significant patient radiation dose reduction.

Pulse-progressive DF is essential for reducing patient radiation dose and should be routinely used. The Alliance for Radiation Safety in Adult Patient Imaging—"Image Wisely"—endorses "pause and pulse" during fluoroscopy. This means carefully planning and preparing before starting fluoroscopy and pulsing the fluoroscopic x-ray beam at the lowest frame rate. This approach has also been adopted by the "Image Gently" campaign for pediatric imaging.

IMAGE RECEPTOR

For DF imaging, one needs a digital image receptor. Two types are employed.

Charge-Coupled Device

A major change from conventional fluoroscopy to DF is the use of a charge-coupled device (CCD) instead of a TV camera tube, as was shown in Fig. 19.13. The CCD was developed in the 1970s for military applications, especially for night vision devices. Today CCDs are used in digital camera, commercial television, security surveillance, astronomy, and all of the new smartphones and tablets.

The demands of medical imaging are much more rigorous than these other applications. That is why the application of the CCD in fluoroscopy is a recent development.

The sensitive component of a CCD is a layer of crystalline silicon (Fig. 20.6). When this silicon is illuminated, electric charge is generated, which is then sampled, pixel by pixel, and manipulated to produce a digital image.

The CCD is mounted on the output phosphor of the image intensifier tube and is coupled through fiber optics (Fig. 20.7) or lens systems (Fig. 20.8). In fact, such coupling is far more complex than that shown in Fig. 20.8.

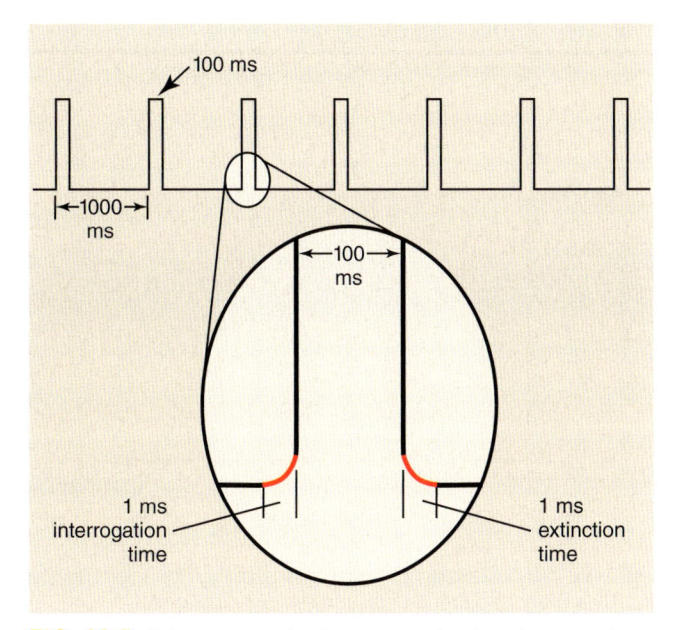

FIG. 20.5 Pulse-progressive fluoroscopy involves terms such as duty cycle, interrogation time, and extinction time.

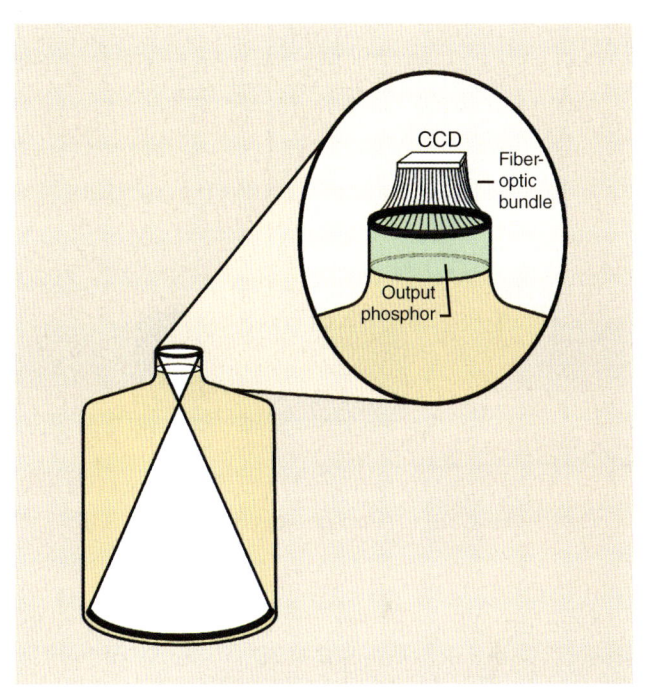

FIG. 20.7 Manner in which a charge-coupled device (*CCD*) can be coupled to the image-intensifier tube.

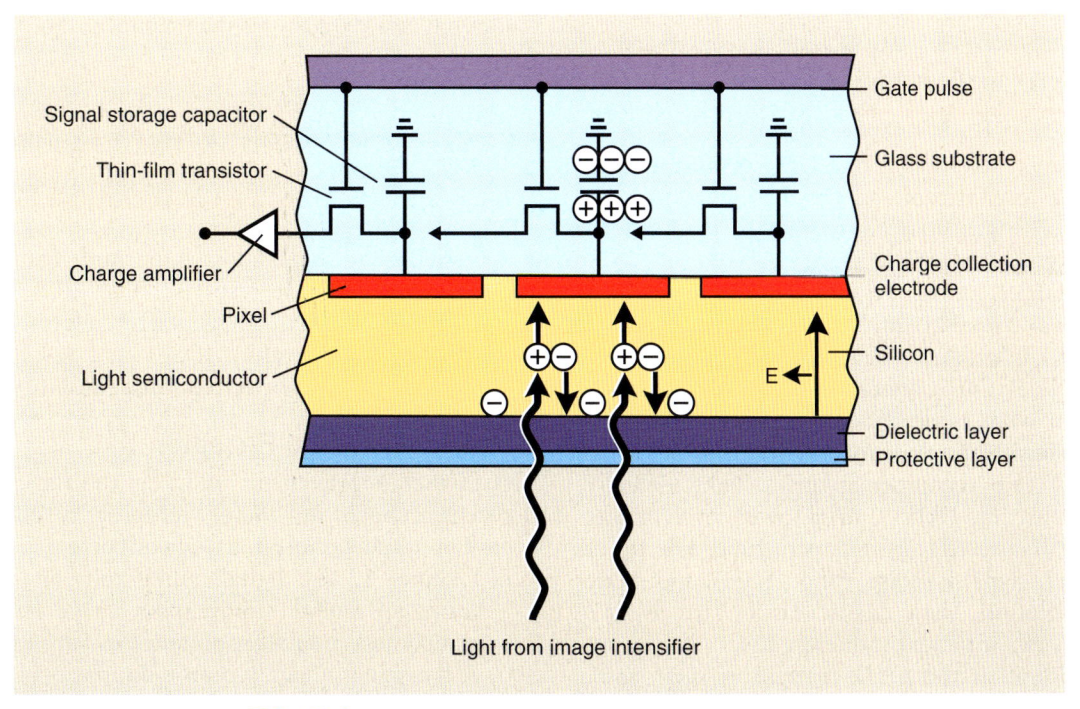

FIG. 20.6 Cross-sectional view of a charge-coupled device.

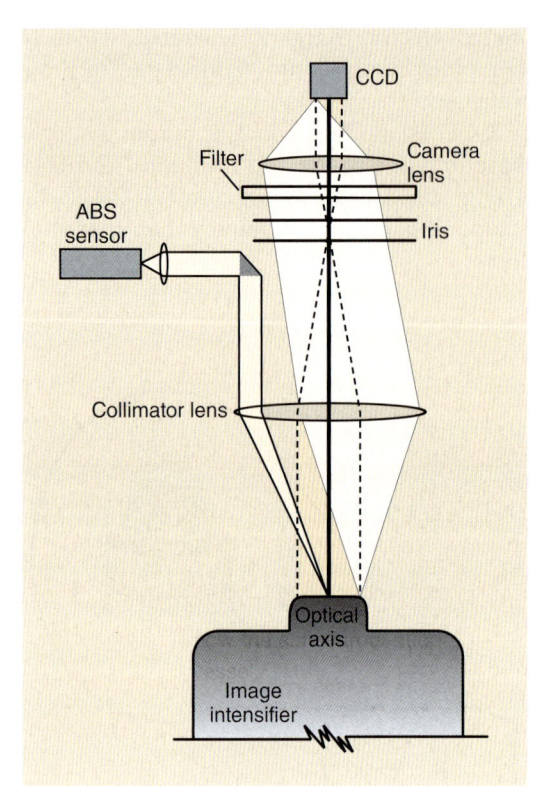

FIG. 20.8 An example of a lens-coupling system for a charge-coupled device (CCD) to an image intensifier.

TABLE 20.1 Advantages of Charge-Coupled Devices for Medical Imaging

- High spatial resolution
- High SNR
- High DQE
- No warm-up required
- No lag or blooming
- No spatial distortion
- No maintenance
- Unlimited life
- Unaffected by magnetic fields
- Linear response
- Lower patient radiation dose

DQE, Detective quantum efficiency; *SNR*, signal-to-noise ratio.

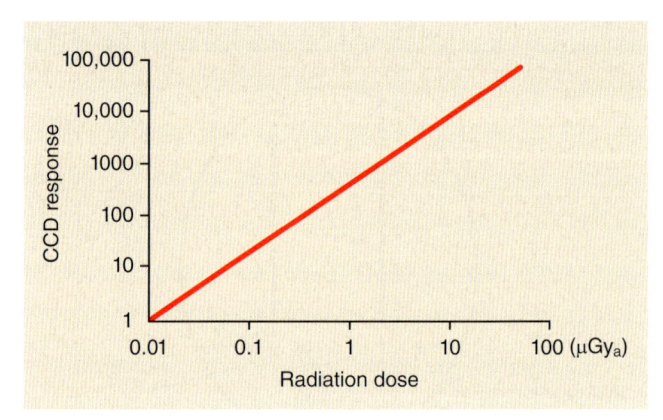

FIG. 20.9 The response to light of a charge-coupled device (CCD) is linear and can be electronically manipulated.

Note the device in Fig. 20.8 that is labeled "ABS sensor." With a lens-coupled CCD, a sample of light is measured and is used to drive the automatic brightness control (ABC) system.

> When the CCD is directly coupled to the image intensifier, the entire CCD signal is sampled and drives the ABC system.

The principal advantages of CCDs in most applications, such as digital cameras, are their small size and ruggedness. The principal advantages of their use for medical imaging are listed in Table 20.1.

The spatial resolution of a CCD is determined by its physical size and pixel count. Systems that incorporate a 1024 matrix can produce images with 10 lp/mm spatial resolution. Television camera tubes can show spatial distortion in what is described as "pincushion" or "barrel" artifacts. No such distortion occurs with a CCD.

The CCD has greater sensitivity to light (detective quantum efficiency, DQE) and a lower level of electronic noise than a television camera tube. The results are a higher signal-to-noise ratio (SNR) and better contrast resolution. These characteristics also result in substantially lower patient radiation dose.

The response of the CCD to light is very stable. Warm-up of the CCD is not required. Neither image lag nor blooming is present. It has essentially an unlimited lifetime and requires no maintenance.

> DF with CCD results in wider dynamic range and better contrast resolution than conventional fluoroscopy.

Perhaps the single most important feature of CCD imaging is its linear response (Fig. 20.9). The linear response feature is particularly helpful for digital subtraction angiography (DSA) and results in wider dynamic range and better contrast resolution.

Flat-Panel Image Receptor

A further improvement of DF is the flat-panel image receptor. Such an image receptor is composed of cesium iodide/amorphous silicon pixels, as described in Chapter 12 for digital radiography. It is essentially a flat-panel digital radiographic image receptor with extremely fast interrogation and extinction times.

A flat-panel image receptor fluoroscopic system has several helpful features. The flat-panel image receptor

TABLE 20.2	Advantages of Flat-Panel Image Receptors Over Charge-Coupled Device Image Intensifiers in Digital Fluoroscopy

- Distortion-free images
- Constant image quality over the entire image
- Improved contrast resolution over the entire image
- High DQE (see Chapter 13) at all radiation dose levels
- Rectangular image area coupled to similar image monitor
- Unaffected by external magnetic fields

DQE, Detective quantum efficiency.

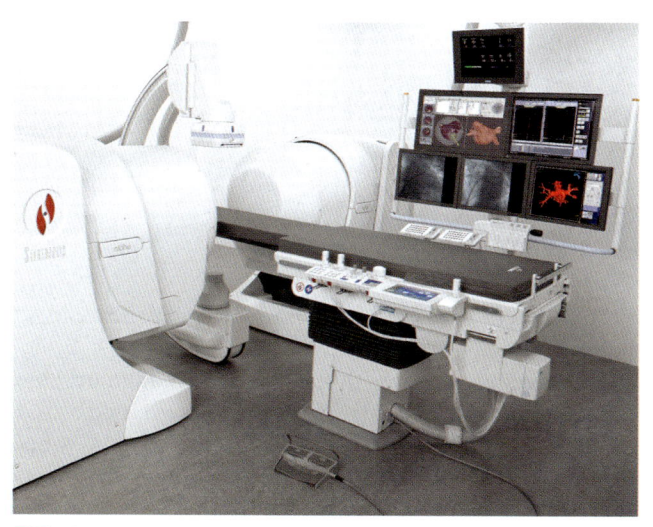

FIG. 20.10 Flat-panel image receptor fluoroscopy makes magnetic steering possible. (Courtesy Siemens Healthcare.)

is much smaller and lighter and is manipulated more easily than an image intensifier. The flat-panel image receptor imaging suite provides easier patient manipulation, and radiologist and interventional radiology technologist movement, because there are no radiographic cassettes. Table 20.2 lists some advantages of flat-panel image receptors over image-intensified fluoroscopy.

In contrast to an image-intensifier tube, the flat-panel image receptor is insensitive to external magnetic fields. This has made possible a new area of IR: image-guided catheter navigation (Fig. 20.10).

A special catheter with a magnetic tip is introduced into the patient vasculature. This catheter is manipulated remotely through tortuous vessels by two large steering magnets that are located on either side of the patient. This technology will find additional application in IR.

IMAGE DISPLAY

The DF image receptor has two alternatives: CCD and flat panel. So does the image display—video and flat panel, or digital display device.

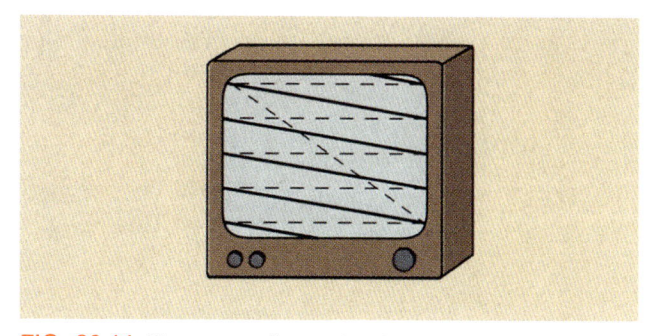

FIG. 20.11 The progressive mode of reading a video signal.

Video System

The video system used in conventional fluoroscopy is usually a 525-line system. Such a system is inadequate for DF.

Conventional video has two limitations that restrict its application in digital techniques. First, the interlaced mode of reading the target of the television camera tube can significantly degrade a digital image. Second, conventional television camera tubes are relatively noisy. They have an SNR of about 200:1; an SNR of 1000:1 is necessary for DF.

> The progressive mode of reading the digital signal produces a sharper image with less flicker.

In DF, the TV camera tube reads in progressive mode. When the video signal is read in the progressive mode, the electron beam of the TV camera tube sweeps the target assembly continuously from top to bottom in 33 ms (Fig. 20.11).

Because conventional television camera tubes have an SNR of about 200:1, the maximum output signal will be 200 times greater than the background electronic noise. An image with an SNR of 5:1 is minimally visible.

An SNR of 200:1 is not sufficient for DF because the video signal is rarely at maximum, and lower signals become even more lost in the noise. This is especially true when subtraction techniques are used. Image contrast resolution is severely degraded by a system with low SNR.

Fig. 20.12 illustrates the difference between the output of a 200:1 SNR television camera tube and that of a 1000:1 tube. At 200:1, the dynamic range is less than 2^8, and at 1000:1, it is approximately 2^{10}. The tube with a 1000:1 SNR provides five times the useful information and is more compatible with computer-assisted image enhancement.

Flat-Panel Image Display

Flat-panel digital display technology is rapidly replacing the cathode ray tube (CRT) in all applications.

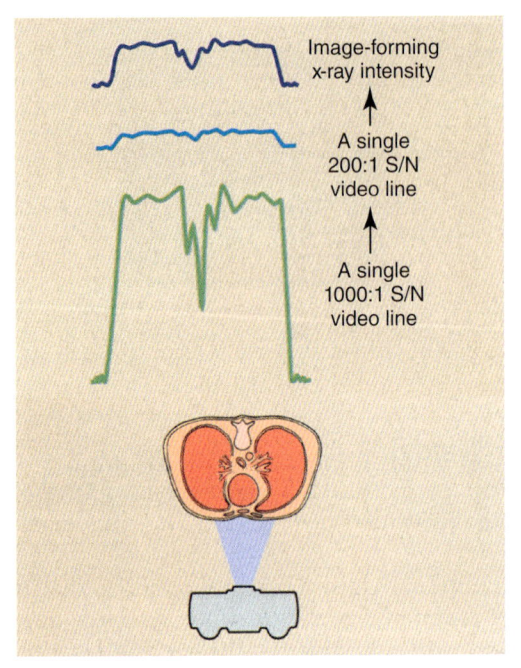

FIG. 20.12 The information content of a video system with a high signal-to-noise ratio (S/N) is greatly enhanced. Shown here are a single video line through an object and the resultant signal at 200:1 and 1000:1 SNRs.

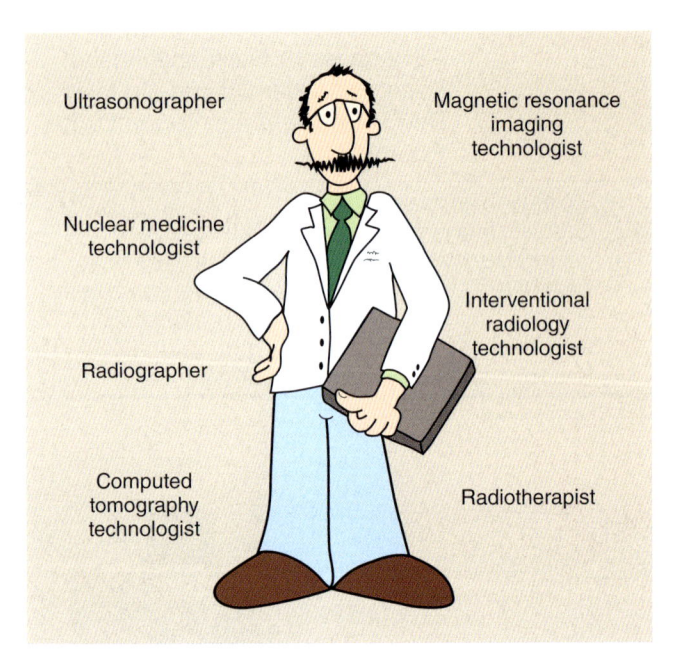

FIG. 20.13 A radiologic technologist can specialize in many types of imaging modalities.

Flat-panel digital displays for television become ever more popular as the price of such devices shrinks.

> Flat-panel digital display devices are easier to view and easier to manipulate, and they provide better images.

The flat-panel display is similarly and rapidly replacing CRTs in radiography and fluoroscopy as well. This advance in image monitoring will be discussed in greater detail in Chapter 24.

TYPES OF INTERVENTIONAL RADIOLOGY PROCEDURES

As medical imaging has developed, so has our identity. First, we were called x-ray operators, then technicians, and now radiologic technologists. A radiologic technologist can be a radiographer, a mammographer, a nuclear medicine technologist, a radiotherapist, or another imaging technologist (Fig. 20.13).

In the same way that radiologic technology has been more precisely divided into disciplines, so has our imaging task. We used to do special procedures, such as pneumoencephalography, myelography, and neuroangiography. The rapid development of vascular imaging as aggressive therapeutic intervention through vessels has resulted in rooms and equipment designed especially for interventional radiology radiologic procedures. The radiographers involved are interventional radiologic technologists.

IR procedures began in the 1930s with **angiography**; needles and contrast media were used to enter and highlight an artery. In the early 1960s, Mason Jones pioneered **transbrachial selective coronary angiography**—entering select coronary arteries through an artery of the arm.

Also during the 1960s, transfemoral angiography—entering an artery in the thigh—of selective visceral, heart, and head arteries was developed. Melvin Judkins introduced coronary angiography, and Charles Dotter introduced visceral angiography.

Angiography refers to the opacification of vessels through injection of contrast media. Angioplasty, thrombolysis, embolization, vascular stents, and biopsy are IR procedures that are conducted in and through vessels. Table 20.3 lists the types of imaging and interventional procedures that are likely to be conducted in an IR suite.

Digital Subtraction Angiography

Minicomputers and microprocessors are used in DF. The capacity of the computer is an important factor in determining image quality, the manner and speed of image acquisition, and the means of image processing and manipulation. Important characteristics of a DF system that are computer controlled include the **image matrix size**, the **system dynamic range**, and the **image acquisition rate**.

The output signal from the image-intensified digital image receptor is transmitted to an **analog-to-digital converter (ADC)**. The ADC accepts the continuously

TABLE 20.3	Representative Procedures Conducted in an Interventional Radiology Suite
Imaging Procedures	**Interventional Procedures**
Angiography	Stent placement
Aortography	Embolization
Arteriography	Intravascular stent
Cardiac catheterization	Thrombolysis
Myelography	Balloon angioplasty
Venography	Atherectomy
	Electrophysiology

TABLE 20.4	Comparison of Temporal Subtraction and Energy Subtraction
Temporal Subtraction	**Energy Subtraction**
A single kVp setting is used.	Rapid kVp switching is required.
Normal x-ray beam filtration is adequate.	X-ray beam filter switching is preferred.
Contrast resolution of 1 mm at 1% is achieved.	Higher x-ray intensity is required for comparable contrast resolution.
Simple arithmetic image subtraction is necessary.	Complex image subtraction is necessary.
Motion artifacts are a problem.	Motion artifacts are greatly reduced.
Total subtraction of common structures is achieved.	Some residual bone may survive subtraction.
Subtraction possibilities are limited by the number of images.	Many more types of subtraction images are possible.

varying signal—the analog signal—and digitizes it. The signal from a flat-panel image receptor is already digital.

To be compatible with the computer, the ADC must have the same dynamic range as the DF system. An 8-bit ADC would convert the analog signal into values between 0 and 256. A 10-bit ADC would be more precise, with an ADC range from 0 to 2^{10} or 0 to 1024. The output of the ADC is then transferred to the main memory and is manipulated so that a digital image in matrix form is stored.

> The dynamic range of each pixel, the number of pixels, and the method of storage determine the speed with which the image can be acquired, processed, and transferred to an digital display device.

If image storage occurs in primary memory, which is usually the case, then data acquisition and transfer can be as rapid as 30 images per second. In general, if the image matrix is doubled (e.g., from 512 to 1024), the image acquisition time will be increased by four.

A representative system might be capable of acquiring 30 images per second in the 512 × 512 matrix mode. However, if a higher spatial resolution image is required and the 1024 × 1024 mode is requested, then only 8 images per second can be acquired. This limitation on data transfer is imposed by the time required to transport enormous quantities of data from one segment of memory to another.

Image Formation

The principal advantages of DF examinations are the image subtraction techniques that are possible and the enhanced visualization of vasculature that results from venous injection of contrast material. Unfortunately an area beam must be used, which reduces image contrast because of associated Compton scatter radiation.

Image contrast, however, can be enhanced electronically. Image contrast is improved by subtraction techniques that provide instantaneous viewing of the subtracted image during passage of a bolus of contrast medium.

> DF provides better contrast resolution through postprocessing of image subtraction.

Temporal subtraction and energy subtraction are the two methods that receive attention in DF. Each has distinct advantages and disadvantages, and these are described in Table 20.4. Temporal subtraction techniques are used most frequently because of high-voltage generator limitations associated with the energy subtraction mode. When the two techniques are combined, the process is called **hybrid subtraction**. Image contrast is enhanced still further by hybrid subtraction because of reduced patient motion between subtracted images.

Temporal subtraction refers to a number of computer-assisted techniques whereby an image obtained at one time is subtracted from an image obtained at a later time. If, during the intervening period, contrast material was introduced into the vasculature, the subtracted image will contain only the vessels filled with contrast material. Two methods are commonly used: the **mask mode** and the **time-interval difference** (**TID**) **mode**.

A typical mask-mode procedure is diagrammed in Fig. 20.14. The patient is positioned under normal

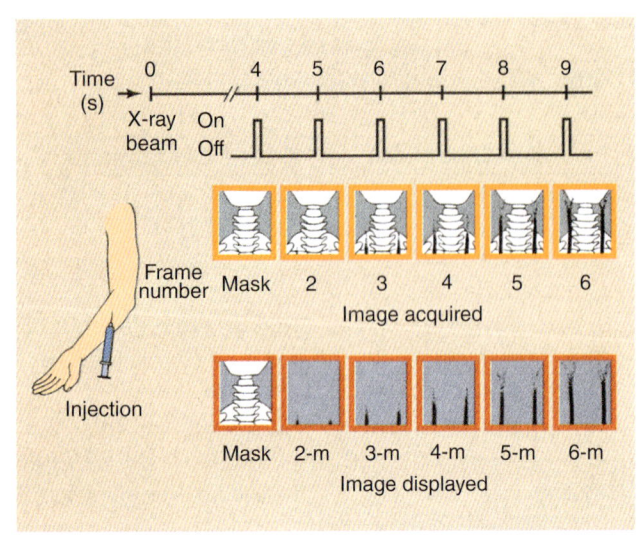

FIG. 20.14 A schematic representation of mask-mode digital fluoroscopy.

fluoroscopic control to ensure that the region of anatomy under investigation is within the field of view.

A power injector is armed and readied to deliver 30 to 50 mL of contrast material at the rate of approximately 15 to 20 mL/s through a venous entry. If an arterial entry is chosen, 10 to 25 mL of diluted contrast material at 10 to 12 mL/s is typical.

The imaging system is changed from the fluoroscopic mode to the DF mode. This requires an increase in x-ray tube current of 20 to 100 times the fluoroscopic mode and the activation of a program of pulse image acquisition.

> Mask mode results in successive subtraction images of contrast-filled vessels.

The injector is fired, and after a delay of 4 to 10 s, before the bolus of contrast medium reaches the anatomic site, an initial x-ray pulsed exposure is made. The image obtained is stored in primary memory and is displayed on video monitor A. This is the **mask image**.

This mask image is followed by a series of additional images that are stored in adjacent memory locations. While these subsequent images are being acquired, the mask image is subtracted from each and the result stored in primary memory. At the same time, the subtracted image is displayed on video monitor B.

Fig. 20.15A shows a preinjection mask lateral view of the base of the skull, an image following contrast injection (see Fig. 20.15B), and a DSA image obtained by subtracting the mask from the injection image (see Fig. 20.15C). The principal result of DSA is improved image contrast.

Digital subtraction of the static object (the skull) allows better analysis of the opacified arteries, especially in their distal parts. The subtracted images appear in real time and are then stored in memory.

> After the examination, each subtracted image can be recalled for closer examination.

As is described here, each image was obtained from a 33-ms x-ray pulse. The time required for one video frame is 33 ms. Because the video system is relatively slow to respond and the video noise may be high, several video frames (usually four or eight) may be summed in memory to create each image. This process is called **image integration**. Although the process improves contrast resolution, it also increases the patient radiation dose because a greater number of image frames are acquired.

In mask-mode DF, the imaging sequence after acquisition of the mask can be controlled manually or preprogrammed. If preprogrammed, the computer controls data acquisition in accordance with the demands of the examination.

To evaluate carotid flow, for example, after a brachial vein injection, the radiologist could inject contrast media and acquire a mask image 2 s after the injection. After another 2-s delay, images are obtained at the rate of 2 per second for 3 s, 1 per second for 5 s, and one every other second for 14 s. If the computer capacity for acquiring images is sufficient, any combination of multiple delays and varying image acquisition rates is possible.

If, on subsequent examination, the initial mask image is inadequate because of patient motion or improper technique or for any other reason, later images may be used as the mask image, a technique termed **remasking**. A typical examination may require a total of 30 images in addition to the mask image.

If the intended mask image is technically inadequate and maximum contrast appears during the 15th image, a better subtraction image may be obtained by using image number 5 as the mask rather than image number 1. The interventional radiologist can even integrate several images (e.g., numbers four through eight) using the composite image as the mask. Unacceptable mask images can be caused by noise, motion, and technical factors.

Some examinations call for each subtracted image to be made from a different mask and follow-up frame (Fig. 20.16). This process is called **time-interval difference (TID)** mode.

In a cardiac study, for example, image acquisition begins 5 s after injection at the rate of 15 images per second for 4 s. A total of 60 images is obtained in such a study. These images are identified as frame numbers 1 through 60. Each image is stored in a separate memory address as it is acquired.

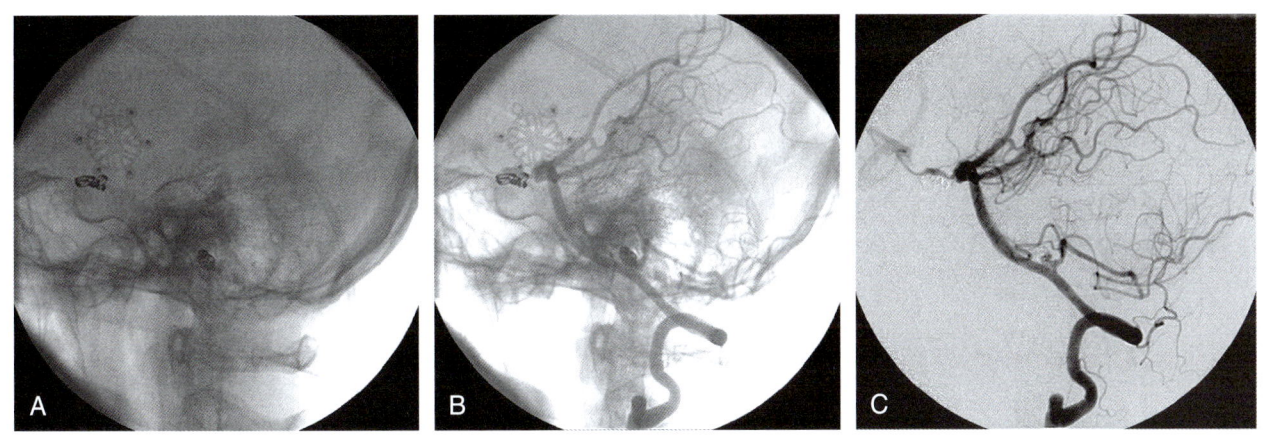

FIG. 20.15 (A) The preinjection mask. (B) A postinjection image. (C) Image produced when the preinjection mask is subtracted from the postinjection image. (Courtesy Charles Trinh, Baylor College of Medicine.)

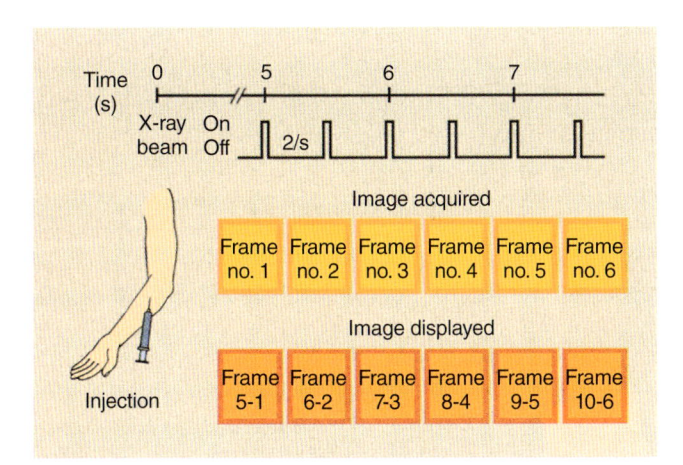

FIG. 20.16 The manner in which sequentially obtained images are subtracted in a time-interval difference study.

If a TID of four images (268 ms) is selected, the first image to appear will be that obtained when frame one is subtracted from frame five. The second image will contain the subtraction of frame two from frame six; the third will contain the subtraction of frame three from frame seven and so forth.

> TID mode produces subtracted images from progressive masks and following frames.

In real time, the images observed convey the flow of contrast medium dynamically. Subsequent closer examination of each TID image shows it to be relatively free of motion artifacts but with less contrast than mask-mode imaging. As a result, TID imaging is applied principally in cardiac evaluation.

Fig. 20.17 shows a typical digital subtraction angiogram of the abdominal aorta. First, a mask image (see Fig. 20.17A) is obtained, then a postinjection image (see Fig. 20.17B), and finally a subtracted image (see Fig. 20.17C).

If patient motion occurs between the mask image and a subsequent image, the subtracted image will contain **misregistration artifacts** (Fig. 20.18). The same anatomy is not registered in the same pixel of the image matrix. This type of artifact frequently can be eliminated by **reregistration** of the mask, that is, by shifting the mask by one or more pixels so that **superimposition** of images is again obtained.

Temporal subtraction techniques take advantage of changing contrast media during the time of the examination and require no special demands on the high-voltage generator. **Energy subtraction**, on the other hand, uses two different x-ray beams alternately to provide a subtraction image that results from differences in photoelectric interaction.

> Energy subtraction is based on the abrupt change in photoelectric absorption at the K edge of contrast media, compared with that for soft tissue and bone.

Fig. 20.19 shows the probability of x-ray interaction with iodine, bone, and muscle as a function of x-ray energy. The probability of photoelectric absorption in all three decreases with increasing x-ray energy. At an energy of 33 keV, an abrupt increase in absorption is noted in iodine and a modest decrease in soft tissue and bone.

This energy corresponds to the binding energy of the two K-shell electrons of iodine. When the incident x-ray energy is sufficient to overcome the K-shell electron binding energy of iodine, an abrupt and large increase in absorption occurs.

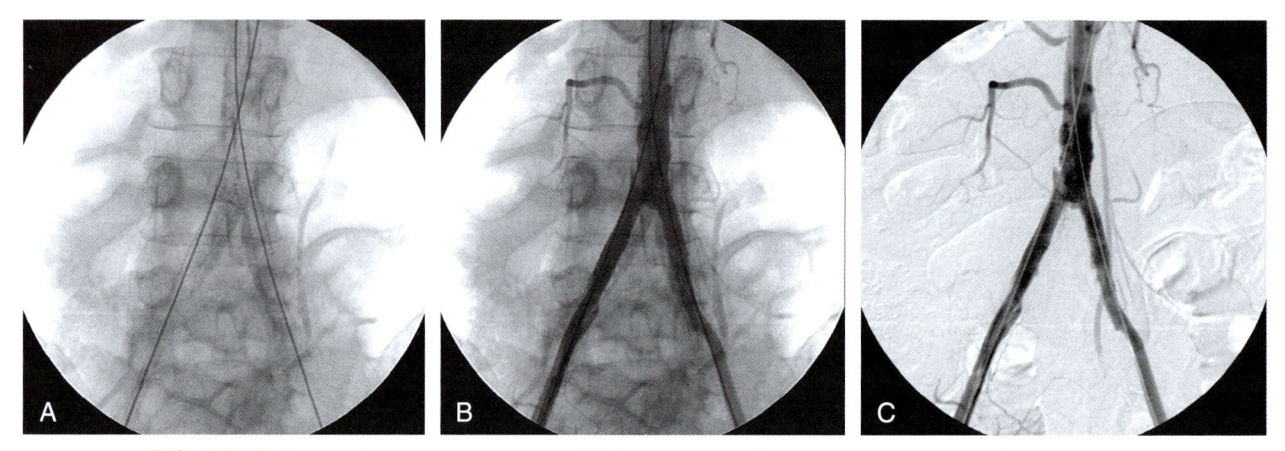

FIG. 20.17 Digital subtraction angiography (DSA) of the aortoiliac area reveals the details of anomalies in the anastomosis region. (Courtesy Dick Fisher, Baylor College of Medicine.)

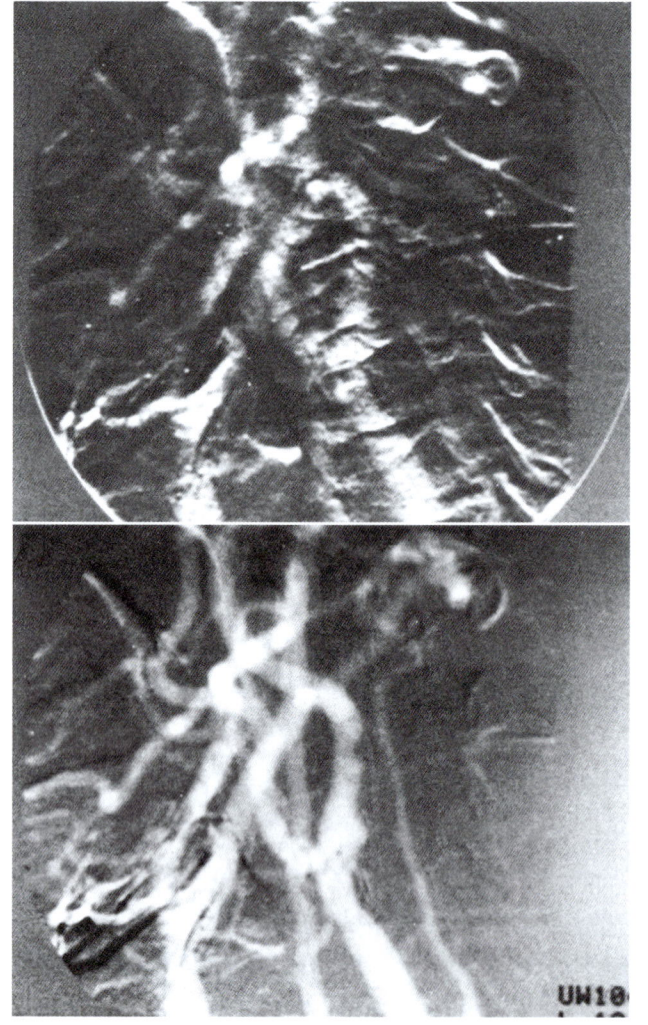

FIG. 20.18 Misregistration artifacts. (Courtesy Ben Arnold, University of California.)

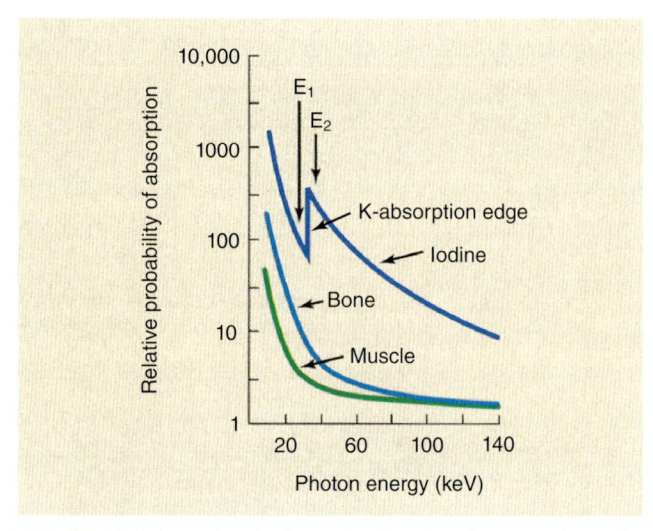

FIG. 20.19 Photoelectric absorption in iodine, bone, and muscle.

> Graphically, this increase is known as the **K-absorption edge**.

If monoenergetic x-ray beams of 32 and 34 keV could be used alternately, the difference in absorption of iodine would be enormous, and resultant subtraction images would have very high contrast. Such is not the case, however, because every x-ray beam contains a wide spectrum of energies.

Energy subtraction has the decided disadvantage of requiring some method of providing an alternating x-ray beam of two different emission spectra. Two methods have been devised: (1) alternately pulsing the x-ray beam at 70 kVp and then 90 kVp and (2) introducing dissimilar metal filters into the x-ray beam alternately on a flywheel.

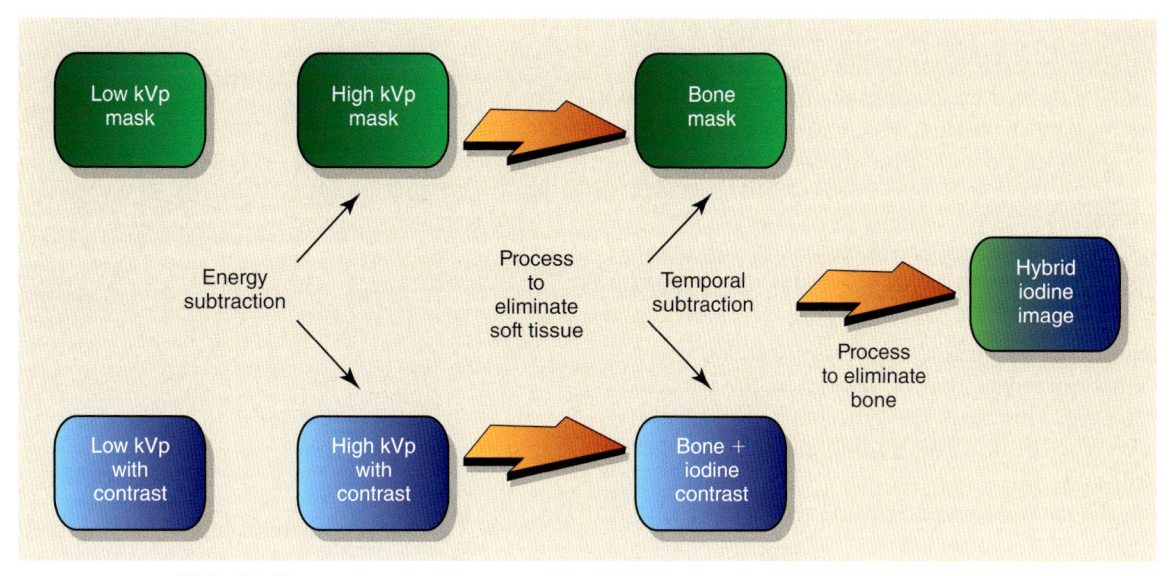

FIG. 20.20 Hybrid subtraction involves temporal and energy subtraction techniques.

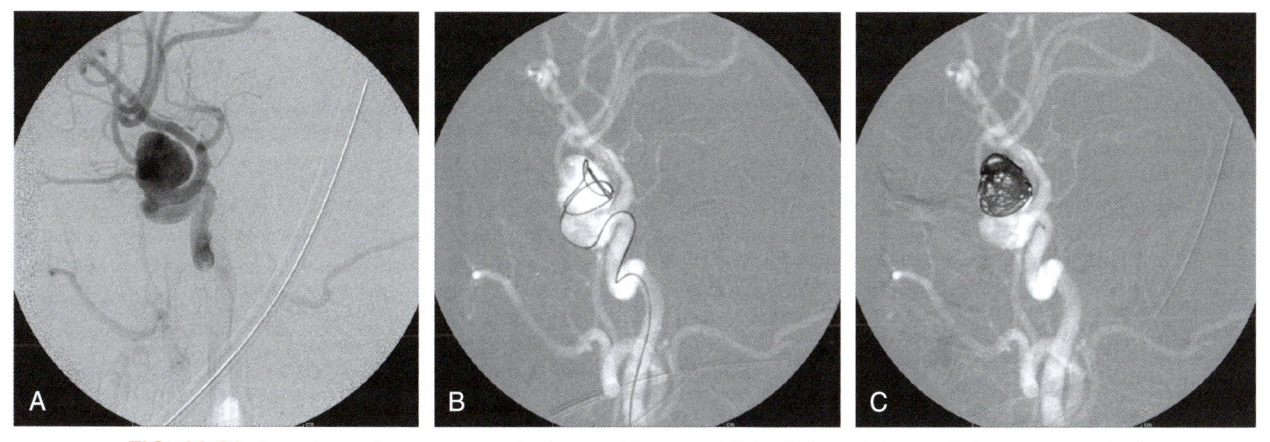

FIG. 20.21 A roadmapping neurovascular image. (Courtesy Michael Mawad, Baylor College of Medicine.)

Some DF systems are capable of combining temporal and energy subtraction techniques into what is called **hybrid subtraction** (Fig. 20.20). Image acquisition follows the mask-mode procedure, as was described previously. Here, however, the mask and each subsequent image are formed by an energy subtraction technique. If patient motion can be controlled, hybrid imaging theoretically can produce the highest contrast DF images.

Roadmapping

Roadmapping is a special application of DSA. A mask image is acquired and stored. The contrast material is injected and subtraction images are acquired as in DSA, as shown in Fig. 20.21A. However, additional steps follow.

As the catheter is fluoroscopically advanced, the image is formed by subtraction from the second mask. The result is shown in Fig. 20.21B—a black guidewire or catheter in a white vessel.

The final DSA image (see Fig. 20.21C) shows the complete vascular tree with good contrast. This last image is inverted and is used as the mask for additional DSA images.

BASIC PRINCIPLES

Arterial Access

In 1953, Sven Ivar Seldinger described a method of arterial access in which a catheter was used. The Seldinger needle is an 18-gauge hollow needle with a stylet. After the Seldinger needle is inserted into the femoral artery and pulsating arterial blood returns, the stylet is removed.

A guidewire then is inserted through the needle into the arterial lumen. With the guidewire in the vessel, the Seldinger needle is removed, and a catheter is threaded onto the guidewire. Under fluoroscopic view, the catheter then is advanced along the guidewire.

In angiography, the common femoral artery is most often used for arterial access. The common femoral artery can be palpated by locating the pulse in the groin below the inguinal ligament, which passes between the symphysis pubis and the anterior superior iliac spine.

Guidewires

After the catheter is in place, the guidewire allows the radiologist to position the catheter within the vascular network.

Guidewires are fabricated of stainless steel and contain an inner core wire that is tapered at the end to a soft, flexible tip. This core wire prevents loss of sections of the wire if it breaks. The trailing end of the guidewire is stiff and allows the guidewire to be pushed and twisted so the catheter can be positioned in the chosen vessel.

> Guidewires allow the safe introduction of the catheter into the vessel.

Conventional guidewires are 145 cm long. Catheters overlaying the guidewire are usually 100 cm long or less. Guidewires are categorized additionally by length to the beginning of the tapered tip, configuration of the tip, stiffness of the guidewire, and coating. They are coated with a hydrophilic material so the catheter slides over the wire more easily. This coating makes guidewires more resistant to thrombus (blood clot) and easier to irrigate while they are in the vascular system.

The J-tip for guidewires is a variation of the tip configuration that was initially designed for use in atherosclerotic vessels filled with plaque. The J-tip deflects off the edges of plaques and helps prevent subintimal dissection of the artery.

The coatings on guidewires are materials that are designed to reduce friction; they include Teflon, heparin coatings, and, more recently, hydrophilic polymers. The latter type, called a **glidewire**, represents a major technologic advance in IR.

Catheters

Similar to guidewires, catheters are designed in many different shapes and sizes. Usually catheter diameter is categorized in French (Fr) sizes, with 3 Fr equaling 1 mm in diameter. Fig. 20.22 illustrates six common catheter shapes.

> The shaped tip of the catheter is required for selective catheterization of openings into specific arteries.

The H1 or headhunter tip designed by Vincent Hinck is used for the femoral approach to the brachiocephalic

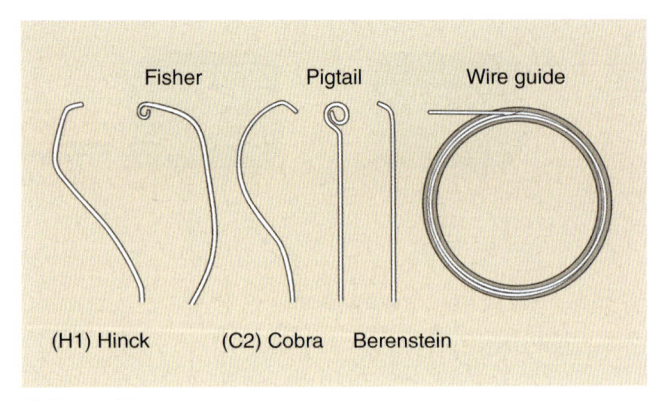

FIG. 20.22 Typical catheter shapes.

vessels. The Fisher catheter is highly curved for approach to sharply angled vessels and was also designed for cerebral angiography. It was later adopted for visceral angiography. The C2 or Cobra catheter has an angled tip joined to a gentle curve and is used for introduction into celiac, renal, and mesenteric arteries.

Pigtail catheters have side holes for ejecting contrast media into a compact bolus. A catheter with side holes helps reduce a possible whiplash effect. The jet effect is minimized with the curved pigtail, which prevents injury to the vessel.

After the catheter is introduced into the vessel, the guidewire is removed. The catheter then must be flushed immediately to prevent clotting of blood within the catheter. Heparinized saline generally is used to flush catheters.

After catheter placement, a test injection is performed under fluoroscopy before static imaging to check that the catheter tip is not wedged and that it is in the correct vessel. Injection rates of the automatic power injector are gauged by the test flow speed.

Contrast Media

Vessels under investigation in angiography are injected with radiopaque contrast media. Initially, ionic iodine compounds were used for contrast injections; however, nonionic contrast media have largely replaced ionic agents.

Nonionic contrast media have a low concentration of ions (low osmolality). The result of using such nonionic contrast media is that physiologic problems and adverse reactions are reduced for patients undergoing angiographic injection.

Patient Preparation and Monitoring

Before angiography is performed, the radiologist visits the patient to establish rapport and to explain the procedure and its risks. A history and physical examination are necessary to assess the patient for allergies and other conditions so the radiologist can conclude whether a procedure is indicated and which route is optimal.

Orders are written for IV hydration and a diet of clear liquids. The patient may be premedicated in the IR suite to reduce anxiety.

During the procedure, monitoring by electrocardiography, automatic blood pressure measurement, and pulse oximetry is mandatory. The code or "crash" cart for life-threatening emergencies must be accessible.

After the procedure has been performed, when the catheter is removed, the femoral puncture site must be manually compressed. The patient then is instructed to remain immobile for several hours after the angiographic procedure has been completed while vital signs are monitored and the puncture site is inspected.

Risks of Arteriography

The most common complication associated with catheter angiography is continued bleeding at the puncture site. Of course, the risk of reaction to contrast media is present, and other risk factors are related to kidney failure.

Minimization of these risks requires a complete patient medical examination and the taking of surgical and allergy histories before any angiographic procedure can be done. Although uncommon, serious adverse reactions related to blood clot formation or catheter or guidewire penetrating injury can occur.

INTERVENTIONAL RADIOLOGY SUITE

Different from radiography and fluoroscopy, IR requires a suite of rooms (Fig. 20.23). The procedure room itself should not be less than 20 ft along any wall and not less than 500 ft². This size is necessary to accommodate the quantity of equipment required and the large number of people involved in most procedures.

Patient access should be available through a door wide enough to accommodate a bed. Access to the procedure room from the control room with the operating console does not usually require a protective door. An open passageway is adequate. Such doors interfere with movement of personnel.

The procedure room should be finished with consideration for maintaining a clean and sterile environment. The floor, walls, and all counter cabinet surfaces must be smooth and easily cleaned.

The control room should be large, perhaps 100 ft². Ideally this room should communicate directly with the viewing areas. It also should have positive air pressure and filtered incoming air.

Personnel

A radiographer can specialize in many different fields. One who specializes in IR requires additional skills. The American Registry of Radiologic Technologists (ARRT) offers examinations in cardiovascular interventional and vascular interventional radiography. After the examination is passed, the radiographer may add (CI) or (VI) after the RT (R).

Two or three interventional radiologic technologists may be present in the IR suite, as well as the interventional radiologist and a radiology nurse, who

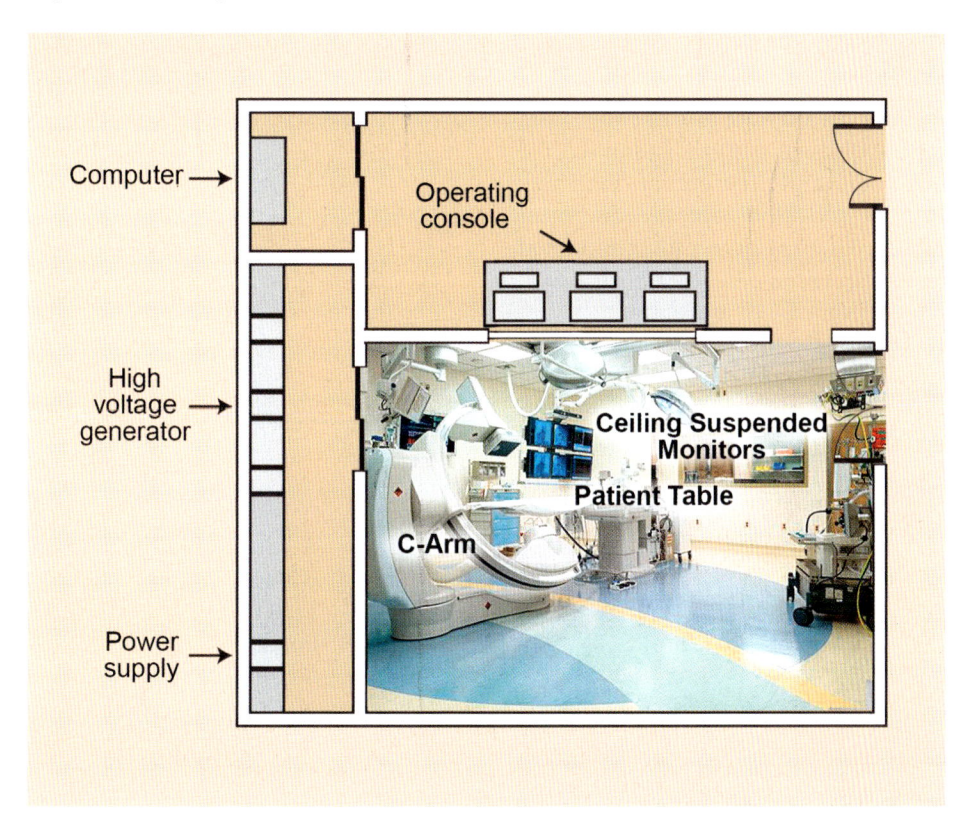

FIG. 20.23 Typical layout of an interventional radiology suite.

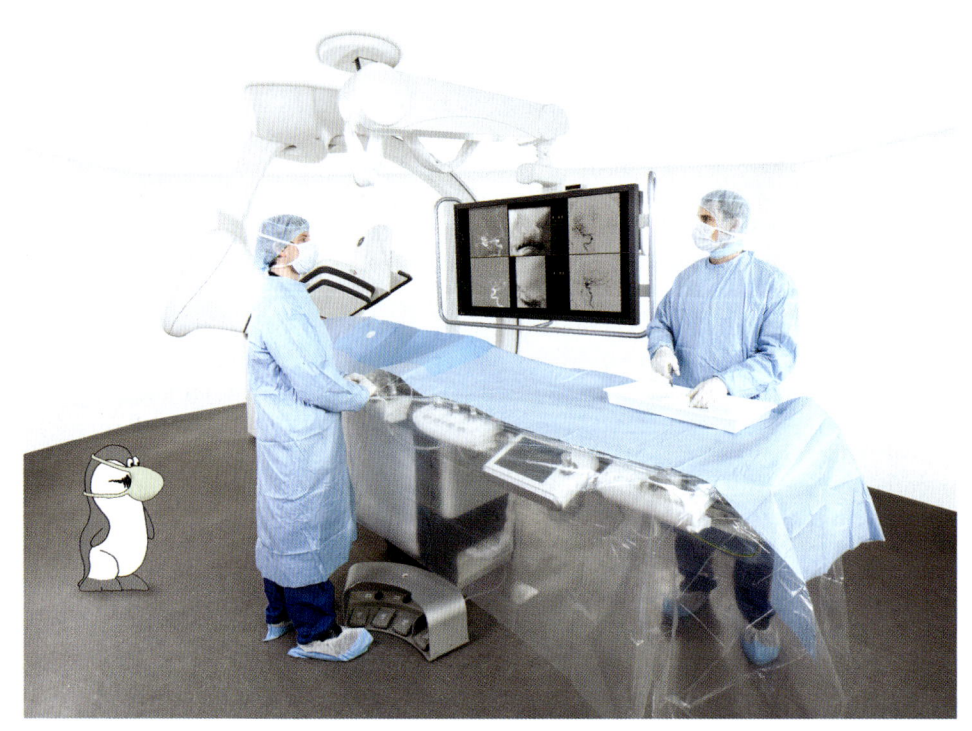

FIG. 20.24 Advanced interventional fluoroscopic equipment. (Courtesy Heidi Seerden, General Electric Healthcare.)

carefully monitors the patient. During procedures that require the patient to be highly medicated, an anesthesiologist also may be present.

Equipment

The x-ray apparatus for an IR suite is generally more massive, flexible, and expensive than that required for conventional radiographic and fluoroscopic imaging. Advanced radiographic and fluoroscopic equipment is required (Fig. 20.24). One or more ceiling-mounted radiographic x-ray tubes are required, along with a digital fluoroscope mounted on a C- or an L-arm.

The **x-ray tube** used for IR procedures has a small target angle, a large-diameter massive anode disc, and cathodes designed for magnification and serial radiography. Table 20.5 describes the specifications for such an x-ray tube.

A small focal spot of not greater than 0.3 mm is necessary for the spatial resolution requirements of small-vessel magnification radiography. Neuroangiography can be performed in contrast-filled vessels as small as 1 mm, with typical selection of geometric factors and careful patient positioning.

When a source-to-image receptor distance (SID) of 100 cm and an object-to-image receptor distance of 40 cm are used, the radiographer can take advantage of the air gap to improve image contrast. A 0.3-mm focal spot results in a focal-spot blur of 0.2 mm.

TABLE 20.5	Specifications for a Typical Interventional Radiology X-ray Tube	
Feature	Size	Why
Focal spot	1.0 mm/0.3 mm	Large for heat load; small for magnification radiography
Disc size	15-cm diameter; 5-cm thick	To accommodate heat load
Power rating	80 kW	For rapid sequence, serial radiography
Anode heat capacity	1 MHU	To accommodate heat load

Question: A left cerebral angiogram is performed with a 0.3-mm focal spot at 100-cm SID. The artery to be imaged is 20 cm from the image receptor. What is the magnification factor (MF) and the focal-spot blur (FSB)?

Answer:
$$MF = \frac{100 \text{ cm SID}}{80 \text{ cm SOD}} = 1.25$$

$$FSB = 0.3 \left(\frac{20 \text{ cm OID}}{80 \text{ cm SOD}} \right) = 0.075 \text{ mm}$$

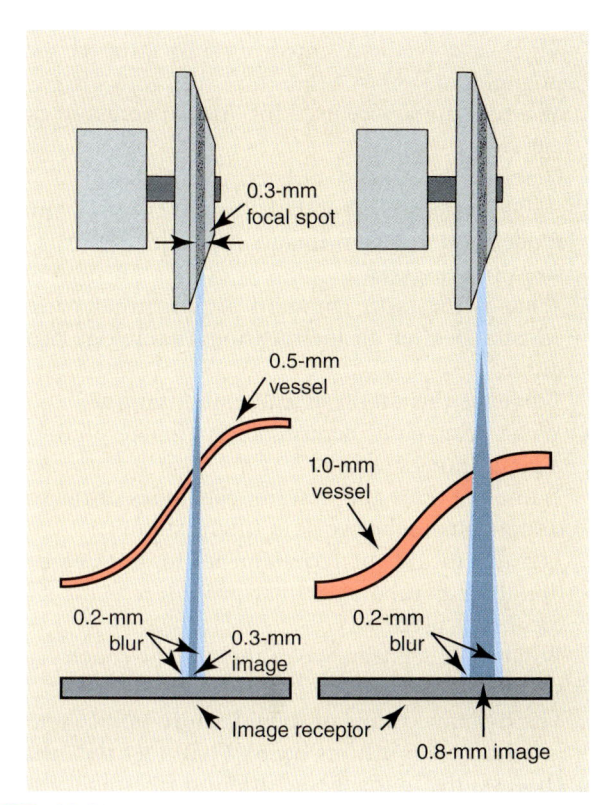

FIG. 20.25 For a given geometry such as this one, which produces a 0.2-mm focal-spot blur, the vessels must be twice the size of the focal-spot blur.

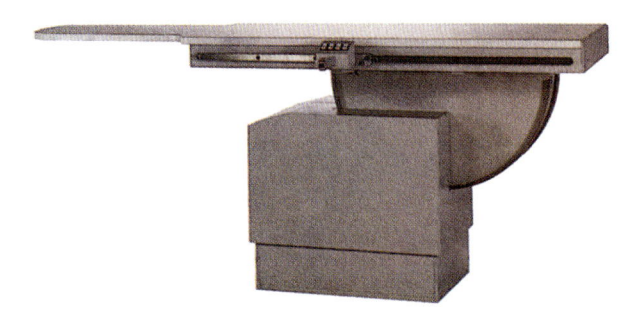

FIG. 20.26 Typical interventional radiology patient couch with a floating, rotating, and tilting top. (Courtesy Odelft.)

Spatial resolution for this procedure can be approximated by multiplying the focal-spot blur by 2. Fig. 20.25 shows geometry that results in 0.2-mm focal-spot blur images of a 1.0-mm vessel. A 0.5-mm vessel will be too blurred to be seen. Any vessel larger than 1.0 mm will be imaged.

All other essential characteristics of an interventional x-ray tube are based on required tube loading. The size and construction of the anode disc determine the anode heat capacity, which in turn influences the power rating. An x-ray tube with a minimum 80-kW rating and 1-MHU heat capacity is required.

High-frequency generators are increasingly popular in all x-ray examinations, including IR procedures. However, some IR procedures require higher power than may be available with high-frequency generators. High-voltage generators with three-phase, 12-pulse power capable of at least 100 kW with low ripple are needed for such high power requirements.

Whereas most general fluoroscopy imaging systems have a tilt table, IR imaging systems do not. General fluoroscopy often requires head-down and head-up tilting of the patient for manipulation of contrast media. Imaging techniques such as myelography require a tilt couch; therefore such procedures are common in general fluoroscopy.

Other imaging and interventional procedures do not require a tilt couch, but a stationary **patient couch** with a floating or movable tabletop is used instead (Fig. 20.26). Controls for couch positioning are located on the side of the table and are duplicated on a floor switch. The floor switch is necessary to accommodate patient positioning while a sterile field is maintained.

The patient couch may have computer-controlled stepping capability. This feature is necessary to allow imaging from the abdomen to the feet after a single injection of contrast medium. An additional requirement of this stepping feature is the ability to preselect the time and position of the patient couch to coincide with the **image receptor**.

> Several different types of digital image receptors can be used in IR procedures.

Flat-panel image receptors are the image receptor of choice for IR. Imaging system advances for IR have been driven largely out of concerns for patient radiation dose, and this is covered more completely in Chapter 41.

Patient Radiation Dose

One potential advantage of DF is reduced patient radiation dose. DF images appear to be continuous, but, in fact, they are discrete. Most DF x-ray beams are pulse progressive; therefore the fluoroscopic dose rate is lower than that for continuous fluoroscopy, even though the mA setting may be higher.

Static images with DF also are made with a lower patient radiation dose per frame than those attained with a spot-film camera. Both the television camera tube and the CCD have greater sensitivity than the spot film. Digital spot images are so easy to acquire that it is possible to make more exposures than are necessary. If the fluoroscopist gets carried away, patient radiation dose savings will disappear.

SUMMARY

DF has added a computer, at least two flat-panel digital display devices, and a complex control panel to conventional fluoroscopic equipment. The minicomputers in DF control the image matrix size, the system dynamic range, and the image acquisition rate.

Subtraction is the process of removing or masking all unnecessary anatomy from an image and enhancing only the anatomy of interest. With DF, subtraction is accomplished by temporal or energy techniques.

Catheter tip designs vary widely, and each is used for specific arteries. The contrast media used are generally nonionic; this reduces the incidence of physiologic problems and adverse reactions in patients.

The typical IR x-ray tube is designed for magnification, high spatial resolution, and massive heat loads. The patient couch is a floating tabletop with a stepping capability that automatically allows imaging from abdomen to feet after a single injection of contrast media.

Digital imaging is used for interventional procedures with power injection of contrast media and imaging synchronized to optimize visualization of the vessel of interest.

CHALLENGE QUESTIONS

1. Define or otherwise identify the following:
   a. ABS
   b. Arteriography
   c. Catheter
   d. CCD
   e. Duty cycle
   f. Flat-panel image receptor
   g. Guidewire
   h. Hybrid subtraction
   i. Interrogation time
   j. Venography
2. What are the principal advantages of digital fluoroscopy over conventional fluoroscopy?
3. Describe the sequence of image acquisition in mask-mode fluoroscopy.
4. What artery is used most often for arterial access in angiography?
5. Why is a guidewire used for arterial access of catheters?
6. Describe the process of energy subtraction.
7. A DF system is operated in a 512 × 512 image mode with a 23-cm image intensifier. What is the size of each pixel?
8. What is the most common problem that patients encounter after an interventional radiology procedure?
9. What are thrombolysis and embolization?
10. What principally determines spatial resolution in digital fluoroscopy?
11. Name the titles and describe the duties of the team of personnel who work in the IR suite.
12. List the focal-spot requirements for the interventional x-ray tube. For what procedure is the small focal spot used?
13. What does it mean when the patient couch has a stepping capability?
14. The dynamic range of digital fluoroscopic systems is described as 12 bits deep. What does this mean?
15. Discuss the patient radiation dose implications associated with DF compared with conventional fluoroscopy.
16. What is transbrachial selective coronary angiography?
17. Why are some catheters fenestrated (pierced with holes)?
18. How does osmolarity affect the action of a contrast agent?
19. How can misregistration artifacts be corrected?
20. What initials may a radiographer with a specialty in vascular interventional radiology place after RT(R)?

The answers to the Challenge Questions can be found by logging on to our website at http://evolve.elsevier.com.

Cartoon image shows two penguins in conversation with a penguin in the background wearing crown. The text at the bottom reads: "Thinks he's a descendant of an Emperor Penguin."

Computed Tomography

CHAPTER 21

OBJECTIVES

At the completion of this chapter, the student should be able to do the following:

1. List and describe the various generations of computed tomography (CT) imaging systems.
2. Relate the CT imaging system components to their functions.
3. Discuss image reconstruction via interpolation, back projection, and iteration.
4. Describe CT image characteristics of image matrix, Hounsfield unit, and sensitivity profile.
5. Understand technique selection in CT.
6. Explain the helical imaging relationships among pitch, index, dose profile, and patient radiation dose.
7. Discuss image quality as it relates to spatial resolution, contrast resolution, noise, linearity, and uniformity.

OUTLINE

Principles of Operation 306
Generations of Computed Tomography 307
Multislice Helical Computed Tomography 309
   Interpolation Algorithms 310
   Pitch 311
   Sensitivity Profile 313
Imaging System Design 313
   Operating Console 313
   Computer 314
   Gantry 314
   Slip-Ring Technology 316
Image Characteristics 316
   Image Matrix 317
   Computed Tomography Numbers 317
   Image Reconstruction 318
   Multiplanar Reformation 319
Image Quality 320
   Spatial Resolution 320
   Contrast Resolution 322
   Noise 324
   Linearity 324
   Uniformity 325
Imaging Technique 325
   Multislice Detector Array 325
   Data Acquisition Rate 326
   Photon Counting 327
Computed Tomography Quality Control 327
   Noise and Uniformity 328
   Linearity 328
   Spatial Resolution 328
   Contrast Resolution 328
   Slice Thickness 329
   Couch Incrementation 329
   Laser Localizer 329
Summary 329
Challenge Questions 330

The computed tomography (CT) imaging system is revolutionary. No ordinary image receptor, such as the interventional radiology flat panel image receptor, is involved. A collimated x-ray beam is directed on the patient, and the attenuated image-forming x-radiation is measured by a radiation detector whose response is transmitted to a computer.

After the signal from the detector is analyzed, the computer reconstructs the image and displays the image on a monitor. Computer reconstruction of the cross-sectional anatomy is accomplished with mathematical equations, **algorithms**, adapted for computer processing.

Helical CT, which has emerged as a new and improved diagnostic tool, provides improved imaging of anatomy compromised by respiratory motion. This chapter introduces the physical principles of multislice helical CT. Special imaging system design features and image characteristics are reviewed.

The components necessary to construct a CT imaging system were available to medical physicists 20 years before Godfrey Hounsfield first demonstrated the technique in 1970. Hounsfield was a physicist and engineer with EMI, Ltd., the British company most famous for recording the Beatles, and both he and his company justifiably have received high acclaim.

Allan Cormack, a Tufts University medical physicist, shared the 1979 Nobel Prize in Physiology or Medicine with Hounsfield. Cormack had earlier developed the mathematics that would be used to reconstruct CT images.

The CT imaging system is an invaluable step forward in medical imaging. Its development and introduction into radiologic practice have assumed an importance comparable with the Coolidge hot-cathode x-ray tube, the Potter-Bucky diaphragm, the image-intensifier tube, and even magnetic resonance imaging. Arguably, no other development in medical imaging over the past 50 years has been as significant.

PRINCIPLES OF OPERATION

When the abdomen is imaged radiographically, the image is created directly on the image receptor (IR) and is low in contrast, principally because of Compton scatter radiation. The intensity of scatter radiation is high because of the large-area x-ray beam. The image is also degraded because of superimposition of all of the anatomical structures in the abdomen.

For better visualization of an abdominal structure, such as the kidneys, conventional tomography was used (Fig. 21.1). In nephrotomography, the renal outline is distinct because the overlying and underlying tissues were blurred. In addition, the contrast of the in-focus structures was enhanced. Yet the image remained rather dull and blurred.

The latest advance in digital radiography is digital radiographic tomosynthesis (see Chapter 22). This imaging technique uses an area x-ray beam to produce multiple digital images. The images form a three-dimensional data set from which any anatomical plane can be reconstructed. The result is even better image contrast.

Conventional tomography is called **axial tomography** because the plane of the image is parallel to the long axis of the body; this results in sagittal and coronal images. A CT image is a transaxial or **transverse** image that is perpendicular to the long axis of the body (Fig. 21.2). Coronal and sagittal images can be reconstructed from the transverse image data set.

The precise method by which a CT imaging system produces a transverse image is extremely complicated, and understanding it requires strong knowledge of physics, engineering, and computer science. The basic principles, however, can be observed if one considers the simplest of CT imaging systems, which consists of a finely collimated x-ray beam and a single detector.

> The x-ray source and the detector move synchronously for computed tomography.

When the source-detector assembly makes one sweep, or **translation**, across the patient, the internal structures of the body attenuate the x-ray beam according to their mass density and effective atomic number, as was discussed in Chapter 10. The intensity of radiation detected varies according to this attenuation pattern, and an intensity profile, or **projection**, is formed (Fig. 21.3).

At the end of this translation, the source detector assembly returns to its starting position, and the entire assembly **rotates** and begins a second translation. During the second translation, the detector signal again will be proportional to the x-ray beam attenuation of anatomical structures, and a second projection will be described.

If this process is repeated many times, many projections are generated. These projections are not displayed visually but are stored in digital form in the computer. Computer processing of these projections involves effective superimposition of each projection to **reconstruct** an image of the anatomical structures within that slice.

CHAPTER 21 Computed Tomography   307

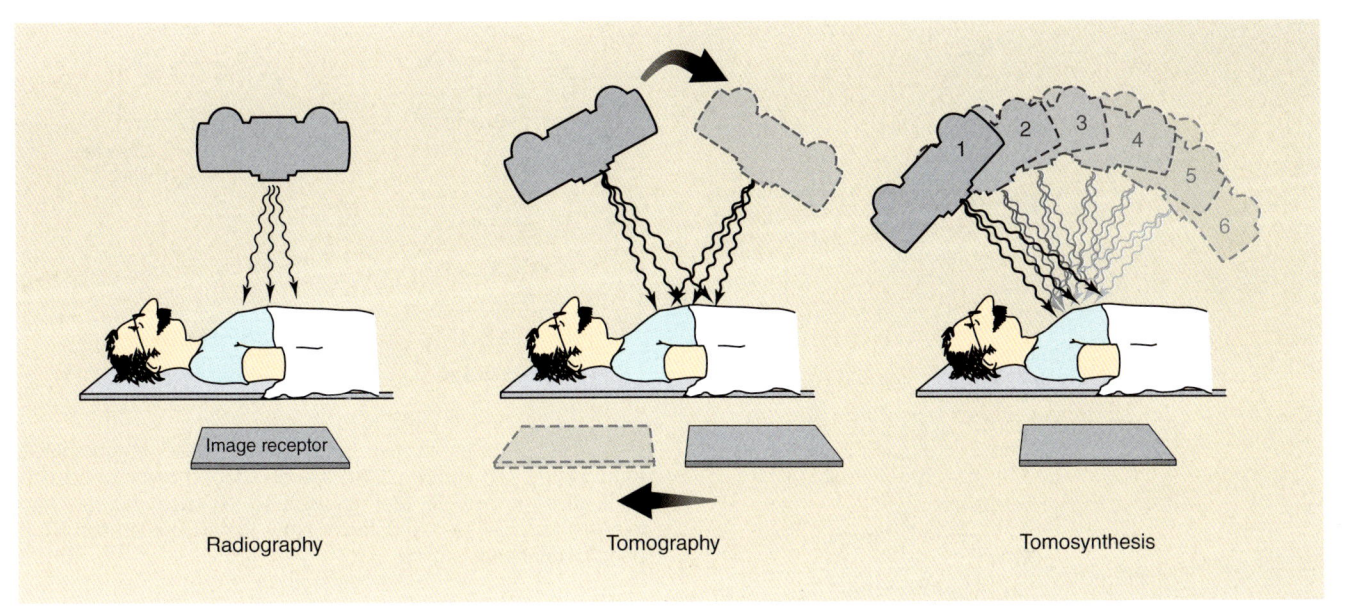

FIG. 21.1 Equipment arrangement for obtaining a radiograph, a conventional tomograph, and a digital radiographic tomosynthesis image set.

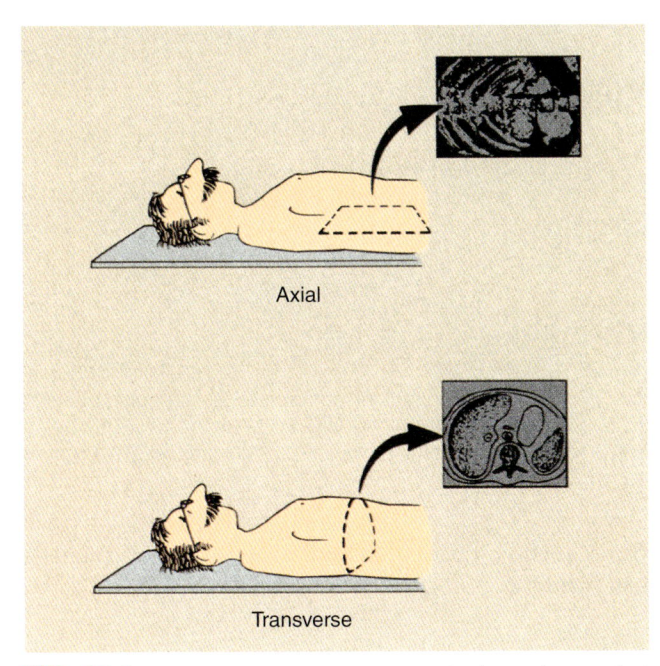

FIG. 21.2 Conventional tomography results in an image that is parallel to the long axis of the body. Computed tomography produces a transverse image.

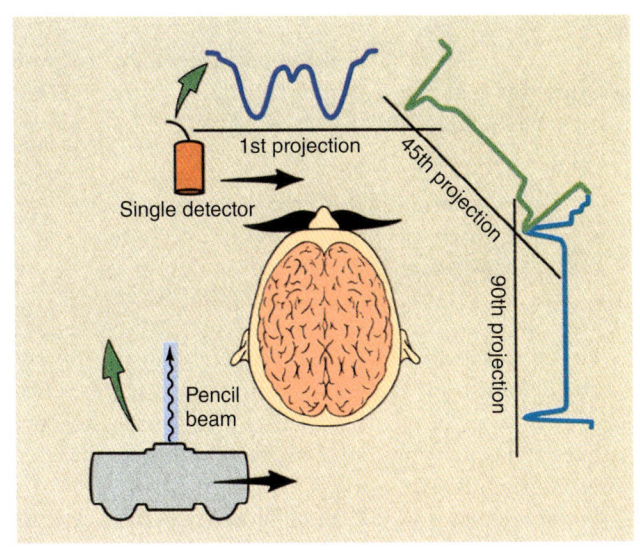

FIG. 21.3 In its simplest form, a computed tomography imaging system consists of a finely collimated x-ray beam and a single detector, both of which move synchronously in a translate-and-rotate fashion. Each sweep of the source-detector assembly results in a projection, which represents the attenuation pattern of the patient profile.

Superimposition of these projections does not occur as one might imagine. The detector signal during each translation has a dynamic range of 12 bits (4096 gray levels). The value for each increment is related to the x-ray attenuation coefficient of the total path through the tissue. Through the use of simultaneous equations, a matrix of values is obtained that represents the transverse cross-sectional anatomy.

GENERATIONS OF COMPUTED TOMOGRAPHY

The previous description of a finely collimated x-ray beam and single detector assembly that translates across the patient and rotates between successive translations is characteristic of **first-generation CT imaging systems.** The original EMI imaging system required 180 translations, which were separated from one another by

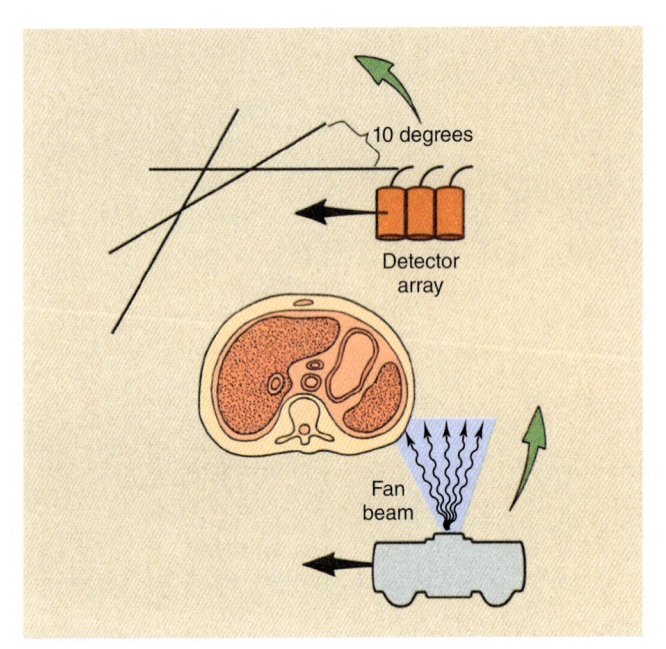

FIG. 21.4 Second-generation computed tomography imaging systems operated in the translate-and-rotate mode with a multiple-detector array intercepting a fan-shaped x-ray beam.

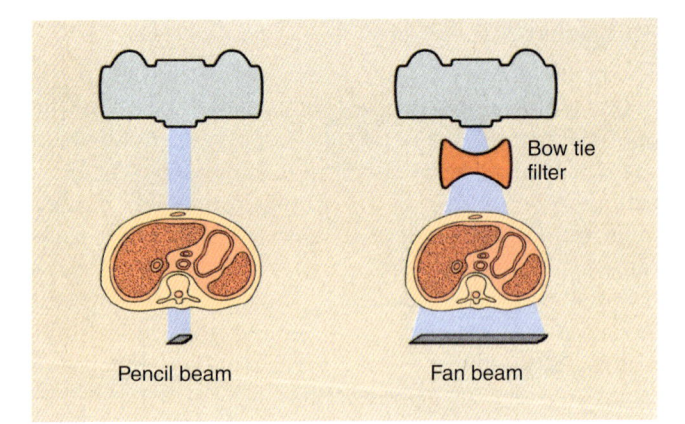

FIG. 21.5 Profiles of two x-ray beams used in computed tomography (CT) imaging. With the fan-shaped beam of second generation, a bow-tie filter is used to equalize the radiation intensity that reaches the detector array. For first-generation CT, a pencil x-ray beam is used.

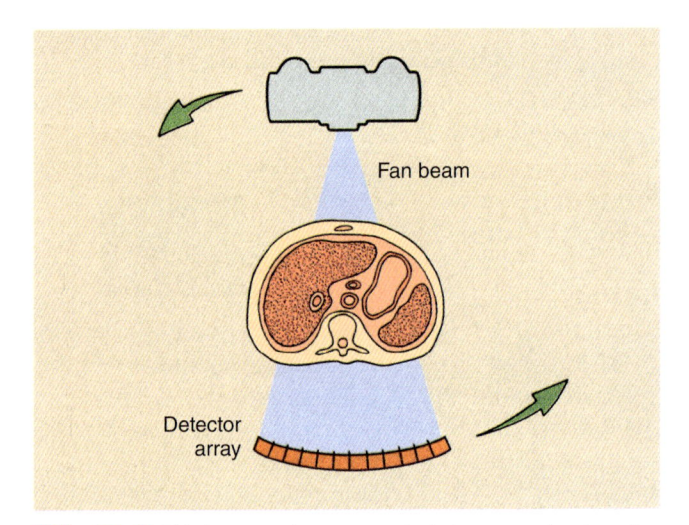

FIG. 21.6 Third-generation computed tomography imaging systems operate in the rotate-only mode with a fan x-ray beam and a multiple-detector array revolving concentrically around the patient.

a 1-degree rotation. The principal drawback to these systems was that nearly 5 minutes was required to complete a single image.

> First-generation imaging system: translate-and-rotate, pencil beam, single detector, 5-minute imaging time.

First-generation CT imaging systems can be considered a demonstration project. They proved the feasibility of the functional marriage of the source-detector assembly, mechanical gantry motion, and the computer to produce an image.

Second-generation CT imaging systems were also of the translate-and-rotate type. These units incorporated the natural extension of the single detector to a multiple-detector assembly while intercepting a fan-shaped rather than a pencil-shaped x-ray beam (Fig. 21.4).

One disadvantage of the fan beam is the increased radiation intensity that occurs toward the edges of the beam because of body shape. This is compensated for with the use of a "bow-tie" filter. These characteristic features of a first- versus a second-generation CT imaging system are shown in Fig. 21.5.

The principal advantage of the second-generation CT imaging system was speed. These imaging systems consisted of 5 to 30 detectors in the detector assembly; therefore shorter imaging times were possible. Because of the multiple-detector array, a single translation resulted in the same number of data points as several translations with a first-generation CT imaging system. Consequently, translations were separated by rotation increments of 5 degrees or more.

> Second-generation imaging system: translate-and-rotate, fan beam, detector array, 30-second imaging time.

Still, the principal limitation of second-generation CT imaging systems was examination time. Because of the complex mechanical motion of translation and rotation and the enormous mass involved in the gantry, most units were designed for imaging times of 20 seconds or longer. This limitation was overcome by **third-generation CT imaging systems**. With these imaging systems, the source and the detector array are rotated about the patient (Fig. 21.6). As rotate-only units,

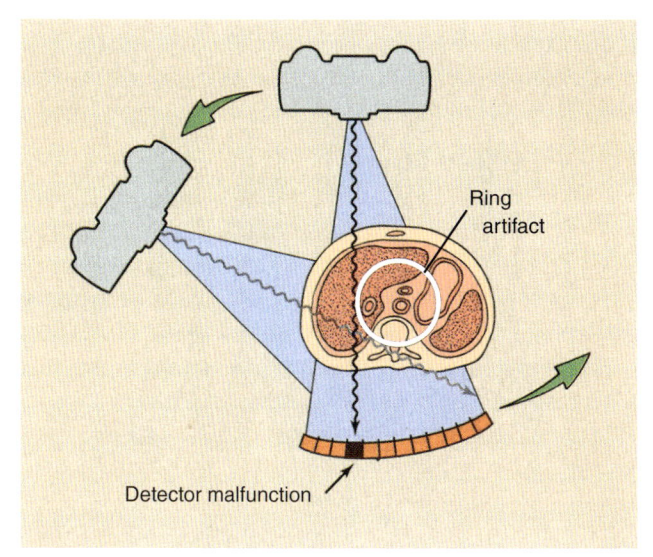

FIG. 21.7 Ring artifacts can occur in third-generation computed tomography imaging systems because each detector views a ring of anatomy during the examination. The malfunction of a single detector can result in the ring artifact.

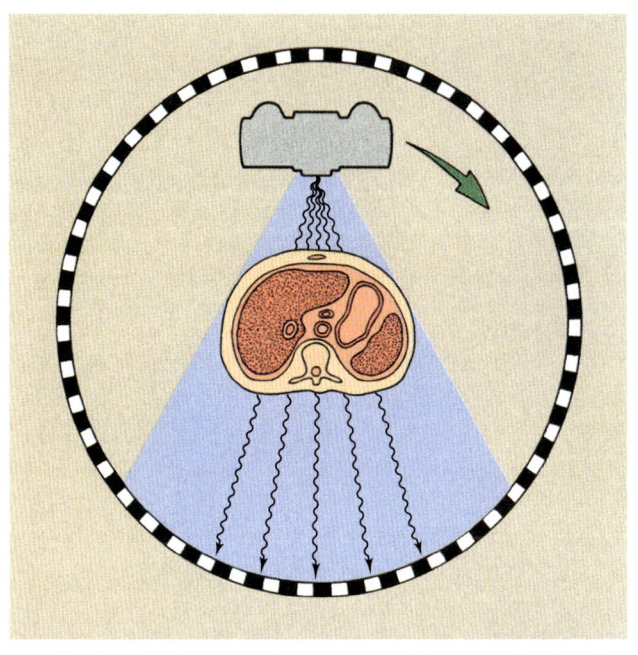

FIG. 21.8 Fourth-generation computed tomography imaging systems operate with a rotating x-ray source and stationary detectors.

third-generation imaging systems can produce an image in less than 100 ms.

The third-generation CT imaging system uses a curvilinear detector array and a fan beam. The number of detectors and the width of the fan beam—between 30 and 60 degrees—are both substantially larger than for second-generation CT imaging systems. In third-generation CT imaging systems, the fan beam and the detector array view the entire patient at all times.

The curvilinear detector array produces a constant source-to-detector path length, which is an advantage for good image reconstruction. This feature of the third-generation detector assembly also allows for better x-ray beam collimation and reduces the effect of scatter radiation.

A disadvantage of third-generation CT imaging systems is the occasional appearance of ring artifacts. If any single detector or bank of detectors malfunctions, the acquired signal or lack thereof results in a ring on the reconstructed image (Fig. 21.7). These ring artifacts were troublesome with early third-generation CT imaging systems. Software-corrected image reconstruction algorithms now remove such artifacts.

> Third-generation imaging system: rotate-and-rotate, fan beam, detector array, subsecond imaging time.

The **fourth-generation CT imaging system** incorporates a rotate-and-stationary configuration. The x-ray source rotates, but the detector assembly does not.

Radiation detection is accomplished through a fixed circular array of detectors (Fig. 21.8), which contains as many as 4000 individual detectors. The x-ray beam is fan shaped with characteristics similar to those of third-generation fan beams.

> Fourth-generation CT imaging system: rotate-and-stationary, fan beam, detector array, subsecond imaging time.

The fixed detector array of fourth-generation CT imaging systems does not result in a constant beam path from the source to all detectors, but it does allow each detector to be calibrated and its signal normalized for each image, as was possible with second-generation imaging systems. Fourth-generation imaging systems were developed because they were free of ring artifacts.

> Today, all CT imaging systems are third generation and have evolved into helical and multislice imaging.

MULTISLICE HELICAL COMPUTED TOMOGRAPHY

Actually, the gantry motion in multislice helical CT is not like a slinky toy; it just appears that way, as seen in Fig. 21.9. Fig. 21.10 shows the difference between spiral and helical.

310 PART IV Advanced Medical Imaging

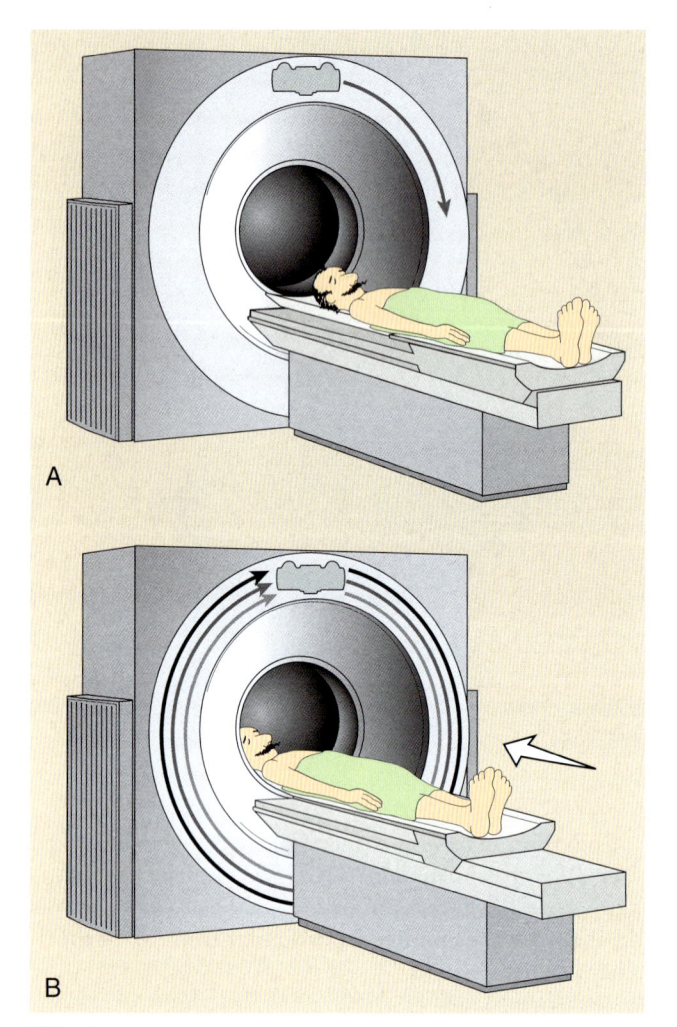

FIG. 21.9 Movement of the x-ray tube is not helical (A). It just appears that way because the patient moves through the plane of rotation during imaging (B).

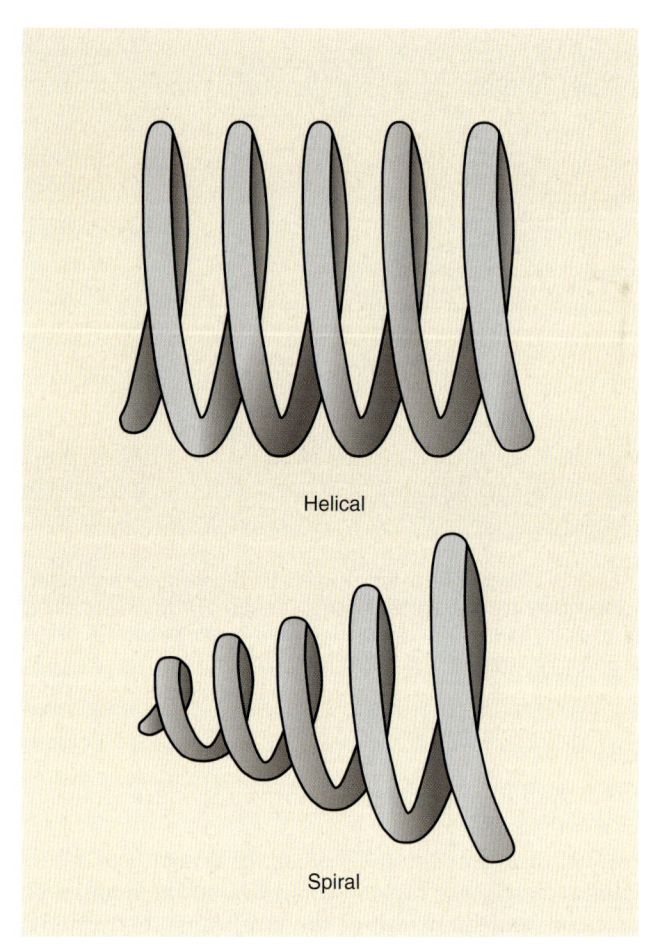

FIG. 21.10 An illustration of the difference between spiral and helical. We image with helical computed tomography.

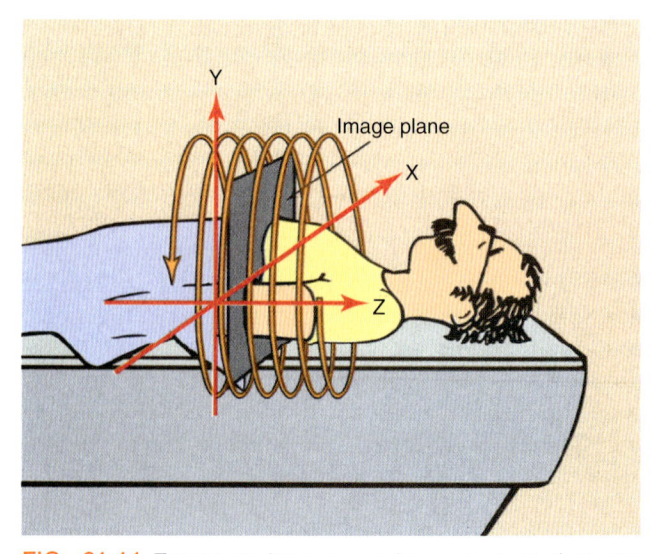

FIG. 21.11 Transverse images can be reconstructed at any plane along the z-axis.

When the examination begins, the x-ray tube rotates continuously. While the x-ray tube is rotating, the couch moves the patient through the plane of the rotating x-ray beam. The x-ray tube is energized continuously, data are collected continuously, and an image then can be reconstructed at any desired z-axis position along the patient (Fig. 21.11).

Interpolation Algorithms

Reconstruction of an image at any z-axis position is possible because of a mathematical process called **interpolation**. Fig. 21.12 presents a graphic representation of interpolation and **extrapolation**. If one wishes to estimate a value between known values, that is interpolation; if one wishes to estimate a value beyond the range of known values, that is extrapolation.

During helical CT, image data are received continuously, as shown by the data points in Fig. 21.13A. When an image is reconstructed, as in Fig. 21.13B, the plane of the image does not contain enough data for reconstruction. Data in that plane must be estimated by interpolation.

Data interpolation is performed by a special computer program called an **interpolation algorithm**. The first interpolation algorithms used 360-degree linear

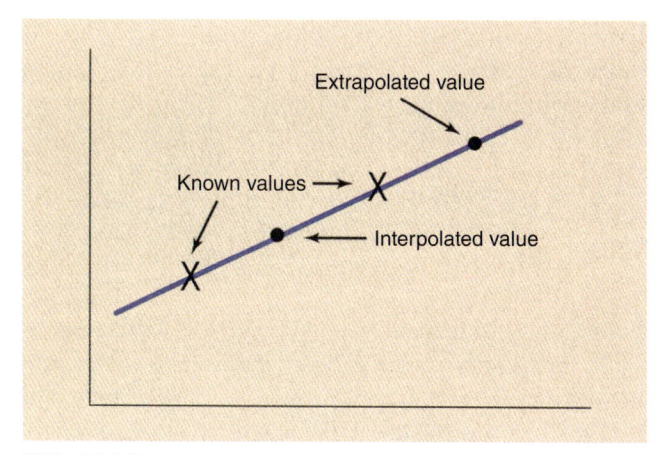

FIG. 21.12 Interpolation estimates a value between two known values. Extrapolation estimates a value beyond known values.

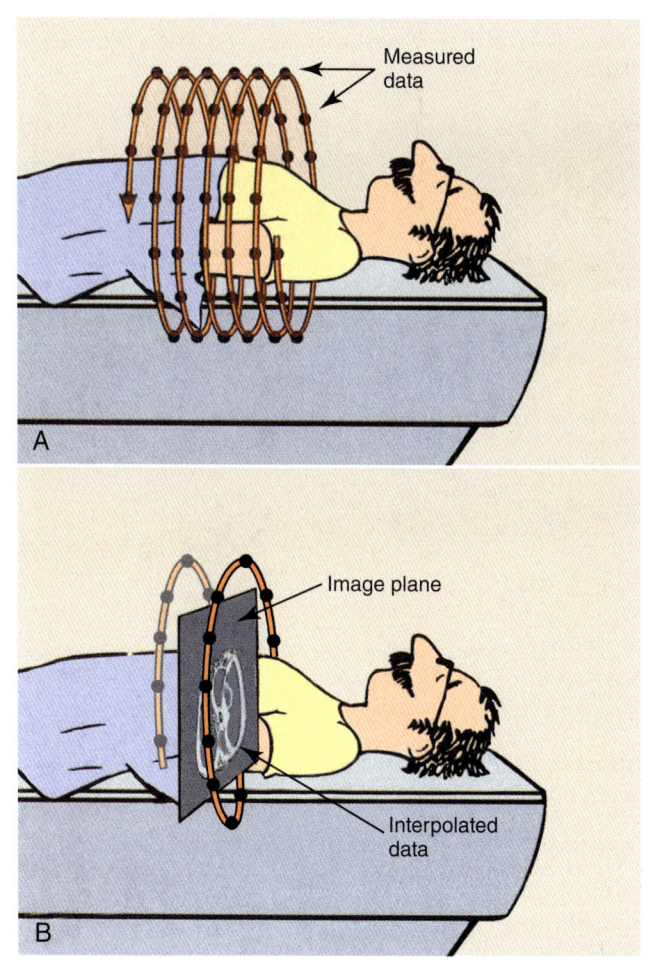

FIG. 21.13 (A) During multislice helical computed tomography, image data are continuously sampled. (B) Interpolation of data is performed to reconstruct the image in any transverse plane.

interpolation. The plane of the reconstructed image was interpolated from data acquired one revolution apart.

When these images are formatted into sagittal and coronal views, blurring can occur. The solution to the blurring problem is interpolation of values separated by 180 degrees—half a revolution of the x-ray tube. This results in improved z-axis resolution and greatly improved reformatted sagittal and coronal views.

> Linear interpolation at 180 degrees improves z-axis resolution.

Pitch

In addition to improved sagittal and coronal reformatted views, 180-degree interpolation algorithms allow imaging at a pitch greater than one. Helical pitch ratio, referred to simply as **pitch**, is the relationship between patient couch movement and x-ray beam width.

> Helical pitch ratio = $\dfrac{\text{Couch movement each 360 degrees}}{\text{Beam width}}$

Pitch is expressed as a ratio, such as 0.5:1, 1.0:1, 1.5:1, or 2:1. A pitch of 0.5:1 results in overlapping images and higher patient radiation dose. A pitch of 2:1 results in extended imaging and reduced patient radiation dose.

Question: During a 360-degree x-ray tube rotation, the patient couch moves 8 mm. Beam width is 5 mm. What is the pitch?

Answer: $\dfrac{8\text{ mm}}{5\text{ mm}} = 1.6:1$

Increasing pitch to above 1:1 increases the volume of tissue that can be imaged at a given time. This is one advantage of multislice helical CT: the ability to image a larger volume of tissue in a single breath-hold. It is particularly helpful in CT angiography, radiation therapy treatment planning, and imaging of uncooperative patients.

> Tissue volume imaged = Beam width × Pitch × Imaging time

Table 21.1 shows this relationship for a fixed imaging time and a fixed beam width.

Question: How much tissue will be imaged if beam width is set to 8 mm, imaging time is 25 s, and pitch is 1.5:1?

Answer: Tissue imaged = 8 mm × 25 s × 1.5 = 300 mm = 30 cm

TABLE 21.1	Tissue Imaged with Changing Pitch			
Beam width (mm)	10	10	10	10
Imaging time (s)	30	30	30	30
Pitch	1.0:1	1.3:1	1.6:1	2.0:1
Tissue imaged (cm)	30	39	48	60

TABLE 21.2	Tissue Imaged with Changing Pitch and a Gantry Rotation Time of 0.5 s		
Beam width (mm)	10	10	10
Scan time (s)	30	30	30
Gantry rotation time (s)	0.5	0.5	0.5
Pitch	1.0:1	1.5:1	2.0:1
Tissue imaged (cm)	60	90	120

What if the gantry rotation time is not 360 degrees in 1 s? In such a situation, the volume of tissue imaged becomes as follows:

$$\text{Tissue volume imaged} = \frac{\text{Beam width} \times \text{Pitch} \times \text{Imaging time}}{\text{Gantry rotation time}}$$

If the gantry rotation time is reduced to 0.5 s, Table 21.1 is changed to Table 21.2. With the availability of such fast multislice helical CT, whole-body imaging is now possible within a single breath-hold.

Question: One wishes to image 40 cm of tissue with a beam width of 8 mm in 25 s. If the gantry rotation time is 1.5 s, what should be the pitch?

Answer:
$$\text{Pitch} = \frac{\text{Tissue image} \times \text{Gantry rotation time}}{\text{Beam width} \times \text{Image time}}$$
$$= \frac{400 \text{ mm} \times 1.5 \text{ s}}{8 \text{ mm} \times 25 \text{ s}}$$
$$= \frac{600}{200}$$
$$= 3.0 : 1$$

In multislice helical CT, the entire width of the multidetector array intercepts the collimated x-ray beam (Fig. 21.14). For example, if all detectors of a 16-slice detector array are used, each of which is 0.5 mm in width, then when the patient couch translates 8 mm, the pitch is 1.0 because the beam width is also 8 mm (Fig. 21.15). If only the central rows of detectors are used, the x-ray beam width is collimated to 4 mm. Now, if the

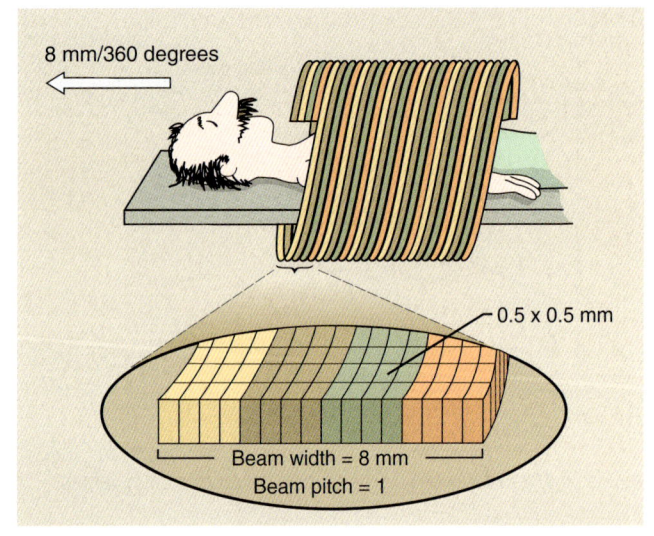

FIG. 21.14 A 16-detector array, each array element 0.5 mm wide, collimated to an 8-mm beam width results in a pitch of 1.0.

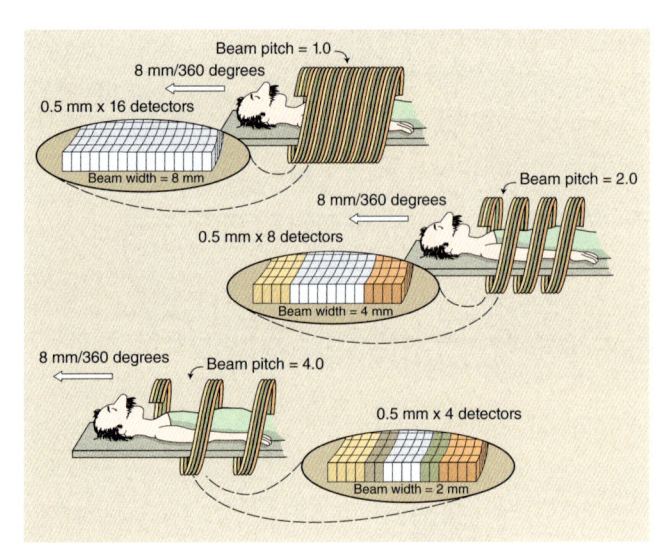

FIG. 21.15 Pitch is patient couch movement divided by x-ray beam width.

patient couch translates 8 mm, an extended helix with a beam pitch of 2.0 is observed.

Question: The beam width during 64-slice helical CT is 32 mm. If the patient couch moves 16 mm per revolution, what is the beam pitch?

Answer: Pitch = 16 mm/32 mm = 0.5
A high data image with double the patient radiation dose

In practice, the pitch for multislice helical CT is usually 1.0. Because multiple slices are obtained and z-axis location and reconstruction width can be selected after imaging, overlapping images are unnecessary.

An exception is CT angiography (CTA), which requires a pitch of less than 1.0:1. Because of multislice capability, more slices are acquired per unit time. This results in a much larger volume of imaged tissue.

Unfortunately, when beam pitch exceeds approximately 1.0:1, the z-axis resolution is reduced because of a wide-section sensitivity profile.

Sensitivity Profile

Consider the sensitivity profile of a 5-mm section obtained with a CT imaging system (Fig. 21.16). If properly collimated, it will have a full width at half maximum (FWHM) of 5 mm. The FWHM is the width of the sensitivity profile. It is also one-half of its maximum value.

IMAGING SYSTEM DESIGN

It is convenient to classify the components of a conventional x-ray imaging system into three major subsystems: the operating console, the generator, and the x-ray tube. It is also convenient to identify the three major components of a CT imaging system: the operating console, the computer, and the gantry (Fig. 21.17). Each of these major components has several subsystems.

Operating Console

Computed tomography imaging systems can be equipped with two or three consoles. One console is used by the CT technologist to operate the imaging system. Another console may be available for a CT technologist to postprocess images and annotate patient data on the image (e.g., hospital identification, name, patient number, age, sex) and to provide identification for each image (e.g., number, technique, couch position).

> The second monitor allows a CT technologist to view images before transferring them to the radiologist's viewing console.

A third console will be available for the radiologist to view the images and manipulate image contrast, size, and general visual appearance. This is in addition to several remote imaging stations available to the radiologist and other physicians.

The operating console contains meters and controls for selection of proper imaging technique factors, for proper mechanical movement of the gantry and the patient couch, and for the use of computer commands that allow image reconstruction and transfer. The radiologist's viewing console accepts the reconstructed image from the operator's console and displays it for viewing and interpretation.

A typical operating console contains controls and monitors for the various technique factors (Fig. 21.18). Operation is usually approximately 120 kVp, although some recent work supports reducing patient radiation dose by using a lower kVp. The maximum mA

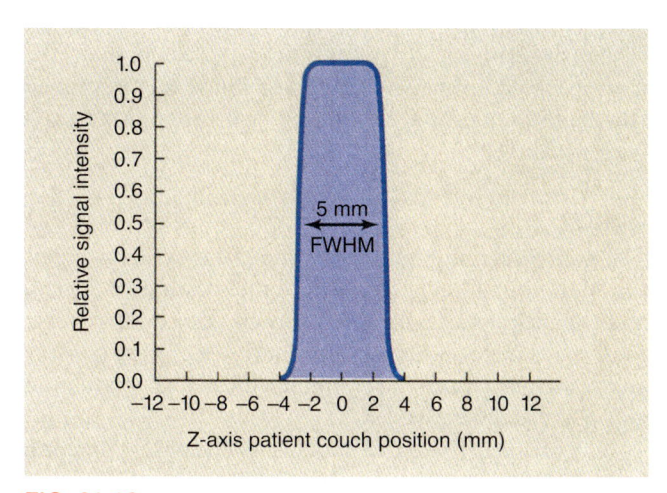

FIG. 21.16 The section sensitivity profile (SSP) for a conventional computed tomography imaging system is nearly rectangular and is identified by its full width at half maximum (*FWHM*). SSP is a fancy name for slice thickness.

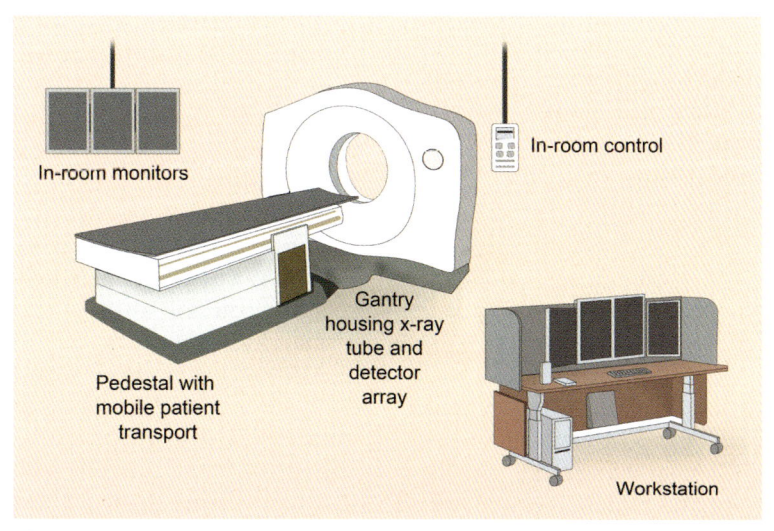

FIG. 21.17 Components of a complete computed tomography imaging system.

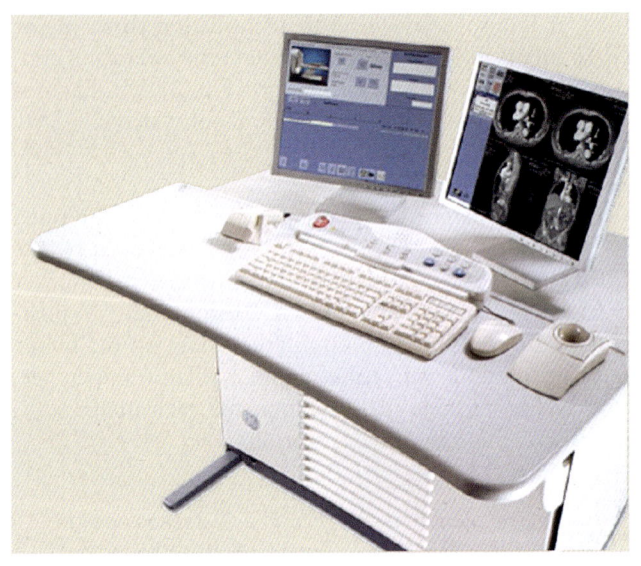

FIG. 21.18 Operator's console for a multislice helical computed tomography imaging system. (Courtesy Reggie Carter, General Electric Healthcare.)

is usually 400 mA and is modulated during imaging according to patient thickness to minimize the patient radiation dose.

The thickness of the tissue slice to be imaged also can be adjusted. Nominal thicknesses are 0.5 to 5 mm. Slice thickness is selected from the console by adjustment of the automatic collimator and by selection of various rows of the detector assembly.

Controls also are provided for automatic movement and for indexing of the patient support couch. This allows the operator to program for Z-axis location, tissue volume to be imaged, and helical pitch.

The radiologist's console allows for retrieving previous images to optimize diagnostic information. The controls provide for contrast and brightness adjustments, magnification techniques, region of interest (ROI) viewing, and use of online computer software packages.

This software may include programs designed to generate plots of CT numbers along any preselected axis, and computation of mean and standard deviation. It can also produce values in a ROI, subtraction techniques, and planar and volumetric quantitative analysis.

> Reconstruction of images along coronal, sagittal, and oblique planes is also possible.

The physician's viewing console is usually remote from the CT suite and is used for postprocessing tasks for all digital images (see Chapter 13). It can also be linked to a picture archiving and communication systems network.

Computer

The computer is a unique subsystem of the CT imaging system. Depending on the image format, as many as 250,000 equations must be solved simultaneously; thus, a large computing capacity is required.

At the heart of the computer used in CT are the microprocessor and the primary memory. These determine the time between the end of imaging and the appearance of an image—the **reconstruction time**. The efficiency of an examination is influenced greatly by reconstruction time, especially when a many image slices are involved.

> Reconstruction time is the time from the end of imaging to appearance of the image.

Many CT imaging systems use an **array processor** instead of a microprocessor for image reconstruction. The array processor does many calculations simultaneously and hence is significantly faster than the microprocessor. The CT computer module is improved constantly. Quantum computing will usher in an even bigger change.

Gantry

The gantry includes the x-ray tube, the detector array, the high-voltage generator, the patient support couch, and the mechanical support for each. These subsystems receive electronic commands from the operating console and transmit data to the computer for image production and postprocessing tasks.

X-ray tubes used in multislice helical CT imaging have special requirements. Multislice helical CT places a considerable thermal demand on the x-ray tube. The x-ray tube can be energized up to 60 s continuously. Although some x-ray tubes operate at relatively low tube current, for many, the instantaneous power capacity must be high.

High-speed rotors are used for the best heat dissipation. Experience has shown that x-ray tube failure is a principal cause of CT imaging-system malfunction and is the principal limitation of sequential imaging frequency.

Focal-spot size is also important in most designs, even though the CT image is not based on direct projection imaging. CT imaging systems designed for high spatial resolution imaging incorporate x-ray tubes with a small focal spot.

Multislice helical CT x-ray tubes are very large. They have an anode heat storage capacity of 8 million heat units (MHUs) or more. They have anode-cooling rates of approximately 1 MHU per minute because the anode disc has a larger diameter, and it is thicker, resulting in much greater mass.

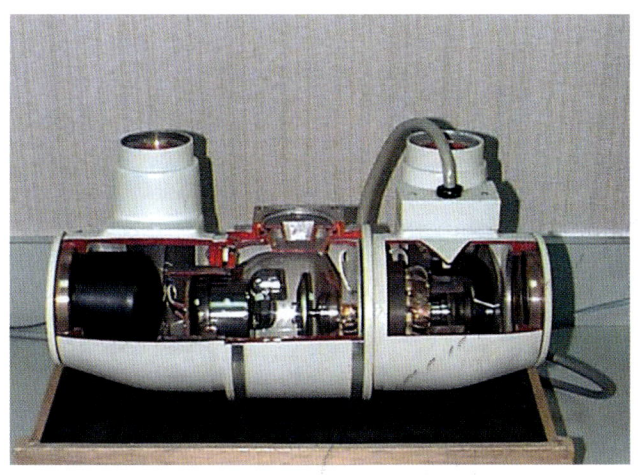

FIG. 21.19 This x-ray tube is designed especially for helical computed tomography. It has a 15-cm-diameter disc that is 5 cm thick with an anode heat capacity of 7 MHU (million heat units). (Courtesy Randy Hood, Philips Medical Systems.)

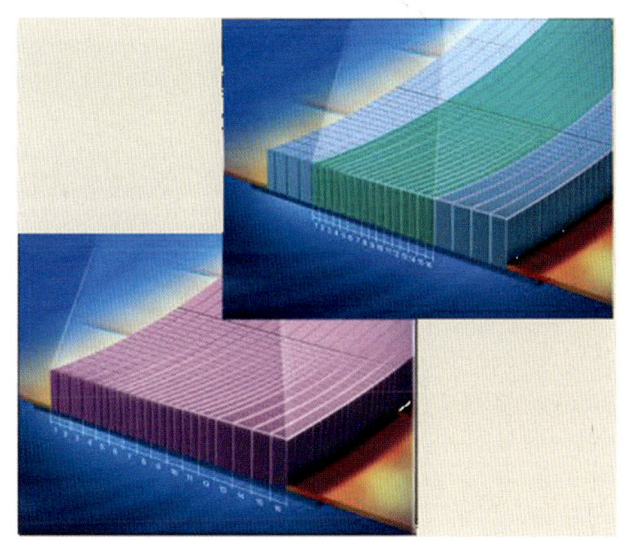

FIG. 21.20 This multidetector array contains 64 rows of 1824 individual detectors, each 0.6 mm wide (116,736 detectors). (Courtesy Andrew Moehring, General Electric Healthcare.)

The limiting characteristics are focal-spot design and heat dissipation. The small focal spot must be especially robust in design. Manufacturers design **focal-spot cooling algorithms** to predict the focal-spot thermal state and to adjust the mA setting accordingly. The x-ray tube in Fig. 21.19 is designed especially for helical CT.

> CT x-ray tubes are expected to last for at least 50,000 exposures.

Multislice helical CT imaging systems have multiple detectors in a **detector array** that can reach tens of thousands (Fig. 21.20). Sodium iodide (NaI) was the detector material used in the earliest imaging systems. This was quickly replaced by bismuth germanate ($Bi_4Ge_3O_{12}$ or BGO) and cesium iodide (CsI). Cadmium tungstate ($CdWO_4$) and special ceramics are the current materials of choice. The concentration of scintillation detectors is an important characteristic of a CT imaging system, which affects the spatial resolution of the system.

Scintillation detectors have high x-ray detection efficiency. Approximately 90% of the x-rays incident on the detector are absorbed, and this contributes to the output signal. It is now possible to pack the detectors so that the space between them is nil. Consequently, overall detection efficiency approaches 90%. The efficiency of the x-ray detector array reduces patient radiation doses, allows faster imaging time, and improves image quality by increasing the signal-to-noise ratio. Detector array design is especially critical for multislice helical CT.

Collimation is required during multislice helical CT imaging for precisely the same reasons as in radiography. Proper collimation reduces patient radiation dose by restricting the volume of tissue irradiated. Even more important is the fact that it improves image contrast by limiting scatter radiation.

In radiography, only one collimator is mounted on the x-ray tube housing. In multislice helical CT imaging, two collimators are used (Fig. 21.21).

One collimator is mounted on the x-ray tube housing or adjacent to it. This collimator limits the area of the patient that intercepts the useful beam and thereby determines the patient radiation dose. This **prepatient collimator** usually consists of several sections, resulting in a nearly parallel x-ray beam.

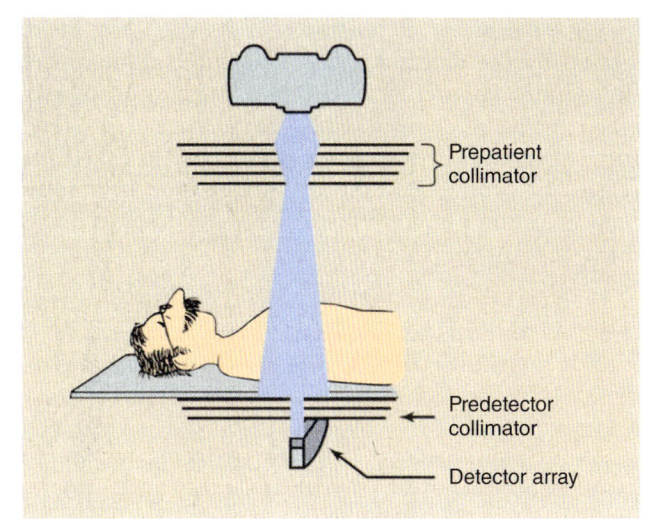

FIG. 21.21 Multislice helical computed tomography imaging systems incorporate both a prepatient collimator and a predetector collimator.

> Prepatient collimation determines the radiation dose profile and patient radiation dose.

The **predetector collimator** restricts the x-ray beam viewed by the detector array. This collimator reduces the scatter radiation incident on the detector array and, when properly coupled with the prepatient collimator, defines the slice thickness, which is also called the **sensitivity profile**. Because the predetector collimator reduces scatter radiation that reaches the detector array, it thereby improves image contrast.

> The predetector collimator determines the sensitivity profile and improves image contrast.

All multislice helical CT imaging systems operate on high-frequency power. A **high-frequency generator** is small because the high-voltage step-up transformer is small, so it can be mounted on the gantry.

The design constraints placed on the high-voltage generator are the same as those for the x-ray tube. In a properly designed multislice helical CT imaging system, the two should be matched to maximum capacity. Approximately 50 kW of power is necessary.

In addition to supporting the patient comfortably, the **patient couch** must be constructed of low-Z material, such as carbon fiber, so it does not interfere with x-ray beam transmission and patient imaging. It should be smoothly and accurately motor-driven to allow precise patient positioning that is unaffected by the weight of the patient.

When patient couch positioning is not exact, the same tissue can be imaged twice, thus doubling the radiation dose, or it can be missed altogether. The patient couch is indexed automatically, so the operator does not have to enter the examination room between imaging sequences. Such a feature reduces the examination time required for each patient.

Slip-Ring Technology

Slip rings are electromechanical devices that conduct electricity and electrical signals through rings and brushes from a rotating surface onto a fixed surface. One surface is a smooth ring and the other a ring with brushes that sweep the smooth ring (Fig. 21.22). Helical CT is made possible by the use of slip-ring technology, which allows the gantry to rotate continuously without interruption.

Early CT imaging was performed with a pause between gantry rotations because high voltage and data cables passed from the gantry. During the pause, the patient couch was moved and the gantry was rewound to a starting position.

> Slip rings eliminate the need for cables, making continuous rotation possible, resulting in multislice helical CT.

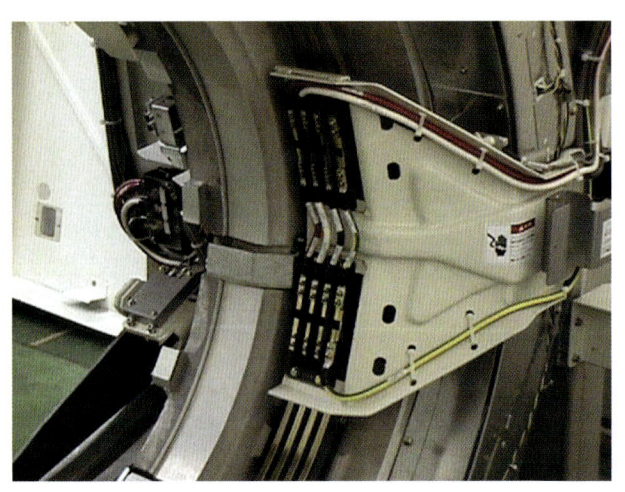

FIG. 21.22 Slip rings and brushes electrically connect the components on the rotating gantry with the rest of the multislice helical computed tomography imaging system. (Courtesy Terry Williams, Toshiba Medical Systems.)

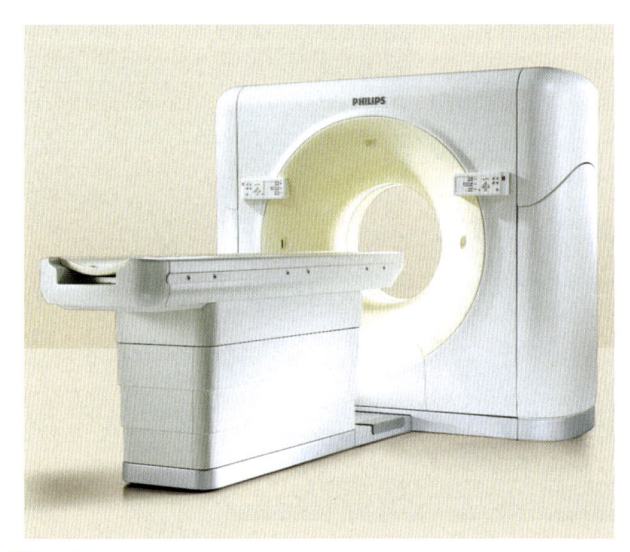

FIG. 21.23 The gantry of this multislice helical computed tomography imaging system contains a high-voltage generator, an x-ray tube, a detector array, and assorted control systems. (Courtesy Philips Healthcare.)

Brushes that transmit power to the gantry components glide in contact grooves on the stationary slip ring. Composite brushes made of conductive material (e.g., silver graphite alloy) are used as a sliding contact. The rings should last for the life of the imaging system. The brushes have to be replaced every year or so during preventive maintenance.

Fig. 21.23 shows how compact a rotating gantry must be.

IMAGE CHARACTERISTICS

The image obtained in CT is different from that obtained in radiography or fluoroscopy. It is created from data received and is not a projected image. In

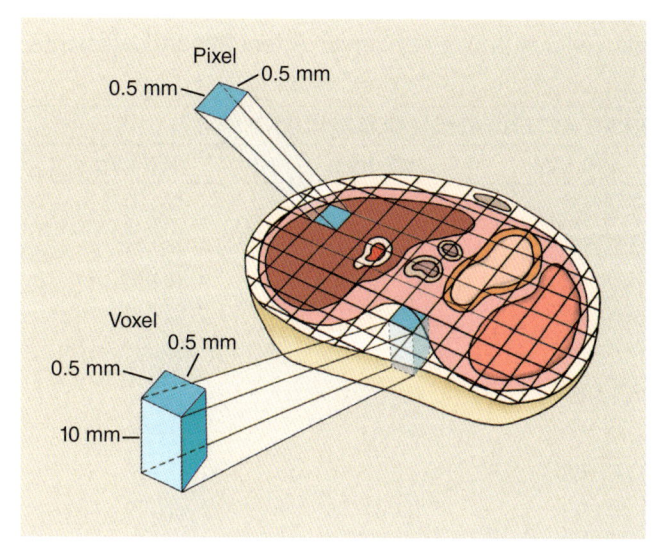

FIG. 21.24 Each cell in a computed tomography image matrix is a two-dimensional representation (pixel) of a volume of tissue (voxel).

radiography and fluoroscopy, x-rays form an image directly on the image receptor. With CT imaging systems, the x-rays form a stored electronic image that is displayed as a matrix of intensities.

Image Matrix

The CT image format consists of many cells, each assigned a number and displayed as a brightness level on the digital display device. The original EMI format consisted of an 80 × 80 matrix for a total of 6400 individual cells of information. Current imaging systems provide matrices of 512 × 512, resulting in 262,144 cells of information.

Each cell of information is a **pixel** (picture element), and the numerical information contained in each pixel is a CT number, or **Hounsfield unit** (**HU**). The pixel is a two-dimensional representation of a corresponding tissue volume (Fig. 21.24).

The diameter of image reconstruction is called the **field of view** (**FOV**). When the FOV is increased for a fixed matrix size, for example, from 12 to 20 cm, the size of each pixel is increased proportionately. When the matrix size is increased for a fixed FOV, for example, 512 × 512 to 1024 × 1024, the pixel size is smaller.

$$\text{Pixel size} = \frac{\text{FOV}}{\text{Matrix size}}$$

Question: Compute the pixel size for the following characteristics of CT images:
  a. FOV 20 cm, 128 × 128 matrix
  b. FOV 20 cm, 512 × 512 matrix
  c. FOV 36 cm, 512 × 512 matrix

Answer:
  a. $\frac{200 \text{ mm}}{128 \text{ pixels}} = 1.6$ mm/pixel
  b. $\frac{200 \text{ mm}}{512 \text{ pixels}} = 0.4$ mm/pixel
  c. $\frac{360 \text{ mm}}{512 \text{ pixels}} = 0.7$ mm/pixel

The tissue volume is known as a **voxel** (volume element), and it is determined by multiplying the pixel size by the thickness of the CT image slice.

$$\text{Voxel size (mm}^3\text{)} = \text{Pixel size (mm}^2\text{)} \times \text{Slice thickness (mm)}$$

Question: If each of the three scans in the preceding question was conducted at a 5-mm slice thickness, what would be the respective voxel sizes?

Answer:
  a. $(1.7 \text{ mm})^2 \times 5 \text{ mm} = 14.5 \text{ mm}^3$
  b. $(0.4 \text{ mm})^2 \times 5 \text{ mm} = 0.8 \text{ mm}^3$
  c. $(0.7 \text{ mm})^2 \times 5 \text{ mm} = 2.5 \text{ mm}^3$

Computed Tomography Numbers

Each pixel is displayed on the digital display device as a level of brightness. These levels correspond to a range of CT numbers from −1000 to +3000 for each pixel. A CT number of −1000 corresponds to air, and a CT number of +3000 corresponds to dense bone. A CT number of zero indicates water. Table 21.3 shows the CT number for various tissues along with respective x-ray linear attenuation coefficients at four kVp values.

The precise CT number of any given pixel is related to the x-ray attenuation coefficient of the tissue contained in the voxel. As discussed in Chapter 10, the degree of x-ray attenuation is determined by the average energy of the x-ray beam and the effective atomic number of the absorber and is expressed by the attenuation coefficient.

The value of a CT number is given by the following:

$$\text{CT number} = k \left(\frac{\mu_t - \mu_w}{\mu_w} \right)$$

where μ_t is the attenuation coefficient of the tissue in the voxel under analysis, μ_w is the x-ray attenuation coefficient of water, and k is a constant that determines the scale factor for the range of CT numbers.

This equation shows that the CT number for water is always zero because for water, $\mu_t = \mu_w$, so that $\mu_t − \mu_w = 0$.

TABLE 21.3 Computed Tomography Number for Various Tissues and X-ray Linear Attenuation Coefficients at Four kVp Techniques

Tissue	CT Number	LINEAR ATTENUATION COEFFICIENT (CM^{-1})			
		75 kVp	100 kVp	125 kVp	150 kVp
Dense bone	3000	0.604	0.528	0.460	0.410
Muscle	50	0.273	0.237	0.208	0.184
White matter	45	0.245	0.213	0.187	0.166
Gray matter	40	0.243	0.212	0.184	0.163
Blood	20	0.241	0.208	0.182	0.163
Cerebrospinal fluid	15	0.240	0.207	0.181	0.160
Water	0	0.239	0.206	0.180	0.160
Fat	−100	0.213	0.185	0.162	0.144
Lungs	−200	0.111	0.093	0.081	0.072
Air	−1000	0.0005	0.0004	0.0003	0.0002

kVp, Kilovolt peak.

For the CT imaging system to operate with precision, detector response must be calibrated continuously so that water is always represented by zero.

> When k is 1000, the CT numbers are called Hounsfield units (HU) and range from −1000 to +1000.

Obviously, an enormous amount of information is wasted when the actual dynamic range of the image is 4096, but it is displayed and viewed as no more than 32 shades of gray. However, completion of postprocessing with window and level adjustment allows the entire dynamic range to be made visible.

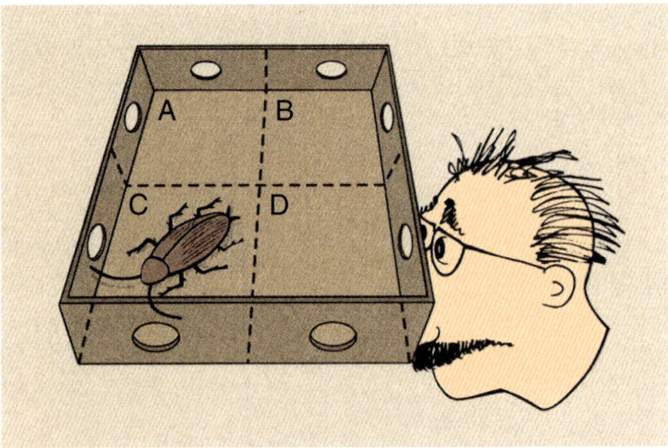

Image Reconstruction

The projections acquired by each detector during CT are stored in computer memory. The image is reconstructed from these projections by a process called **filtered back projection**.

Here, the term **filter** refers to a mathematical function rather than to a metal filter for the x-ray beam. This process is much too complicated to be discussed here, but a simple example helps to explain how it works.

Imagine a box with two holes cut into each side (Fig. 21.25). The box is divided into four cells labeled A, B, C, and D, and a Texas-sized cockroach is found in cell C. If we now cover the box and look through the four sets of holes, we can devise a way of determining precisely in which section the cockroach resides.

Let "1" represent the presence of the cockroach for each viewing. If one sees two empty cells through a hole and the opposite hole, then obviously, the cockroach is

FIG. 21.25 This four-pixel matrix demonstrates the method for reconstructing a computed tomography image by back projection.

not there. We indicate the absence of the cockroach with "0." The path that is being viewed in Fig. 21.25 can be represented symbolically as c + d = 1. Examination of all possible paths shows the following:

$$a + b = 0$$
$$c + d = 1$$
$$a + c = 1$$
$$b + d = 0$$

The result is four equations for which, if solved simultaneously, the solution is C = 1 and A, B, and D = 0.

In CT, we would have not four pixels but rather more than 250,000. Consequently CT image reconstruction requires the solution of more than 250,000 equations simultaneously.

Recently a more robust reconstruction algorithm, iterative reconstruction, has been introduced. Iterative

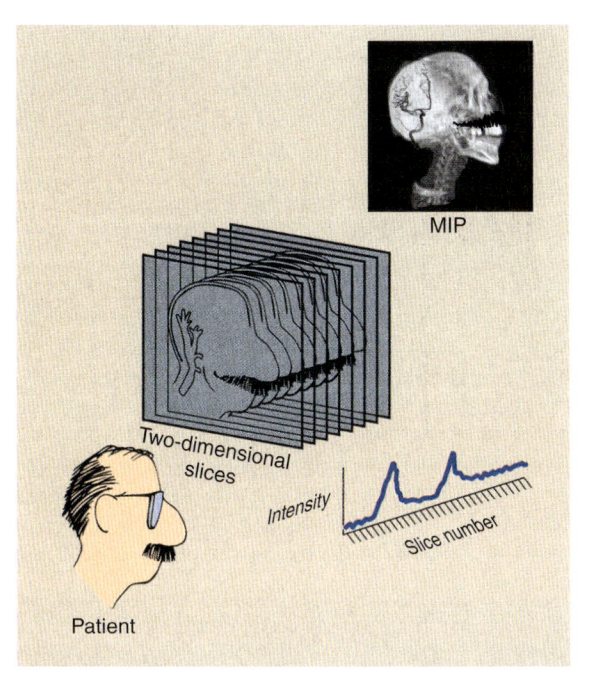

FIG. 21.26 A maximum intensity projection (*MIP*) reconstruction creates a three-dimensional image from multislice two-dimensional data sets. The result is a computed tomography angiogram.

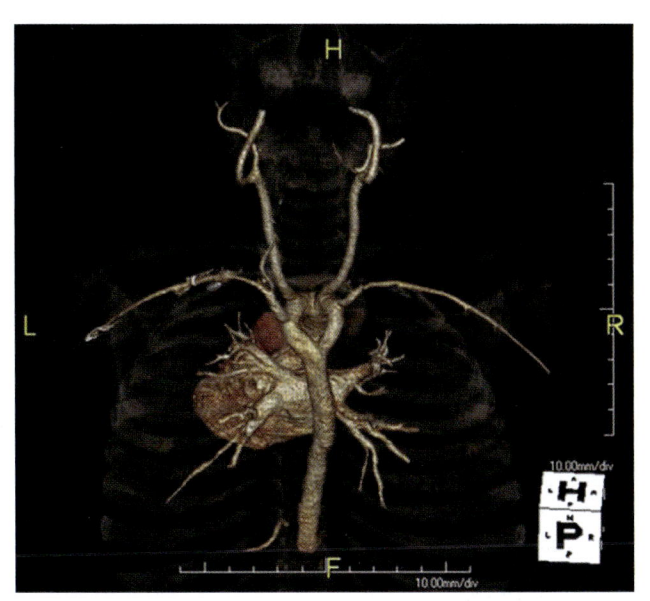

FIG. 21.27 This carotid CT scan was reconstructed from a 64-slice helical computed tomography examination. (Courtesy Lance Blackwell, Tera-Recon Inc.)

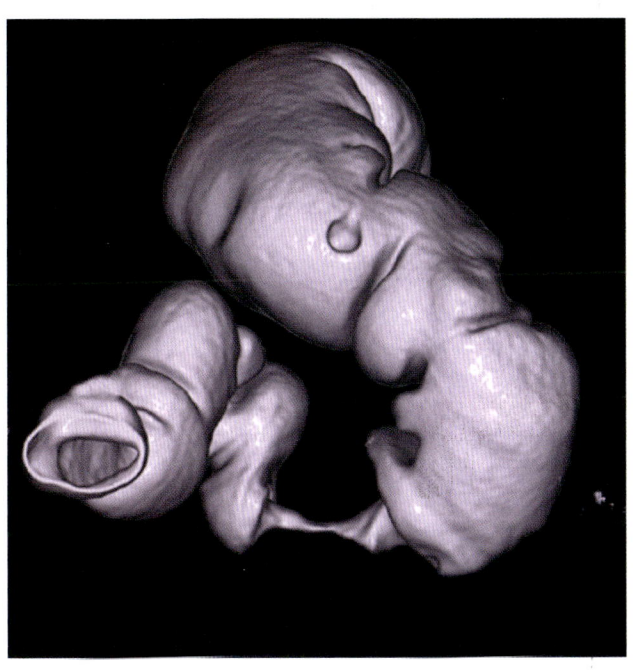

FIG. 21.28 Shaded surface image obtained during virtual colonoscopy reconstructed from a 64-slice spiral computed tomography data set. (Courtesy Lance Blackwell, TeraRecon, Inc.)

reconstruction requires more computer capacity but can result in improved contrast resolution at lower patient radiation dose.

Multiplanar Reformation

Multislice helical CT excels in three-dimensional **multiplanar reformation (MPR)**. Transverse images are stacked to form a three-dimensional data set, which can be rendered as an image in several ways. Three three-dimensional MPR algorithms are used most frequently: **maximum intensity projection (MIP)**, **shaded surface display (SSD)**, and **shaded volume display (SVD)**.

MIP reconstructs an image by selecting the highest value pixels along any arbitrary line through the data set and exhibiting only those pixels (Fig. 21.26). MIP images are widely used in CTA because they can be reconstructed very quickly.

Only approximately 10% of the three-dimensional data points are used. The result can be a very high-contrast three-dimensional image of contrast-filled vessels (Fig. 21.27).

> On computer workstations, the image can be rotated to show striking three-dimensional features.

MIP is the simplest form of three-dimensional imaging. It provides excellent differentiation of the vasculature from surrounding tissue but lacks vessel depth because superimposed vessels are not displayed. This is accommodated somewhat by image rotation. Small vessels that pass obliquely through a voxel may not be imaged because of partial volume averaging.

SSD is a technique that has been borrowed from computer-aided design and manufacturing applications. It was initially applied to bone imaging and now is used regularly for virtual colonoscopy (Fig. 21.28). SSD identifies a narrow range of values as belonging to the object to be imaged and displays that range. The range

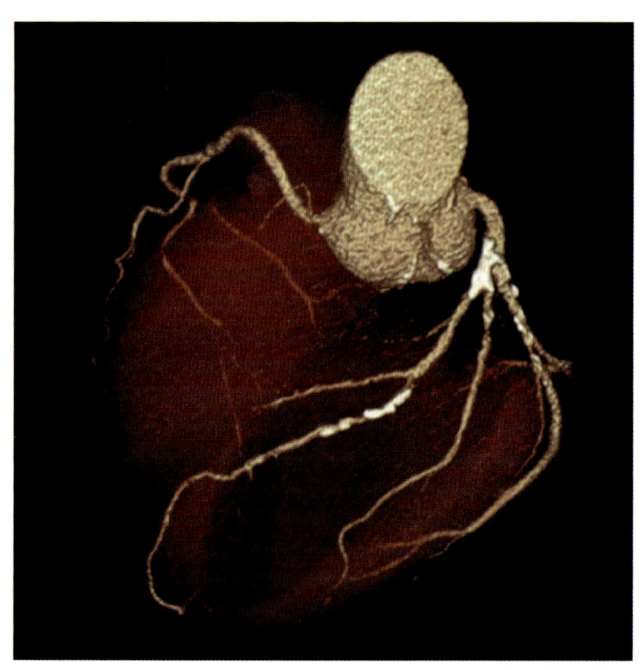

FIG. 21.29 Volume-rendering display of the heart obtained during cardiac computed tomography angiography. This image can be rotated for three-dimensional visualization. (Courtesy Lance Blackwell, TeraRecon, Inc.)

displayed appears as an organ surface that is determined by operator-selected values.

Surface boundaries can be made distinctive and can provide an image that appears very three-dimensional (Fig. 21.29). Such an image is called **volume rendered**. SVD is very sensitive to the operator-selected pixel range; this can make imaging of actual anatomical structures difficult.

IMAGE QUALITY

CT images are composed of discrete pixel values, and therefore image quality is somewhat easy to characterize and quantitate. A number of methods are available for measuring CT image quality, and five principal characteristics are numerically assigned. These include spatial resolution, contrast resolution, noise, linearity, and uniformity.

Spatial Resolution

If one images a regular geometric structure that has a sharp interface, the image at the interface will be somewhat blurred (Fig. 21.30). The degree of blurring is a measure of the spatial resolution of the system and is controlled by a number of factors. Because the image of the interface is a visual rendition of pixel values, these values could be analyzed across the interface to arrive at a measure of spatial resolution.

The image is somewhat blurred owing to limitations of the CT imaging system; the expected sharp edge of CT numbers is replaced with a smoothed range of CT numbers across the interface.

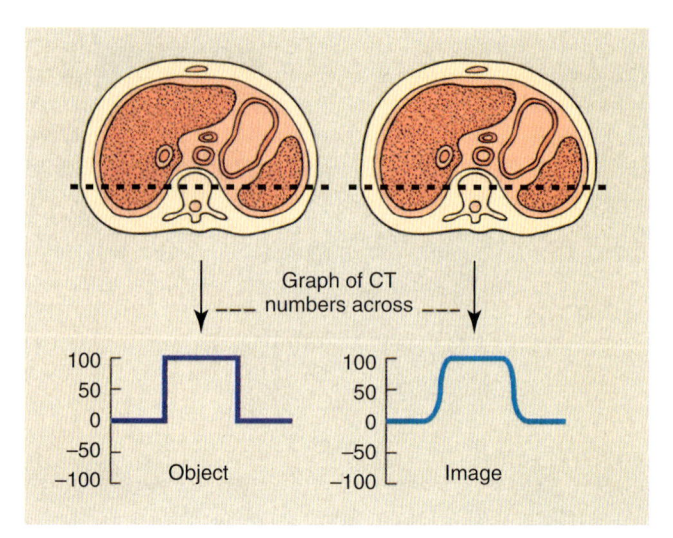

FIG. 21.30 Computed tomography (*CT*) examination of an object organ with distinct borders results in an image with somewhat blurred borders. The actual CT number profile of the object is abrupt, but that of the image is smoothed.

Spatial resolution for all imaging modalities is determined by pixel size. The smaller the pixel, the better the spatial resolution. CT imaging systems allow reconstruction of images followed by postprocessing tasks; this is a powerful way to affect spatial resolution.

Thinner slice thicknesses also allow better spatial resolution. Anatomy that does not lie totally within a slice thickness may result in an artifact called **partial volume averaging**. Therefore voxel size in CT also affects CT spatial resolution.

The ability of the CT imaging system to reproduce with accuracy a high-contrast edge is expressed mathematically as the **edge response function** (ERF). The measured ERF can be transformed into another mathematical expression called the **modulation transfer function** (MTF). The MTF and its graphic representation are most often cited to express the spatial resolution of a CT imaging system.

Although the MTF is a rather complicated mathematical formulation, its meaning is not too difficult to represent. Return to Chapter 13 and review the concept of MTF. Then consider the series of bar patterns that are imaged by CT (Fig. 21.31).

The **spatial frequency** for CT imaging systems is expressed often as line pairs per centimeter (lp/cm) instead of line pair per millimeter (lp/mm).

Question: How does one convert lp/cm to lp/mm?
Answer: 1 lp/cm = 1 lp/10 mm = 0.1 lp/mm

> A low spatial frequency represents large objects and a high spatial frequency represents small objects.

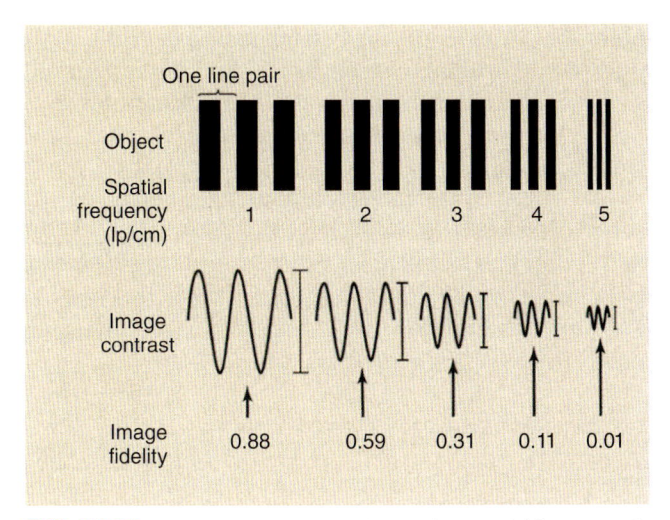

FIG. 21.31 When a bar pattern of increasing spatial frequency is imaged, the fidelity of the image decreases. The tracing of image contrast reveals the reduction in contrast resolution.

FIG. 21.32 The modulation transfer function (*MTF*) is a plot of the image fidelity versus spatial frequency. The six data points plotted here are taken from the analysis of Fig. 21.31.

The image obtained from the low-frequency bar pattern will appear more similar to the object than the image from the high-frequency bar pattern. The loss in faithful reproduction with increasing spatial frequency occurs because of limitations of the imaging system. Characteristics of the CT imaging system that contribute to such image degradation include collimation, pixel size, mechanical and electrical gantry control, and the reconstruction algorithm.

In simplistic terms, the MTF is the ratio of the image to the object as a function of spatial frequency. If the image faithfully represents the object, the MTF of the CT imaging system would have a value of 1. If the image were simply blank and contained no information whatsoever about the object, the MTF would be equal to zero. Intermediate levels of fidelity result in intermediate MTF values.

In Fig. 21.32, image fidelity is measured by determining the image contrast at various spatial frequencies. At a spatial frequency of 1 lp/cm, for instance, the variation in image contrast of the image is 0.88 times that of the object. At 4 lp/cm, it is only 0.11 or 11% that of the object.

> A graph of the image contrast to object contrast at each spatial frequency results in an MTF curve.

Fig. 21.33 shows the MTF for two different CT imaging systems and illustrates how such curves should be interpreted. An MTF curve that extends farther to the right indicates better spatial resolution, which means the imaging system is better able to reproduce very small objects. An MTF curve that is higher at low spatial frequencies indicates better contrast resolution (Fig. 21.34).

Obviously MTF is a complex relationship because it relates the imaging capacity of the system for objects of various sizes. Most CT imaging systems are judged by spatial frequency at an MTF equal to 0.1, sometimes called the **limiting resolution**. As is shown in Fig. 21.33, whereas imaging system A has a 0.1 MTF at 5.2 lp/cm, B can manage only 3.5 lp/cm. Therefore A has better spatial resolution than B.

Although CT image resolution is expressed most often in terms of spatial frequency of the limiting resolution, it is easier to think in terms of the object size that can be reproduced. The absolute object size that can be

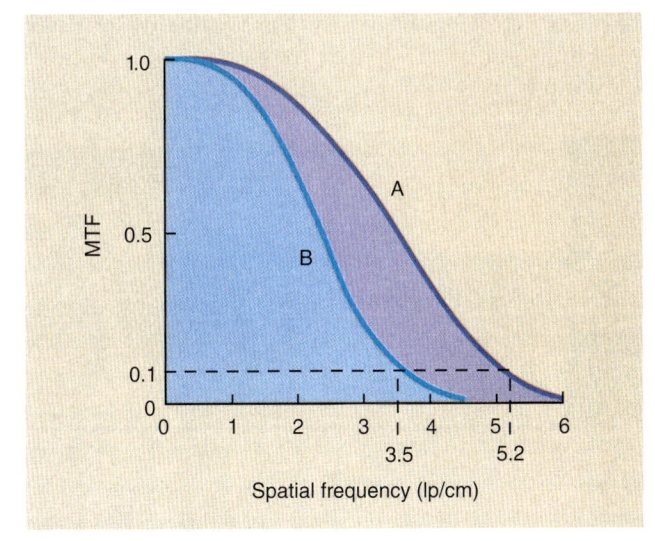

FIG. 21.33 Modulation transfer function (*MTF*) curves for two representative computed tomography imaging systems. Imaging system A has higher spatial resolution than imaging system B.

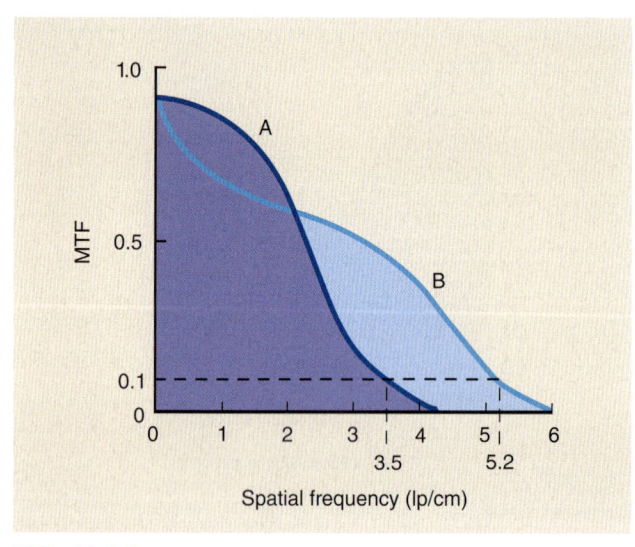

FIG. 21.34 Imaging system A has better contrast resolution. Imaging system B has better spatial resolution. *MTF*, Modulation transfer function.

resolved by a CT imaging system is equal to one-half the reciprocal of the spatial frequency at the limiting resolution.

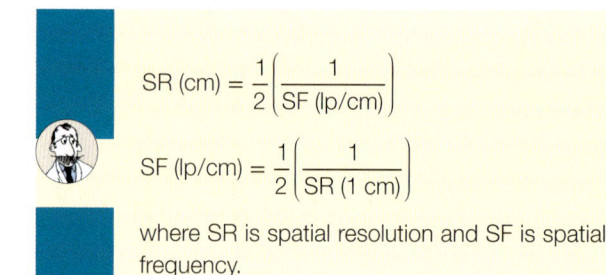

$$SR\ (cm) = \frac{1}{2}\left(\frac{1}{SF\ (lp/cm)}\right)$$

$$SF\ (lp/cm) = \frac{1}{2}\left(\frac{1}{SR\ (1\ cm)}\right)$$

where SR is spatial resolution and SF is spatial frequency.

Question: A CT imaging system is said to be capable of 5 lp/cm resolution. What size object does this represent?

Answer:
The reciprocal of 5 lp/cm = $(5\ lp/cm)^{-1}$
$$= \frac{1}{5\ lp/cm}$$
$$= \frac{1\ cm}{5\ lp}$$
$$= \frac{10\ mm}{5\ lp}$$
$$= \frac{2\ mm}{lp}$$

Because a line pair consists of a bar and an interspace of equal width, 2 mm/lp represents a 1-mm object separated by a 1-mm interspace. The system resolution is therefore 1 mm.

Question: Currently, the best multislice helical CT imaging systems have a limiting resolution of approximately 20 lp/cm. What object size does this represent?

Answer:
The reciprocal of $(20\ lp/cm)^{a-1} = 1$
$$= \frac{1}{20\ lp/cm}$$
$$= \frac{1\ cm}{20\ lp}$$
$$= \frac{10\ mm}{20\ lp}$$
$$= \frac{0.5\ mm}{lp}$$

Therefore the CT resolution is 0.25 mm.

Question: A CT imaging system can resolve a 0.65-mm high-contrast object. What spatial frequency does this represent?

Answer:
0.65-mm object + 0.65-mm interspace
$$= 1.3\ mm/lp$$
$$\frac{1}{1.3\ mm/lp} = 0.77\ lp/mm$$
$$= 7.7\ lp/cm$$

Important measures of imaging-system performance that can be evaluated with test objects include artifact generation, contrast resolution, and spatial resolution. Fig. 21.35 shows the four test sections of the phantom designed by the Physics Commission of the American College of Radiology (ACR) to evaluate a number of CT image quality factors.

> Spatial resolution for a CT image is limited to the size of the pixel.

Although MTF and spatial frequency are used to describe CT spatial resolution, no imaging system can do better than the size of a pixel. In terms of line pairs, one line and its interspace require at least two pixels.

Contrast Resolution

The ability to distinguish one soft tissue from another without regard for size or shape is called **contrast resolution**. This is an area in which multislice helical CT excels.

The absorption of x-rays in tissue is characterized by the x-ray linear attenuation coefficient. This coefficient, as we have seen, is a function of x-ray energy and the atomic number of the tissue. In CT, absorption of x-rays by the patient is determined also by the mass density of the body part.

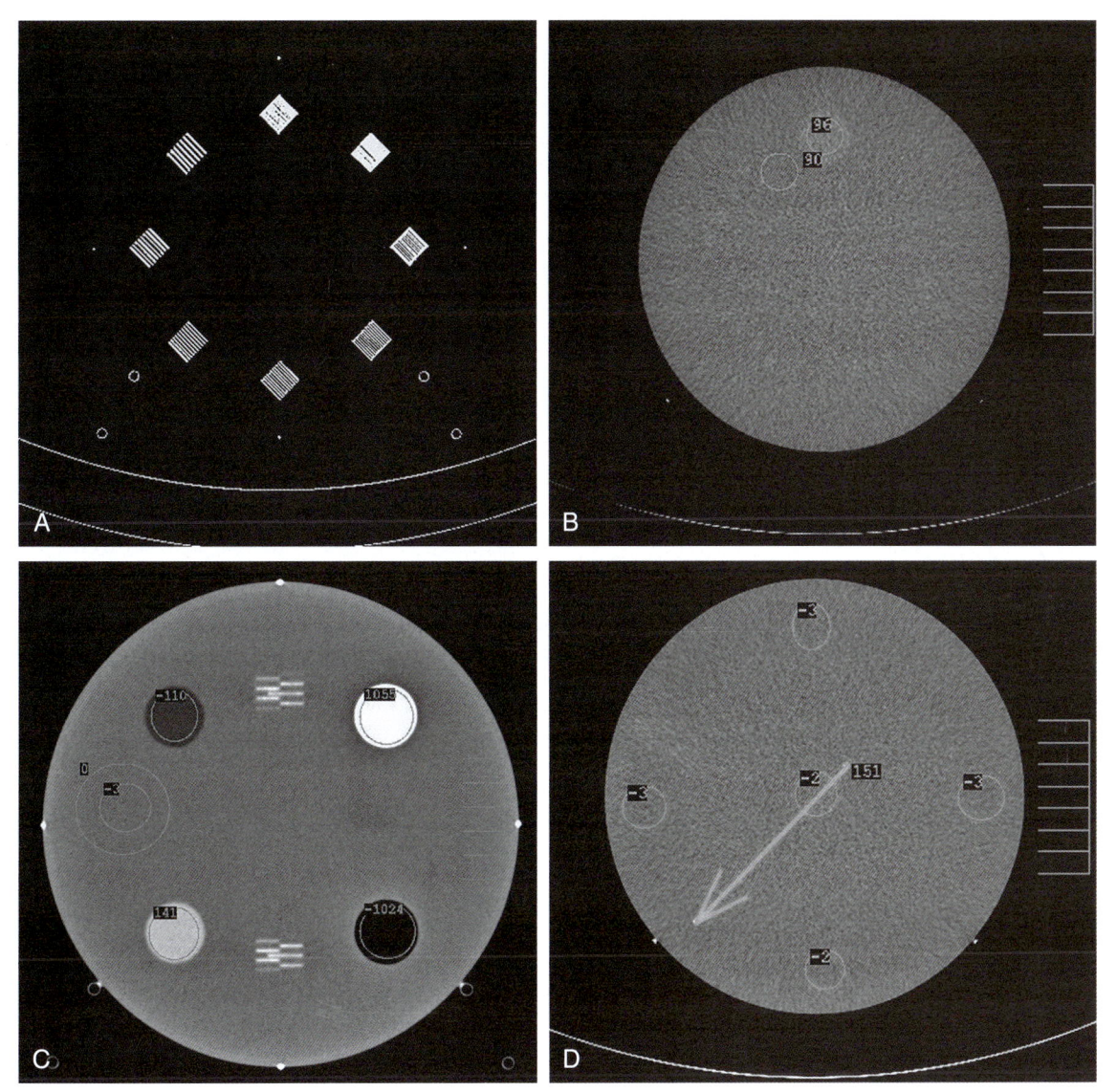

FIG. 21.35 The phantom for evaluating computed tomography image quality contains test objects designed to measure spatial resolution (A), contrast resolution (B), linearity (C), and other image-quality factors (D). (Courtesy Priscilla Butler, American College of Radiology.)

Consider the situation outlined in Fig. 21.36, a fat-muscle-bone structure. Not only are the atomic numbers somewhat different (Z = 6.8, 7.4, and 13.8, respectively), but the mass densities are also different (ρ = 0.91, 1.0, and 1.85 g/cm^3, respectively). Although these differences are measurable, they are not imaged well radiographically, principally because an area x-ray beam is used in radiography.

The CT imaging system is able to amplify these differences in subject contrast so the image contrast is high. The range of CT numbers for these tissues is approximately −100, 50, and 1000, respectively. This amplified contrast scale allows CT to better resolve adjacent structures that are similar in composition.

> Contrast resolution is superior in CT principally because of x-ray beam collimation and postprocessing.

The contrast resolution provided by CT is considerably better than that available in radiography principally because of the scatter radiation rejection of the prepatient and predetector collimators. The ability to image low-contrast objects with CT is limited by the size and uniformity of the object and by the noise of the system.

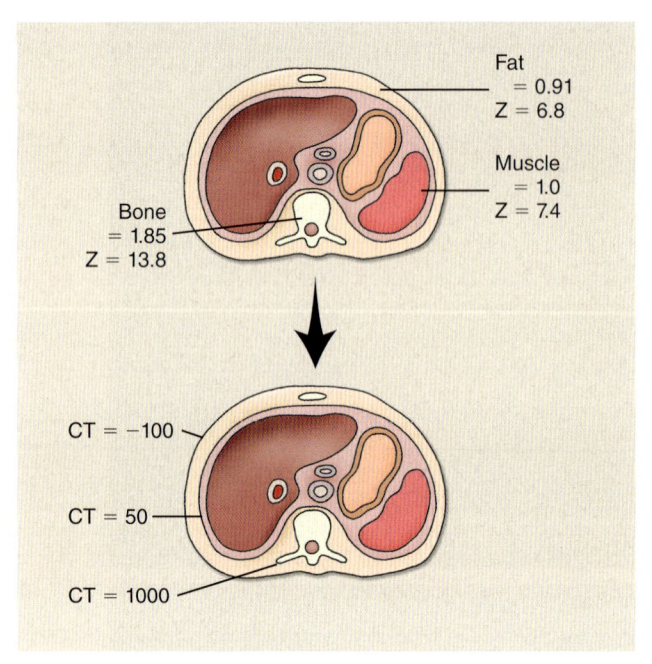

FIG. 21.36 No large differences are noted in mass density and effective atomic number among tissues, but the differences are greatly amplified by computed tomography imaging.

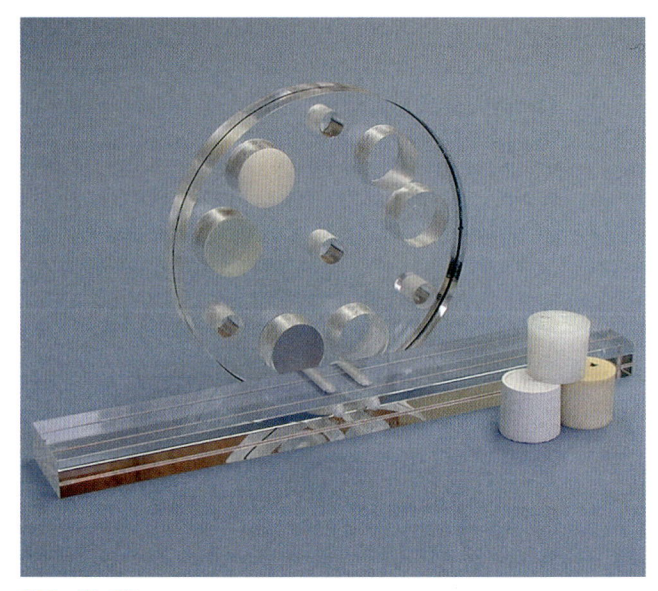

FIG. 21.37 A version of the five-pin test object designed by the American Association of Physicists in Medicine. The attenuation coefficient for each pin is known precisely, and the computed tomography number is computed. (Courtesy Cardinal Health.)

Noise

If a homogeneous medium such as water is imaged, each pixel should have a value of zero. Of course, this never occurs because the contrast resolution of the system is not perfect; therefore the CT numbers may average zero, but a range of values greater than or less than zero exists.

This variation in CT numbers above or below the average value is the **noise** of the system. If all pixel values were equal, the noise would be zero.

> A large variation of pixel values represents high image noise.

Noise is the percent standard deviation of a large number of pixels obtained from a water image. It should be clearly understood that noise depends on many factors:
- kVp and filtration
- Pixel size
- Slice thickness
- Detector efficiency
- Patient radiation dose

Ultimately, the patient radiation dose and the number of x-rays used by the detector to produce the image control noise.

> $$\text{Noise }(\sigma) = \sqrt{\frac{\Sigma(x_i - \bar{x})^2}{n-1}}$$
> where x_i is each CT number, $\bar{x}$ is the average of at least 100 number, and n is the number of CT numbers averaged.

In statistics, noise is called a **standard deviation** and is symbolized by σ.

Noise appears on the image as graininess. Low-noise images appear very smooth to the eye, and high-noise images appear spotty or blotchy.

> The resolution of low-contrast objects is limited by the noise of a CT imaging system.

Noise should be evaluated daily through imaging of a 20-cm-diameter water test object. All CT imaging systems have the ability to identify an ROI on the digital image and to compute the mean and standard deviation of the CT numbers in that ROI. When the CT technologist measures noise, the ROI must encompass at least 100 pixels. Such noise measurements should include five determinations—four on the periphery and one in the center.

Linearity

CT imaging systems must be calibrated frequently so that water is consistently represented by CT number zero and other tissues by the appropriate CT numbers. A check calibration that can be made daily uses the five-pin performance test object of the American Association of Physicists in Medicine (AAPM) (Fig. 21.37). Each of

TABLE 21.4 Characteristics of the Five-Pin American College of Radiology Accreditation Phantom

Material		Mass Density (g/cm³)	Linear Attenuation Coefficient (cm⁻¹) at 60 keV	Computed Tomography Number
Polyethylene	C_2H_4	0.94	0.185	−85
Polystyrene	C_8H_8	1.05	0.196	−85
Nylon	$C_6H_{11}NO$	1.15	0.222	100
Lexan	$C_{16}H_{14}O$	1.20	0.223	115
Plexiglas	$C_5H_8O_2$	1.19	0.229	130
Water	H_2O	1.00	0.206	0

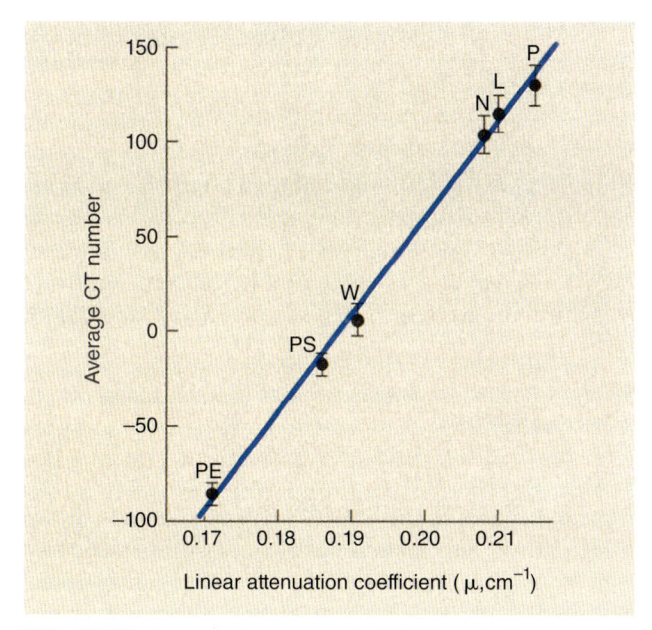

FIG. 21.38 Computed tomography (*CT*) linearity is acceptable if a graph of average CT number versus the linear attenuation coefficient is a straight line that passes through 0 for water.

> The CT value for water may drift from day to day or even from hour to hour.

At any time that water is imaged, the pixel values should be constant in all regions of the reconstructed image. Such a characteristic is called **spatial uniformity**.

Spatial uniformity can be tested easily with an internal software package that allows the plotting of CT numbers along any axis of the image as a histogram or as a line graph. If all values of the histogram or line graph are within two standard deviations of the mean value (±2σ), the system is said to exhibit acceptable spatial uniformity.

X-ray beam hardening may cause a decrease in CT numbers so that the middle of the image appears darker than the periphery. This is the "cupping" artifact, and it can be clearly demonstrated by imaging the water bath inside a Teflon ring to simulate bone.

IMAGING TECHNIQUE

Multislice Detector Array

Multislice helical CT imaging systems have two principal distinguishing features. First, instead of a detector array, multislice helical CT requires several parallel detector arrays that contain thousands of individual detectors (see Fig. 21.20). Second, quickly energizing such a large detector array for large-volume imaging requires a very fast large-capacity computer.

After the initial demonstration of dual-slice imaging in the early 1990s, the number of detector arrays has steadily increased to 320 image slices simultaneously that are now available.

A simple approach to multislice helical CT imaging is the use of four detector arrays, each of equal width. This design is shown in Fig. 21.39 with a beam pitch of 2.0:1—the x-ray beam width is half the patient couch movement. The width of each detector array is 0.5 mm, resulting in four slices, each of 0.5-mm width.

the five pins is made of a different plastic material that has known physical and x-ray attenuation properties and is positioned in water (Table 21.4).

After this test object is imaged, the CT number for each pin should be recorded and its mean value and standard deviation plotted (Fig. 21.38). The plot of CT number versus linear attenuation coefficient should be a straight line that passes through CT number 0 for water.

Uniformity

When a uniform object such as water is imaged, each pixel should have the same value because each pixel represents precisely the same object. Furthermore, if the CT imaging system is properly adjusted, that value should be zero. Because the CT imaging system is an extremely complicated electronic mechanical device, however, such precision is not consistently possible.

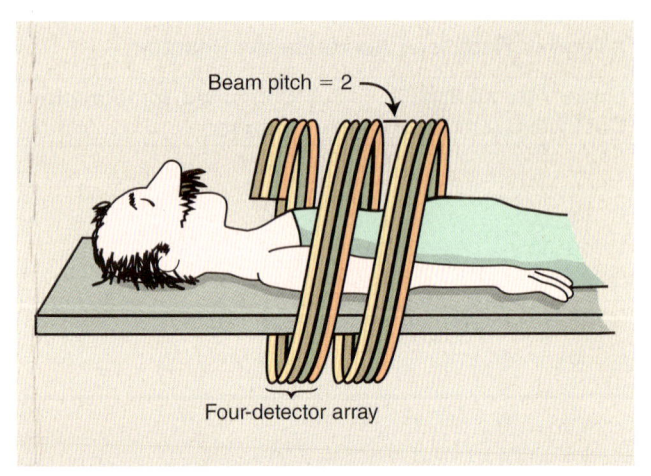

FIG. 21.39 A four-slice helical computed tomography (CT) scan with a pitch of 2.0 covers eight times the tissue volume of single-slice helical CT.

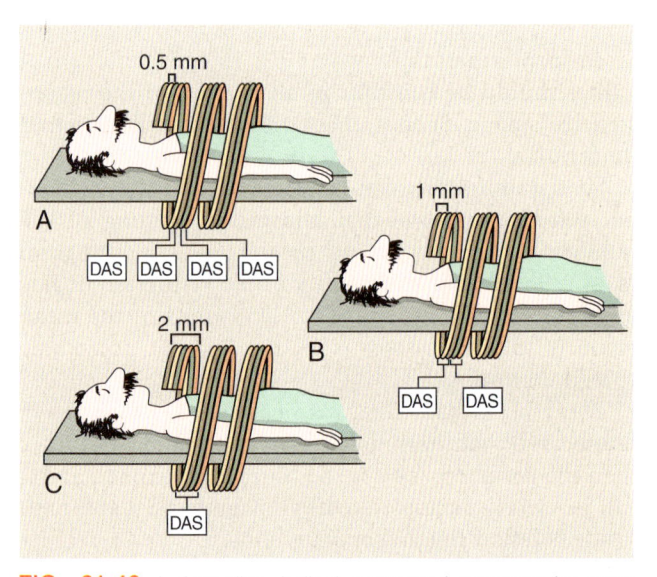

FIG. 21.40 A four-slice helical computed tomography scan allows changes to be made in slice thickness. (A) Four slices of 0.5 mm each. (B) Two 0.5-mm slices can be combined to make two 1-mm slices. (C) Four 0.5-mm slices can be combined to make one 2-mm slice. *DAS*, Data acquisition system.

The design of such a multislice CT imaging system usually allows detected signals from adjacent arrays to be combined to produce two slices of 1 mm width or one slice of 2 mm width (Fig. 21.40). Wider slice imaging results in better contrast resolution at the same mA setting because the detected signal is higher.

> Wider multislices allow imaging of greater tissue volume.

This improvement in contrast resolution is accompanied by a slight reduction in spatial resolution because of increased voxel size. Alternatively a larger tissue volume can be imaged with original contrast resolution at a reduced mA setting.

This discussion of multislice helical CT has used four slices for simplicity as an example. In fact, multislice helical CT progressed to 320 slices in a very short time.

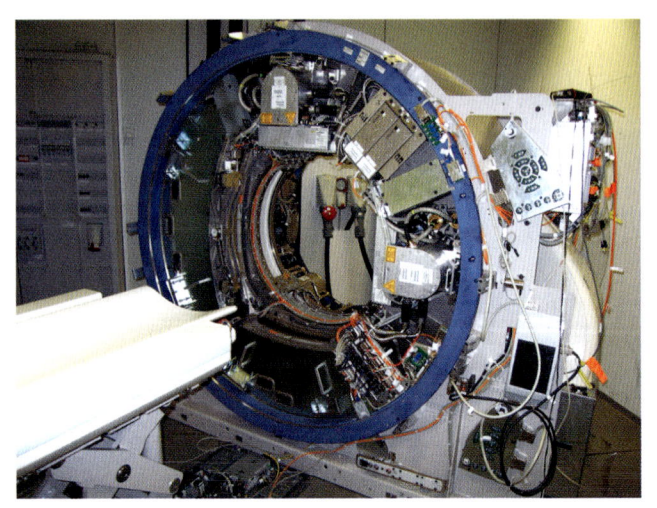

FIG. 21.41 A dual-source multislice helical computed tomography imaging system. (Courtesy of Siemens Medical Solutions USA, Inc.)

> Smaller detector size results in better spatial resolution.

A dual-source multislice CT imaging system is shown in Fig. 21.41. This system has two x-ray tubes and two detector arrays mounted on the revolving gantry. Imaging speed is its principal advantage; 80-ms imaging is possible.

Data Acquisition Rate

Multislice helical CT results in acquisition of multiple slices in the same time previously required for a single slice. The slice acquisition rate (SAR) is one measure of the efficiency of the multislice helical CT imaging system.

$$SAR = (\text{Slices acquired per 360 degrees/Rotation time})$$
$$= (64/0.5) = 128$$

Question: A 64-slice multidetector array is used for 0.5-s multislice imaging. What is the SAR?

Answer: SAR = Slices acquired per 360 degrees
SAR = 64/0.5 = 128

The principal advantage of multislice helical CT is that a larger volume of tissue can be imaged. At the limit, it is now possible to image the entire body—from head to toe—in a single breath-hold. Although a volume of tissue is being imaged, this volume is represented by z-axis coverage as follows:

> Z-axis coverage = SAR × W × T × B
>
> where SAR is the slice acquisition rate, W is the slice width, T is the imaging time, and B is the pitch.

Question: A 64-slice examination is performed with a 32-mm x-ray beam width and a 20-s examination at 0.5 s per revolution. What z-axis coverage is obtained? The patient couch translates 32 mm each revolution.

Answer: Z = (N/R) × W × T × B, where N = 64, R = 0.5 s, W = 0.5 mm (64 ÷ 32 = 0.5 mm), T = 20 s, and B = 1.0.
Z = (64/0.5) × 0.5 × 20 × 1 = 1280 mm = 128 cm

The advantages and limitations of multislice helical CT are summarized in Table 21.5.

Photon Counting

In 2021 the USFDA approved the first photon counting CT (PCCT) for clinical use. The principal advantage to this approach is to improve further the contrast resolution of the CT imaging system. PCCT is one way of detecting and identifying the energy of each individual x-ray photon and assigning it to a bin in the x-ray energy spectrum. This is much the same way that gamma rays have been handled for years in nuclear medicine.

By measuring individual x-ray energy, those that are Compton scattered are removed. Those that contribute only electrostatic noise are also removed from the image-forming data bank. This results in improved signal-to-noise ratio and contrast-to-noise ratio and an increase the contrast resolution of the imaging system. At the same time, this results in lower patient radiation dose.

PCCT basically allows determination of the composition of tissue in each voxel. Previously the voxel represented linear attenuation coefficient as measured by the CT number.

Another potential advantage to PCCT is the ability to remove artifacts. With PCCT, the need for a reference image before the injection of contrast medium is unnecessary. Because of the increased contrast resolution, less contrast medium is required while at the same time patient radiation dose is reduced. PCCT has shown great application in computed tomography angiography (CTA).

With the help of the rapidly advancing artificial intelligence and the upcoming quantum computing (see Chapter 28), PCCT should become the next-generation CT scanning modality.

COMPUTED TOMOGRAPHY QUALITY CONTROL

Computed tomography imaging systems are subject to all the misalignment, miscalibration, and malfunction difficulties of radiographic and fluoroscopic x-ray imaging systems. They have the additional complexities of the multimotional gantry, the interactive console, and the associated computers.

Each of these subsystems increases the risk of drift and instability, which could result in degradation of image quality. Consequently, a dedicated quality control (QC) program is essential for each CT imaging system. Such a program includes daily, weekly, monthly, and

TABLE 21.5 Features of Multislice Helical Computed Tomography

	What	How and Why
Advantages	No motion artifacts	Removes respiratory misregistration
	Improved lesion detection	Reconstructs at arbitrary z-axis intervals
	Reduced partial volume	Reconstructs at overlapping z-axis intervals
		Reconstructs smaller than image interval
	Optimized intravenous contrast	Data obtained during peak of enhancement
		Reduces volume of contrast agent
	Multiplanar images	Higher-quality reconstruction
	Improved patient throughput	Reduces imaging time
Limitations	Increased image noise	Bigger x-ray tubes needed
	Reduced z-axis resolution	Increases with pitch
	Increased processing time	More data and more images needed

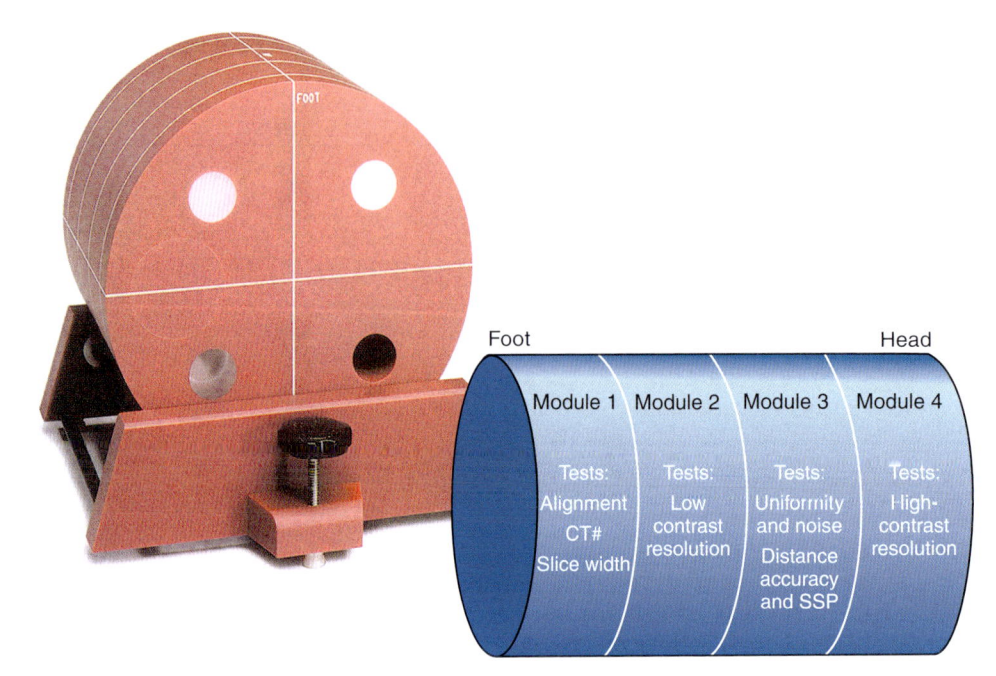

FIG. 21.42 This computed tomography (*CT*) test object is used to evaluate noise, spatial resolution, contrast resolution, slice thickness, linearity, and uniformity. *SSP*, Section sensitivity profile. (Courtesy Priscilla Butler, American College of Radiology.)

annual monitoring in addition to an ongoing preventive maintenance program.

Fig. 21.42 shows a popular test object for CT measurements—the ACR CT accreditation phantom. The measurements specified for an annual performance also should be conducted for all new equipment and for all existing equipment after replacement or repair of a major component.

Noise and Uniformity

A 20-cm water test object should be imaged weekly; the average value for water should be within ±10 CT numbers of zero. Furthermore uniformity across the image should not vary by more than ±10 CT numbers from the center to the periphery.

Nearly all CT imaging systems easily meet these performance specifications. If a system is used for quantitative CT, however, tighter specifications may be appropriate. When this assessment is performed, one should change one or more of the following: CT scan parameters, slice thickness, reconstruction diameter, or reconstruction algorithm.

Linearity

Linearity is assessed with an image of the AAPM five-pin insert. Analysis of the values of the five pins should show a linear relationship between the CT number and electron density. The coefficient of correlation for this linear relationship should be at least 0.96%, or two standard deviations.

This assessment should be conducted semiannually. It is particularly important for systems used for quantitative CT, which requires precise determination of the value of tissue in CT numbers.

Spatial Resolution

Monitoring of spatial resolution is the most important component of this QC program. Constant spatial resolution ensures proper performance of the detector array, reconstruction electronics, and the mechanical components.

> Spatial resolution is assessed by imaging a wire or an edge to obtain the edge response function.

The edge response function (ERF) is then mathematically transformed to obtain the MTF. However, determining the MTF requires considerable time and attention. Most medical physicists find it acceptable to image a bar pattern or a hole pattern. Spatial resolution should be assessed semiannually and should be within the manufacturer's specifications.

Contrast Resolution

CT excels as an imaging modality because of its superior contrast resolution. The performance specifications of the various CT imaging systems differ from one manufacturer to another and from one model to another, depending on the design of the imaging system.

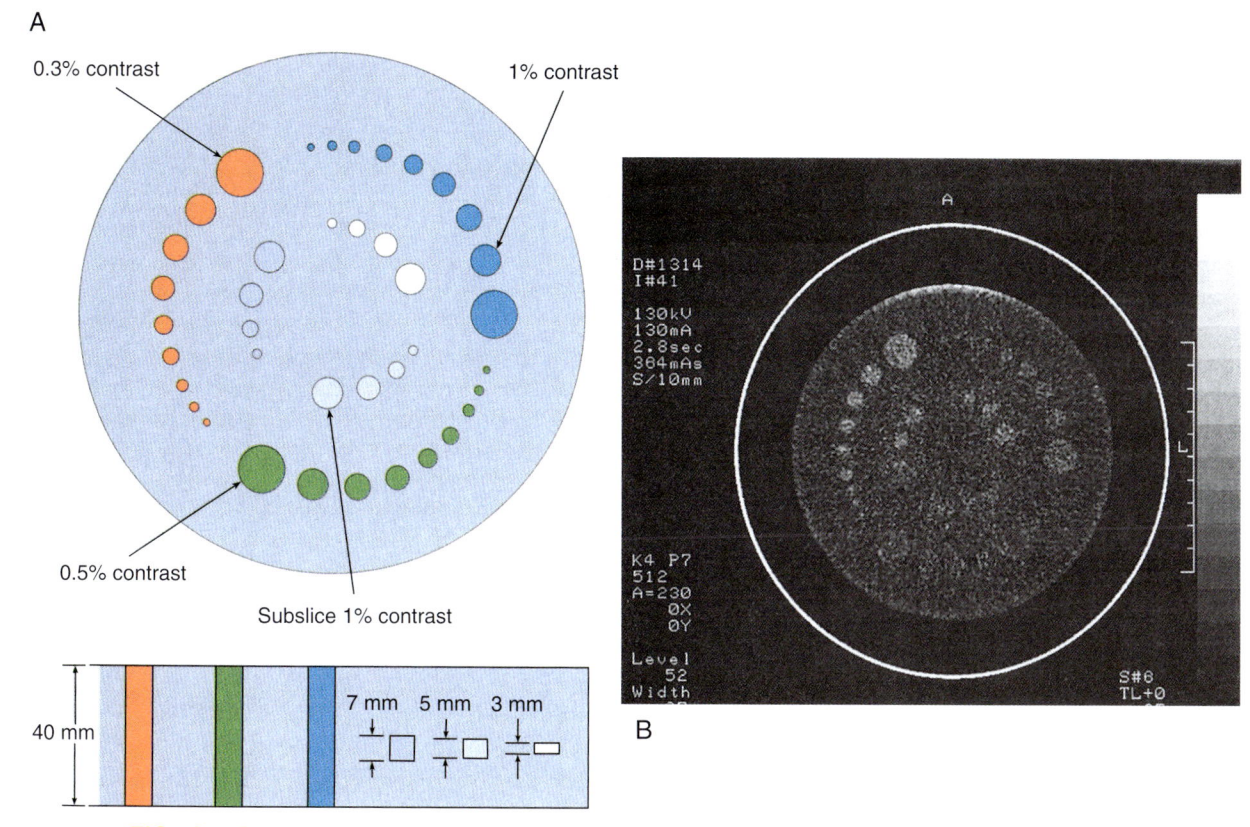

FIG. 21.43 Schematic drawing (A) of a low-contrast computed tomograpghy (CT) test object and (B) its image. This test object is designed especially for multislice helical CT. (Courtesy Josh Levy, Phantom Laboratory.)

> All CT imaging systems should be capable of resolving 5-mm objects at 0.5% contrast.

Contrast resolution should be assessed semiannually. This is done with any of a number of low-contrast test objects with the built-in analytic schemes that are available on all CT imaging systems (Fig. 21.43).

Slice Thickness

Slice thickness (sensitivity profile) is measured with the use of a specially designed test object that incorporates a ramp, a spiral, or a step wedge. This assessment should be done semiannually; the slice thickness should be within 1 mm of the intended slice thickness for a thickness of 5 mm or greater. For an intended slice thickness of less than 5 mm, the acceptable tolerance is 0.5 mm.

Couch Incrementation

With automatic maneuvering of the patient through the CT gantry, the patient must be precisely positioned. This evaluation should be done monthly. During a clinical examination with a patient-loaded couch, note the position of the couch at the beginning and at the end of the examination with the use of a tape measure and a straightedge on the couch rails. Compare this with the intended couch movement. It should be within ±2 mm.

Laser Localizer

Most CT imaging systems have internal and/or external laser-localizing lights for patient positioning. The accuracy of these lasers can be determined with any number of specially designed test objects. Their accuracy should be assessed at least semiannually; this is usually done at the same time as the evaluation of couch incrementation.

SUMMARY

The multislice helical CT imaging system does not record an image, as in radiography or fluoroscopy. The collimated x-ray beam is directed to the patient; the attenuated image-forming x-ray beam is measured by a detector array; the signal from the detector array is analyzed by a computer; the image is reconstructed in the computer; and, finally, the image is interpreted on a digital display device.

Multislice helical CT acquires transverse images, which are sections of anatomy that are perpendicular to the long axis of the body. The resultant computer image is an electronic matrix of intensities. The matrix size is usually 512 × 512 pixels. Each pixel contains numeric information called a CT number. The pixel is a two-dimensional representation of a corresponding tissue volume or voxel.

Contrast resolution of the CT imaging system is excellent because of scatter radiation rejection resulting from x-ray beam collimation. The ability to image low-contrast anatomy is limited by the noise of the system. System noise is determined by the number of x-rays used by the detector array to produce the image.

Multislice helical CT offers the following advantages over earlier step-and-shoot CT. When the examination begins, the x-ray tube rotates continuously, and the patient couch moves through the plane of the rotating beam. The data collected are reconstructed at any desired z-axis position by interpolation.

Pitch is the ratio of patient couch movement to x-ray beam width. Increasing the pitch to above 1:1 increases the volume of tissue that can be imaged, and at a reduced patient radiation dose.

The volume of tissue imaged is determined by examination time, couch travel, pitch, and beam width. Improvement in z-axis spatial resolution is noted with helical CT because no gaps in data are apparent, and reconstruction images can even overlap.

CHALLENGE QUESTIONS

1. Define or otherwise identify the following:
   a. Algorithm
   b. Transverse image
   c. Projection
   d. Interpolation
   e. Pixel
   f. Spatial frequency
   g. CT number
   h. Slip ring
   i. MTF
   j. PCCT
2. Name the individual who, in 1970, first demonstrated CT.
3. Explain the phrase "linear interpolation at 180 degrees."
4. What are the components in the gantry portion of the multislice helical CT imaging system?
5. What are the special requirements of the x-ray tube as used in multislice helical CT imaging?
6. Write the formula for the multislice helical CT pitch.
7. What is the volume of tissue imaged with beam width thickness of 10 mm, scan time of 30 s, and pitch of 1.6:1?
8. Describe the two collimators used in CT imaging.
9. What material makes up the patient support couch?
10. Explain how slip-ring technology contributed to the development of helical CT.
11. What is the voxel size of a CT imaging system with a 320 × 320 matrix size, a 20-cm reconstruction diameter, and a 0.5-cm slice thickness?
12. The volume of tissue imaged during helical CT is determined by which technique selections?
13. What generation CT currently prevails with what principal features?
14. Explain the mathematics of the multislice helical CT image reconstruction process.
15. What type of high-voltage generator is used for multislice helical CT?
16. A multislice helical CT imaging system can resolve a 0.65-mm high-contrast object. What spatial frequency does this represent?
17. A 10-s multislice helical CT examination is conducted with a 1.5:1 pitch and 5-mm beam width. How much tissue is imaged?
18. Why is multislice helical CT pitch greater than 2:1 rarely used?
19. What determines in-plane spatial resolution?
20. What does the CT linearity describe?

The answers to the Challenge Questions can be found by logging on to our website at http://evolve.elsevier.com.

Tomosynthesis

CHAPTER 22

OBJECTIVES

At the completion of this chapter, the student should be able to do the following:

1. Describe the various x-ray tube and image receptor movements during digital radiographic tomosynthesis.
2. Identify the several image reconstruction algorithms available for digital radiographic tomosynthesis.
3. Recognize some image artifacts associated with digital radiographic tomosynthesis.
4. Relate quality control measures for digital radiographic tomosynthesis.
5. Understand how application of digital radiographic tomosynthesis in clinical areas can result in reduced patient radiation dose.

OUTLINE

Digital Radiographic Tomosynthesis 332
X-ray Source 333
   X-ray Tube Motion 333
   Sweep Angle 334
   Projections 334
Image Receptors 334
Image Reconstruction 334
Artifacts 335
Quality Control 336
Patient Radiation Dose 336
   Breast 337
   Chest 339
   Emergency Department 339
Summary 340
Challenge Questions 340

IN THE EARLY 1930s, about the time that the rotating anode x-ray tube began to appear, an understanding of the importance of contrast resolution entered the discussion. By that time, spatial resolution had been well described. Spatial resolution was viewed as principally geometric—focal spot size, source-to-object distance, and source-to-image receptor distance.

It had been only a decade since Compton scattering was discovered and the need for radiographic grids became apparent. The concept of tomography emerged, and radiographic tomography was demonstrated by several radiographers. The principal investigators in those early days were radiographers.

Tomography was the inspiration for computed tomography (CT) in the 1970s. CT was the first demonstration of a digital medical image. Digital radiography appeared at the turn of the 21st century and resulted in the rapid disappearance of screen/film as an image receptor. Digital image receptors made possible digital radiographic tomosynthesis (DRT) or simply tomosynthesis. The introduction of CT buried radiographic tomography because the contrast resolution of CT was superior to any previous imaging modality.

The principal advantage of tomography, which developed first with screen-film image receptors in the 1920s, followed in this century with digital radiographic image receptors, as shown in Fig. 22.1, is better image contrast. The joined movement of the x-ray tube and screen/film image receptor blurred tissue on either side of the plane of the fulcrum (Fig. 22.2).

Some described the blurring of tissue out of the fulcrum plane as bringing the tissue in the plane of the fulcrum "into focus." There was no focusing at all, but the procedure did improve the image contrast of tissue in the fulcrum plane. Tomography increased image contrast, but normally, several tissue sections were imaged, and this required additional patient positioning time and much increased patient radiation dose.

DIGITAL RADIOGRAPHIC TOMOSYNTHESIS

Tomosynthesis, like so many medical terms, has its roots in Greek. *Tomos*, in Greek, means "slice, a cutting, or a section." *Synthesis* means "a process" or "the combination of ideas to form a theory or system." The first DRT appeared in digital mammography as digital breast tomosynthesis (DBT). DBT is currently fundamental for screening mammography and diagnostic mammography. DRT is set to replace much of CT as the imaging modality of choice for many patient conditions.

> The main image characteristic to DRT is improved image contrast.

One reason for change is cost. A DRT imaging system is only a little more expensive than a radiographic imaging system. More importantly, in addition to considerably less cost, DRT results in much lower patient radiation dose than CT.

The following discussion of DRT applies equally to DBT, which will be engaged more fully later. It is early

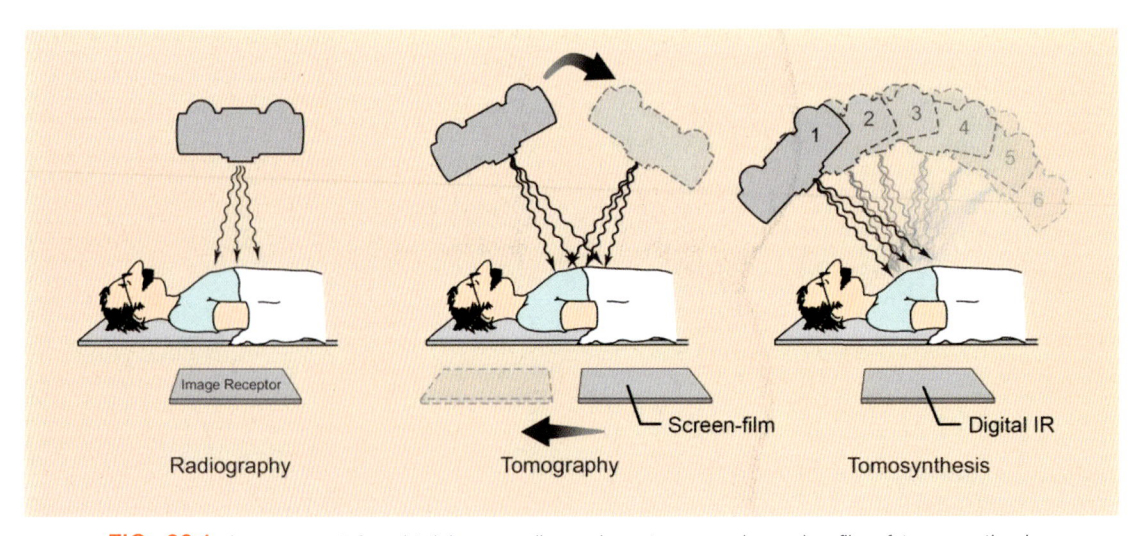

FIG. 22.1 Arrangement for obtaining a radiograph, a tomograph, and a file of tomosynthesis images.

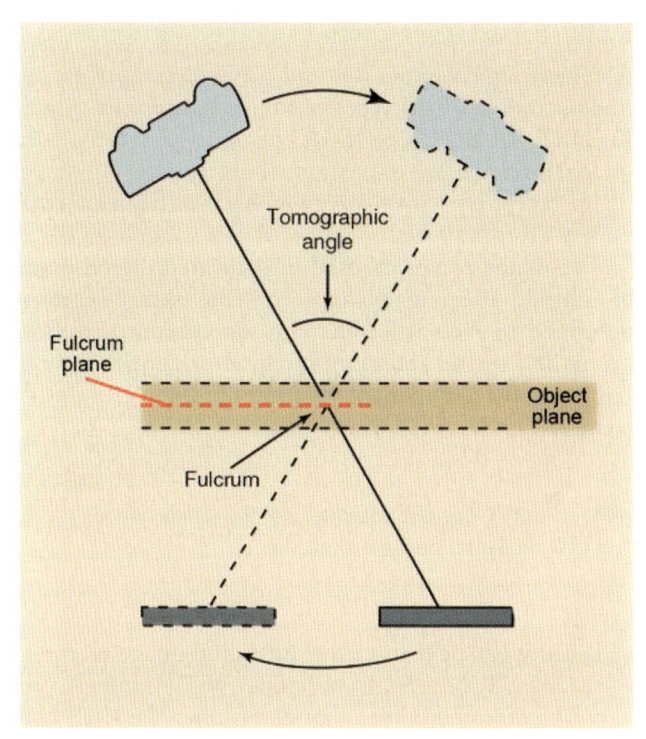

FIG. 22.2 Relationship of the x-ray tube travel, the fulcrum plane, and the movement of the image receptor during tomography.

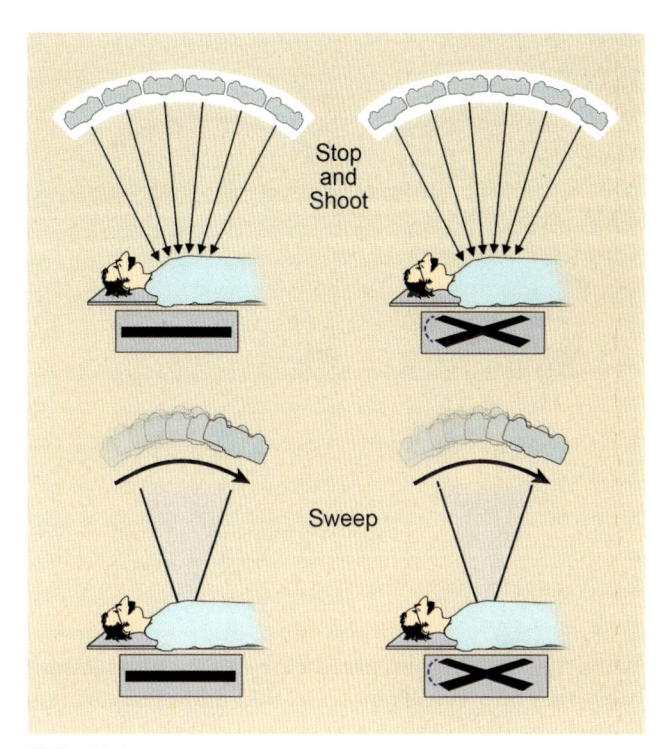

FIG. 22.3 Two approaches to x-ray tube movement and image receptor movement during digital radiographic tomosynthesis.

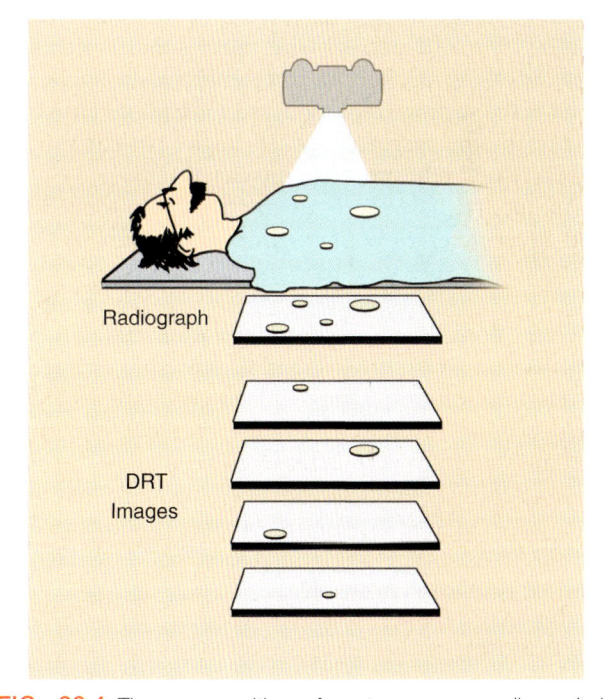

FIG. 22.4 The superposition of anatomy on a radiograph is removed with digital radiographic tomosynthesis (*DRT*).

in the clinical application of DRT, so we should anticipate rapid changes in vendor development. One change is for sure—rapid, increasing clinical application. The image acquisition parameters important to understand are x-ray tube motion, sweep angle, and number of projections.

X-RAY SOURCE

Any x-ray tube engaged for DRT must be robust. All are tungsten (W) anode with various thicknesses of aluminum (Al) filtration. All are rotating anode x-ray tubes with high heat capacity. The x-ray tube may be energized up to approximately 20 seconds, thus requiring heat capacity to 500,000 heat units or more.

X-ray Tube Motion

There are two approaches to the motion of the x-ray tube during DRT (Fig. 22.3). Some systems will drive the x-ray tube in a **continuous** sweep ranging from ±5 to ±25 degrees. The other approach is to interrupt the arc sweep in a **stop-and-shoot** fashion. Note that during either approach, the image receptor will either remain fixed or change angle position so that it is always perpendicular to the central x-ray.

When the stop-and-shoot technique is used, additional measures may be necessary to avoid motion blur. One such approach is to pulse the x-ray tube with a short, 100-ms pulse width.

> Continuous sweep and stop-and-shoot are the two methods to produce a DRT image.

The principal advantage to DRT is to reduce or eliminate tissue superimposition, as shown in Fig. 22.4.

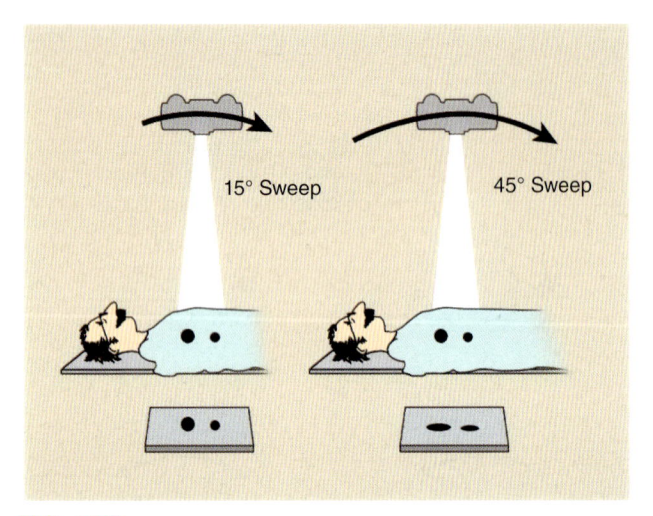

FIG. 22.5 A large sweep angle results in reduced spatial resolution and contrast resolution; both resolutions, however, are better than digital radiography.

When multiple areas of interest are imaged radiographically, they are superimposed. DRT allows separation of such areas, resulting in increased image contrast of each area.

Sweep Angle

The sweep angle design for DRT ranges from approximately 10 to 50 degrees and, with some systems, is selectable (Fig. 22.5). The larger the sweep angle, the better is the section resolution and separation. However, because of the increased sweep angle, patient motion and increased blur must be considered.

An important sweep angle metric is scan time. Short scan time increases patient throughput. Perhaps more importantly, short scan time minimizes patient motion blur.

When considering section resolution, think about out-of-section resolution (spatial and contrast) versus in-section resolution. Using wide sweep angle improves out-of-section resolution. There is a reduction of in-section resolution with increasing sweep angle.

An additional characteristic of sweep angle that must be considered for in-plane resolution is illustrated in Fig. 22.5. As sweep angle increases, both spatial and contrast resolution are worse.

Projections

The number of data projections that are sampled has a significant impact on any DRT examination. This characteristic is usually expressed as projections sampled per degree sweep angle. More projections will usually lead to better image quality.

Too few projections will result in undersampling and can lead to image reconstruction artifacts. Too many projections divide a fixed total image receptor radiation dose. That results in a low dose per projection and possible increased image noise.

IMAGE RECEPTORS

A review of Chapters 11 and 12 will reinforce your understanding of the types of image receptors available for DRT. All have been tried, but none has been settled on exclusively. An important characteristic of digital image receptors is pixel size, which varies from approximately 70 to 150 μm.

The image receptors used in dedicated digital mammographic imaging systems are the same as those described in the earlier chapters on computed radiography and digital radiography. Interestingly, the use of DRT is still accompanied by a radiographic grid during some DRT examinations.

> DRT was not possible until the digital image receptor became available.

It is not yet clear if one of the digital image receptors (i.e., CsI, GdOS, a-Se, BaFl halide) will ultimately prevail. The atomic number that determines the K-absorption edge energy and the capture element thickness both determine the detective quantum efficiency and therefore image receptor speed and patient radiation dose.

A generalization for projection radiography is that smaller is better. The smaller the pixel size, the better is the spatial resolution of the system. Unfortunately, smaller pixel size requires higher patient radiation dose. This pixel size association with spatial resolution and with patient radiation dose is not as important with DRT as it is with digital radiography.

IMAGE RECONSTRUCTION

A number of reconstruction algorithms are in use or under investigation for DRT. Filtered back projection and iterative reconstruction are methods developed for CT that have found a home in DRT. Other algorithms identified as algebraic reconstruction and maximum likelihood are also considered. With each of these reconstruction algorithms, section thickness and section separation as low as 1 mm are possible. Appropriate thickness and separation are determined principally by the body part that is being imaged.

Filtered back projection is a faster image reconstruction method than iterative reconstruction. The algorithms of iterative reconstruction allow a wider selection of image appearance. Filtered back projection is particularly useful for screening examinations because of the shorter reconstruction time.

> Computer-aided detection (CAD) is an early application of artificial intelligence (AI) in DRT.

TABLE 22.1	Characteristics of Clinical Digital Radiographic Tomosynthesis
Source-to-image receptor distance	60–100 cm
Source-to-center of rotation distance	60–100 cm
X-ray tube angular range	±5 to ±25 degrees
X-ray tube motion	Stop-and-shoot or continuous
Number of projections	9–25
Scan time	3–25 s
Detector pixel size	70–100 μm

DRT image reconstruction will be considerably impacted by the continuing advances of AI and quantum computing (see Chapter 28 and 29). CAD has already found its way into some DRT procedures. The transition to AI will be quick and will help radiologists be faster and more accurate during image interpretation. Table 22.1 shows some of the evolving characteristics of DRT.

ARTIFACTS

There are a number of image artifacts that are unique to DRT. You will need to recognize and understand these artifacts.

The **blurred-ripple** artifact (Fig. 22.6) occurs if too few projections are acquired. Blurred-ripple artifacts appear perpendicular to the x-ray tube sweep direction. Blurred-ripple artifacts are less noticeable with iterative reconstruction than with filtered back projection.

High-mass-density surgical clips or calcifications affect the blurred-ripple artifact by distance from the reconstructed image plane. The blurred-ripple artifact is seen perpendicular to the x-ray tube sweep direction. The tomosynthesis section containing the object will show no blurring. Sections close to the object plane will produce ripples equal in number to the number of projections.

Theoretically, blurred-ripple artifacts decrease with increasing number of projections. Blurred-ripple artifacts disappear when the number of projections equals the number of DRT sections reconstructed.

Truncation in mathematics is the discarding of the least significant digits to the right of the decimal point. Truncation artifacts in DRT deal with tissue that is not imaged because of the limited sweep angle. Examine Fig. 22.7 and notice the tissue not totally within the widest sweep angle. To truncate is to shorten or reduce. In physics, it means approximating an infinite sum with a finite number. Fig. 22.8 is an example of a truncation artifact.

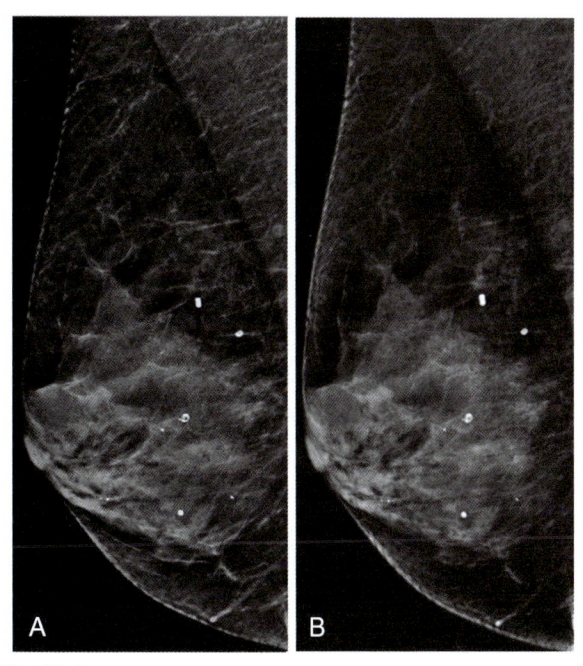

FIG. 22.6 Blurred-ripple artifact from a biopsy clip in the superior right breast seen on a synthesized 2D mammogram (A). This artifact is not present on a 2D full-field digital mammogram (B). (Courtesy Robert Edward Lynch, Baylor College of Medicine.)

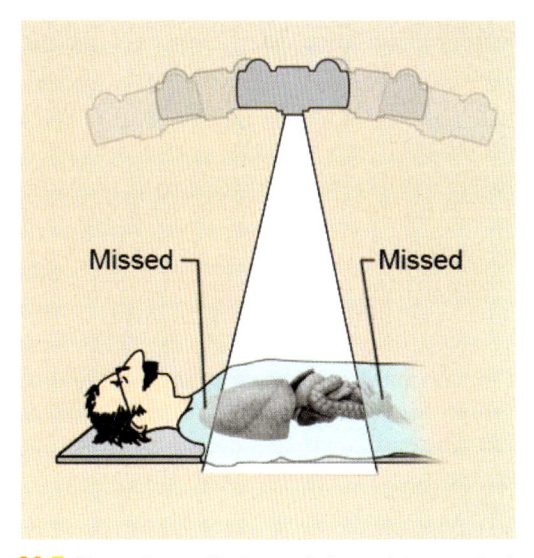

FIG. 22.7 Truncation artifacts result from data acquired at the extremes of x-ray tube sweep. The result is missed anatomy on some digital radiographic tomosynthesis image sections.

> DRT has its own artifacts—blurred ripple and truncation.

One type of artifact that is not exclusively associated with DRT is a motion artifact. Motion artifacts occur because of patient movement, large sweep angle, long exposure time, and poor positioning.

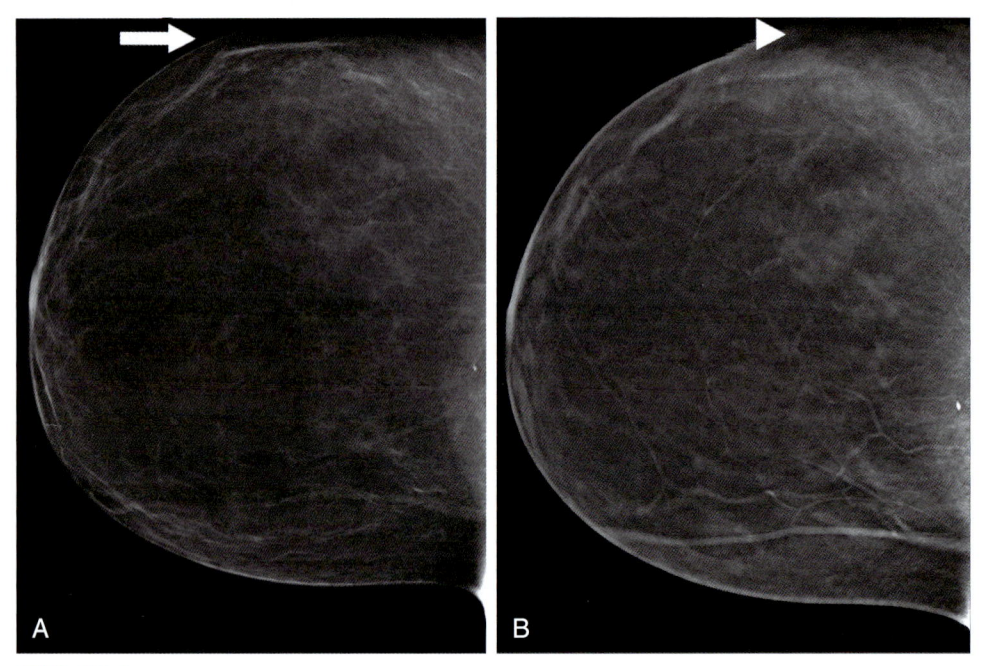

FIG. 22.8 Examples of truncation artifacts, which usually appear as a "stair-step" effect or a "bright-edge" effect on digital breast tomosynthesis images. (Courtesy Tamara Ortiz-Perez, Baylor College of Medicine.)

As with radiography, when there is a malfunction of a pixel or column or row of pixels, artifacts can appear. However, these are relatively easy to correct with postprocessing.

QUALITY CONTROL

Quality control (QC) in DRT is similar in many ways to that engaged for other imaging modalities. QC programs are designed to ensure optimal image quality that remains consistent over time.

The image characteristics of spatial resolution, contrast resolution, and artifacts must be a part of any QC program. The daily, weekly, and longer QC observations or tests must be tailored to the specific DRT imaging system.

Each imaging system vendor will suggest an appropriate QC program. Test objects like those shown in Fig. 22.9 and Fig. 22.10 can be easily used in any QC program. Any QC program must also have "as low as reasonably achievable" (ALARA) as its goal regarding patient radiation dose.

PATIENT RADIATION DOSE

We will visit patient radiation dose more completely during Chapter 41. For the time being, consider patient radiation dose from DRT to be the same as that from radiography. Depending on the sweep angle and time of sweep, it will likely be 10% to 20% higher, but for our purposes it may be considered equal.

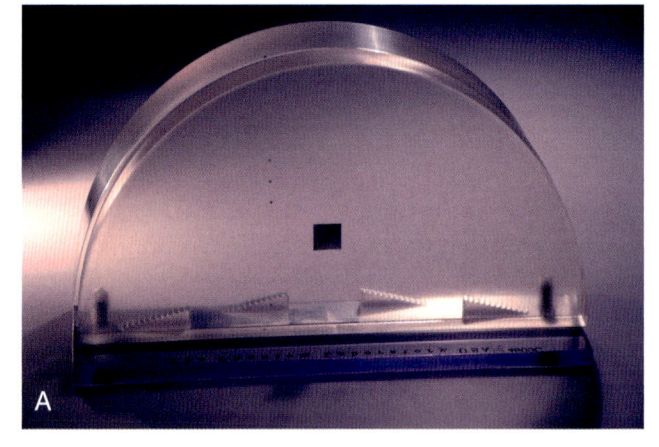

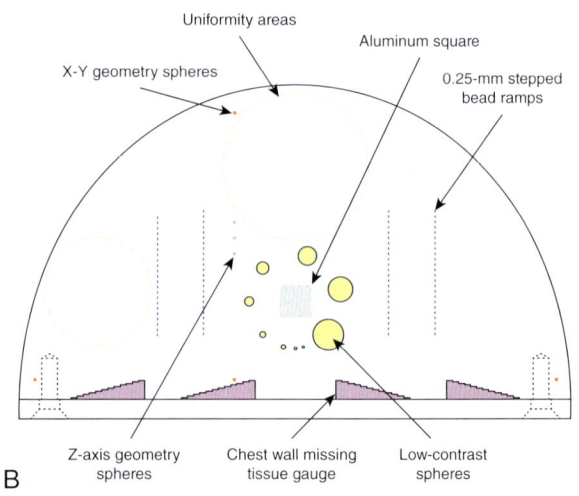

FIG. 22.9 Digital radiographic tomosynthesis quality control evaluation. (A) Test object. (B) Test object inserts. (Courtesy Megan Stalter, The Phantom Laboratory.)

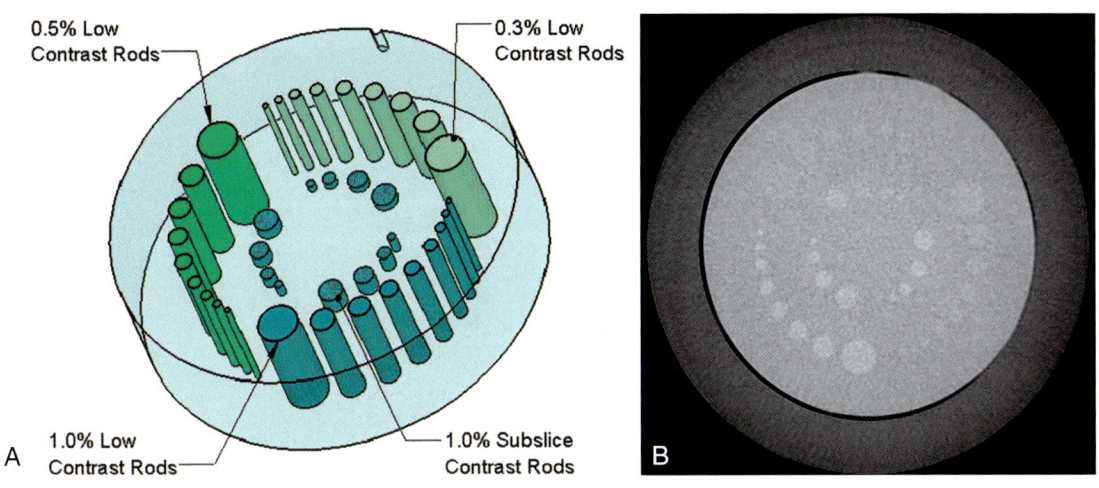

FIG. 22.10 A test object (A) and image (B) for evaluating spatial resolution and contrast resolution for several digital imaging modalities. (Courtesy Jonathan Gerdes, The Phantom Laboratory.)

It is likely that DRT will replace CT imaging for many clinical situations. That will result in a very large reduction in patient radiation dose. On the other hand, when DRT is the examination of choice over MRI, the patient radiation dose rises from zero to low.

If our experience with DRT is the same as our DBT experience, DRT could become a replacement for digital radiography. DBT has shown to result in fewer patient recalls and increased sensitivity in detecting disease compared with digital mammography. This is especially so when imaging a breast with high mass density.

Should DRT replace DRT plus radiography, we will see a significant patient radiation dose reduction. This will surely happen when DRT **synthesized radiography** replaces radiography. A synthesized radiographic image is produced by reformatting the DRT images into a single radiographic image without exposing the patient to x-radiation again.

Breast

When DRT was first introduced in 2011, it was added as a supplement to mammography. The application as DBT has been very successful, but application to other parts of the body is exploding. Let us review DBT first.

Mammography has received wide attention and success since the 1950s (see Chapter 18). Following establishment by the US Food and Drug Administration (US FDA) of the Mammography Quality Standards Act (MQSA) in 1994, any mammography equipment changes must be certified and approved by the US FDA.

Since the findings of the Digital Mammography Imaging Study Trial (DMIST) in 2006, the availability, complexity, and use of mammographic imaging systems has soared.

> Spatial resolution in digital mammography is limited by pixel size.

The DMIST was designed to compare the efficiency of digital mammography with that of screen/film mammography, with which we had 40 years of experience. The result was that digital mammography was equal to screen-film mammography for mature, fatty breasts, but it was superior when imaging younger, denser breasts.

> Digital mammography has superior contrast resolution principally because of postprocessing. DBT is even better.

The US FDA approved a Hologic imaging system in 2011 as the first DBT system. Many additional DBT systems have since been certified. The principal purpose of tomography and therefore DBT is to improve the contrast resolution of the imaging system and increase image contrast, as shown in Fig. 22.11.

> DMIST showed without question that contrast resolution is more important than spatial resolution for diagnostic efficacy.

It was the introduction of the digital image receptor that made DBT possible. It cannot be done with a screen-film image receptor.

Fig. 22.12 shows the relationships of x-ray source, breast, and image receptor that is used to produce a mammogram. Then, with the breast and image receptor fixed, additional images are obtained with various sweep angles of the x-ray tube.

Each of these additional images, including the first, are obtained at 10% or less of the normal mammography technique so that patient dose is approximately the same as a screening mammogram. Each view produces a digital image matrix.

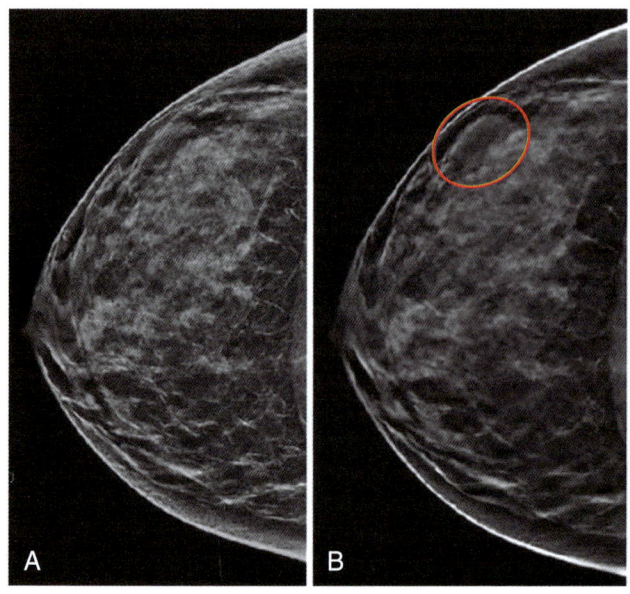

FIG. 22.11 The synthesized 2D mammogram (A) and digital breast tomosynthesis (DBT) (B) illustrate the improved image contrast with DBT. The DBT image better demonstrates an oval mass in the outer right breast at an anterior depth *(red circle)*. (Courtesy Robert Edward Lynch, Baylor College of Medicine.)

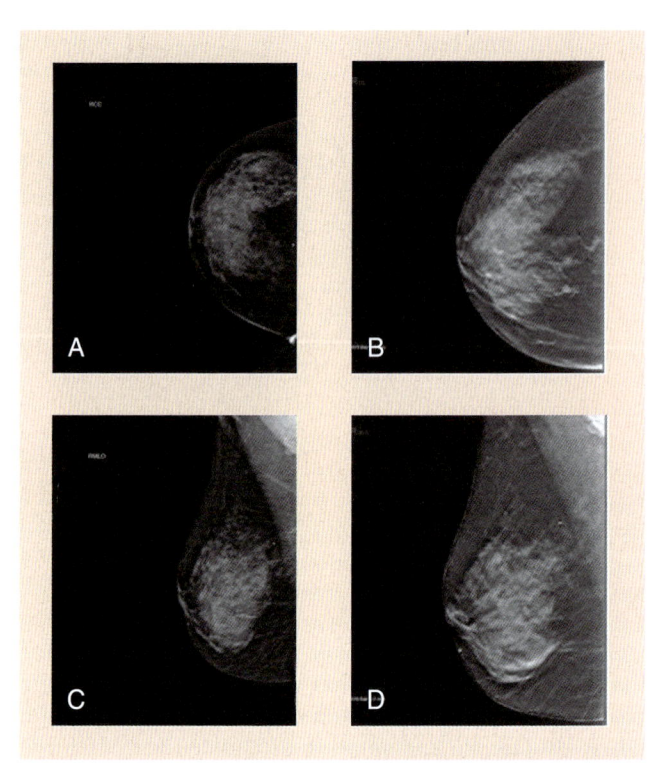

FIG. 22.13 Three axis reconstructed images showing improved image contrast resolution when performing digital breast tomosynthesis (same patient). (A) and (C), Diagnostic images. (B) and (D), Tomosynthesis images showing architectural distortion in the right upper outer quadrant suspicious for malignancy. (Courtesy Elizabeth Shields, Presbyterian Medical Center, Charlotte, North Carolina.)

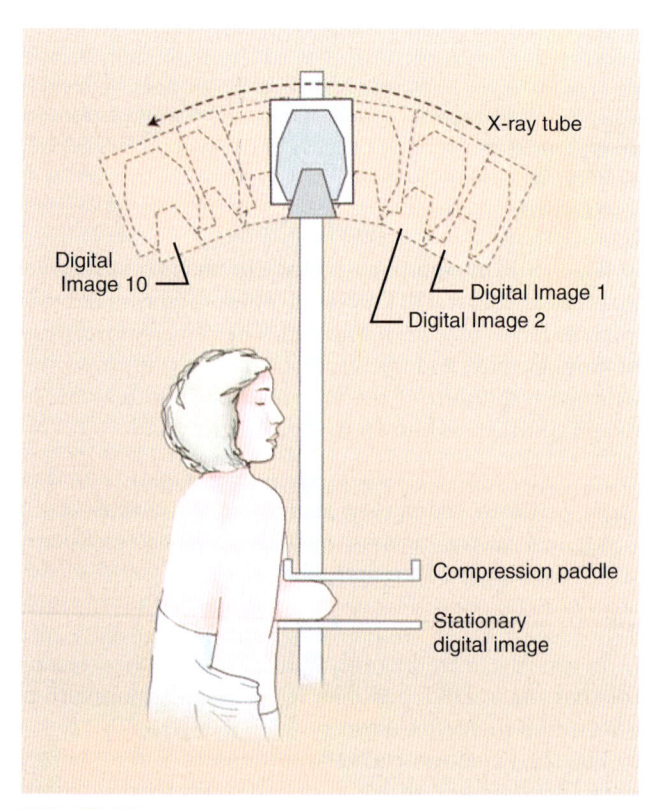

FIG. 22.12 The movements of an x-ray mammography system that produce digital mammographic tomosynthesis images.

At the end of the examination, one has a three-dimensional matrix of values that can be reconstructed in any plane—coronal, sagittal, or transverse. The result is improved image contrast and even more precise diagnostic images, as seen in Fig. 22.13.

The American College of Radiology instituted the Tomosynthesis Mammographic Imaging Screening Trial. This is a voluntary reporting program designed to evaluate how far we can go in replacing the screening mammogram with DBT.

MQSA currently requires that breast imaging facilities engaging in DBT obtain a separate certification. All personnel—radiologists, mammographers, medical physicists—must complete 8 hours of initial DBT training and 15 hours of category 1 continuing medical education credits.

Several considerations come to mind when performing mammography. What is the level of mass density? Is there tissue distortion? What is the morphology and distribution of microcalcifications? What is the additional breast radiation dose?

There is not a simple answer to any of these questions. The quick answer is that DBT is an improvement to each of these questions. Consider breast radiation dose.

MQSA contains a number of breast dose limits. The simplest dose limit is 3 mGy_t to the breast per examination. This limit applies to both screening mammography and diagnostic mammography.

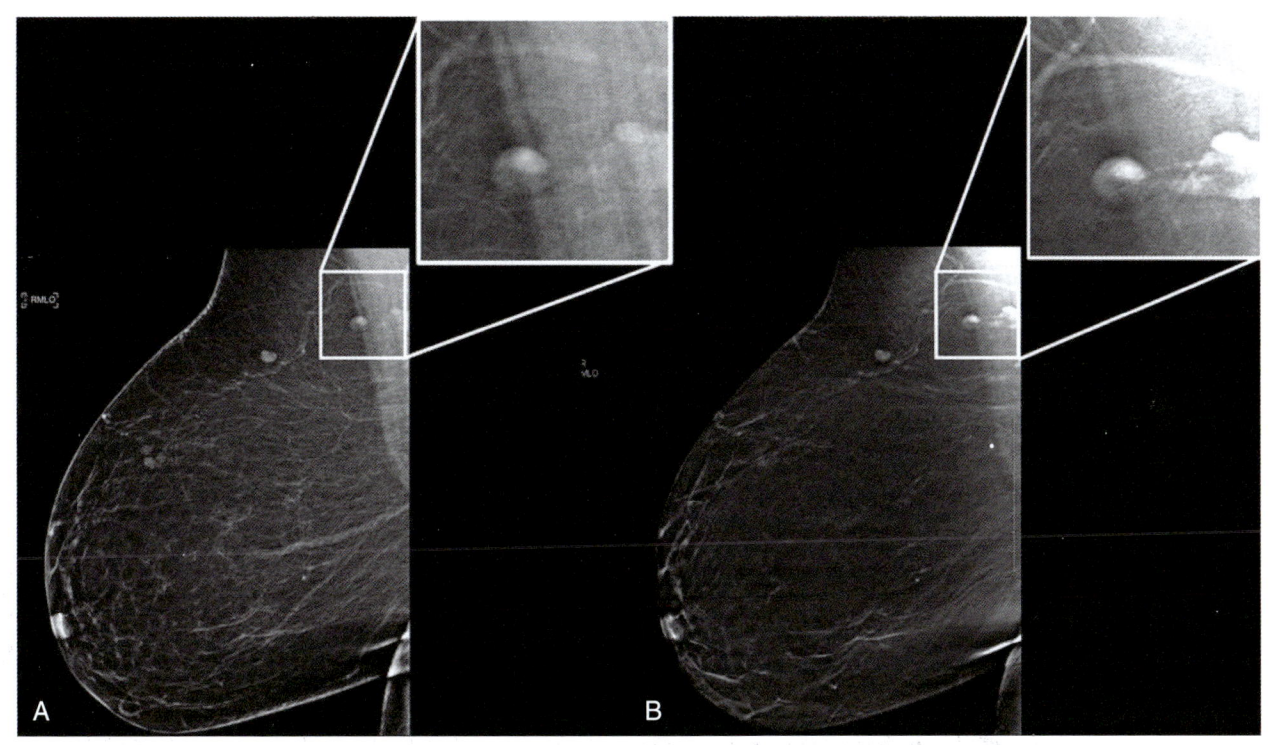

FIG. 22.14 Full-field digital mammogram of a 39-year-old female (A) and bright-edge artifact in digital breast tomosynthesis (B) at periphery of image manifests as falsely increased attenuation in axilla. (Courtesy Shawn P. Quillin, Mecklenburg Radiology Associates.)

The radiation dose to the average 4-inch compressed breast is 1 to 2 mGy_t. Add DBT to the examination, and the breast dose is still within regulatory limits.

The latest development in DRT is termed **image synthesis**. If one performs DBT without the usual full-field mammogram but would like to view a single image instead of leafing through all of the DBT images, construct a synthetic image (see Fig. 22.11).

Several algorithms have been developed to synthesize a full-field mammogram from the DBT projections. With slight exceptions, the synthetic image has the same appearance as the mammogram, and the total breast radiation dose is halved because the mammogram was avoided. Following the incorporation of DBT in medical imaging, the reduction in radiologist interpretation time is significant.

DBT occasionally manifests different artifacts. Fig. 22.14 is an example of a *bright-edge* artifact. Fig. 22.15 illustrates a *stop-and-shoot* artifact.

Chest

As was described for breast imaging, it may not be necessary for a standard chest radiograph. The synthetic chest image reconstructed from DRT may be satisfactory. The radiation dose saving is small but in keeping with ALARA.

Table 22.2 shows some specific lung conditions that may be properly managed with chest DRT instead of CT. That patient radiation dose reduction is significant.

Emergency Department

Just a few years ago, all emergency department (ED) imaging was radiographic. Slowly, CT scanners were installed in the ED. Quickly, the use of CT in the ED dramatically increased, as shown in Fig. 22.16. Trauma radiographs are becoming a thing of the past.

However, that is changing as DRT imaging systems are installed in the ED. The examination and image reconstruction times associated with DRT are much shorter than CT. DRT is also adaptable to interventional procedures.

DRT has an advantage over radiography when it comes to localizing swallowed objects. Fractures presented in the ED are delineated better with DRT, especially blow-out fractures.

A patient visit to your local ED can result in imaging of all areas of the body. When you have a stomachache severe enough to send you to the ED, the diagnosis of urinary stones, pancreatitis, or any of many gastrointestinal tract disorders is possible. Most of these abdominal issues are better managed with DRT compared with radiography. All eligible abdominal issues may be managed at much less patient radiation dose compared with CT.

Another area of radiography served in the ED by DRT is orthopedic imaging. DRT has been shown superior to radiography for subtle fractures, occult fractures, articular surfaces, and posttrauma follow-up.

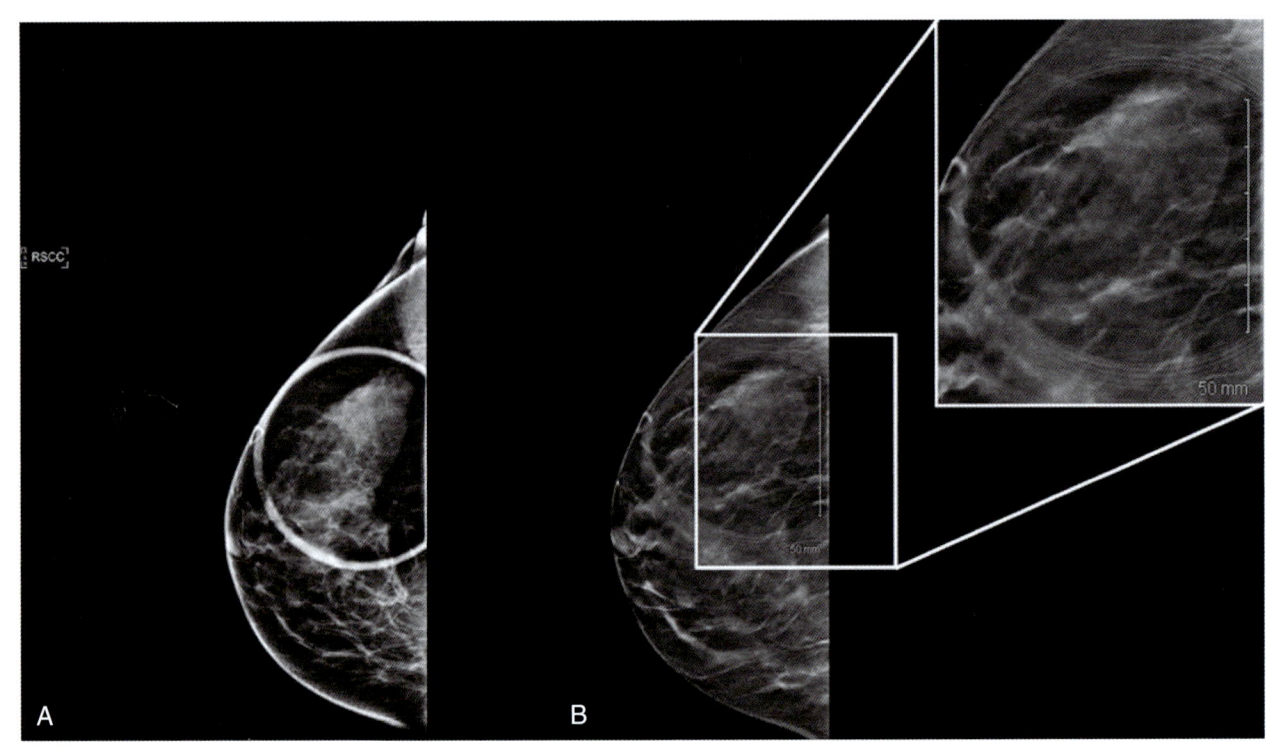

FIG. 22.15 Full-field digital mammography with spot compression of a 39-year-old female (A) and stop-and-shoot artifact from compression paddle in spot compression digital breast tomosynthesis (B). (Courtesy Shawn P. Quillin, Mecklenburg Radiology Associates.)

TABLE 22.2	Clinical Conditions Amenable to Chest Digital Radiographic Tomosynthesis Rather Than Chest Computed Tomography

- Airway changes
- Cardiac calcifications
- Cystic fibrosis
- Immune compromised patients
- Interstitial lung disease
- Metastatic disease
- Osseous lesions
- Pulmonary mycobacterial disease
- Subtle pneumothoraces

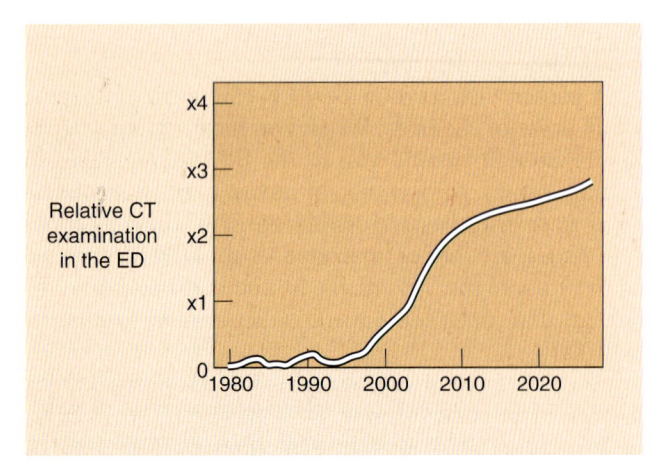

FIG. 22.16 Posteroanterior chest versus chest digital radiographic tomosynthesis. *ED*, Emergency department.

Many patients visiting the ED require head and neck imaging. If DRT is not available, CT will be ordered and a substantially higher patient radiation dose will be required. DRT for paranasal sinus imaging will replace CT as we gain more clinical experience with DRT. The various positioning views—Waters, Caldwell, lateral projections—are avoided with DRT, saving the time required for the precise patient positioning. Using DRT properly will lower eye lens radiation dose.

SUMMARY

DRT has been developed in just the past 15 years and is already making a considerable impact in all areas of medical imaging. DRT was not possible until the introduction of the digital image receptor.

The principal advantage to DRT is improved image contrast. As DRT replaces CT, we will experience further reduction in patient radiation dose.

Image artifacts generated during DRT are unique and require a deeper understanding of this image production method. QC is essential with DRT, and appropriate QC test objects are available.

CHALLENGE QUESTIONS

1. Define or otherwise identify the following:
   a. Tomography
   b. Computer-aided detection
   c. Image contrast

d. Contrast resolution
   e. Fulcrum
   f. Blurred ripple
   g. Continuous sweep
   h. Synthesized image
   i. Tomosynthesis
   j. Reconstruction algorithm
2. For what does DMIST stand?
3. Describe the relationship between imaging system contrast resolution and postprocessing.
4. What imaging modality was first to produce a digital image?
5. Why can we not perform DRT with screen-film image receptors?
6. What is the required radiation dose limit to the breast according to MQSA?
7. What is the difference between continuous sweep and stop-and-shoot x-ray tube motion? Which is better?
8. Who is credited with the first tomography imaging?
9. Name three advantages of digital radiographic tomosynthesis over radiography.
10. What is detective quantum efficiency, and why is it important in digital radiographic tomosynthesis?
11. Has the use of computed tomography leveled off in the emergency department?
12. Define tomographic angle.
13. What happens to image quality as tomosynthesis sweep angle increases?
14. List three image artifacts associated specifically with DRT.
15. What is the difference between image contrast and contrast resolution?
16. Why is a digital image receptor (IR) necessary for DRT?
17. What is meant by image synthesis?
18. What does truncation mean and why is it important to DRT?
19. A principal advantage to DRT is reduced tissue superimposition. What does that mean?
20. What pixel size is associated with DRT?

The answers to the Challenge Questions can be found by logging on to our website at http://evolve.elsevier.com.

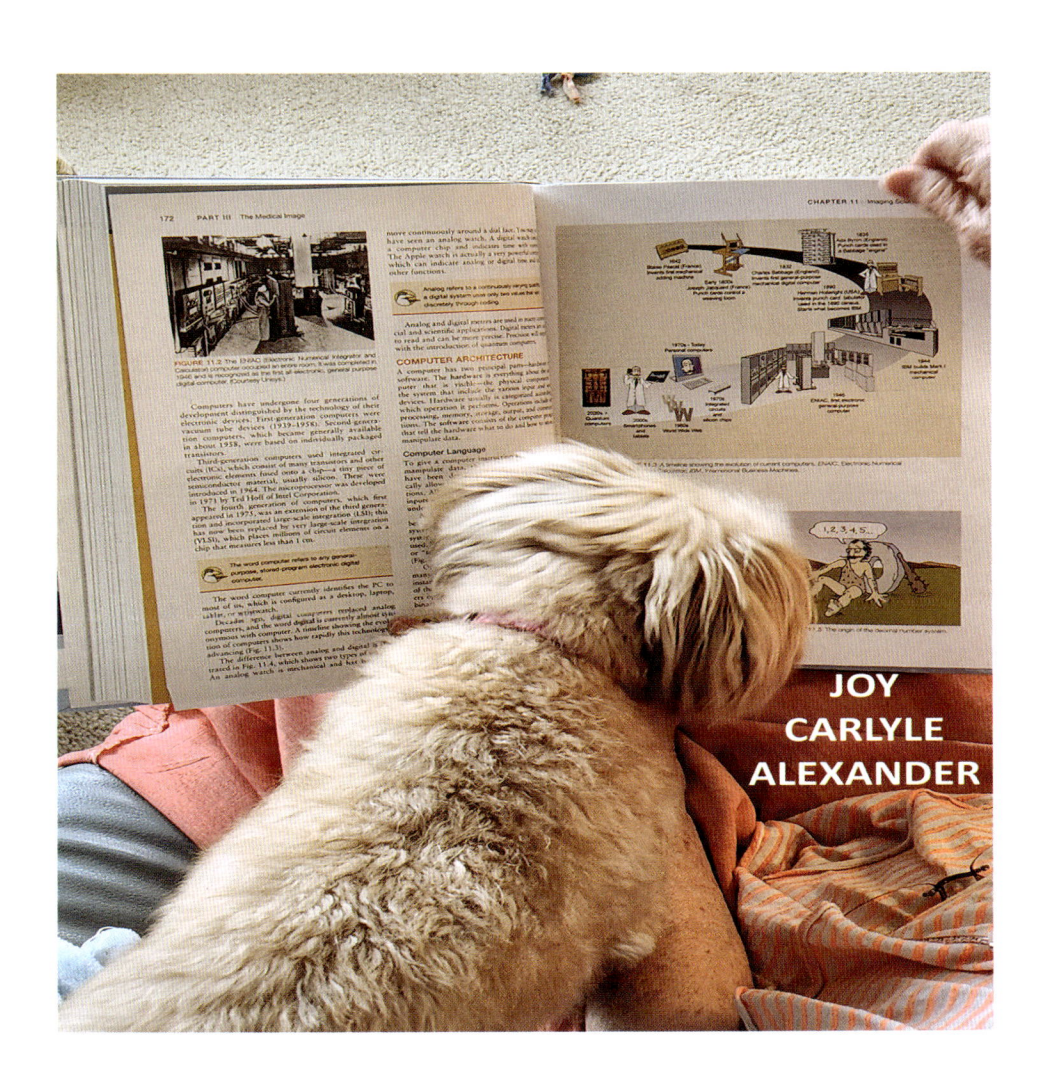

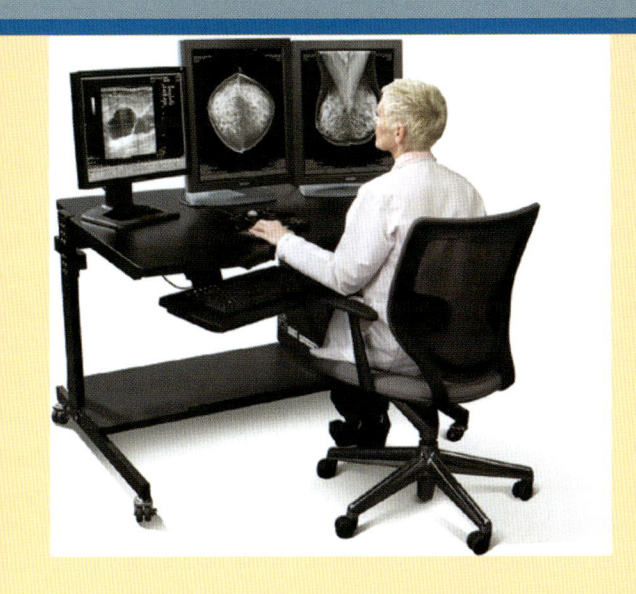

PART V

MEDICAL IMAGE DISPLAY

CHAPTER 23

Patient-Image Optimization

OBJECTIVES

At the completion of this chapter, the student should be able to do the following:
1. Discuss the body habitus patient factors and how they influence imaging factors.
2. Describe the relationships among spatial resolution/contrast resolution and image detail.
3. Identify types of distortion.
4. Define image artifact.
5. Describe magnification radiography and its uses.

OUTLINE

Patient Factors 345
　Thickness 345
　Composition 346
　Pathology 346
Image-Quality Factors 347
Image Detail 347
Distortion 347
Image Artifacts 348
Summary 348
Challenge Questions 348

CHAPTER 23 Patient-Image Optimization

IN TODAY'S digital imaging environment, the radiographer is the professional closest to the patient. The radiologist may have some patient interaction, but no interaction is more likely. The radiologist may be in Australia interpreting images via teleradiology of a patient in Houston.

The radiographer is the person who welcomes the patient to the imaging room, performs the imaging task, and bids the patient farewell, perhaps with instructions or information regarding how the results and interpretive reports are handled.

Such patient contact requires observational skill on the part of the radiographer. The patient's appearance, body habitus, medical history, and current medical condition may have a considerable effect on the imaging modality requested and its specific application techniques.

PATIENT FACTORS

Radiographic technique may be described by identifying three groups of factors. One group includes **patient factors**, such as anatomical thickness and body composition. A second group consists of **image-quality factors**, such as image receptor (IR) response, contrast resolution, spatial resolution, and distortion. Also of importance is how these image-quality factors are influenced by the patient characteristics.

The final group includes the **exposure technique factors**, such as kVp, milliamperage, exposure time, and source-to-image receptor distance (SID), as well as grids, screens, focal spot size, and filtration. These factors determine the basic characteristics of radiation exposure of the IR and patient radiation dose. They also provide the radiographer with a specific and orderly means of producing, evaluating, and comparing radiographs. These tasks were discussed in Chapter 14.

Perhaps the most difficult task for radiographers involves evaluation of the patient. The patient's size, shape, and physical condition greatly influence the required radiographic technique.

The general size and shape of a patient is called **body habitus**. Four such states have been described (Fig. 23.1).

Sthenic—meaning "strong, active"—patients are average patients.

Hyposthenic patients are thin but healthy appearing; these patients generally require less radiographic technique.

Hypersthenic patients are big in frame and usually overweight.

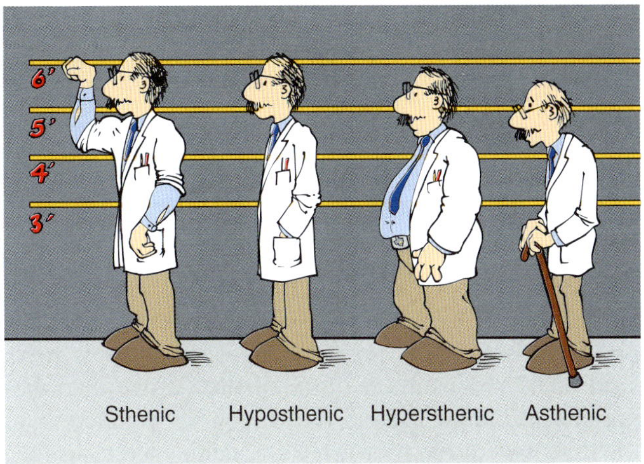

FIG. 23.1 The four general states of body habitus.

TABLE 23.1	Fixed Kilovolt Peak (kVp) Technique for an Anteroposterior Abdominal Examination								
kVp	80	80	80	80	80	80	80	80
Patient thickness (cm)	16	18	20	22	24	26	28	30
mAs	12	15	22	30	45	60	90	120

mAs, Milliampere seconds.

Asthenic patients are small, frail, sometimes emaciated, and often elderly.

> Radiographic technique charts embedded in the operating console are based on sthenic patients.

Recognition of body habitus is essential to radiographic technique selection. Most operating consoles have a positive or negative technique based on normal, sthenic anatomy. After this has been established, the thickness and composition of the anatomy being examined must be determined more precisely by the radiographer.

Thickness

The thicker the patient, the more x-radiation is required to penetrate the patient to expose the IR. For this reason, **calipers** are available to the radiographer for use to measure the thickness of the anatomy being imaged.

> Patient thickness should not be guessed!

Depending on the type of radiographic technique practiced, the mAs setting or the kVp will be altered as a function of the thickness of the part. Table 23.1 shows

TABLE 23.2	Variable Kilovolt Peak Technique (kVp) for an Anteroposterior Pelvis Examination							
mAs	100	100	100	100	100	100	100	100
Patient thickness (cm)	15	16	17	18	19	20	21	22
kVp	56	58	60	62	64	66	68	70

mAs, Milliampere seconds.

an example of how the mAs setting changes when the abdomen is imaged if a fixed kVp technique is used. Table 23.2 shows an example of the change in radiographic technique factors that occurs as a function of the thickness of the part when a variable kVp technique is used. Measurement of the patient thickness with calipers should follow, along the central ray.

Composition

Measurement of the thickness of the anatomic part does not release the radiographer from exercising some additional judgment when selecting a proper radiographic technique. The thorax and the abdomen may have the same thickness, but the radiographic technique used for each will be considerably different. The radiographer must estimate the mass density of the anatomical part and the range of mass densities involved.

In general, when only soft tissue is being imaged, low kVp and high mAs are used. With an extremity that consists of soft tissue and bone, low kVp is used because the body part is thin.

When imaging the chest, the radiographer takes advantage of the high subject contrast. Lung tissue has very low mass density, the bony structures have high mass density, and the mediastinal structures have intermediate mass density. Consequently, high kVp and low mAs can be used to good advantage. This results in an image with satisfactory contrast and low patient radiation dose.

> The chest has high subject contrast; the abdomen has low subject contrast.

These various tissues are often described by their degree of **radiolucency** or **radiopacity** (Fig. 23.2). Radiolucent tissue attenuates few x-rays and appears black on the radiograph. Radiopaque tissue absorbs x-rays and appears white on the radiograph. Table 23.3 shows the relative degree of radiolucency for various types of body habitus and tissue.

Pathology

The type of pathology, its size, and its composition influence radiographic technique selection. In this case, the patient examination request form and previous images may be of some help. The radiographer should

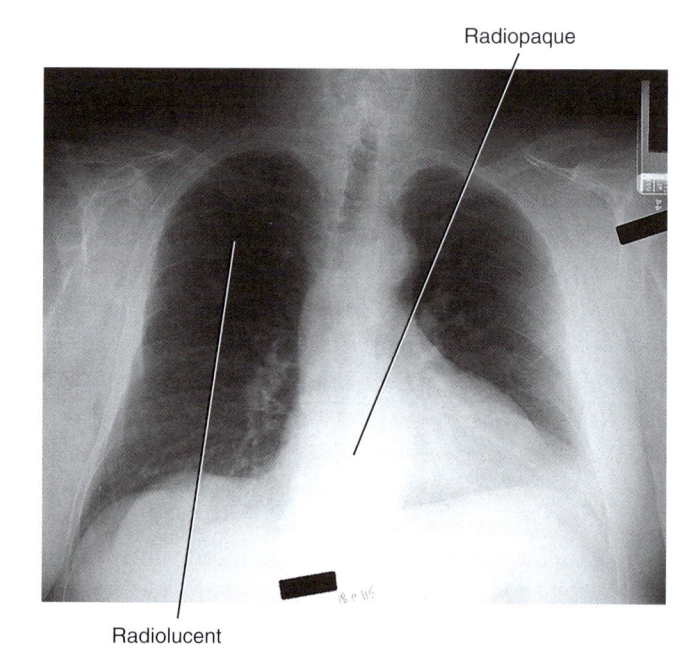

FIG. 23.2 Relative radiolucency is shown on this radiograph. (Courtesy Bette Shans, Colorado Mesa University.)

TABLE 23.3	Relative Degrees of Radiolucency		
	Appearance	Body Habitus	Tissue Type
Radiolucent ↓ Radiopaque	Black ↓ White	Asthenic Hyposthenic Sthenic Hypersthenic	Lung Fat Muscle Bone

not hesitate to seek more information from the referring physician, the radiologist, or the patient regarding the suspected pathology.

> Pathology can appear with increased radiolucency or radiopacity.

Some pathology is destructive by decreasing thickness, mass density, or average atomic number, causing the tissue to be more radiolucent. Other pathology

TABLE 23.4 Classifying Pathology

Radiolucent (Destructive)	Radiopaque (Constructive)
Active tuberculosis	Aortic aneurysm
Atrophy	Ascites
Bowel obstruction	Atelectasis
Cancer	Cirrhosis
Degenerative arthritis	Hypertrophy
Emphysema	Metastases
Osteoporosis	Pleural effusion
Pneumothorax	Pneumonia
	Sclerosis

can be constructive, causing the tissue to be more radiopaque. Practice and experience will guide the radiographer's clinical judgment, but Table 23.4 presents a beginning classification scheme.

IMAGE-QUALITY FACTORS

Image-quality factors refer to characteristics of the radiographic image. These include spatial resolution, contrast resolution, distortion, and image artifacts. These factors provide a means for the radiographer to produce, review, and evaluate radiographs. Image quality factors are considered the "language" of radiography. Often, it is difficult to separate one factor from another.

Refer to Chapter 13 to refresh your understanding of spatial resolution and contrast resolution, which are the two principal image-quality factors. Also recall that spatial resolution is limited by pixel size and that contrast resolution can be improved with postprocessing.

> **5% RULE**
> An increase of 5% in kVp may be accompanied by a 30% reduction in mAs to produce the same IR response.

Image Detail

Historically, *image detail* was a term sometimes used to describe the appearance of anatomic structures on the image. Image detail was characterized by two measures: **sharpness of image detail** and **visibility of image detail**.

Sharpness of image detail was an attempt to describe **spatial resolution**. Similarly, visibility of image detail was related to **contrast resolution** and image contrast.

These terms have largely disappeared from the radiographer's vocabulary. They were the best use of the English language at that time. This situation is one of many where the understanding of a physics principle is confounded by English. Substitute the discussion of Chapter 13 for this information.

> Sharpness of image detail is best measured by spatial resolution.

Visibility of image detail describes the ability to see the detail on the radiograph and is best measured by contrast resolution. Loss of visibility refers to any factor that causes deterioration or obscuring of image detail. For example, fog reduces the ability to observe structural lines and soft tissue abnormalities on the image.

> Visibility of image detail is best measured by contrast resolution.

The assumption is that any factor that affects IR response, such as collimation, use of grids, and other methods that prevent scatter radiation from reaching the IR, affects the contrast resolution of the imaging system.

Distortion

Another image quality factor is distortion, the misrepresentation of object size and shape in the image. Because of the position of the x-ray tube, the anatomic part, and the IR, the final image may misrepresent the object.

Poor alignment of the IR or the x-ray tube can result in **elongation** of the image—the anatomic part of interest appears bigger than normal. Poor alignment of the anatomical part may result in **foreshortening** of the image—the anatomic part appears smaller than normal.

> Distortion is reduced by positioning the anatomic part of interest in a plane parallel to that of the IR and the central ray perpendicular to both.

Fig. 23.3 provides examples of elongation and foreshortening. Many body parts are naturally foreshortened as a result of their shape (e.g., ribs, facial bones).

Distortion can be minimized through proper alignment of the tube, the anatomic part, and the IR. The central ray of the x-ray beam should be perpendicular to both the anatomic part and to the IR. This alignment is fundamentally important for patient positioning.

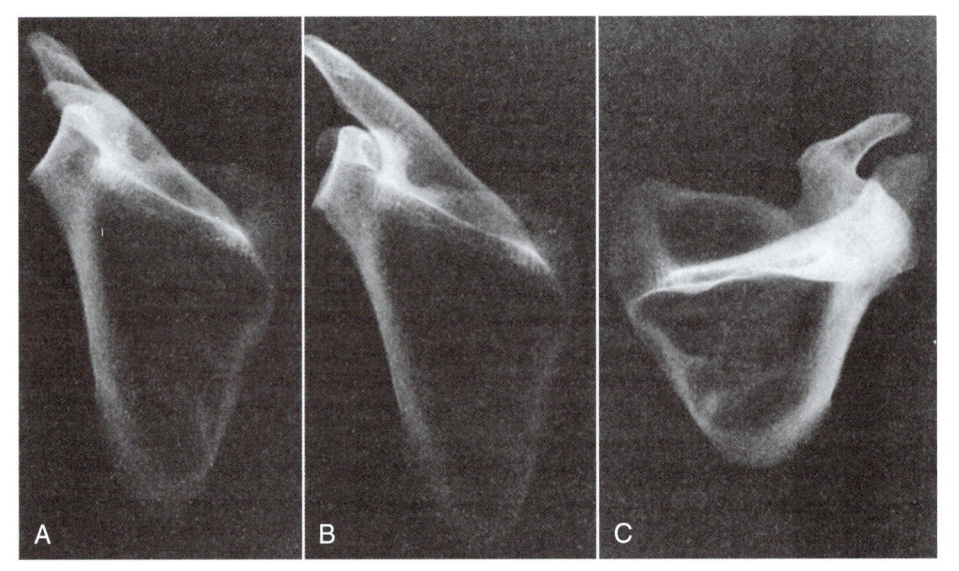

FIG. 23.3 (A) Normal projection of the scapula. (B) Elongation of the scapula. (C) Foreshortening of the scapula. (Courtesy Lynn Davis, Houston Community College.)

Image Artifacts

Each imaging modality has characteristic image artifacts. Image artifacts associated with magnetic resonance imaging, diagnostic ultrasound, and nuclear medicine are specific to each imaging modality.

Similarly, radiographic artifacts are unique to x-ray imaging. Such artifacts are categorized as IR artifacts, software artifacts, and object artifacts. Refer to Chapter 17 to refresh your understanding of radiographic artifacts.

SUMMARY

Patient factors include anatomic thickness, body composition, and any pathology that is present. Radiographers recognize sthenic, asthenic, hyposthenic, and hypersthenic body habitus types as a way to determine body composition and thus to select proper radiographic technique. Pathology in the body may be destructive and therefore radiolucent, which requires a reduction in radiographic technique. Constructive pathology is radiopaque and requires an increase in radiographic technique.

Image quality factors include spatial resolution, contrast resolution, distortion, and artifacts. To produce the best spatial resolution, the smallest focal spot, the longest SID, and the least object-image distance should be used. Distortion refers to the misrepresentation of object size or shape on the radiograph.

CHALLENGE QUESTIONS

1. Define or otherwise identify the following:
   a. Calipers
   b. Constructive pathology
   c. 5% rule
   d. Spatial resolution
   e. Foreshortening
   f. Software artifacts
   g. Body habitus
   h. Radiolucent pathology
   i. Subject contrast
   j. Contrast resolution
2. When a variable kVp technique is used, what happens to mAs as patient thickness increases?
3. A radiolucent appears black on an image. What is the corresponding body habitus and tissue example?
4. Investigate and list five types of digital radiographic artifacts.
5. With what body parts are low kVp technique usually used?
6. List the principal image-quality factors.
7. What is the advantage of increasing kVp according to the 5% rule?
8. Sharpness of image detail should be replaced by what physics term?
9. The use of collimation and grids principally affects what image-quality factor?

10. Define image artifact.
11. Why is it important to keep exposure time as short as possible?
12. The use of a small x-ray tube focal spot principally affects what image-quality factor?
13. Visibility of image detail should be replaced by what physics term?
14. What is meant by subject contrast?
15. What is your body type?
16. Name a few tissue types that suggest constructive pathology and appear radiopaque on the image.
17. How does body habitus affect the selection of technical factors?
18. When fixed kVp is used, what happens to mAs as patient thickness increases?
19. Define contrast. Give examples of tissues with high contrast and with low contrast.
20. Identify a tissue type associated with each of the four degrees of body habitus.

The answers to the Challenge Questions can be found by logging on to our website at http://evolve.elsevier.com.

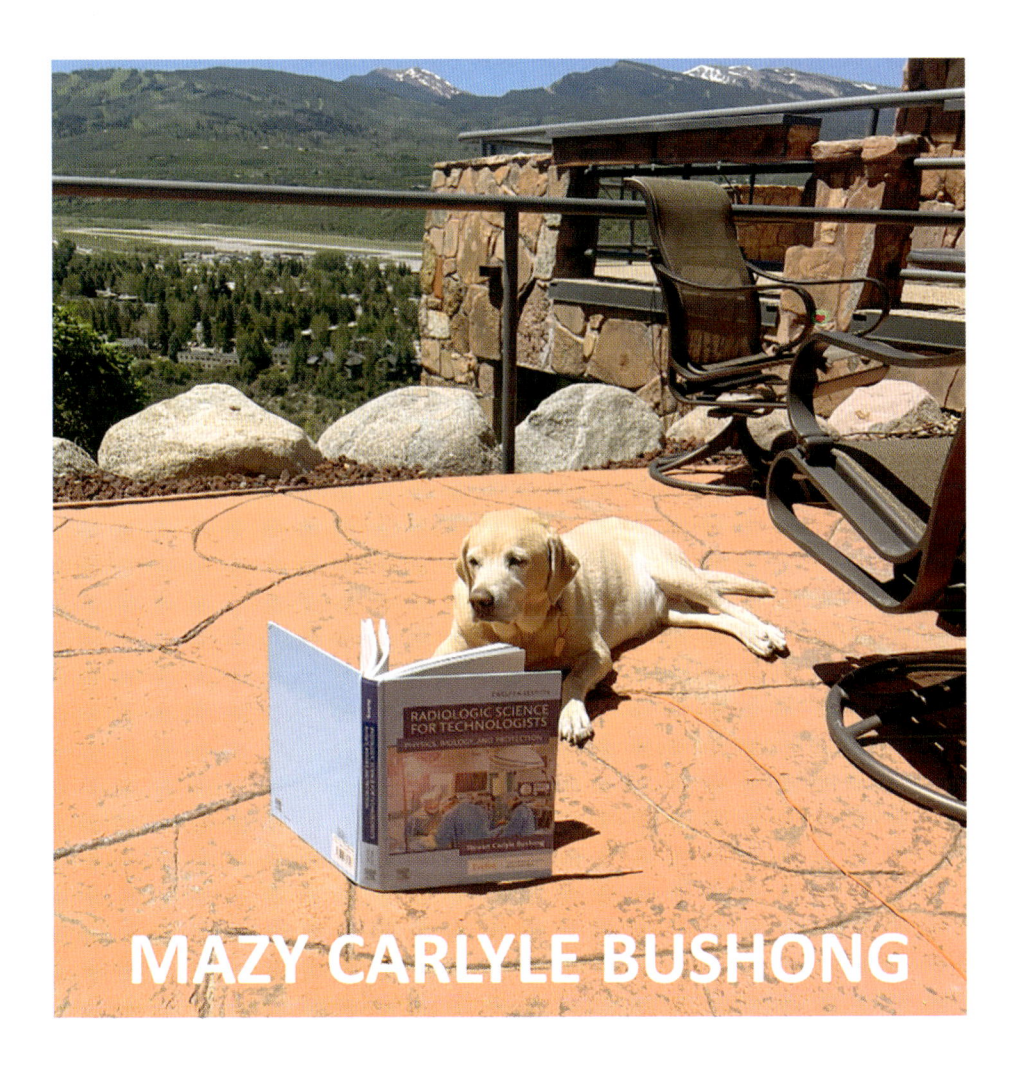

CHAPTER 24

Viewing the Medical Image

OBJECTIVES

At the completion of this chapter, the student should be able to do the following:

1. Identify quantities and units used in photometry.
2. Explain the variation in luminous intensity of digital display devices.
3. Describe differences in hard copy and soft copy and the interpretation of each.
4. Discuss the features of liquid crystal display and light-emitting diode digital display devices.
5. Describe the features of preprocessing and postprocessing.

OUTLINE

Photometric Quantities 351
  Response of the Eye 351
  Photometric Units 351
  Cosine Law 351
Hard Copy-Soft Copy 352
Liquid Crystal Display 353
  Display Characteristics 353
  Image Luminance 353
Light-Emitting Diode Display 354
  Backlight 355
  Ambient Light 355
Preprocessing the Digital Image 356
Postprocessing the Digital Image 356
Summary 358
Challenge Questions 359

TO THIS point in digital imaging, understanding the physical concepts and associated quantities of energy and ionizing radiation has been necessary. The adoption of digital imaging and the "soft read" of images on a digital display device requires an understanding of an additional area of physics—**photometry**.

Photometry is the science of the response of the human eye to visible light. Refer to the discussion in Chapter 19 for an overview of human vision and a brief description of the anatomy of the eye.

PHOTOMETRIC QUANTITIES

A description of human visual response is exceptionally complex and involves psychology, physiology, and physics, among other disciplines. The first attempt to quantify human vision was made in 1924 by the newly formed Commission Internationale de l'Éclairage (CIE) and included a definition of light intensity, the candle, the footcandle (fc), and candle power.

Response of the Eye

The CIE recognized the difference between **photopic**; bright-light vision with cones; and **scotopic**, dim-light vision with rods. This resulted in the standard CIE photopic and scotopic response curves shown in Fig. 24.1. Bright vision is best at 555 nm, and dim vision is best at 505 nm.

Photometric Units

Radiographers must have some familiarity with the units used to express photometric quantities. The basic unit of photometry is the **lumen**. It is scaled to the maximum photopic eye response at 555 nm.

> The basic photometric unit is the lumen.

Luminous flux is expressed in lumens (lm). Luminous flux is the total intensity of light from a source. Household lamps are rated by the power they consume in watts. An equally important value found on each lamp package is its luminous flux in lumens. Check it out the next time you go shopping.

Illuminance describes the intensity of light incident on a surface. One lumen of luminous flux incident on a single square foot is a footcandle (fc). This English unit, the fc, is still in use. The International System of Units (SI) equivalent is 1 lumen per square meter, which is a lux (lx): 1 fc = 10.8 lx.

Luminance intensity is a property of the source of light, such as a digital display device. Luminance intensity is the luminous flux that is emitted into the entire viewing area; it is measured in lumens per steradian or **candela**. The steradian is the SI solid angle. A solid angle is a three-dimensional version of an angle, as shown in Fig. 24.2.

Luminance is a quantity that is similar to luminance intensity. Luminance is another measure of the brightness of a source, such as a digital display device expressed in units of candela per square meter or **nit**, the SI unit.

Table 24.1 summarizes these photometric quantities and their associated units. Table 24.2 shows the range of illuminance for several familiar situations. Most indoor work and play areas are illuminated to 100 to 200 fc.

Cosine Law

Two fundamental laws are associated with photometry. Luminous intensity decreases in proportion to the

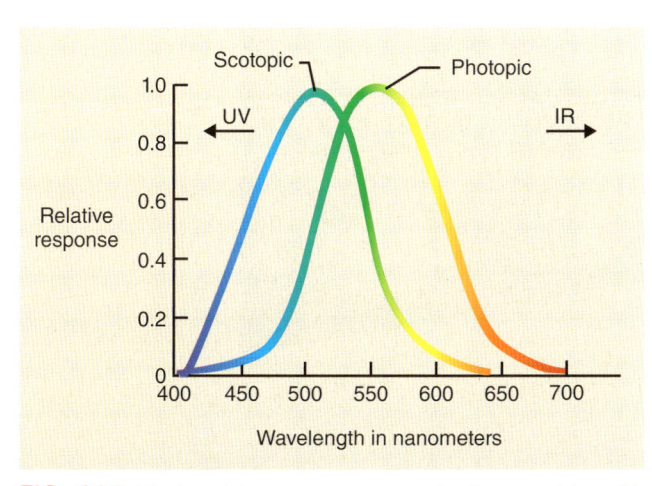

FIG. 24.1 Photometric response curves for human vision. *IR*, Infrared; *UV*, ultraviolet.

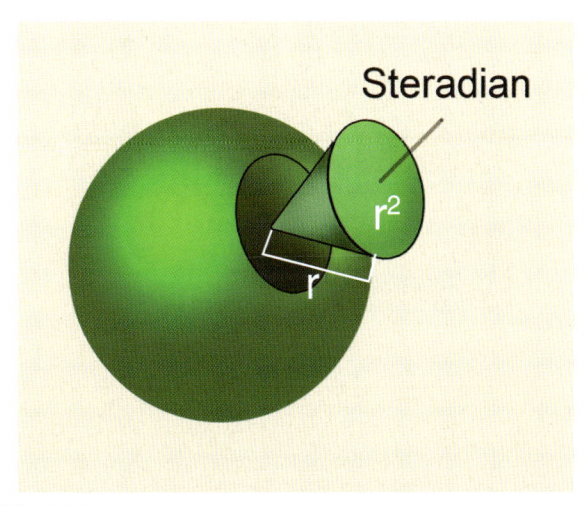

FIG. 24.2 The steradian is the solid angle with radius r. One lumen per steradian is one candela, the measure of luminance intensity.

inverse square of the distance from the source. This is the famous **inverse square law** (see Chapter 4).

The **cosine law** is important for describing the luminous intensity of a digital display device. When a monitor is viewed straight on, the luminous intensity is maximum. When a monitor is viewed from an angle, the contrast and the luminous intensity, as seen in Fig. 24.3, are reduced.

TABLE 24.1	Photometric Quantities and Units	
Quantity	**Units**	**Abbreviation**
Luminous flux	Lumen	lm
Illuminance	Lumen/ft^2	fc
	Lumen/m^2	lx
Luminous intensity	Lumen/steradian	cd
Luminance	Candela/m^2	nit

> The best viewing of a digital display device is straight on.

This reduced projected surface area follows a mathematical function called a *cosine*. Luminous intensity falls off rapidly as one views a digital display device at larger angles from perpendicular.

HARD COPY-SOFT COPY

Until approximately 2000, essentially all medical images were "hard copy"—that is, the images were presented to the radiologist on film. The image was interpreted from the film, which was positioned on a lighted viewbox.

Computed tomography (1974) and magnetic resonance imaging (1980) were the first widespread digital images. However, earlier, even these digital images were interpreted from film placed on a lighted viewbox.

Now all medical images are digital and all digital images are interpreted from presentation on a digital display device. The knowledge required of a radiographer regarding the viewing of a film image on a viewbox is rather simple. The knowledge required for viewing on a digital display device is not only different but ever more difficult.

TABLE 24.2	Illuminance in Modern Lighting	
Scene	**fc**	**lx**
Radiology reading room	1	10.8
Twilight	5	0.54
Corridor	20	216
Waiting room	30	324
Laboratory	100	1080
Tennis court	200	2160
Cloudy day	1000	10,800
Surgery	3000	32,400
Sunny day	10,000	108,000

fc, Footcandle; *lx*, lux.

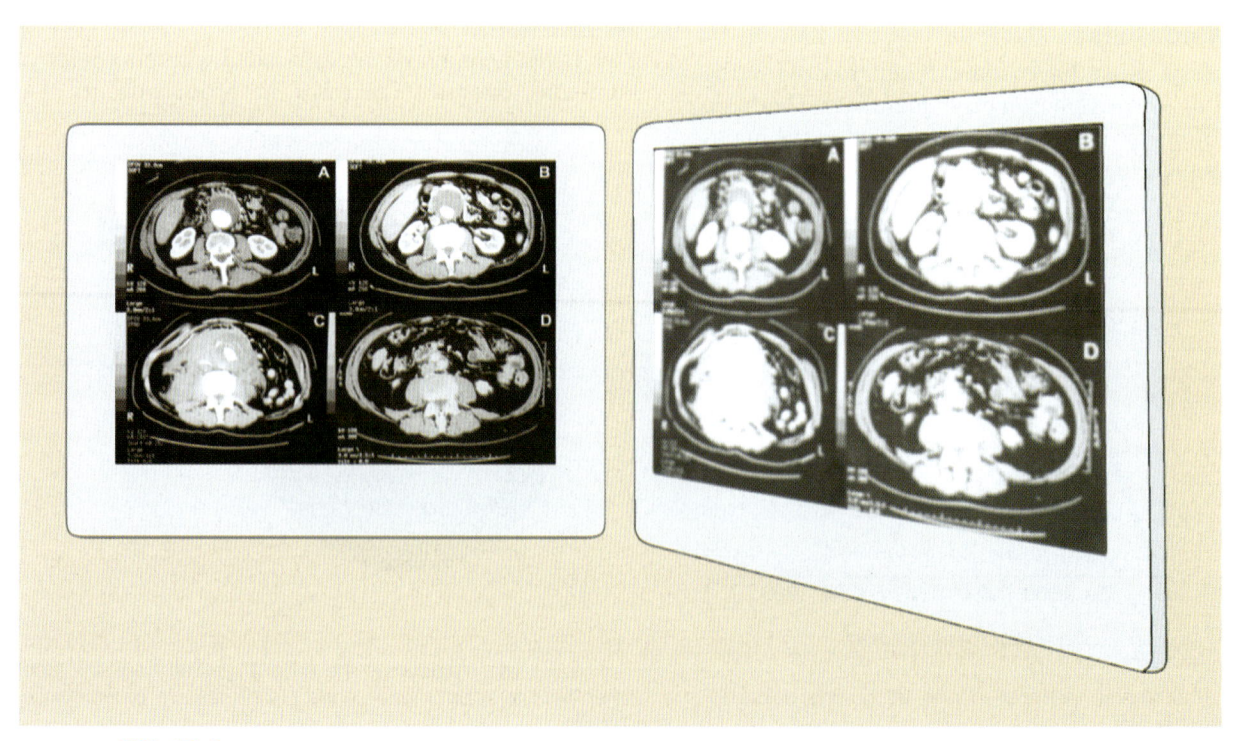

FIG. 24.3 When a digital display device is viewed from the side, illumination and image contrast are reduced.

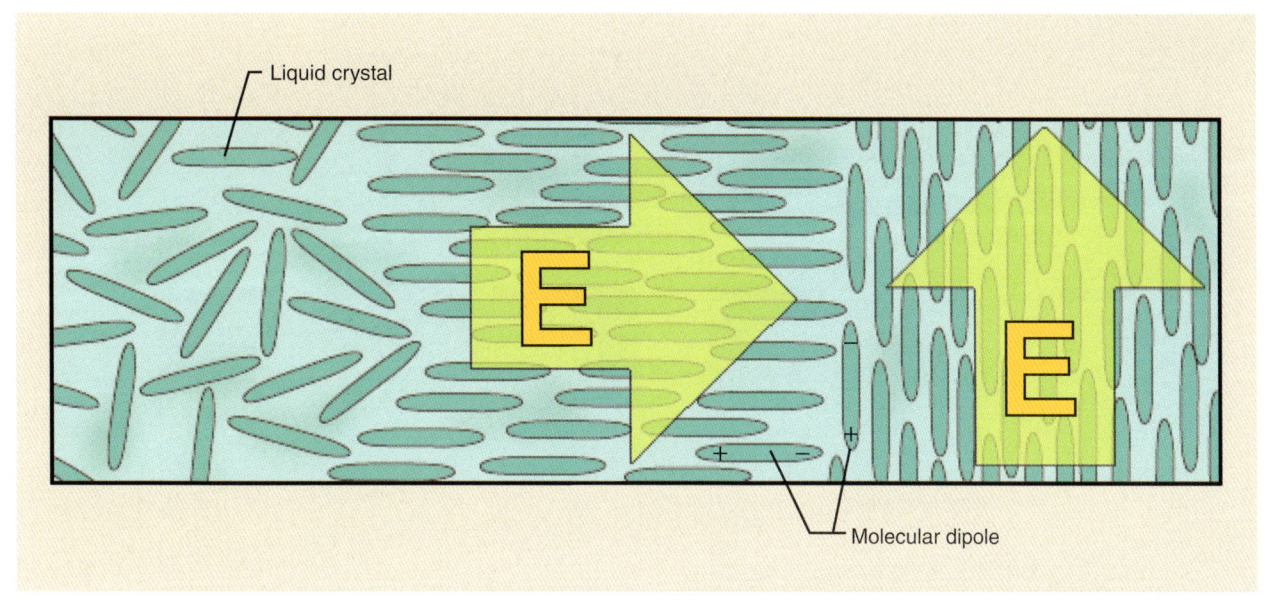

FIG. 24.4 Liquid crystals are randomly oriented in the natural state and are structured under the influence of an external electric field.

Soft copy viewing is performed on a liquid crystal display (LCD) or a light-emitting diode display (LED). The essentials of the cathode ray tube (CRT) are no longer relevant, having been replaced by LCD and LED monitors.

LIQUID CRYSTAL DISPLAY

We all know that matter takes the form of gas, liquid, or solid. A liquid crystal is a material state between that of a liquid and a solid.

A liquid crystal has the property of a highly ordered molecular structure (a crystal) and the property of viscosity (a fluid). Liquid crystal materials are linear organic molecules (Fig. 24.4) that are electrically charged, forming a natural molecular dipole. Consequently, the liquid crystals can be aligned through the action of an external electric field.

Display Characteristics

LCDs are fashioned pixel by pixel. The LCD has a very intense white backlight that illuminates each pixel. Each pixel contains light-polarizing filters and films to control the intensity and color of light transmitted through the pixel.

The differences between color and monochrome LCDs involve the design of the filters and films. Color LCDs have red-green-blue filters within each pixel fashioned into subpixels, each with one of these three filters.

Most medical flat panel digital display devices are color LCDs. Fig. 24.5 illustrates the design and operation of a single pixel. A **backlight** illuminates the pixel and is blocked or transmitted by the orientation of the liquid crystals.

The pixel consists of two glass plate substrates that are separated by embedded spherical glass beads of a few microns in diameter that act as spacers. In addition, bus lines—electric conductors—control each pixel with a thin-film transistor (TFT).

> Spatial resolution improves with the use of higher megapixel digital display devices.

Medical flat panel digital display devices are identified by the number of pixels in the LCD. A 1-megapixel display will have a 1000 × 1000 pixel arrangement. A high-resolution monitor will have an 8-megapixel display or a 2160 × 3840 pixel arrangement. Table 24.3 reports the matrix array for popular medical flat panel digital display devices.

Image Luminance

The LCD is a very inefficient device. Only approximately 10% of the backlight is transmitted through a monochrome monitor and half of that through a color monitor. This inefficiency is partly attributable to light absorption in the filters and polarizers. Because a substantial portion of each pixel is blocked by the TFT and the bus lines, efficiency is reduced still further.

The portion of the pixel face that is available to transmit light is the "aperture ratio." Aperture ratio is to a digital display device as "fill factor" is to a digital image receptor. Aperture ratios of 50% to 80% are characteristic of medical LCDs.

> Aperture ratio is a measure of image luminance of LCDs.

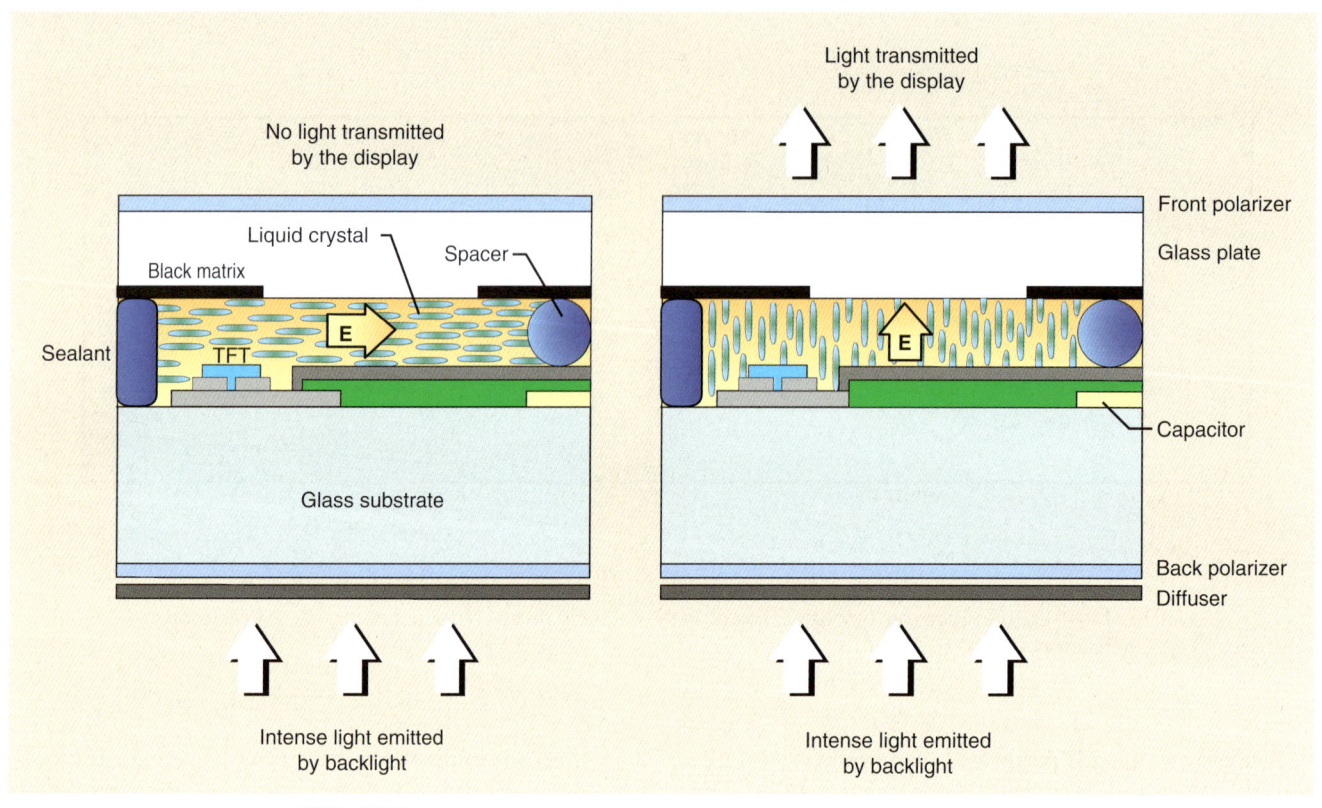

FIG. 24.5 Cross-sectional rendering of one pixel of an active-matrix LCD.

TABLE 24.3	Standard Sizes of Medical Flat Panel Digital Display Devices
Description of Size (MP)	**Matrix Array (Pixels)**
1	1000 × 1000
2	1200 × 1800
3	1500 × 2000
5	2000 × 2500
8	2160 × 3840

LCDs have good grayscale definition. LCDs are not limited by veiling glare or reflections in the glass faceplate; thus good contrast resolution is attained. The intrinsic noise of an LCD is low, and this also results in better contrast resolution.

LIGHT-EMITTING DIODE DISPLAY

Any material that emits light in response to an outside stimulus is called a **phosphor** and the resulting visible light is called **luminescence**. A number of stimuli, including electric current (the fluorescent lamp), biochemical reactions (a lightning bug), visible light (a watch dial), and x-rays (Roentgen's discovery), cause luminescence in materials.

Luminescence is similar to characteristic x-ray emission. However, luminescence involves outer shell electrons. When a luminescent material is stimulated, the outer shell electrons are raised to excited energy levels.

This situation effectively creates a hole in the outer-electron shell, which is an unstable condition for the atom. The hole is filled when the excited electron returns to its normal state. This transition is accompanied by the emission of a visible light photon.

The range of excited energy states for an outer shell electron is narrow, and these states depend on the structure of the phosphor. The wavelength of emitted light is determined by the level of excitation to which the electron was raised and is characteristic of a given phosphor.

Two types of luminescence have been identified. If visible light is emitted only while the phosphor is stimulated, the process is called **fluorescence**. If, on the other hand, the phosphor continues to emit light after stimulation, the process is called **phosphorescence**. There is yet a third, more recently engaged luminescence: **electroluminescence**.

Electroluminescence was first described early in the 20th century and developed into a commercial product as a **light-emitting diode (LED)** by Texas Instruments in the 1960s. A diode is an electronic device that allows electric current flow in one direction only.

Solid-state semiconductor diodes appeared before transistors and integrated circuits and helped in the discovery of LEDs, which are in widespread use today. The symbol for an LED is shown in Fig. 24.6.

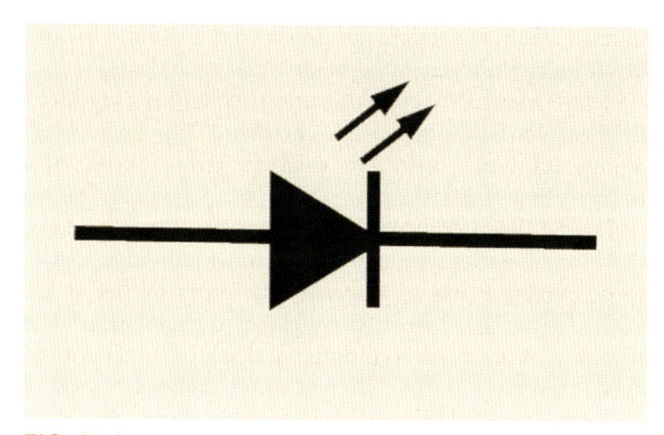

FIG. 24.6 Symbol for a light-emitting diode.

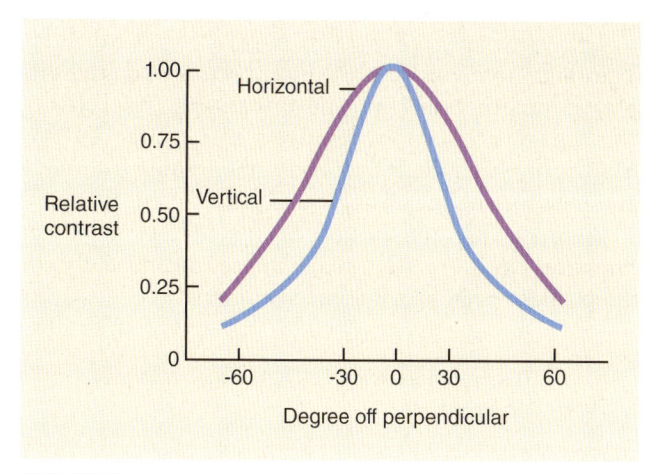

FIG. 24.7 Loss of image contrast as a function of off-perpendicular viewing of a light-emitting diode.

> An LED emits light when electrically stimulated.

The first LED semiconductor material was gallium arsenide (GaAs), and it emitted infrared photons. Newer semiconductors are employed in the commercial production of LEDs that emit photons spanning across the ultraviolet, visible, and infrared spectrum of radiation. The use of blue, green, and red LEDs is widespread today in many lighting products, including black/white and color digital display devices.

Backlight

In addition to digital display devices and video monitors, LEDs are now commonly found in general lighting applications, automobile headlights, traffic signals, and instrument panels. High-power white-light LEDs are rapidly replacing incandescent and fluorescent lighting and LCD medical image monitoring.

Actually, the LED does not replace the LCD digital display monitor; it simply provides the backlight for such a monitor. The LED replaces the fluorescent lamp in earlier LCDs.

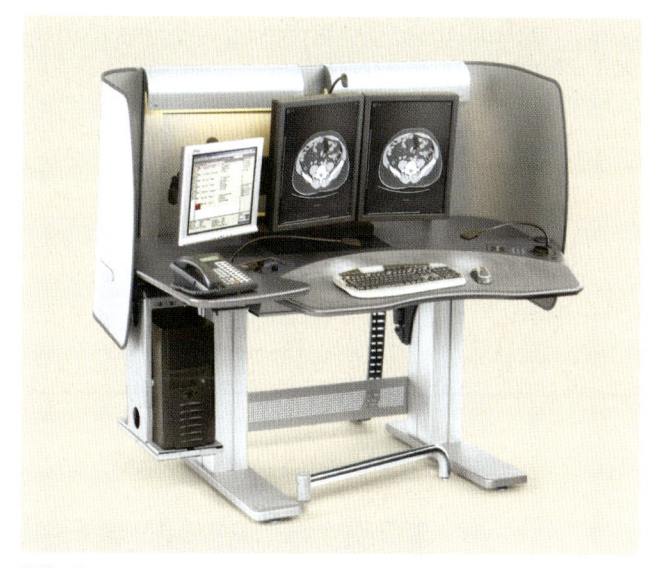

FIG. 24.8 An ergonomically designed digital image workstation. (Courtesy Melissa Gasser, Anthro Corporation.)

> All video monitors today are really LCDs with a more intense backlight, the LED.

There are a number of advantages to the use of LEDs as the backlight. Such digital display devices are thinner and have a larger active area for the visual screen. They have inspired the newest generation of curved video screens and ever-larger video screens.

LED monitors have a longer life by at least a factor of two over fluorescent backlit digital display devices. They have lower power consumption, which is registered as a reduced electric power bill for the hospital. They produce measurably less heat, which is reflected in the hospital power bill as well as increased radiology reading room comfort.

Ambient Light

LCDs are designed to better reduce the influence of ambient light on image contrast. The principal disadvantage of an LCD is the angular dependence of viewing. Fig. 24.7 shows that the image contrast falls sharply as the viewing angle increases.

This characteristic of flat panel digital display devices has led to considerable ergonomic design of digital workstations. **Ergonomics** is the act of matching a worker to the work environment for maximum efficiency.

Fig. 24.8 shows an example of an ergonomically designed digital image workstation. Levels of ambient light at the workstation must be reduced to near darkness for best viewing.

PREPROCESSING THE DIGITAL IMAGE

The ability to manipulate the image before and after display is **preprocessing** and **postprocessing**, respectively. The image acquisition described in Chapter 14 has historically been identified as a radiographic technique and is becoming increasingly automatic in engagement.

Preprocessing and postprocessing following patient radiation exposure alter image appearance, usually for the purpose of improving image contrast.

> The preprocessing of digital images is largely automatic.

Preprocessing actions are outlined in Table 24.4. Preprocessing is designed to produce artifact-free digital images. In this regard, preprocessing provides electronic calibration to reduce pixel-to-pixel, row-to-row, and column-to-column response differences. The processes of pixel interpolation, lag correction, and noise correction are automatically applied.

Offset images and **gain images** are automatic calibration images designed to make the response of the image receptor uniform. Gain images are generated every few months, and offset images are generated many times each day.

These preprocessing calibration techniques are identified as **flatfielding** and are shown in Fig. 24.9. Averaging techniques also are used to reduce noise and improve image contrast.

Digital IRs and display devices have millions of pixels; therefore it is reasonable to expect some individual pixels to be defective and to respond differently or not at all. Such defects are corrected by **signal interpolation**. The response of pixels surrounding the defective pixel is averaged, and that value is assigned to the defective pixel.

Each type of digital IR generates an electronic latent image that may not be made visible completely. What remains is **image lag**, and this can be troublesome when one is switching from high-dose to low-dose techniques, such as switching from digital subtraction angiography (DSA) to fluoroscopy. The solution is application of an **offset voltage** before the next image is acquired.

Some voltage variations may be seen along the buses that drive each pixel. This defect, called **line noise**, can cause linear artifacts to appear on the final image. The solution is to apply a voltage correction from a row or a column of pixels in a dark, unirradiated area of the IR.

POSTPROCESSING THE DIGITAL IMAGE

Postprocessing is where digital imaging shines and we will address this in several following chapters. In contrast to preprocessing, which is largely automatic, postprocessing requires intervention by the radiographer and the radiologist. Postprocessing refers to anything

TABLE 24.4 Digital Image Preprocessing

Problem	Solution
Defective pixel	Interpolate adjacent pixel signals
Image lag	Offset correction
Line noise	Correct from dark reference zone

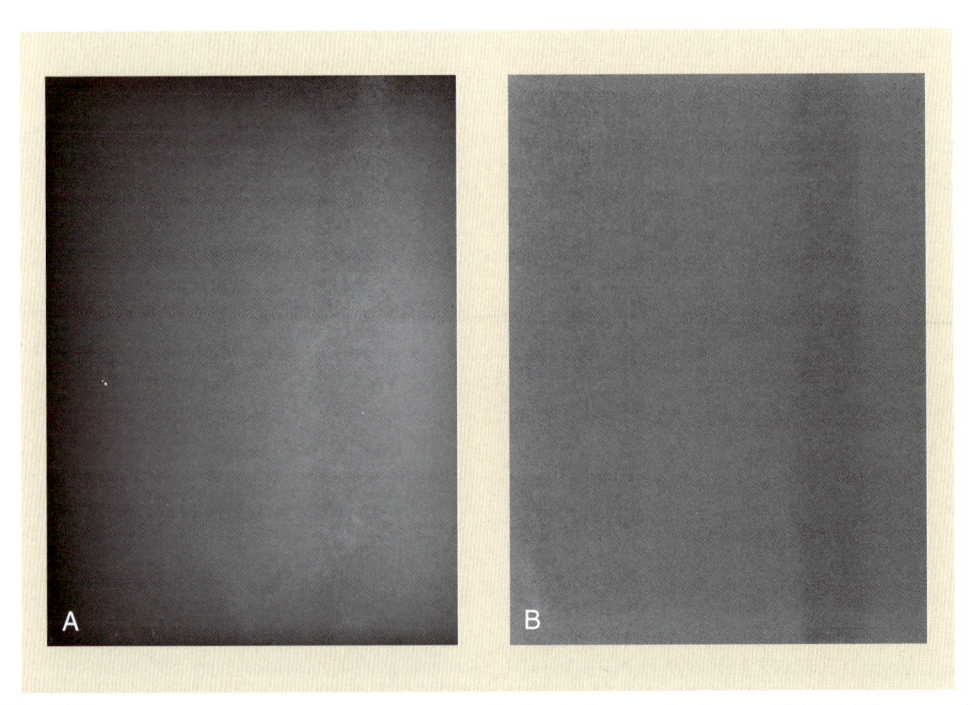

FIG. 24.9 (A) Exposure to a raw x-ray beam shows the heel effect on the image. (B) Flatfielding corrects this defect and makes the image receptor response uniform. (Courtesy Anthony Siebert, University of California, Davis.)

that can be done to a digital image after it is acquired by the imaging system.

> The postprocessing of digital images requires operator manipulation.

TABLE 24.5 Digital Image Postprocessing

Process	Results
Annotation	Label the image
Window and level	Expand the digital grayscale to visible
Magnification	Improve visualization and spatial resolution
Image flip	Reorient image presentation
Image inversion	Make white-black and black-white
Subtraction (DSA)	Improve image contrast
Pixel shift	Reregister an image to correct for patient motion
Region of interest	Determine average pixel value for use in quantitative imaging

DSA, Digital subtraction angiography.

Postprocessing of the digital image is performed to optimize the appearance of the image for the purpose of improved image interpretation. Table 24.5 lists the more useful postprocessing functions.

Annotation is the process of adding text to an image. In addition to patient identification, annotation is often helpful in informing the clinician about anatomy and diagnosis.

Digital images have dynamic ranges up to 16-bit, 65,536-gray levels. However the human visual system can visualize only approximately 30 shades of gray. By **window** and **level adjustment**, the radiographer can make all 65,536 shades of gray visible. This amplification of image contrast may be the most important feature of digital imaging.

The larger matrix size digital display devices have better spatial resolution because they have smaller pixels. This allows, among other properties, **magnification** of a region of an image to render the smallest anatomic objects visible. Magnification in digital imaging is similar to using a magnifying glass on a printed page.

At times, multiple digital images must be flipped horizontally or vertically. This process, called **image flip,** is used to bring images into standard viewing order.

Most digital images are viewed through the classical contrast rendition that depicts bone as white and soft tissue as black. However sometimes pathology can be made more visible with **image inversion**, which results in a black appearance of bone and a white appearance of soft tissue (Fig. 24.10).

Image subtraction, as used in DSA, was discussed in Chapter 20. Subtraction of digital radiographic images obtained months apart—temporal subtraction—is used to amplify changes in anatomy or disease.

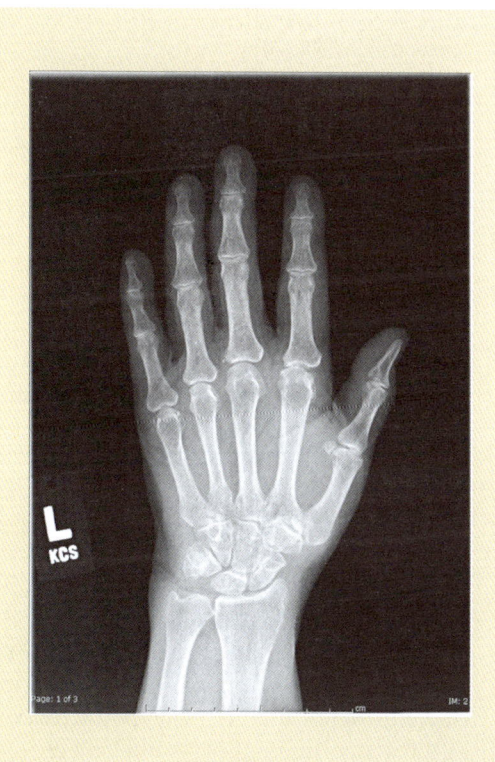

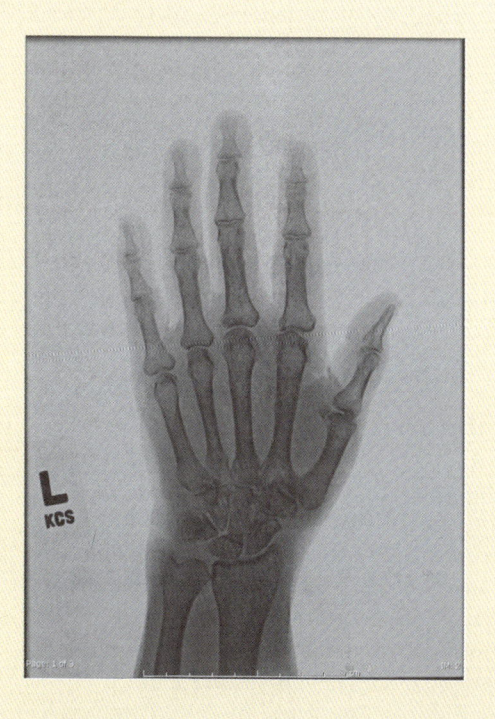

FIG. 24.10 Digital image inversion is sometimes helpful in making disease more visible, as in this case of a digital hand image. (Courtesy Colin Bray, Baylor College of Medicine.)

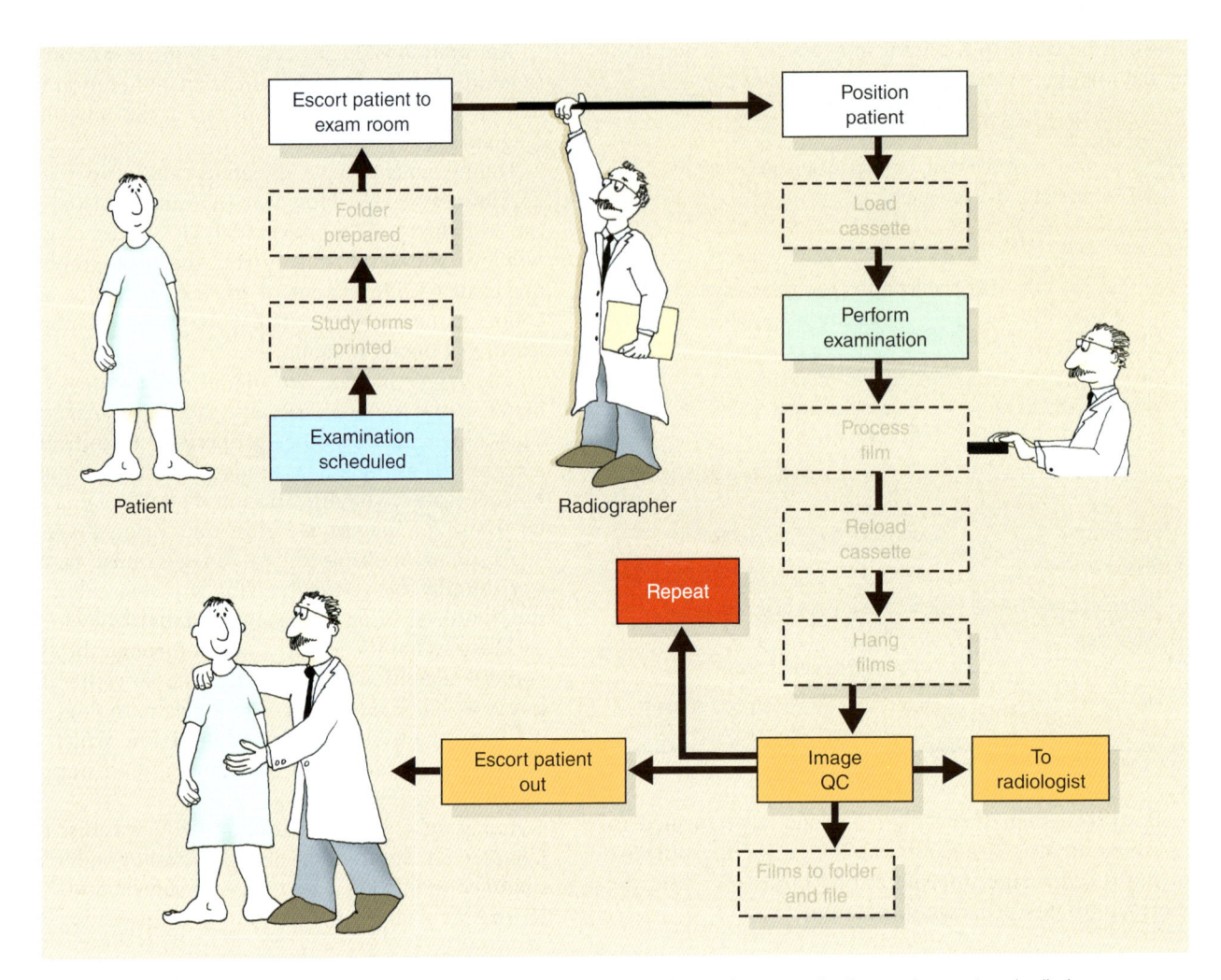

FIG. 24.11 Combining digital images with a picture archiving and communication system network eliminates even more steps in medical imaging workflow and enhances efficiency.

> The purpose of image subtraction is to enhance image contrast.

Misregistration of a subtraction image occurs when the patient moves during serial image acquisition. This can be corrected by reregistering the image through a technique called **pixel shift**.

Greater use is being made of quantitative imaging—that is, use of the numeric value of pixels to assist in diagnosis. This requires identifying a **region of interest (ROI)** and computing the mean pixel value for that ROI. This is an area of digital imaging that has been identified as quantitative radiology; it is finding application in bone mineral assay, calcified lung nodule detection, and renal stone identification.

Edge enhancement is effective for fractures and small, high-contrast tissues. **Highlighting** can be effective in identifying diffuse, nonfocal disease. **Pan, scroll,** and **zoom** allow for careful visualization of precise regions of an image.

The engagement of artificial intelligence (AI) and quantum computing (QC), as introduced in Chapters 28 and 29, will certainly continue to accelerate. As this 13th edition becomes available, the impact of AI and QC will be evident more to the radiologist than to the radiographer.

But get ready and pay attention to the change as the radiographer also becomes more engaged. Already the workflow chart is greatly reduced, as shown in Fig. 4.11. This leads to much-improved imaging efficiency.

SUMMARY

The viewing of digital images requires that radiographers have an introductory knowledge of photometry. Knowledge of photometric units and concepts is essential to successful digital imaging. Photopic vision and scotopic vision are used for the viewing of digital images.

The active-matrix LCD is the principal system for viewing digital images. The characteristics of an LCD affect image luminance. Ambient light is also of great consideration with the use of LCD. The LCD has been replaced by LED digital display devices.

Preprocessing and postprocessing of the digital image are the properties that propel digital imaging to be superior to previous analog medical imaging and soon to be assisted by AI.

CHALLENGE QUESTIONS

1. Define or otherwise identify the following:
   a. Lumen
   b. Ambient light
   c. Photometry
   d. Scotopic
   e. Pixel shift
   f. Footcandle
   g. Interpolation
   h. Candela
   i. CRT, LCD, LED
   j. Backlight
2. What is image registration, and how is it used?
3. Describe the effect of off-axis viewing of a digital display system.
4. What photometric quantity best describes image brightness?
5. Describe the properties of a liquid crystal.
6. How much digital capacity is required to store a 2000 × 2500 digital mammogram with a 16-bit grayscale?
7. How is interpolation used to preprocess a digital image?
8. What is the difference between bright vision and dim vision?
9. What is the approximate illumination of an office, major league night baseball, and a sunny snow scene?
10. Briefly, how does an active-matrix LCD work?
11. What is the difference between monochrome and polychrome?
12. Describe image inversion.
13. What is the aperture ratio of a medical LED?
14. What ergonomic properties are incorporated into a digital image workstation?
15. What are the four major photometric quantities?
16. Describe the difference between soft copy and hard copy.
17. Relate the visible light spectrum from short to long wavelength. Where is visual perception best?
18. What is the luminous flux of one of your household lightbulbs?
19. The cosine law deals with what area of image viewing?
20. What is the difference between a monochrome monitor and a color monitor?

The answers to the Challenge Questions can be found by logging on to our website at http://evolve.elsevier.com.

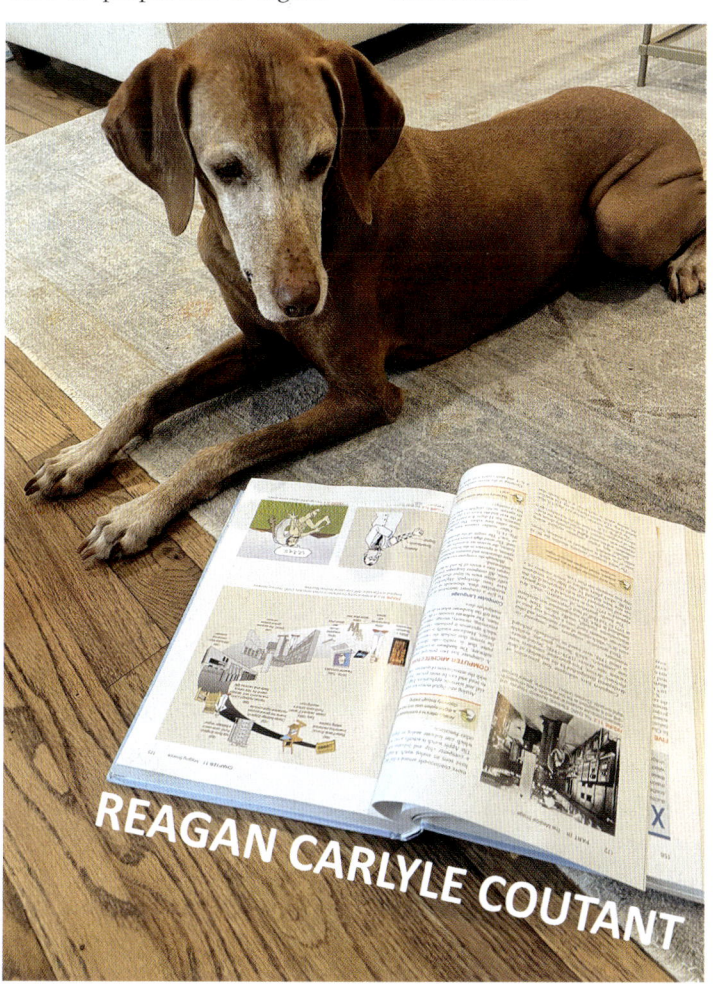

REAGAN CARLYLE COUTANT

CHAPTER 25

Medical Image Informatics

OBJECTIVES

At the completion of this chapter, the student should be able to do the following:

1. Identify several of the organizations associated with digital medical imaging.
2. Relate the order sequence from patient arrival to archiving the digital image.
3. Describe the function of the Picture Archiving and Communication System in digital imaging.
4. Discuss the changing role of the radiographer in digital imaging today.
5. Explain the difference between a header and a tag on a digital image.

OUTLINE

Electronic Programs 361
   Network 361
   Teleradiology 362
   Storage System 363
   Electronic Medical Record 363
   Informatics
     Communication 364

Medical Information
   Organizations 365
Radiographer
   Responsibilities 365
Summary 366
Challenge Questions 367

THE 21st century brought forth a revolution in medical imaging—the conversion to digital imaging. The revolution began with the introduction of computed tomography (CT) in 1974 and, some might say, finished in the year 2000 with the first commercial digital radiography (DR) systems. However, as reported in Chapters 28 and 29, this revolution continues with the introduction of artificial intelligence (AI) and quantum computing (QC) to medical imaging.

Radiology adopted digital imaging very rapidly, so that today all medical images are digital.

These digital images come from every area, including nuclear medicine, diagnostic ultrasonography, radiography, fluoroscopy, CT, and magnetic resonance imaging. These changes result in new challenges for the radiographer.

ELECTRONIC PROGRAMS

In earlier times, the radiographer was primarily responsible for the chemical processing of film and positioning the film (hanging) for the radiologist to interpret. The radiologist would write or dictate a diagnostic report, and a transcriptionist would process the report and pass the paper document on to the referring clinician.

All of that has changed and has been replaced with various electronic modalities. A good place to start is Table 25.1. It is not necessary for you to know each of these modalities—just that they exist as you become more involved.

Of the imaging team, the radiologist is ultimately responsible for the interpretation of images, but each of the other members of the team, particularly the radiographer, has specific responsibilities. Radiologists and radiographers interact most directly with Picture Archiving and Communication System (PACS) and Radiology Information System (RIS). The RIS deals with schedules, protocol descriptors, diagnostic conclusions, and billing. PACS deals strictly with image manipulation and document storage.

PACS, when fully implemented, allows not only the acquisition but also the interpretation and storage of each digital image without resorting to hard copy (film). The efficiencies in time and cost are enormous, but so are the new responsibilities of both the radiologist and radiographer.

> PACS implements and speeds image processing, viewing, interpretation, storage, and recall.

The four principal components of a PACS are the image acquisition system, the display system, the network, and the data storage system. Earlier chapters introduced digital image acquisition and the digital display system.

Network

To be truly effective, each of these image-processing modes must be quick and easy to use. This requires that each workstation be microprocessor controlled and interact with each imaging system and with the central computer. To provide for such interaction, a network is required.

Computer scientists use the term **network** to describe the manner in which many computers can be connected to interact with one another. In a business office, for instance, each secretary might have a microprocessor-based workstation, which is interfaced with a central office computer, so that information can be transferred from one workstation to another or to and from a main computer or server.

Any hospital at any time can enter the unique identifier and access the medical records for that patient. Because of PACS/RIS, the network includes digital images.

In radiology, in addition to secretarial workstations, the network may consist of various types of devices that allow storage, retrieval, and viewing of digital images, PACS workstations, remote PACS workstations, a departmental mainframe, and a hospital mainframe (Fig. 25.1). Each of these devices is called a **client** of the network.

> Clients are interconnected by wire among buildings, and by microwave or satellite transmission to remote facilities.

TABLE 25.1 Digital Imaging Programs

- ACR-AAPM-SIIM Technical Standard
- DICOM—Digital Imaging and Communication
- CAD—Computer-Aided Detection/Diagnosis
- EMR—Electronic Medical Record
- HIS—Hospital Information Systems
- HL7—Health Level Seven
- IAC—Intersocietal Accreditation Commission
- IHE—Integrating the Healthcare Enterprise
- PACS—Picture Archiving and Communication System
- RIS—Radiology Information System

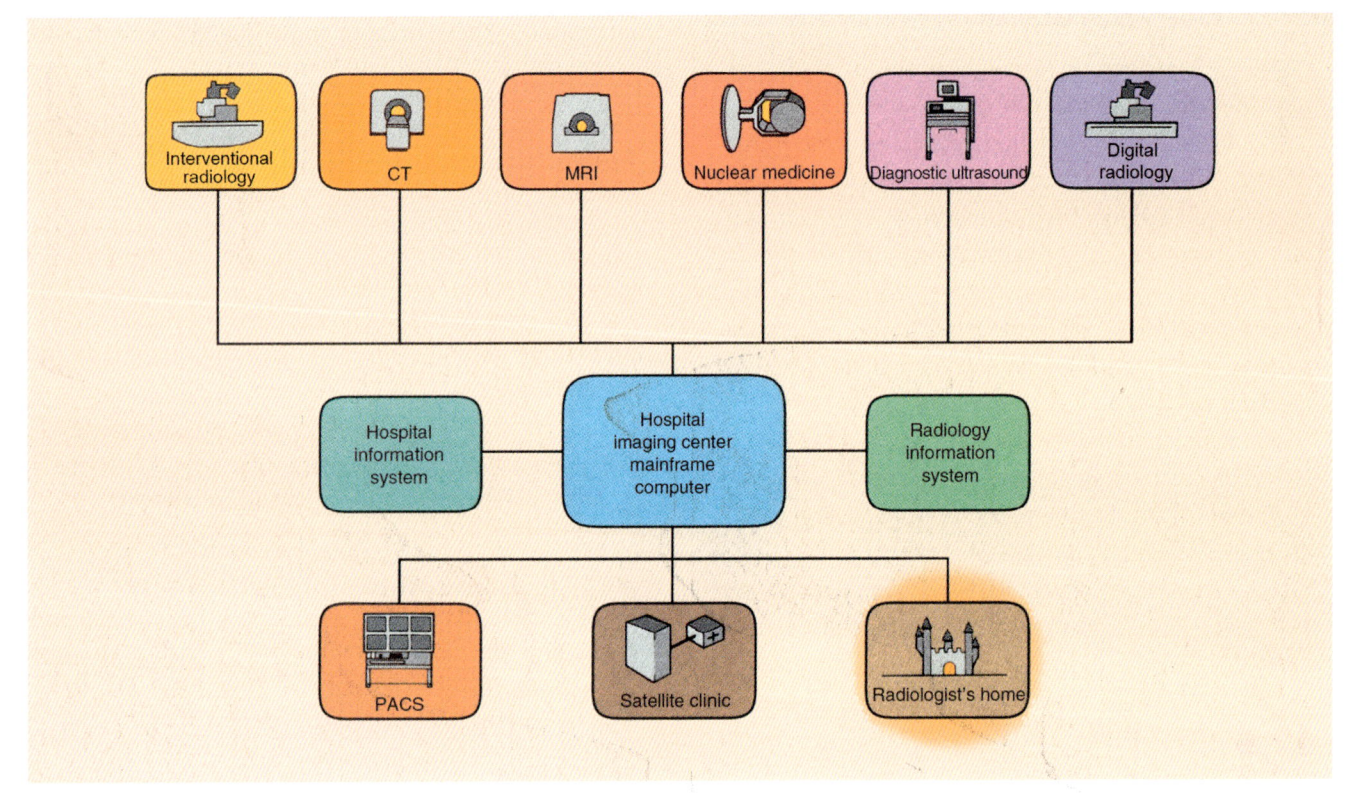

FIG. 25.1 The Picture Archiving and Communication System (*PACS*) network allows interaction among various modes of data acquisition, digital image processing, and digital image archiving. *CT*, Computed tomography; *MRI*, magnetic resonance imaging.

Teleradiology

The process of remote transmission and viewing of digital images is termed **teleradiology**. To ensure adaptability among different imaging systems, the American College of Radiology (ACR), in cooperation with the National Electrical Manufacturers Association (NEMA), has produced a standard imaging and interface format called Digital Imaging and Communications in Medicine (DICOM).

The network begins at the digital imaging system, where data are acquired. Images reconstructed from the original data are processed at the console of the imaging system and transmitted to a PACS workstation for additional processing.

> Teleradiology allows for image interpretation remotely, even intercontinentally.

At any time, such images can be transferred to other clients within or outside the hospital or imaging center. Instead of running films up to surgery for viewing on a viewbox, as previously done, one simply transfers the digital images electronically to the PACS workstation in surgery.

When a radiologist is not immediately available for image interpretation, the image can be transferred to a PACS workstation in the radiologist's home. Time is essential when one is considering image manipulation; therefore fast computers and networks with broad bandwidth are required for this task.

These requirements are relaxed for the information management and database portion of PACS, which is the RIS. Such lower-priority RIS functions include message and mail utilities, calendar reporting, storage of text data, financial accounting, and planning.

From the RIS workstation, any number of coded diagnostic reports can be initiated and transferred to a secretarial workstation for report generation. The secretarial workstation, in turn, can communicate with the main hospital computer for patient identification, billing, accounting, and interaction with other departments.

Such interconnection allows for the "prefetching" of images from the archive. The moment a patient reports to any reception desk anywhere in the facility, the process of recovering archived records commences automatically. By the time the patient reaches the x-ray examination room, all previous images and reports are available.

Similarly, a secretarial workstation at the departmental reception desk can interact with a departmental computer for scheduling of patients, radiographers, and radiologists and for analysis of departmental statistics. Finally, at the completion of an examination, PACS allows for more efficient image archiving.

Many applications now exist for electronic notepads and mobile phones that allow these devices to serve as viewing stations. Concerns for patient confidentiality continue, but clearly remote mobile digital image viewing is here.

Storage System

One motivation for PACS is archiving. In the past, films were checked out of the file room and sometimes never returned. How many films disappeared from jackets? How many jackets disappeared? How often were films copied for clinicians?

> Just the cost of the hospital space to accommodate a film-file room was sufficient to justify PACS.

Image storage requirements are determined by the number of digital images and the digital image data file size. Digital image file size is the product of the matrix size and the dynamic range or grayscale bit depth. The following examples should help with this understanding.

Question: How much computer capacity is required to store an MRI examination that consists of 120 images, each with an image matrix size of 256 × 256 and 256 shades of gray?

Answer:
Size of Matrix		Shades of Gray
256 × 256	×	256
256 × 256	×	8 bit
65,536	×	1 byte
		= 65,536 bytes

120 × 65,536 = 7,864,320 bytes, or ≈8 MB

Question: How much computer capacity is required to store a single chest image with a 4096 × 4096 matrix size and a 12-bit dynamic range?

Answer: This is a 4096 × 4096 matrix with 1024 shades of gray.

Size of Matrix	Shades of Gray
4096 × 4096	12 bit
16,777,216	1.5 byte
	= 25,165,824 bytes, or ≈25 MB

Because of the dynamic range of DR and digital mammography (DM), the storage system is stretched. Table 25.2 shows the file sizes for various medical images.

TABLE 25.2 Approximate File Size for Various Digital Images

Digital Image	Image Size (MB)	Examination Size (MB)
Nuclear medicine	0.25	5
Diagnostic ultrasonography	0.25	8
Magnetic resonance imaging	0.25	12
Computed tomography	0.5	20
Digital radiography	5	20
Digital mammography	10	60

MB, Megabyte.

Today, the previous hospital film-file room is accommodated by a data storage device the size of a desk. Electronically, digital images can be recalled from this archival system to any workstation in seconds. Backup image storage is accommodated offsite at a digital data storage vendor—in the cloud—in case the main file is corrupted.

One of the disappointing features of PACS/RIS applications in digital imaging is the reduced, if not totally absent, face time between the radiologist and the radiographer. During the 20th century, there was hourly contact and communication between the radiologist and radiographer. Now, the radiologist can be totally remote in Australia when interpreting images, while the radiographer is stationed at a local imaging system (Fig. 25.2). The ability of one to learn from the other has been lost.

Electronic Medical Record

When the patient checks into the hospital or imaging center, a document is prepared to properly identify the patient. This document, the electronic medical record (EMR), is incorporated with a similar document, the Hospital Information System (HIS), which is integrated with other documents for information transfer and storage. In this arrangement, RIS is specific within radiology and requires PACS. HIS is the principal component of the EMR, both of which are routinely changed during a patient stay.

In some countries, national networks are used for medical data. Regardless, all patients have a unique identifier—a number that is exclusively theirs for life.

A new patient, on arrival, will be registered in the EMR, which may, if appropriate, lodge a request for a medical image. Such a request is relayed to the RIS, where a specific protocol, the **Protocol Worklist**, is opened and the request filed with a specific **Imaging Modality Worklist**.

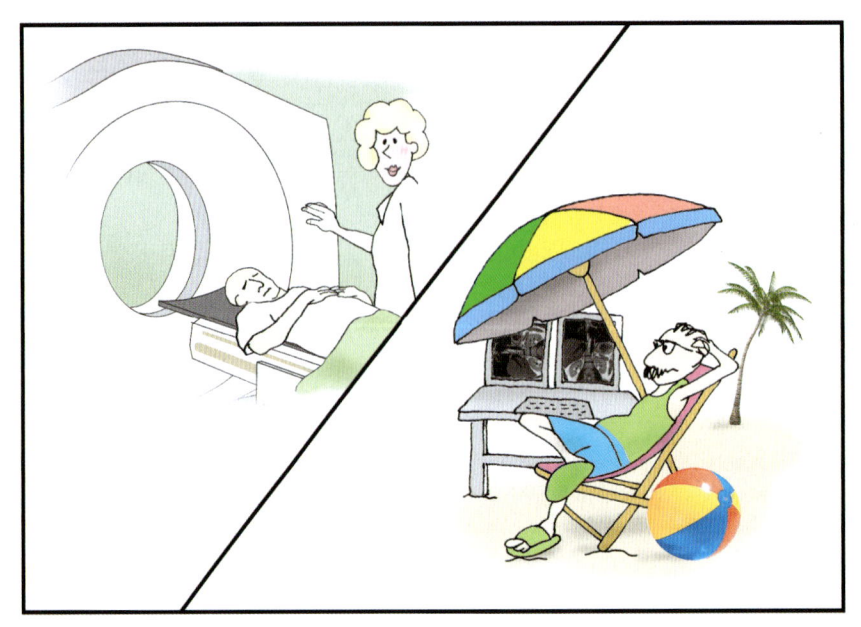

FIG. 25.2 The radiographer is normally at a fixed station with an imaging system while the radiologist is at a Picture Archiving and Communication System/Radiology Information System workstation, which can be remote (and even across the ocean).

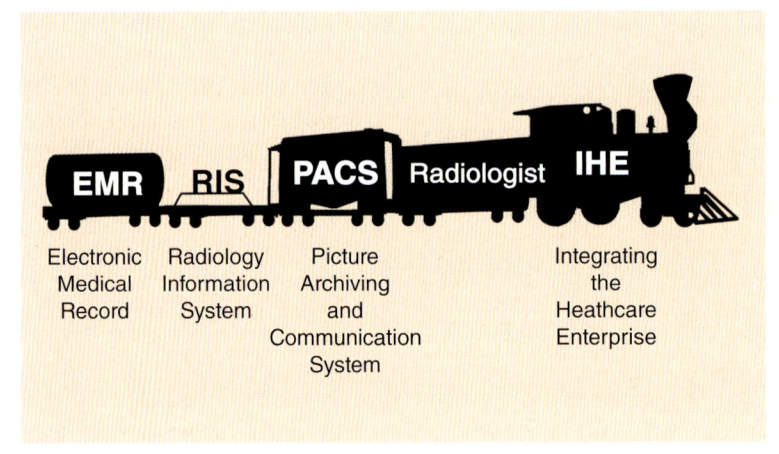

FIG. 25.3 On completion of digital imaging, the images and data flow from the radiographer to the radiologist through the various digital stations are shown.

The radiographer retrieves the imaging request from the imaging modality worklist, performs the examination, and transfers the results to PACS/RIS for attention by the radiologist, as shown in Fig. 25.3. There are several steps taken by the radiologist before the diagnostic report becomes clinically available. However, these steps take very little time, regardless of the location of the radiologist.

For the final steps, the diagnostic report is returned through PACS/RIS to the EMR for billing, education, research, and quality improvement.

Informatics Communication

It is critical that the data and digital images assembled in PACS/RIS be quickly and easily shared with those who need this information. The requirement for efficient communication among various computers and physical sites is managed by the DICOM standard and the Health Level Seven (HL7) standard. Integrating the Healthcare Enterprise (IHE) is a project that manages these connections, as shown in Fig. 25.4.

DICOM is revised regularly to accommodate new medical imaging techniques by a committee whose membership includes national and international representatives of scientific societies, commercial vendors, and individual vendors. DICOM has expanded beyond the scope of radiology into additional medical specialties.

The DICOM image **header metadata** is specific for each type of imaging system modality, and the

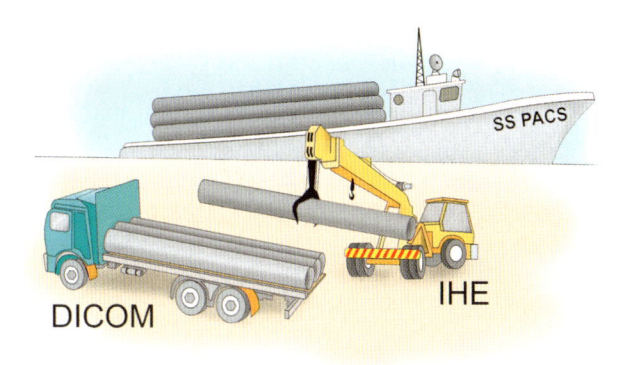

FIG. 25.4 Integrating the Healthcare Enterprise (*IHE*) manages data flow between Digital Imaging and Communications (*DICOM*) and Picture Archiving and Communication System (*PACS*).

TABLE 25.3	The ACR-AAPM-SIIM Technical Standard

- Personnel
- Equipment specifications
- Documentation
- Credentialing and liability
- Radiation safety
- Quality and safety
- Patient education

AAPM, American Association of Physicists in Medicine; *ACR*, American College of Radiology; *SIIM*, Society for Imaging Informatics in Medicine.

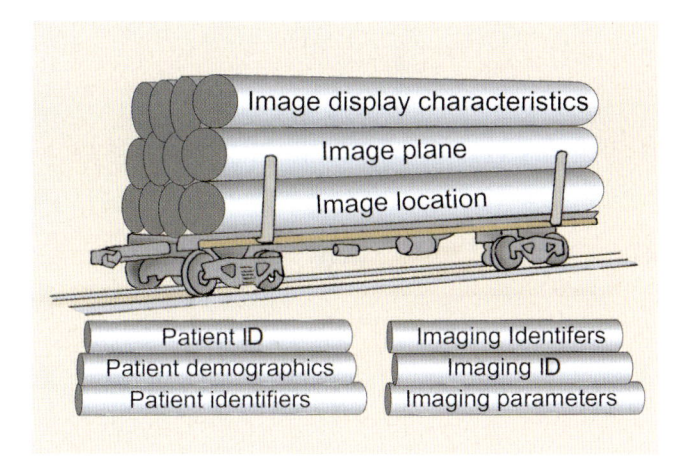

FIG. 25.5 The Digital Imaging and Communication header metadata include each of the labeled pipes.

radiographer should become familiar with such information, as shown in Fig. 25.5. Much of the header metadata is automatic, but some are input by the radiographer. Accuracy of input is imperative and that responsibility falls on the radiographer.

The DICOM standard identifies documents of data that link to digital images. Such documents as "X-Ray Radiation Dose Structured Report," "CAD Structured Reports," structured reports of measurements in obstetrical and vascular ultrasound, and Breast Imaging—Reporting and Data System (BI-RADS) require understanding by the attending radiographer to take full advantage of DICOM. Applications of AI algorithms continue to shape this area of digital imaging.

MEDICAL INFORMATION ORGANIZATIONS

The standardized approach to digital imaging programs is continually improved by the efforts of organizations dedicated to the standardization of vocabulary. The goal is for constancy and uniformity in describing medical symptoms, procedures, and results.

Standardized vocabulary, the **lexicon**, and standardized term relationships, the **ontology**, are undergoing constant development. During clinical exposure, the radiologist and radiographer will become more aware of and familiar with the properties assigned to digital images.

The Current Procedural Terminology (CPT codes) is a lexicon developed by the American Medical Association, which now numbers over 15,000 items. Each CPT code refers to a specific clinical situation. Personnel identified as **coders** in the billing office deal with CPT codes to produce the invoice presented as the patient bill.

The International Classification of Diseases codes were developed by the Center for Medicare and Medicaid Services (CMS) for identifying diseases and symptoms of diseases.

RadLex is a recent creation of the RSNA (Radiological Society of North America). RadLex is a language ontology of image descriptors for each of the imaging modalities. RadLex is principally for the use of the radiologist to arrive at clear, unambiguous diagnostic reports.

There are DICOM, HL7, and IHE working groups meeting regularly to create and update standards dealing with everything discussed in this chapter and more. Imaging modality vendors must pledge conformance with the evolving DICOM standard. There could be a place for you on one of these working groups. Consider the ACR Dose Index Registry as we continually work to make patient radiation dose ALARA (as low as reasonably achievable).

RADIOGRAPHER RESPONSIBILITIES

The evolution of digital imaging requires that the radiographer gain skills unheard of just a few years ago. Three organizations—the ACR, American Association of Physicists in Medicine (AAPM), and Society for Imaging Informatics in Medicine (SIIM), as identified in Table 25.1—have joined to produce an important document called "The Technical Standard for Electronic Practice of Medical Imaging."

A quick look at this document identifies the medical imaging team and the responsibilities of each. Table 25.3 identifies the various parts of the ACR-AAPM-SIIM Technical Standard.

Regardless of the tasks associated with image acquisition and interpretation, the radiologist is responsible

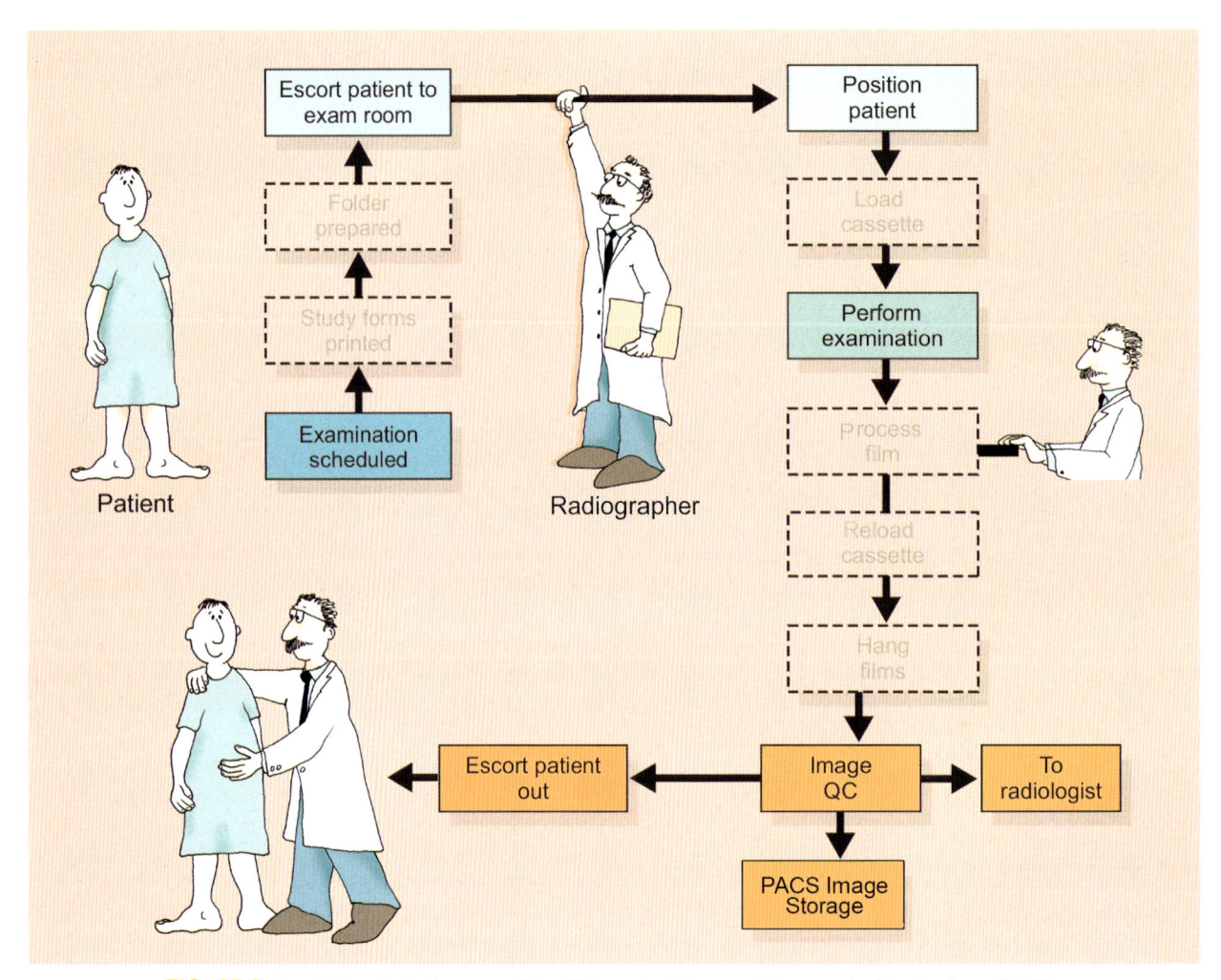

FIG. 25.6 Combining digital images with a Picture Archiving and Communication System (PACS) network eliminates even more steps in the medical imaging workflow and enhances efficiency. *QC,* Quality control.

for every step in the process and the personnel actions required.

During earlier years, a radiographer would aspire, with age and experience, to be promoted to the position of Chief Technologist. The Chief Technologist was the Department Administrator, but that position has been abandoned to the job of department administrator, which is now filled by someone with an MBA, educated in the administration of a medical department.

A radiographer can now become a radiology assistant (RA) and work more closely with the radiologist in implementing all of the areas previously described for digital imaging. The RA does not perform examinations using the various imaging modalities. Rather, the RA helps the radiologist make better use of time by managing patients through the imaging procedure and assisting in the PACS/RIS read by the radiologist. The RA must be well versed in PACS/RIS and DICOM.

The radiographer is principally engaged in performing the examination on the various imaging modalities. This requires skill in both operating the imaging modality and managing the PACS/RIS electronic data and images. Both the RA and radiographer must be credentialed by the American Registry of Radiologic Technologists.

Using PACS/RIS with digital imaging, the workflow chart is greatly reduced, as is shown in Fig. 25.6. This leads to greatly improved imaging efficiency.

SUMMARY

PACS and several computer-based programs have fundamentally changed the way we perform digital imaging. PACS and RIS have replaced film files, film-file rooms, and film folders. Digital image manipulation has streamlined medical imaging temporarily and accurately.

The adoption of DR at the turn of the 21st century is now complete. All medical imaging is now digital. PACS can be considered the digital format for image acquisition, image display, image storage, and retrieval. The entire process is more effective and increasingly more accurate.

CHALLENGE QUESTIONS

1. Define or otherwise identify the following:
   a. Network
   b. EMR
   c. Protocol worklist
   d. Header metadata
   e. Imaging ontology
   f. Coder
   g. Imaging lexicon
   h. Imaging modality worklist
   i. HIS
   j. Teleradiology
2. Describe the interaction of the various imaging modes provided by PACS.
3. What electronic stations are visited by an image traveling from radiographer to radiologist?
4. Identify three advantages of combining PACS with digital images.
5. What is included in the DICOM header metadata?
6. Approximately how many MB are required for a nuclear medicine examination report?
7. What is the ACR-AAPM-SIIM technical standard?
8. The next generation of computer technology will involve new terminology based on what new computer science?
9. Which station of the digital medical record deals with image manipulation and document storage?
10. Approximately how many CPT codes does a coder use?
11. How are ACR-NEMA-DICOM connected?
12. What is a network client?
13. There are four principal components of PACS. What are they?
14. During the 20th century, one responsibility of the radiographer was to hang films on the viewbox for interpretation by the radiologist. What analogous responsibility does the radiographer have today?
15. When did the first digital image modality appear, and what is it?
16. Approximately how many MB are required for a mammography examination?
17. List medical image size by modality from smallest to largest.
18. How many digital medical imaging programs can you recall? What are their acronyms?
19. The phrase "Integrating the Healthcare Enterprise" carries what meaning?
20. What imaging modes are necessary for teleradiology?

The answers to the Challenge Questions can be found by logging on to our website at http://evolve.elsevier.com.

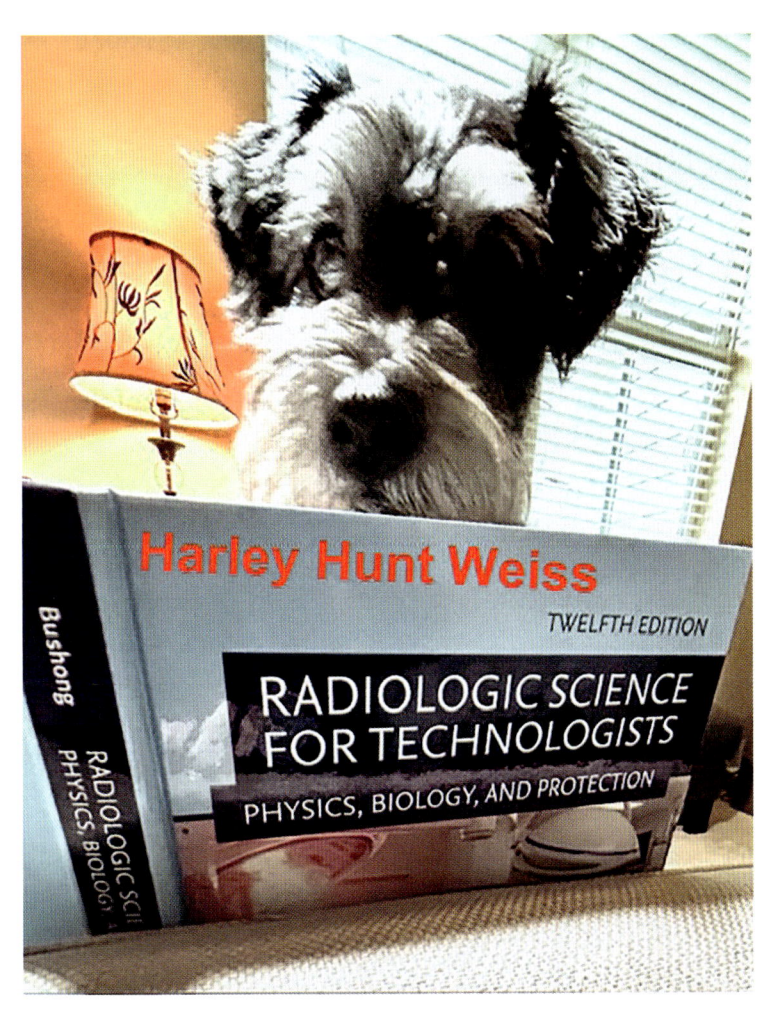

CHAPTER 26

Digital Display Device

OBJECTIVES

At the completion of this chapter, the student should be able to do the following:

1. Describe various factors associated with the performance of digital display devices.
2. Identify AAPM TG 18 and its importance to the radiographer.
3. Explain the various test patterns suggested by AAPM TG 18 on digital display device performance assessment.
4. Connect the concept of luminance to grayscale to *P*-values.
5. Discuss the quality control tests and schedule used for digital display devices.

OUTLINE

Performance Assessment Standards 369
   SMPTE 369
   NEMA-DICOM 369
   DIN 2001 369
   VESA 369
   AAPM TG 18 370
Luminance Meter 370
Digital Display Device Quality Control 371
   Geometric Distortion 371
   Reflection 372
   Luminance Response 372
   Display Spatial Resolution 374
   Display Noise 374
Quality Control by the Radiographer 374
Summary 375
Challenge Questions 376

WITH THE advent of digital imaging, the scope of quality control (QC) protocols has expanded beyond the previous areas of medical imaging with screen-film radiographic image receptors. QC procedures for the support of screen-film radiographic imaging were directed to wet chemistry processors, screens, and film view boxes.

The QC requirements for digital imaging involves the reading environment and the digital imaging display device.

In the current radiology reading room, multiple digital display devices are carefully positioned for image review and interpretation. Any malfunctioning component in the digital display device can produce image degradation that can simulate or obscure disease or abnormality. To ensure proper functioning of digital display devices, it is essential that a comprehensive QC program be implemented under the supervision of a qualified medical physicist with the daily assistance of a QC radiographer.

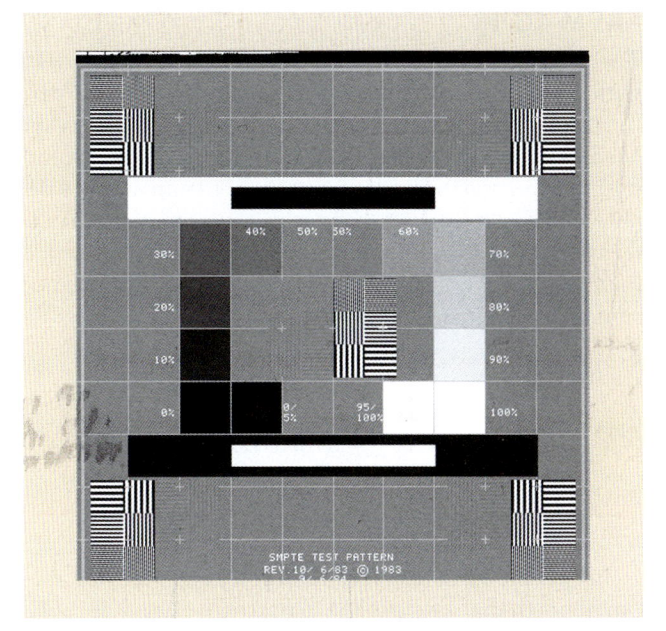

FIG. 26.1 The SMPTE pattern was developed by the Society of Motion Picture and Television Engineers.

PERFORMANCE ASSESSMENT STANDARDS

Assessing the performance of digital display devices requires that we have some understanding of the field of photometry. This was covered in Chapter 24, where an additional system of units was introduced and described.

Numerous initiatives have been developed to standardize soft copy digital display device performance standards.

SMPTE

The Society of Motion Picture and Television Engineers (SMPTE) has described the format, dimensions, and contrast characteristics of a pattern used to make measurements of the resolution of display systems. One outcome of these performance recommendations is what is commonly referred to as the SMPTE pattern (Fig. 26.1).

Among other characteristics that the SMPTE pattern provides, the most common is the observation of 5% and 95% luminance patches. This helps to point out any gross deviations in luminance adjustments. We will deal with luminance again later in this chapter.

NEMA-DICOM

The American College of Radiology (ACR) and the National Electrical Manufacturers Association (NEMA) formed a committee that generated a standard for Digital Imaging and Communication in Medicine that is referred to as the DICOM standard. They presented their work as a document known as the Grayscale Display Function (GSDF). The intent of this standard was to allow digital images which were transferred according to the DICOM standard to be displayed on any DICOM-compatible digital display device with a consistent grayscale appearance.

The consistent appearance was achieved in keeping with the principle of perceptual linearization, wherein equal changes in digital values associated with an image translate into equal changes in perceived brightness on the display. GSDF is currently mandated for all digital display devices.

DIN 2001

In 2001 the German standards institution, Deutsches Institut für Normung (DIN), published a document titled "Image Quality Assurance in X-Ray Diagnostics; Acceptance Testing for Image Display Devices" (DIN 2001). DIN 2001 was developed as an acceptance testing standard to address the requirements for digital display devices. It called for joint performance evaluation of the imaging modality and the digital display device.

VESA

In 1998 the Flat Panel Display Measurement standard, version 1.0, was released by the Video Electronics Standard Association (VESA). This standard provides a set of instructions that can be used to help in the evaluation of system performance according to a compliance standard.

AAPM TG 18

To evaluate a digital display device comprehensively with the goal of ensuring acceptable clinical performance, the American Association of Physicists in Medicine (AAPM) developed a set of test patterns and outlined related procedures in Task Group Report 18 (TG 18). The following sections explain the various patterns recommended by the AAPM along with prescribed methods for use. TG 18 is currently the performance standard recognized worldwide.

> AAPM TG 18 measurements and observations should be routinely instituted for all digital display devices.

In its standards for teleradiology, the ACR has recommended that the AAPM patterns be used for QC purposes as well. Most digital imaging equipment vendors provide the patterns in a format such that they can be displayed on the digital display device for evaluation purposes.

Particular emphasis is placed on the details of associated patterns that can be used by a radiographer to perform checks to ensure proper system performance. We begin with an introduction to the test tools that are used by medical physicists for comprehensive testing of digital display devices. The QC radiographer is responsible for frequent and regular assessment of digital display devices with the use of the AAPM TG 18 QC test pattern.

LUMINANCE METER

Recall from Chapter 24 that luminance is a measure of the brightness of a digital display device expressed in units of candela per square meter (cd/m^2). A typical display device has a luminance of 50 to 300 cd/m^2.

> Luminance is the measure of the brightness of a digital display device.

Luminance should not be confused with illuminance, which is a measure of how much light is incident on a surface. Illuminance is measured in lumens per square meter (l/m^2) or **lux**. Table 26.1 shows various levels of illuminance.

> Illuminance is the measure of the intensity of light incident on a surface.

TABLE 26.1 Illuminance Levels

Full moon	1 lux
Reading room	10 lux
Hallway	200 lux
Waiting room	300 lux
Tennis court	2000 lux
Cloudy day	10,000 lux
Surgery	30,000 lux
Sunny day	100,000 lux

The luminance response of digital display devices and luminance uniformity measurements require the use of a properly calibrated **photometer**. Two types of photometers are commonly used: near-range and telescopic photometers.

> Photometric evaluation of digital display devices and ambient light levels is essential to digital image QC.

Near-range photometers (Fig. 26.2) are used in close proximity to digital display devices; telescopic photometers are used to test from a distance of 1 m.

The response from the two types of photometers may be slightly different, depending on the contribution made by stray sources of light. However, the readings from both types are acceptable as long as measurements are performed in a consistent manner. Contributions from ambient light should be kept constant when either photometer is used.

The luminance meter should use a calibration method that is traceable to the National Institute of Standards and Technology (NIST) and should be able to measure luminance in the range of 0.05 to 1000 cd/m^2 with better than 5% accuracy and a precision of at least 0.01. The photometer also should comply with the Commission Internationale de l'Éclairage (CIE) standard photopic spectral response within a range of 3%.

To evaluate digital display device reflection and to assess ambient light conditions, an **illuminance meter**, or lux meter, is used. The illuminance meter should be calibrated according to NIST standards; response to better than 5% at a 50-degree angulation should be required.

It is important to quantify the color tint of various grayscale displays to match multiple digital display devices that may be used at a single workstation. **Colorimeters** are used to measure CIE-specified color coordinates of a digital display device. These are available in near-range and telescopic styles.

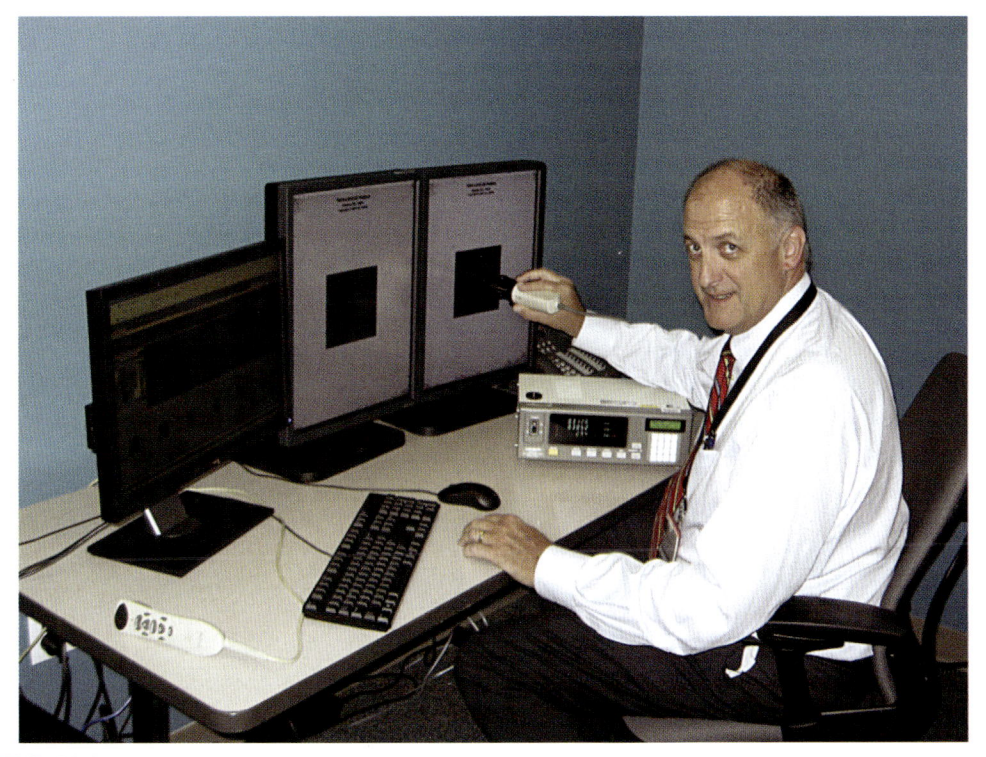

FIG. 26.2 Use of a near-range photometer during digital display device evaluation. (Courtesy John Hazle, MD Anderson Cancer Center.)

DIGITAL DISPLAY DEVICE QUALITY CONTROL

To carefully evaluate the comprehensive characteristics of the digital display device, a range of tests are performed. For most of these, AAPM TG 18 patterns are used to perform qualitative and quantitative tests. For a few tests, no test patterns are required.

Geometric Distortion

Geometric distortion arises from problems that cause the displayed image to be geometrically different from the original image. This can affect the relative size and shape of image features.

Visual assessment of geometric distortion can be carried out with the use of TG 18 QC (Fig. 26.3) and TG 18 LPV/LPH test patterns. By filling the entire screen with the test pattern, one can look for pincushion and barrel-like distortions. These types of distortions are common in cathode ray tube-based display devices but rare in digital display devices. All lines in the pattern should generally appear straight.

By measuring distances in the square areas of the pattern with the help of a flexible plastic ruler, one can quantify the level of distortion in the images. Measurements are performed in various quadrants to look at variations in geometric distortion in different areas of the digital display device.

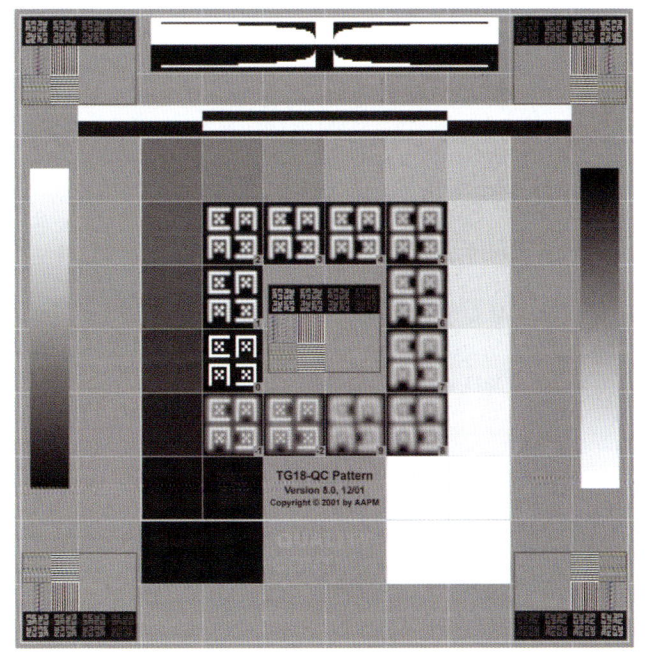

FIG. 26.3 AAPM TG 18 QC test pattern.

With primary class devices, the acceptable level of distortion in various quadrants in either direction is 2%. The corresponding criterion for secondary class devices is 5%.

Reflection

An ideal digital display device has a luminance that is based on the light generated only by the device itself. In reality, the ambient light significantly contributes to the light reflected by the digital display device, which in turn depends on the reflection characteristics of the digital display device. It is important to understand these reflection characteristics of the digital display device.

Usually, the digital display device reflection is characterized as **specular** and **diffuse**. Specular reflection results in the generation of mirror images of light sources surrounding the digital display device. In diffuse reflection, light is randomly scattered on the digital display device.

> Reflection from a digital display device appears as specular or diffuse.

A simple test to assess specular reflection is to simply turn off the digital display device and look for sources of illumination within a 15-degree angle of observation at an approximate distance of 30 to 50 cm. Look for images of various light sources and any high-contrast patterns from the viewers' clothing or surroundings. Digital display devices (see Fig. 26.4) exhibit very little reflection. That is why such viewing is now the norm.

The TG 18 AD pattern (Fig. 26.5) consists of uniformly varying low-contrast patterns. To evaluate diffuse reflection, one has to observe the threshold of visibility for low-contrast patterns under ambient lighting conditions and in total darkness. Under both conditions, the threshold of visibility should be the same. If the ambient lighting changes the threshold, then the ambient lighting should be reduced.

Luminance Response

The image acquired by a digital imaging modality is stored as an array of pixel values. These pixel values are also called **grayscale values**, and they are sent to a digital display device as presentation values or **P-values**.

The *P*-values then are transformed into digital driving levels (DDLs) that then are transformed into luminance values through a look-up table (LUT). Transformation of presentation values to DDLs is performed according to the DICOM standard, which ensures that when these DDLs are displayed as luminance levels, corresponding equal changes in perceived brightness correspond to equal changes in *P*-values.

> Digital image data arrive at the digital display device as *P*-values transformed into digital driving levels and viewed as luminance levels.

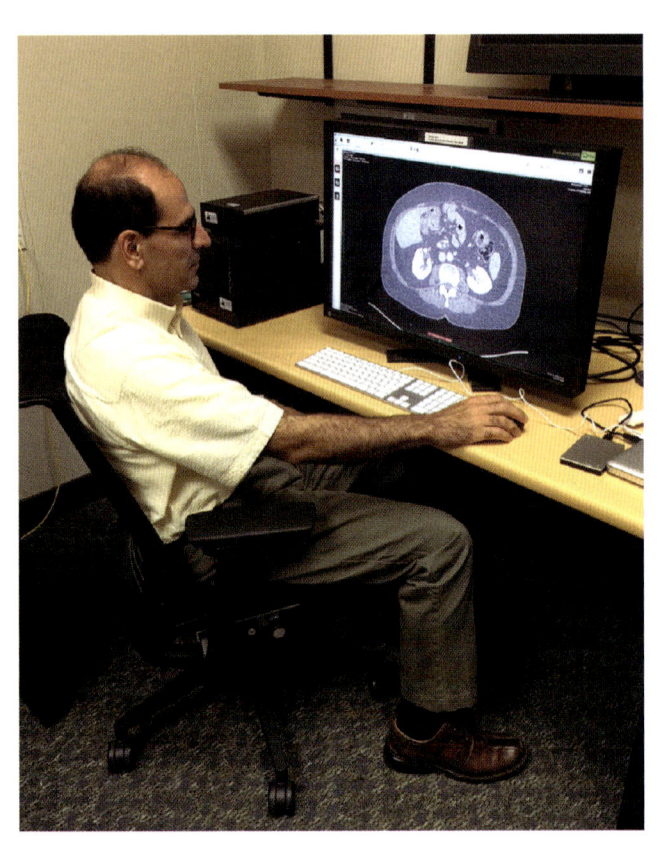

FIG. 26.4 Even in a well-lit reading area (not recommended), there is little reflection, diffuse or specular, from a medical image display device. (Courtesy Ehsan Samei, Duke University, North Carolina.)

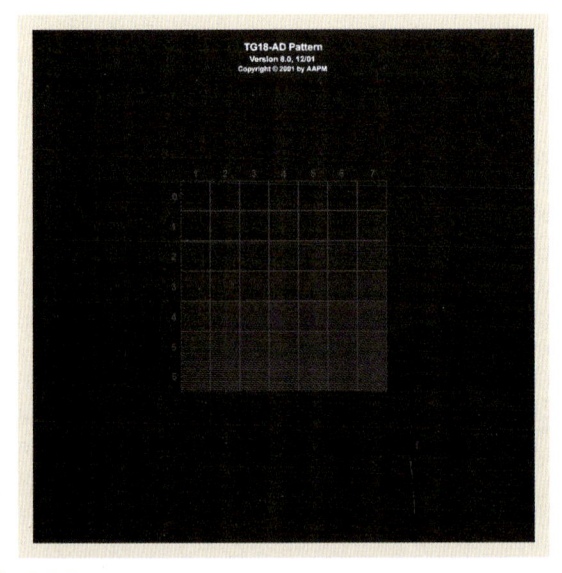

FIG. 26.5 AAPM TG 18 AD pattern used for evaluating diffuse reflection.

The luminance response of a digital display device refers to the relationship between displayed luminance and input values of a standardized display system. Displayed luminance consists of light produced by the digital display device; it varies between L_{min} and L_{max} and receives a fixed contribution from diffusely reflected ambient light, L_{amb}.

The TG 18 CT test pattern (Fig. 26.6) is used to perform a qualitative evaluation of the luminance response of a digital display device. This pattern has low-contrast targets that should be visible in all 16 regions of the pattern. The pattern should be evaluated from a distance of approximately 30 cm. A common failure is the inability to see targets in one or two of the dark regions.

With the use of an external photometer and TG 18 LN test patterns (Fig. 26.7), the luminance in the test region should be recorded for the 18 DDLs. Ambient lighting conditions should be reduced to minimum levels. The maximum luminance value should be greater than 171 cd/m^2. Maximum luminance values should be verified against the manufacturer's quoted value.

The luminance response of a digital display device varies as a function of location on the display surface. The contrast behavior is a function of the viewing angle as well. The maximum variation of luminance across the display area when a uniform pattern is displayed is referred to as **luminance nonuniformity**.

The TG 18 UN test patterns (Fig. 26.8) can be used for visual evaluation of nonuniformity. By observing the patterns across the display screen, one can observe any gross variations in uniformity. No luminance variations with dimensions on the order of 1 cm or larger should be observed.

For qualitative or visual assessment of angular dependence, the TG 18 CT test pattern is used. By first observing the half-moon targets straight on-axis and then comparing them with viewing angles in which the visibility of half-moon targets is altered, one can gain an understanding of viewing angle dependency of a particular digital display device.

> The best image viewing is straight on.

The viewing angle within which the digital display device shows no variation in viewed patterns will define a conelike region and is the region in which the display device should be viewed clinically. Established viewing angle limits may be clearly labeled on the front of the digital display device. For multiple light-emitting diode monitor workstations, displays should be adjusted in such a way that each display optimally faces the user.

For quantitative evaluation of luminance uniformity, one measures the luminance in different regions of TG

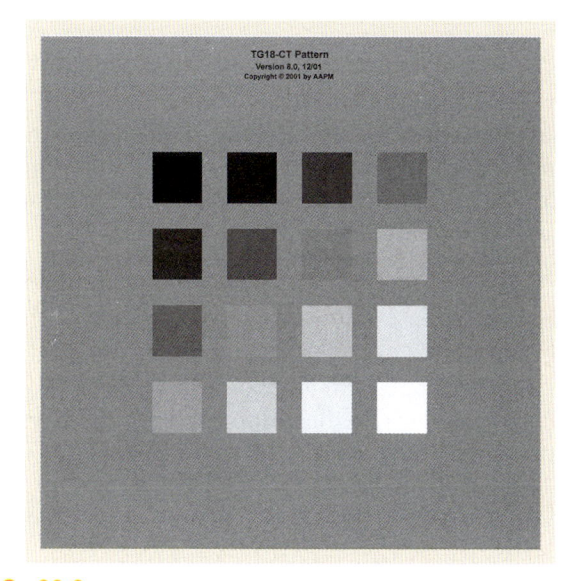

FIG. 26.6 AAPM TG 18 CT pattern with half-16 area of half-moon targets.

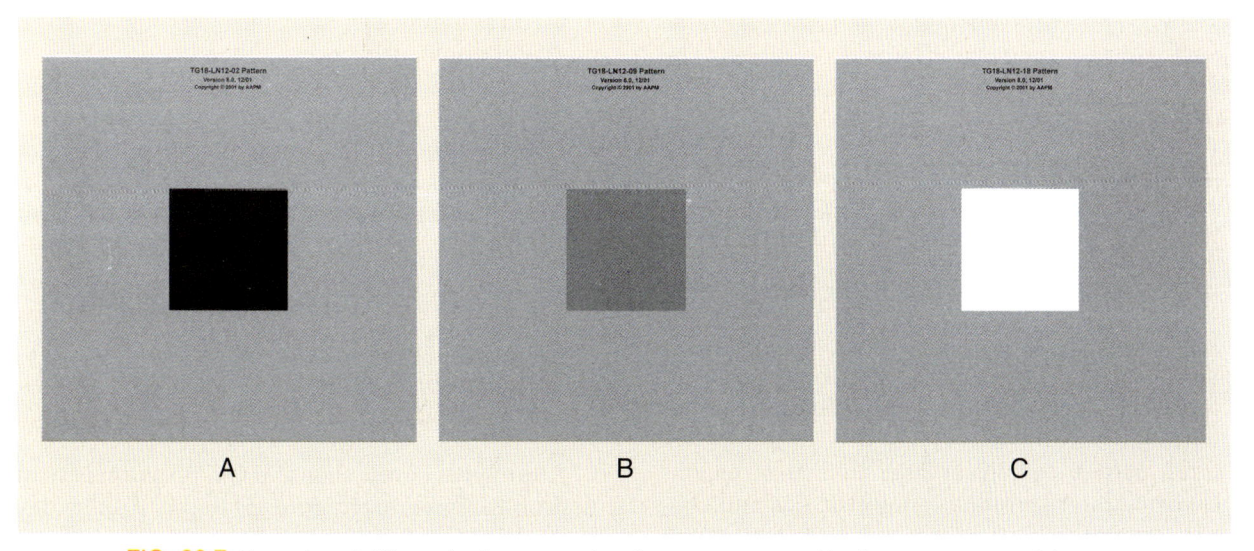

FIG. 26.7 Examples of different luminance patches for measurement of luminance response of the system, using AAPM TG 18 LN test patterns.

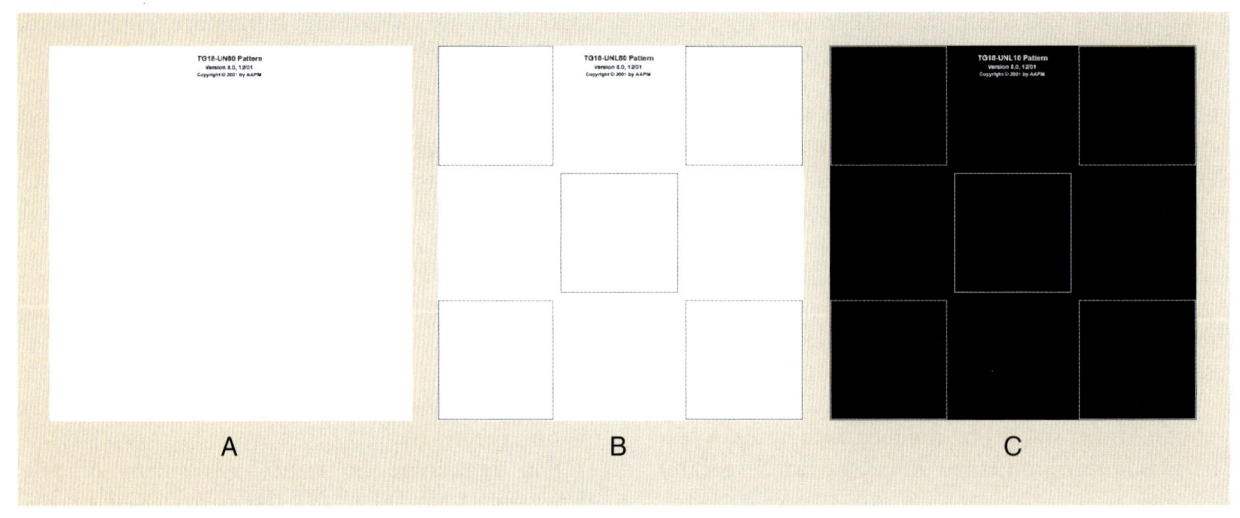

FIG. 26.8 AAPM TG 18 UN and TG 18 UNL patterns for luminance uniformity assessment.

18 UNL10 and TG 18 UNL80 patterns with an external photometer. Luminance is measured at five different locations of the digital display device.

Maximum deviation in uniformity is calculated as the percentage of difference between maximum and minimum luminance values relative to their average value as follows:

$$200 \times (L_{max} - L_{min})/(L_{max} + L_{min})$$

Maximum nonuniformity for an individual digital display device should be less than 30%.

Display Spatial Resolution

Spatial resolution is the quantitative measure of the ability of the digital display device to produce separable images of different points of an object with high fidelity.

TG 18 CX (Fig. 26.9) and TG 18 QC (see Fig. 26.5) patterns can be used to evaluate display spatial resolution. The CX patterns in the middle and corners can be evaluated with a magnifying glass and compared. The TG 18 PX (Fig. 26.10) pattern can be used to evaluate spatial resolution uniformity.

Display Noise

Noise in an image, along with image contrast and size, is an important factor in determining the visibility of an object. Any high-frequency fluctuations or patterns that interfere with detection of the true signal are classified as noise. Noise can be quantified with the TG 18 AFC test pattern (Fig. 26.11), which is based on the method used to determine just noticeable luminance difference as a function of size.

The test pattern contains a large number of regions with changing target positions. However, size and contrast are constant in four of the quadrants into which the pattern is subdivided.

In addition to all the AAPM TG 18 patterns that have been described here, other patterns are designed to evaluate characteristics such as veiling glare and display chromaticity. In addition, several reference anatomic images, such as the digital chest image shown in Fig. 26.12, are available for overall digital display system evaluation.

QUALITY CONTROL BY THE RADIOGRAPHER

The digital display device QC described in this chapter is principally the responsibility of the medical physicist. However, QC radiographers should learn how to acquire the TG 18 QC test pattern (see Fig. 26.5) and use it on each digital display device regularly.

To ensure proper operation of each digital display device, it is important to develop a continuous QC program. This should include the following:

- Medical physicist's acceptance testing of any new digital display devices
- Routine QC tests by the QC radiographer using the TG 18 QC test pattern
- Periodic review of QC program by a qualified medical physicist
- Annual and postrepair medical physics performance evaluations

> The AAPM Task Group Report 18 (TG 18) QC test pattern should be viewed regularly.

Although a comprehensive QC program is strongly desirable, regular evaluation of digital display devices with the TG 18 QC test pattern is important and takes just a few minutes. QC records are essential. A quick review of the pattern should give the radiographer an idea about any gross changes in system

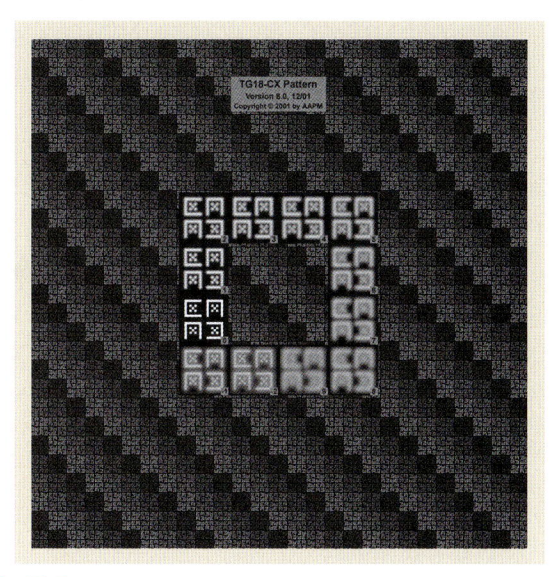

CHAPTER 26 Digital Display Device   375

FIG. 26.9 AAPM TG 18 CX pattern for display resolution evaluation.

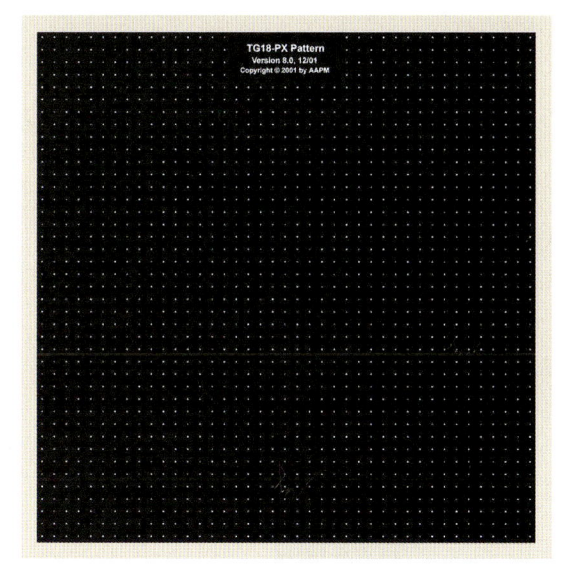

FIG. 26.10 AAPM TG 18 PX pattern for resolution uniformity evaluation. TG 18 CX pattern shows equidistant white dots marked in horizontally and vertically on a black background.

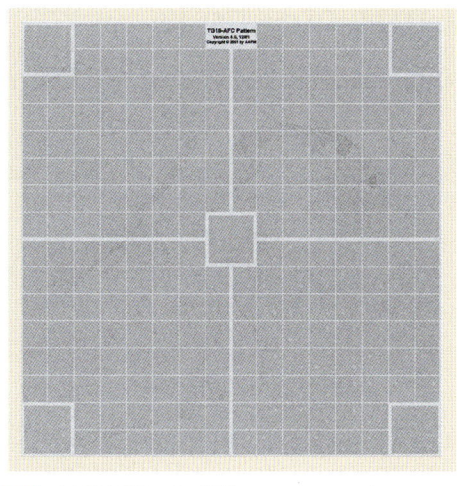

FIG. 26.11 AAPM TG 18 AFC pattern used to assess digital display device noise.

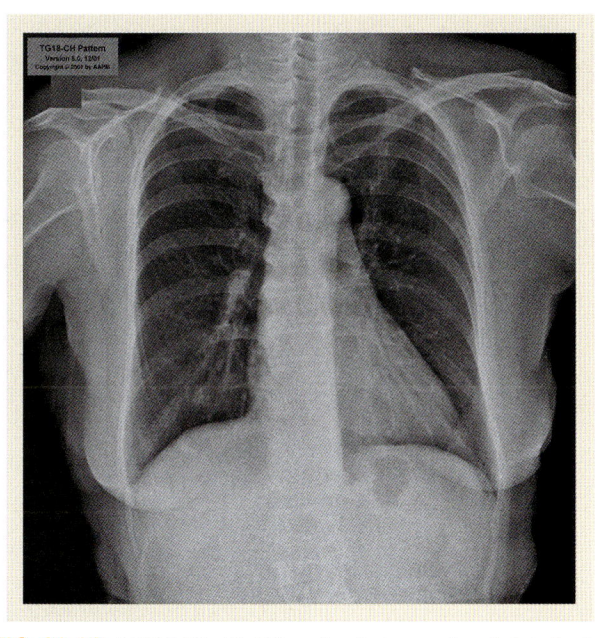

FIG 26.12 AAPM TG 18-CH anatomic image for digital display device evaluation.

performance. For example, a change in contrast detail of "QUALITY CONTROL" letters may be indicative of a malfunctioning system; this may necessitate further testing by a medical physicist and the engineering staff.

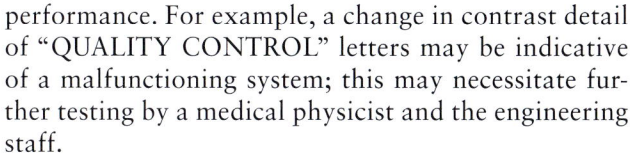

All of the performance assessment evaluations described in this chapter are under significant reduction in time and effort by radiologists, radiographers, and medical physicists through the application of artificial intelligence (AI). AI application is improving digital display device performance assessment. Chapter 28 discusses this further.

SUMMARY

Several national and international scientific organizations have published protocols that are based on electronic test patterns for assessing the quality of a digital display device. Assessment requires visual interpretation of a test pattern and photometric measurement of emitted light intensity and stray light intensity.

A spatial electronic display pattern should be used for the evaluation of various digital display device characteristics. The AAPM TG 18 QC test pattern should be used regularly for overall digital display device evaluation.

376 PART V Medical Image Display

CHALLENGE QUESTIONS

1. Define or otherwise identify the following:
   a. SMPTE pattern
   b. Specular reflection
   c. GSDF
   d. cd/m^2
   e. Veiling glare
   f. Presentation value
   g. VESA
   h. AAPM TG 18
   i. NIST
   j. Pincushion distortion
2. Which AAPM TG 18 test pattern is used to evaluate diffuse reflection, and how does the pattern appear?
3. What type of device is used to evaluate diffuse reflection?
4. What are the time requirements on radiographer QC of a digital display device?
5. Which TG 18 test pattern is used to evaluate digital display resolution, and how does the pattern appear?
6. What luminance range should be measurable?
7. What does L_{amb} represent, and what is its preferred value?
8. Which AAPM TG 18 test pattern is used to evaluate digital display device noise, and how does it appear?
9. What is the principle of perceptual linearization?
10. When should a medical physicist perform digital display device quality control?
11. What AAPM TG 18 test pattern is used to evaluate contrast resolution of a digital display device, and how does it appear?
12. What is threshold of visibility?
13. What are the standard descriptions for digital display devices?
14. What is digital display device noise?
15. Which AAPM TG 18 test pattern is used for luminance uniformity assessment, and how does it appear?
16. What is the approximate illumination level in your kitchen?
17. What is the purpose of the GSDF = Grayscale Display Function?
18. An instrument called a photometer is used for what purpose in digital imaging?
19. Explain the difference between luminance and illuminance.
20. SMPTE is the acronym for what organization?

The answers to the Challenge Questions can be found by logging on to our website at http://evolve.elsevier.com.

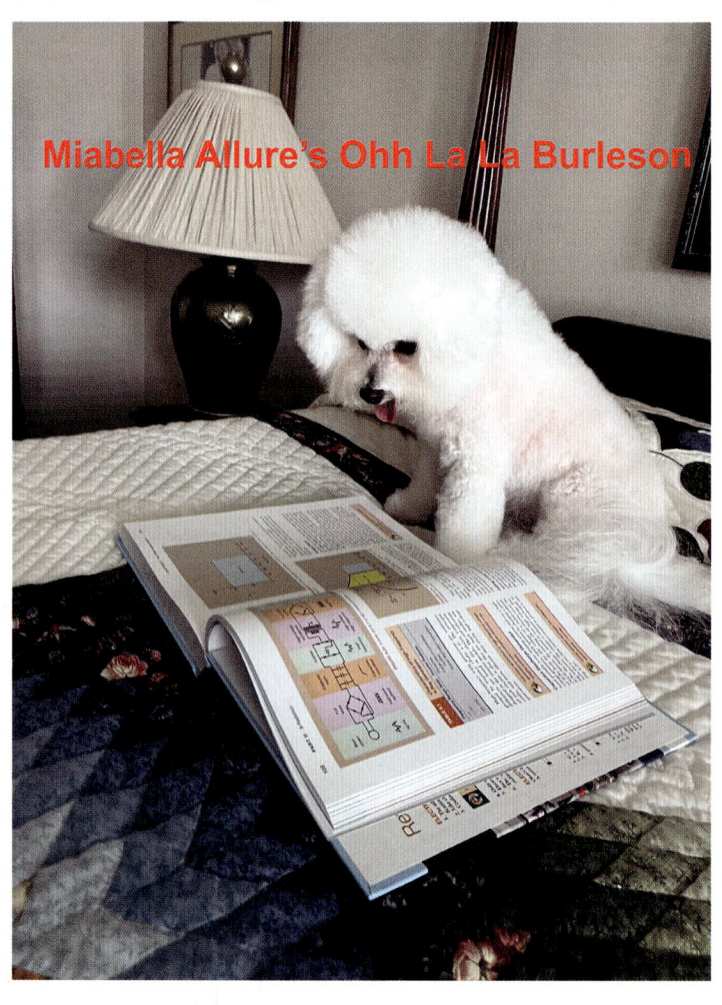

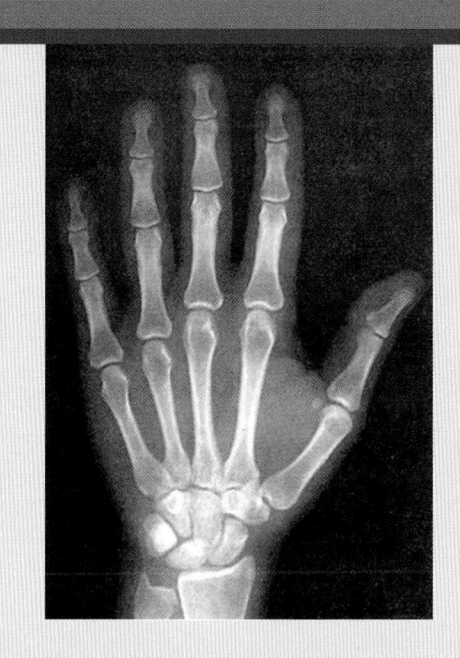

PART VI

THE MEDICAL IMAGE

CHAPTER 27

Imaging Science

OBJECTIVES

At the completion of this chapter, the student should be able to do the following:

1. Discuss the history of computers and the role of the transistor and microprocessor.
2. Define bit, byte, and word as used in computer terminology.
3. List and explain various computer languages.
4. Contrast the two classifications of computer programs, systems software, and applications programs.
5. List and define the components of computer hardware.

OUTLINE

History of Computers 379
Computer Architecture 380
   Computer Language 380
   Components 386
Applications to Digital Imaging 390

The Cloud 390
Teleradiology 390
Summary 393
Challenge Questions 393

TODAY, THE word **computer** primarily refers to the personal computer (PC), which is responsible for the current explosion in computer applications. In addition to scientific, engineering, and business applications, the computer has become evident in everyday life. For example, we know that computers are involved in video games, automatic teller machines, and highway toll systems. Other everyday uses include supermarket checkouts, ticket reservation centers, industrial processes, smartphones, tablets, traffic lights, and automobile ignition and guidance systems.

Computer applications in radiology also continue to grow. The first large-scale radiology application was computed tomography (CT) back in the 1970s. Magnetic resonance imaging (MRI), diagnostic ultrasonography, and nuclear medicine imaging use computers similarly to the way CT imaging systems do. Computers control high-voltage x-ray generators and radiographic control panels, making digital fluoroscopy and digital radiography now routine.

Telecommunication systems have provided for the development of teleradiology, which is the transfer of digital images and patient data to remote locations for interpretation. Teleradiology has changed the way human resources are allocated for all digital imaging stages: acquisition, interpretation, and data management. Future applications of **artificial intelligence** (AI) and **quantum computing** will further extend the value of imaging science in all areas of health care.

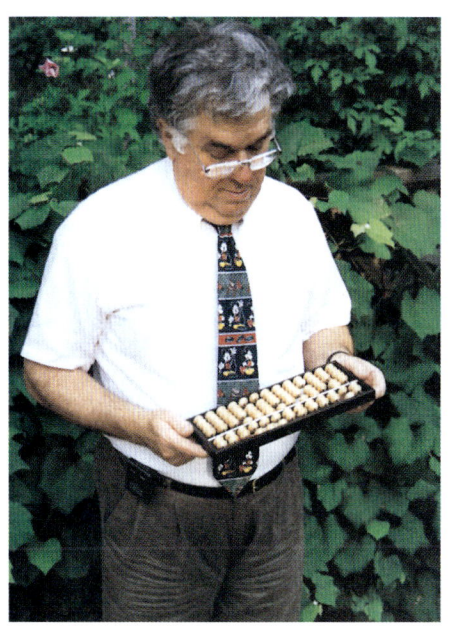

FIG. 27.1 The abacus was the earliest calculating tool. (Courtesy Robert J. Wilson, University of Tennessee.)

> In 1939 John Atansoff and Clifford Berry designed and built the first electronic digital computer.

HISTORY OF COMPUTERS

The earliest calculating tool, the abacus (Fig. 27.1), was invented thousands of years ago in China and is still used in some parts of Asia. In the 17th century, two mathematicians, Blaise Pascal and Gottfried Leibniz, built mechanical calculators using pegged wheels that could perform the four basic arithmetic functions of addition, subtraction, multiplication, and division.

In 1842 Charles Babbage designed an analytic engine that performed general calculations automatically. Herman Hollerith designed a tabulating machine to record census data in 1890. The tabulating machine stored information as holes on cards that were interpreted by machines with electrical sensors. Hollerith's company later grew to become IBM (International Business Machines).

In December of 1943 the British built the first fully operational working computer, called Colossus, which was designed to crack encrypted German military codes. Colossus was very successful, but because of its military significance, it was given the highest of all security classifications, and its existence was known only to relatively few people. That classification remained until 1976, which is why it is rarely acknowledged.

The first general-purpose modern computer was developed in 1944 at Harvard University. Originally called the Automatic Sequence Controlled Calculator (ASCC), it is now known simply as the Mark I. It was an electromechanical device that was exceedingly slow and was prone to malfunction.

The first general-purpose **electronic computer** was developed in 1946 at the University of Pennsylvania by J. Presper Eckert and John Mauchly at a cost of $500,000. This computer, called ENIAC (Electronic Numerical Integrator and Calculator), contained more than 18,000 vacuum tubes that failed at an average rate of once every 7 minutes (Fig. 27.2). Neither the Mark I nor the ENIAC had instructions stored in a memory device.

In 1948 scientists led by William Shockley at the Bell Telephone Laboratories developed the transistor. A transistor is an electronic switch that alternately allows or does not allow electronic signals to pass. It made possible the development of the "stored-program" computer and thus the continuing explosion in computer science.

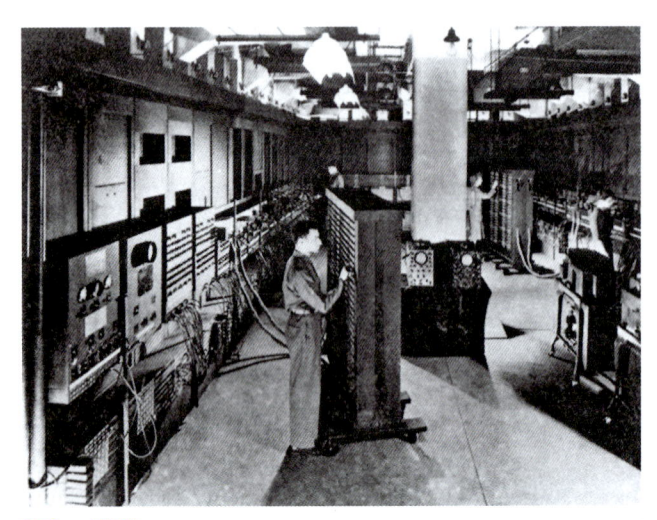

FIG. 27.2 The ENIAC (Electronic Numerical Integrator and Calculator) computer occupied an entire room. It was completed in 1946 and is recognized as the first all-electronic, general-purpose digital computer. (Courtesy Unisys.)

The transistor allowed Eckert and Mauchly of the Sperry-Rand Corporation to develop UNIVAC (UNIVersal Automatic Computer), which appeared in 1951 as the first commercially successful general-purpose, stored program electronic digital computer.

Computers have undergone four generations of development distinguished by the technology of their electronic devices. First-generation computers were vacuum tube devices (1939–58). Second-generation computers, which became generally available in about 1958, were based on individually packaged transistors.

Third-generation computers used integrated circuits (ICs), which consist of many transistors and other electronic elements fused onto a chip, a tiny piece of semiconductor material, usually silicon. These were introduced in 1964. The microprocessor was developed in 1971 by Ted Hoff of Intel Corporation.

The fourth generation of computers, which first appeared in 1975, was an extension of the third generation and incorporated large-scale integration (LSI); this has now been replaced by very large-scale integration, which places millions of circuit elements on a chip that measures less than 1 cm.

> The word computer refers to any general-purpose, stored-program electronic digital computer.

The word computer is currently identified as the PC to most of us and is configured as a desktop, laptop, tablet, or wristwatch.

Decades ago, digital computers replaced analog computers, and the word **digital** is currently almost synonymous with computer. A timeline showing the evolution of computers shows how rapidly this technology is advancing (Fig. 27.3).

The difference between analog and digital is illustrated in Fig. 27.4, which shows two types of watches. An analog watch is mechanical and has hands that move continuously around a dial face. You may never have seen an analog watch. A digital watch contains a computer chip and indicates time with numbers. The smart watch, first introduced by Apple, is actually a very powerful computer which can indicate analog or digital time and many other functions.

> Analog refers to a continuously varying quantity; a digital system uses only two values that vary discretely through coding.

Analog and digital meters are used in many commercial and scientific applications. Digital meters are easier to read and can be more precise. Precision will improve further with the introduction of quantum computers.

COMPUTER ARCHITECTURE

A computer has two principal parts: hardware and software. The **hardware** is everything about the computer that is visible, including the physical components of the system that include the various input and output devices. Hardware usually is categorized according to which operation it performs. Operations include input processing, memory, storage, output, and communications. The **software** consists of the computer programs that tell the hardware what to do and how to store and manipulate data.

Computer Language

To give a computer instruction on how to store and manipulate data, thousands of computer languages have been developed. Higher-level languages typically allow users to input short English-based instructions. All computer languages translate what the user inputs into a series of 1s and 0s, digits, that the computer can understand.

Although the computer can accept and report alphabetic characters and numeric information in the decimal system, it operates in the binary system. In the decimal system, which we normally use, 10 digits (0–9) are used. The word **digit** comes from the Latin for "finger" or "toe." The origin of the decimal system is obvious (Fig. 27.5).

Other number systems have been formulated to many other base values. The duodecimal system, for instance, has 12 digits. It is used to describe the months of the year and the hours in a day and night. Computers operate on the simplest number system of all: the binary number system.

> The binary number system has only two digits: 0 and 1.

CHAPTER 27 Imaging Science   381

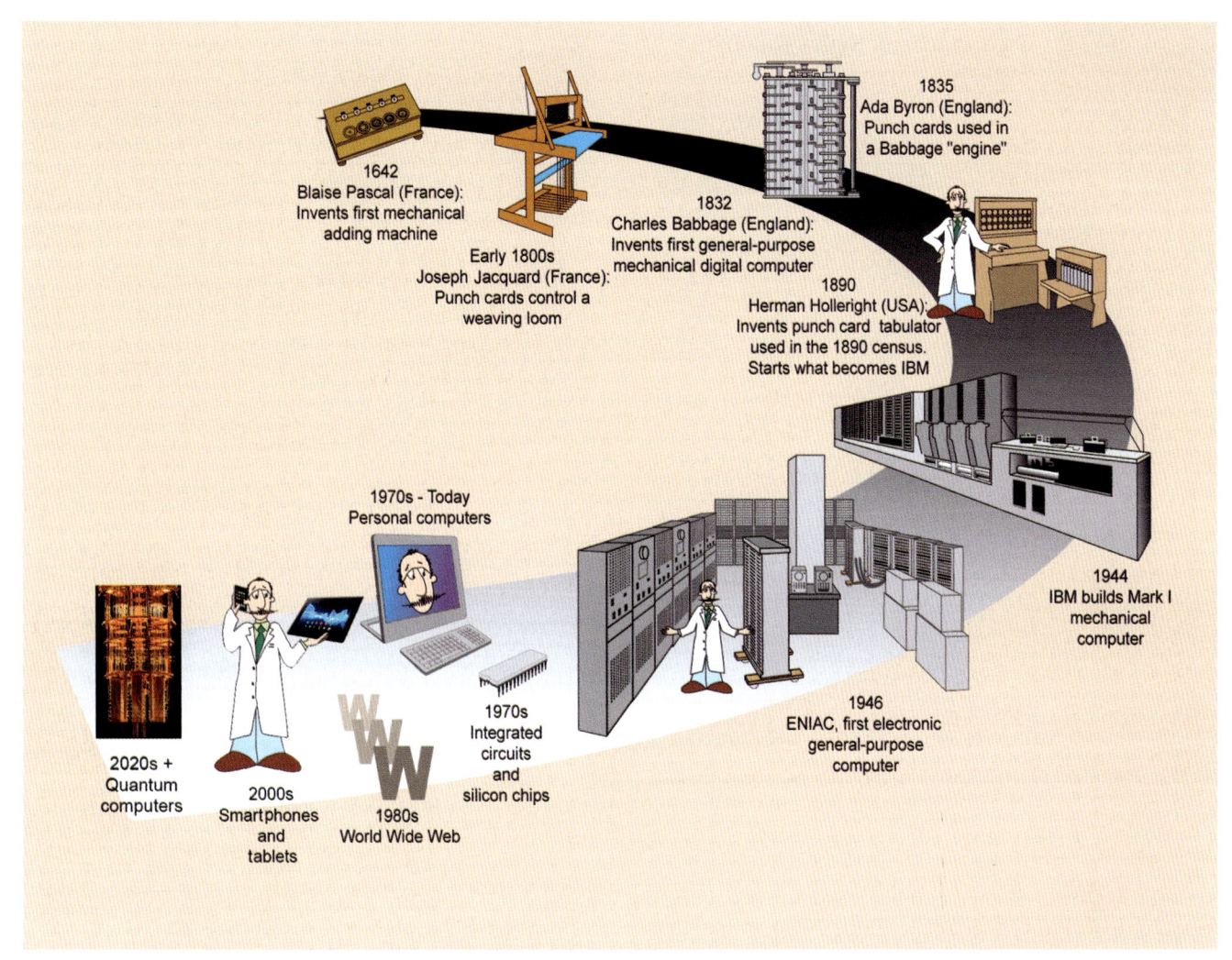

FIG. 27.3 A timeline showing the evolution of current computers. *ENAIC*, Electronic Numerical Integrator and Calculator; *IBM*, International Business Machines.

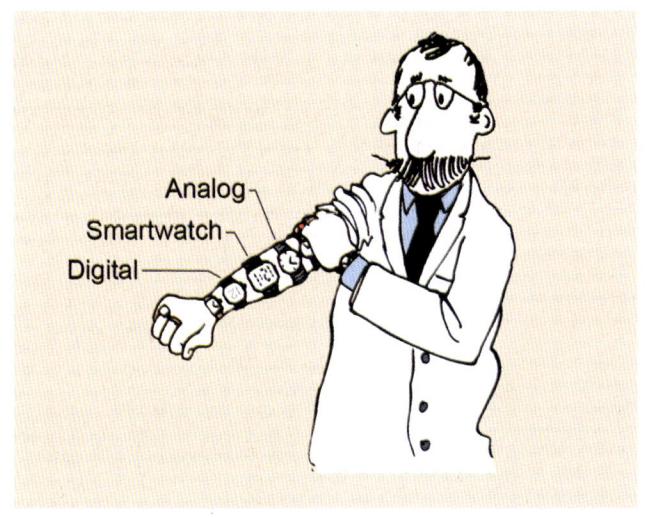

FIG. 27.4 Two styles of wristwatches demonstrate analog versus digital.

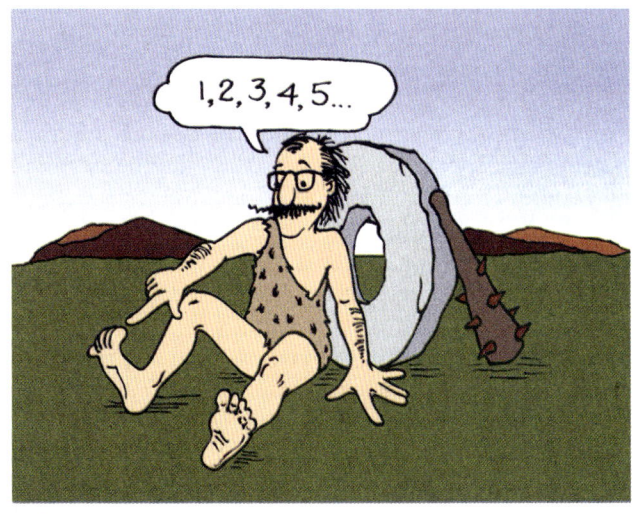

FIG. 27.5 The origin of the decimal number system.

TABLE 27.1 Organization of Binary Number System

Decimal Number	Binary Equivalent	Binary Number
0	0	0
1	2^0	1
2	$2^1 + 0$	10
3	$2^1 + 2^0$	11
4	$2^2 + 0 + 0$	100
5	$2^2 + 0 + 2^0$	101
6	$2^2 + 2^1 + 0$	110
7	$2^2 + 2^1 + 2^0$	111
8	$2^3 + 0 + 0 + 0$	1000
9	$2^3 + 0 + 0 + 2^0$	1001
10	$2^3 + 0 + 2^1 + 0$	1010
11	$2^3 + 0 + 2^1 + 2^0$	1011
12	$2^3 + 2^2 + 0 + 0$	1100
13	$2^3 + 2^2 + 0 + 2^0$	1101
14	$2^3 + 2^2 + 2^1 + 0$	1110
15	$2^3 + 2^2 + 2^1 + 2^1$	1111
16	$2^4 + 0 + 0 + 0 + 0$	10000

TABLE 27.2 Power of Ten, Power of Two, and Binary Notation

Power of Ten	Power of Two	Binary Notation
$10^0 = 1$	$2^0 = 1$	1
$10^1 = 10$	$2^1 = 2$	10
$10^2 = 100$	$2^2 = 4$	100
$10^3 = 1000$	$2^3 = 8$	1000
$10^4 = 10,000$	$2^4 = 16$	10000
$10^5 = 100,000$	$2^5 = 32$	100000
$10^6 = 1,000,000$	$2^6 = 64$	1000000
	$2^7 = 128$	
	$2^8 = 256$	
	$2^9 = 512$	
	$2^{10} = 1024$	
	$2^{12} = 4096$	
	$2^{14} = 16,384$	
	$2^{16} = 65,536$	

Counting in the binary number system starts with 0 to 1 and then counts over again (Table 27.1). It includes only two digits, 0 and 1, and the computer performs all operations by converting alphabetic characters, decimal values, and logic functions to binary values.

Even the computer's instructions are stored in binary form. In this way, although binary numbers may become exceedingly long, computation can be handled by properly adjusting the thousands of flip-flop circuits in the computer.

In the binary number system, 0 is 0 and 1 is 1, but there, the direct relationship with the decimal number system ends. It ends at 1 because the 1 in binary notation comes from 2^0. Recall that any number raised to the zero power is 1; therefore 2^0 is 1.

In binary notation, the decimal number 2 is equal to 2^1 plus 0. This is expressed as 10. The decimal number 3 is equal to 2^1 plus 2^0 or 11 in binary form; 4 is 2^2 plus no 2^1 plus no 2^0 or 100 in binary form. Each time it is necessary to raise 2 to an additional power to express a number, the number of binary digits increases by one.

Just as we know the meaning of the power of 10, it is necessary to recognize the power of 2. Power of 2 notation is used in digital imaging to describe image size, image dynamic range, and image storage capacity. Table 27.2 reviews these power notations. Note the following similarity. In both power notations, the number of 0s to the right of 1 equals the value of the exponent.

Question: Express the number 193 in binary form.

Answer: The number 193 falls between 2^7 and 2^8. Therefore it is expressed as 1 followed by seven binary digits. Simply add the decimal equivalent of each binary digit from left to right:

Yes 2^7 = 1 = 128
Yes 2^6 = 1 = 64
Yes 2^5 = 1 = No 32
No 2^4 = 1 = No 16
No 2^3 = 1 = No 8
No 2^2 = 1 = No 4
No 2^1 = 1 = No 2
Yes 2^0 = 1 = 1
11000001 = 193

Question: What is the decimal value of the binary number 100110011?

Answer: Follow the previous process by first listing the binary number and then computing each power of 2.

1 = 2^8 Yes = 256
0 = 2^7 No = 0
0 = 2^6 No = 0
1 = 2^5 Yes = 32
1 = 2^4 Yes = 16
0 = 2^3 No = 0
0 = 2^2 No = 0
1 = 2^1 Yes = 2
1 = 2^0 Yes = 1
= 307

Digital images are made of discrete **picture elements**, **pixels**, arranged in a matrix. The size of the image is described in the binary number system by power of 2 equivalents. Most radiologic images measure 256 × 256 (2^8) to 1024 × 1024 (2^{10}) for CT and MRI. The 1024 × 1024 matrix is used in digital fluoroscopy. Matrix sizes of 2048 × 2048 (2^{11}) and 4096 × 4096 (2^{12}) are used in digital radiography and digital mammography.

> In computer language, a single binary digit, 0 or 1, is called a **bit**.

The computer uses as many bits as necessary to express a decimal digit, depending on how it is programmed. The 26 characters of the alphabet and other special characters are usually encoded by 8 bits.

Bits are grouped into bunches of eight called **bytes**. Computer capacity is expressed by the number of bytes that can be accommodated. Depending on the microprocessor, a string of 8, 16, 32, or 64 bits is manipulated simultaneously.

> To encode is to translate from ordinary characters to computer-compatible characters, which are binary digits.

One kilobyte (kB) is equal to 1024 bytes. Note that **kilo** is not metric in computer use. Instead, it represents 2^{10}, or 1024. The computers typically used in digital radiologic imaging have capacities measured in gigabytes (GB), where 1 GB = 1 kB × 1 kB × 1 kB = 2^{10} × 2^{10} × 2^{10} = 2^{30} = 1,099,511,627,776 bytes and 1 GB = 1024 MB.

Question: How many bits can be stored on a 64-kB chip?

Answer:
$$\frac{1024 \text{ bits}}{\text{k bytes}} \times 64 \text{ k bytes} \times \frac{8 \text{ bits}}{\text{byte}}$$
$$2^{10} \times 2^6 \times 2^3 = 2^{19} = 524{,}288 \text{ bits}$$

Depending on the computer configuration, 2 bytes usually constitute a **word**. In the case of a 16-bit microprocessor, a word would consist of 16 consecutive bits of information that are interpreted and shuffled about the computer as a unit. Each word of data in memory has its own address. In most computers, a 32-bit or 64-bit word is the standard word length.

The sequence of instructions developed by a software programmer is called a **computer program**. It is useful to distinguish two classifications of computer programs: **application programs** and **systems software**. Application programs are designed to run on a mobile device such as a tablet, phone, or watch. There are currently millions of such software application programs.

Systems software consists of programs that make it easy for the user to operate a computer to its best advantage.

> Computer programs are the software of the computer.

The computer program most closely related to the system hardware is the **operating system**. The operating system is that series of instructions that organizes the course of data through the computer to the solution of a particular problem.

Commands such as "open file" to begin a sequence or "save file" to store some information in secondary memory are typical of operating system commands. MAC-OS and Windows are popular operating systems.

Computers ultimately understand only 0s and 1s. To relieve humans from the task of writing programs in this form, other programs called **assemblers, compilers**, and **interpreters** have been written. These types of software provide a computer language that can be used to communicate between the language of the operating system and everyday language.

An assembler is a computer program that recognizes symbolic instructions such as "subtract (SUB)," "load (LD)," and "print (PT)" and translates them into the corresponding binary code. Assembly is the translation of a program written in symbolic, machine-oriented instructions into machine language instructions.

Compilers and interpreters are computer programs that translate an application program from its high-level language, such as Java, BASIC, C++, or Pascal, into a form that is suitable for the assembler or into a form that is accepted directly by the computer. Interpreters make program development easier because they are interactive. Compiled programs run faster because they create a separate machine language program.

Application programs are those written in a higher-level language expressly to carry out some user function. Most computer programs as we know them are application programs, now known as **apps**. Computer programs that are written by a computer manufacturer, by a software manufacturer, or by the users themselves to guide the computer to perform a specific task are called apps.

> Word, Excel, iTunes, and Spider Solitaire are apps.

Application programs allow users to print mailing lists, complete income tax forms, evaluate financial statements, or reconstruct images from x-ray

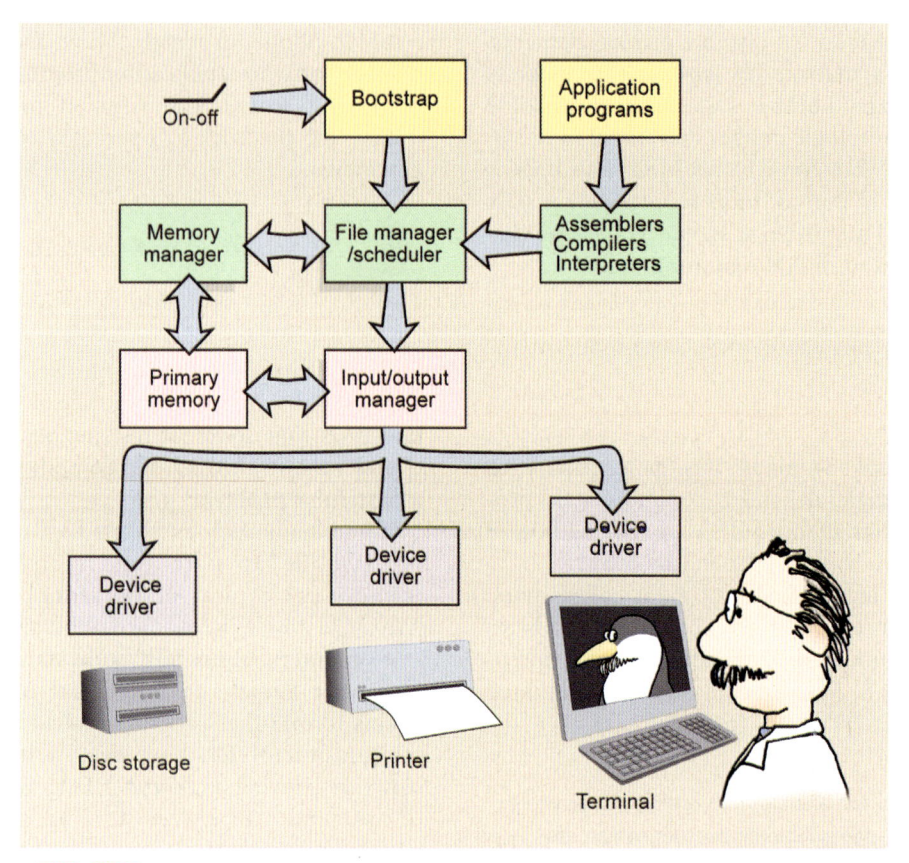

FIG. 27.6 The sequence of software manipulations required to complete an operation.

transmission patterns. They are written in one of many high-level computer languages and then are translated through an interpreter or a compiler into a corresponding machine language program that subsequently is executed by the computer.

The diagram in Fig. 27.6 illustrates the flow of the software instructions from turning the computer on to completing a computation. When the computer is first turned on, a program called a **bootstrap**, frozen permanently in read-only memory (ROM), automatically opens. The bootstrap program is capable of transferring other necessary programs into the computer memory.

The bootstrap program loads the operating system into primary memory, which in turn controls all subsequent operations. A machine language application program likewise can be copied into primary memory, where prescribed operations occur. After completion of the program, results are transferred from primary memory to an output device under the control of the operating system.

> The hexadecimal number system is used by assembly-level applications.

As you have seen, assembly language acts as a midpoint between the computer's binary system and the user's human language instructions. The set of hexadecimal numbers is 0, 1, 2, 3, 4, 5, 6, 7, 8, 9, A, B, C, D, E, and F. Each of these symbols is used to represent a binary number or, more specifically, a set of 4 bits. Therefore because it takes 8 bits to make a byte, a byte can be represented by two hexadecimal numbers. The set of hexadecimal numbers corresponds to the binary numbers for 0 to 15, as is shown in Table 27.3.

High-level programming languages allow the programmer to write instructions in a form that approaches human language, with the use of words, symbols, and decimal numbers rather than the 1s and 0s of machine language. A brief list of the more popular programming languages is given in Table 27.4. With the use of one of these high-level languages, a set of instructions can be written that will be understood by the system software and will be executed by the computer through its operating system.

> The oldest language for scientific, engineering, and mathematical problems is FORTRAN.

FORTRAN (FORmula TRANslation) was the prototype for current algebraic languages, which are oriented toward computational procedures for solving mathematical and statistical problems.

Problems that can be expressed in terms of formulas and equations are called **algorithms**. An algorithm is a step-by-step process used to solve a problem, much in the way a recipe is used to bake a cake, except that the algorithm is more detailed; that is, it would include instructions to remove the egg from the shell. FORTRAN was developed in 1956 by IBM in conjunction with some major computer users.

Developed at Dartmouth College in 1964 as a first language for students, **BASIC** (Beginners All-purpose Symbolic Instruction Code) is an algebraic programming language. It is an easy-to-learn, interpreter-based language. BASIC contains a powerful arithmetic facility, several editing features, a library of common mathematical functions, and simple input and output procedures.

Microsoft developed BASIC into a powerful programming language that can be used for commercial applications and for quick, single-use programs.

One high-level, procedure-oriented language designed for coding business data processing problems is **COBOL** (COmmon Business Oriented Language). A basic characteristic of business data processing is the existence of large files that are updated continuously. COBOL provides extensive file-handling, editing, and report-generating capabilities for the user.

Pascal is a high-level, general-purpose programming language that was developed in 1971 by Nicklaus Wirth of the Federal Institute of Technology at Zürich, Switzerland. A general-purpose programming language is one that can be put to many different applications. Currently, Pascal is the most popular programming language for teaching programming concepts, partly because its syntax is relatively easy to learn and closely resembles that of the English language in usage.

TABLE 27.3 The Hexadecimal Number System

Decimal	Binary	Hexadecimal
0	0000	0
1	0001	1
2	0010	2
3	0011	3
4	0100	4
5	0101	5
6	0110	6
7	0111	7
8	1000	8
9	1001	9
10	1010	A
11	1011	B
12	1100	C
13	1101	D
14	1110	E
15	1111	F

TABLE 27.4 Programming Languages

Language	Date Introduced	Description
FORTRAN	1956	First successful programming language; used for solving engineering and scientific problems
COBOL	1959	Minicomputer and mainframe computer applications in business
ALGOL	1960	Especially useful in high-level mathematics
BASIC	1964	Most frequently used with microcomputers and minicomputers; science, engineering, and business applications
BCPL	1965	Development-stage language
B	1969	Development-stage language
C	1970	Combines the power of assembly language with the ease of use and portability of high-level language
Pascal	1971	High-level, general-purpose language; used for teaching structured programming
ADA	1975	Based on Pascal; used by the US Department of Defense
VisiCalc	1978	First electronic spreadsheet
C++	1980	Response to complexity of C; incorporates object-oriented programming methods
QuickBASIC	1985	Powerful high-level language with advanced user features
Visual C	1992	Visual language programming methods; design environments
Visual BASIC	1993	Visual language programming methods; design environments; advanced user-friendly features

C is considered by many to be the first modern "programmer's language." It was designed, implemented, and developed by real working programmers and reflects the way they approached the job of programming. C is thought of as a middle-level language because it combines elements of high-level languages with the functionality of an assembler (low-level) language. In response to the need to manage greater complexity, C++ was developed by Bjarne Stroustrup in 1980, who initially called it "C with Classes."

When a program exceeds approximately 30,000 lines of code, it becomes so complex that it is difficult to grasp as a single object. Therefore **OOP** (object-oriented programming) is a method of dividing up parts of the program into groups, or objects, with related data and applications, in the same way that a book is broken into chapters and subheadings to make it more readable.

Visual programming languages are more recent languages, and they are under continuing development. They are designed specifically for the creation of Windows applications with minimal effort from the programmer.

In theory, the most inexperienced programmer should be able to create complex programs with visual languages. The idea is to have the programmer design the program in a design environment without ever really writing extensive code. Instead the visual language creates the code to match the programmer's design.

Most spreadsheet and word processing applications offer built-in programming commands called **macros**. These work in the same way as commands in programming languages, and they are used to carry out user-defined functions or a series of functions in the application.

One application that offers a very good library of macro commands is Excel, a spreadsheet program. The user can create a command to manipulate a series of data by performing a specific series of steps.

Other program languages have been developed for other purposes. **LOGO** is a language that was designed for children. **ADA** is the official language approved by the US Department of Defense for software development. It is used principally for military applications and AI. **Java** is a language that was developed in 1995 and has become very useful in web application programming as well as application software. In addition, **HTML** (HyperText Markup Language) is the predominant language used to format web pages.

Components

Central Processing Unit. The central processing unit (CPU) in a computer is the primary element that allows the computer to manipulate data and carry out software instructions. An example of currently available CPUs is the Intel Core vPro. In microcomputers, this is often referred to as the **microprocessor**. The

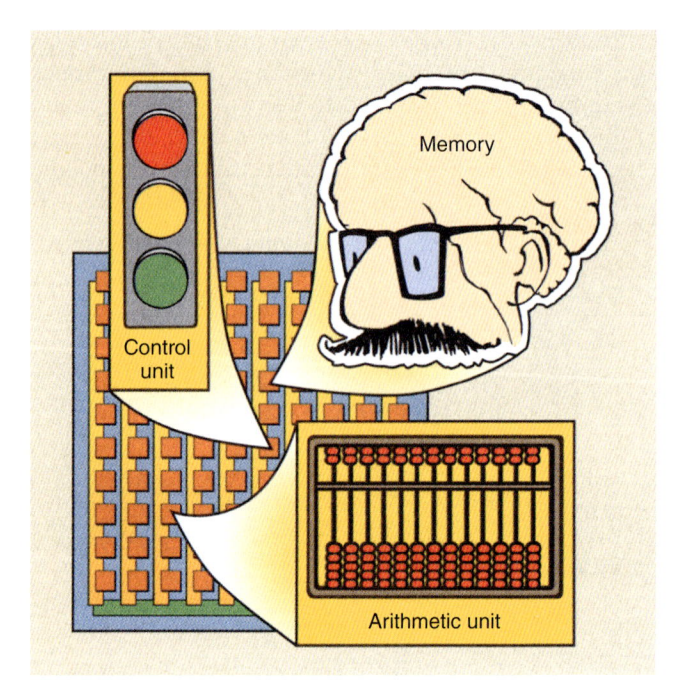

FIG. 27.7 The central processing unit contains a control unit, an arithmetic unit, and sometimes memory.

Pentium microprocessor is manufactured by the Intel Corporation and is designed for large, high-performance, multiuser or multitasking systems.

A computer's CPU consists of a **control unit** and an **arithmetic/logic unit** (ALU). These two components and all other components are connected by an electrical conductor called a **bus** (Fig. 27.7). The control unit tells the computer how to carry out software instructions, which direct the hardware to perform a task. The control unit directs data to the ALU or to memory. It also controls data transfer between the main memory and the input and output hardware (Fig. 27.8).

> The electronic circuitry that does the actual computations and the memory that supports this together are called the *processor*.

The speed of these tasks is determined by an internal system clock. The faster the clock, the faster is the processing. Microcomputer processing speeds usually are defined in megahertz (MHz), where 1 MHz equals 1 million cycles per second. Current microcomputers commonly run at up to several gigahertz (GHz; 1 GHz = 1000 MHz).

Computers typically measure processing speed as **MIPS** (millions of instructions per second). Typical speeds range up to 200,000 MIPS. However, MIPS is an older term that has become obsolete because there is no standard for measuring MIPS. Now many computer scientists say MIPS stands for **M**eaningless **I**ndicator of **P**erformance.

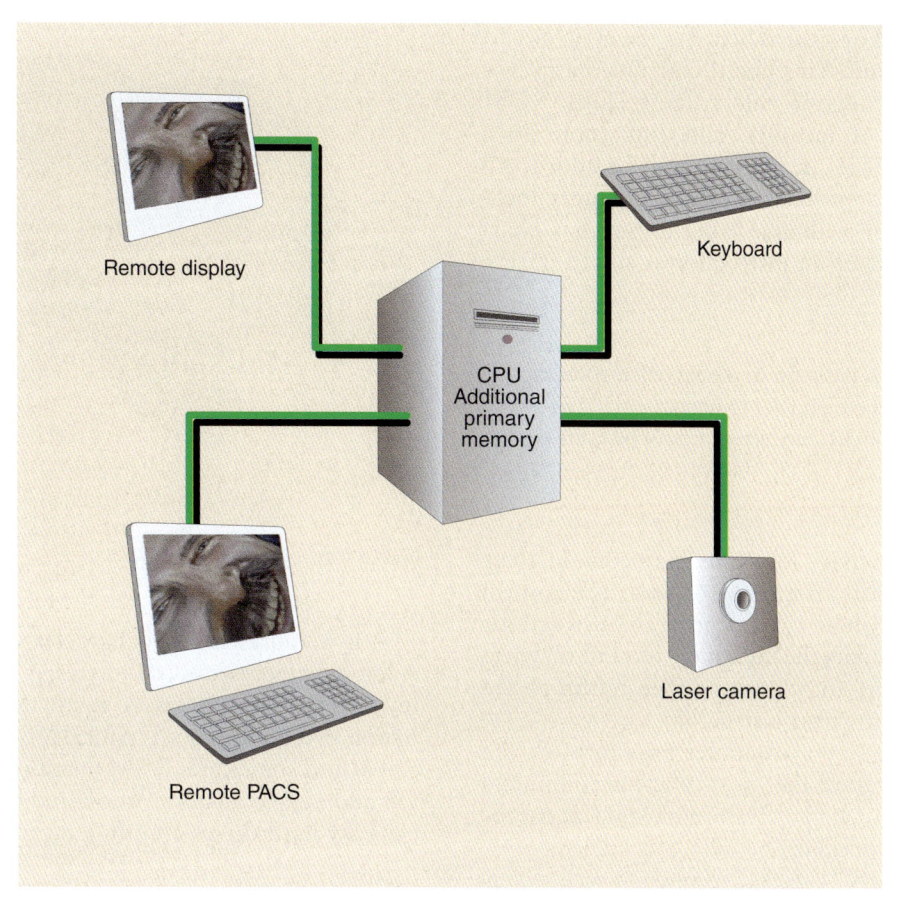

FIG. 27.8 The control unit is a part of the central processing unit (*CPU*) that is directly connected with additional primary memory and various input/output devices. *PACS*, Picture archiving and communication system.

The ALU performs arithmetic or logic calculations, temporarily holds the results until they can be transferred to memory, and controls the speed of these operations. The speed of the ALU is controlled by the system clock.

Primary Memory. Computer memory is distinguished from storage by its function. Memory is more active, whereas storage is more archival. This active storage is referred to as memory, primary storage, internal memory, or random access memory (RAM). **Random access** means data can be stored or accessed at random from anywhere in main memory in approximately equal amounts of time, regardless of where the data are located.

The contents of RAM are temporary, and RAM capacities vary widely in different computer systems. RAM capacity usually is expressed as megabytes (MB), gigabytes (GB), or terabytes (TB), referring to millions, billions, or trillions of characters stored, respectively.

> Main memory is the working storage of a computer.

RAM chips are manufactured with the use of complementary metal-oxide semiconductor (CMOS) technology. These chips are arranged as **single in-line memory modules** (SIMMS).

Special high-speed circuitry areas called **registers** are found in the control unit and the ALU. Registers are contained in the processor that hold information that will be used immediately. Main memory is located outside the processor and holds material that will be used "a little bit later."

ROM chips contain information supplied by the manufacturer, called **firmware** that cannot be written on or erased. One ROM chip contains instructions that tell the processor what to do when the system is first turned on and the bootstrap is initiated. Another ROM chip helps the processor to transfer information among the screen, the printer, and other peripheral devices to ensure that all units are working correctly. These instructions are called ROM BIOS (basic input/output system). ROM is also one of the factors involved in making a "clone" PC; for instance, to be a true Dell clone, a computer must have the same ROM BIOS as a Dell computer.

The motherboard or system board is the main circuit board in a system unit. This board contains the microprocessor, any coprocessor chips, RAM chips, ROM chips, other types of memory, and expansion slots, which allow additional circuit boards to be added. All main memory is addressed; that is, each memory location is designated by a unique label in which a character of data or part of an instruction is stored during processing.

> Each address is similar to a post office address that allows the computer to access data at specific places in memory without disturbing the rest of the memory.

A sequence of memory locations may contain steps of a computer program or a string of data. The control unit keeps track of where current program instructions are stored, which allows the computer to read or write data to other memory locations and then return to the current address for the next instruction.

All data processed by a computer pass through the main memory. Therefore the most efficient computers have enough main memory to store all data and programs needed for processing.

Secondary Memory. Usually, secondary memory is required in the form of compact discs (CDs), digital video discs (DVDs), hard drives, and solid-state storage devices such as flash drives. Secondary memory functions similarly to a filing cabinet; you store information there until you need to retrieve it.

After the appropriate file has been retrieved, it is copied into primary memory, where the user works on it. An old version of the file remains in secondary memory while the copy of the file is being edited or updated. When the user is finished with the file, it is taken out of primary memory and is returned to secondary memory (the filing cabinet), where the updated file replaces the old file.

The word **file** is used to refer to a collection of data or information that is treated as a unit by the computer. Each computer file has a unique name, and PC-based file names have extension names added after a period. For example, .docx is added by a word processing program to files that contain word processing documents (e.g., report.docx).

Common file types are program files, which contain software instructions; data files, which contain data, not programs; image files, which contain digital images; audio files, which contain digitized sound; and video files, which contain digitized video images.

To understand memory, it is necessary to understand the terms used to measure the capacity of memory devices. A **bit** describes the smallest unit of measure, a binary digit 0 or 1. Bits are combined into groups of 8 bits, called a **byte**.

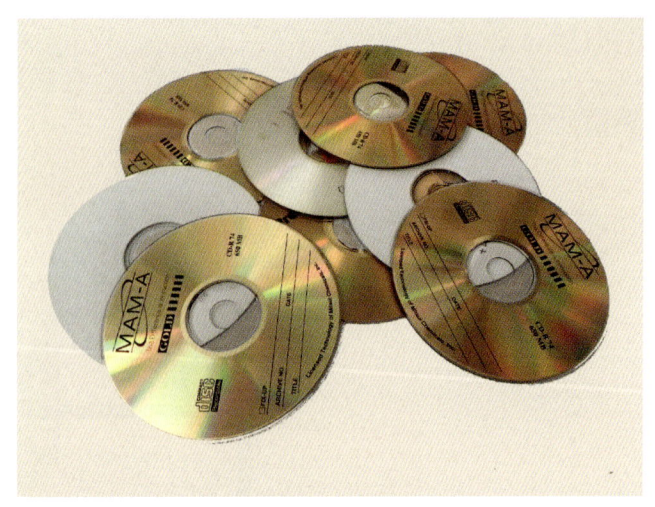

FIG. 27.9 Compact discs can store up to approximately 700 MB of data.

A byte represents one character, digit, or other value. A **kilobyte** represents 1024 bytes. A **megabyte** is approximately 1 million bytes. A **gigabyte** is approximately 1 billion bytes and is used to measure the capacity of hard drives and sometimes RAM memory. A **terabyte** is 1024 GB and approximately 1 thousand billion bytes; higher-capacity hard drives are often measured in terabytes.

> Storage is an archival form of memory.

The most common types of secondary memory are CDs, DVDs, hard drives, flash drives, and cloud-based storage services such as Dropbox, Google Drive, and iCloud Drive. Magnetic tape and the floppy disc are now history.

The CD stores data and programs as tiny indentions or pits on a disc-shaped, flat piece of Mylar plastic. These "pits" are read by a laser while the disc is spinning. The CD is removable from the computer and transferable (Fig. 27.9).

The most common CD is nearly 5 inches in diameter; however, smaller CDs are also available. Data are recorded on a CD in rings called **tracks**, which are invisible, closed concentric rings.

CDs also are defined by their capacity, which ranges to several GB. A **CD drive** is the device that holds, spins, reads data from, and writes data to a CD. DVDs operate in the same manner as CDs but offer higher capacity. These devices are commonly known as optical storage devices.

A flash drive is the smallest, easiest to handle, portable memory device (Fig. 27.10). The flash drive has a capacity of several GB; it connects through a USB port and transfers data rapidly. The drives operate using solid-state technology and are one of the most durable forms of storage.

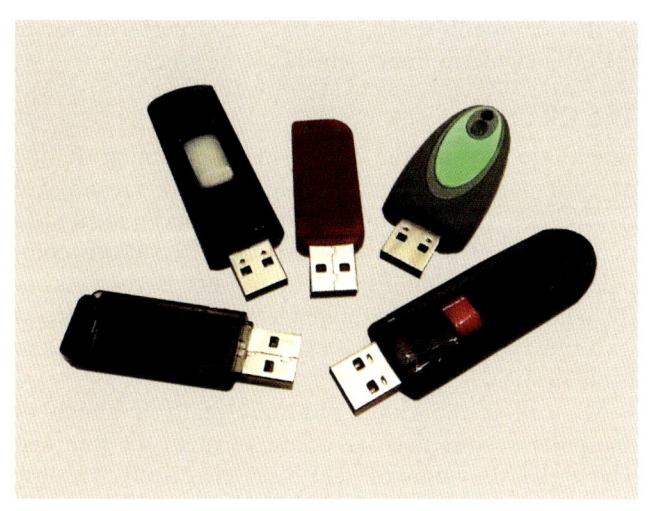

FIG. 27.10 A flash drive is a small, solid-state device that is capable of storing in excess of 1 TB of data.

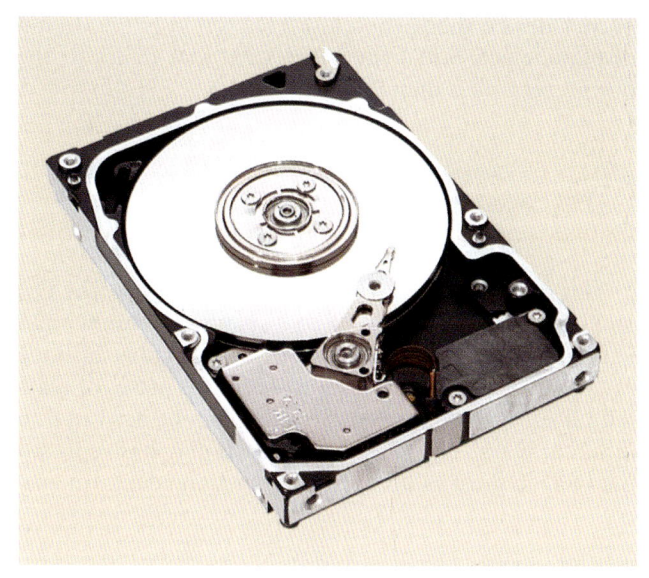

FIG. 27.11 This disc driver reads all formats of optical compact discs and reads, erases, writes, and rewrites to a 1-TB optical cartridge. (Courtesy Hitachi Medical Systems.)

> A flash drive is also called a jump drive or jump stick.

In contrast to CDs, hard drives are thin, rigid glass or metal platters. Each side of the platter is coated with a recording material that can be magnetized. Hard drives are tightly sealed in a hard disc drive, and data can be recorded on both sides of the disc platters. Hard drives are typically located inside the computer but can also be attached externally.

Another form of internal data storage is a solid-state drive (SSD). These drives are typically of lower capacity than hard drives and more expensive. However, they store data based on solid-state principles and therefore allow for much faster access to data and are more durable.

Compared with CDs and flash drives, hard drives can have thousands of tracks per inch. Storage systems that use several hard discs use the cylinder method to locate data (Fig. 27.11). Hard drives have greater capacity and speed than optical storage devices and SSDs.

A redundant array of independent discs (RAID) system consists of two or more hard drives in a single cabinet that collectively act as a single storage system. RAID systems have greater reliability because if one disc drive fails, others can take over.

A single CD-ROM (compact disc-ROM) typically can hold 1 TB of data. CD-ROM drives used to handle only one disc at a time, but now, multidisc drives called **jukeboxes** can handle up to 2000 discs. The optical disc jukebox now replaces the film file room (Fig. 27.12) in some radiology digital imaging departments.

Computer Output. Output devices include plotters, multifunction devices, and audio output devices. The

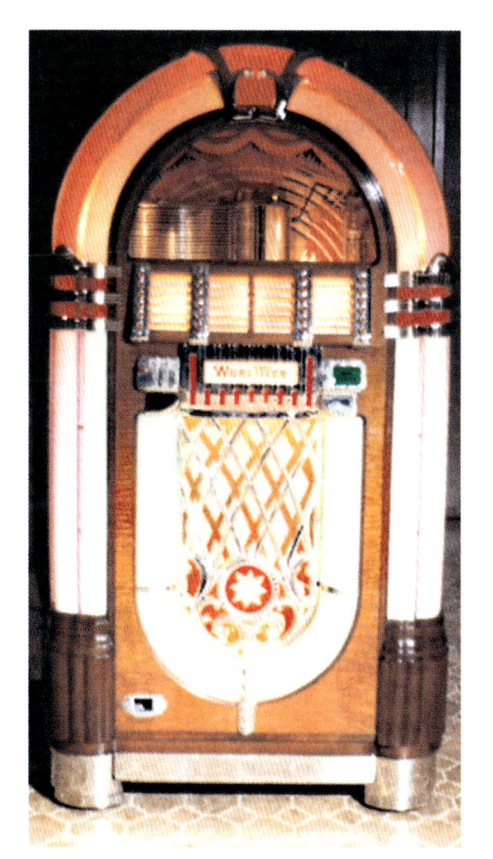

FIG. 27.12 This 1946 Wurlitzer jukebox with its 78-rpm platters serves as a model for the optical disc jukebox of the picture archiving and communication system network. (Courtesy Raymond Wilenzek[†], Tulane University.)

output device that people use most often is the digital display device. **Soft copy** is the term that refers to the output seen on a digital display device.

> Common output devices are the digital display device and printers.

Flat-panel displays (liquid crystal displays [LCDs] and light-emitting diode [LED] displays) are thinner and lighter and consume less power than previous cathode ray tubes. These displays are made of two plates of glass with a substance between them that can be activated in different ways. The LED flat-panel display has replaced the LCD in most radiology digital imaging departments.

> Output hardware consists of devices that translate computer information into a form that humans can understand.

A **terminal** is an input/output device that uses a keyboard for input and a digital display device for output. Terminals can be dumb or intelligent.

A dumb terminal cannot do any processing on its own; it is used only to input data or receive data from a main or host computer. Airline agents at ticketing and check-in counters are usually connected to the main computer system through dumb terminals.

An intelligent terminal has built-in processing capability and RAM but does not have its own storage capacity.

Printers are another form of output device and are categorized by the manner in which the print mechanism physically contacts the paper to print. Impact printers such as dot matrix and high-speed line printers have direct contact with the paper. Such printers have largely been replaced by **inkjet printers**.

Inkjet printers form images with little dots. These printers electrically charge small drops of ink that are then sprayed onto the page. Inkjet printers are quiet and inexpensive and can print in color. Printing up to 20 ppm for black text and 10 ppm for color images is possible with even modestly priced inkjet printers. Epson, Hewlett-Packard (HP), and Canon, among others, offer inexpensive printers for home use and large multitalented printers for offices and facilities.

Other specialized output devices serve specific functions. For example, plotters are used to create documents such as architectural drawings and maps. Multifunction devices deliver several capabilities, such as printing, imaging, copying, and faxing, through one unit.

APPLICATIONS TO DIGITAL IMAGING

Radiologic science continues to expand and extend computer applications along many avenues. Each contributes to the increasing speed, accuracy, and performance of digital imaging to improvements in healthcare.

The Cloud

When one accesses the cloud, one is obtaining the use of a computer server or multiple computer servers over the Internet. These computer servers can be located at many different data centers operated by various companies. The individual user, you, do not have access to the computer servers to manage, but rather the access is to run applications. This arrangement is illustrated in Fig. 27.13.

We call it the cloud but it is really a bunch of computer servers that we access through the Internet. The cloud allows us to deal more effectively with big data and run various software applications that would encumber the use of our personal computer.

We can log on to the cloud by mobile phone, regardless of where we are on the planet. And then we can work on any number of **Big Data** files and any number of applications that can be addressed quickly with ease.

As with so many other areas of life today, the cloud is really a virtual technology. Once we access the cloud, it behaves as though it were our own personal computer. In fact, it is a virtual computer and really a virtual computer server.

Teleradiology

Telecommunications describes the transfer of data from a sender to a receiver across a distance. A computer network is any system of two or more computers that are linked together. The practice of teleradiology involves the transfer of medical images and patient data.

Electric current, radio frequency, or light is used to transfer data through a physical medium, which may be a cable, a wire, or even the atmosphere (i.e., wireless). Many communications lines are still analog; therefore a computer needs a **modem** (**mo**dulate/**dem**odulate) to convert digital information into analog. The receiving computer's modem converts analog information back into digital.

> Teleradiology is the transfer of images and patient reports to remote sites.

In addition to modems, the transfer of imaging data may require a **router** to deliver the images and reports to several terminals simultaneously. Transmission speed, the rate at which data are moved across a communications channel, is measured in bits per second (bps) or kilobits per second (kbps), or megabits per second (Mbps).

Advances in technology have allowed for the development of faster and faster teleradiology devices. The term **broadband** commonly refers to high-speed Internet

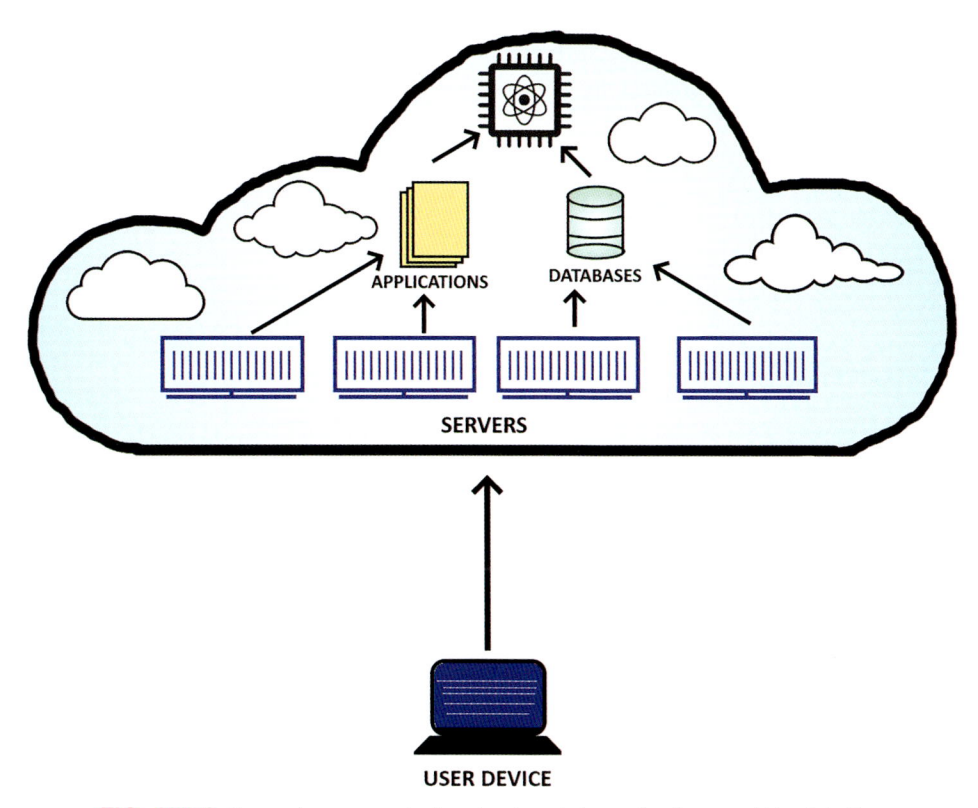

FIG. 27.13 Computer servers in the cloud contain applications and big data files.

access that is always on and faster than traditional dial-up access. Broadband includes several high-speed transmission technologies, such as:
- Digital subscriber line (DSL)
- Cable modem
- Fiber
- Wireless
- Satellite

Integrated services digital network transmits over regular phone lines up to five times faster than basic modems. DSLs transmit at speeds in the middle range of the previous two technologies. DSLs also use regular phone lines. Currently, the fastest available type of digital communication is a fiber-optic line that transmits signals digitally. These lines can range in speed from 5 Mbps to 100 Gbps, which at the fastest is approximately 1 million times faster than the original dial-up modems used with a telephone line.

In 1990 Tim Berners-Lee invented the World Wide Web, which has profoundly connected us and shrunk our planet communications-wise. Telecommunications in the form of teleradiology is changing the way we allocate human resources to improve the speed of interpretation, reporting, and archiving of images and other patient data. Fig. 27.14 is a good summary of the increasing speed and capacity of microprocessors designed to support teleradiology and digital image file sizes.

Input hardware includes keyboards, mice, trackballs, touchpads, and source data entry devices. A keyboard includes standard typewriter keys that are used to enter words and numbers and function keys that enter specific commands.

> Input hardware converts data into a form that the computer can use.

Source data entry devices include scanners, fax machines, imaging systems, audio and video devices, electronic cameras, voice-recognition systems, sensors, and biologic input devices. **Scanners** translate images of text, drawings, or photographs into a digital format recognizable by the computer. **Barcode readers**, which translate the vertical black-and-white–striped codes on retail products into digital form, are a type of scanner.

QR Code. Approximately 75 years ago, several graduate school science programs with exceptional students began toying with the idea of producing a geometrical pattern that would be machine readable. The first such device was patented in the early 1950s, termed a **barcode** (Fig. 27.15).

It was somewhat based on Morse code interpreted by an optical scanner called a **barcode reader**. It went through several stages of development and finally became commercially successful in the 1970s when

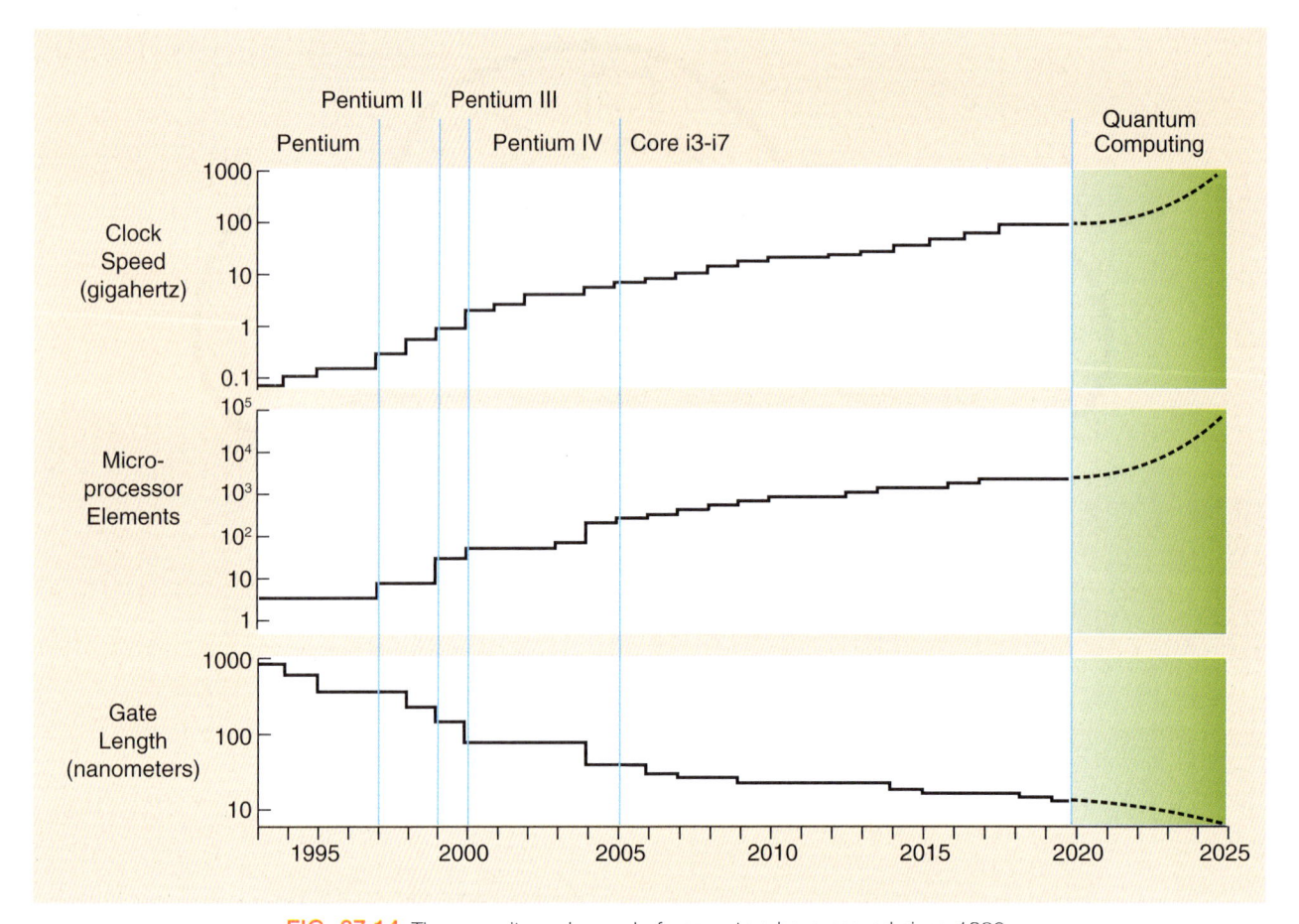

FIG. 27.14 The capacity and speed of computers have soared since 1990.

FIG. 27.15 A barcode is a series of lines and spaces of different widths.

FIG. 27.16 A quick response code, better known as the QR code, is shown.

used to automate the checkout at a grocery store or supermarket.

During this time of development, the barcode went from a linear form (1D) to a form consisting of different width bars and interspaces (2D) to the current matrix codes that are now being replaced with QR codes (Fig. 27.16) that can be read and interpreted by a mobile device such as a smartphone.

The QR code (quick response code) is the latest development of the matrix barcode. The QR code consists of a matrix of black squares of different sizes positioned on a white background. There are fiducial markers variously positioned on the code to assist in locating and identifying various items. The numeric and alpha-numeric encoding allows for accessing stored data and for web browsing with your smart device.

An **audio input device** translates analog sound into digital format. Similarly, video images, such as those from a VCR or camcorder, are digitized by a special video card that can be installed in a computer. Digital cameras and video recorders capture images in digital format that can easily be transferred to the computer for immediate access.

Voice-recognition systems add a microphone and an audio sound card to a computer and can convert speech into digital format. Radiologists use these systems to produce rapid diagnostic reports and to send findings to remote locations by teleradiology.

Computers play a large role in radiologic imaging, and the practice of digital imaging would not be possible without them. A digital image stored in a computer is rectangular in format and made up of small squares called **pixels**. A typical digital chest x-ray might contain

2000 columns of pixels and 2500 rows of pixels for a total of 5 million pixels.

As discussed previously, computers at the most basic level read in binary format. This is the case in a digital image. Each pixel contains a series of 1s and 0s defining the gray scale or shade of that particular point on a digital x-ray image. Each space available for a 1 or 0 is called a bit. A group of 8 bits is called a byte.

> A digital mammogram has a 16-bit dynamic range, which means that the image is capable of displaying 65,536 shades of gray.

Question: How much storage space do you think a 16-bit 2000 × 2500 pixel x-ray image would take?

Answer: (1 byte/8 bits) × 16 bits × 2000 × 2500 pixels = 10,000,000 bytes
10,000,000 bytes × 1 kB/1024 byte × 1 MB/1024 kB = 9.5 MB

In addition to the pixel information contained in the image, a medical image contains information about the patient, type of examination, and place of examination. This information is stored in the image in what is called the **header**. The addition of a header requires that the image be stored in a slightly more complex way than just a series of pixels and their associated values.

The American College of Radiology, along with the National Electrical Manufacturers Association, has developed a standard method of image storage for diagnostic medical images. This is known as the Digital Imaging and Communications in Medicine (DICOM) standard.

One problem with digital medical images is that they take up a relatively large amount of storage space and need to be transferred from the examination room to the radiologist and then need to be archived. The picture archiving and communication system (PACS) takes care of all of these tasks (see Chapter 25). PACS has made digital image interpretation and report extremely convenient from any location. This has expanded the practice of teleradiology.

> Teleradiology is the practice in which radiologists remotely interpret digital images and report the results.

A radiologist might be in Sydney, Australia; read an examination that was performed in Houston, Texas; and complete the diagnosis in the same amount of time as a radiologist who was on-site.

Computers have become so advanced that smartphones and tablets today are more powerful than earlier large computers. By 2010 more mobile smartphones were sold than PCs (101 million vs. 92 million). In 2022, approximately 1.4 billion smartphones were sold worldwide. This is changing the practice of teleradiology.

The US Food and Drug Administration approved the first application that allows for the viewing of medical images on a mobile phone in 2011. The radiologist of the future will be so much more efficient and correct. An image will arrive at the radiologist's workstation on whatever continent having been preprocessed by AI algorithms with a suggested diagnostic report.

SUMMARY

The word computer is used as an abbreviation for any general-purpose, stored-program electronic digital device. General purpose means the computer can solve problems. Stored program means the computer has instructions and data stored in its memory. Electronic means the computer is powered by electrical and electronic devices. Digital means that the data are in discrete values.

A computer has two principal parts: the hardware and the software. The computer's nuts and bolts are the hardware. The computer's programs, which tell the hardware what to do, are the software.

Hardware consists of several types of components, including a CPU, a control unit, an arithmetic unit, memory units, input and output devices, a video terminal display, secondary memory devices, a printer, and a modem.

The basic parts of the software are the bits, bytes, and words. In computer language, a single binary digit, either 0 or 1, is called a bit. Bits grouped in bunches of eight are called bytes. Computer capacity is typically expressed in gigabytes or terabytes.

Computers use a specific language to communicate commands in software systems and programs. Computers operate on the simplest number system of all, the binary system, which includes only two digits: 0 and 1. The computer performs all operations by converting alphabetic characters, decimal values, and logic functions into binary values. Other computer languages allow programmers to write instructions in a form that approaches human language.

Two developments that promise even greater advances in imaging science are AI and quantum computing.

CHALLENGE QUESTIONS

1. Define or otherwise identify the following:
   a. Logic function
   b. Central processing unit
   c. Modem

d. Flash drive
   e. Byte
   f. Operating system
   g. Bootstrap
   h. Algorithm
   i. BASIC
   j. RAM
2. Name three operations in radiology departments that are computerized.
3. The acronyms ASCC, ENIAC, and UNIVAC stand for what?
4. What is the difference between a calculator and a computer?
5. How many megabytes are in 1 TB?
6. What are the two principal parts of a computer and the distinguishing features of each?
7. List and define the several components of computer hardware.
8. Define bit, byte, and word as used in computer terminology.
9. Distinguish systems software from applications programs.
10. List several types of computer languages.
11. What is the difference between a CD and a DVD?
12. A memory chip is said to have 256 MB of capacity. What is the total bit capacity?
13. What is high-level computer language?
14. What computer language was the first modern programmers' language?
15. List and define the four computer processing methods.
16. Calculate the amount of storage space needed for a 32-bit 1024 × 1024 pixel digital image.
17. What is teleradiology?
18. What input/output devices are commonly used in radiology?
19. Describe the cloud-server complex.
20. What is the difference between a barcode and a QR code?

The answers to the Challenge Questions can be found by logging on to our website at http://evolve.elsevier.com.

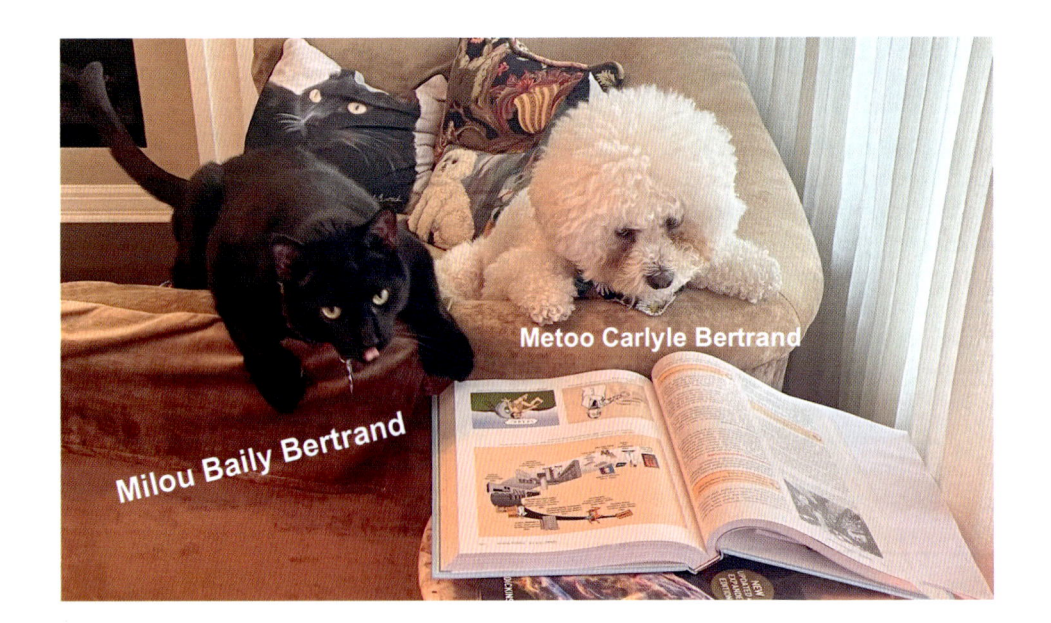

Artificial Intelligence

CHAPTER 28

OBJECTIVES

At the completion of this chapter, the student should be able to do the following:

1. Identify and define many artificial intelligence (AI) terms.
2. Understand the terms data file, data storage, training data, and Big Data.
3. Differentiate between machine learning and deep learning.
4. Discuss the predicted changes in imaging workflow.
5. List areas of radiologic AI algorithms that cause radiology to be the AI leader among medical specialties.
6. Describe how image quality control will be impacted by AI.

OUTLINE

Basic Concepts 396
   Vectors 396
   Terms 398
Machine Learning 399
   Supervised 400
   Unsupervised 400
Deep Learning 400
Imaging Workflow 401
Ethics and Artificial Intelligence 402
   Representativeness Bias 403
   Algorithmic Bias 403
   Cognitive Bias 403
Summary 404
Challenge Questions 405

> A QUESTION every student asks themselves, or their teacher, is "Why must I learn about this?" In the case of **artificial intelligence (AI)**, the answer is "Because you are, for the patient, the primary, often only, person representing radiology. You are the one who assures the patient that everything that follows will be safe, effective, beneficial, and properly controlled."
>
> AI functions are in virtually every element of digital imaging today. While device manufacturers provide you with excellent training materials, it will often be up to you to describe to a patient what is happening.

The adaptation of computer technology to mimic the human mind in cognitive activities such as learning and problem solving is termed artificial intelligence. Although the concept of AI surfaced in the middle of the 20th century, it was not until the 21st century that machine learning (ML) algorithms, such as optical character recognition, autonomous automobiles, drones, and games, were described as AI.

When Deep Blue, the IBM computer, beat Garry Kasarov in chess in 1997, the public was first introduced to AI. AI sometimes goes by the names "Augmented Intelligence" or even "Arbitrary Intelligence," but when connected to radiologic imaging it is artificial intelligence. The English language associated with AI is imprecise and changing rapidly. Most terms are defined for convenience and lack of a more extensive vocabulary.

> Artificial intelligence is a descriptor for applications that function as a simulation of human intelligence.

At the end of this chapter you will discover artificial intelligence (AI) ethics. You may be responsible for assuring everyone that the data of this patient has been ethically collected, its privacy is assured, and that future uses of it have been explained to the patient.

BASIC CONCEPTS

The first futuristic application of AI occurred in cosmology, the science of the cosmos. Telescopic images have been digitized and analyzed with AI techniques to discover and identify exoplanets in distant galaxies.

When we talk about AI used in digital imaging today, it is reasonable to limit the description to analog, digital, and quantum computing devices where chips, algorithms, and data have been brought together. Such systems are faster, with more memory capacity and function following known principles of physics. It was in late 2023 that the company OpenAI made publicly available one class of AI systems: **large language models (LLMs)**.

> OpenAI produced the first LLM available: ChatGPT.

As had been the case in the development of all computing technology, LLMs were made possible by innovations in hardware design that came from graphical processing units (**GPUs**) and central processing units (**CPUs**), in natural language processing (**NLP**), and **Big Data** in organization, manipulation, and quantity. **Algorithms** remain the heart and soul of building AI systems and reveal the genealogy of AI from its roots in physics, mathematics, logic, and engineering.

The first of the US Food and Drug Administration (USFDA) designations of "Software as Medical Devices" were awarded to radiology equipment vendors. Radiologic applications have always dominated the FDA's list.

Early in 2023, there were hundreds of such medical device approvals. Digital imaging devices continue to represent the largest percentage of all such approved devices. Of the four computer models (analog, digital, quantum, and hybrids), the creativity curve is unabated.

Vectors

Vectors play a fundamental role in AI, particularly in ML and deep learning (DL) algorithms, serving as a cornerstone for data representation, analysis, and processing. Understanding their nature and importance is essential for grasping how AI models function and learn from data.

Nature of Vectors in AI. In the context of AI, a vector is essentially an array of numbers. These numbers can represent various features or attributes of data points. For example, in NLP, words or phrases can be converted into vectors using techniques like Word2Vec or GloVe. In image processing, an image can be represented as a vector of pixel values.

Represent Data. Vectors transform real-world information into a format that algorithms can process. Each dimension of a vector can represent a different feature of the data, such as color intensity in images or word occurrence in text data.

Measure Similarity. By calculating distances or angles between vectors (using metrics like Euclidean distance or cosine similarity), vectors can determine the similarity of two data points. This is crucial for tasks like clustering, recommendation systems, and classification.

Performance Calculations. Operations on vectors, such as addition, subtraction, and dot products, are fundamental in the mathematical formulations of ML algorithms, including optimization and prediction functions.

> The Importance of vectors is essential for AI understanding.

Efficient Data Representation. Vectors enable the efficient and compact representation of complex data in a form that AI models can easily manipulate and learn from. This is crucial for handling high-dimensional data, such as images and text.

Facilitates Machine Learning Operations. Many ML algorithms, especially in DL, rely on linear algebra operations that are naturally applied to vectors. This includes operations within neural networks, such as the activation functions and back project propagation.

Enables Advanced Techniques. Vectors are foundational for implementing advanced techniques in AI, such as embeddings in NLP, where words or phrases are mapped to vectors of real numbers, capturing semantic similarity in a high-dimensional space.

Scalability and Performance. Vectorized operations are highly scalable and can be efficiently executed, especially on modern hardware designed for parallel processing, like GPUs. This scalability is vital for training complex models on large data sets.

Universality and Interoperability. The vector-based representation of data is a universal format that facilitates interoperability between different AI models and systems. This means that the same data representation can be used across different tasks and models, enhancing the modular development of AI applications.

In summary, vectors are integral to AI for representing data, performing mathematical operations, and enabling the algorithms to learn from data. Their efficient, scalable, and versatile nature makes them indispensable in the field, underlying the success of many AI applications and advancements. However, having read this section once, the radiologist or radiographer does not need to return to this discussion. Concentrate on the rest of this chapter.

AI is currently impacting many areas of life, as shown in Table 28.1 games, finance, manufacturing (robotics), recognition (language and image), self-driving cars, education, law, and many areas of healthcare, including digital imaging. Virtual personal assistants such as Apple's Siri and Microsoft's Alexa have become common for producing digital imaging reports (Table 28.2) as will AI as a service (AIaaS), a few examples of which are shown in Table 28.3. Face recognition is replacing fingerprints.

AI is now competing in healthcare in many ways, and the potential change to digital imaging is astounding.

TABLE 28.1 Daily Impact of Artificial Intelligence

Games—video
Finance
Oil and gas exploration
Scientific research
Manufacturing—robotics
Recognition—language, image, face
Autonomous—automobiles, trucks, appliances
Education
Law
Healthcare—digital imaging, pathology, patient services
Meteorology
Cryptography

TABLE 28.2 Artificial Intelligence Machine Learning

IBM	Deep Blue
	Watson
Google	Alpha GO
	Translate

IBM, International Business Machines.

TABLE 28.3 Virtual Personal Assistants (VPAs)

VPA	Sponsor
Siri	Apple
Google Assistant	Google
Alexa	Amazon
Cortana	Microsoft

The AI subsets of ML and DL, which enable functions such as pattern recognition to be possible, are being applied to digital images.

The adoption of AI cannot come soon enough. The current population of radiologists cannot keep up with the ever-increasing workload produced by many radiology departments. Such an increase is due to more images per examination, as in digital breast tomosynthesis, and the effect that our aging population has placed on healthcare in the United States. AI makes image interpretation more efficient in many ways, such as detecting and removing motion, noise, and artifacts in an image.

In addition to efficiency, AI will improve the performance of radiologists and radiographers in providing excellent patient care. This was tried in the 1990s with some success using computer-assisted diagnosis (CADx). The objection was that CADx predicted the end of radiologists, and it was changed to computer-assisted

TABLE 28.4	Artificial Intelligence as a Service

- Amazon AI
- IBM Watson Assistant
- Microsoft Cognitive Services
- Google AI

AI, Artificial intelligence; *IBM*, International Business Machines.

detection! The job security concerns expressed by some radiologists are also voiced by professionals in several of the areas covered in Table 28.4.

> The term CADx was in radiologic use way before AI.

In 2019 the first program titled "Artificial Intelligence" convened at the annual Radiological Society of North America (RSNA) meeting, and 2019 marked the first year of a new journal titled *Radiology: Artificial Intelligence*. It is challenging, but necessary, that radiologists and radiographers acquire an understanding of AI and the changes in professional practice that it will inevitably bring.

The cognitive functions, such as teaching, learning, and decision-making that we in radiology— radiologists, radiographers, and medical physicists—use regularly are about to profoundly change every area of digital imaging. The application of data mining to increasingly larger big data imaging files will be used to improve the quality of radiologic images, reduce patient radiation dose, and improve quality control using phantoms and test objects designed for AI evaluation.

> Radiology leads all of medicine in the adoption of AI.

As many have expressed, AI will not take over the radiologist's job, but it will make that job more productive and accurate. However, if the radiologist does not learn to embrace AI, they could be replaced by one who has learned.

Currently there are over 100 companies involved in AI for radiology. The USFDA has approved hundreds of AI algorithms for applications in radiology. In addition to all else described for radiologic AI algorithms, they have been shown capable of passing the ABR CORE certification examination. Radiology leads the way for AI in medicine.

Virtual assistance has already become important in many areas of daily life. Virtual assistance will become ever more valuable to the radiologist and radiographer in teaching, image manipulation, report writing, and all intellectual activities.

Terms

With the rapid introduction of AI into all facets of life, particularly digital imaging, there are many old and new English words applied to AI. Understanding the physics of AI requires first an understanding of the meaning of the English words. The following terms are identified according to their AI use. Many of these terms are identified and defined in other chapters. There are many synonyms to each of these terms, but those presented here are brief for review as the terms that the Penguin prefers.

> The Penguin prefers the following terms and definitions when discussing AI:
>
> **Algorithm**—A set of step-by-step mathematical instructions used in AI to solve a problem or reach an explanation. It is to AI as a recipe is to cooking.
>
> **AI**—Computer science that deals with the interpretation of radiologic images by simulating human intelligence.
>
> **Big Data**—Large data files in size (number of patients) and in content (patient description, imaging description).
>
> **Classification**—An algorithmic technique for identifying a category to which something belongs (e.g., anomaly identification, patient triage, outcome prediction).
>
> **Clinical decision**—Clinical decision support is usually provided at the patient's bedside to help provide proper decisions regarding a patient's care.
>
> **Cloud-based computing**—The cloud is basically remote computer access to the internet. Many organizations now offer computing services including storage, networking analytics, and intelligence with fast, free, and flexible resources.
>
> **Clustering**—Clustering is particularly important to digital imaging. It is a method to segment data, identifying boundaries of an anomaly or mass.
>
> **Data file**—The data file is a digital file of data to be used in a computer application. The data file does not normally contain instructions or code. Some files are identified as Big Data.
>
> **Data mining**—Unsupervised training of Big Data files to discover incidentalomas.
>
> **Data storage**—Data storage refers to digital devices in the form of file storage, block storage, and object storage, each designed for a particular application.
>
> **Decision tree**—A hierarchy or model that uses a tree-like model to describe the consequences of decisions, including chance event outcomes. It is one way to display an algorithm that contains clinical decision statements.

Deep neural network—The foundation of DL. The digital image is the input, and there are many hidden layers between the input layer, and the output layer with the diagnosis as the output.

Generative pretrained transformer—GPT is a type of language model that uses deep learning to generate human-like text. It has advanced natural language processing (NLP) capabilities and is used in AI algorithms to produce radiology reports.

Graphics processing unit—GPU is a digital module that can perform AI algorithm calculations much faster than the CPU (central processing unit) and has better Big Data capability.

Machine learning—Use of AI algorithms that teach the machine (computer) to recognize data patterns.

Metrology—Experimental or theoretical measurements of uncertainty.

Neural network—Another name for AI algorithms grouped for supervised and unsupervised applications. A layered set of networks through which data is processed.

Practice standards—Practice standards are statements established by professional societies for judging the quality of practice, service, and education. Practice standards change regularly as a result of technological advances in economic and market forces.

Predictive algorithm—A major function of ML that is a critical decision function in digital imaging.

Radiomics—The use of AI algorithms to extract features of digital images and assist diagnosis and patient care suggestions.

Supervised—The use of training data that has known answers. AI functions on data that proves the data, its structure, and the results.

Training data—A large data file used to develop the many algorithms required to go from input, the image, to output, the diagnosis. Usually a portion of the data is set aside as training data while a larger portion is retained for testing and evaluation.

Unsupervised—The use of training data that does not include answers. Uses even larger data files to recognize and correlate similar data patterns.

Virtual technology—Several companies, such as Meta, have provided new ways to assist teachers at every level of education. Virtual technology provides a 3D experience in time and place that can be a helpful teaching environment.

There are many subsets to AI, but the two most important for medical imaging purposes are **machine learning** and **deep learning**. Both of these terms are examples of the developing English used to describe AI. Both machine learning and deep learning deal with special computers, not autonomous machines, and meticulously designed computer algorithms. They were probably introduced by Alan Turing in a 1950 paper titled "Computing Machinery and Intelligence."

MACHINE LEARNING

A machine (computer) is taught or "trained" to learn by providing it with a large collection of training data or information (Fig. 28.1). The training data sets would be composed of digital images. There are many classifications of AI algorithms, such as a support vector machine, k-nearest-neighbor, regression algorithms, and iterative algorithms such as clustering. A discussion of such AI algorithms is beyond the scope of this textbook. Besides, the acceleration in radiologic algorithms is exponential.

> Machine learning (ML) is training with supervised and unsupervised methods.

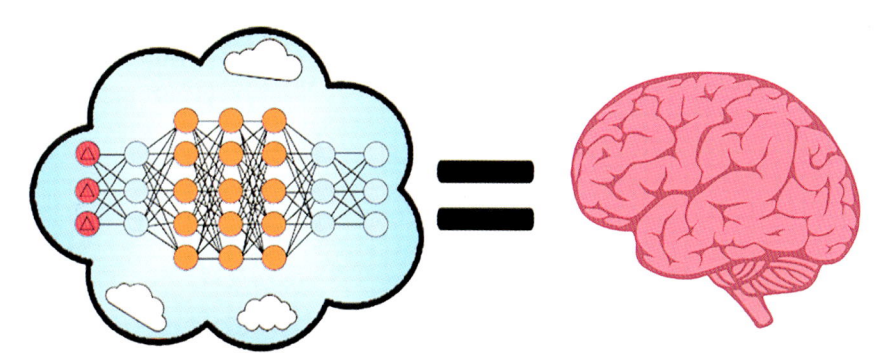

FIG. 28.1 Deep learning with computers mimics the anatomy of the human brain.

There are two categories of training methods for ML systems: **supervised** and **unsupervised**. With supervised learning, the ML system is provided a large set of training data that includes the normal and abnormal information, and the programmer identifies the abnormality. Unsupervised machine learning uses larger training data and lets the AI algorithms arrive at a decision of normal or abnormal that includes a percentile accuracy value.

Supervised

If a programmer wants to build and train the ML algorithm to detect pneumonia on frontal view chest radiographs, the programmer would provide the system with a large set of anteroposterior chest images with and without pneumonia. The exact number of required images is not known for accurate results, but would likely require thousands of images to be accurate. After the ML system receives all of the information provided by the programmer, it "learns" and correlates distinct features on each image and identifies areas it considers "abnormal."

After the initial training process, the programmer can adjust parameters within the AI algorithms to increase the accuracy in the analytical process where the end result, or output, is as close to the ground truth as possible. This ground truth is already known by the programmer. The system is quite literally led in a direction to provide an answer that is already known. Supervised learning is a laborious process for the programmer as each piece of training data must be labeled as normal or abnormal.

Unsupervised

Unsupervised learning is similar to the supervised method. The ML system is still provided a large set of training data; however, the normal and abnormal information is withheld throughout the training process and the system is left to identify abnormalities in the data set on its own.

Through density estimation, dimensionality reduction, and clustering, the unsupervised ML system is eventually able to classify abnormalities in the training data. For the previous example of detecting pneumonia on frontal chest radiographs, the unsupervised system will categorize its finding as a percentage of normal and abnormal.

An early application of both clustering and data mining is prediction modeling with a **decision tree**, as seen in Fig. 28.2. The decision tree algorithms begin with a branch, cluster, through smaller branches, to a leaf, and finally to the diagnosis.

> Digital imaging AI algorithms form the decision tree that results in diagnosis and in detection of incidentalomas.

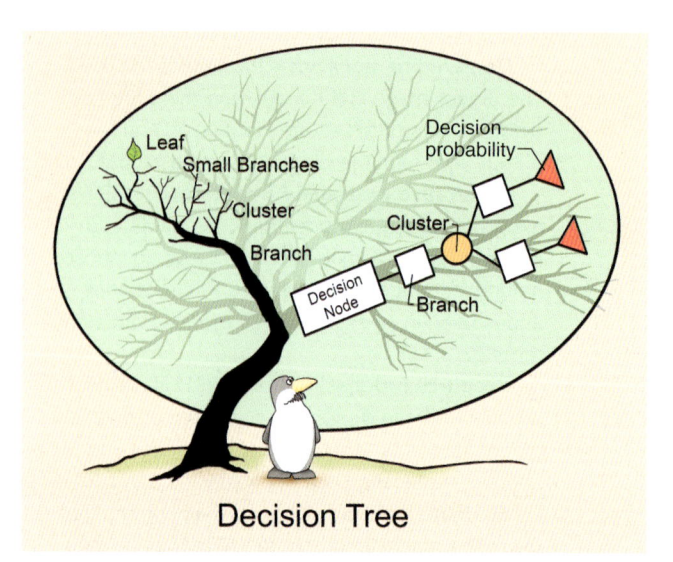

FIG. 28.2 The decision tree is an application of prediction modeling machine learning. The leaf is the diagnosis.

Supervised training includes the set of digital images and the known abnormality, and its location and appearance. Unsupervised training has no known output, but contains algorithms to identify and describe similar **clustering** of data, resulting in pattern recognition. Unsupervised training is a form of **data mining** that has the ability to discover previously unknown patterns leading to diagnosis. This area of data mining is termed **anomaly detection**, which relates to **incidentalomas** in digital imaging.

LLMs are a form of data mining applied with the patient's electronic medical record (EMR) to identify incidentalomas. Patient care is improved by automatic referral of such cases to the referring physician.

DEEP LEARNING

The term deep learning did not appear until approximately half a century after machine learning, and when it did there was, and still is, confusion within the English language. It can be visualized as a co-set or a subset to ML, as shown in Fig. 28.3.

Deep learning is similar to machine learning in network design and function. However, deep learning is distinctly different from machine learning when viewing the depth of the neural network and the near exclusive use of unsupervised training. The "deep" in deep learning refers to the number of hidden layers used to analyze the input data.

> When compared to machine learning (ML), deep learning (DL) has many more hidden layers of AI algorithms.

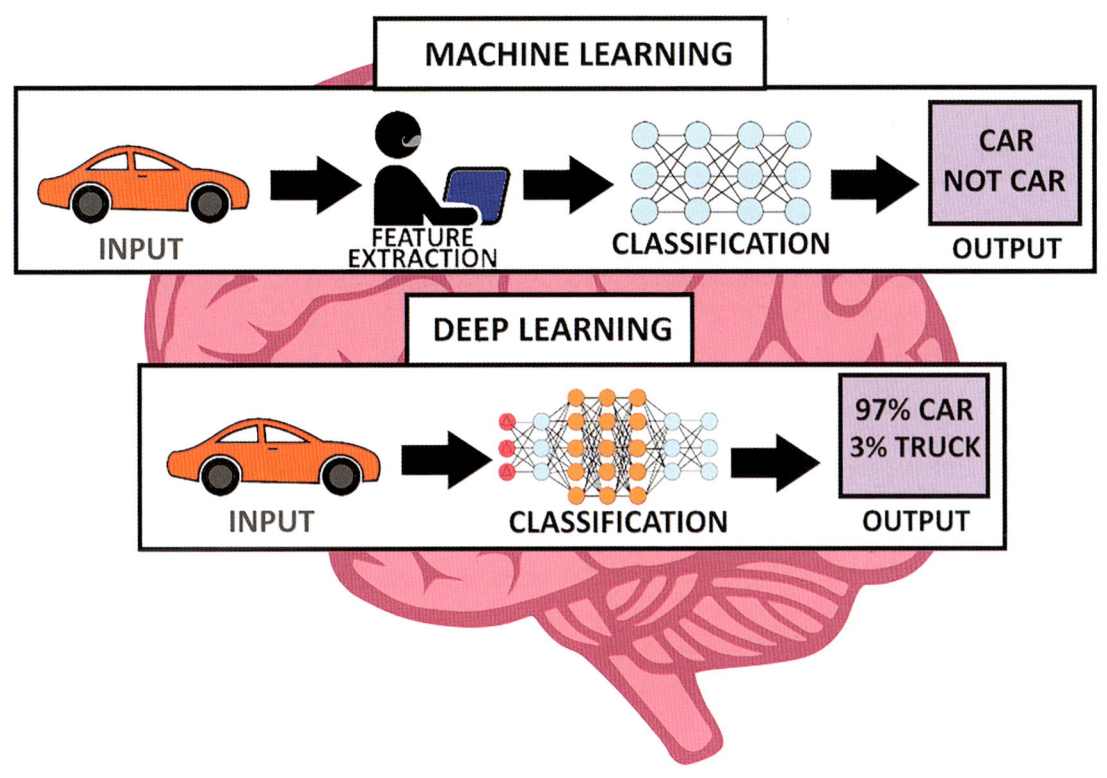

FIG. 28.3 Artificial intelligence results in faster interpretation and more accurate diagnosis, coupled with a probability coefficient.

Although both ML and DL use **artificial neural networks** (ANNs) for processing and analyzation purposes, deep neural networks contain many more layers than the basic neural networks used for machine learning. ANNs are aptly named because they closely resemble the structure and function of the biologic human brain.

Deep learning can be thought of as a computer representation of the human brain. The human brain contains billions of neurons connected by synapses where information is transmitted from the senses so we can recognize and understand the world around us. ANNs also contain connected neurons (**nodes**) that transmit information from one layer of the network to the next.

> ANNs behave like the neuron-synapse structure of the human brain.

Nodes are connected at both edges and can have robust numeric descriptors that are AI algorithm driven. The deep is getting deeper and deeper and also better. When quantum computing arrives clinically, watch out!

As with ML, there is supervised training and unsupervised training. Most current applications of ANN are unsupervised and are listed in Table 28.5. One result is that the diagnosis will be produced with a probability factor.

TABLE 28.5 AI Benefits to Radiologist and Patient Care

Extensive differential diagnosis
Control repetitive tasks
Provide a second opinion
Reduce report variability
Combine with clinical service reports
Use the digital image as input
Produce a more easily understood report
Correct speech recognition errors

IMAGING WORKFLOW

There is much current hype regarding the replacement of radiologists with AI machine learning tools. Such is not likely, but the use of AI to improve the speed, accuracy, and diagnosis of digital images is sure to transform digital imaging as it was transformed from analog to digital at the turn of the 21st century.

> Digital imaging AI algorithms are likely to have more impact on imaging workflow than on diagnosis.

A good place to start in trying to understand the changes coming in the applications of AI in patient care is RadLex, an RSNA (Radiological Society of North America) website to assist the radiologist and radiographer. First, a little English lesson. An **ontology** is a formal way of connecting different knowledge concepts and relationships among these concepts in a mathematically acceptable format. The use of an ontology is to predict relationships among concepts that are not obvious or readily available. Ontology is often described as an application of metaphysics.

The concepts in terms just referred to as belonging to a particular knowledge domain is called a **lexicon**. RadLex (www.rsna.org/radlex) was first announced in 2023 and included 46,000 appropriate and useful terms in radiologic practice.

Digital imaging workflow involves many steps that can be adequately described with the four shown in Fig. 28.4. The clinician requests patient imaging and that request is evaluated by the radiologist or radiographer for appropriateness. Changes in the request may result in the imaging request being transferred to the appropriate imaging modality workstation.

> There are four stages involved in imaging workflow: image acquisition, image processing, image interpretation, and report communication/follow-up.

During the first stage, the image is acquired by a radiographer at a particular imaging modality workstation. The acquisition of the image and its associated data files are manipulated by way of existing programs, such as PACS and DICOM; see Chapter 25.

The second stage is image processing at a workstation available to both the radiologist and radiographer and often even remotely. Image processing is conducted with the use of radiologic AI algorithms. There was already extensive preprocessing. Now postprocessing is most important because it leads to the third stage of human image interpretation.

Image interpretation is the traditional radiologist's role. Radiographers are involved by preparing the images for such interpretation. The role of radiologic AI algorithms in this stage of the imaging workflow continues to increase.

At this stage, machine learning and deep learning may be involved and engaged by the radiologist or radiographer. With this information at hand, the radiologist, with the help of AI, generates a report of analysis and interpretation that is then transmitted via phone, email, and the EMR to the requesting clinician.

Table 28.5 is a list of what are perceived to be the benefits to the radiologist and to the patient's healthcare. A more extensive differential diagnosis with percentile accuracy values will be produced. This could be followed by a second opinion and cause the radiologist to reconsider. We know that different radiologists produce different types of written reports.

Even the same radiologist will experience variability depending on the time of day or the previous night's party! Such variability will be reduced, making the reports more readable by the clinician and patient. AI will do a better job of combining the radiologic report with other clinical service reports. It will also detect and correct speech recognition errors, which are verbal errors in the dictated radiology report.

Follow-up is an activity performed by both the radiologist and the radiographer. Follow-up ensures that the diagnostic interpretation was properly delivered and properly understood by the referring clinician and perhaps also the patient. Follow-up includes placing the radiologist's report onto a website such as MyChart for patient use.

ETHICS AND ARTIFICIAL INTELLIGENCE

There is considerable ethical concern for the application of AI into the daily activity of radiologic practice. The AI learning tools are only as smart as the data we give them, which can be flawed or biased.

Unlike computer-aided diagnosis (CAD) that was developed before the turn of the 21st century. Most

Image Acquisition → **Image Processing** → **Image Interpretation** → **Follow-Up**

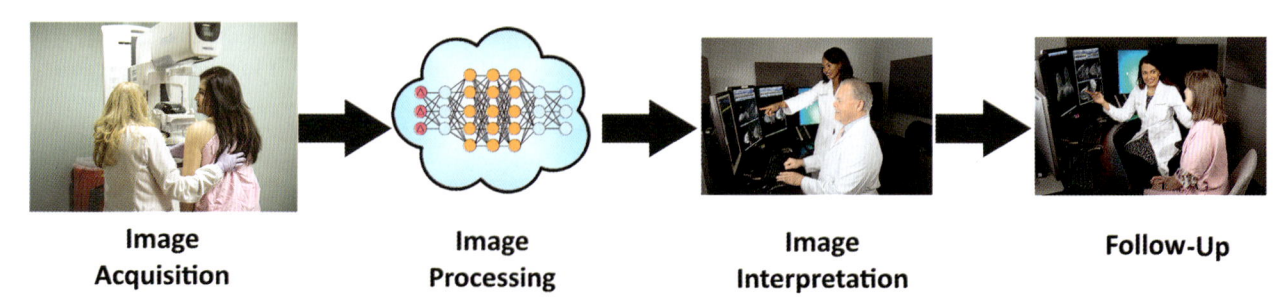

FIG. 28.4 A workflow analysis for digital imaging contains at least four steps: image acquisition, image processing, image interpretation, and report communication/followup. (Image Interpretation and Follow up: Courtesy Mecklenburg Radiology Associates. Image Acquisition: Courtesy Samsung Healthcare.)

agree that AI will be a very positive additional tool, particularly those algorithms based on the deep learning of ANNs.

> We must constantly consider the ethical application of AI algorithms: representative bias, algorithmic bias, cognitive bias, and do no harm.

AI systems are not naturally ethical. The systems have no learned set of rules for the ethics of their behavior or their results. There is an absence of guardrails in AI. Thus concerns about replacing the radiologist or the radiographer are unwarranted.

More, and better, data are needed for training, clinical research, and for the ground-truth analyses. There are several consequences. The value of patient data increases and has a monetary worth that challenges existing ethical codes and regulations concerning privacy, ownership, and consent. Such value has become so great that medical care organizations are favorite targets of cybercriminals.

Besides being able to answer patients' questions, there are specific things that might need to be addressed. If presented with a request to sell patient information, the radiographer should know the organization's data security contact and report the offer. The radiographer needs to know whether the procedure or its results are part of a clinical trial and whether the patient read, understood, and consented to the terms of both the procedure and its role in a clinical trial. The differences in rights accorded by informed consent for treatment versus experimentation are important.

Currently, there is a major challenge to those responsible for quality assurance in the practices, procedures, personal, and outcomes of radiologic services. The challenge is that LLMs, particularly, are built of data that is unfettered by evaluations of truth or falseness unless labeled and structured specifically for that. In an LLM, the text concerning a medical condition or a procedure (think vaccine injection) from a social media site can have nearly the same vector value as text from a reputable medical text. Again, the ethical and practical consequences are that there will always be a need for human judgment and evaluation by the radiologist and radiographer.

The earliest manifestation of a significant problem with existing AI Big Data has been that of bias. There are three principal forms of bias called **representativeness bias, algorithmic bias,** and **cognitive bias.**

Representativeness Bias

Many of the Big Data sets for medical analytic use are from patient populations not representative of the population as a whole. This, of course, has always been a challenge in clinical trials and is a major reason statistical techniques have been developed to estimate how well the data fit a theoretical distribution.

Big Data in LLMs is undifferentiated as to whether it came from a unique hospital or medical practice, a public health system database, or a narrowly defined clinical trial sample. The consequence is that when used as training data, the Big Data set does not represent features of race, age, gender, sexual orientation, and other relevant factors. Concerns with equity, equality, inclusiveness, and sheer accuracy of estimates of benefits inflict bias on the results.

Representative bias is not something that can be addressed directly or immediately. It should, however, always treat results from an AI system as outcomes that are modeled using data that may be unrepresentative. Always assume, like the "Warning: Choking Hazard" label on plastic packaging, AI results come with a "Warning: Bias Hazard."

Algorithmic Bias

Algorithmic bias is found when the mathematics or the ensemble of algorithms may introduce bias. The risk of algorithmic bias increases significantly when the AI model is based on an ensemble of algorithms.

In situations where there is transfer of learning taking place between models, AI algorithm verification is the responsibility of the radiologist and radiographer. Both should be actively engaged in continuous AI algorithm monitoring.

Cognitive Bias

Accepting that AI resembles "cognition," cognitive bias is an appropriate ethical AI bias. Cognitive bias is that arising from the humans who create the AI and those who are users. There seems, at this point, to be little written about how technology alters our existing, evolutionary bent toward cognitive bias.

Some decision theory and behavioral economics show how cognitive bias can come into play in the decisions we make. A simple example of cognitive bias would be in the role it might come to play in the critical radiological decision about triage. If the AI system has successfully predicted the distinction between a true positive and a false negative, the radiologist might develop a cognitive bias toward accepting the AI's first call and not remain appropriately skeptical until all evidence is present.

Cognitive bias that every radiologist, indeed every one of us, might exercise can be a concern. How much information about the patient is essential when making a determination from a digital image? For example, how much would knowing the gender of the patient invoke an inherent cognitive bias of the image

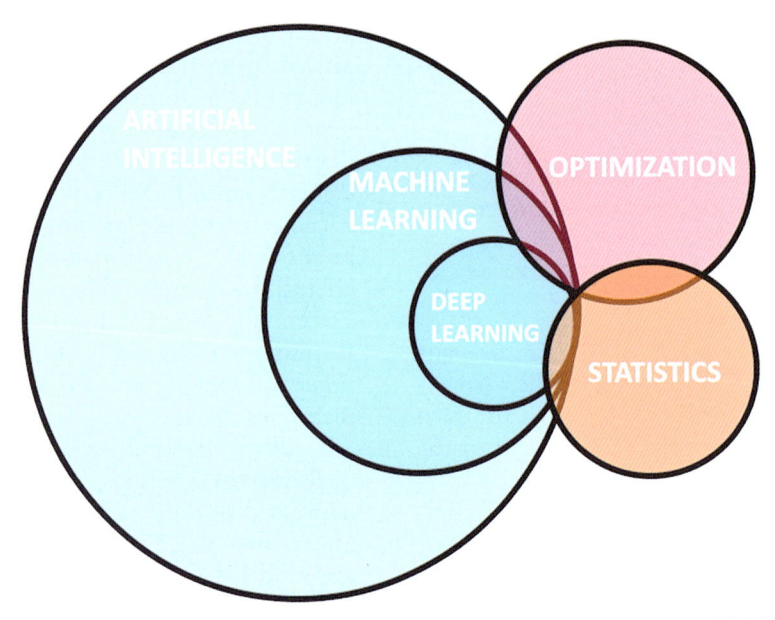

FIG. 28.5 An attempt to properly combine the new physics terms associated with artificial intelligence.

interpretation? The neurosciences will be helping us understand far more about the decision-making going into image interpretation.

AI algorithms are in clinical use to speed up image interpretation by identifying a region of interest (ROI) for the radiologist's concentration. AI has shown a preliminary benefit in interpretation of breast, lung, and brain images by directing the attention of the radiologist to an ROI and then suggesting a diagnosis. Fig. 28.5 is a version of a widely used attempt to properly combine the various new terms of AI.

In 2021, the American Board of Radiology (ABR) added AI to its Core Examination, the certification examination for radiologists. In 2022, the American Society of Radiologic Technologists (ASRT) added AI to the optional content in the Radiography Curriculum.

The future of AI in digital imaging is enormous and progressing rapidly. It will require the close involvement of radiologists and radiographers to achieve its great potential. With AI assistance, digital imaging will be quicker and more accurate.

SUMMARY

The adaption of computer technology to mimic the human mind in cognitive activities such as learning and problem-solving is termed artificial intelligence (AI). Our English language is not able to properly describe the mathematics associated with AI. The most rapid application of AI in medicine is in diagnostic digital imaging.

The first large language model became available through OpenAI and resulted in ChatGPT, which is universally employed and has advanced. The result has been the availability of GPUs (graphical processing units), CPUs (central processing units), and NLP (natural language processing). The first several hundred USFDA medical device software applications were awarded for radiology applications. Vectors serve as a cornerstone for data representation, analysis and processing. They play a fundamental role in the adoption of AI to accelerate the ability of radiologists and radiographers to provide excellent patient care.

In 2019 the first new RSNA journal appeared: *Radiology: Artificial Intelligence*. The cognitive functions of teaching, learning, and decision-making using AI will make the radiologist and radiographer more productive in less time. Machine learning (ML) is a term to describe the use of digital imaging information. Supervised and unsupervised ML leads to more effective radiology algorithms.

ML was overcome by deep learning (DL) a long time later. DL is a subset of ML; however, DL is distinctively different because the deep in DL refers to the number of ANNs used to analyze input data. Both ML and DL use ANNs for processing. RadLex, which is an ontology and lexicon, has impacted the workflow of digital imaging and improved radiologist and radiographer performance. There is considerable concern about the ethics associated with the use of AI topics, such as representative bias, algorithmic bias, and cognitive bias. We now must be concerned that such bias can slip into patient data, clinical trials, quality assurance procedures, and AI algorithms.

CHALLENGE QUESTIONS

1. Define or otherwise identify the following:
   a. Training data
   b. Virtual assistant
   c. CAD
   d. Cognitive functions
   e. Data mining
   f. LUT
   g. AI algorithm
   h. ANN
   i. The last step of imaging workflow
   j. AI ethics
2. What is the difference between machine learning and deep learning?
3. How many games can you recall that are powered by AI?
4. Identify the cognitive functions that you use daily in your radiologic science activity.
5. Describe your understanding of an AI algorithm.
6. How does sensitivity differ from specificity? Which is more important?
7. Explain the difference between supervised and unsupervised learning.
8. As a computer programmer, which would be more difficult, developing supervised or unsupervised AI algorithms, and why?
9. What does the "deep" in deep learning refer to? How does it work?
10. What is the difference between the English words lexicon and ontology as they are used in digital imaging?
11. How do you communicate best with the patient following an imaging study?
12. When viewing the four stages of digital imaging, identify the level of activity of the radiologist, radiographer, and medical physicist in each.
13. A human brain cell, the neuron, is identified with what AI term? If the neuron is in the brain, where is the AI term located?
14. What is the relationship between large language models (LLMs) and generative AI?
15. What is the purpose of including a percentile accuracy score with unsupervised learning?
16. What does it mean when one expresses that the availability of digital imaging AI algorithms is accelerating exponentially?
17. How many pixels are in a CT image size 1024 and bit depth 24?
18. What are you doing now to improve your understanding of artificial intelligence?
19. Are we generating more or fewer images per patient? Name some examples of imaging modality.
20. List AI synonyms for artificial intelligence.

The answers to the Challenge Questions can be found by logging on to our website at http://evolve.elsevier.com.

CHAPTER 29

Quantum Computing

OBJECTIVES

At the completion of this chapter, the student should be able to do the following:
1. Define and describe how qubits differ from digits.
2. Discuss the terms employed to describe quantum mechanics.
3. Understand the potential for quantum computing in radiologic science.
4. Identify the 20th-century history of physics leading to the quantum computer.
5. Diagram the concept of quantum superposition and quantum entanglement.

OUTLINE

What is Quantum Mechanics? 407
  Wave-Particle Duality 408
  The Uncertainty Principle 408
  Quantum Tunneling 409
  Quantum Superposition 409
  Quantum Entanglement 409

Quantum Computer 412
  The Unit of Information 412
  Quantum Algorithms 413
  Quantum Applications 414
Summary 416
Challenge Questions 416

MODERN PHYSICS was born on July 5, 1687, when Sir Isaac Newton published *Principia Mathematica*. In this work, Newton laid out, for the first time, concise mathematical formulas that describe the motion of everything from a baseball to the planets. For the next 200 years, his insights perfectly described everything that happened in the physical world. This became known as **classical physics**.

This changed in the late 1800s as scientists began to explore the underlying nature of the physical world. In 1895 William Roentgen discovered x-rays. Other discoveries followed that identified the nature of the atom; the fact that it consisted of a tiny nucleus orbited by electrons. Furthermore these atoms and their components did not seem to follow the rules of classical physics.

Modern Physics Universe

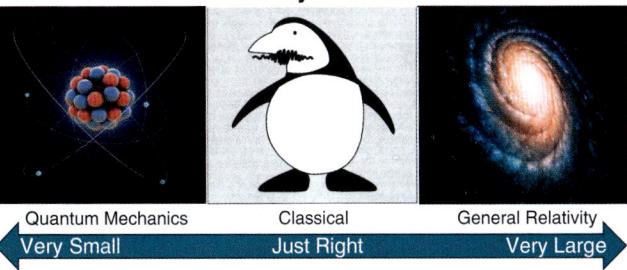

FIG. 29.1 Modern physics extends from atoms and smaller (quantum mechanics) to galaxies and larger (general relativity). (Courtesy Richard Weber, Carnegie-Mellon University.)

While classical physics worked well for activities and interactions in the ordinary everyday world with which we normally deal, it became obvious that these rules did not work for systems at extreme scales, large or small. In the early 1900s, two groups of scientists began developing formal mathematical descriptions of how the universe works at these extreme scales.

One group, led by Niels Bohr, Werner Heisenberg, Erwin Schrödinger, Wolfgang Pauli, and others, developed a comprehensive mathematical description for how forces and particles interact at the extremely small scale of atoms. Their work is now referred to as **quantum mechanics**. Quantum mechanics deals with probability and uncertainty, not the fixed reality of everyday life, classical physics. The mathematics of quantum mechanics describes in precise detail how atoms, elementary particles, and the fundamental forces of nature, except gravity, interact.

Another group, led by Albert Einstein, Satyendra Nath Bose, and others, developed a concise explanation of the force of gravity and the relationship between matter and energy. Their work is now referred to as **general relativity**.

While Newton's laws describe the effect of gravity on objects at "short" distances, it could not explain what gravity is or how it would behave over extremely large-distance scales such as between galaxies. General relativity describes not only what gravity is—the curvature of space/time caused by any object that has mass—but also predicts the effects of gravity at large distances and at high speeds. The three "legs" of modern physics are shown in Fig. 29.1.

Both of these groups, seen in Fig. 29.2, came together at the Fifth Solvay Conference in 1927 in Brussels, where the mathematics of quantum mechanics was debated and formalized.

There were 29 attendees and 17 were, or would become, Nobel Prize winners.

> The Solvay Conference combined the efforts of many leading physicists into quantum mechanics.

While the effects described by general relativity do not directly impact us, the effects described by quantum mechanics affect us in almost everything we do every day. All of the devices we use—from cell phones to computers to sophisticated clinical equipment—depend on quantum mechanical effects for their operation.

Even though the mathematics of quantum mechanics is beyond the scope of this text, it is important to understand some of the quantum mechanical phenomena and how they impact the devices we use, especially those of digital imaging. It is also important to understand how these effects might provide significantly enhanced capabilities in the future.

WHAT IS QUANTUM MECHANICS?

One of the great revelations that emerged as scientists began to unravel the mysterious behavior of atoms and their constituents was that, at the tiniest scales, the universe is not "smooth." Instead, the properties of these tiny particles could only have specific discrete values. In other words, the inhabitants of this tiny world are "quantized." This realization led to the discovery of a number of other strange properties of elementary particles.

We humans simply do not have the intuition to describe the physics concepts of quantum mechanics; however, the mathematics that describes quantum mechanics is very clear and very descriptive but also beyond the scope of this textbook. Nothing in our daily lives even approaches the thought processes involved with quantum mechanics.

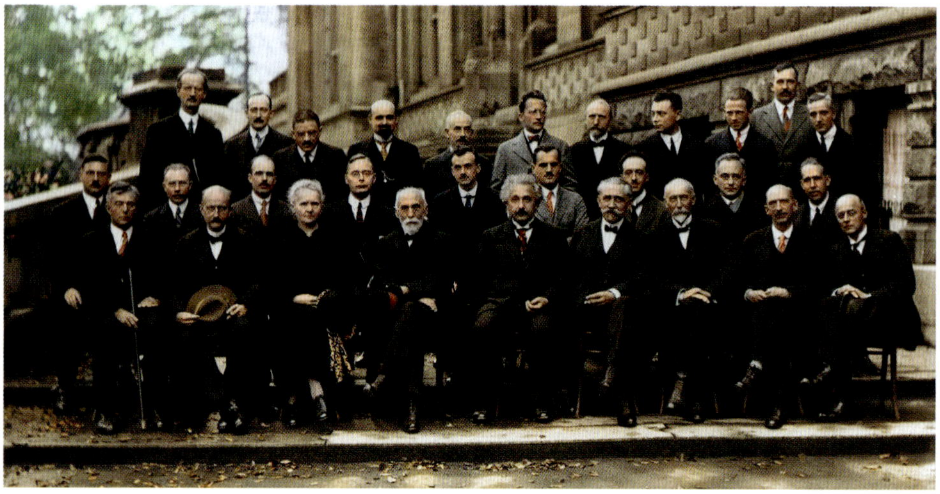

FIG. 29.2 *The Wall Street Journal* called this group of scientists The Quantum Physics Club. Max Planck, Marie Currie, and Albert Einstein are in the front row.

The topic titles that follow were all engaged separately by many physicists during the first two decades of the 20th century. Albert Einstein, of course, is the most famous because of his theory of relativity; however, the theory of relativity is not a contributor to quantum mechanics. Einstein's description of the photoelectric effect is part of quantum mechanics and for that he won the Nobel Prize in Physics in 1921.

Wave-Particle Duality

A principal feature of quantum mechanics is that subatomic particles can be described as either waves or as particles. Max Planck, in about 1900, was the first to describe the **wave-particle duality** of subatomic particles.

On the one hand, there were many experiments at that time showing that the atom, subsequently known as the Bohr atom for the Danish physicist Niels Bohr, consisted of electrons in fixed orbits circling a dense and heavy nucleus. The electrons, and subsequently subnuclear particles, were shown to be particles by the way they were observed to interact.

The "wave nature" of matter was first identified by Thomas Young in 1801. Using an oil lamp and a piece of cardboard with two thin slits, he showed that light generates a wave-like interference pattern. Other experiments clearly demonstrated that light also acts as a particle. So, depending on how the question is asked, light can exhibit properties of either a particle or a wave. This same dual nature has been demonstrated with all the other elementary particles and with photon radiation.

> Subatomic particles and photons interact with matter as both particles and waves.

At the same time, such particles were also shown to mirror the wave-like interactions of visible light. Visible light was also shown to behave and interact as a particle; hence wave-particle duality is a fundamental concept in quantum physics. The x-ray photon was described by Roentgen as a wave, but was also shown to have particle-like interactions with matter.

To describe the wave nature of objects in a quantum system, Erwin Schrodinger developed a "wave function." By tradition, the wave function is represented by the Greek letter psi = Ψ (pronounced "sigh"). There is no truth to the rumor that he decided on this letter based on how his students reacted when he assigned a problem to them.

English words such as superposition, entanglement, tunneling, and probability are not able to properly describe the mathematics involved in quantum physics. We are not even going to approach such mathematics. However, before continuing, please accept one small example, the symbol Ψ that is shown in Fig. 29.3 illustrates a qubit in the discussions that follow.

The Uncertainty Principle

One consequence of the wave nature of elementary particles is that they do not have specific properties until they are measured. The best that can be said is that there is a probability that a particular property will have a certain value. Quantum mechanics is intrinsically probabilistic, not precise.

Anytime a property of a system is measured, the act of measuring will result in a change to the system. The easiest way to demonstrate this is when you test the pressure in a tire. When you take the measurement, a small amount of air is released from the tire into the pressure gauge. If you do the measurement many times, you will see the pressure decrease.

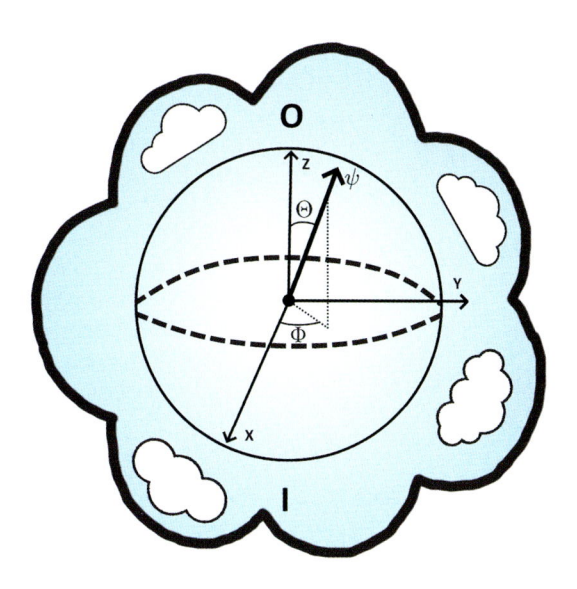

FIG 29.3 A qubit can be represented by an arrow inside of an imaginary sphere.

This principle also applies to elementary particles. Furthermore, the more precise a measurement is made of one property, for example its position, the less precise its other properties, such as velocity, can be measured. In fact, there is a precisely defined minimum value for the uncertainty in the measurements. This is a direct consequence of the fact that, in the quantum world, everything is expressed as probabilities.

When one attempts to measure a subatomic particle or a photon, the action of the measurement interferes with the measurement. The position and the state of the particle or photon that is being measured is probably not exactly correct. Uncertainty exists regarding all such subatomic particle and photon measurements because of the method of measurement.

By the time such a measurement is made, the particle or photon is in a different position. Because of this difference, by the time the physicist has made an observation, a probability coefficient must be attached to the observation.

> The effort to measure a particle or photon affects the certainty of that measurement.

Max Born, another physicist at that time, migrated from Germany to Britain and was responsible for expressing the probability as a quantum mechanical feature that he termed the **probability density function**. Each of these advances in describing quantum physics required the introduction of new English terms.

Quantum Tunneling

In classical physics, when a particle or photon arrives at a barrier, it cannot penetrate or cross it. It is trapped on one side of that barrier. Quantum mechanics allows a particle or photon that does not have sufficient energy to penetrate such a barrier to tunnel under that barrier and reappear on the other side. Quantum tunneling is connected with radioactive decay, nuclear fusion, and even some commercial applications such as scanning tunneling microscopy.

Quantum Superposition

In 1935 Erwin Schrodinger used a cat in a box, which has become a classic thought experiment, to describe the paradox of **quantum superposition**. The box is closed. The observer does not know if the cat is dead or alive.

> A particle or photon can exist in multiple states at the time of measurement.

Schrodinger elegantly described this hypothetical cat in a box with a poison flask, a radioactive source, a Geiger counter, and a hammer ready to smash the poison flask (Fig. 29.4). If the Geiger counter detects radiation, it releases the hammer to smash the poison flask and kill the cat. The cat is simultaneously alive or dead depending on when the observation is made. The result is quantum superposition. This was an interesting use of a Geiger counter and radioactive source, both new to the physics world. Fig. 29.5 is a copy of the WANTED sign posted in many towns.

Quantum Entanglement

Digital computing is based on the binary number system and bits. Quantum computing is based on quantum mechanics and qubits (**quantum bits**). Furthermore, the manipulation of qubits is based on **superposition** and **entanglement**, two of many properties embedded deeply in the physics of quantum mechanics.

Bits, as we have shown in Chapter 27, are in a 0 or 1 state. Qubits are also in a 0 or 1 state, but they can also be in a 0 or 1 superposition state, resulting in many more values. Furthermore, the superposition of qubits is simultaneous; instead of two states, many states are possible simultaneously. Measurements on a particle will simultaneously impact the state of a similar particle separated by a long distance. That is entanglement. Spooky, yes, but true.

> Quantum entanglement is a recognized property of quantum mechanics from years ago.

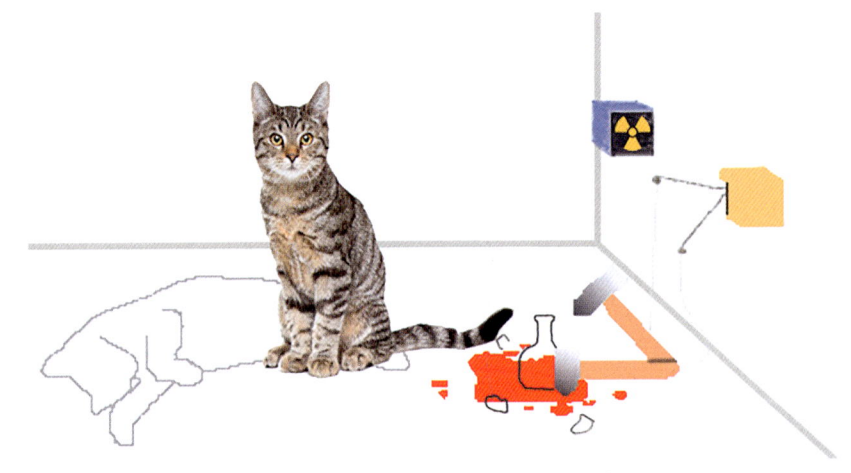

FIG. 29.4 Erwin Schrodinger used a now-famous cat to explain the state of superposition. The cat was both alive and dead.

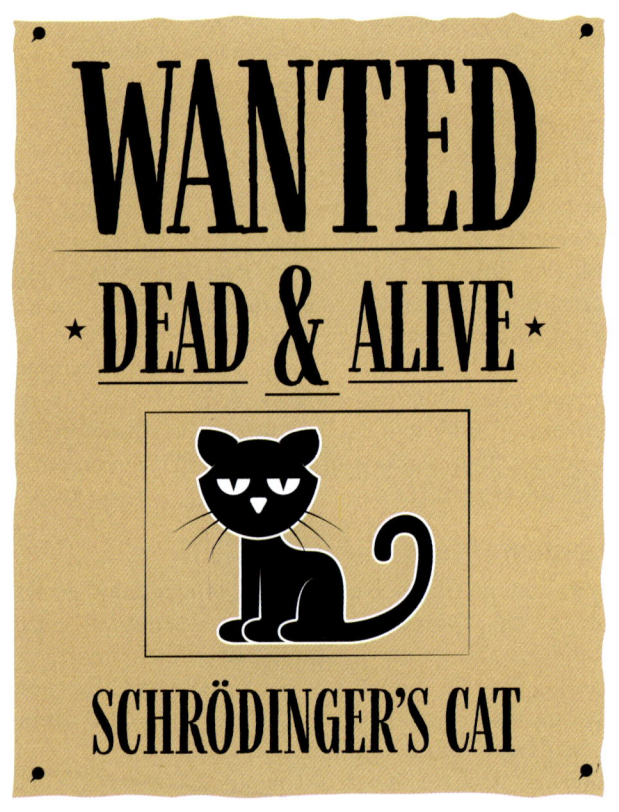

FIG. 29.5 This WANTED sign has been posted in many towns. (Courtesy Richard Weber, Carnegie-Mellon University.)

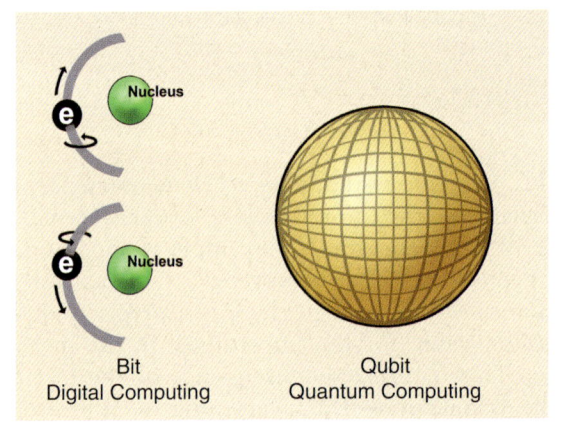

FIG. 29.6 A qubit can exist in many different energy states simultaneously.

Fig. 29.6 shows another representation of a qubit. In classical physics, bits are precise. In quantum mechanics, a probability function is applied to qubits and therefore any quantum computer algorithm will be probabilistic. Wineland and Haroche received the 2012 Nobel Prize in Physics for helping us understand this quantum superposition and entanglement.

The 2024 Nobel Prize in Physics went to Hopfield and Hinton for their work on artificial neural networks which are essential to quantum computing. They have been called the "godfathers of AI". Their research was fundamental to the development and availability of Open AI's ChatGPT in late 2023 as discussed in Chapter 28.

The promise of quantum computing is a leap forward in computing speed and capacity. We will likely see this in a few years with the introduction of quantum computers into daily life.

Quantum entanglement mathematically describes what happens when quantum systems interact. It is the release mechanism for classical mechanics to transition to quantum mechanics to transition to a quantum computer. Fig. 29.7 is a quick summary of the differences to be expected as we progress in the development of quantum computers.

The 2023 Nobel Prize in Physics was awarded to three theoretical physicists who described the movement

CHAPTER 29 Quantum Computing

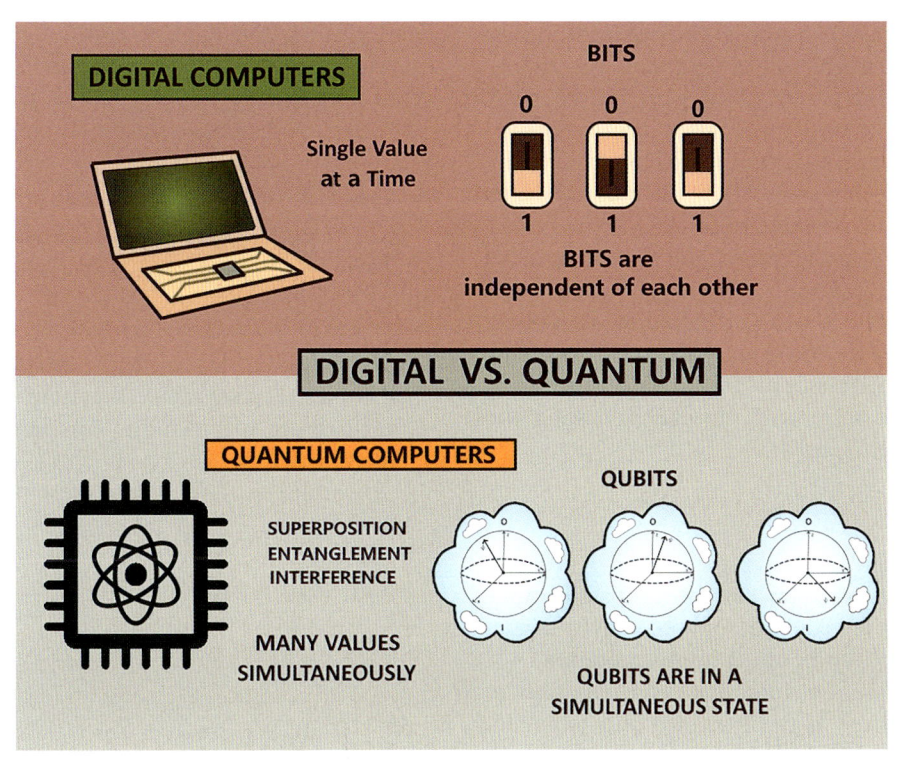

FIG. 29.7 Major differences between digital computers and quantum computers.

TABLE 29.1	The Travel Distance of Light During Different Periods of Time

Travel Distance of Light

One second (1 s): Earth to moon
One millisecond (1 ms = 10^{-3} s): National Collegiate Athletic Association football field
One microsecond (1 μs = 10^{-9} s): A bowling lane
One nanosecond (1 ns = 10^{-9} s): This page
One attosecond (1 as = 10^{-12} s): One biologic molecule

of electrons in one attosecond (1 as = 10^{-18}s). That is the time frame for engaging quantum entanglement and for the concept of quantum tunneling. Table 29.1 relates the distance a photon of light travels during different time periods to give you a reference to the magnitude of the prefix atto.

Quantum entanglement describes the manner in which one qubit can become engaged with other qubits. Two or more qubits can influence other qubits instantly, regardless of position or the distance of separation. Quantum entanglement considerations are beyond the capacity of current digital computers. We will certainly become involved in future episodes of qubital time travel, even back in time as in the 1985 science-fiction thriller *Back to the Future*.

It might be worth your time to view that classic movie to better understand quantum tunneling and quantum entanglement. Keep in mind that this is using English to describe very difficult mathematics.

> Mathematics is the language of quantum physics.

Quantum entanglement can be described with a penguin tale. I travel to the Antarctic and capture two penguins living together, a little blue penguin and an emperor penguin (see Fig. 17.10). I call and tell you that I am sending you two penguins for your collection. When the crate arrives, it has only the little blue penguin! I still have the emperor penguin with me. But the penguins are family and continue to interact as such. They are in a state of superposition but still entangled no matter their separation in space.

Refer to the previous chapter and the list of terms. Review the definition of measurement called **metrology**. Quantum metrology, when coupled with quantum tunneling and quantum entanglement, will apply with future access to quantum computers. Entanglement will allow instant influence of one qubit with another regardless of distance. Tunneling suggests that return to an earlier time might be possible.

> Quantum tunneling and entanglement allow repetition via time reversal.

Quantum tunneling and quantum entanglement suggest that in the future one might be able to retroactively change the outcome of previous events. All we need as a takeaway is that the future of quantum mechanics, because of tunneling and entanglement, has the potential to revolutionize decision making in many areas of life, such as gambling, investing, cooking, and scientific research.

Consider cooking on the attosecond time scale as an example. You have prepared a most delicious cherry pie and tasted it, but you are disappointed, wishing it had more sweetness. You engage culinary tunneling and culinary entanglement to the earlier pie-making stage. You adjust the recipe and repeat the cooking and WOW!!! A much better result.

QUANTUM COMPUTER

Quantum computing was first predicted by Richard Feynman, a physicist and educator of the past century. There is currently an incredible amount of activity engaging in the future application of quantum computing.

The resulting quantum computers are expected to be exponentially faster in performance and exponentially larger in big data management. The speed of such management will be the exceptional characteristic of the quantum computer. Fig. 29.8 is a photograph of the IBM Quantum System One installed at Cleveland Clinic.

With the expectations described, what is actually accomplished and when, is very much unknown. The predictions at the turn of the 20th century had quantum computing available at the time of this Golden Anniversary edition. That obviously did not happen. The future ability to purchase a quantum computer and place it into service at home or at the office is now anyone's guess.

The Unit of Information

The **qubit** (Fig. 29.3) is to the quantum computer what a bit is to the digital computer. Both deal with electrons and employ the English words of position, spin, and phase by applying the two digits 0 and 1. Bits come in two sizes, 0 and 1. Qubits come in many sizes and are described as having metastable states in addition to the states of 0 and 1.

> Digital computers operate with two-stage digits. Quantum computers require multistage qubits.

In classical physics, bits are precise. In quantum mechanics, a probability function is applied to qubits and therefore any quantum computer algorithm will be probabilistic.

An additional, simpler representation of a qubit is shown in Fig. 29.9 where the direction of the arrow Ψ indicates the metastable state of the qubit at that instant. Recall that the symbol Ψ is that which physicists use when describing a quantum state or solving a quantum physics problem.

> Digits are fixed at 0 or 1. Qubits have many values and a probability function.

The concept of superposition permits a single qubit to exist in many different states simultaneously, as shown in Fig. 29.9 If the qubit arrow is horizontal, left or right, there is a 50% chance of observing a 0 or 1, as shown in Fig. 29.10.

Extend this approach to that shown in Fig. 29.11 and we have an example of entanglement. When two qubits are entangled, the position of the metastable arrow is

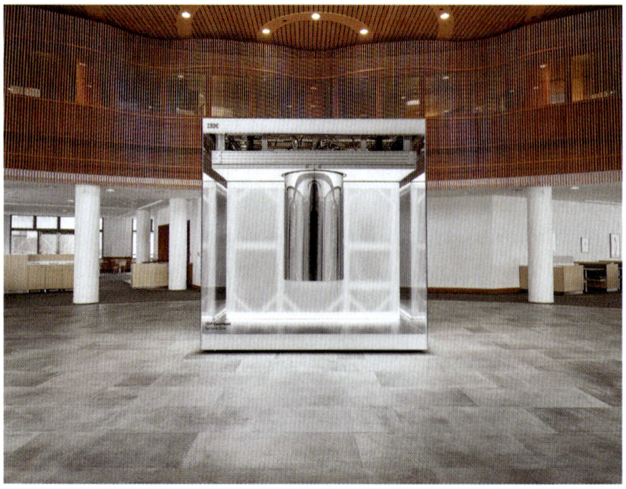

FIG. 29.8 An IBM Q System One is a quantum computer with 20 superconducting qubits. (Ryan Lavine for IBM, reprint Courtesy of IBM Corporation © 2024.)

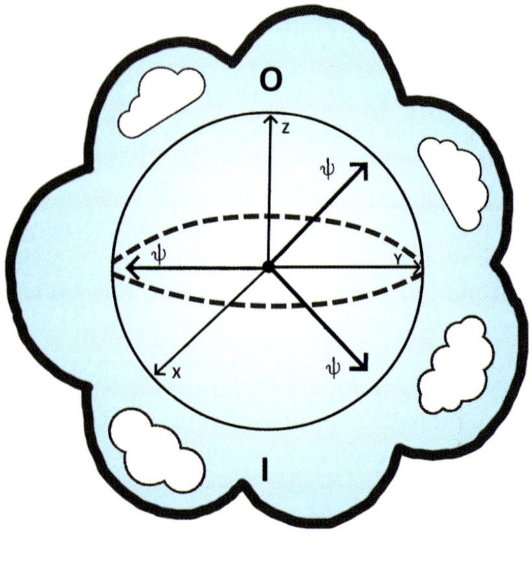

FIG. 29.9 A way of showing the metastable state of a qubit, which changes every attosecond.

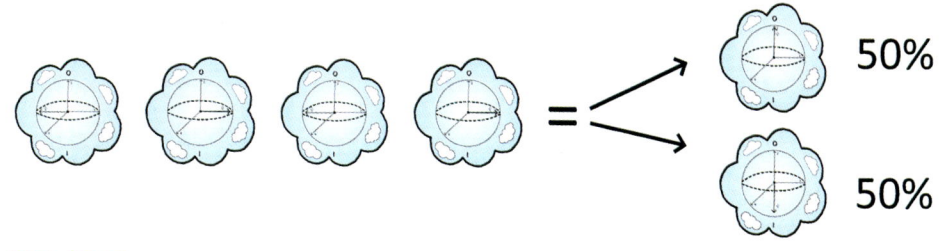

FIG. 29.10 These qubits each have a 50% chance of being detected at the time of observation.

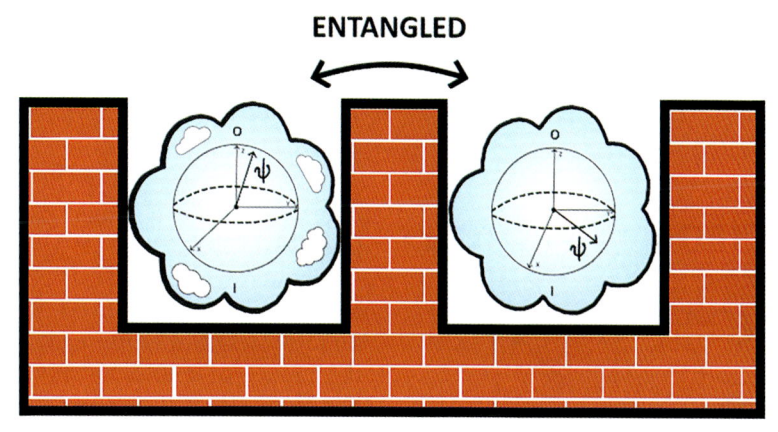

FIG. 29.11 When qubits are entangled, they are represented as shown.

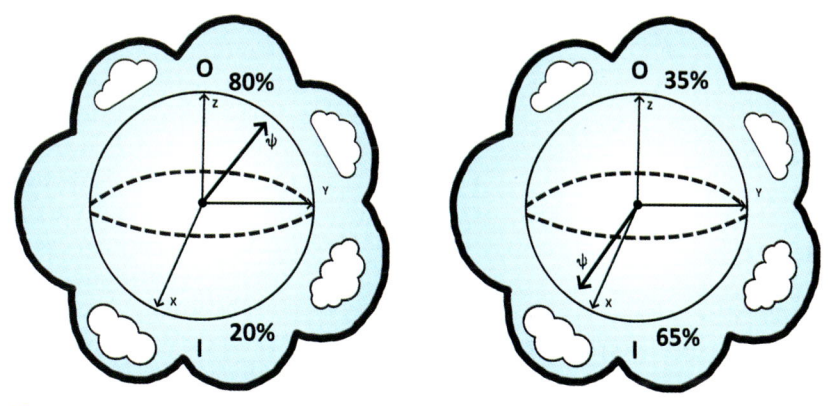

FIG. 29.12 When qubits are entangled, there is a constantly changing probability of the position of the metastable arrow with the percent entanglement as shown at that instant.

constantly changing, as shown in Fig. 29.12. This leads to the probability density function mentioned earlier in this chapter and is shown graphically in Fig. 29.13.

But what exactly is a qubit besides an arrow in a sphere? Qubits are either an atom, an electron, or a photon. Each of these can be considered to have the multilevel energy states described by Ψ. These qubits are shown in Fig. 29.14.

Quantum Algorithms

The previous chapter explained AI algorithms as digital or digital imaging algorithms. As we engage quantum computing, we will not be so aware of quantum algorithms. Quantum algorithms control how qubits deal with the various environmental and design features influencing them.

An algorithm is a deep mathematical description of how to do something. It is a mathematical recipe. A recipe lists what materials to use and how much of each. Then, it lists how to prepare them: sift, sort, stir. Finally, it lists how to use them.

Quantum algorithms are designed to control qubital errors, such as noise, decoherence, and fault tolerance. If not controlled, qubital errors accumulate, slow the quantum computer, and limit its data management size. Digital computer AI algorithms will continue to run on

PROBABILITY DISTRIBUTION

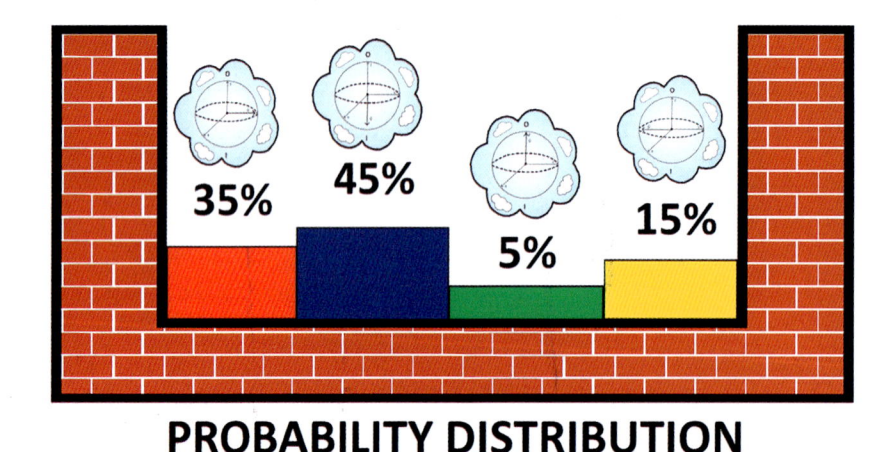

FIG. 29.13 The probability density function can be displayed as shown.

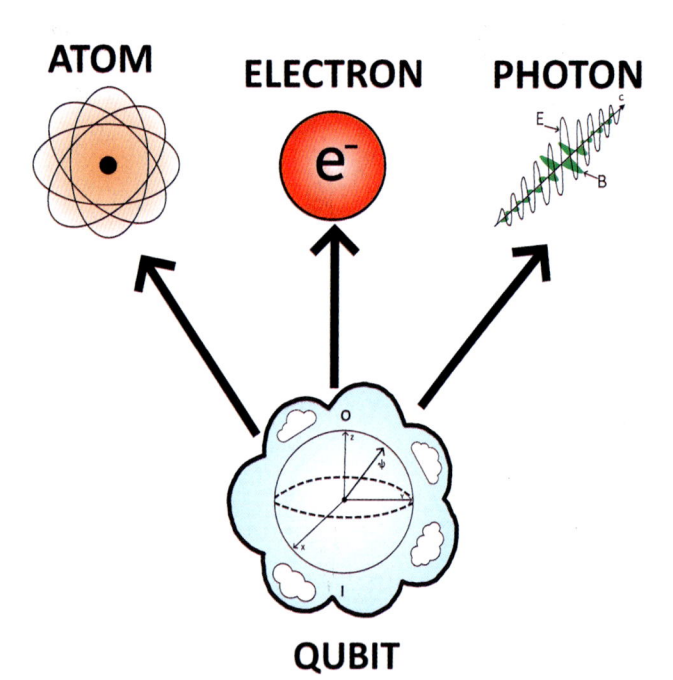

FIG. 29.14 Qubits can be atoms, nuclear particles, electrons, or photons.

quantum computers but for total success in speed and data management, quantum algorithms will be required to be continuously developed.

There are currently many quantum algorithms up and running on small hybrid quantum computers. Thus far, many algorithms are named for the scientists involved in that algorithm development: Shore, Feynman, Turing, Douche, Simons, Bernstein, Diffie, Grover, Lloyd, and more coming.

When qubits entangle, as illustrated in Fig. 29.11, the entanglement will experience **decoherence** because of environmental noise such as cosmic rays and heat. Much effort is in place to produce **fault-tolerant** quantum computers. That task requires many entangled qubits to make a single perfect fault-tolerant qubit (Fig. 29.15).

The arrow used to describe the qubit in Fig. 29.3 is in a random position at every instant of time. To produce a fault-tolerant quantum computer, we need to arrange the family of qubits as though they were the minute hands on a display of wristwatches. These minute hands on the watches would all be set at precisely the same position, at the same time.

Better yet, consider a waddle of penguins on an iceberg, as in Fig. 29.16. If there are 10 penguins to be positioned in line, by the time you have penguin no. 10 in position, the earlier penguins will have already left the line. They are not coherent but rather experience decoherence. The waddle is not fault tolerant!

There are currently many approaches to producing a quantum computer and the main efforts are listed in Table 29.2. It is too early to even guess which effort will prevail, but the superconducting quantum computer is probably in the lead.

An early approach to producing a quantum computer is addressed by Quantinuum (Fig. 29.17). It is a classical digital computer with just a few qubits embedded for some very limited practice to help us get started. Multiple new vendors are on the way.

> Quantum computers will be at least 10 times faster, managing 10 times the data.

The promise of quantum computing is a leap forward in computing speed and capacity. We will likely see this in the next few years with the introduction of quantum computers.

Quantum Applications

Algorithms are mathematical, but they instruct the quantum computer when and how to apply. Algorithms are the cooking instructions and they are being developed

FAULT-TOLERANT QUBITS

FAULTY QUBITS

"PERFECT" QUBIT

FAULT-TOLERENT QUBIT

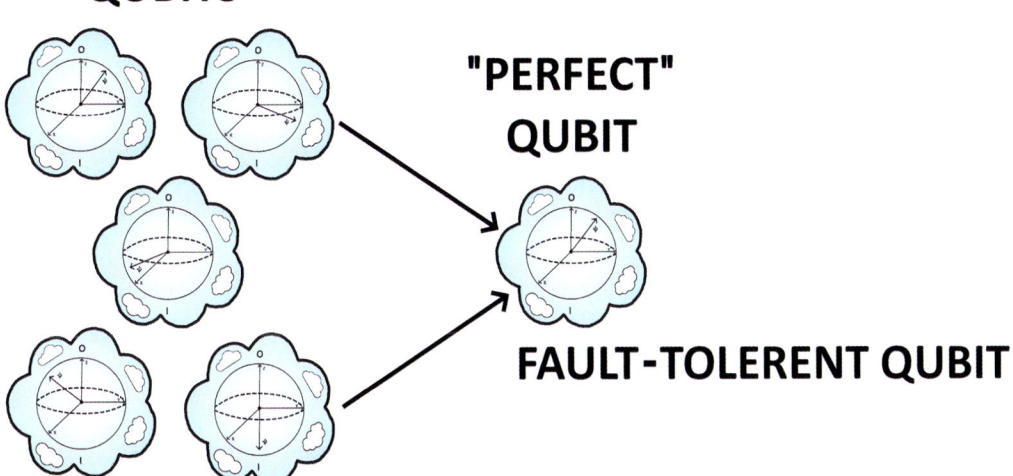

FIG. 29.15 Quantum fault correction for a single perfect qubit.

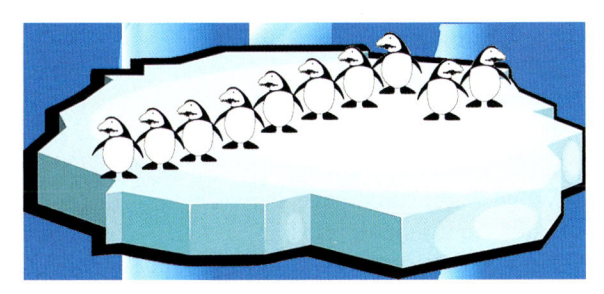

FIG. 29.16 A waddle of penguins on an iceberg to demonstrate a fault-tolerant qubit.

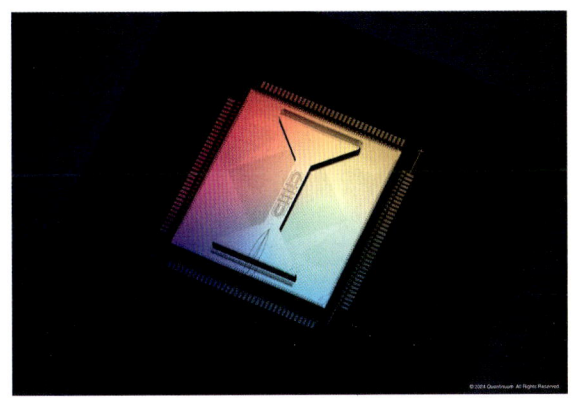

FIG. 29.17 A hybrid quantum computer. (Courtesy Quantinuum.)

TABLE 29.2	Types of Quantum Computers
Types)	**Description**
Color Center Quantum Computer	Spin coherence timed with optical transition
Hybrid Computer	Both digital and analog
Linear Optical Quantum Computer	Uses photons and optical instruments
Quantum Dot Quantum Computer	Nanometer size semiconductors with various optical properties
Superconducting Quantum Computer	Uses superconducting qubits as quantum dots
Trapped Ion Quantum Computer	Charges atoms, ion, confined to electromagnetic fields

rapidly for specific tasks such as cryptography, digital image interpretation, and for what some see as a future quantum internet—a **quantumnet**.

The promise of quantum computing is based principally on speed and data. Both computational speed and data management are promised to be at least an order of magnitude greater, 10 times, than that of the digital computer. The likely measure of success for a quantum computer will be speed, in terms of how much faster than the digital computer the quantum computer will access large data files, process the data, and compute the result.

SUMMARY

Quantum computing is the latest physics accomplishment that began with Isaac Newton 400 years ago. Physics has progressed through classical physics to general relativity and to quantum mechanics.

Quantum mechanics was formalized in 1927 at the Solvay Conference. At that time, the wave-particle duality was described with ever-deeper mathematics. Subatomic particles can interact as waves, and electromagnetic waves can interact as particles.

Schrödinger's uncertainty principle introduced the symbol φ to our physics vocabulary. It states that there is considerable uncertainty in a physical measurement because the measurement disturbs the object.

Quantum mechanics introduced us to quantum tunneling, quantum superposition, and quantum entanglement. We do not need to understand the mathematics but rather the English descriptions of these quantum mechanics features.

Quantum mechanics has also introduced us to the qubit, which is to quantum computing what the digit is to digital computing. Digits exist with only two values: 0 and 1. Qubits exist with many metastable values simultaneously, and they change in attoseconds. The result is that quantum computers have greater speed and greater data management than digital computers.

Algorithms have been used for many years with digital computers. They instruct the computer how to manipulate data. Quantum algorithms are designed to do the same but much faster, managing much larger data files and controlling qubital errors. Qubital errors such as noise, decoherence, and fault tolerance are controlled by quantum algorithms in order that the quantum computer will not be limited in speed or data management.

The likely future of computer applications communication and connection will be also exponentially faster on the future quantumnet.

The answers to the Challenge Questions can be found by logging on to our website at http://evolve.elsevier.com

CHALLENGE QUESTIONS

1. Define or otherwise identify the following:
   a. A quantum bit
   b. Classical physics
   c. The Solvay Conference
   d. The Bohr atom
   e. Schrodinger's cat
   f. *Back to the Future*
   g. Probability
   h. Ψ
   i. Quantum physics
   j. Quantum computing
2. Describe quantum superposition.
3. List the different types of qubits.
4. What is the difference between quantum mechanics and quantum physics?
5. Explain the meaning of wave-particle duality.
6. What do you think about time reversal *Back to the Future*?
7. If there are 5 qubits in a quantum algorithm, how many states are there?
8. How many values can a qubit have?
9. What causes decoherence of qubits?
10. How will we describe the internet of the future?
11. What group photograph has been described as The Quantum Physics Club?
12. What is the difference between special relativity and general relativity?
13. What is quantum entanglement, and how does it differ from quantum superposition?
14. What is the difference between an AI algorithm and a quantum algorithm?
15. How many qubits will be required to engage a single fault-tolerant qubit?
16. Identify a few possible types of quantum computers.
17. Is an x-ray photon a wave, a particle, or a packet of energy?
18. What language best describes quantum physics?
19. How would you describe classical physics?
20. What does quantum tunneling mean?

Image Perception

CHAPTER 30

OBJECTIVES

At the completion of this chapter, the student should be able to do the following:

1. List and discuss the several special requirements of a radiographer in support of image interpretation by a radiologist.
2. Describe the difference between photopic vision and scotopic vision.
3. Discuss the concept of visual acuity.
4. Draw and explain a receiver operating characteristic curve for an experienced radiographer versus an experienced radiologist.
5. Identify several ergonomic requirements for digital image interpretation.

OUTLINE

Special Demands of Digital Imaging 418
  Illumination 418
  Visual Physiology 418
  Contrast Sensitivity 420
Interpretation 421
Receiver Operating Characteristic Curves 422
  Ergonomics 424
Summary 424
Challenge Questions 425

THE INVENTION of the fluoroscope by Thomas A. Edison in 1896 brought with it the classic feature of motion imaging with x-rays and also a challenge for the radiologist in interpreting very dim images. **Image perception** has always been a distinct challenge for fluoroscopy. It returns in this 21st century as a challenge in terms of the interpretation of digital medical images.

Image perception is a scientific term for what we call visual **sensitivity**. Image perception in medical imaging relates to how well we can visualize an image, and although the radiographer is not normally involved in image interpretation, it is the radiographer's responsibility to produce a quality image that can be properly interpreted.

> Image perception is the visual sensitivity required for proper image interpretation.

Fluoroscopic images are relatively dim, have low intensity, and exhibit low contrast. Therefore the perception of anatomy is restricted by the human visual anatomy. Such restrictions do not exist with digital imaging because of the various postprocessing features available. Window and level allow all shades of gray to be observed, but such image manipulation brings additional challenges for the radiographer.

Image interpretation is the principal responsibility of the radiologist and continues to be a primary source of error—**false negative**, missing a lesion or abnormality, and **false positive**, calling an abnormality when there is none.

Radiographers need a basic understanding of the physiological ability of the human eye, described as **visual acuity** and **contrast sensitivity**. This, in turn, requires an understanding of foveal and peripheral vision. Visual acuity is closely connected with spatial resolution. It is the ability to distinguish shapes and details in a digital image. Contrast sensitivity is related to contrast resolution and digital image postprocessing. It deals with shades of gray.

Image perception and cognition are part of this basic understanding and involve many aspects, such as **visual search** and **visual training**. Visual training is required of both the radiologist and radiographer.

Many human-computer interactions come into play with digital imaging, requiring expertise on the part of the radiographer. Some of these interactions were discussed in previous chapters. Consider this an extension, emphasizing the special visual demands of digital imaging.

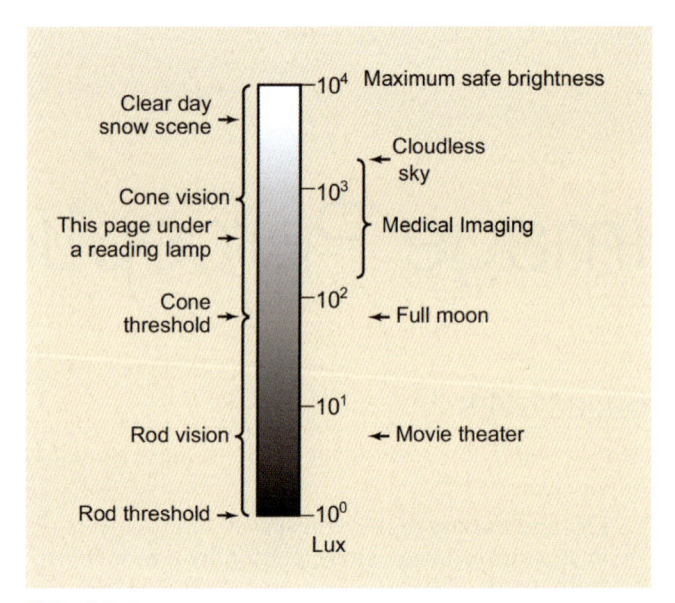

FIG. 30.1 The range of human vision is wide; it covers four orders of visual illuminance.

SPECIAL DEMANDS OF DIGITAL IMAGING

The special demands of digital imaging are postprocessing and numerical analysis. These require some knowledge of image illumination and visual physiology.

Illumination

A principal advantage of digital imaging over earlier analog imaging is image brightness. Just as it is much more difficult to read a book in dim light, it is much harder to interpret a dim image than a bright one.

Illumination levels are measured in units of lumen per square meter or lux. It is not necessary to know the precise definition of lux; its importance lies in the wide range of illumination levels over which the human eye is sensitive. Fig. 30.1 lists approximate illumination levels for familiar objects.

Digital images are visualized under illumination levels of 100 to 1000 lux. (You may want to return to the discussion of photometric quantities in Chapter 24 to reinforce your understanding.)

Visual Physiology

The structures of the eye that are responsible for the sensation of vision are called **rods** and **cones**. Fig. 30.2 is a cross-section of the human eye that reveals its principal parts and its appearance on a magnetic resonance image (MRI). Light incident on the eye must first pass through the cornea, a transparent protective covering, and through the lens, where the light is focused onto the retina.

Between the cornea and the lens are the pupil and iris, which behave similarly to the diaphragm of a

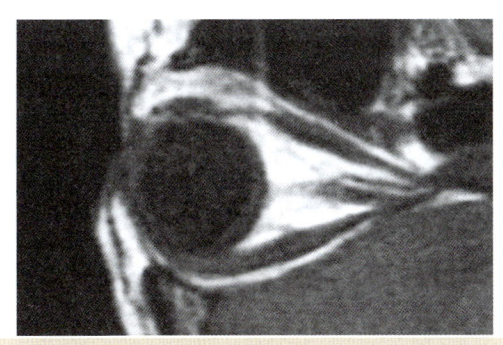

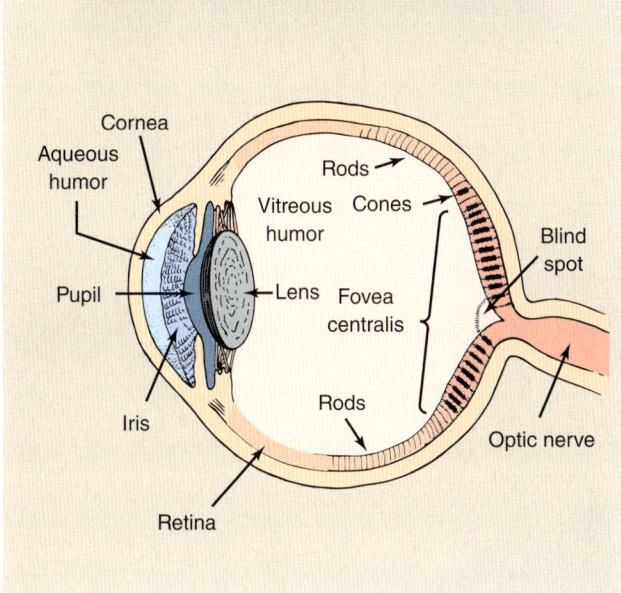

FIG. 30.2 The appearance of the human eye on a magnetic resonance image and the parts responsible for vision.

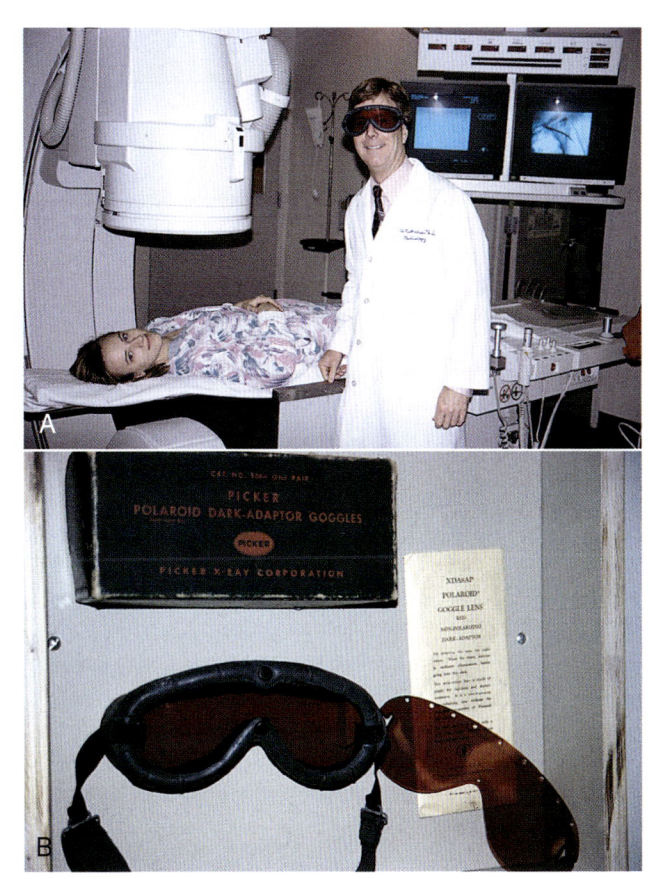

FIG. 30.3 Red goggles were used to dark adapt for conventional screen fluoroscopy. This radiologist is "**Back to the Future**." (Courtesy Ben Archer, Baylor College of Medicine.)

photographic camera in controlling the amount of light that is admitted to the eye. The pupil is basically a hole in the iris. The iris controls the size of the center of the hole.

In the presence of bright light, the iris contracts the pupil and allows only a small amount of light to enter. During low-light conditions, such as the dimly lit digital image reading area, the iris dilates the pupil (i.e., it opens up) and allows more light to enter.

Visual **adaption** was very important to early radiologists, who had to dark adapt for at least 10 minutes, sometimes wearing red glasses (Fig. 30.3) before performing a fluoroscopic procedure. The same situation holds today when a radiologist enters a digital image reading room with ambient light levels of 25 to 50 lux from a well-lit hallway, although the dark adaption is not nearly as severe.

Visual **accommodation** is a term related to changes we make voluntarily and involuntarily in order to improve our image perception. We view an image at a distance of approximately 40 to 50 cm (voluntary). It takes about 200 ms for the eye to focus and converge on an object (involuntary). This temporal accommodation, 200 ms, restricts the frame rate for digital fluoroscopy to 5 images/s (200 ms/image = 1 s/5 images).

> When light arrives at the retina, it is detected by the rods and the cones.

Rods and cones are small structures; more than 100,000 of them are found per square millimeter of retina. The cones are concentrated at the center of the retina in an area called the **fovea centralis** (see Fig. 30.2). Rods, on the other hand, are more numerous on the periphery of the retina. No rods are found at the fovea centralis.

The rods are sensitive to low-light levels and are stimulated during dim-light situations such as a dark motion picture theater or the radiology reading room.. The threshold for rod vision is approximately 2 lux. Cones, on the other hand, are less sensitive to light; their threshold is approximately 100 lux, but cones are capable of responding to intense light levels, rods cannot.

When light falls on rods and cones, pigments in these cells convert light into an electrical signal energizing various nerve cells. These nerve cells communicate

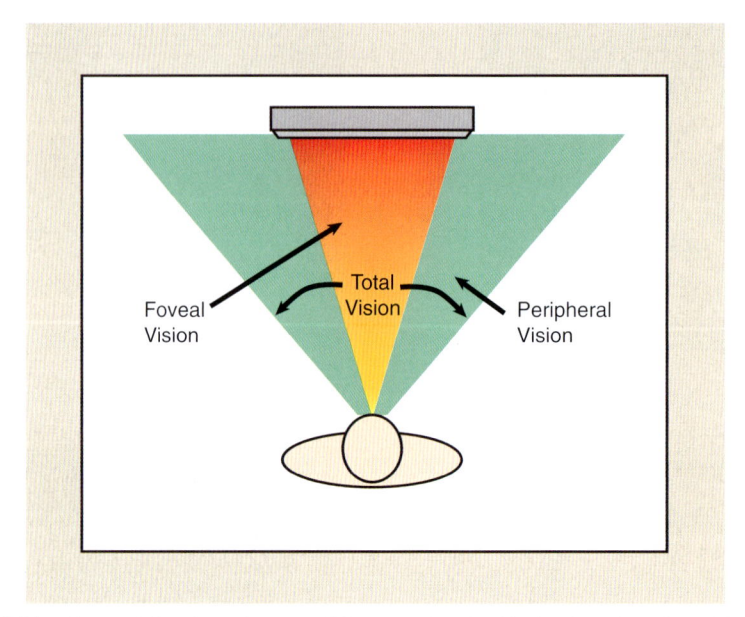

FIG. 30.4 Visual search involves the sensitivity associated with the foveal and peripheral vision. There is a blind spot where the optic nerve becomes the retina.

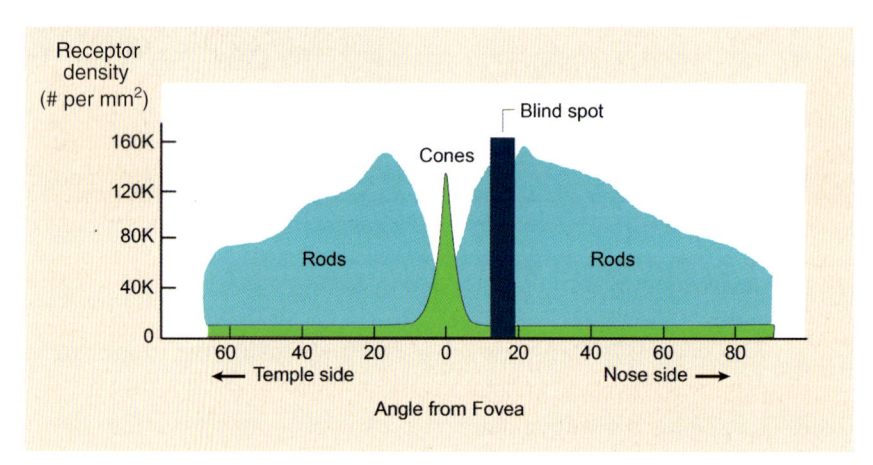

FIG. 30.5 Distribution of rods and cones on the retina and the location of the blind spot.

through the optic nerve and beyond to the visual cortices of the brain.

Consequently, cones are used primarily for daylight vision, called **photopic vision**, and rods are used for night vision, called **scotopic vision**. This aspect of visual physiology explains why dim objects are viewed more readily if they are not looked at directly. Astronomers and radiologists are familiar with the fact that a dim object is best viewed peripherally, where rod vision predominates.

Visual acuity is highest in the central portion of the retina where the cones are concentrated (Fig. 30.4). This region is the fovea centralis, and the view registered without an eye or head movement is **foveal vision**. When the radiologist moves the eyes around the image in order to see different areas better, **visual search** is engaged. There is a small blind spot because there are no rods or cones on that part of the retina where the optic nerve enters.

Peripheral vision is associated with the distribution of rods shown in Fig. 30.5 and illustrated by field size in Fig. 30.4. Peripheral vision is somewhat better for high-contrast image areas and for the motion associated with scrolling through many CT or MRI images on a multiple-image display workstation.

Contrast Sensitivity

Cones perceive small objects better than rods. This ability to perceive fine detail is called **visual acuity**. The parallel to digital imaging is spatial resolution. Cones are also much better at detecting differences in brightness levels. This property of vision is called **contrast sensitivity** and is related to contrast resolution.

Cones are sensitive to a wide range of wavelengths of light; they are very color sensitive. Both visual acuity and contrast sensitivity improve with higher luminance levels of the image.

> Higher object contrast is required for image perception under low illuminance.

A recently introduced metric is JND (Just Noticeable Difference). JND is beyond this discussion; just know that it exists. It deals with why we see stars at night but not in the daytime. It deals with why it is easier to view a bright breast mass on a fatty breast than on a dense breast when interpreting a digital mammogram.

Digital images do not have uniform luminance images do not have uniform luminance. A single image may have very dark and very bright luminance, ranging from 200 to 2000 lux. In such a situation, the contrast sensitivity is best at the average luminance of the image and falls off significantly in brighter and darker regions.

INTERPRETATION

Both the radiologist and the radiographer should become a little aware of the psychology of digital image interpretation. This awareness is particularly important with the rapid adoption of artificial intelligence (AI) (see Chapter 28) with digital images.

The interpretation of a digital image by a radiologist can be considered a two-step process. First, the radiologist will glance at an image and quickly form a **global impression**.

The global impression by the radiologist can be completed within 400 ms and principally uses rod-stimulated peripheral vision. This is enough time to identify the type of image—CT, MRI, positron emission tomography, and so forth—and plan the next thought process. Global impression allows a faint glimpse at image content and maybe even a hint at diagnosis.

Following this global impression, there is a **visual search** employing the cones and foveal vision. It is during this visual search that a diagnosis is formed. This, of course, can take many minutes on the part of the radiologist.

A visual search will quickly result in a normal versus suspicious anatomy interpretation. This phase of interpretation surely will be reduced in terms of time and improved in terms of the decisions made with the continued application of AI.

One of the many AI algorithms designed for visual search is shown in Fig. 30.6. AI procedures are also underway to speed up the process by identifying areas of abnormality and identifying them with a mark or region of interest.

The time a radiologist dwells on an area of an image is called **fixation time**. Fixation times of a second or longer indicate that a visual search is in progress. Short fixation time is associated with the correct diagnosis of an abnormality. However, even longer fixation times may result in diagnosing an abnormality when there actually is none—a false positive (FP).

Normally, the radiologist will conduct the visual search as shown in Fig. 30.7. Each circle in this figure shows where the foveal vision fixes when the eye stops.

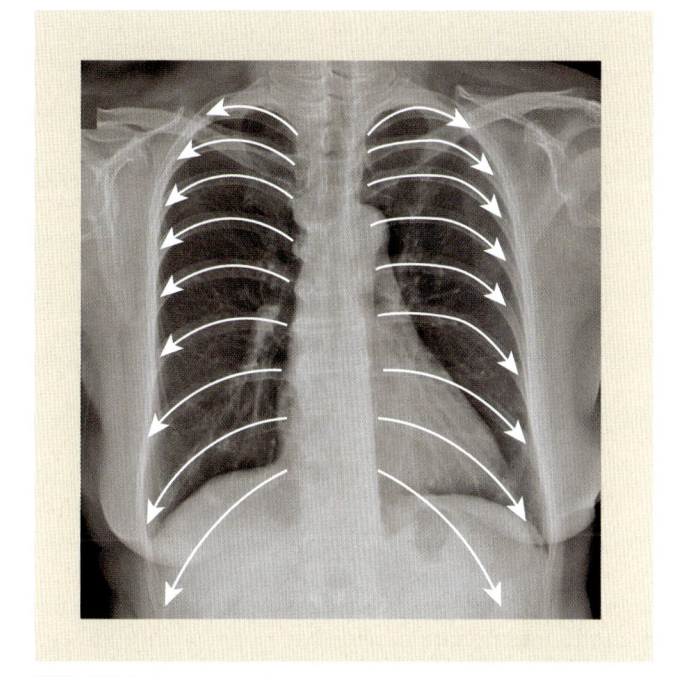

FIG. 30.6 An early artificial intelligence algorithm is designed to perform this visual search pattern for evaluation of the lungs.

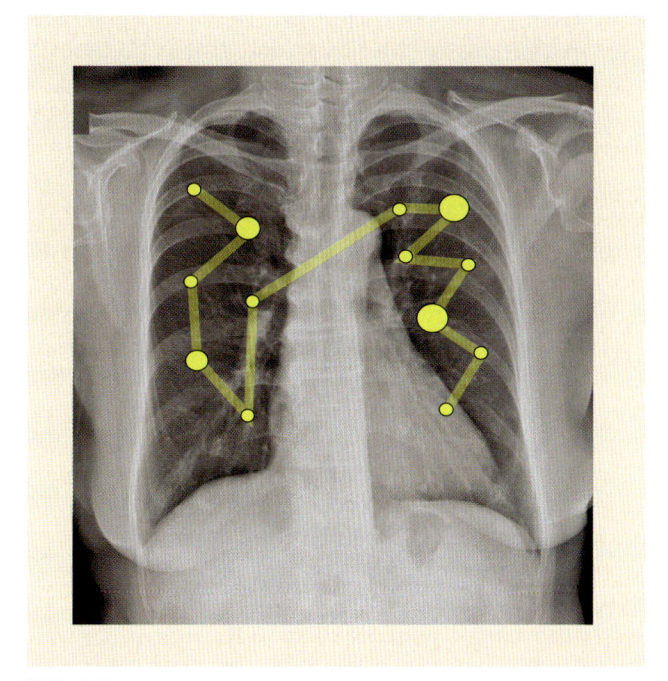

FIG. 30.7 An example of visual search when interpreting a chest radiograph.

The size of the circle represents the relative length of time for each fixation. The lines show the path for each visual search fixation.

This is where the radiographer's involvement is particularly important—image quality. The radiographer should continually focus on producing an image with good **spatial resolution** and good **contrast resolution**, consistent with the digital imaging modality.

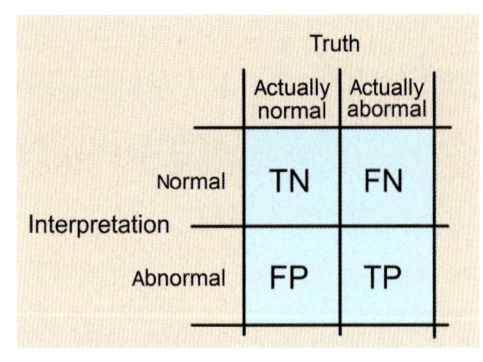

FIG. 30.8 This 2 × 2 decision matrix is basic to constructing a receiver operating characteristic curve. *FN*, False negative; *FP*, false positive; *TN*, true negative; *TP*, true positive.

TABLE 30.1 Four Basic Components of Receiver Operating Characteristic Curves

True positive (TP)—accurate diagnosis of disease/abnormality
True negative (TN)—accurate diagnosis of normal image/anatomy
False positive (FP)—diagnosed as disease/abnormality when in fact it turned out to be normal
False negative (FN)—diagnosed as normal when in fact it turned out to be diseased/abnormal

The secondary features of a digital image that require a radiographer's attention are reduced **noise** and reduced **artifacts**. Reducing noise and artifacts will be improved with AI. Good image quality is essential for accurate interpretation, and that responsibility falls to the radiographer.

With assured image quality, the presentation of the image is also a responsibility of the radiographer. If you become the quality control (QC) radiographer, you will also need to understand DICOM (Digital Imaging and Communications in Medicine) and GSFD (Grayscale Standard Display Function).

The next and final step should be the radiologist's decision.

Receiver Operating Characteristic Curves

There is a growing area of education that attempts to evaluate various areas of decision-making. This area is summarized with what is called an **ROC** (receiver operating characteristic) curve. It is not necessary that the radiographer should be trained in this area, but it is helpful if one understands the various associated English meanings of words, terms, and phrases.

Image quality is most important because it determines how well digital image information is conveyed to the radiologist. This concept of conveyance, as well as the skill of the radiologist, can be evaluated with ROC curves.

We can start to understand an ROC curve by considering the 2 × 2 matrix in Fig. 30.8. This matrix contains two columns labeled "truth" and two rows labeled "interpretation." Each of these four cells represents a decision by the radiologist. In order to validate the diagnosis in each, confirmation usually requires specimen pathology or long-term follow-up.

Table 30.1 presents the various components of this four-cell matrix for reference. Notice that true positive (TP) and true negative (TN) represent accurate diagnoses. False positive (FP) and false negative (FN) represent misdiagnoses or diagnostic errors.

The four cells of the **decision matrix** (Fig. 30.8) are reduced to two—normal or abnormal—by the radiologist for each digital image. If an image were interpreted by many radiologists, the results would be a normal distribution for each such decision, as seen in Fig. 30.9. The ordinate scale (y-axis) would represent the number of radiologists participating. The abscissa scale (x-axis) has values of x centered about the average, x, and σ, the standard deviation.

These normal distributions can be positioned along the x-axis when labeled **decision threshold** (%), as in Fig. 30.9. The area under the normal curve is usually about 10 times that under the abnormal curve. Accurate diagnosis by the radiologist is more than 90% of all interpretations. Don't put much on that percentage, because it varies widely by digital imaging modality and anatomic site.

The larger normal distribution curve centered at approximately 40% decision threshold represents all of the TP and TN truths. The smaller curve centered at approximately 60% represents all of the FP and FN misdiagnoses.

Consider the additional metrics associated with an ROC curve, given in Table 30.2. Beginning with TP, TN, FP, and FN, and assuming a decision threshold, one can compute the true positive fraction (TPF), which is termed **sensitivity**. The true negative fraction (TNF) is termed **specificity**.

> You will be so proud of yourself once you study and understand the ROC curve.

The ROC curve shown in Fig. 30.10 is a plot of true positive fraction (TPF) versus false positive fraction (FPF). Two dots are shown on this ROC curve. Dot A is at a decision threshold of 50% and has a value of TPF = 0.7 and FPF = 0.3. When we move the decision threshold to the lower value of Dot B at 30%, now the TPF = 0.3 and the FPF = 0.1.

By sweeping the decision threshold over the entire width of the normal and abnormal distributions—many pairs of TPF and FPF—the ROC curve is produced. The construction of an ROC curve is not an easy task. In the case of describing the interpretive performance of a

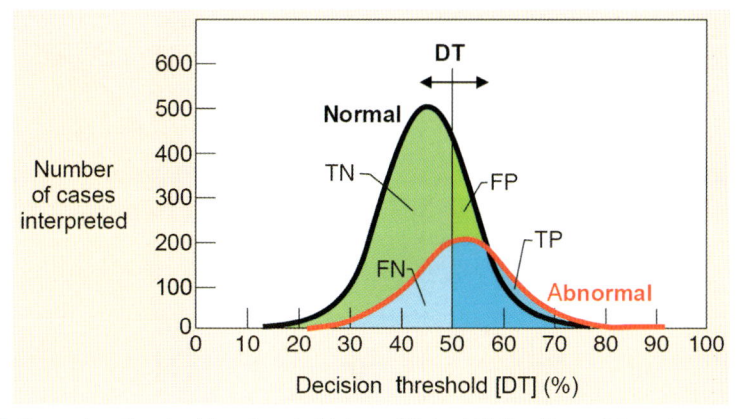

FIG. 30.9 Sweeping the decision threshold from 0% to 100% will result in ordered pairs, which can then be used to construct a receiver operating characteristic curve and estimate sensitivity and specificity. *FN*, False negative; *FP*, false positive; *TN*, true negative; *TP*, true positive.

TABLE 30.2 Terms Used in Analysis With an Receiver Operating Characteristic Curve

Sensitivity—TPF
Specificity—(1 − FPF)
True positive fraction (TPF) = TP/(TP+FN)
True negative fraction (TNF) = TN/(TN+FP)
False positive fraction (FPF) = FP/(TN+FP)
False negative fraction (FNF) = FN/(FN+TP)

FN, False negative; *FP*, false positive; *TN*, true negative; *TP*, true positive.

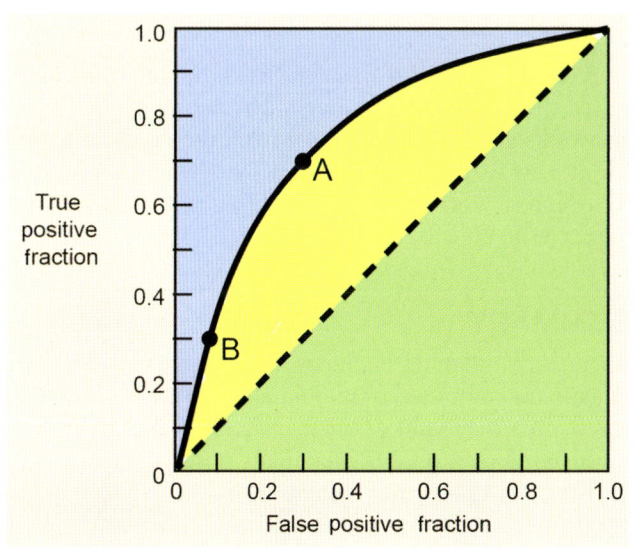

FIG. 30.10 The receiver operating characteristic curve is a plot of true positive fraction versus false positive fraction. Points *A* and *B* were obtained from the sweeping decision threshold.

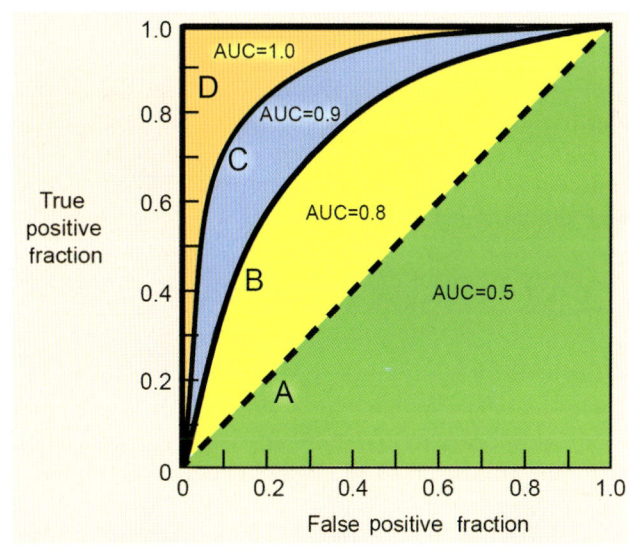

FIG. 30.11 Area under the curve *(AUC)* is a single metric to evaluate a decision process. Curve *A* is guessing. Curve *D* is completely correct.

The ROC curve is plotted on a square of area 1.0. The dashed straight line labeled A, from lower left to upper right, represents the total set of responses, each given as a guess. The AUC for pure guessing is 0.5. Next, consider the ROC curve labeled D. This represents perfect decision-making always and results in an AUC of 1.0.

> Radiologists interpreting digital images produce AUC values of greater than 0.90.

ROC curves B and C represent real-life decisions. When evaluating image interpretation, the larger the AUC (curve C), the more accurate the decisions. For example, curve C might represent a radiologist interpreting mammograms, while curve B represented a pathologist interpreting the same images.

radiologist, it requires specially designed question sets and lots of computer attention.

When the ROC analysis is finally completed, we typically will evaluate the data using a single metric AUC (area under the curve). Fig. 30.11 presents four ROC curves with the associated AUC values.

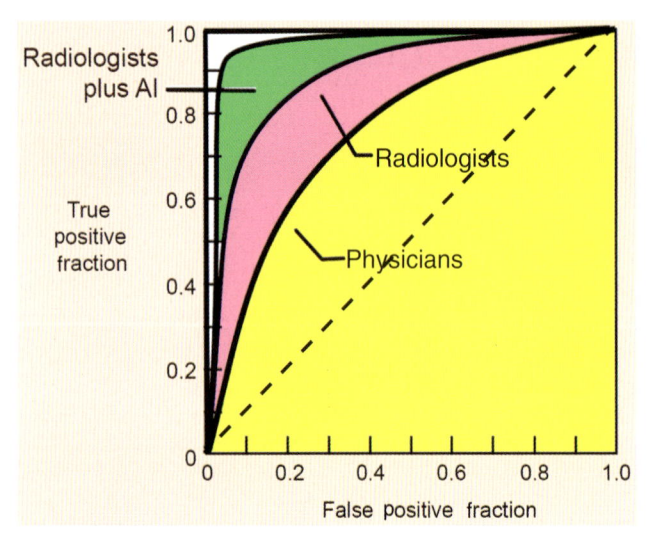

FIG. 30.12 Artificial intelligence *(AI)* is expected to improve the decision process significantly while reducing interpretation time.

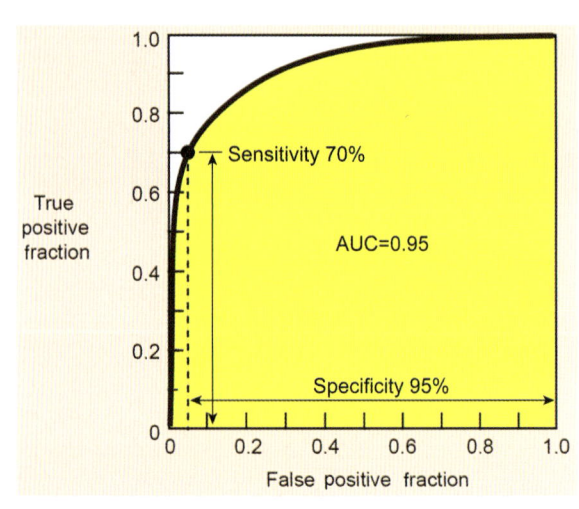

FIG. 30.13 Sensitivity is the value of the true positive fraction, 70%. Specificity is the value of the true negative fraction, 95%. *AUC*, Area under the curve.

A glimpse at the future is illustrated in Fig. 30.12, which shows three ROC curves and the relationship of each to the AUC. This is one example of how AI is expected to revolutionize and improve patient health with digital imaging.

Fig. 30.13 shows the relationship of sensitivity and specificity to the ROC curve. Sensitivity is the TPF. Specificity is (1 − FPF).

Ergonomics

The process of matching any worker to the work environment in order to maximize efficiency is **ergonomics**. With the transition to all-digital imaging, ergonomics becomes an ever-more important feature in radiology. Table 30.3 lists the areas of ergonomics of which we should have some knowledge.

For a properly designed, multidisplay workstation, the chair and desk must be adjustable to the size of the radiologist. The chair must be designed for good lumbar support by having adjustable pads. Five-roller-wheel manipulation has been found minimally acceptable.

The desk must be adjustable to the individual radiologist and customized for various manual input devices and multiple displays. This will help avoid injury or adverse effects on upper extremity joints—fingers, hands, wrists, elbows, and shoulders.

Lights in the reading area should never be turned off or turned up to maximum brightness. This will minimize radiologist eye accommodation. Ambient levels of illumination in the reading area should be in the 10 to 50 lux range and should be provided by indirect sources to reduce glare and reflection.

Noise can be a distraction in a reading area. Moveable walls and partitions made of sound-absorbing material should be used. Some radiologists find noise-canceling headphones helpful.

TABLE 30.3 Ergonomics of Medical Image Interpretation

Posture—chair, desk, walkaround
Workstation—one size does not fit all
Lighting—10–50 lux
Noise—<40 dB
Temperature—20°C–25°C (68°F–76°F)
Humidity—20%–60%

A most successful exercise used by radiologists is called the **20-20-20 rule**. Every 20 minutes, the radiologist looks at least 20 feet away from the digital displays for at least 20 seconds. Radiographers who are required to attend a workstation should also acknowledge and observe the 20-20-20 rule.

SUMMARY

All medical imaging is digital in form. That is, medical images are composed of individual pixels, each of which has a numerical value. One principal advantage of digital imaging over analog imaging is postprocessing.

The principal disadvantage of digital imaging is the additional demand it places on our understanding of visual perception. We now must have a better knowledge of the physics of photometry and the biology of visual physiology and perception.

To meet these new knowledge requirements, an understanding of an area of electrical engineering, the ROC curve, is introduced. AI promises interpretation advances best described by ROC.

Ergonomics is used to develop the workstations of both the radiologist and the radiographer.

CHALLENGE QUESTIONS

1. Define or otherwise identify the following:
   a. Visual sensitivity
   b. Ergonomics
   c. False positive
   d. Visual search
   e. Decision threshold
   f. ROC
   g. Visual adaption
   h. Scotopic vision
   i. 20-20-20 rule
   j. Global impression
2. What is your understanding of image perception?
3. Digital imaging is superior to analog imaging because of what single characteristic?
4. Describe the vision difference between rods and cones.
5. What is the approximate illumination in your area right now?
6. How does JND fit into a reading room?
7. As the AUC of an ROC increases, what happens?
8. How much time is required for involuntary visual accommodation?
9. What is the unit used to describe image brightness?
10. What are the two most important digital image characteristics?
11. What is the difference between sensitivity and specificity?
12. Image perception is important for both the radiographer and radiologist. What is image perception?
13. When a radiologist interprets an image as normal when, in fact, there is an abnormality on the image, what is this situation is called?
14. What is the meaning of contrast sensitivity?
15. What visual structures are concentrated at the fovea centralis?
16. Is foveal vision good or bad?
17. Which structure in the eye controls the intensity of light admitted to the retina of the eye?
18. What is the meaning of visual acuity?
19. Digital imaging has been universally adopted because of what property?
20. Can you report the ergonomic requirements for a radiologist workstation?

The answers to the Challenge Questions can be found by logging on to our website at http://evolve.elsevier.com.

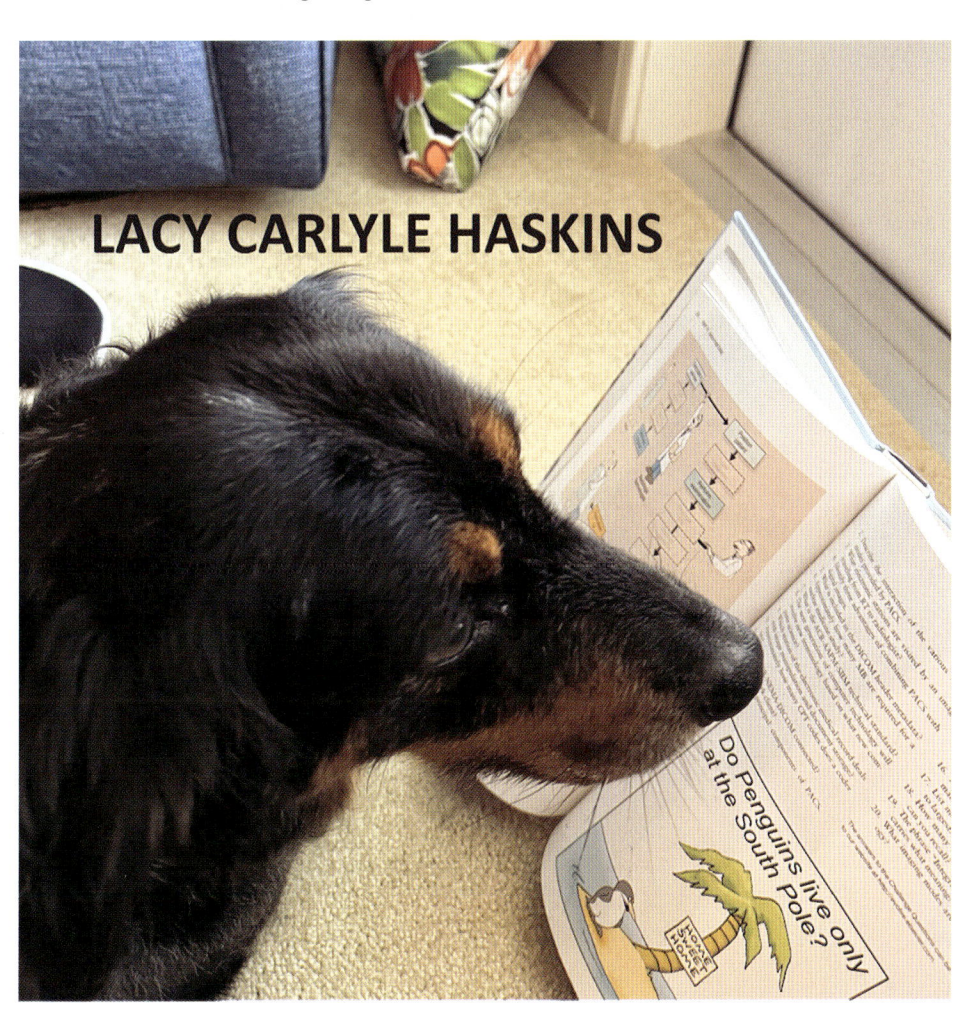

LACY CARLYLE HASKINS

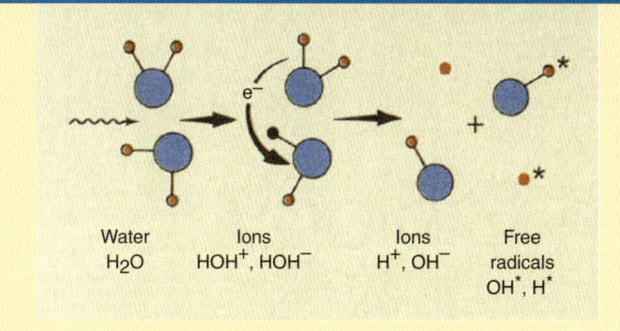

PART VII

RADIOBIOLOGY

CHAPTER 31

Human Biology

OBJECTIVES

At the completion of this chapter, the student should be able to do the following:

1. Discuss the cell theory of human biology.
2. List and describe the molecular composition of the human body.
3. Explain the parts and functions of the human cell.
4. Describe the processes of mitosis and meiosis.
5. Evaluate the radiosensitivity of tissues and organs.

OUTLINE

Human Radiation Response 429
**Composition of the Human
   Body** 430
   Cell Theory 431
   Molecular Composition 431
The Human Cell 434
   Cell Function 435
   Mitosis 436
   Meiosis 436
Tissues and Organs 438
Summary 439
Challenge Questions 439

CHAPTER 31 Human Biology

IT IS known beyond the shadow of a doubt that x-rays are harmful. If sufficiently intense, x-rays can cause skin burns, cataracts, cancer, leukemia, and other harmful effects. What is not known for certain is the degree of effect, if any, after exposure to diagnostic levels of radiation.

The benefits derived from digital imaging with x-rays are enormous. It is the job of radiographers, radiologists, and medical physicists to produce high-quality digital images with minimal radiation exposure. This approach results in the greatest benefit with the lowest risk to patients and radiation workers. This is the practice known as **ALARA**—"as low as reasonably achievable."

This chapter examines the concepts of human biology and discusses the known radiosensitivity of tissues, organs, and cells.

HUMAN RADIATION RESPONSE

The effect of x-rays on humans is the result of interactions at the atomic level (see Chapter 10). These atomic interactions take the form of ionization or excitation of orbital electrons and result in the deposition of energy in tissue.

Deposited energy can produce a molecular change, the consequences of which can be measurable if the molecule involved is critical. Fig. 31.1 summarizes the sequence of events between radiation exposure and resultant human injury.

When an atom is ionized, its chemical binding properties change. If the atom is a constituent of a large molecule, ionization may result in breakage of the molecule or relocation of the atom within the molecule. The abnormal molecule may in time function improperly or cease to function, which can result in serious impairment or death of the cell.

> At nearly every stage in the sequence, it is possible to repair radiation damage and to recover.

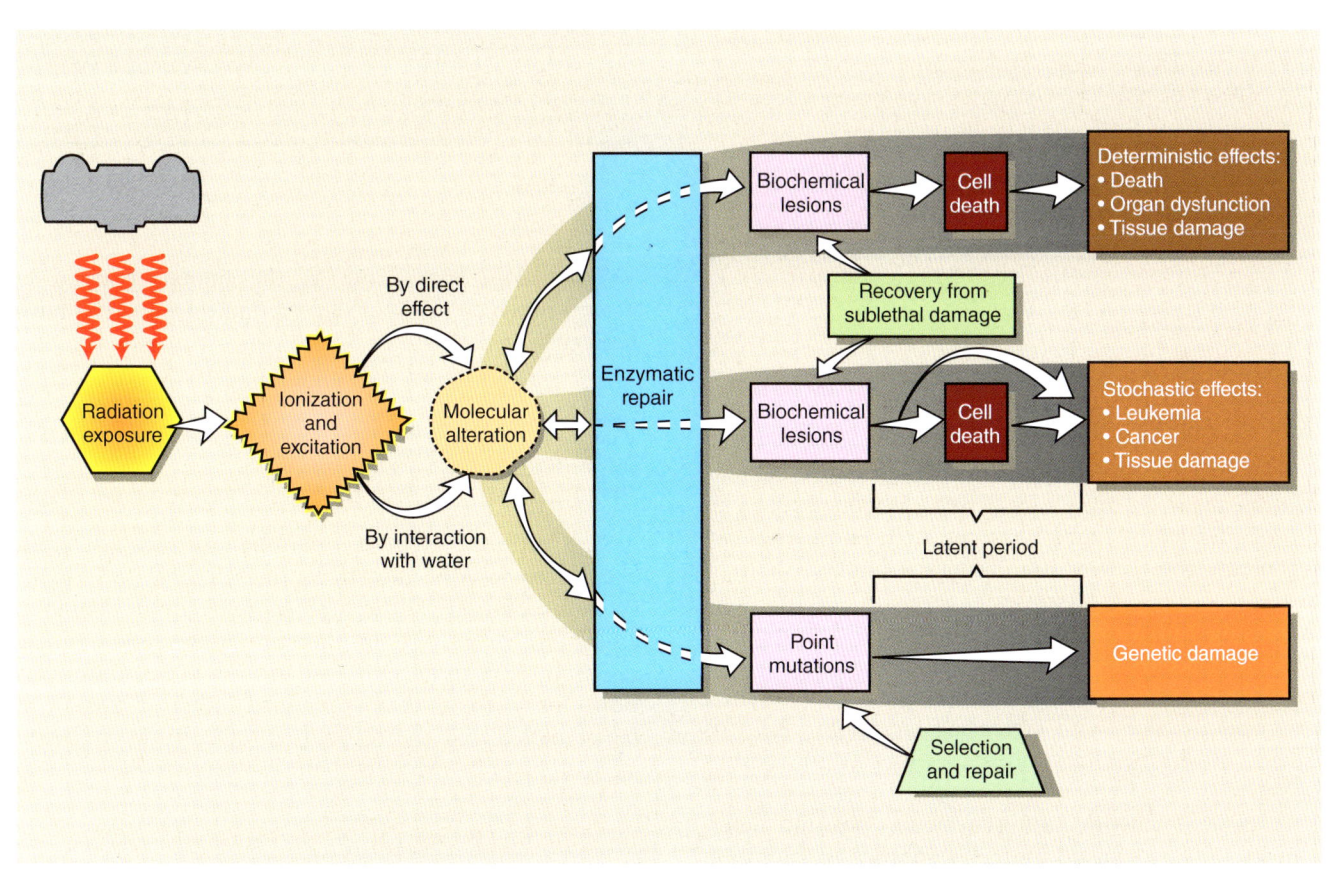

FIG. 31.1 The sequence of events after radiation exposure of humans can lead to several radiation responses. At nearly every step, mechanisms for recovery and repair are available.

TABLE 31.1 Human Responses to Ionizing Radiation

- Deterministic Effects of Radiation on Humans
  1. Acute radiation syndrome
     a. Hematologic syndrome
     b. Gastrointestinal syndrome
     c. Central nervous system syndrome
  2. Local tissue damage
     a. Skin
     b. Gonads
     c. Extremities
     d. Eyes
  3. Hematologic depression
  4. Cytogenetic damage
- Stochastic Effects of Radiation on Humans
  1. Leukemia
  2. Other malignant disease
     a. Bone cancer
     b. Lung cancer
     c. Thyroid cancer
     d. Breast cancer
     e. Skin cancer
  3. Shortening of life span
  4. Genetic damage
     a. Cytogenetic damage
     b. Doubling dose
     c. Genetically significant dose
- Effects of Fetal Irradiation
  1. Prenatal death
  2. Neonatal death
  3. Congenital malformation
  4. Childhood malignancy
  5. Diminished growth and development

TABLE 31.2 Human Populations in Whom Radiation Effects Have Been Observed

Population	Effect
American radiologists	Leukemia, reduced life span
Atomic bomb survivors	Malignant disease
Radiation accident victims (e.g., Chernobyl, SL-1)	Acute lethality
Marshall Islanders	Thyroid cancer
Uranium miners	Lung cancer
Radium watch-dial painters	Bone cancer
Patients treated with ^{131}I	Thyroid cancer
Children treated for enlarged thymus	Thyroid cancer
Children of Belarus (downwind from Chernobyl)	Thyroid cancer
Patients with ankylosing spondylitis	Leukemia
Patients who underwent Thorotrast studies	Liver cancer
Irradiation in utero	Childhood malignancy
Volunteer convicts	Fertility impairment
Cyclotron workers	Cataracts

This process is reversible. Ionized atoms can become neutral again by attracting a free electron. Molecules can be mended by repair enzymes. Cells and tissues can regenerate and recover from radiation injury.

If the radiation response increases in **severity** with increasing radiation dose, it is called a **deterministic effect** and occurs within days after the radiation exposure. On the other hand, if the **incidence** of the radiation response increases with increasing radiation dose, it is called a **stochastic effect** and is not observed for months or years.

A general classification scheme of possible deterministic and stochastic human responses to radiation is shown in Table 31.1. In addition, many other radiation responses have been experimentally observed in animals. Most human responses have been observed to occur after exposure to rather large radiation doses. However, we are cautious and assume that even small radiation doses may be harmful.

Table 31.2 lists some of the human population groups in which many of these radiation responses have been observed.

> Radiobiology is the study of the effects of ionizing radiation on biologic tissue.

The ultimate goal of radiobiologic research is to accurately describe the effects of radiation on humans so that radiation can be used more safely in diagnosis and more effectively in therapy. Most radiobiologic research seeks to develop radiation dose-response relationships so the effects of planned radiation doses can be predicted and the response to accidental radiation exposure can be managed better.

COMPOSITION OF THE HUMAN BODY

At its most basic level, the human body is composed of atoms; radiation interacts at the atomic level. The atomic composition of the body determines the character and degree of the radiation interaction that occurs.

The molecular and tissue composition defines the nature of the radiation response. Table 31.3 summarizes

TABLE 31.3	Atomic Composition of the Human Body

- 60.0% hydrogen
- 25.7% oxygen
- 10.7% carbon
- 2.4% nitrogen
- 0.2% calcium
- 0.1% phosphorus
- 0.1% sulfur
- 0.8% trace elements

TABLE 31.4	Molecular Composition of the Human Body

- 80% water
- 15% protein
- 2% lipids
- 1% carbohydrates
- 1% nucleic acid
- 1% other

the atomic composition of the body and shows that more than 85% of the body consists of hydrogen and oxygen.

Cell Theory

Radiation interaction at the atomic level results in molecular change, which can produce a cell that is deficient in terms of normal growth and metabolism. Robert Hooke, the English schoolmaster, first named the **cell** as the biologic building block in 1665. Shortly thereafter, in 1673, Anton van Leeuwenhoek accurately described a living cell on the basis of his microscopic observations.

It was more than 100 years later, however, in 1838, that Schneider and Schwann showed conclusively that in all plants and animals, cells are the basic functional units. This is the **cell theory**.

The 1953 Watson and Crick description of the molecular structure of deoxyribonucleic acid (DNA) as the genetic substance of the cell was a major accomplishment. Precise mapping of the 40,000 human genes, which was the result of the Human Genome Project completed in the year 2000, promises exceptional solutions to the detection and management of human disease.

Molecular imaging is already making significant contributions to human health.

Molecular Composition

Five principal types of molecules are found in the human body (Table 31.4). Four of these molecules—proteins, lipids (fats), carbohydrates (sugars and starches), and nucleic acids—are macromolecules.

Macromolecules are very large molecules that sometimes consist of hundreds of thousands of atoms.

Proteins, lipids, and carbohydrates are the principal classes of **organic molecules**. An organic molecule is life supporting and contains carbon. One of the rarest molecules—a nucleic acid concentrated in the nucleus of a cell, DNA—is considered to be the most critical and radiosensitive target molecule.

Water is the most abundant molecule in the body, and it is the simplest. Water, however, plays a particularly important role in delivering energy to the target molecule, thereby contributing to radiation effects. In addition to water and the macromolecules, some trace elements and inorganic salts are essential for proper metabolism.

Water consists of two atoms of hydrogen and one atom of oxygen (H_2O) and constitutes approximately 80% of human tissue. Humans are basically made of structured water.

The water molecules exist both in the free state and in the bound state—that is, bound to other molecules. They provide some form and shape, assist in maintaining body temperature, and enter into some biochemical reactions.

During vigorous exercise, body water is lost through perspiration to stabilize temperature and respiration. Water loss must be replaced to maintain **homeostasis**, which is the concept of the relative constancy of the internal environment of the human body.

Water and carbon dioxide are end products in the **catabolism** (breaking down into smaller units) of macromolecules. **Anabolism**, the production of large molecules from small molecules, and catabolism collectively are referred to as **metabolism**. Some athletes use anabolic steroids to build muscle mass, but harmful adverse effects may occur.

Metabolism = Anabolism + Catabolism

Approximately 15% of the molecular composition of the body is **protein**. Proteins are long-chain macromolecules that consist of a linear sequence of **amino acids** connected by **peptide bonds**. Twenty-two amino acids are used in **protein synthesis**, the metabolic production of proteins. The linear sequence, or arrangement, of these amino acids determines the precise function of the protein molecule.

Protein = AA * AA * AA * AA ...
where AA is the amino acid and * is the peptide bond.

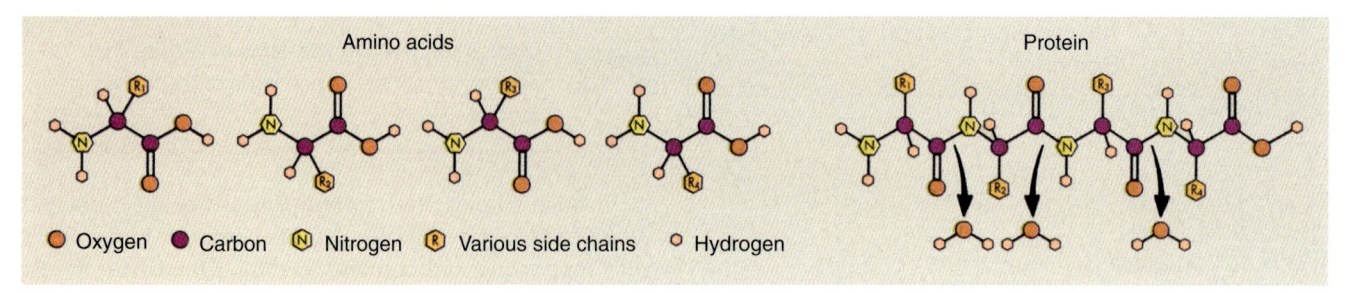

FIG. 31.2 Proteins consist of amino acids linked by peptide bonds. The creation of the peptide bond requires the removal of a molecule of water.

Fig. 31.2 shows the chemical form of a protein molecule. The generalized formula for a protein is $C_nH_nO_nN_nT_n$, where the subscript "n" refers to the number of atoms of each element in the molecule; T represents trace elements. In general, 50% of the mass of a protein molecule is carbon, 20% oxygen, 17% nitrogen, 7% hydrogen, and 6% other elements.

Proteins have a variety of uses in the body. They provide structure and support. Muscles are very high in protein content. Proteins also function as enzymes, hormones, and antibodies.

Enzymes are molecules that are necessary in small quantities to allow a biochemical reaction to continue even though they do not directly enter into the reaction.

Hormones are molecules that exercise regulatory control over some body functions, such as growth and development. Hormones are produced and secreted by the **endocrine glands**—the pituitary, adrenal, thyroid, parathyroid, pancreas, and gonads.

Antibodies constitute a primary defense mechanism of the human body against infection and disease. The molecular configuration of an antibody may be precise and designed for attacking a particular type of invasive or infectious agent, the **antigen**.

Lipids are organic macromolecules composed solely of carbon, hydrogen, and oxygen. They are represented by the general formula, $C_nH_nO_n$. Structurally, lipids are seen in the form shown in Fig. 31.3, and it is this structure that distinguishes them from carbohydrates. In general, lipids are composed of two types of smaller molecules: **glycerol** and **fatty acid**. Each lipid molecule is composed of one molecule of glycerol and three molecules of fatty acid.

Lipids are present in all tissues of the body and are the structural components of cell membranes. Lipids often are concentrated just under the skin and serve as a thermal insulator from the environment. Penguins, for instance, have a particularly thick layer of subcutaneous fat (blubber) that protects them from the cold.

Lipids also serve as fuel for the body by providing energy stores. It is more difficult, however, to extract energy from lipids than from the other major fuel source, carbohydrates; this relationship, of course, is

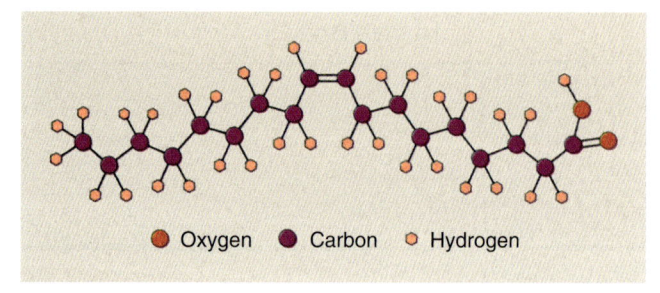

FIG. 31.3 The structural configuration of a lipid is represented by a molecule of oleic acid: $CH_2(CH_2)_7CH = CH(CH_2)_7COOH$.

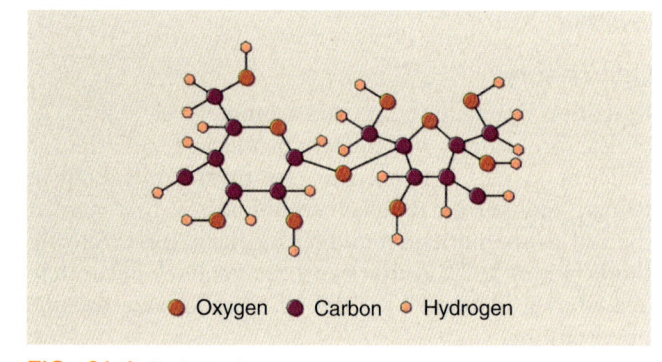

FIG. 31.4 Carbohydrates are structurally different from lipids, even though their composition is similar. This is a molecule of sucrose, or ordinary table sugar: $(C_{12}H_{22}O_{11})$.

associated with one of the major dilemmas in modern nutrition: obesity.

Carbohydrates, similar to lipids, are composed solely of carbon, hydrogen, and oxygen, but their structure is different (Fig. 31.4). This structural difference determines the contribution of the carbohydrate molecule to human biochemistry. The ratio of the number of hydrogen atoms to oxygen atoms in a carbohydrate molecule is 2:1 (as in water), and a large fraction of this molecule consists of these atoms. Consequently, carbohydrates were first considered to be watered, or hydrated, carbons; hence, their name.

Carbohydrates also are called **saccharides**. **Monosaccharides** and **disaccharides** are sugars. The chemical formula for glucose, a simple sugar, is $C_6H_{12}O_6$. These

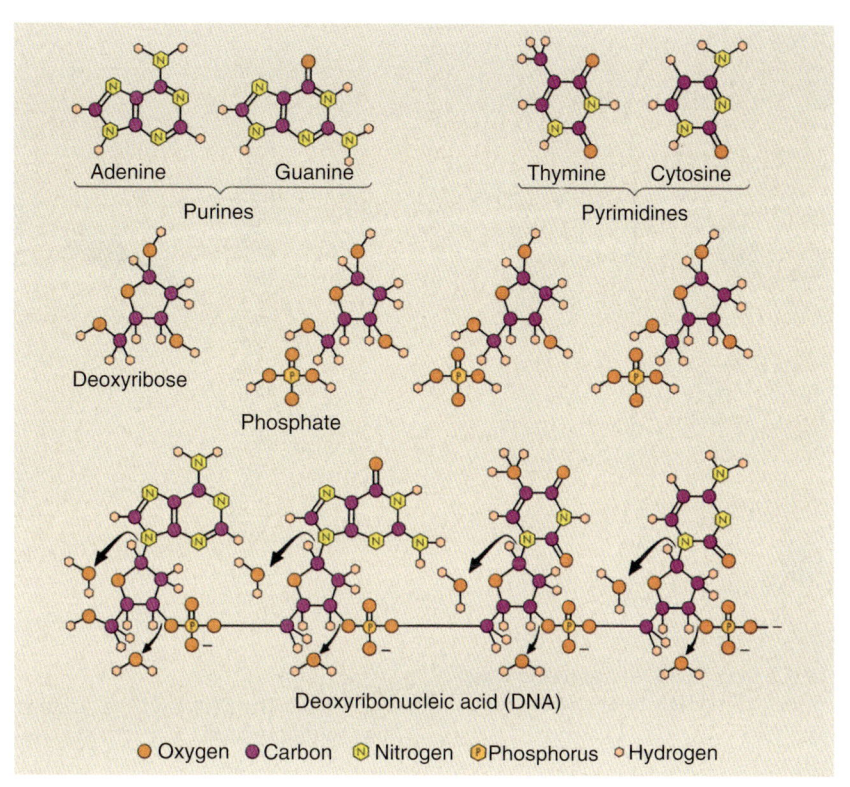

FIG. 31.5 DNA is the control center for life. A single molecule consists of a backbone of alternating sugar (deoxyribose) and phosphate molecules. One of the four organic bases is attached to each sugar molecule.

molecules are relatively small. **Polysaccharides** are large and include plant **starches** and animal **glycogen**. The chemical formula for a polysaccharide is $(C_6H_{10}O_5)_n$, where "n" is the number of simple sugar molecules in the macromolecule.

> The chief function of carbohydrates in the human body is to provide fuel for cell metabolism.

Some carbohydrates are incorporated into the structure of cells and tissues to provide shape and stability. The human polysaccharide, glycogen, is stored in the tissues of the body and is used as fuel only when quantities of the simple sugar, glucose, are inadequate.

Glucose is the ultimate molecule that fuels the human body. Lipids can be catabolized into glucose for energy but only with great difficulty. Polysaccharides are much more readily transformed into glucose. This explains why a chocolate bar, which is high in glucose, can provide a quick burst of energy for an athlete.

Two principal **nucleic acids** are important to human metabolism: **DNA** and **ribonucleic acid (RNA)**. Located principally in the nucleus of the cell, DNA serves as the command and control molecule for cell function. DNA contains all the hereditary information that represents a cell and, of course, if the cell is a **germ cell**, all the hereditary information of the individual.

Located principally in the cytoplasm, RNA also is found in the nucleus. Two types of RNA have been identified: messenger RNA (mRNA) and transfer RNA (tRNA). These are distinguished according to their biochemical functions. These molecules are involved in the growth and development of the cell through a number of biochemical pathways—most notably, protein synthesis.

The nucleic acids are very large and extremely complex macromolecules. Fig. 31.5 shows the structural composition of DNA and reveals how the component molecules are joined. DNA consists of a backbone composed of alternating segments of deoxyribose (a sugar) and phosphate. For each deoxyribose-phosphate conjugate formed, a molecule of water is removed.

> DNA is the radiation-sensitive target molecule.

Attached to each deoxyribose molecule is one of four different nitrogen-containing or nitrogenous organic bases: **adenine, guanine, thymine,** or **cytosine**. Adenine and guanine are **purines**; thymine and cytosine are **pyrimidines**.

The base sugar-phosphate combination is called a nucleotide, and the **nucleotides** are strung together in one long-chain macromolecule. Human DNA exists as two of these long chains attached together in ladder

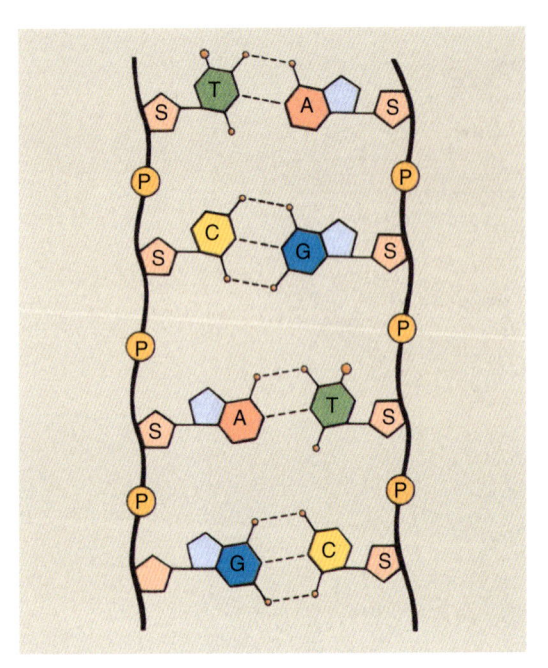

FIG. 31.6 DNA consists of two long chains of alternating sugar and phosphate molecules fashioned similarly to the side rails of a ladder with pairs of bases as rungs.

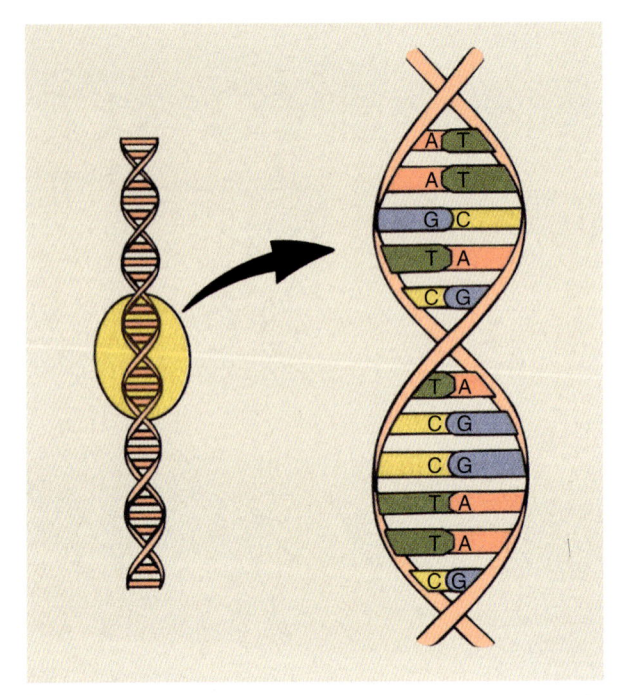

FIG. 31.7 The DNA ladder is twisted about an imaginary axis to form a double helix.

fashion (Fig. 31.6). The side rails of the ladder are the alternating sugar-phosphate molecules, and the rungs of the ladder consist of bases joined together by hydrogen bonds.

To complete the picture, the ladder is twisted about an imaginary axis, much like a slinky toy. This produces a molecule with the **double-helix** configuration (Fig. 31.7). The sequence of base bonding is limited to adenines bonded to thymines and cytosines bonded to guanines.

> Only adenine-thymine and cytosine-guanine base bonding is possible in DNA.

Structurally, RNA resembles DNA. In RNA, the sugar component is ribose rather than deoxyribose, and uracil replaces thymine as a base component. In contrast, RNA forms a single helix, not a double helix.

THE HUMAN CELL

The principal molecular components of the human body are made of intricate cellular structures. The distribution of these structures throughout the cell is reminiscent of the way the parts of an automobile are assembled. This assembly of the cell ensures proper growth, development, and function of the cell. Fig. 31.8 is a cutaway view of a human cell, with its principal structures labeled.

The two major structures of the cell are the **nucleus** and **cytoplasm**. The principal molecular component

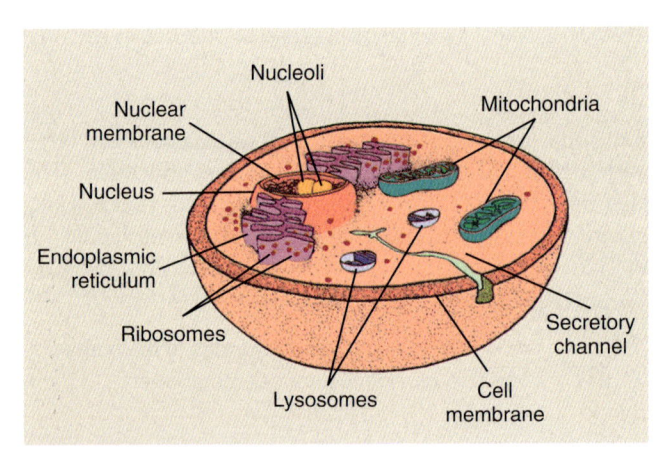

FIG. 31.8 Schematic view of a human cell that shows the principal structural components.

of the nucleus is DNA—the genetic material of the cell. The nucleus also contains some RNA, protein, and water.

Most of the RNA is contained in a rounded structure, the **nucleolus**. The nucleolus often is attached to the nuclear membrane, a double-walled structure that at some locations is connected to the endoplasmic reticulum. This connection, by its nature, controls the passage of molecules, particularly RNA, from the nucleus to cytoplasm.

The cytoplasm makes up the bulk of the cell and contains great quantities of all molecular components except DNA. A number of intracellular structures are found in the cytoplasm. The **endoplasmic reticulum** is a channel or a series of channels that allows the nucleus to communicate with the cytoplasm.

The large bean-shaped structures are **mitochondria**. Macromolecules are digested in the mitochondria to produce energy for the cell. The mitochondria are therefore called the engine of the cell.

The small, dot-like structures are **ribosomes**. Ribosomes are the site of protein synthesis and therefore are essential to normal cellular function. Ribosomes are scattered throughout the cytoplasm and the endoplasmic reticulum.

The small pea-like sacs are **lysosomes**. The lysosomes contain enzymes capable of digesting cellular fragments and sometimes the cell itself. Lysosomes help control intracellular contaminants.

All of these structures, including the human cell itself, are surrounded by membranes. These membranes consist principally of lipid-protein complexes that selectively allow small molecules and water to diffuse from one side to the other.

> Cellular membranes provide structure and form for the human cell and its components.

When the critical macromolecular cellular components are irradiated by themselves, a dose of approximately 10 kGy$_t$ is required to produce a measurable change in any physical characteristic of the molecule.

When a macromolecule is incorporated into the apparatus of a living cell, only a few mGy$_t$ are necessary to produce a measurable biologic response. The lethal dose in some single-cell organisms, such as human cells, is measured in Gy$_t$. Human cells can be killed with a dose of less than 1 Gy$_t$.

A number of experiments have shown that the nucleus is much more sensitive than the cytoplasm to the effects of ionizing radiation. Such experiments are conducted with the use of precise microbeams of high-energy electrons that can be focused and directed to a particular cell part or through incorporation of the radioactive isotopes tritium (^{3}H) and carbon-14 (^{14}C) into cellular molecules that localize exclusively to the cytoplasm or to the nucleus.

Cell Function

Every human cell has a specific function in supporting the total body. Some differences are obvious, as in nerve cells, blood cells, and muscle cells. Similarities are also somewhat obvious.

In addition to its specialized function, each cell to some extent absorbs all molecular nutrients through the cell membrane and uses these nutrients in energy production and molecular synthesis. If this molecular synthesis is damaged by radiation exposure, the cell may malfunction and die.

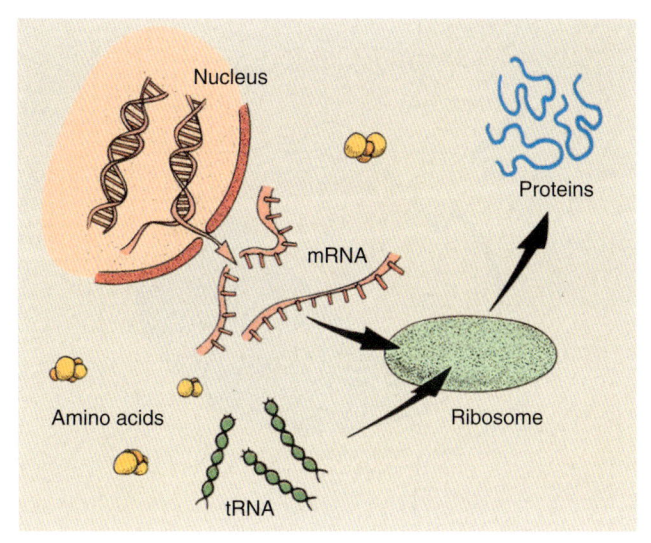

FIG. 31.9 Protein synthesis is a complex process that involves many different molecules and cellular structures.

Protein synthesis is a good example of a critical function necessary for cell survival (Fig. 31.9). DNA, located in the nucleus, contains a molecular code that identifies which proteins the cell will make. This code is determined by the sequence of base pairs (adenine-thymine and cytosine-guanine).

> A series of three base pairs, called a **codon**, identifies 1 of the 22 human amino acids available for protein synthesis.

This genetic message is transferred within the nucleus to a molecule of mRNA: messenger RNA. mRNA leaves the nucleus by way of the endoplasmic reticulum and makes its way to a ribosome, where the genetic message is transferred to yet another RNA molecule tRNA: transfer RNA.

tRNA searches the cytoplasm for the amino acids for which it is coded. It attaches to the amino acid and carries it to the ribosome, where it is joined with other amino acids in sequence by peptide bonds to form the required protein molecule.

Interference with any phase of this procedure for protein synthesis could result in damage to the cell. Radiation interaction in which the molecule has primary control over protein synthesis (DNA) is more effective in producing a response than radiation interaction with other molecules involved in protein synthesis.

Although a high dose of ionizing radiation is necessary to produce physically measurable disruption of macromolecules in vitro, single ionizing events at a particularly sensitive site of a critical target molecule are thought to be capable of disrupting cell proliferation.

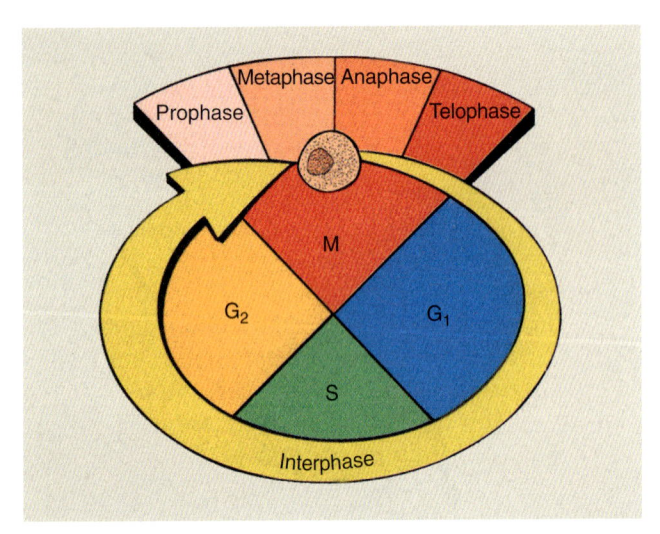

FIG. 31.10 Progress of the cell through one cycle involves several phases.

> Cell proliferation is the act of a single cell or group of cells reproducing and multiplying in number.

The human body consists of two general types of cells: **somatic cells** and **genetic cells**. The genetic cells include the oogonium of the female and the spermatogonium of the male. All other cells of the body are somatic cells. When somatic cells divide and proliferate, they undergo **mitosis**. Genetic cells undergo **meiosis**.

Mitosis

Cell biologists and geneticists view the cell cycle differently (Fig. 31.10). Each cell cycle includes the various states of cell growth, development, and division. Geneticists consider only two phases of the cell cycle: mitosis (M) and **interphase**.

Mitosis, the division phase, is characterized by four subphases: **prophase, metaphase, anaphase,** and **telophase**. The portion of the cell cycle between mitotic events is interphase, the period of growth of the cell between divisions.

Cell biologists usually identify four phases of the cell cycle: M, G_1, S, and G_2. These phases of the cell cycle are characterized by the structure of the chromosomes, which contain the genetic material DNA. The **gap** in cell growth between M and S is G_1. G_1 is the pre-DNA synthesis phase.

The DNA synthesis phase is S. During this period, each DNA molecule is replicated into two identical daughter DNA molecules.

During the S phase, the chromosome is transformed from a structure with two chromatids attached to a centromere to a structure with four chromatids attached to a centromere (Fig. 31.11). The result is two pairs of homologous chromatids; that is, chromatids with precisely the same DNA content and structure.

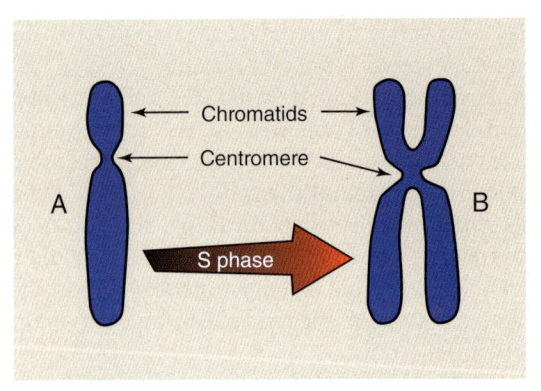

FIG. 31.11 During the synthesis portion of interphase, the chromosomes replicate from a two-chromatid structure (A) to a four-chromatid structure (B).

The G_2 phase is the post-DNA synthesis gap of cell growth.

During interphase, the chromosomes are not visible; however, during mitosis, the DNA slowly takes the form of the chromosomes, as seen microscopically. Fig. 31.12 schematically depicts the process of mitosis.

During **prophase**, the nucleus swells and the DNA becomes more prominent and begins to take structural form. At **metaphase**, the chromosomes appear and are lined up along the equator of the nucleus. It is during metaphase that mitosis can be stopped and chromosomes can be studied carefully under the microscope.

> Radiation-induced chromosome damage is analyzed during metaphase.

Anaphase is characterized by the splitting of each chromosome at the centromere so that a centromere and two chromatids are connected by a fiber to the poles of the nucleus. These poles are called **spindles**, and the fibers are called **spindle fibers**. The number of chromatids per centromere has been reduced by half, and these newly formed chromosomes migrate slowly toward the spindle.

The final segment of mitosis, **telophase**, is characterized by the disappearance of structural chromosomes into a mass of DNA and the closing off of the nuclear membrane, like a dumbbell, into two nuclei. At the same time, the cytoplasm is divided into two equal parts, each of which accompanies one of the new nuclei.

Cell division is now complete. The two daughter cells look precisely the same as the parent cell and contain exactly the same genetic material.

Meiosis

Genetic material can change during the division process of genetic cells, which is called **meiosis**.

Genetic cells begin with the same number of chromosomes as somatic cells: 23 pairs (46 chromosomes).

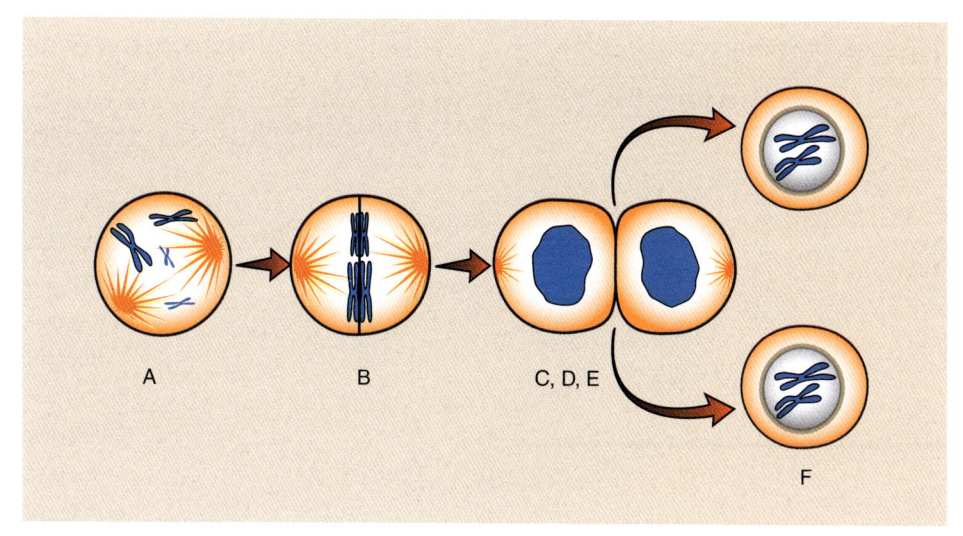

FIG. 31.12 Mitosis is the phase of the cell cycle during which the chromosomes become visible, divide, and migrate to daughter cells. (A) Interphase. (B) Prophase. (C) Metaphase. (D) Anaphase. (E) Telophase. (F) Interphase.

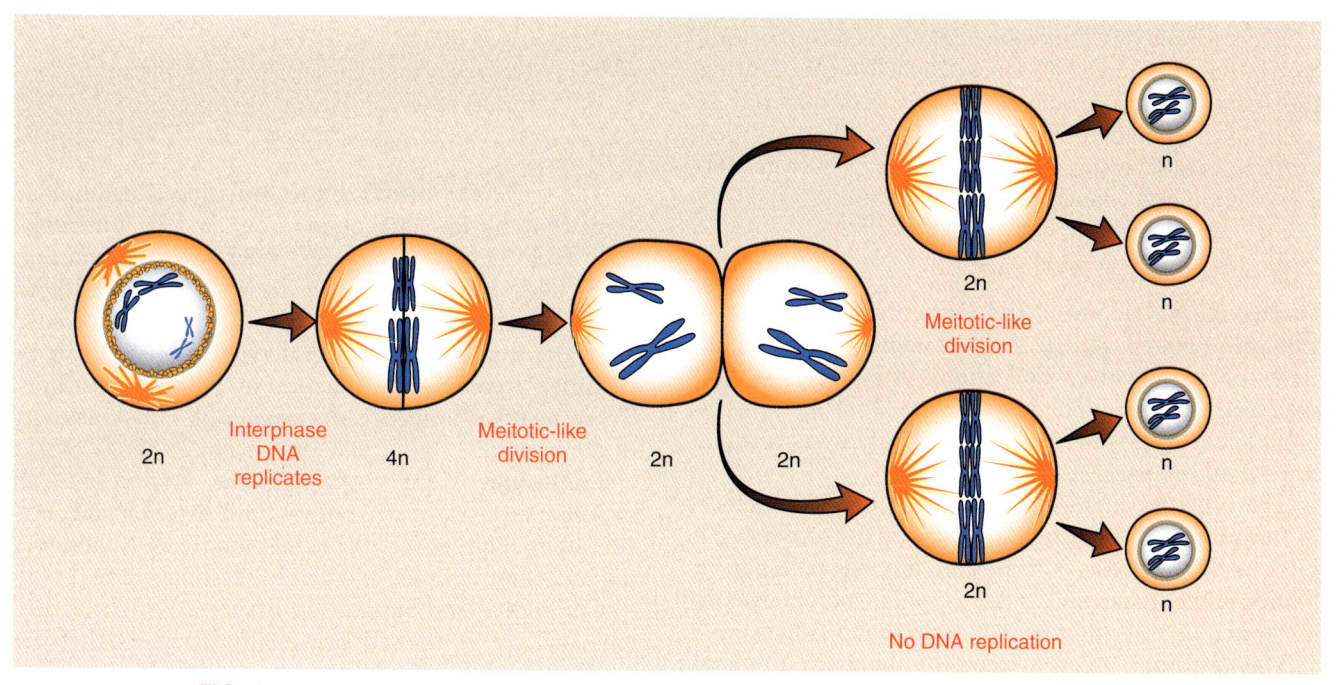

FIG. 31.13 Meiosis is the process of reduction division, and it occurs only in reproductive cells. n, Number of similar chromosomes.

However, for a genetic cell to be capable of marriage to another genetic cell, its complement of chromosomes must be reduced by half to 23, so that after conception and the union of two genetic cells, the daughter cells again will contain 46 chromosomes (Fig. 31.13).

> Meiosis is the process whereby genetic cells undergo **reduction division**.

The genetic cell begins meiosis with 46 chromosomes that appear the same as in a somatic cell that has completed the G_2 phase. The cell then progresses through the phases of mitosis into two daughter cells, each containing 46 chromosomes of two chromatids each. The names of the subphases are the same for meiosis and mitosis.

Each of the daughter cells of this first division now progresses through a second division in which all cellular material, including chromosomes, is divided.

TABLE 31.5 Tissue Composition of the Body

Tissue	Abundance (%)
Muscle	43
Fat	14
Organs	12
Skeleton	10
Blood	8
Subcutaneous tissue	6
Bone marrow	4
Skin	3

TABLE 31.6 Response to Radiation Is Related to Cell Type

Radiosensitivity	Cell Type
High	Lymphocytes
	Spermatogonia
	Erythroblasts
	Intestinal crypt cells
Intermediate	Endothelial cells
	Osteoblasts
	Spermatids
	Fibroblasts
Low	Muscle cells
	Nerve cells

However, the second division is not accompanied by an S phase. Therefore no replication of DNA occurs; consequently, no chromosomes are duplicated. Each of the resulting granddaughter cells contains only 23 chromosomes.

Each parent has undergone two division processes, which have resulted in four daughter cells. During the second division, some chromosomal material is exchanged among chromatids through a process called **crossing over**. Crossing over results in changes in genetic constitution and changes in inheritable traits.

TISSUES AND ORGANS

During the development and maturation of a human from two united genetic cells, a number of different types of cells evolve. Collections of cells of similar structure and function form **tissues**. Table 31.5 is a breakdown of the composition of the body according to its tissue constituents.

These tissues in turn are precisely bound together to form **organs**. The tissues and the organs of the body serve as discrete units with specific functional responsibilities. Some tissues and organs combine into an overall integrated organization known as an **organ system**.

The principal organ systems of the body are the nervous system, digestive system, endocrine system, respiratory system, and reproductive system. Effects of radiation that appear at the whole-body level result from damage to these organ systems that occurs as the result of radiation injury to the cells of that system.

> Organ Systems = Nervous, Reproductive, Digestive, Respiratory, and Endocrine.

The cells of a tissue system are identified by their rate of proliferation and their stage of development. Immature cells are called **stem cells**. As a cell matures through growth and proliferation, it can pass through various stages of differentiation into a fully functional and mature cell.

> Stem cells are more sensitive to radiation than mature cells.

The sensitivity of the cell to radiation is determined somewhat by its state of maturity and its functional role. Table 31.6 lists a number of different types of cells in the body according to their degree of radiosensitivity.

The tissues and organs of the body include both stem cells and mature cells. Several types of tissue can be classified according to structural or functional features. These features influence the degree of radiosensitivity of the tissue.

Epithelium is the covering tissue, and it lines all exposed surfaces of the body—both exterior and interior. Epithelium covers the skin, blood vessels, abdominal and chest cavities, and gastrointestinal tract.

Connective and **supporting tissues** are high in protein and are composed principally of fibers that are usually highly elastic. Connective tissue binds tissues and organs together. Bone ligaments and cartilage are examples of connective tissue.

Muscle is a special type of tissue that can contract. It is found throughout the body and is high in protein content.

Nervous tissue consists of specialized cells called **neurons** that have long, thin extensions from the cell to distant parts of the body. Nervous tissue is the avenue by which electrical impulses are transmitted throughout the body for control and response.

When these various types of tissue are combined to form an organ, they are identified according to two parts of the organ. The **parenchymal** part contains tissues that represent that particular organ. The **stromal**

TABLE 31.7 Relative Radiosensitivity of Tissues and Organs Based on Clinical Radiation Oncology

Level of Radiosensitivity[a]	Tissue or Organ	Effects
High: 2–10 Gy_t	Lymphoid tissue	Atrophy
	Bone marrow	Hypoplasia
	Gonads	Atrophy
Intermediate: 10–50 Gy_t	Skin	Erythema
	Gastrointestinal tract	Ulcer
	Cornea	Cataract
	Growing bone	Growth arrest
	Kidney	Nephrosclerosis
	Liver	Ascites
	Thyroid	Atrophy
Low: >50 Gy_t	Muscle	Fibrosis
	Brain	Necrosis
	Spinal	Transection

[a]The minimum dose delivered at the rate of approximately 2 Gy_t/day that will produce a response.

part is composed of connective tissue and vasculature that provide structure to the organ.

The deterministic effects of high-dose radiation may include observable organ damage. The various organs of the body exhibit a wide range of sensitivity to radiation. This radiosensitivity is determined by the function of the organ in the body, the rate at which cells mature within the organ, and the inherent radiosensitivity of the cell type.

Precise knowledge of these various organ radiosensitivities is unnecessary; however, knowledge of general levels of radiosensitivity is helpful toward understanding the effects of whole-body radiation exposure, particularly in the acute radiation syndrome (Table 31.7).

SUMMARY

After radiation exposure, the human body responds in predictable ways. Radiobiology is the study of the effects of ionizing radiation on humans conducted to define knowledge of the expected response to radiation.

If the intensity of the response increases with increasing radiation dose, it is called a deterministic response and occurs within days of exposure. If the frequency of the response increases with increasing radiation dose, it is called a stochastic effect and is not observable for years.

The cell is the basic functional unit of all plants and animals. At the molecular level, the human body is composed primarily of water, protein, lipid, carbohydrate, and nucleic acid. The two important nucleic acids in human metabolism are DNA and RNA.

DNA contains all the hereditary information in the cell. If the cell is a genetic cell, the DNA contains the hereditary information of the whole individual. DNA is a macromolecule that is made up of two long chains of base sugar-phosphate combinations twisted into a double helix.

Major cellular function consists of protein synthesis and cell division. Mitosis is the growth, development, and division of cells. *Meiosis* is the term applied to the division of genetic cells.

Cells of similar structure bind together to form tissue. Tissues bind together to form organs. An overall integrated organization of tissue and organs is called an *organ system*.

The principal organ systems of the body are the nervous, digestive, endocrine, and reproductive systems. The radiosensitivity of various tissue and organ systems varies widely. Reproductive cells are highly radiosensitive; nerve cells are least radiosensitive.

CHALLENGE QUESTIONS

1. Define or otherwise identify the following:
    a. ALARA
    b. Cell theory
    c. Anabolism
    d. Carbohydrate
    e. M, G_1, S, G_2
    f. Epithelium
    g. Cytoplasm
    h. Enzyme
    i. Organic molecule
    j. Late effect of radiation

2. At what structural level do x-rays interact with humans to produce a radiation response?
3. How does ionizing radiation affect an atom within a large molecule?
4. List five human groups in which radiation effects have been observed.
5. What are the effects of radiation on the populations mentioned in Question 4?
6. What is the most abundant atom and the most abundant molecule in the body?
7. What is a stem cell?
8. Why do we say that humans are basically a structured aqueous suspension?
9. What is the meaning of epithelium?
10. How do proteins function in the human body?
11. What do carbohydrates do for us?
12. DNA is the abbreviation for what molecule?
13. Which molecule is considered the genetic material of the cell?
14. What is the function of the endoplasmic reticulum?
15. What is the approximate radiation dose required to produce a measurable physical change in a macromolecule?
16. List the stages of cell division of a somatic cell.
17. List the stages of cell reduction division of a genetic cell.
18. What cell type is the most radiosensitive?
19. What type of tissue is the least radiosensitive?
20. List three early radiation effects and three late radiation effects in humans.

The answers to the Challenge Questions can be found by logging on to our website at http://evolve.elsevier.com.

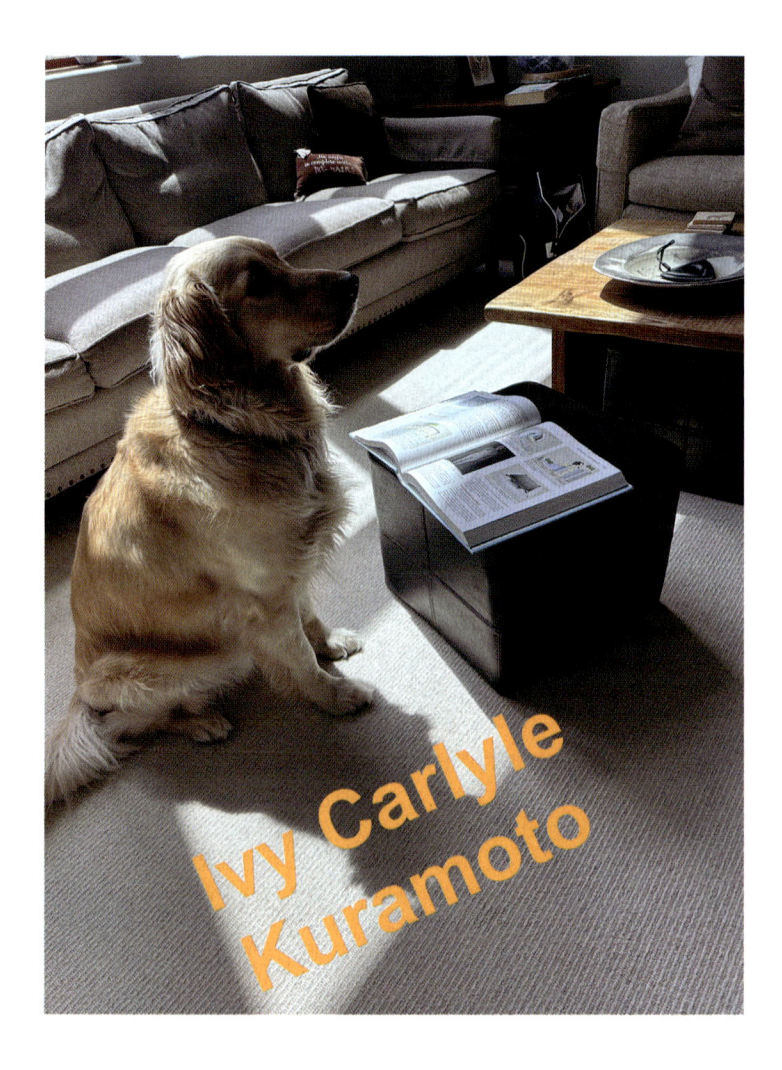

Fundamental Principles of Radiobiology

CHAPTER 32

OBJECTIVES

At the completion of this chapter, the student should be able to do the following:

1. State the law of Bergonie and Tribondeau.
2. Describe the physical factors that affect radiation response.
3. Describe the biological factors that affect radiation response.
4. Explain radiation dose-response relationships.
5. Describe five types of radiation dose-response relationships.

OUTLINE

Law of Bergonie and Tribondeau 442
Physical Factors That Affect Radiosensitivity 442
  Linear Energy Transfer 442
  Relative Biologic Effectiveness 442
  Protraction and Fractionation 443
Biologic Factors That Affect Radiosensitivity 443
  Oxygen Effect 443
  Age 444
  Recovery 444
  Chemical Agents 444
  Hormesis 445
Radiation Dose-Response Relationships 445
  Linear Dose-Response Relationships 445
  Nonlinear Dose-Response Relationships 446
  Constructing a Dose-Response Relationship 446
Summary 447
Challenge Questions 448

SOME TISSUES are more sensitive than others to radiation exposure. Such tissues usually respond more rapidly and to lower doses of radiation.

Physical factors and biological factors affect the radiobiologic response of tissue. Knowledge of these radiobiologic factors is essential for understanding the positive effects of radiation oncology and the potentially harmful effects of the low-dose radiation exposure of digital imaging.

The principal aim of the study of radiobiology is to understand radiation dose-response relationships. A dose-response relationship is a mathematical and graphic function that relates radiation dose to observed response.

LAW OF BERGONIE AND TRIBONDEAU

In 1906 two French scientists, Jean Alban Bergonie and Louis Tribondeau, theorized and observed that reproductive cells are more sensitive than nerve cells. They theorized that radiosensitivity was a function of the metabolic state of the tissue being irradiated. This has come to be known as the law of Bergonie and Tribondeau and has been verified many times. Basically, the law states that the radiosensitivity of living tissue varies with maturation and metabolism (Table 32.1).

This law is principally interesting as a historical note in the development of radiobiology. It has found some application in radiation oncology. In digital imaging, the law serves to remind us that fetuses are considerably more sensitive to radiation exposure, as are children, compared with mature adults.

PHYSICAL FACTORS THAT AFFECT RADIOSENSITIVITY

When one irradiates tissue, the response of the tissue is determined principally by the amount of energy deposited per unit mass—the radiation dose in Gy_t. Even under controlled experimental conditions, however, when equal doses are delivered to equal specimens, the response may not be the same because of other modifying factors. A number of physical factors affect the degree of radiation response.

Linear Energy Transfer

Linear energy transfer (**LET**) is a measure of the rate at which energy is transferred from ionizing radiation to soft tissue. It is another method of expressing radiation energy and determining the value of the **radiation weighting factor** (**WR**) used in radiation protection (see Chapter 37). LET is expressed in units of kiloelectron volt of energy transferred per micrometer of track length in soft tissue (keV/μm).

> The LET of diagnostic x-rays is approximately 3 keV/μm.

The ability of ionizing radiation to produce a biologic response increases as the LET of radiation increases. When LET is high, ionizations occur frequently, increasing the probability of interaction with a target molecule.

Relative Biologic Effectiveness

As the LET of radiation increases, the ability to produce biologic damage also increases. This effect is described by the relative biologic effectiveness (**RBE**). RBE is the ratio of radiation dose from a standard radiation necessary to produce a given effect to the dose from a test radiation to produce the same effect.

> RBE is the ratio of a standard radiation dose to produce the same response as that following a test radiation dose.

The standard radiation, by convention, is x-radiation in the range of 200 to 250 kVp. This type of x-ray beam was used for many years in radiation oncology and in essentially all early radiobiologic research.

Diagnostic x-rays have an RBE of 1. Whereas radiations with lower LET than diagnostic x-rays have an RBE less than 1, radiations with higher LET have a higher RBE.

> The RBE of diagnostic x-rays is 1.

Fig. 32.1 shows the relationship between RBE and LET and identifies some of the more common types of radiation. Table 32.2 lists the approximate LET and RBE of various types of ionizing radiation.

TABLE 32.1 Law of Bergonie and Tribondeau

- Stem cells are radiosensitive; mature cells are radioresistant.
- Younger tissues and organs are radiosensitive.
- Tissues with high metabolic activity are radiosensitive.
- A high proliferation rate for cells and a high growth rate for tissues result in increased radiosensitivity.

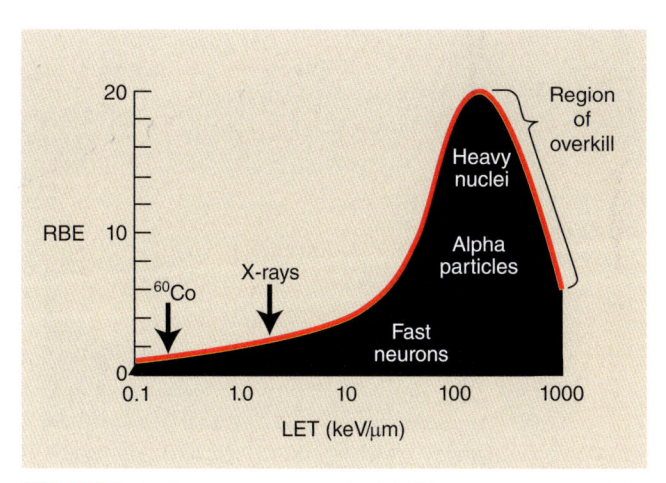

CHAPTER 32 Fundamental Principles of Radiobiology

FIG. 32.1 As linear energy transfer (*LET*) increases, relative biologic effectiveness (*RBE*) also increases, but a maximum value is reached followed by a lower RBE because of overkill.

TABLE 32.2 Linear Energy Transfer and Relative Biologic Effectiveness of Various Types of Radiation

Type of Radiation	LET (keV/μm)	RBE
25 MV x-rays	0.2	0.8
^{60}Co gamma rays	0.3	0.9
1 MeV electrons	0.3	0.9
Diagnostic x-rays	3.0	1.0
10 MeV protons	4.0	5.0
Fast neutrons	50.0	10
5 MeV alpha particles	100.0	20
Heavy nuclei	1000.0	30

LET, Linear energy transfer; *RBE*, relative biologic effectiveness.

Question: When mice are irradiated with 250-kVp x-rays, death occurs at 6.5 Gy$_t$. If similar mice are irradiated with fast neutrons during a cyclotron experiment, death occurs at only 2.1 Gy$_t$. What is the RBE for the fast neutrons?

Answer:
$$\text{RBE} = \frac{6.5 \text{ Gy}_t}{2.1 \text{ Gy}_t} = 3.1$$

Protraction and Fractionation

If a dose of radiation is delivered over a long period of time rather than quickly, the effect of that radiation dose is less. Stated differently, if the time of irradiation is lengthened, a higher dose is required to produce the same effect. This lengthening of time can be accomplished in two ways.

If the radiation dose is delivered continuously but at a lower dose rate, it is said to be **protracted**. Six gray delivered in 3 minutes at a dose of 2 Gy$_t$/min is lethal for a mouse. However, when 6 Gy$_t$ is delivered at the rate of 10 mGy$_t$/hr for a total time of 600 hours, the mouse will survive.

> Dose protraction and fractionation cause less effect because the longer irradiation time allows for intracellular repair and tissue recovery.

If the 6-Gy$_t$ dose is delivered at the same dose rate, but in 12 equal fractions of 500 mGy$_t$, all separated by 24 hours, the mouse will survive. In this situation, the radiation dose is said to be **fractionated**.

Radiation dose fractionation reduces effect because cells undergo repair and recovery between doses. Dose fractionation is used routinely in radiation oncology to reduce the response of normal nonmalignant tissue adjacent to the tumor.

BIOLOGIC FACTORS THAT AFFECT RADIOSENSITIVITY

In addition to these physical factors, a number of biologic conditions alter the radiation response of tissue. Some of these factors, such as age and metabolic rate, have to do with the inherent state of tissue. Other factors are related to artificially introduced modifiers of the biologic system.

Oxygen Effect

Tissue is more sensitive to radiation when irradiated in the oxygenated state than when irradiated under anoxic (without oxygen) or hypoxic (low-oxygen) conditions. This characteristic of tissue radiation response is called the **oxygen effect** and is described numerically by the oxygen enhancement ratio (**OER**).

The OER is the ratio of the radiation dose necessary to produce a given effect under anoxic tissue conditions to that required to produce the same effect under aerobic conditions.

> OER is the ratio of radiation doses under anoxic conditions to produce the same response as that following irradiation under oxygenated conditions.

In general, tissue irradiation is conducted under conditions of full oxygenation. Hyperbaric (high-pressure) oxygen has been used in radiation oncology in an attempt to enhance the radiosensitivity of nodular, avascular tumors, which are less radiosensitive than tumors with an adequate blood supply.

> Diagnostic digital imaging is performed under conditions of full oxygenation.

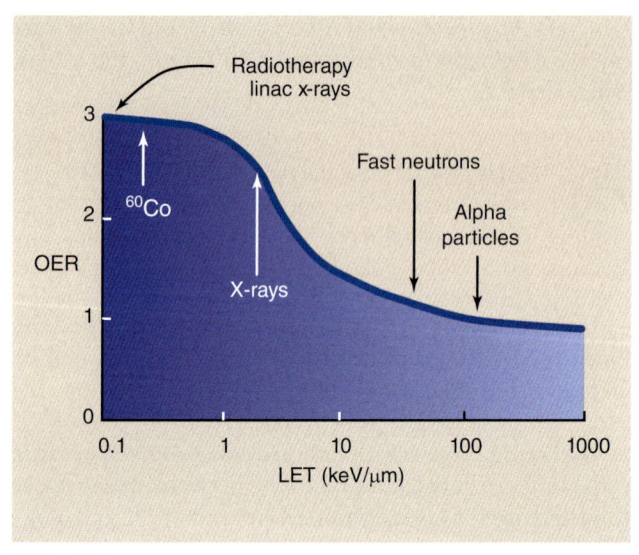

FIG. 32.2 The oxygen enhancement ratio (*OER*) is high for low linear energy transfer (*LET*) radiation and decreases in value as the LET increases.

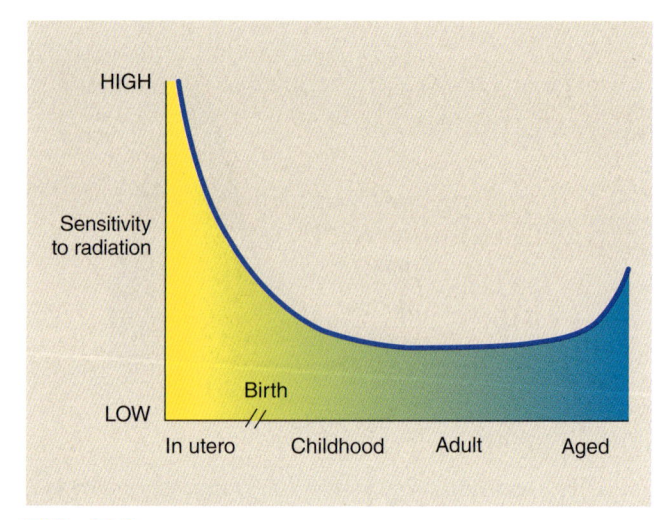

FIG. 32.3 Radiosensitivity varies with age. Experiments with animals have shown that very young and very old individuals are more sensitive to radiation.

Question: When experimental mouse mammary carcinomas are clamped and irradiated under hypoxic conditions, the tumor control dose is 106 Gy_t. When these tumors are not clamped and are irradiated under aerobic conditions, the tumor control dose is 40.5 Gy_t. What is the OER for this system?

Answer: $OER = \dfrac{106}{40.5} = 2.6$

The OER is LET dependent (Fig. 32.2). The OER is highest for low-LET radiation, with a maximum value of approximately 3 that decreases to approximately 1 for high-LET radiation.

Age

The age of a biologic structure affects its radiosensitivity. The response of humans is characteristic of this age-related radiosensitivity (Fig. 32.3). Humans are most sensitive before birth.

After birth, sensitivity decreases until maturity, at which time humans are most resistant to the effects of radiation. In old age, humans again become somewhat more radiosensitive.

Recovery

In vitro experiments show that human cells can recover from radiation damage. If the radiation dose is not sufficient to kill the cell before its next division (**interphase death**), then given sufficient time, the cell will recover from the sublethal radiation damage it has sustained.

> Interphase death occurs when the cell dies before replicating.

This intracellular recovery is attributable to a **repair** mechanism inherent in the biochemistry of the cell. Some types of cells have greater capacity than others for the repair of sublethal radiation damage. At the whole-body level, this recovery from radiation damage is assisted through **repopulation** by surviving cells.

If a tissue or organ receives a sufficient radiation dose, it responds by shrinking. This is called **atrophy**, and it occurs because some cells die and disintegrate, and are carried away as waste products.

> The combined processes of intracellular repair and repopulation contribute to recovery from radiation damage.

If a sufficient number of cells sustain only sublethal damage and survive, they may proliferate and repopulate the irradiated tissue or organ.

Chemical Agents

Some chemicals can modify the radiation response of cells, tissues, and organs. For chemical agents to be effective, they must be present at the time of irradiation. Postirradiation application does not usually alter the degree of radiation response.

Agents that enhance the effect of radiation are called **radiosensitizers**. Examples include halogenated pyrimidines, methotrexate, actinomycin D, hydroxyurea, and vitamin K.

The halogenated pyrimidines become incorporated into the DNA of the cell and amplify the effects of radiation on that molecule. All radiosensitizers have an effectiveness ratio of approximately 2—that is, if 90% of a cell culture is killed by 2 Gy_t, then in the presence of a sensitizing agent, only 1 Gy$_t$ is required for the same percentage of lethality.

Radioprotective compounds include molecules that contain a sulfhydryl group (sulfur and hydrogen bound together), such as cysteine and cysteamine. Hundreds of others have been tested and found effective by a factor of approximately 2. For example, if 6 Gy$_t$ is a lethal dose to a mouse, then in the presence of a radioprotective agent, 12 Gy$_t$ would be required to produce lethality.

Radioprotective agents have not found human application because, to be effective, they must be administered at toxic levels. The protective agent can be worse than the radiation!

Hormesis

A separate and small body of radiobiologic evidence suggests that a little bit of radiation is good for you. Some studies have shown that animals given low radiation doses live longer than unirradiated controls. The prevailing explanation is that a little radiation stimulates hormonal and immune responses to other toxic environmental agents.

Many nonradiation examples of hormesis can be found. In large quantities, fluoride is deadly. In small quantities, it is a known tooth preservative.

Regardless of radiation hormesis, we continue to practice ALARA ("as low as reasonably achievable") vigorously as a known safe approach to radiation management.

RADIATION DOSE-RESPONSE RELATIONSHIPS

Although some scientists were working with animals to observe the effects of radiation a few years after the discovery of x-rays, these studies were not experimentally sound, nor were their results applied. With the advent of the age of the atomic bomb in the 1940s, however, interest in radiobiology increased enormously.

The object of nearly all radiobiologic research is the establishment of radiation dose-response relationships. A radiation dose-response relationship is a mathematical relationship between various radiation dose levels and the magnitude of the observed response.

Radiation dose-response relationships have two important applications in radiology. First, these experimentally determined relationships are used to design therapeutic treatment routines for cancer patients.

Radiobiologic studies also have been designed to yield information on the effects of low-dose irradiation. These studies and the dose-response relationships that were revealed provide the basis for radiation management activities and are particularly significant for diagnostic radiology.

TABLE 32.3 Characteristics of Stochastic and Deterministic Radiation Responses

Stochastic	Nonthreshold dose-response relationship
	Linear dose-response relationship
	Incidence of response increases with radiation dose
Deterministic	Threshold dose-response relationship
	Nonlinear dose-response relationship
	Severity of response increases with radiation dose

Human responses to radiation exposure fall into two types: deterministic or stochastic.

Deterministic radiation responses usually follow high-dose radiation exposure and appear as an early response. They exhibit a radiation dose threshold; there is a dose below which no such response occurs. As radiation dose increases, the **severity** of the response increases. Radiation-induced skin burns represent a deterministic response.

Stochastic responses are cancer, leukemia, and genetic effects. Such responses usually follow low radiation exposure and appear years later as a late radiation response. There is no dose threshold, and as radiation dose increases, the **incidence** of response in a population increases.

Every radiation dose-response relationship has two characteristics. It is either linear or nonlinear, and it is either threshold or nonthreshold (Table 32.3). These characteristics can be described mathematically or graphically. The following discussion avoids the math.

Linear Dose-Response Relationships

Fig. 32.4 shows examples of the linear dose-response relationship, which is so named because the response is directly proportional to the radiation dose. When the radiation dose is doubled, the response to radiation likewise is doubled.

In Fig. 32.4, dose-response relationships *A* and *B* intersect the dose axis at zero or below. These relationships are thus the **linear, nonthreshold (LNT)** type. In a nonthreshold dose-response relationship, any dose, regardless of its size, is expected to produce a response.

At zero dose, relationship *A* exhibits a measurable response, R$_N$. The level R$_N$, called the **natural response level**, indicates that even without radiation exposure, that type of response, such as cancer, occurs.

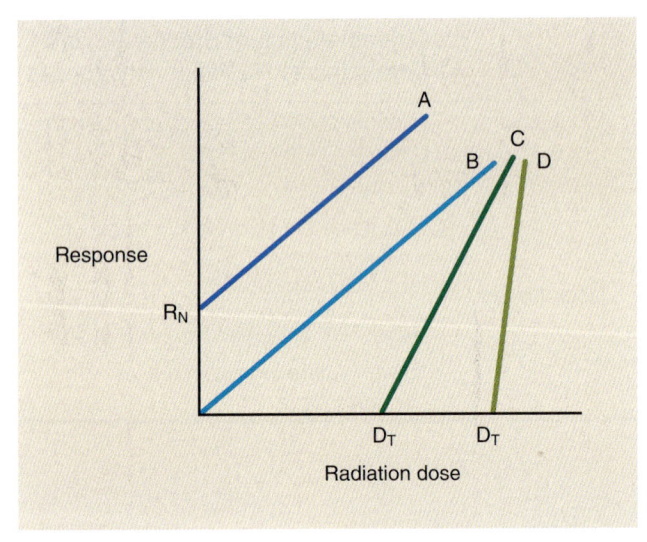

FIG. 32.4 Linear dose-response relationships A and B are nonthreshold types. C and D are threshold types. R_N is the normal incidence or response with no radiation exposure.

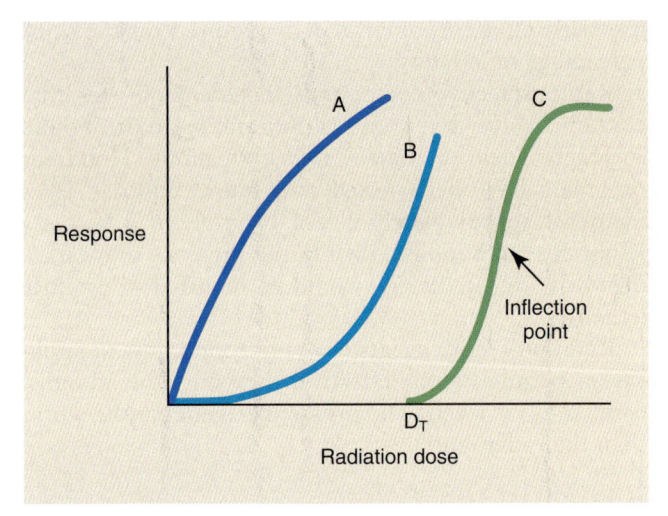

FIG. 32.5 Nonlinear dose-response relationships can assume several shapes. Curves A and B are nonthreshold. Curve C is nonlinear, threshold. D_T, Threshold dose.

> Radiation-induced cancer, leukemia, and genetic effects follow a linear, nonthreshold dose-response relationship.

Dose-response relationships C and D are identified as **linear, threshold** because they intercept the dose axis at some value greater than zero. Radiation dose-response relationships C and D are radiologically unimportant. The threshold dose for C and D is D_T.

At radiation doses below D_T, no response is observed. Relationship D has a steeper slope than C; therefore, above the threshold dose, any increment of dose produces a larger response if that response follows relationship D rather than C.

Nonlinear Dose-Response Relationships

All other radiation dose-response relationships are nonlinear (Fig. 32.5). Curves A and B are **nonlinear, nonthreshold**. Curve A shows that a large response results from a very small radiation dose. At high-dose levels, radiation is not so efficient because an incremental dose at high levels results in less relative response than the same incremental dose at low levels.

The dose-response relationship represented by curve B is just the opposite. Incremental radiation doses in the low-dose range produce very little response. At high doses, however, the same increment of dose produces a much larger response.

Curve C is a **nonlinear, threshold** relationship. At doses below D_T, no response is measured. As the dose is increased to above D_T, it becomes increasingly effective per increment of dose until the dose that corresponds to the inflection point of the curve is reached. This type of dose-response relationship is characteristic of a deterministic response.

The inflection point occurs when the curve stops bending up and begins bending down. Above this level, incremental doses become less effective. Relationship C is sometimes called a **sigmoid-type**, radiation dose-response relationship.

> Skin effects resulting from high-dose fluoroscopy follow a sigmoid-type dose-response relationship.

We will refer to these general types of radiation dose-response relationships when discussing the type and degree of human radiation injury. Diagnostic radiology is concerned almost exclusively with the late effects of radiation exposure and therefore with linear, nonthreshold radiation dose-response relationships. For completeness, however, Chapter 35 briefly discusses early radiation damage.

Constructing a Dose-Response Relationship

Determining the radiation dose-response relationship for a whole-body response is tricky. It is very difficult to determine the degree of response, even that of early effects, because the number of experimental animals that can be used is usually small. It is nearly impossible to measure low-dose, stochastic effects—the area of greatest interest in digital imaging.

Therefore, we resort to irradiating a limited number of animals to very large doses of radiation in the hope of observing a statistically significant response. Fig. 32.6 shows the results of such an experiment in which four groups of animals were irradiated to a different radiation dose. The observations on each group result in an

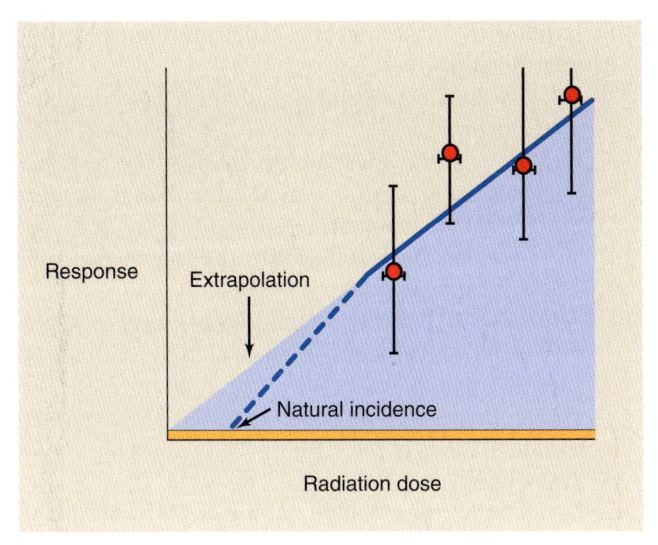

FIG. 32.6 A dose-response relationship is produced when high-dose experimental data are extrapolated to low doses.

FIG. 32.7 Dose-response relationship for radiation hormesis.

ordered pair of data: a radiation dose and the associated biologic response.

The error bars in each ordered pair indicate the confidence associated with each data point. Error bars on the dose measurements are very narrow because we can measure radiation dose very accurately. Error bars on the response, however, are very wide because of biologic variability and the limited number of observations at each dose.

The principal interest in digital imaging is to estimate the response at very low radiation doses. Because this cannot be done directly, we **extrapolate** the dose-response relationship from the high-dose, known region into the low-dose, unknown region.

This extrapolation invariably results in a **linear, nonthreshold** dose-response relationship. Such an extrapolation, however, may not be correct because of the many qualifying conditions on the experiment. As seen in Fig. 32.6, the natural incidence may be higher, and there is always natural background radiation dose.

The radiation dose-response relationship that demonstrates radiation hormesis is shown in Fig. 32.7. At very low doses, irradiated subjects experience less response than control participants. The existence of radiation hormesis is a highly controversial topic in radiologic science.

> No human radiation responses have been observed after radiation doses less than 100 mGy_t.

Many radiation scientists today believe that the dose-response relationship associated with digital imaging falls in between the LNT and hormesis (see Fig. 36.1). Indeed, regardless of our concern for low radiation doses to large populations, patient radiation doses less than approximately 50 mSv are totally acceptable in medical imaging, considering the benefit to the patient. Nevertheless, we need to be particularly aware of pediatric patient radiation dose.

SUMMARY

In 1906 two French scientists first theorized that radiosensitivity was a function of the metabolic state of tissue being irradiated. Their theory, known as the law of Bergonie and Tribondeau, states that (1) stem cells are radiosensitive, and mature cells are less so; (2) young tissue is more radiosensitive than older tissue; (3) high metabolic activity is radiosensitive, and low metabolic rate is radioresistant; and (4) increases in proliferation and growth rates of cells make them more radiosensitive.

Physical and biological factors affect tissue radiosensitivity. Physical factors include LET, RBE, fractionation, and protraction. Biological factors that affect radiosensitivity include the oxygen effect, the age-related effect, and the recovery effect.

Some chemicals can modify cell response. These are called *radiosensitizers* and *radioprotectors*.

Radiobiologic research concentrates on radiation dose-response relationships. In linear dose-response relationships, the response is directly proportional to the dose. In nonlinear dose-response relationships, varied doses produce varied responses.

The threshold dose is the level below which there is no response. The nonthreshold dose-response relationship means that any dose is expected to produce a response. For establishing radiation protection guidelines for digital imaging, the linear, nonthreshold dose-response model is used.

CHALLENGE QUESTIONS

1. Define or otherwise identify the following:
   a. Linear energy transfer
   b. Standard radiation
   c. Oxygen enhancement ratio
   d. Repopulation
   e. Extrapolation
   f. Threshold dose
   g. Interphase death
   h. Dose protraction
   i. Radiation weighting factor
   j. Hormesis
2. Write the formula for relative biologic effectiveness.
3. Give an example of fractionated radiation.
4. Why is high-pressure (hyperbaric) oxygen used in radiation oncology?
5. Write the formula for the oxygen enhancement ratio.
6. How does age affect the radiosensitivity of tissue?
7. When a radiobiologic experiment is conducted in vitro, what does this mean?
8. Name three agents that enhance the effects of radiation.
9. Name three radioprotective agents.
10. Are radioprotective agents used for human application?
11. Explain the meaning of a radiation dose-response relationship.
12. What occurs in a nonlinear radiation dose-response relationship?
13. Explain why the linear, nonthreshold dose-response relationship is used as a model for digital imaging radiation management.
14. State two of the corollaries to the law of Bergonie and Tribondeau.
15. Approximately 8 Gy_t of 220 kVp x-rays is necessary to produce death in an armadillo. Cobalt-60 gamma rays have a lower LET than 220 kVp x-rays; therefore 9.4 Gy_t is required for armadillo lethality. What is the RBE of ^{60}CO compared with 220 kVp?
16. Under fully oxygenated conditions, 90% of human cells in culture will be killed by 1.5 Gy_t x-rays. If cells are made anoxic, the dose required for 90% lethality is 4 Gy_t. What is the OER?
17. What are the units of LET?
18. Describe how RBE and LET are related.
19. Is occupational radiation exposure fractionated, protracted, or continuous?
20. Describe how OER and LET are related.

The answers to the Challenge Questions can be found by logging on to our website at http://evolve.elsevier.com.

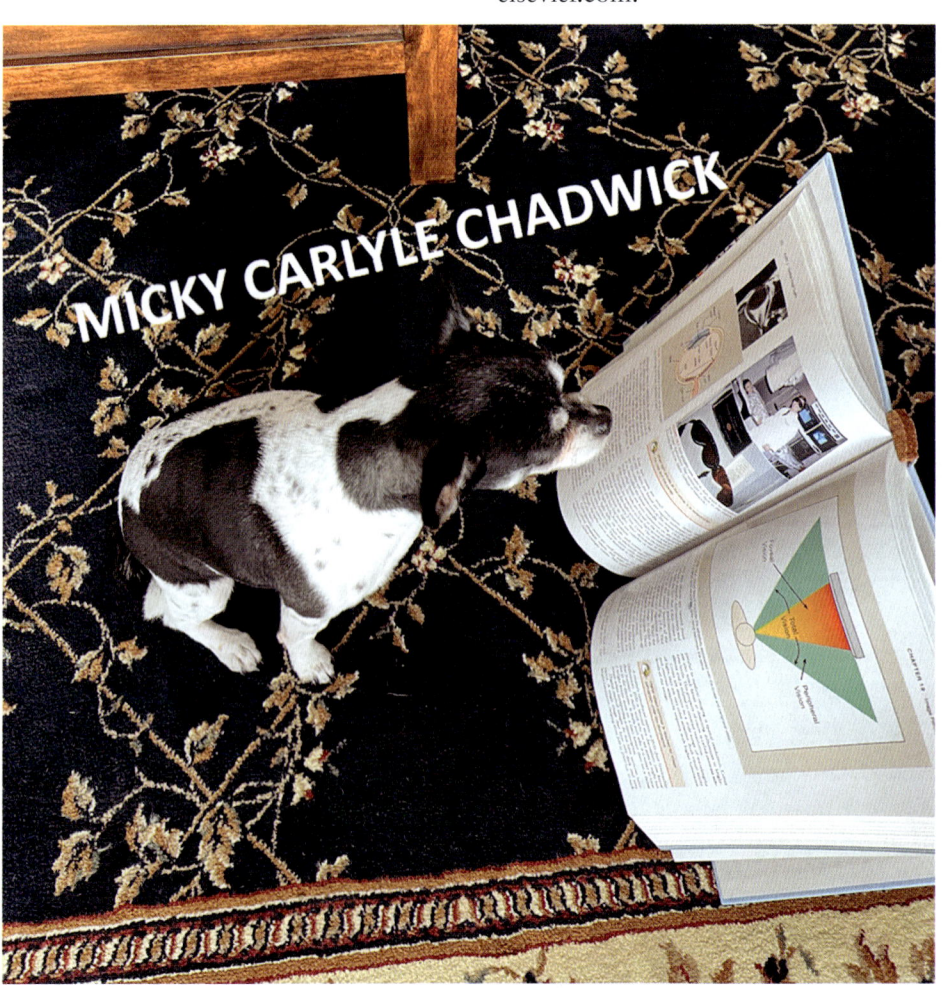

Molecular Radiobiology

CHAPTER 33

OBJECTIVES

At the completion of this chapter, the student should be able to do the following:

1. Discuss three effects of in vitro irradiation of macromolecules.
2. Explain the effects of radiation on DNA.
3. Identify the chemical reactions involved in the radiolysis of water.
4. Define direct effect and indirect effect, and identify the importance of each.

OUTLINE

Irradiation of Macromolecules 450
Main-Chain Scission 450
Cross-Linking 450
Point Lesions 450
Macromolecular Synthesis 450
Radiation Effects on DNA 451
Radiolysis of Water 452
Direct and Indirect Effects 454
Summary 454
Challenge Questions 454

EVEN THOUGH the initial interaction between radiation and tissue occurs at the electron level, observable human radiation response results from change at the molecular level. The occurrence of molecular lesions is identified by effects on macromolecules and on water. This chapter discusses the irradiation of macromolecules and the radiolysis of water.

Because the human body is an aqueous solution that contains 80% water molecules, radiation interaction with water is the principal molecular radiation interaction in the body. However, the ultimate damage occurs to the target molecule, DNA, which controls cellular metabolism and reproduction.

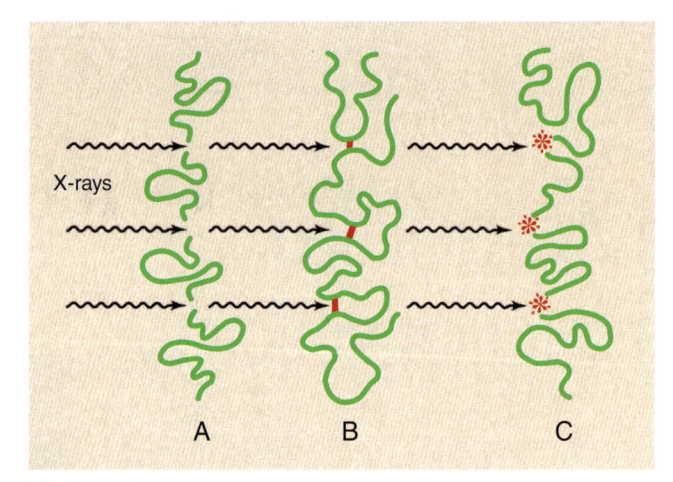

FIG. 33.1 The results of irradiation of macromolecules: (A) Main-chain scission. (B) Cross-linking. (C) Point lesions.

The effect of irradiation of macromolecules is quite different from that of irradiation of water. When macromolecules are irradiated **in vitro**—that is, outside the body or outside the cell, a considerable radiation dose is required to produce a measurable effect. Irradiation **in vivo**—that is, within the living cell, demonstrates that macromolecules are considerably more radiosensitive in their natural state.

> In vitro is irradiation outside of the cell or body. In vivo is irradiation within the cell.

IRRADIATION OF MACROMOLECULES

A **solution** is a liquid that contains dissolved substances. A mixture of fluids, such as water and alcohol, is also a solution. When macromolecules are irradiated in solution in vitro, three major effects occur: main-chain scission, cross-linking, and point lesions (Fig. 33.1).

Main-Chain Scission
Main-chain scission is the breakage of the backbone of the long-chain macromolecule. The result is the reduction of a long, single molecule into many smaller molecules, each of which may still be macromolecular.

Main-chain scission reduces not only the size of the macromolecule but also the **viscosity** of the solution. A viscous solution is one that is very thick and slow to flow, such as cold maple syrup. Tap water, on the other hand, has low viscosity. Measurements of viscosity determine the degree of main-chain scission.

Cross-Linking
Some macromolecules have small, spurlike side structures that extend off the main chain. Others produce these spurs as a consequence of irradiation.

These side structures can behave as though they have a sticky substance on the end, and they attach to a neighboring macromolecule or to another segment of the same molecule. This process is called **cross-linking**. Radiation-induced molecular cross-linking increases the viscosity of a macromolecular solution.

Point Lesions
Radiation interaction with macromolecules can also result in disruption of single chemical bonds, producing **point lesions**. Point lesions are not detectable, but they can cause a minor modification of the molecule, which in turn can cause it to malfunction within the cell.

> Point lesions can result in the stochastic radiation effects observed at the whole-body level.

Laboratory experiments have shown that all these types of radiation effects on macromolecules are reversible through intracellular repair and recovery.

Macromolecular Synthesis
Modern molecular biology has developed a generalized scheme for the function of a normal human cell. Molecular nutrients are brought to the cell and are diffused through the cell membrane, where they are broken down (**catabolism**) into smaller molecules with an accompanying release of energy.

This energy is used in several ways, but one of the more important ways is in the **synthesis** of macromolecules from smaller molecules (**anabolism**). The synthesis of proteins and nucleic acids is critical to the survival of the cell and to its reproduction.

> Metabolism consists of catabolism and anabolism.

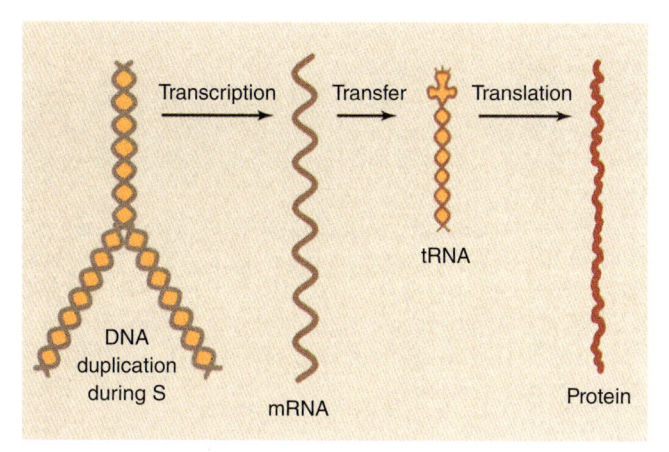

FIG. 33.2 The genetic code of DNA is transcribed by messenger RNA (mRNA) and is transferred to transfer RNA (tRNA), which translates it into a protein.

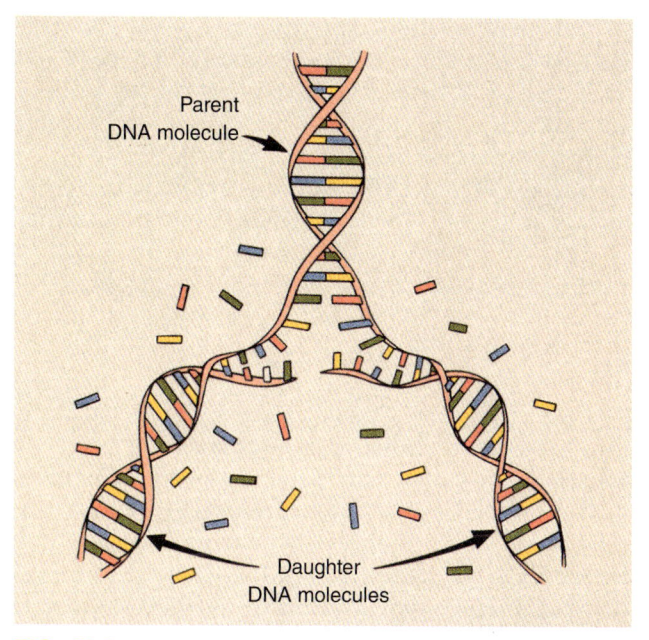

FIG. 33.3 During S phase, the DNA separates like a zipper, and two daughter DNA molecules are formed, each alike and each a replicate of the parent molecule.

Chapter 31 describes the scheme of protein synthesis and its dependence on nucleic acids. Proteins are manufactured by **translation** of the genetic code from transfer RNA (tRNA), which has been **transferred** from messenger RNA (mRNA). The information carried by the mRNA was in turn **transcribed** from DNA. This chain of events is shown schematically in Fig. 33.2.

Radiation damage to any of these macromolecules may result in cell death or late stochastic effects. Proteins are continuously synthesized throughout the cell cycle and occur in much more abundance than nucleic acids. Furthermore, multiple copies of specific protein molecules are always present in the cell. Consequently, proteins are less radiosensitive than nucleic acids.

Similarly, multiple copies of both types of RNA molecules are present in the cell, although they are less abundant than protein molecules. On the other hand, the DNA molecule, with its unique assembly of bases, is not so abundant.

> DNA is the most radiosensitive molecule in the human body.

DNA is synthesized somewhat differently from proteins. During the G_1 portion of interphase, the deoxyribose, phosphate, and base molecules accumulate in the nucleus. These molecules combine to form a single large molecule that, during the S portion of interphase, is attached to an existing single chain of DNA (Fig. 33.3). During G_1, molecular DNA is in the familiar double-helix form.

> Half as much DNA is present in G_1 as in G_2.

As the cell moves into S phase, the ladder begins to open up in the middle of each rung, much like a zipper. Now the DNA consists of only a single chain, and no pairing of bases occurs.

This state does not exist long, however, because the combined base sugar–phosphate molecule attaches to the single-strand DNA sequence, as determined by permitted base pairing. Consequently, where one double-helix DNA molecule was present, now two similar molecules exist, each a duplicate of the original. Parent DNA is said to be replicated into two duplicate DNA daughter molecules.

Radiation Effects on DNA

DNA is the most important molecule in the human body because it contains the genetic information for each cell. DNA is the radiation **target molecule**. Each cell has a nucleus that contains DNA complexed with other molecules in the form of chromosomes. Chromosomes thus control the growth and development of the cell; these, in turn, determine the characteristics of the individual (Fig. 33.4).

If radiation damage to the DNA is severe enough, visible chromosome aberrations may be detected. Fig. 33.5 is a representation of a normal chromosome and several distinct types of chromosome aberrations. Radiation-induced **chromosome aberrations** or **cytogenetic damage** are discussed more completely in Chapter 35.

The DNA molecule can be damaged without the production of a visible chromosome aberration. Although such damage is reversible, it can lead to cell death. If enough cells of the same type respond similarly, then a particular tissue or organ can be destroyed. That describes the cause of a **deterministic effect**.

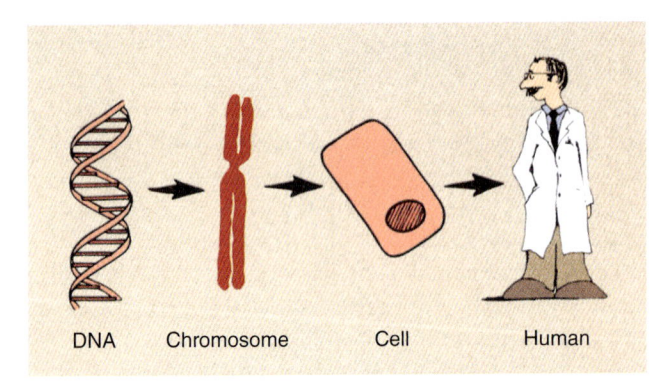

FIG. 33.4 DNA is the target molecule for radiation damage. It forms chromosomes and controls cell and human growth and development.

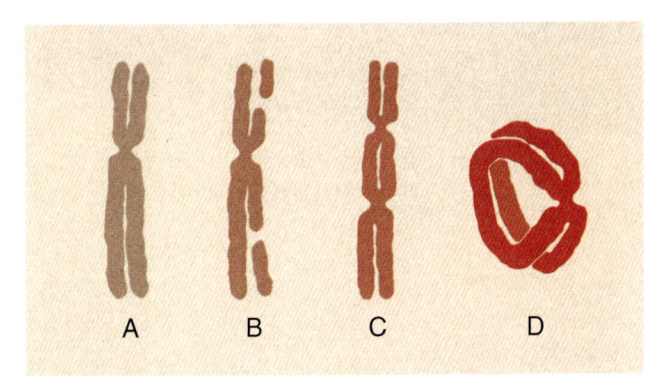

FIG. 33.5 Normal and radiation-damaged human chromosomes: (A) Normal. (B) Terminal deletion. (C) Dicentric formation. (D) Ring formation.

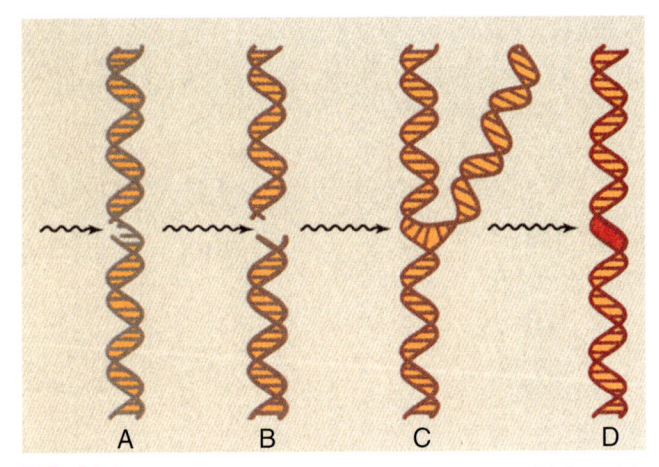

FIG. 33.6 Types of damage that can occur in DNA: (A) One side rail severed. (B) Both side rails severed. (C) Cross-linking. (D) Rung breakage.

Damage to the DNA also can result in abnormal metabolic activity. Uncontrolled rapid proliferation of cells is the principal characteristic of radiation-induced malignant disease. That describes the cause of a **stochastic effect**.

If damage to the DNA occurs within a germ cell, then it is possible that the response to radiation exposure will not be observed until the following generation or even later. This describes the cause of a genetic effect, which has all the characteristics of a stochastic effect.

The chromosome contains miles of DNA; therefore when a visible aberration does appear, it signifies a considerable amount of radiation damage. Unobserved damage to the DNA also can produce responses at cellular and whole-body levels.

> **RADIATION RESPONSE OF DNA**
> - Main-chain scission with only one side rail severed
> - Main-chain scission with both side rails severed
> - Main-chain scission and subsequent cross-linking
> - Rung breakage causing a separation of bases
> - Change in or loss of a base

The gross structural radiation response of DNA is diagrammed schematically in Fig. 33.6. Although each of these effects results in a structural change in the DNA molecule, they are all reversible. In some of these types of damage, the sequence of bases can be altered; therefore the triplet code of codons may not remain intact. This represents a genetic mutation at the molecular level.

> Cell death, malignant disease, and genetic effects result from irradiation of DNA.

The fifth type of damage, the change or loss of a base, also destroys the triplet code and may not be reversible. This type of radiation damage is a molecular lesion of the DNA. These molecular lesions are called **point mutations**, and they can be of minor or major importance to the cell. One critical consequence of point mutations is the transfer of the incorrect genetic code to one of the two daughter cells. This sequence of events is shown in Fig. 33.7.

RADIOLYSIS OF WATER

Because the human body is an aqueous solution that contains approximately 80% water molecules, the irradiation of water represents the principal radiation interaction in the body. When water is irradiated, it dissociates into smaller molecules; this action is called the **radiolysis of water** (Fig. 33.8).

When an atom of water (H_2O) is irradiated, it is ionized and dissociates into two ions—an ion pair, as shown by the following:

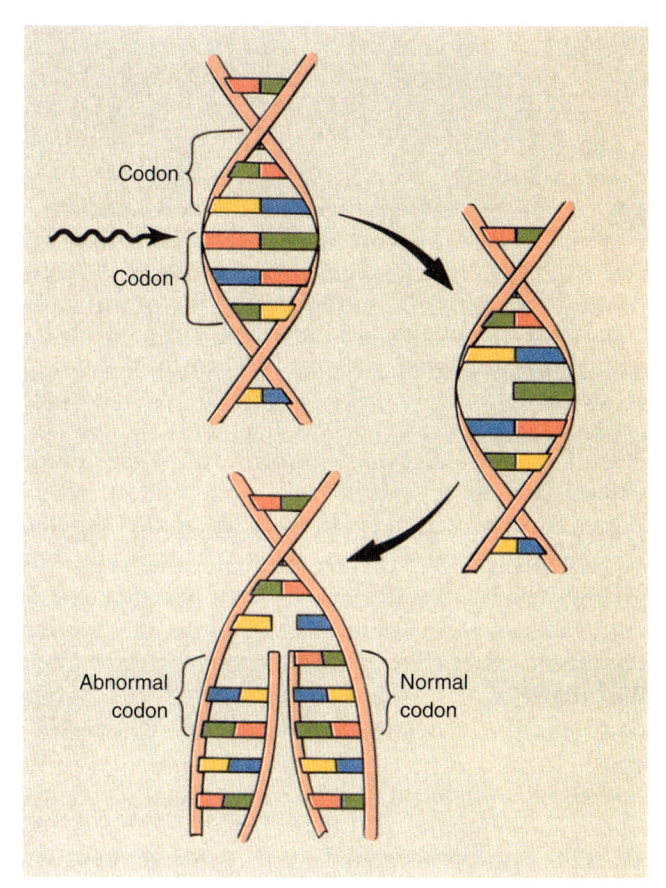

FIG. 33.7 A point mutation results in the change or loss of a base, which creates an abnormal gene. This is therefore a genetic mutation that is passed to one of the daughter cells.

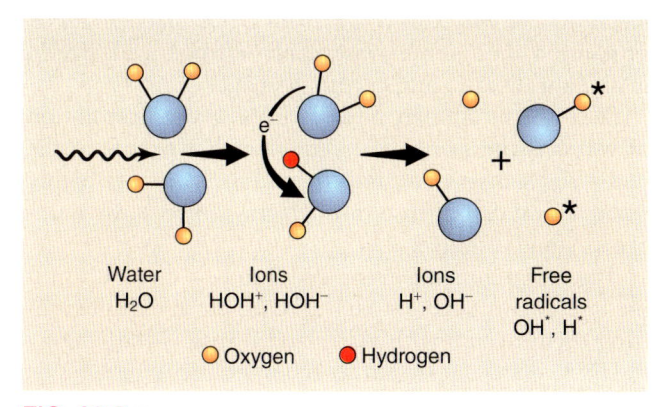

FIG. 33.8 The radiolysis of water results in the formation of ions and free radicals.

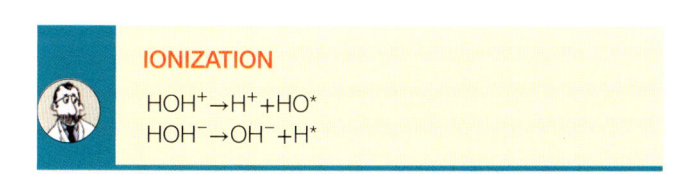

> **IONIZATION**
> $HOH^+ \rightarrow H^+ + HO^*$
> $HOH^- \rightarrow OH^- + H^*$

After this initial ionization, a number of reactions can occur. First, the ion pair may rejoin into a stable water molecule. In this case, no damage occurs. Second, if these ions do not rejoin, it is possible for the negative ion (the electron) to attach to another water molecule through the following reaction to produce yet a third type of ion.

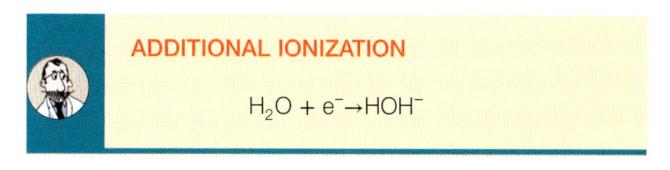

> **ADDITIONAL IONIZATION**
> $H_2O + e^- \rightarrow HOH^-$

The HOH^+ and HOH^- ions are relatively unstable and can dissociate into still smaller molecules, as follows.

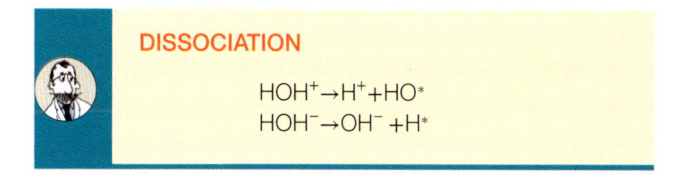

> **DISSOCIATION**
> $HOH^+ \rightarrow H^+ + HO^*$
> $HOH^- \rightarrow OH^- + H^*$

The final result of the radiolysis of water is the formation of an ion pair, H^+ and OH^-, and two **free radicals**, H^* and OH^*. The ions can recombine; therefore no biologic damage would occur.

These types of ions are not unusual. Many molecules in aqueous solution exist in a loosely ionized state because of their structure. Salt (NaCl), for instance, easily dissociates into Na^+ and Cl^- ions. Even in the absence of radiation, water can dissociate into H^+ and OH^- ions.

> A free radical is an uncharged molecule that contains a single unpaired electron in the outer shell.

Free radicals are another story. They are highly reactive. Free radicals are unstable and therefore exist with a lifetime of less than 1 ms. During that time, however, they are capable of diffusion through the cell and interaction at a distant site. Free radicals contain excess energy that can be transferred to other molecules to disrupt bonds and produce point lesions at some distance from the initial ionizing event.

The H^* and OH^* molecules are not the only free radicals that are produced during the radiolysis of water. The OH^* free radical can join with a similar molecule to form hydrogen peroxide.

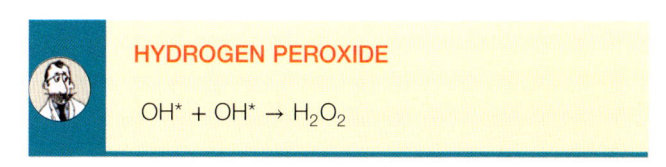

> **HYDROGEN PEROXIDE**
> $OH^* + OH^* \rightarrow H_2O_2$

Hydrogen peroxide is poisonous to the cell and therefore acts as a toxic agent.

The H* free radical can interact with molecular oxygen to form the hydroperoxyl radical.

> **HYDROPEROXYL FORMATION**
> $H^* + O_2 \rightarrow HO^*_2$

The hydroperoxyl radical, along with hydrogen peroxide, is considered to be the principal damaging product after the radiolysis of water. Hydrogen peroxide also can be formed by the interaction of two hydroperoxyl radicals.

> **HYDROGEN PEROXIDE FORMATION**
> $HO^*_2 + HO^*_2 \rightarrow H_2O_2 + O_2$

Some organic molecules, symbolized as RH, can become reactive free radicals, as follows.

> **FREE RADICAL FORMATION**
> $RH + \uparrow \rightarrow RH^* \rightarrow H^* + R^*$

When oxygen is present, yet another species of free radical is possible, as follows.

> **ORGANIC FREE RADICAL FORMATION**
> $R^* + O_2 \rightarrow RO^*_2$

Free radicals are energetic molecules because of their unique structure. This excess energy can be transferred to DNA, and this can result in bond breaks.

DIRECT AND INDIRECT EFFECTS

When biologic material is irradiated in vivo, the harmful effects of irradiation occur principally because of damage to a particularly sensitive molecule, such as DNA. Evidence for the **direct effect** of radiation comes from in vitro experiments wherein various molecules can be irradiated in solution. The effect is produced by the ionization of the target molecule.

> When the ionizing event occurs on the target molecule, the effect of radiation is direct.

On the other hand, if the initial ionizing event occurs on a distant, noncritical molecule, which then transfers the energy of ionization to the target molecule, an **indirect effect** has occurred. Free radicals, with their excess energy of reaction, are the intermediate molecules. They migrate to the target molecule and transfer their energy, which results in damage to that target molecule.

> The principal effect of radiation on humans is indirect.

It is not possible to identify whether a given interaction with the target molecule resulted from a direct or indirect effect. However, because the human body consists of approximately 80% water and less than 1% DNA, it is concluded that essentially all of the effects of irradiation in vivo result from indirect effect. When oxygen is present, as in living tissue, the indirect effects are amplified because of the additional types of free radicals that are formed.

SUMMARY

When macromolecules are irradiated in vitro, three major effects occur: (1) main-chain scission, (2) cross-linking, and (3) disruption of single chemical bonds, causing point lesions. All three types of damage are reversible through intracellular repair and recovery.

DNA, with its unique assembly of bases, is not abundant in the cell. As a result, DNA is the most radiosensitive of all macromolecules and is called the target molecule. Chromosome aberrations or abnormal metabolic activity can result from DNA damage. DNA irradiation has three observable effects: cell death, malignant disease, and genetic damage.

Because the human body is 80% water, irradiation of water is the principal interaction that occurs in the body. Water dissociates into free radicals that are highly reactive and can diffuse through the cell to cause damage at some distance.

The initial ionizing event is said to be a direct effect if the interaction occurs with a DNA molecule. If the ionizing event occurs with water and transfers that energy to DNA, the event is said to be an indirect effect.

CHALLENGE QUESTIONS

1. Define or otherwise identify the following:
   a. In vitro
   b. Cytogenetic damage
   c. Point mutation
   d. Free radical
   e. Target theory
   f. Viscosity
   g. Cross-linking
   h. Radiation hit
   i. Catabolism
   j. Stochastic effect

2. List the effects of irradiation of macromolecules in solution in vitro.
3. How is solution viscosity used to determine the degree of radiation macromolecular damage?
4. What is the difference between catabolism and anabolism?
5. In what phase of the cell cycle does the DNA ladder open up in the middle of each rung and consist of only a single chain?
6. Name the three principal observable effects of DNA irradiation.
7. Differentiate among transcription, transfer, and translation when applied to molecular genetics.
8. Draw a diagram that illustrates the point mutations of DNA that transfer the incorrect genetic code to one of the two daughter cells.
9. Write the formula for the radiolysis of water, in which the atom of water is ionized and dissociates into two ions.
10. What happens to radiation-induced free radicals within the cell?
11. Describe the molecular cause of a deterministic effect.
12. What happens to the quantity of DNA as the cell progresses from G_1 and G_2?
13. Chromosome aberrations are an example of what type of cell damage?
14. When a single nucleotide base is lost, what happens?
15. Complete the following chemical equations:
    a. H_2O + Radiation →?
    b. HOH^+ (dissociation) →?
    c. HOH^- (dissociation) →?
16. What molecular change results in a stochastic effect?
17. Describe the characteristics of a free radical.
18. What is the difference between direct effect and indirect effect?
19. How much DNA is in a cell?
20. Discuss the difference in radiation responses in vivo compared with in vitro.

The answers to the Challenge Questions can be found by logging on to our website at http://evolve.elsevier.com.

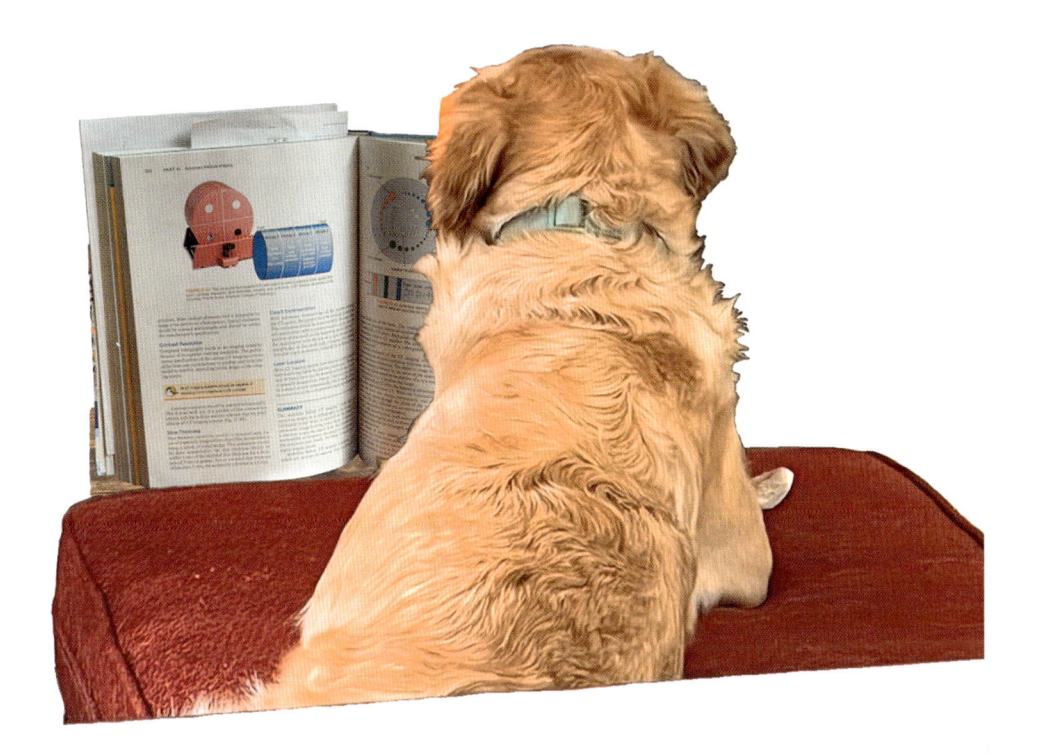

GERALDINE CARLYLE MILLER

CHAPTER 34

Cellular Radiobiology

OBJECTIVES

At the completion of this chapter, the student should be able to do the following:

1. Describe the effects of in vivo irradiation.
2. Describe the principles of target theory.
3. Discuss the kinetics of cell survival after irradiation.
4. Identify the cell survival model that best describes human cells.
5. Name the most radiation-sensitive stage of the human cell.

OUTLINE

Target Theory 457
Cell-Survival Kinetics 457
  Single-Target, Single-Hit Model 458
  Multitarget, Single-Hit Model 459
  Recovery 461
Cell-Cycle Effects 462
Radiation Effect Modification 463
Summary 464
Challenge Questions 464

THE EFFECT of radiation on cells results from an ionizing event that changes the target molecule, DNA. The response of the cell is either cellular transformation or cell death.

Cellular transformation can result in a late stochastic effect at the human level. Cell death can result in an early deterministic effect at the human level.

Most effects on cells result in no response because of metabolic recovery and repair processes. This chapter deals primarily with cell death as a radiation response.

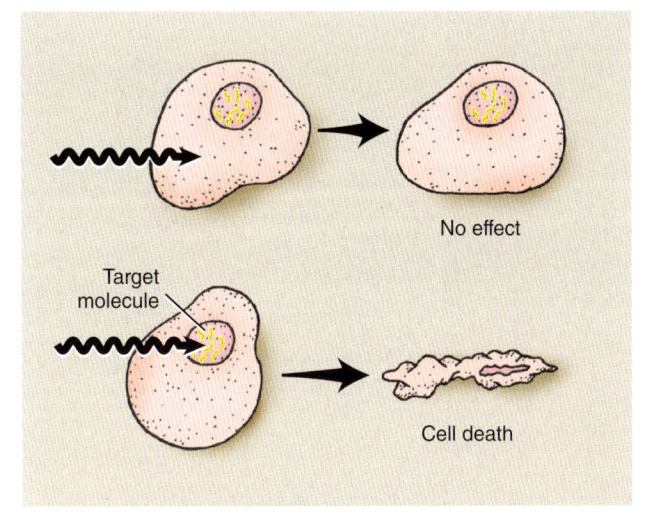

FIG. 34.1 According to target theory, cell death will occur only if the target molecule is inactivated. DNA, the target molecule, is located within the cell nucleus.

TARGET THEORY

The cell contains many species of molecules, most of which exist in overabundance. Radiation damage to such molecules probably would not result in noticeable injury to the cell because similar molecules would be available to continue to support the cell.

On the other hand, some molecules in the cell are considered to be particularly necessary for normal cell function. These molecules are not abundant; in fact, there may be only one such molecule. Radiation damage to such a molecule could affect the cell severely because no similar molecules would be available as substitutes.

This concept of a sensitive key molecule serves as the basis for the **target theory**. According to the target theory, for a cell to die after radiation exposure, its target molecule must be inactivated (Fig. 34.1).

> DNA is the target molecule.

Originally, the target theory was used to represent cell lethality. However, it can be used equally effectively to describe nonlethal radiation-induced cell abnormalities.

The target in target theory is considered to be an area of the cell occupied by the target molecule or by a sensitive site on the target molecule. This area changes position with time because of intracellular molecular movement.

The interaction between radiation and cellular components is random; therefore when an interaction does occur with a target, it occurs randomly. There is no favoritism by ionizing radiation to the target molecule. The sensitivity of the target molecule to radiation occurs simply because of its vital function in the cell.

When radiation does interact with the target, a **hit** is said to have occurred. Radiation interaction with molecules other than the target molecule also can result in a hit. It is not possible to distinguish between a direct and an indirect hit.

> Hits occur through both direct and indirect effects.

When a hit occurs through indirect effect, the size of the target appears considerably larger because of the mobility of the free radicals. This increased target size contributes to the importance of the indirect effect of radiation.

Fig. 34.2 illustrates some of the consequences of using target theory to explain the relationships among linear energy transfer (LET), the oxygen effect, and direct versus indirect effect. With low-LET radiation, in the absence of oxygen, the probability of a hit on the target molecule is low because of the relatively large distances between ionizing events.

If oxygen is present, free radicals are formed and the volume of effectiveness surrounding each ionization is enlarged. Consequently, the probability of a hit is increased.

When high-LET radiation is used, the distance between ionizations is so close that the probability of a hit by direct effect is high. When oxygen is added to the system and high-LET radiation is used, the added sphere of influence for each ionizing event, although somewhat larger, does not result in additional hits. The maximum number of hits has already been produced by direct effect with high-LET radiation.

CELL-SURVIVAL KINETICS

Early radiation experiments at the cell level were conducted with simple cells, such as bacteria. It was not until the mid-1950s that laboratory techniques were

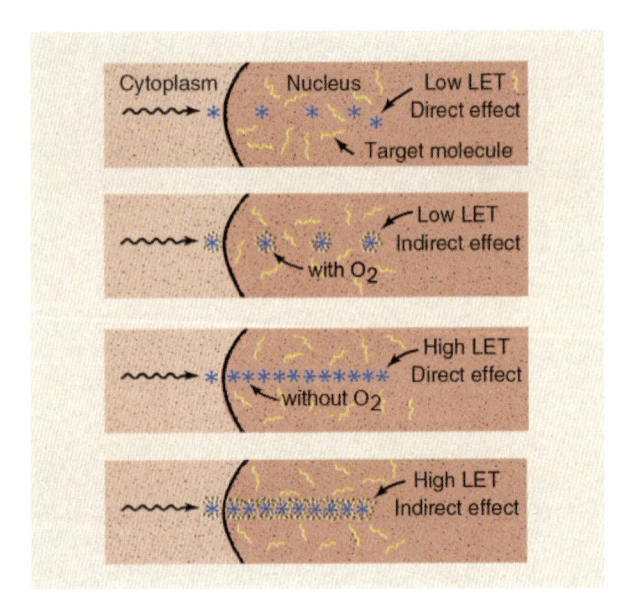

FIG. 34.2 In the presence of oxygen, the indirect effect is amplified and the volume of action for low-linear energy transfer (*LET*) radiation is enlarged. The effective volume of action for high-LET radiation remains unchanged in that maximum injury will have been inflicted by direct effect.

developed to allow the growth and manipulation of human cells in vitro.

One technique for measuring the lethal effects of radiation on cells is shown in Fig. 34.3. If normal cells are planted individually in a Petri dish and are incubated for 10 to 14 days, they divide many times and produce a visible colony that consists of many cells. This is cell **cloning**.

After irradiation of such single cells, some do not survive; therefore fewer colonies are formed. A higher radiation dose leads to the formation of fewer colonies.

> The lethal effects of radiation are determined by observing cell survival, not cell death.

When a mathematical extension of target theory is used, two models of cell survival result. The **single-target, single-hit** model applies to biologic targets, such as enzymes, viruses, and simple cells such as bacteria. The **multitarget, single-hit** model applies to more complicated biologic systems, such as human cells.

The following discussion concerns the equation of these models. The mathematics of these models is relatively unimportant, but is given here for interested students.

Single-Target, Single-Hit Model

Consider the situation illustrated in Fig. 34.4. It is raining on a large concrete runway that contains 100 squares. A square is considered wet when one or more raindrops have fallen on it.

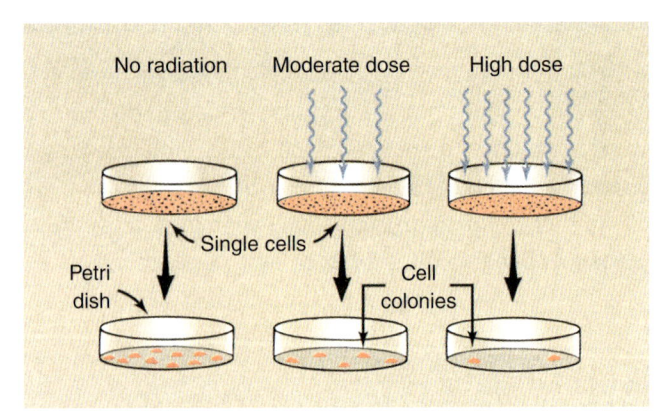

FIG. 34.3 When single cells are planted in a Petri dish, they grow into visible colonies. Fewer colonies develop if the cells are irradiated.

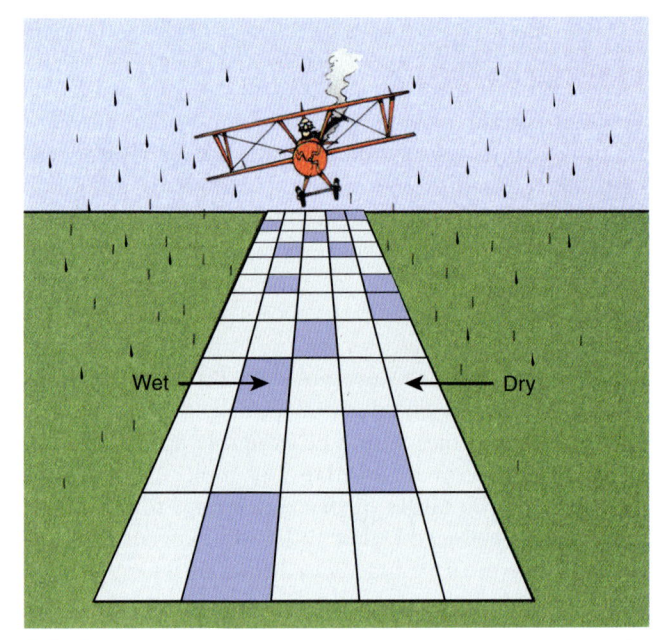

FIG. 34.4 When rain falls on a dry pavement that consists of a large number of squares, the number of squares that remains dry decreases exponentially as the number of raindrops increases.

When the first raindrop falls on the pavement, 1 of the 100 squares becomes wet. When the second raindrop falls, it will probably fall on a dry square and not on the one that is already wet. Consequently, 2 of 100 squares will be wet.

When the third raindrop falls, there will probably be 3 wet and 97 dry squares. As the number of raindrops increases, however, it becomes more probable that a given square will be hit by two or more drops.

Because the raindrops are falling **randomly**, the probability that a square will become wet is governed by a statistical law called the **Poisson distribution**. According to this law, when the number of raindrops is equal to the number of squares (100 in this case), 63% of the squares will be wet and 37% of the squares will be dry.

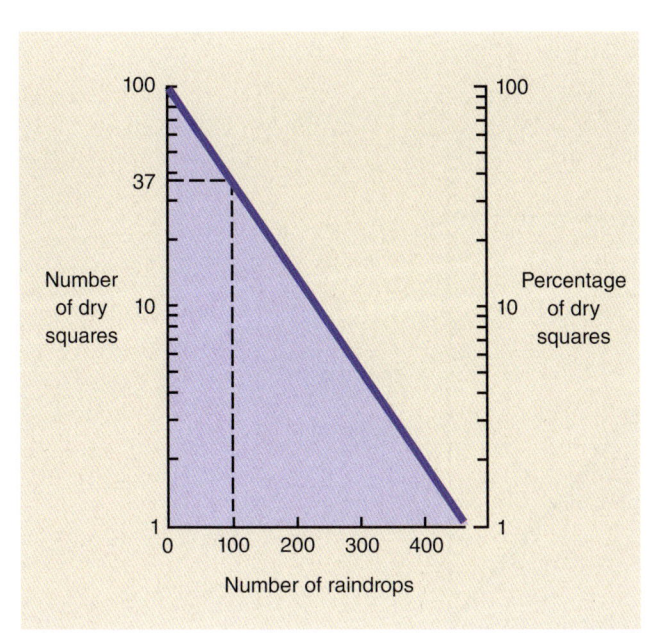

FIG. 34.5 When the number of dry squares is plotted semilogarithmically as a function of the number of raindrops, a straight line results because when a few drops fall, some squares will be hit more than once.

If the raindrops had fallen **uniformly**, all 100 squares would become wet with 100 raindrops.

> Radiation interacts randomly with matter.

Obviously, many of the 63 squares in this example have been hit two or more times. When the number of raindrops equals twice the number of squares, then 14 squares will be dry. After 300 raindrops, only five squares will remain dry.

Examine a graph of the number of dry squares as a function of the number of raindrops (Fig. 34.5). If the number of squares exposed to the rain was large or unknown, the scale on the right, expressed in a percentage, would be used. Note that the y-axis is logarithmic.

The wet squares analogy can be extended to the irradiation of a large number of biologic specimens—for example, 1000 bacteria. Bacteria presumably contain a single sensitive site, or target, that must be inactivated for the cell to die. As 1000 bacteria are irradiated with increasing increments of dose, a greater number are killed (Fig. 34.6).

Just as with the wet squares, however, as the dose increases, some cells will sustain two or more hits. All hits per target in excess of one represent a wasted radiation dose because the bacteria had been killed already by the first hit.

> A hit is not simply an ionizing event but rather an ionization that inactivates the target molecule.

When the radiation dose reaches a level sufficient to kill 63% of the cells (37% survival), it is called D_{37}. After a dose equal to $2 \times D_{37}$, 14% of the cells would survive ($0.37 \times 0.37 = 0.1369$). D_{37} is a measure of the radiosensitivity of the cell. A low D_{37} indicates a highly radiosensitive cell, and a high D_{37} reveals radioresistance.

> If the radiation were uniform (no wasted radiation), D_{37} would be sufficient to kill 100% of the cells.

The equation that describes the dose-response relationship represented by the graph in Fig. 34.6 is the **single-target, single-hit** model of radiation-induced lethality.

SINGLE-TARGET, SINGLE-HIT MODEL

$$S = N/N_0 = e^{-D/D_{37}}$$

where S is the surviving fraction, N is the number of cells surviving a dose (D), N_0 is the initial number of cells, and D_{37} is a constant dose related to cell radiosensitivity.

Multitarget, Single-Hit Model

Returning to the wet squares analogy, suppose that each pavement square were divided into two equal parts, two targets (Fig. 34.7). By definition, each half now must be hit with a raindrop for the square to be considered wet. The first few raindrops probably will hit only one-half of any given square; therefore after a very light rain, no squares may be wet.

Many raindrops must fall before any single square suffers a hit in both halves so that it can be considered wet. This represents a **threshold** because, according to our definition, a number of raindrops can fall and all squares will remain dry. As the number of raindrops increases, eventually some squares will have both halves hit and therefore will be considered wet. This portion of the curve is represented by region A in Fig. 34.8.

When a large number of raindrops have fallen, region C will be reached, where every square will be at least half wet. When this occurs, each additional raindrop will produce a wet square. In region C, the relation between the number of raindrops and wet squares is that described by the single-target, single-hit model. The intermediate region B is the region of accumulation of hits.

> Complex biologic specimens, such as human cells, are thought to have more than a single critical target.

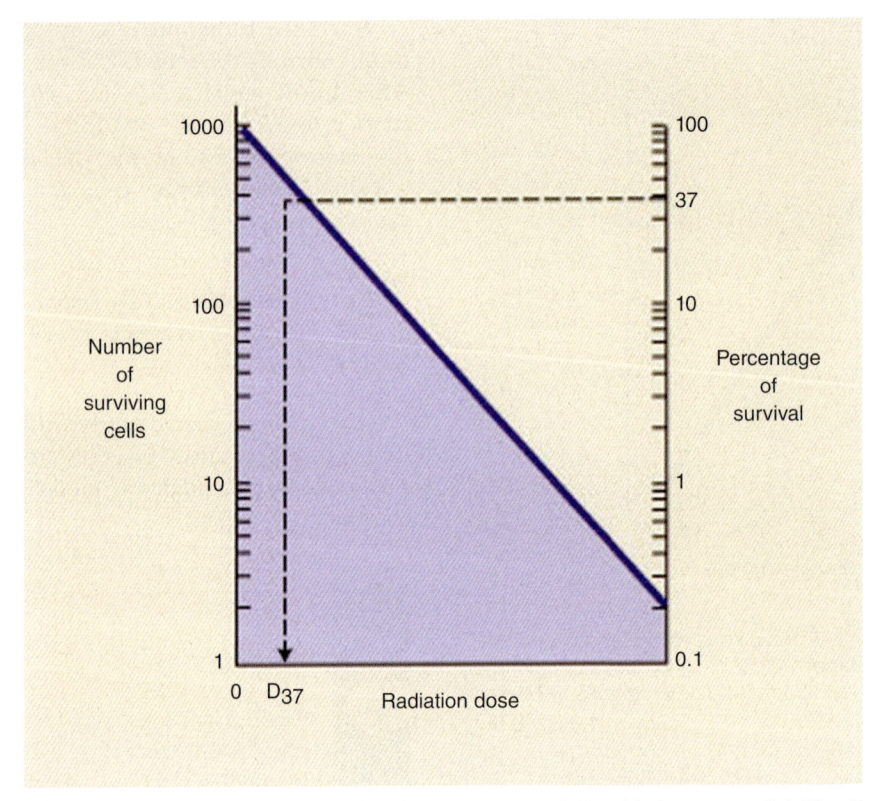

FIG. 34.6 After irradiation of 1000 cells, the dose-response relationship is exponential. The D_{37} is the dose that results in 37% survival.

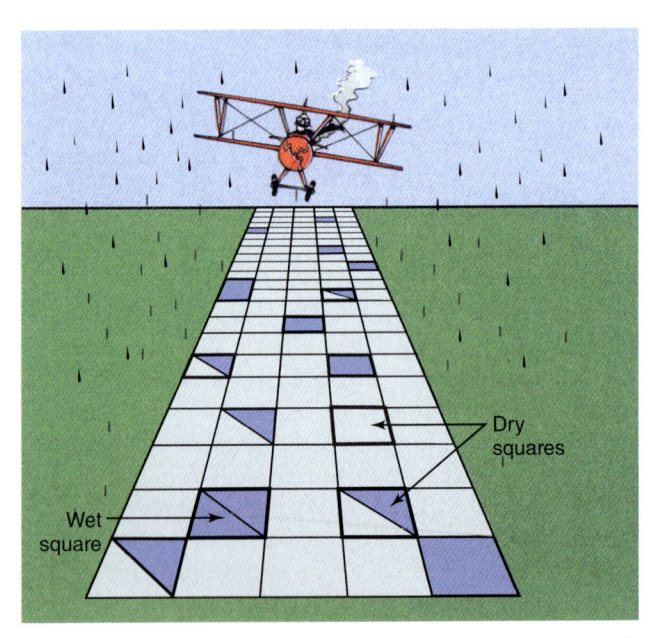

FIG. 34.7 If each pavement square has two equal parts, each part must be hit for the square to be considered wet.

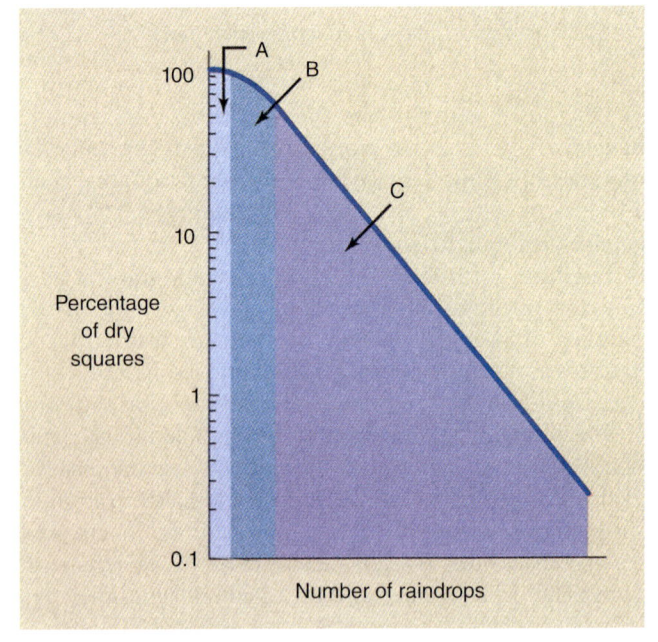

FIG. 34.8 When a square contains two equal parts, both of which have to be hit to be considered wet, three regions of the dry square versus raindrops relationship can be identified.

Suppose that the human cell has two targets, each of which has to be inactivated for the cell to die. This would be analogous to the square having two halves, each of which had to be hit by rain for it to be considered wet. Fig. 34.9 is a graph of single-cell survival for human cells that have two targets.

At very low radiation doses, cell survival is nearly 100%. As the radiation dose increases, fewer cells survive because more sustain a hit in both target molecules.

At a high radiation dose, all cells that survive have one target hit. Therefore at still higher doses, the

CHAPTER 34 Cellular Radiobiology

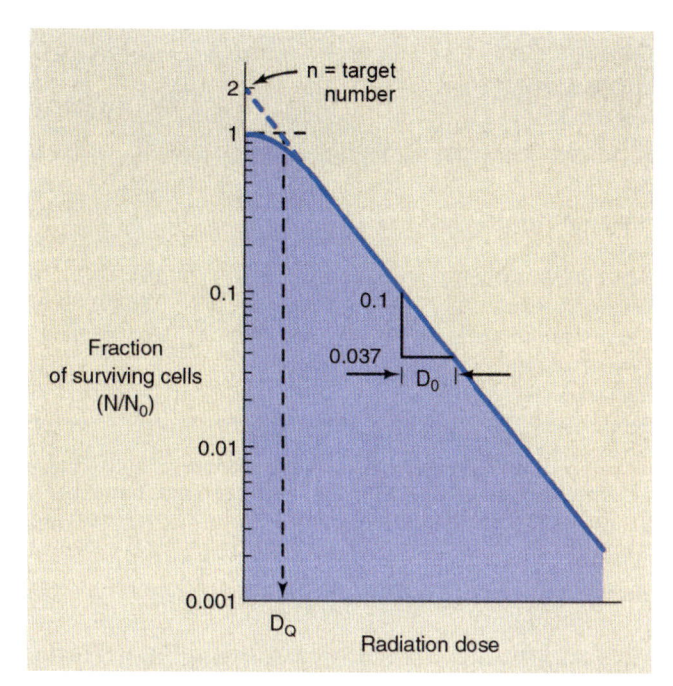

FIG. 34.9 The multitarget, single-hit model of cell survival is characteristic of human cells that contain two targets.

TABLE 34.1 Doses for Various Experimental Mammalian Cell Lines

Cell Type	D_0 (Gy$_a$)	D_Q (Gy$_a$)
Mouse oocytes	0.91	0.62
Mouse skin	1.35	3.50
Human bone marrow	1.37	1.00
Human fibroblasts	1.50	1.60
Mouse spermatogonia	1.80	2.70
Chinese hamster ovary	2.00	2.10
Human lymphocytes	4.00	1.00

D_0, Mean lethal dose; D_Q, threshold dose.

dose-response relationship would appear as the single-target, single-hit model.

The model of cell survival just described is the **multitarget, single-hit** model.

MULTITARGET, SINGLE-HIT MODEL

$$S = N/N_0 = 1 - (1 - e^{D/D_0})^n$$

where S is the surviving fraction, N is the number of cells surviving a dose (D), N_0 is the initial number of cells, D_0 is the dose necessary to reduce survival to 37% in the straight-line portion of the graph, and n is the extrapolation number.

The D_0 is called the **mean lethal dose** and is a constant related to the radiosensitivity of the cell. It is equal to D_{37} in the linear portion of the graph and therefore represents the dose that would result in one hit per target in the straight-line portion of the graph if no radiation were wasted.

> A large D_0 indicates radioresistant cells. A small D_0 is characteristic of radiosensitive cells.

The **extrapolation number** is also called the **target number**. When this type of experiment was first conducted with human cells, the observed extrapolation number was 2. That result agreed with the hypothesis that similar regions on two homologous chromosomes (an identical pair) had to be inactivated to produce cell death. Because chromosomes come in pairs, the experimental results confirmed the hypothesis.

Subsequent experiments, however, have resulted in extrapolation numbers ranging from 2 to 12, and therefore the precise meaning of **n** is unknown.

The D_Q is called the **threshold dose**. It is a measure of the width of the shoulder of the multitarget, single-hit model and is related to the capacity of the cell to recover from sublethal damage. Table 34.1 lists reported values for D_0 and D_Q for various experimental cell lines.

> A large D_Q indicates that the cell can recover readily from sublethal radiation damage.

Recovery

The shoulder of the graph of the multitarget, single-hit model shows that for mammalian cells, some damage must be accumulated before the cell dies. This accumulated damage is called **sublethal damage**. The wider the shoulder, the more sublethal damage that can be sustained and the higher the value of D_Q.

Fig. 34.10 demonstrates the results of a split-dose irradiation designed to describe the capacity of a cell to recover from sublethal damage. This illustration shows a rather typical human cell survival curve with $D_0 = 1.6$ Gy$_t$, $D_Q = 1.1$ Gy$_t$, and n = 2. If one takes those cells that survive any large dose (e.g., 4.7 Gy$_t$) and reincubates them in a growth medium, they will grow into another large population.

This new population of cells then can be used to perform a second cell survival experiment. When the cells that survived the first dose are subsequently subjected to additional incremental radiation doses, a second dose-response curve is generated that has precisely the same shape as the first.

After such a split occurs, the extrapolation number is the same, the mean lethal dose is the same, and the second dose-response curve is separated along the dose axis from the first dose-response curve by D_Q. For full recovery to occur, the time between such split doses must be at least as long as the cell generation time, usually 24 hours.

Such experiments show that cells that survive an initial radiation insult exhibit precisely the same characteristics as nonirradiated cells; therefore the surviving cells have fully recovered from the sublethal damage produced by the initial irradiation.

> D_Q is a measure of the capacity to accumulate sublethal damage and the ability to recover from sublethal damage.

Question: From Fig. 34.10, estimate the overall surviving fraction for a cell receiving a split dose of 4 Gy_t followed by 4 Gy_t.

Answer: At a dose of 4 Gy_t, approximately 0.15 of the cells survive. Therefore at a split dose of 4 Gy_t and 4 Gy_t, the surviving fraction should equal $0.15 \times 0.15 = 0.023$.

The total dose is 8 Gy_t, and the surviving fraction on the split-dose curve at 8 Gy_t should equal 0.023—and it does. If the 8 Gy_t had been delivered at one time, the surviving fraction would have been 0.012, as is shown by the single-dose curve of Fig. 34.10.

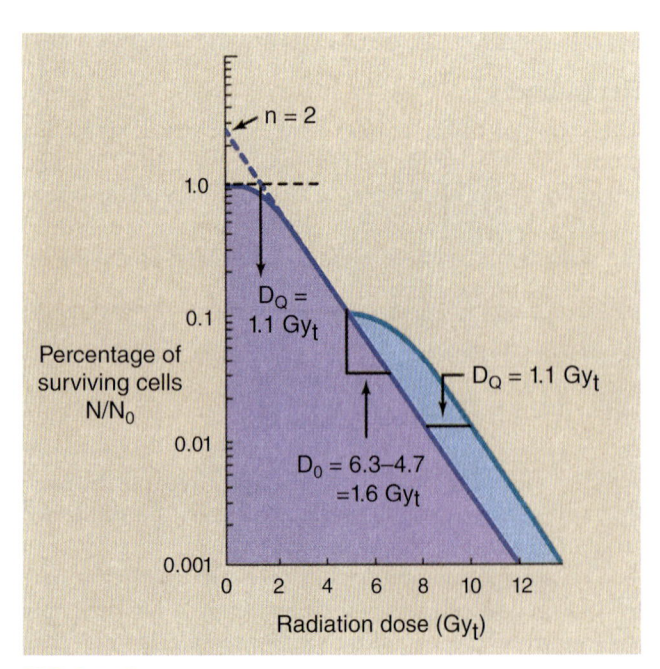

FIG. 34.10 Split-dose irradiation results in a second cell survival curve with the same characteristics as the first and displaced along the dose axis by D_Q.

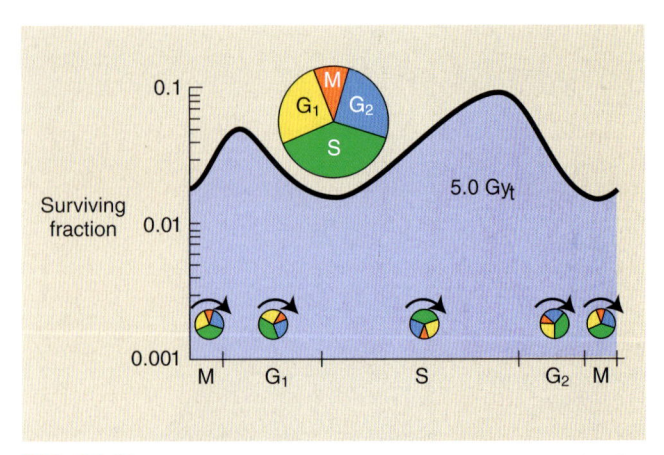

FIG. 34.11 The age response of human fibroblasts after irradiation shows minimum survival during the M phase and maximum survival during the late S phase. Such cells are most radiosensitive during mitosis and most radioresistant during the late S phase.

CELL-CYCLE EFFECTS

When human cells replicate by mitosis, the average time from one mitosis to another is called the **cell-cycle time**. Most human cells that are in a state of normal proliferation have cell-cycle times of approximately 24 hours.

Some specialized cells have cell-cycle times that extend to hundreds of hours, and other cells, such as neurons (nerve cells), do not normally replicate. Longer cell-cycle times primarily result from the lengthening of the G_1 phase of the cell cycle.

> G_1 is the most time variable of cell phases.

A randomly growing population of cells that are uniformly distributed in position throughout the cell cycle can be **synchronized** in various ways. A population of synchronized cells then can be subdivided into smaller populations and irradiated sequentially as they pass through the phases of the cell cycle.

Fig. 34.11 represents results obtained from human fibroblasts. The fraction of cells that survive a given dose can vary by a factor of 10 from the most sensitive to the most resistant phase of the cell cycle.

> Human cells are most radiosensitive in M and most radioresistant in late S.

This pattern of change in radiosensitivity as a function of phase in the cell cycle is the **age-response function**, and it varies among cells. Cells in mitosis are always most sensitive. The fraction of surviving cells is lowest in this phase. The next most sensitive phase of the cell cycle occurs at the G_1-S transition. The most resistant portion of the cell cycle is the late S phase.

RADIATION EFFECT MODIFICATION

Mammalian cell survival experiments have been used extensively to measure the effects of various types of radiation and to determine the magnitude of various dose-modifying factors, such as oxygen. Because the mean lethal dose, D_0, is related to radiosensitivity, the ratio of D_0 for one condition of irradiation compared with another is a measure of the effectiveness of the dose modifier, whether it is physical or biological.

If the same cell type is irradiated by two different radiations under identical conditions, results may appear as shown in Fig. 34.12. At a very high LET (as with alpha particles and neutrons), cell-survival kinetics follow the single-target, single-hit model. With low-LET radiation (x-rays), the multitarget, single-hit model applies.

> Irradiation of mammalian cells with high-LET radiation follows the single-target, single-hit model.

The mean lethal dose after low-LET irradiation is always greater than that after high-LET irradiation. If the low-LET D_0 represents x-rays, then the ratio of one D_0 to another equals the relative biologic effectiveness (RBE) for the high-LET radiation as follows:

> **RELATIVE BIOLOGIC EFFECTIVENESS**
>
> $$\text{RBE} = \frac{D_0 \text{ (x-radiation) to produce an effect}}{D_0 \text{ (test radiation) to produce the same effect}}$$

Question: Fig. 34.12 shows the radiation dose-response relationship of human fibroblasts exposed to x-rays and those exposed to 14 MeV neutrons. The D_0 after x-radiation is 1.7 Gy_t, and the D_0 for neutron irradiation is 1 Gy_t. What is the RBE of 14 MeV neutrons relative to x-rays?

Answer:
$$\text{RBE} = \frac{1.7 \text{ Gy}_t}{1.00 \text{ Gy}_t} = 1.7$$

The most completely studied dose modifier is oxygen. The presence of oxygen maximizes the effect of low-LET radiation. When anoxic cells are exposed, a considerably higher dose is required to produce a given effect.

With high-LET radiation, little difference is noted between the response of oxygenated cells and that of anoxic cells. Fig. 34.13 shows typical cell-survival curves for each of these combinations of LET and oxygen. The value of D_0 for each condition is shown in Table 34.2.

Such experiments are designed to measure the magnitude of the oxygen effect. The OER determined from single-cell survival experiments is illustrated as follows:

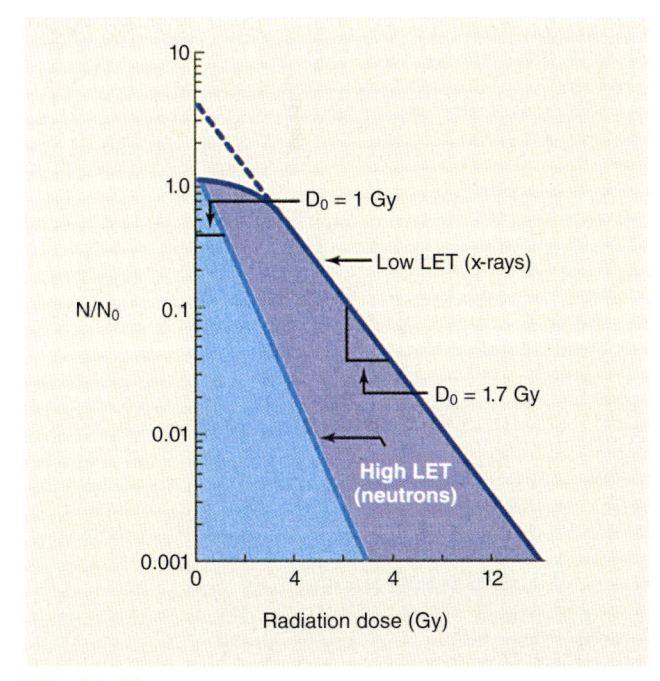

FIG. 34.12 Representative cell-survival curves after exposure to 200-kVp x-rays and 14-MeV neutrons.

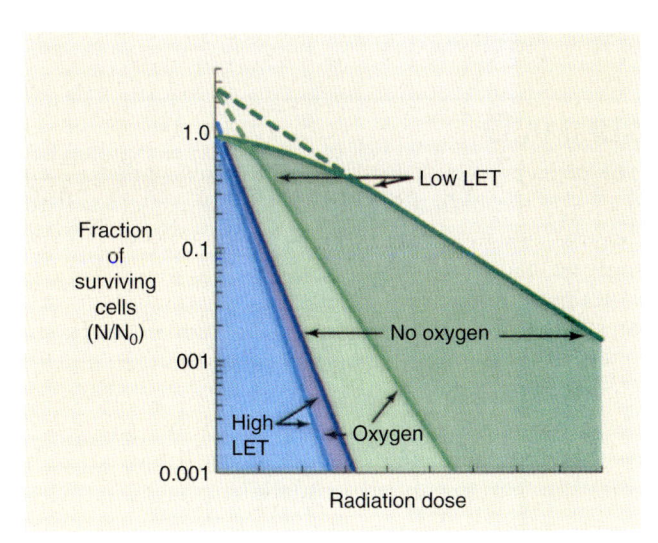

FIG. 34.13 Cell-survival curves for human cells irradiated in the presence and the absence of oxygen with high- and low-linear energy transfer (*LET*) radiation.

TABLE 34.2	Mean Lethal Dose for the Cell Irradiations as Shown in Fig. 34.13	
D_0	**Aerobic**	**Anaerobic**
Low LET	1.4	3.4
High LET	0.7	0.9

LET, Linear energy transfer.

OXYGEN ENHANCEMENT RATIO

$$\text{OER} = \frac{D_0 \text{ (anoxic) to produce an effect}}{D_0 \text{ (oxygenated) to produce the same effect}}$$

Question: With reference to Fig. 34.13, what is the estimated OER for human cells exposed to low-LET radiation and to high-LET radiation?

Answer: Low LET, no oxygen $D_0 = 3.40$ Gy_t

Low LET, oxygen $D_0 = 1.40$ Gy_t

$$\text{OER} = \frac{3.40 \text{ Gy}_t}{1.40 \text{ Gy}_t} = 2.4$$

High LET, no oxygen $D_0 = 0.90$ Gy_t

High LET, oxygen $D_0 = 0.70$ Gy_t

$$\text{OER} = \frac{0.90 \text{ Gy}_t}{0.70 \text{ Gy}_t} = 1.3$$

The interrelationships among LET, RBE, and OER are complex. However, LET determines the magnitude of RBE and OER.

SUMMARY

The concept of a sensitive key molecule within a cell serves as the basis for the target theory. For a cell to die after radiation exposure, the target molecule, DNA, must be inactivated.

Radiation exposure results in two models of cell survival. The single-target, single-hit model applies to simple cells such as bacteria. The multitarget, single-hit model implies a dose threshold. However, at higher doses, the relationship becomes a single-hit, single-target model. Experiments in cell recovery show that cells can recover from sublethal radiation damage.

CHALLENGE QUESTIONS

1. Define or otherwise identify the following:
   a. In vitro
   b. Cytogenetic damage
   c. Oxygen enhancement ratio
   d. High-LET radiation
   e. Target theory
   f. D_{37}
   g. Mean lethal dose
   h. Radiation hit
   i. Target number
   j. D_Q
2. What type of interaction with tissue results in a hit?
3. What are the phases of the cell cycle?
4. If x-rays interacted uniformly and $D_0 = 1$ Gy_t, how many cells would survive 1 Gy_t?
5. Why do radiobiologists synchronize human cells?
6. Instead of cell survival, why do we not measure cell death?
7. What are the three numerical parameters attendant to multitarget, single-hit kinetics?
8. What single-cell survival parameter best represents the number of targets in a cell?
9. Describe the relationship between RBE and OER.
10. What happens to radiation-induced free radicals within the cell?
11. What is the target theory of radiobiology?
12. Does radiation interact with tissue uniformly or randomly?
13. Draw cell-survival curves to show the difference between irradiation with low-LET and high-LET radiation.
14. What is the difference between in vitro and in vivo?
15. Which single-cell survival parameter best represents a cell's ability to recover from sublethal damage?
16. The D_{37} of a cellular species that follows the single-target, single-hit model is 1.5 Gy_t. What percentage of cells will survive 4.5 Gy_t?
17. What is the RBE of alpha radiation if the D_0 is 400 mGy_t compared with 1.8 Gy_t for x-rays?
18. What is the difference between direct effect and indirect effect?
19. How does the radiosensitivity of human cells vary with stages of the cell cycle?
20. Draw cell-survival curves to show the difference between low-LET irradiation of aerobic cells and anoxic cells.

The answers to the Challenge Questions can be found by logging on to our website at http://evolve.elsevier.com.

Deterministic Effects of Radiation

CHAPTER 35

OBJECTIVES

At the completion of this chapter, the student should be able to do the following:

1. Describe the three acute radiation syndromes.
2. Identify the two stages that lead to acute radiation lethality.
3. Define $LD_{50/60}$.
4. Discuss local tissue damage after high-dose irradiation.
5. Review the cytogenetic effects of radiation exposure.
6. Describe the three features of a deterministic radiation effect.

OUTLINE

Acute Radiation Lethality 466
   Prodromal Period 467
   Latent Period 467
   Manifest Illness 467
   $LD_{50/60}$ 468
   Mean Survival Time 469
Local Tissue Damage 470
   Effects on the Skin 470
   Effects on the Gonads 471
   Effects on the Eyes 473
Hematologic Effects 474
   Hemopoietic System 474
   Hemopoietic Cell Survival 475

Cytogenetic Effects 475
   Normal Karyotype 477
   Single-Hit Chromosome
      Aberrations 477
   Multihit Chromosome
      Aberrations 478
   Kinetics of Chromosome
      Aberrations 478
The Human Genome 479
   Summary 479
Challenge Questions 480

DURING THE 1920s and the 1930s, it would not have been unusual for a radiologist or radiographer to visit the hematology laboratory once a week for a routine blood examination. Before the introduction of personnel radiation monitors, periodic blood examination was the only way to monitor x-ray workers for occupational radiation exposure.

Today's occupational radiation exposures are quite low. Unfortunately patient radiation dose remains high, including doses high enough to cause injury. That is why the radiologist and radiographer must understand the deterministic effects of high radiation doses.

This chapter explores such deterministic effects from the most severe (death) to the most worrisome today (skin burns). The chapter also reviews hematologic and cytogenetic effects.

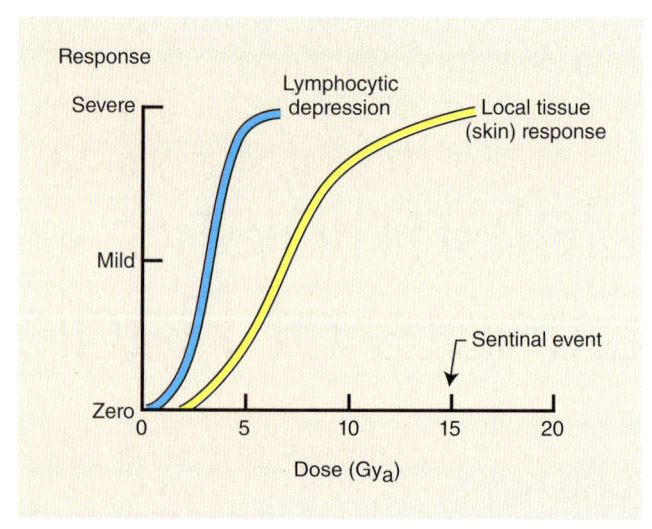

FIG. 35.1 The dose-response curve for deterministic effects is threshold, nonlinear. The two shown here could possibly result from medical imaging.

TABLE 35.1 Principal Deterministic Effects of Radiation Exposure on Humans and the Approximate Threshold Dose

Effect	Anatomic Site	Threshold Dose
Death	Whole body	2 Gy_t
Hematologic depression	Whole body	250 mGy_t
Skin erythema	Small field	2 Gy_t
Epilation	Small field	3 Gy_t
Chromosome aberration	Whole body	50 mGy_t
Gonadal dysfunction	Local tissue	100 mGy_t

To produce a radiation response in humans within a few days to months, the dose must be substantial. Such a response is called an **early effect** of radiation exposure. A dose of this magnitude is rare in diagnostic radiology.

Deterministic radiation effects are those that exhibit increasing severity with increasing radiation dose. Furthermore, there is a dose threshold, and the dose-response relationship is nonlinear (Fig. 35.1).

These early effects have been studied extensively with laboratory animals, and some data have been obtained from observations of humans. This chapter considers only the more important effects as identified in Table 35.1, along with the minimum radiation dose necessary to produce each.

ACUTE RADIATION LETHALITY

Death, of course, is the most devastating human response to radiation exposure. No cases of death after diagnostic x-ray exposure have ever been recorded, although some early x-ray pioneers died from the stochastic effects of x-ray exposure. In each of these cases, however, the total radiation dose was extremely high by today's standards.

Acute radiation-induced human lethality is of only academic interest in diagnostic radiology. Diagnostic x-ray beams are neither intense enough nor large enough to cause death.

> Diagnostic x-ray beams always result in partial-body exposure, which is less harmful than whole-body exposure.

Some accidental exposures of persons in the nuclear weapons and nuclear energy fields have resulted in immediate death, but the number of such accidents has been small, considering the length and activity of the atomic age. The unfortunate incidents at the SL-1 in January 1961, at Chernobyl in April 1986 and at Fukushima in March 2011 are notable exceptions.

Thirty people at Chernobyl experienced acute radiation syndrome and died. A number of minor late effects have been observed. No one died or was even seriously exposed in the March 1979 incident at the nuclear power reactor at Three Mile Island, Pennsylvania.

No acute lethality was observed at the tsunami-induced meltdown of three nuclear reactors at Fukushima, Japan. However, the dispersal of TBq (terabecquerel) quantities of radioactive material to the environment caused the evacuation of more than 150,000 neighboring residents.

CHAPTER 35 Deterministic Effects of Radiation 467

> Employment in the nuclear power industry is a safe occupation.

The sequence of events that follow high-level radiation exposure, leading to death within days or weeks is called the **acute radiation syndrome**. There are, in fact, three separate syndromes that are dose related and that follow a rather distinct course of clinical responses.

These syndromes are **hematologic death, gastrointestinal (GI) death,** and **central nervous system (CNS) death**. The clinical signs and symptoms of each are outlined in Table 35.2. CNS death requires radiation doses in excess of 50 Gy_t and results in death within hours. Hematologic death and GI death follow lower exposures and require a longer time for death to occur.

In addition to the three lethal syndromes, two periods are associated with acute radiation lethality. The **prodromal period** consists of acute clinical symptoms that occur within hours of exposure and continue for up to a day or two. After the prodromal period has ended, there may be a **latent period**, during which the subject is free of visible effects.

Prodromal Period

At radiation doses above approximately 1 Gy_t delivered to the total body, signs and symptoms of radiation sickness may appear within minutes to hours. The symptoms of early radiation sickness most often take the form of nausea, vomiting, diarrhea, and a reduction in the white blood cells of the peripheral blood (leukopenia).

> The immediate response of radiation sickness is the prodromal period.

The prodromal period may last from a few hours to a couple of days. The severity of the symptoms is dose related; at doses in excess of 10 Gy_t, symptoms can be violent. At still higher doses, the duration of the prodromal syndrome becomes shorter until it is difficult to separate the prodromal syndrome from the period of manifest illness.

Latent Period

After the prodromal period, the period of initial radiation sickness, a period of apparent well-being occurs, which is called the **latent period**. The latent period extends from hours or less (at doses in excess of 50 Gy_t) to weeks (at doses from 1–5 Gy_t).

> The latent period is the time after radiation exposure during which there is no sign of radiation sickness.

The latent period is sometimes mistakenly thought to indicate an early recovery from a moderate radiation dose. It may be misleading, however, because it gives no indication of the extensive radiation effect yet to follow.

Manifest Illness

The dose necessary to produce a given syndrome and the mean survival time are the principal quantitative measures of human radiation lethality (see Table 35.2). Although ranges of dose and resultant mean survival times are given, there is rarely a precise difference in the dose and time-related sequence of events associated with each syndrome. At very high radiation doses, the latent period disappears altogether. At very low radiation doses, there may be no prodromal period at all.

Radiation doses in the range of approximately 2 to 10 Gy_t produce the **hematologic syndrome**. The patient initially experiences mild symptoms of the prodromal syndrome, which appear in a matter of a few hours and may persist for several days.

The latent period that follows can extend as long as 4 weeks and is characterized by a general feeling of

TABLE 35.2 Summary of Acute Radiation Lethality

Period	Approximate Dose (Gy_t)	Mean Survival Time (Days)	Clinical Signs and Symptoms
Prodromal	>1	—	Nausea, vomiting, diarrhea
Latent	1–100	—	None
Hematologic	2–10	10–60	Nausea, vomiting, diarrhea, anemia, leukopenia, hemorrhage, fever, infection
Gastrointestinal	10–50	4–10	Same as hematologic plus electrolyte imbalance, lethargy, fatigue, shock
Central nervous system	>50	0–3	Same as gastrointestinal plus ataxia, edema, system vasculitis, meningitis

wellness. There are no obvious signs of illness, although the number of cells in the peripheral blood declines during this time.

> The hematologic syndrome is characterized by a reduction in white blood cells, red blood cells, and platelets.

The period of **manifest illness** is characterized by possible vomiting, mild diarrhea, malaise, lethargy, and fever. Each of the types of blood cells follows a rather characteristic pattern of cell depletion. If the dose is not lethal, recovery begins in 2 to 4 weeks, but as long as 6 months may be required for full recovery.

If the radiation injury is severe enough, the reduction in blood cells continues unchecked until the body's defense against infection is nil. Just before death, hemorrhage and dehydration may be pronounced. Death occurs because of generalized infection, electrolyte imbalance, and dehydration.

Radiation doses of approximately 10 to 50 Gy_t result in the **gastrointestinal (GI) syndrome**. The prodromal symptoms of vomiting and diarrhea occur within hours of exposure and persist for hours to as long as a day. A latent period of 3 to 5 days follows, during which no symptoms are present.

The manifest illness period begins with a second wave of nausea and vomiting, followed by diarrhea. The victim experiences a loss of appetite and may become lethargic. The diarrhea persists and becomes more severe, leading to loose and then watery and bloody stools. Supportive therapy cannot prevent the rapid progression of symptoms that ultimately leads to death within 4 to 10 days of exposure.

> GI death occurs principally because of severe damage to the cells lining the intestines.

Intestinal cells are normally in a rapid state of proliferation and are continuously being replaced by new cells. The turnover time for this cell renewal system is normally 3 to 5 days.

Radiation exposure kills the most sensitive cells—stem cells. This controls the length of time until death. When the intestinal lining is completely denuded of functional cells, fluids pass uncontrollably across the intestinal membrane, electrolyte balance is destroyed, and conditions promote infection.

At doses consistent with the GI syndrome, measurable and even severe hematologic changes occur. It takes a longer time for the cell renewal system of the blood to develop mature cells from the stem cell population; therefore there is not enough time for maximum hematologic effects to occur.

After a radiation dose in excess of approximately 50 Gy_t or higher is received, a series of signs and symptoms occur that lead to death within a matter of hours to days. This is the **central nervous system (CNS) syndrome**.

First, severe nausea and vomiting begin, usually within a few minutes of exposure. During this initial onset, the patient may become extremely nervous and confused, may describe a burning sensation in the skin, may lose vision, and can even lose consciousness within the first hour. This may be followed by a latent period that lasts up to 12 hours, during which earlier symptoms subside or disappear.

The latent period is followed by the period of manifest illness, during which symptoms of the prodromal stage return but are more severe. The person becomes disoriented; loses muscle coordination; has difficulty breathing; may go into convulsive seizures; experiences loss of equilibrium, ataxia, and lethargy; lapses into a coma; and dies.

Regardless of the medical attention given to the patient, the symptoms of manifest illness appear rather suddenly and always with extreme severity. At radiation doses high enough to produce CNS effects, the outcome is always death within a few days of exposure.

> The ultimate cause of death in CNS syndrome is the elevated fluid content of the brain.

The CNS syndrome is characterized by increased intracranial pressure, inflammatory changes in the blood vessels of the brain (vasculitis), and inflammation of the meninges (meningitis). At doses sufficient to produce CNS damage, damage to all other organs of the body is equally severe. The classic radiation-induced changes in the GI tract and the hematologic system cannot occur because there is insufficient time between exposure and death for them to appear.

LD$_{50/60}$

If experimental animals are irradiated with varying doses of radiation from 1 to 10 Gy_t, the plot of the percentage that dies as a function of radiation dose would appear as shown in Fig. 35.2. This figure illustrates the radiation dose-response relationship for acute human lethality.

> The LD$_{50/60}$ is the whole-body radiation dose that causes 50% of irradiated subjects to die within 60 days.

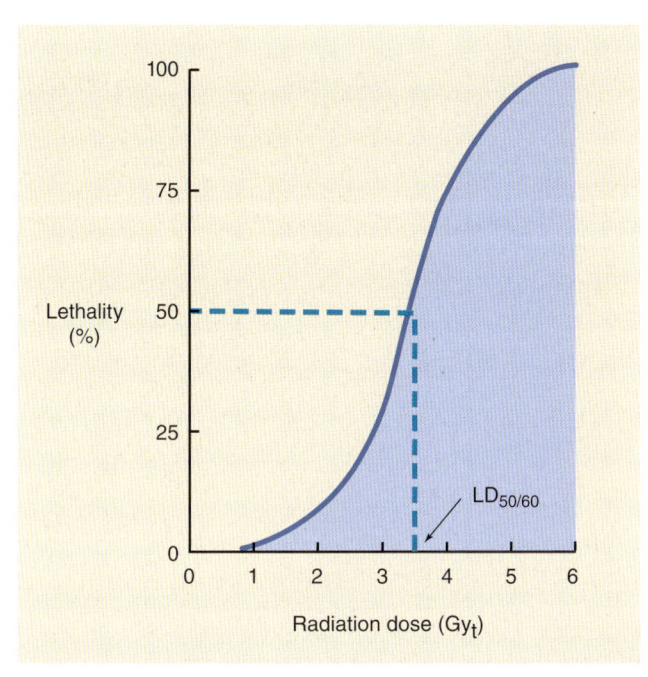

CHAPTER 35 Deterministic Effects of Radiation   469

FIG. 35.2 Radiation-induced death in humans follows a nonlinear, threshold dose-response relationship.

TABLE 35.3	Approximate LD$_{50/60}$ for Various Species After Whole-Body Radiation Exposure
Species	**LD$_{50/60}$ (Gy$_t$)**
Pig	2.5
Dog	2.8
Human	3.5
Guinea pig	4.3
Monkey	4.8
Opossum	5.1
Mouse	6.2
Goldfish	7.0
Hamster	7.0
Rat	7.1
Rabbit	7.3
Gerbil	10.5
Turtle	15
Armadillo	20
Newt	30
Cockroach	100

LD$_{50/60}$, Dose of radiation to the whole body that causes 50% of irradiated subjects to die within 60 days.

At the lower dose of approximately 1 Gy$_t$, no one is expected to die. Above approximately 6 Gy$_t$, all those irradiated die unless vigorous medical support is available. Above 10 Gy$_t$, even vigorous medical support does not prevent death.

> Acute radiation lethality follows a nonlinear, threshold dose-response relationship.

If death is to occur, it usually happens within 60 days of exposure. Acute radiation lethality is measured quantitatively by the LD$_{50/60}$, which is approximately 3.5 Gy$_t$ for humans. With clinical support, humans can tolerate much higher doses; the maximum is reported to be 8.5 Gy$_t$. Table 35.3 lists the values of LD$_{50/60}$ for various species.

Question: From Fig. 35.2, estimate the radiation dose that will produce 25% lethality in humans within 60 days.

Answer: First, draw a horizontal line from the 25% level on the y-axis until it intersects the S curve. Now, drop a vertical line from this point to the x-axis. This intersection with the x-axis occurs at LD$_{25/60}$, which is approximately 2.5 Gy$_t$.

Mean Survival Time

As the whole-body radiation dose increases, the average time between exposure and death decreases. This time is

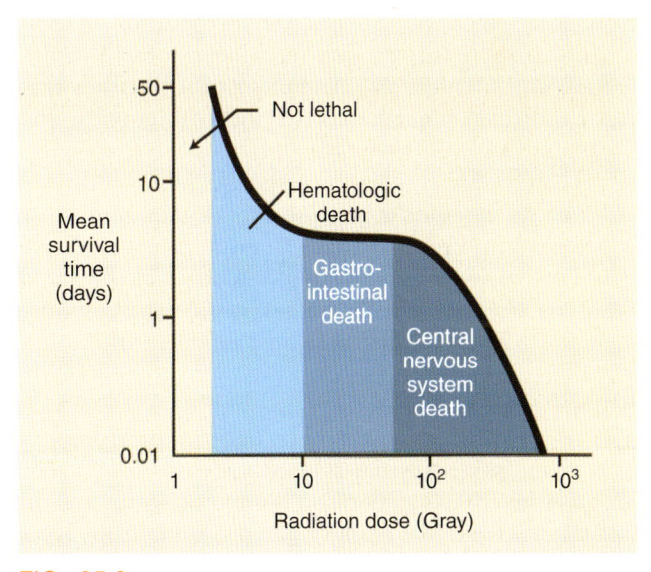

FIG. 35.3 Mean survival time after radiation exposure shows three distinct regions. If death is attributable to hematologic or central nervous system effects, the mean survival time will vary with dose. If gastrointestinal effects cause death, it occurs in approximately 4 days.

known as the **mean survival time**. A graph of radiation dose versus mean survival time is shown in Fig. 35.3. This graph depicts three distinct regions associated with the three radiation syndromes.

As the radiation dose increases from 2 to 10 Gy_t, the mean survival time decreases from approximately 60 to 4 days; this region is consistent with death resulting from the hematologic syndrome. Mean survival time is dose dependent with the hematologic syndrome.

In the dose range associated with GI syndrome, however, the mean survival time remains relatively constant at 4 days. With larger doses, those associated with CNS syndrome, the mean survival time is again dose dependent, varying from approximately 3 days to a matter of hours.

LOCAL TISSUE DAMAGE

When only part of the body is irradiated, in contrast to whole-body irradiation, a higher dose is required to produce a response. Every organ and tissue of the body can be affected by partial-body irradiation. The effect is cell death, which results in shrinkage of the organ or tissue. This effect can lead to a total lack of function for that organ or tissue, or it can be followed by recovery.

> Atrophy is the shrinkage of an organ or tissue caused by cell death.

There are many examples of local tissue damage immediately after radiation exposure. In fact, if the dose is high enough, any local tissue will respond. The manner in which local tissues respond depends on their intrinsic radiosensitivity and the kinetics of cell proliferation and maturation. Examples of local tissues that can be affected immediately are the skin, gonads, and bone marrow.

All deterministic radiation responses follow a **threshold-type** dose-response relationship. A minimum dose is necessary to produce a deterministic response. Local tissue damage is a good example. When that threshold dose has been exceeded, the **severity** of the response increases with increasing dose, in a nonlinear fashion.

Effects on the Skin

The tissue with which we have had the most experience is the skin. Normal skin consists of three layers: an outer layer (the epidermis), an intermediate layer of connective tissue (the dermis), and a subcutaneous layer of fat and connective tissue.

The skin has additional accessory structures, such as hair follicles, sweat glands, and sensory receptors (Fig. 35.4). All cell layers and accessory structures participate in the response to radiation exposure.

The skin, similar to the lining of the intestine, represents a continuing cell renewal system, only with a much slower rate than that experienced by intestinal cells. Almost 50% of the cells lining the intestine are replaced every day, but skin cells are replaced at a rate of only approximately 2% per day.

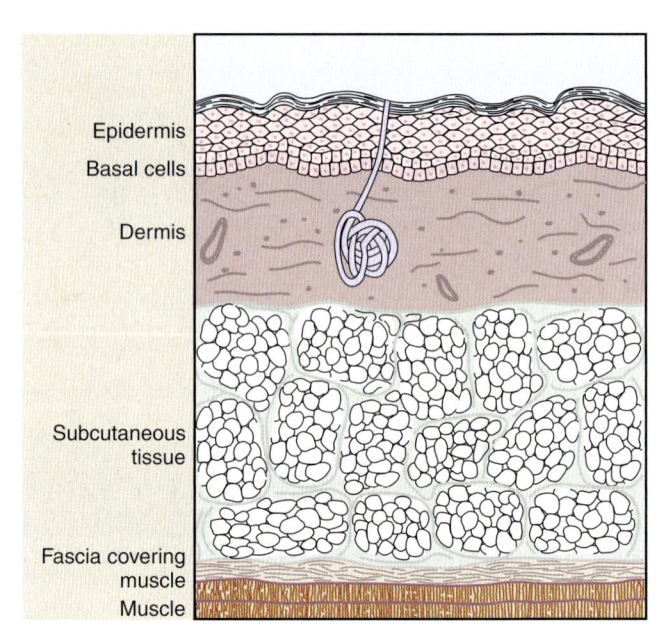

FIG. 35.4 A cross-sectional view of the anatomic structures of the skin. The basal cell layer is most radiosensitive.

The outer skin layer, the epidermis, consists of several layers of cells; the lowest layer consists of **basal cells**. Basal cells are the **stem cells** that mature as they migrate to the surface of the epidermis. When these cells arrive at the surface as mature cells, they are slowly lost and need to be replaced by new cells from the basal layer.

> Damage to basal cells results in the earliest manifestation of radiation injury to the skin.

In earlier times, the tolerance of the patient's skin determined the limitations of radiation oncology with orthovoltage x-rays (200–300 kVp x-rays). The object of x-ray therapy was to deposit energy in the tumor while sparing the surrounding normal tissue. Because the x-rays had to pass through the skin to reach the tumor, the skin was necessarily subjected to higher radiation doses than the tumor.

The resultant skin damage was seen as **erythema** (a sunburn-like reddening of the skin) followed by **desquamation** (ulceration and denudation of the skin), which often required interruption of treatment.

After a single dose of 3 to 10 Gy_t, an initial mild erythema may occur within the first or second day. This first wave of erythema then subsides, only to be followed by a second wave that reaches maximum intensity in about 2 weeks.

At higher doses, this second wave of erythema is followed by a moist desquamation, which in turn may lead to a dry desquamation. Moist desquamation is known as **clinical tolerance** for radiation oncology.

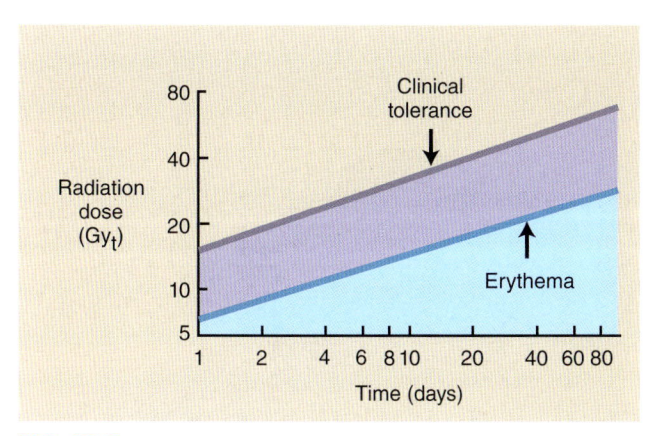

FIG. 35.5 These isoeffect curves show the relationship between the number of daily fractions and the total radiation dose that will produce erythema or moist desquamation. As the fractionation of the dose increases, so does the total dose required.

TABLE 35.4	Potential Radiation Responses of Skin from High-Dose Fluoroscopy		
Potential Radiation Response	**Threshold Dose (Gy$_t$)**	**Approximate Time of Onset**	
Early transient erythema	2	Hours	
Main erythema	6	10 days	
Temporary epilation	3	3 weeks	
Permanent epilation	7	3 weeks	
Moist desquamation	15	4 weeks	

During radiation oncology, the skin is exposed according to a fractionated scheme, usually approximately 2 Gy$_t$/day, 5 days a week. To assist the radiation oncologist in planning patient treatment, isoeffect curves have been generated that accurately project the dose necessary to produce skin erythema or clinical tolerance after a prescribed treatment routine (Fig. 35.5). Contemporary radiation oncology uses high-energy x-radiation from linear accelerators or protons from cyclotrons. Both protect the skin from radiation damage.

Erythema was perhaps the first observed biologic response to radiation exposure. Many of the early x-ray pioneers, including Roentgen, sustained skin burns induced by x-rays.

One of the hazards to the patient during the early years of radiology was also x-ray–induced erythema. During those years, x-ray tube potentials were so low that it was usually necessary to position the tube very close to the patient's skin; exposures of 10 to 30 minutes were required. Often the patient would return several days later with an x-ray burn.

These skin effects follow a nonlinear, threshold dose-response relationship similar to that described for radiation-induced lethality. Small doses of x-radiation do not cause erythema. Extremely high doses of x-radiation cause erythema in all people so irradiated.

Whether intermediate radiation doses produce erythema depends on the individual's radiosensitivity, the dose rate, and the size of the irradiated skin field. Analysis of persons irradiated therapeutically with superficial x-rays has shown that the skin erythema dose required to affect 50% of those irradiated is about 5 Gy$_t$.

Before the Roentgen was defined and accurate radiation-measuring apparatus was developed, the skin was observed, and its response to radiation was used in formulating radiation protection practices. The unit used was the SED$_{50}$ (skin erythema dose) and permissible occupational radiation exposures were specified in fractions of SED$_{50}$.

Another response of the skin to radiation exposure is epilation, or loss of hair. For many years, soft x-rays (10–20 kVp), called **Grenz rays**, were used as the treatment of choice for persons with skin diseases, such as ringworm (tinea capitis).

Tinea capitis of the scalp, which is common in children, was successfully treated by Grenz radiation; unfortunately, the patient's hair would fall out for weeks or even months. Sometimes an unnecessarily high dose of Grenz rays results in permanent epilation.

High-dose fluoroscopy has focused more attention on the response of the skin to x-rays. The longer fluoroscopy times required for cardiovascular and interventional procedures, coupled with allowed exposure rates twice the previous normal, are of great concern. Injuries to patients have been reported, and steps are being taken to establish better control over such exposures. Table 35.4 summarizes the potential effects of high-dose fluoroscopy.

Effects on the Gonads

Human gonads are critically important target organs. As an example of local tissue effects, they are particularly sensitive to radiation. Responses to doses as low as 100 mGy$_t$ have been observed. Because these organs produce the germ cells that control fertility and heredity, their response to radiation has been studied extensively.

Much of what is known about the types of radiation response and dose-response relationships has been derived from numerous animal experiments. Significant data are also available from human populations. Radiotherapy patients, radiation accident victims, and volunteer convicts all have provided data; this has resulted in a rather complete description of the gonadal response to radiation.

The cells of the testes (the male gonads) and the ovaries (the female gonads) respond differently to radiation because of differences in progression from the stem cell to the mature cell. Fig. 35.6 illustrates this

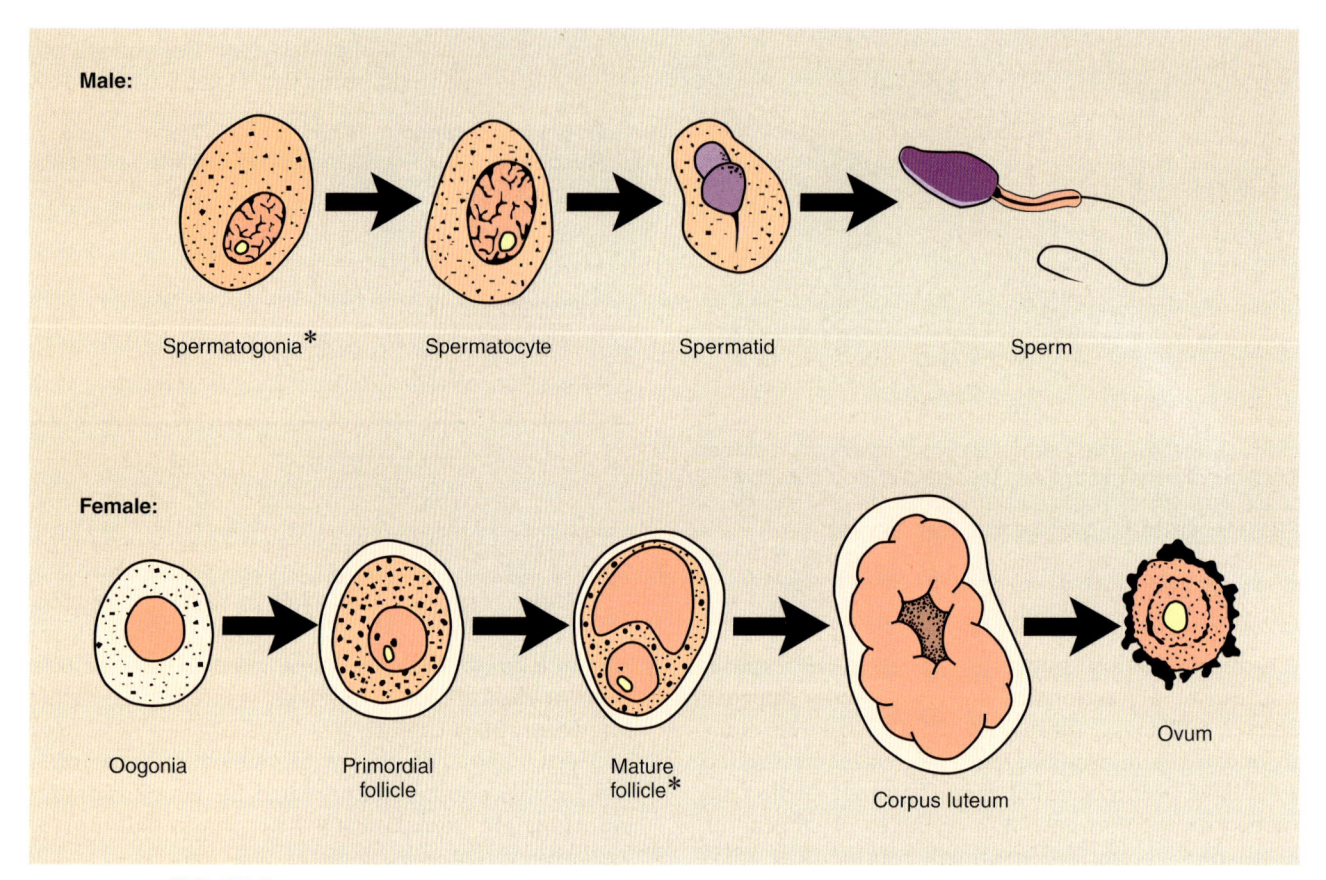

FIG. 35.6 Progression of germ cells from the stem cell phase to the mature cell. Asterisks indicate the most radiosensitive cells.

progression, indicating the most radiosensitive phase of cell maturation.

> Ovaries and testes produce oogonia and spermatogonia, which mature into ovum and sperm, respectively.

Germ cells are produced by both ovaries and testes, but they develop from the stem cell phase to the mature cell phase at different rates and at different times. This process of development is called **gametogenesis**.

The stem cells of the ovaries are the **oogonia**, and they multiply in number only before birth during fetal life. The oogonia reach a maximum number of several million and then begin to decline because of spontaneous degeneration.

During late fetal life, many **primordial follicles** grow to encapsulate the oogonia, which become **oocytes**. These follicle-containing oocytes remain in a suspended state of growth until puberty. By the time of prepuberty, the number of oocytes has been reduced to only several hundred thousand.

Commencing at puberty, the follicles rupture with regularity, ejecting a mature germ cell, the **ovum**. Only 400 to 500 such ova are available for fertilization (number of years of menstruation times 13 per year).

The germ cells of the testes are continually being produced from stem cells progressively through a number of stages to maturity, and similar to the ovaries, the testes provide a sustaining cell renewal system.

The male stem cell is the **spermatogonia**, which matures into the **spermatocyte**. The spermatocyte in turn multiplies and develops into a **spermatid**, which finally differentiates into the functionally mature germ cell, the **spermatozoa** or **sperm**. The maturation process from stem cells to spermatozoa requires 3 to 5 weeks.

Irradiation of the **ovaries** early in life reduces their size (atrophy) through germ cell death. After puberty, such irradiation also causes suppression and delay of menstruation.

> The most radiosensitive cell during female germ cell development is the oocyte in the mature follicle.

Radiation effects on the ovaries depend somewhat on age. At fetal life and in early childhood, the ovaries are especially radiosensitive. They decline in radiosensitivity, reaching a minimum in the age range of 20 to 30 years, and then increase continually with age.

Doses as low as 100 mGy$_t$ may delay or suppress menstruation in a mature female. A dose of approximately 2 Gy$_t$ produces temporary infertility; approximately 5 Gy$_t$ to the ovaries results in permanent sterility.

In addition to the destruction of fertility, irradiation of the ovaries of experimental animals has been shown to produce genetic mutations. Even moderate doses, such as 250 to 500 mGy$_t$, have been associated with measurable increases in genetic mutations. Evidence also indicates that oocytes that survive such a modest dose can repair some genetic damage as they mature into ova.

The **testes**, similar to the ovaries, atrophy after high doses of radiation. A large volume of data on testicular damage has been gathered from observations of volunteer convicts and patients treated for carcinoma in one testis while the other was shielded. Many investigators have recorded normal births in such patients, whose remaining functioning testis received a radiation dose up to 3 Gy$_t$.

The spermatogonial stem cells signify the most sensitive phase in the gametogenesis of the spermatozoa. After irradiation of the testes, maturing cells, spermatocytes, and spermatids are relatively radioresistant and continue to mature. Consequently, no significant reduction in spermatozoa occurs until several weeks after exposure; therefore fertility continues throughout this time, during which irradiated spermatogonia would have developed into mature spermatozoa, had they survived.

Radiation doses as low as 100 mGy$_t$ can reduce the number of spermatozoa (Table 35.5) in a manner reminiscent of the radiation response of the ovaries. With increasing dose, the depletion of spermatozoa increases and extends over a longer period.

Two gray produces temporary infertility, which commences approximately 2 months after irradiation and persists for up to 12 months. Five gray to the testes produces permanent sterility. Even after doses sufficient to produce permanent sterility, the male patient normally retains his ability to engage in sexual intercourse.

TABLE 35.5	Response of Ovaries and Testes to Radiation
Approximate Dose (mGy$_t$)	**Response**
100	Minimal detectable response
2000	Temporary infertility
5000	Sterility

> Male gametogenesis is a self-renewing system.

After testicular irradiation of doses exceeding approximately 100 mGy$_t$, the male patient should refrain from procreation for 2 to 4 months until all cells that were in the spermatogonial and postspermatogonial stages at the time of irradiation have matured and disappeared.

This reduces but probably does not eliminate any increase in genetic mutations caused by the persistence of the stem cell. Evidence from animal experiments suggests that genetic mutations undergo some repair even when the stem cell is irradiated.

Effects on the Eyes

In 1932, Ernest O. Lawrence of the University of California developed the first cyclotron, a 12-cm-diameter device capable of accelerating charged particles to very high energies. These charged particles are used as "bullets" that are shot at the nuclei of target atoms in the study of nuclear structure. By 1940, every university physics department of any worth had built its own cyclotron and was engaged in what has become high-energy physics.

The modern cyclotron is used principally to produce radionuclides for use in nuclear medicine, especially fluorine-18 for positron emission tomography.

Interestingly, E.O. Lawrence's brother, John Lawrence, MD, was the first physician to apply radionuclides (from his brother's cyclotron) on humans. E.O. Lawrence received the 1939 Nobel Prize in Physics. His brother is considered the Father of Nuclear Medicine.

The largest particle accelerators in the world are located at Argonne National Laboratory in the Unites States and at CERN in Switzerland. These accelerators are used to discover the ultimate fine structure of matter and to describe exactly what happened at the moment of creation of the universe.

Early cyclotrons were located in one room, and a beam of high-energy particles was extracted through a tube and steered and focused by electromagnets onto the target material in an adjacent room. At that time, sophisticated equipment was not available for controlling this high-energy particle beam.

Cyclotron physicists used a tool of the radiographer, the radiographic intensifying screen, to aid them in locating the high-energy beam. Unfortunately, in doing so, these physicists received high radiation doses to the lens of their eyes because they looked directly into the beam.

In 1949, the first paper reporting cataracts in cyclotron physicists appeared. This was particularly tragic because there were few high-energy physicists.

> Radiation-induced cataracts occur on the posterior pole of the lens.

Based on these observations and on animal experimentation, several conclusions can be drawn regarding radiation-induced cataracts. The radiosensitivity of the lens of the eye is age dependent. As the age of the individual increases, the radiation effect becomes greater and the latent period becomes shorter.

Latent periods ranging from 5 to 30 years have been observed in humans, and the average latent period is approximately 15 years. High-LET radiation, such as neutron and proton radiation, has a high relative biologic effectiveness (RBE) for the production of cataracts.

> The dose-response relationship for radiation-induced cataracts is non-linear, threshold.

If the lens dose is high enough, in excess of approximately 10 Gy_t, cataracts develop in nearly 100% of those who are irradiated. The precise level of the threshold is difficult to access.

Most investigators would suggest that the threshold after an acute x-ray exposure is approximately 2 Gy_t. The threshold after fractionated exposures, such as that received in radiology, is probably in excess of 10 Gy_t. Occupational exposures to the lens of the eye are too low to require protective lens shields for the radiologists or radiographers.

> It is nearly impossible for a radiologist or radiographer to reach the threshold radiation dose for cataracts.

Radiation administered to patients who are undergoing head and neck examination by fluoroscopy or computed tomography (CT) can be significant. In CT, the lens dose can be 50 mGy_t. In either case, protective lens shields are not normally required. However, in CT, it is common to modify the examination to reduce the dose to the eyes.

HEMATOLOGIC EFFECTS

If you were a radiologist or radiographer in practice during the 1920s and 1930s, you might have visited the hematology laboratory once a week for a routine blood examination. Before the introduction of personnel radiation monitors, periodic blood examination was the only monitoring performed on x-ray and radium workers. This examination included total cell counts and a leukocyte differential count.

Most institutions had a radiation safety regulation such that if the leukocytes were depressed by more than 25% of normal level, the employee was given time off or was assigned to nonradiation activities until the count returned to normal.

> Under no circumstances is a periodic blood examination recommended as a feature of any current radiation protection program.

What was not entirely understood at that time was that the minimum whole-body dose necessary to produce a measurable hematologic depression was approximately 250 mGy_t. These workers were being heavily irradiated by today's standards.

Hemopoietic System

The hemopoietic system consists of bone marrow, circulating blood, and lymphoid tissue. Lymphoid tissues are the lymph nodes, spleen, and thymus. With this system, the principal effect of radiation is a depressed number of blood cells in the peripheral circulation. Time- and dose-related effects on the various types of circulating blood cells are determined by the normal growth and maturation of these cells.

All cells of the hemopoietic system develop from a single type of stem cell (Fig. 35.7). This stem cell is called a **pluripotential stem cell** because it can develop into several different types of mature cells.

Although the spleen and the thymus manufacture one type of leukocyte (the lymphocyte), most circulating blood cells, including lymphocytes, are manufactured in the bone marrow. In a child, the bone marrow is rather uniformly distributed throughout the skeleton. In an adult, the active bone marrow responsible for producing circulating cells is restricted to flat bones, such as the ribs, sternum, and skull, and the ends of long bones.

> From the single pluripotential stem cell, a number of cell types are produced.

The products of bone marrow stem cells are **lymphocytes** (those involved in the immune response), **granulocytes** (scavenger type of cells used to fight bacteria), **thrombocytes** (also called **platelets** and involved in the clotting of blood to prevent hemorrhage), and **erythrocytes** (red blood cells that are the transportation agents for oxygen). These cell lines develop at different rates in the bone marrow and are released to the peripheral blood as mature cells.

While in the bone marrow, the cells proliferate in number, differentiate in function, and mature. Developing granulocytes and erythrocytes spend about 8 to 10 days in the bone marrow. Thrombocytes have a lifetime of approximately 5 days in the bone marrow.

Lymphocytes are produced over varying times and have varying lifetimes in the peripheral blood. Some have lives measured in terms of hours, and others have lives measured in years. In the peripheral blood, granulocytes have a lifetime of only a couple of days.

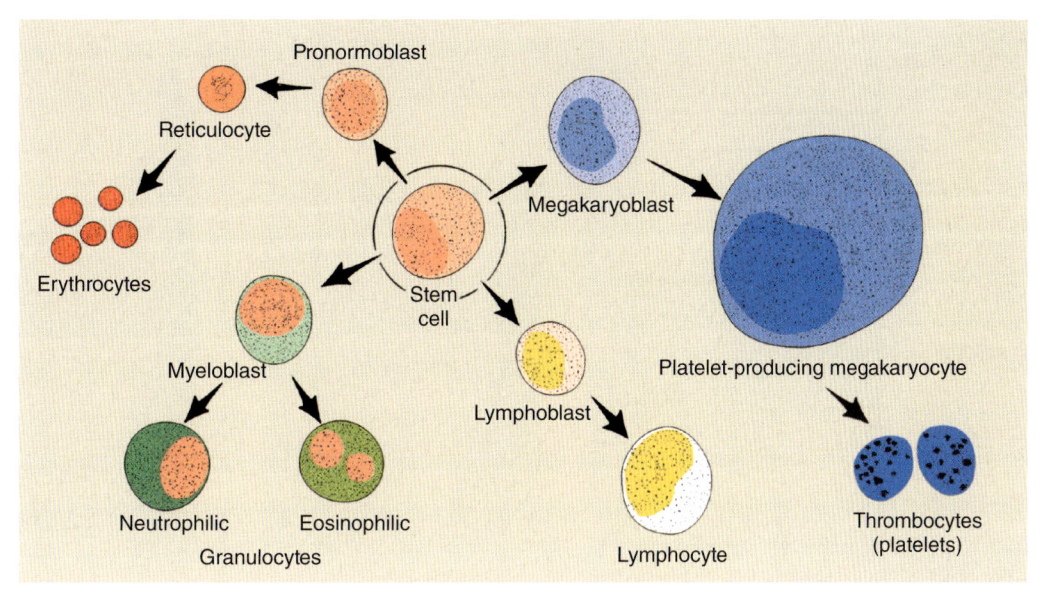

FIG. 35.7 Four principal types of blood cells—lymphocytes, granulocytes, erythrocytes, and thrombocytes—develop and mature from a single pluripotential stem cell.

Thrombocytes have a lifetime of approximately 1 week, and erythrocytes have a lifetime of nearly 4 months.

The hemopoietic system, therefore, is another example of a cell renewal system. Normal cell growth and development determine the effects of radiation on this system.

Hemopoietic Cell Survival

The principal response of the hemopoietic system to radiation exposure is a decrease in the numbers of all types of blood cells in the circulating peripheral blood. Lethal injury to the stem cells causes depletion of these mature circulating cells.

Fig. 35.8 shows the radiation response of three circulating cell types. Examples are given for low, moderate, and high radiation doses, showing that the degree of cell depletion increases with increasing dose. These figures are the results of observations on experimental animals, radiotherapy patients, and the few radiation accident victims.

After exposure, the first cells to become affected are the lymphocytes. These cells are reduced in number within minutes or hours after exposure, and they are very slow to recover. Because the response is so immediate, the radiation effect is apparently a direct one on the lymphocytes themselves rather than on the stem cells.

> The lymphocytes and the spermatogonia are the most radiosensitive cells in the body.

Granulocytes experience a rapid rise in number (granulocytosis) followed first by a rapid decrease and then a slower decrease in number (granulocytopenia). If the radiation dose is moderate, then an abortive rise in granulocyte count may occur 15 to 20 days after irradiation. Minimum granulocyte levels are reached approximately 30 days after irradiation. Recovery, if it is to occur, takes approximately 2 months.

The depletion of platelets (thrombocytopenia) after irradiation develops more slowly, again because of the longer time required for the more sensitive precursor cells to reach maturity. Thrombocytes reach a minimum in about 30 days and recover in approximately 2 months, similar to the response of granulocytes.

Erythrocytes are less sensitive than the other blood cells, apparently because of their very long lifetime in the peripheral blood. Injury to these cells is not apparent for a matter of weeks. Total recovery may take 6 months to a year.

CYTOGENETIC EFFECTS

A technique developed in the early 1950s contributed enormously to human genetic analysis and radiation genetics. The technique calls for a culture of human cells to be prepared and treated so that the chromosomes of each cell can be easily observed and studied. This has resulted in many observations on radiation-induced chromosome damage.

> Cytogenetics is the study of the genetics of cells, particularly cell chromosomes.

The photomicrograph depicted in Fig. 35.9 shows the chromosomes of a human cancer cell after radiation oncology. The many chromosome aberrations represent a high degree of damage.

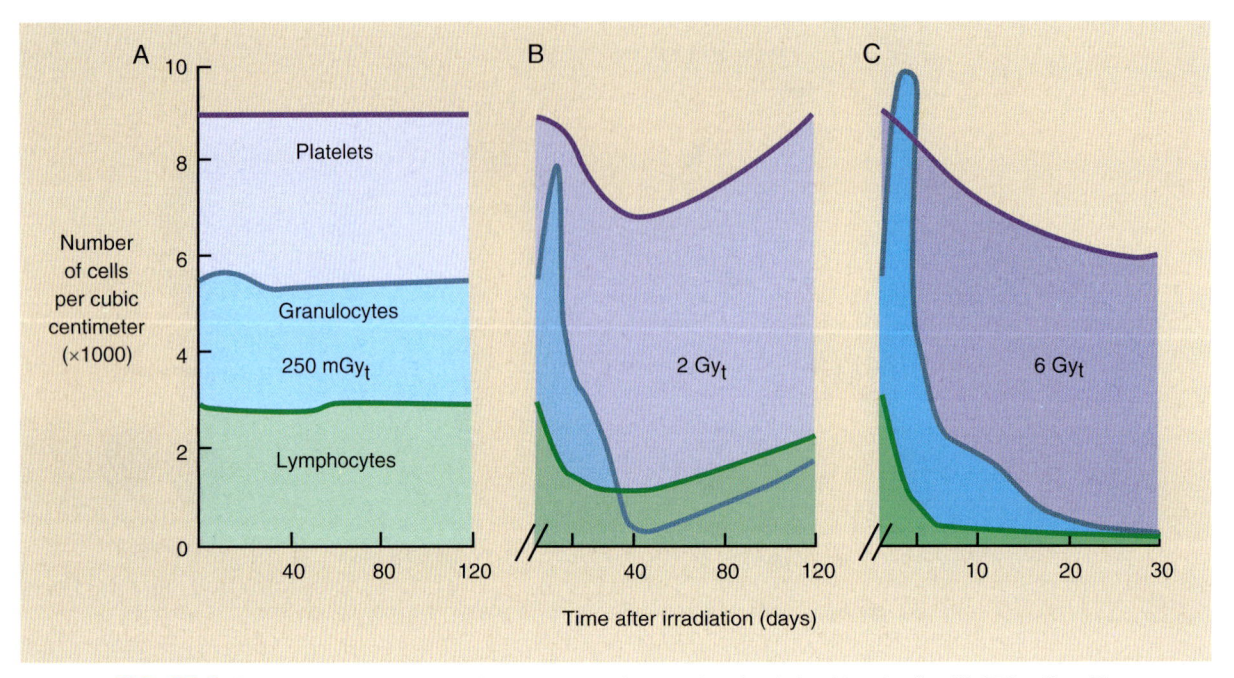

FIG. 35.8 Graphs showing the radiation response of the major circulating blood cells. (A) 250 mGy$_t$. (B) 2 Gy$_t$. (C) 6 Gy$_t$.

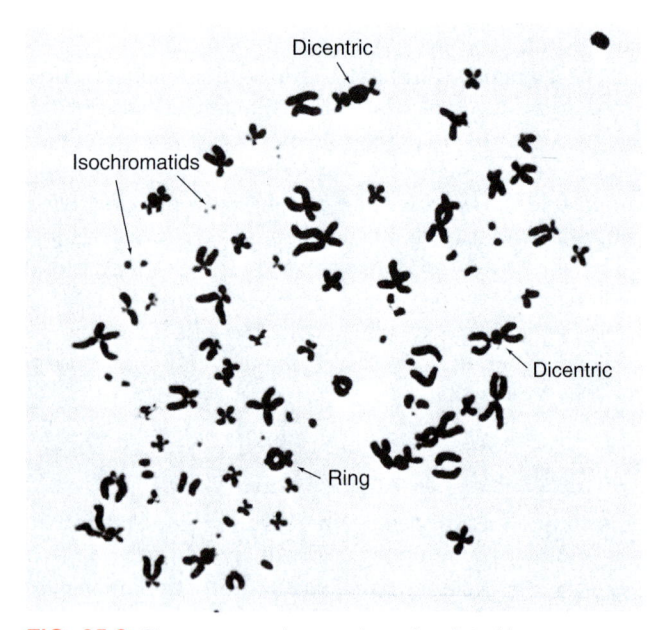

FIG. 35.9 Chromosome damage in an irradiated human cancer cell. Microscopic view of chromosome shows three types of damages labeled as ring, dicentric, and isochromatids. (Courtesy Neil Wald†, University of Pittsburgh.)

Radiation cytogenetic studies have shown that nearly every type of chromosome aberration can be radiation induced and that some aberrations may be specific to radiation. The rate of induction of chromosome aberrations is related in a complex way to the radiation dose and differs among the various types of aberrations.

Attempts to measure chromosome aberrations in patients after diagnostic x-ray examination have been largely unsuccessful. However, some studies involving high-dose fluoroscopy have shown radiation-induced chromosome aberrations soon after the examination was performed.

> Radiation-induced chromosome aberrations follow a nonthreshold dose-response relationship.

Without question, high doses of radiation cause chromosome aberrations. Low doses no doubt also do, but it is technically difficult to observe aberrations at doses that are less than approximately 100 mGy$_t$. An even more difficult task is to identify the link between radiation-induced chromosome aberrations and latent illness or disease.

When the body is irradiated, all cells can sustain cytogenetic damage. Such damage is classified here as an early response to radiation because if the cell survives, the damage is manifested during the next mitosis after the radiation exposure.

Human peripheral lymphocytes are most often used for cytogenetic analysis, and these lymphocytes do not move into mitosis until stimulated in vitro by an appropriate laboratory technique.

Although cytogenetic damage occurs at the time of irradiation, it can be months and even years before the damage is measured. For this reason, chromosome abnormalities in circulating lymphocytes persist in some workers who were irradiated in industrial accidents 20 years ago.

Normal Karyotype

The human chromosome consists of many long strings of DNA mixed with a protein and folded back on itself many times. Refer to Fig. 31.11, which shows a normal chromosome as it would appear in the G_1 phase of the cell cycle when only two chromatids are present and in the G_2 phase of the cell cycle after DNA replication. The chromosome structure of four chromatids represented for the G_2 phase is that which is visualized in the metaphase portion of mitosis.

For certain types of cytogenetic analysis, photographs are taken and enlarged so that each chromosome can be cut out like a paper doll and paired with its sister into a chromosome map, which is called a **karyotype** (Fig. 35.10).

> Each cell has 22 pairs of autosomes and one pair of sex chromosomes—the female X chromosome and the male Y chromosome.

Structural radiation damage to individual chromosomes can be visualized without constructing a karyotype. These are the single- and double-hit chromosome aberrations. Reciprocal translocations require a karyotype for detection. Point genetic mutations are undetectable, even with karyotype construction.

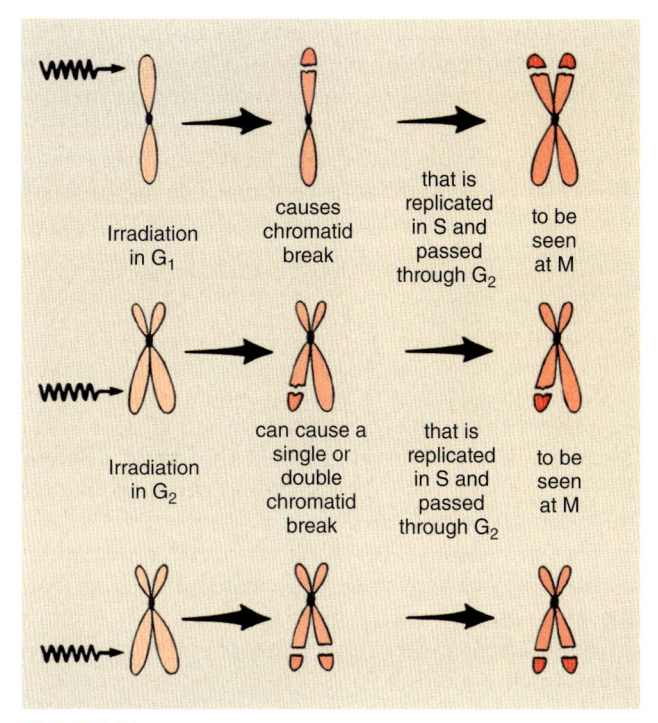

FIG. 35.11 Single-hit chromosome aberrations after irradiation in G_1 and G_2. The aberrations are visualized and recorded during the M phase.

Single-Hit Chromosome Aberrations

When radiation interacts with chromosomes, the interaction can occur through direct or indirect effect. In either mode, these interactions result in a **hit**. This hit, however, is somewhat different from the hit described previously in radiation interaction with DNA.

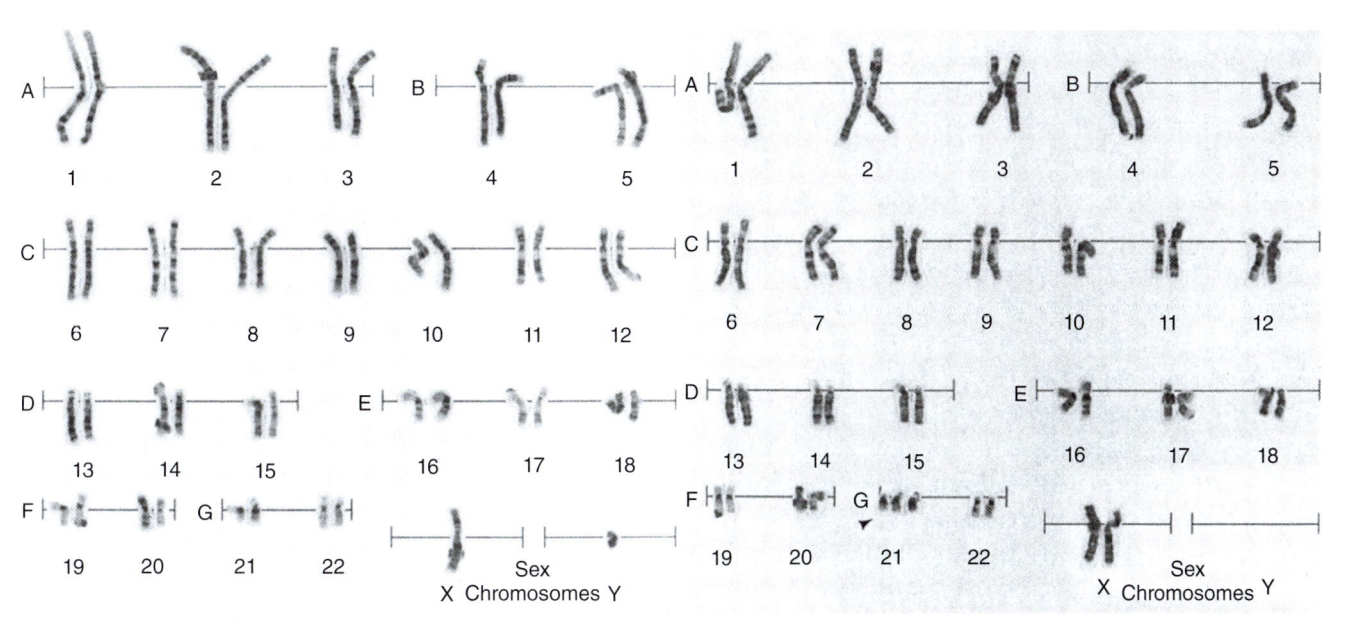

FIG. 35.10 A photomicrograph of the human cell nucleus at metaphase shows each chromosome distinctly. The karyotype is made by cutting and pasting each chromosome, similar to paper dolls, and aligning them, largest to smallest. The left karyotype is male, and the right is female. (Courtesy Caroline Caskey Goodner, Identigene, Inc.)

The DNA hit results in an invisible disruption of the molecular structure of the DNA. A chromosome hit, on the other hand, produces a visible derangement of the chromosome. Because the chromosomes contain DNA, this indicates that such a hit has disrupted many molecular bonds and has severed many chains of DNA.

> A chromosome hit represents severe damage to the DNA.

Single-hit effects produced by radiation during the G_1 phase of the cell cycle are shown in Fig. 35.11. The breakage of a chromatid is called **chromatid deletion**. During S phase, both the remaining chromosome and the deletion are replicated.

The chromosome aberration visualized at metaphase consists of a chromosome with material missing from the ends of two sister chromatids and two acentric (without a centromere) fragments. These fragments are called **isochromatids**.

Chromosome aberrations also can be produced by single-hit events during the G_2 phase of the cell cycle (see Fig. 35.11). The probability that ionizing radiation will pass through sister chromatids to produce isochromatids is low. Usually radiation produces a chromatid deletion in only one arm of the chromosome. The result is a chromosome with an arm that is obviously missing genetic material and a chromatid fragment.

Multihit Chromosome Aberrations

A single chromosome can sustain more than one hit. Multihit aberrations are not uncommon (Fig. 35.12).

In the G_1 phase of the cell cycle, ring chromosomes are produced if the two hits occur on the same chromosome. Dicentrics are produced when adjacent chromosomes each sustain one hit and recombine. The

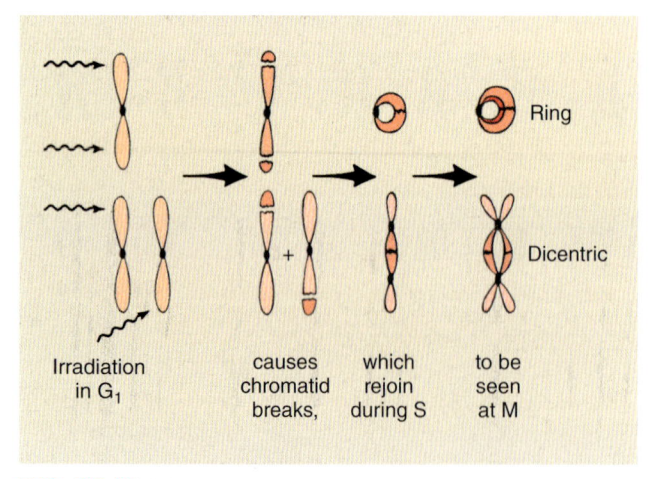

FIG. 35.12 Multihit chromosome aberrations after irradiation in G_1 result in ring and dicentric chromosomes, in addition to chromatid fragments. Similar aberrations can be produced by irradiation during G_2, but they are rarer.

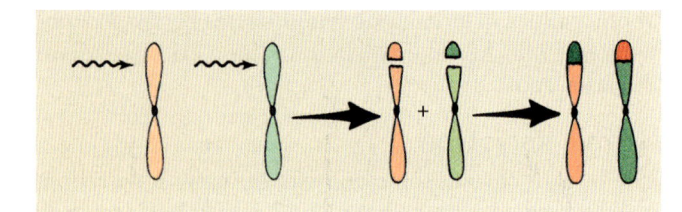

FIG. 35.13 Radiation-induced reciprocal translocations are multihit chromosome aberrations that require karyotypic analysis for detection.

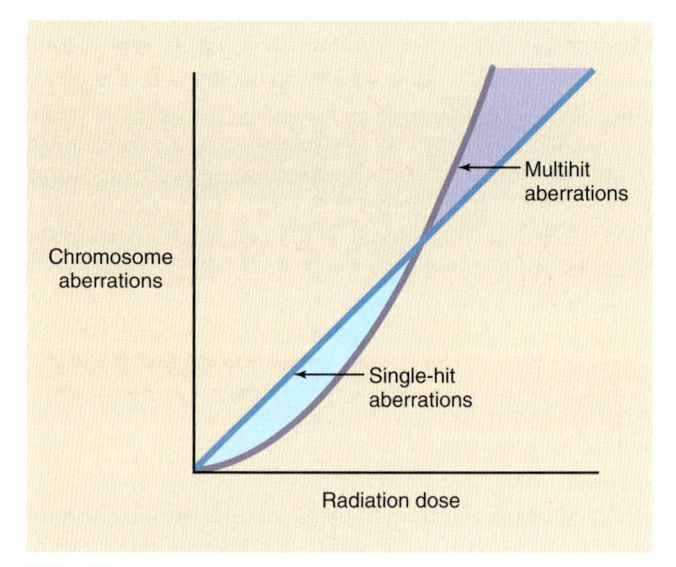

FIG. 35.14 Dose-response relationships for single-hit aberrations are linear, nonthreshold, but those for multihit aberrations are nonlinear, nonthreshold.

mechanism for the joining of chromatids depends on a condition called **stickiness** that is radiation-induced and appears at the site of the severed chromosome.

Similar aberrations can be produced in the G_2 phase of the cell cycle; however, such aberrations again require that either (1) the same chromosome be hit two or more times or (2) adjacent chromosomes be hit and joined together. However, these events are rare.

The multihit chromosome aberrations previously described represent rather severe damage to the cell. At mitosis, the acentric fragments are lost or are attracted to only one of the daughter cells because they are unattached to a spindle fiber. Consequently, one or both of the daughter cells can be missing considerable genetic material.

Reciprocal translocations are multihit chromosome aberrations that require karyotypic analysis for detection (Fig. 35.13). Radiation-induced reciprocal translocations result in no loss of genetic material—simply a rearrangement of the genes. Consequently, all or nearly all genetic codes are available; they simply may be organized in an incorrect sequence.

Kinetics of Chromosome Aberrations

At very low doses of radiation, only single-hit aberrations occur. When the radiation dose exceeds approximately

1 Gy_t, the frequency of multihit aberrations increases more rapidly.

The general dose-response relationship for production of single-hit and multihit aberrations is shown in Fig. 35.14. Single-hit aberrations are produced with a **linear, nonthreshold** dose-response relationship. Multihit aberrations are produced following a **nonlinear, nonthreshold** relationship. A number of investigators have experimentally characterized these relationships.

> **RADIATION DOSE-RESPONSE RELATIONSHIPS FOR CYTOGENETIC DAMAGE**
>
> Single–hit: $Y = a + bD$
>
> Multihit: $Y = a + bD + cD^2$
>
> where Y is the number of single-hit or multihit chromosome aberrations, a is the naturally occurring frequency of chromosome aberrations, and b and c are radiation dose (D) coefficients of damage for single-hit and multihit aberrations, respectively.

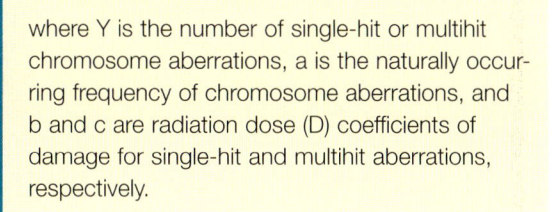

Multihit aberrations are considered to be the most significant in terms of later human response. If the radiation dose is unknown yet is not life threatening, the approximate chromosome aberration frequency is two single-hit aberrations per 10 mGy_t per 1000 cells and one multihit aberration per 100 mGy_t per 1000 cells.

Recently cytogenetic analysis has claimed more attention because of the increasing application of medical genetics and neuroscience. Patient management can now involve both medical genetics and neuroscience as routine.

THE HUMAN GENOME

After many years of scientific investigation, in 2000, the human genome was mapped. This was a worldwide project involving many different laboratories. Humans have about 35,000 genes distributed along the DNA of the 46 chromosomes.

Many human health effects have now been associated with aberrations identified for specific genes, and researchers are finding ways to correct these genetic defects or replace them. Perhaps as many as 50 different health conditions are now identified with a specific genetic defect.

A great example is BrCa1 and BrCa2, located on chromosomes 17 and 13, respectively, which are associated with breast cancer. Many other examples are available, not only with cancer but also with other health conditions, such as heart disease and mental health.

It is now possible to perform molecular genetic counseling and advise patients of their risk for breast cancer, other cancers, and other health risks. With the help of artificial intelligence and quantum computing we will be able to identify radiation-induced aberrations and alert patients and radiation workers to possible future risks.

SUMMARY

After exposure to a high radiation dose, humans can experience a response within a few days to a few weeks. This immediate response is called a deterministic effect. Such early effects are deterministic because the severity of response is dose related, there is a dose threshold, and the dose-response relationship is nonlinear.

The sequence of events that follows high-dose radiation exposure leading to death within days or weeks is called acute radiation syndrome, which includes hematologic syndrome, GI syndrome, and CNS syndrome. These syndromes are dose related.

$LD_{50/60}$ is the dose of radiation to the whole body after which 50% of subjects will die within 60 days. For humans, this dose is estimated at 3.5 Gy_t. As radiation dose increases, the time between exposure and death decreases.

When only part of the body is irradiated, higher doses are tolerated. Examples of local tissue damage include effects on the skin, gonads, eyes, and bone marrow. The first manifestation of radiation injury to the skin is damage to the basal cells. Resultant skin damage occurs as erythema, desquamation, or epilation.

Radiation of the male testes can result in a reduction of spermatozoa. A dose of 2 Gy_t produces temporary infertility. A dose of 5 Gy_t to the testes produces permanent sterility. In males as in females, the stem cell is the most radiosensitive phase.

Radiation induced cataracts require a threshold dose of at least 10 Gy_t. In digital imaging, it is not possible to get to that level of lens exposure for patients or radiographers.

The hemopoietic system consists of bone marrow, circulating blood, and lymphoid tissue. The principal effect of radiation on this system is fewer blood cells in the peripheral circulation. Radiation exposure decreases the numbers of all precursor cells; this reduces the number of mature cells in the circulating blood. Lymphocytes and spermatogonia are considered the most radiosensitive cells in the body.

The study of chromosome damage from radiation exposure is called radiocytogenetics. Chromosome damage takes on the following different forms: (1) chromatid deletion, (2) dicentric chromosome aberration, and (3) reciprocal translocations.

CHALLENGE QUESTIONS

1. Define or otherwise identify the following:
    a. GI death
    b. Latent period
    c. LD$_{50/60}$
    d. Erythema
    e. Clinical tolerance
    f. Primordial follicle
    g. Erythrocyte
    h. Karyotype
    i. Epilation
    j. Multihit aberration
2. What is the minimum dose that results in reddening of the skin?
3. Explain the prodromal syndrome.
4. Clinical signs and symptoms of the manifest illness stage of acute radiation lethality are classified into which three groups?
5. During which stage of the acute radiation syndrome is recovery stimulated?
6. What dose of radiation results in the GI syndrome?
7. Why can death occur following the GI syndrome?
8. Identify the cause of death from the CNS syndrome.
9. Describe the stages of gametogenesis in a female. Identify the most radiosensitive phases.
10. What cells of the hemopoietic system arise from pluripotential stem cells?
11. Discuss the maturation of basal cells in the epidermis.
12. What two cells are the most radiosensitive cells in the human body?
13. Describe the changes in mean survival time associated with increasing doses.
14. What is the approximate value of LD$_{50/60}$ in humans?
15. What are the four principal blood cell lines, and what is the function of each?
16. Diagram the mechanism for the production of a reciprocal translocation.
17. List the clinical signs and symptoms of the hematologic syndrome.
18. What mature cells form from the omnipotential stem cell?
19. If the normal incidence of single hit–type chromosome aberrations is 0.15 per 100 cells and the dose coefficient is 0.0094, how many such aberrations would be expected after a dose of 380 mGy$_t$?
20. If the normal incidence of multihit chromosome aberrations is 0.082 and the dose coefficient is 0.0047, how many dicentrics per 100 cells would be expected after a whole-body dose of 160 Gy$_t$?

The answers to the Challenge Questions can be found by logging onto our website at http://evolve.elsevier.com.

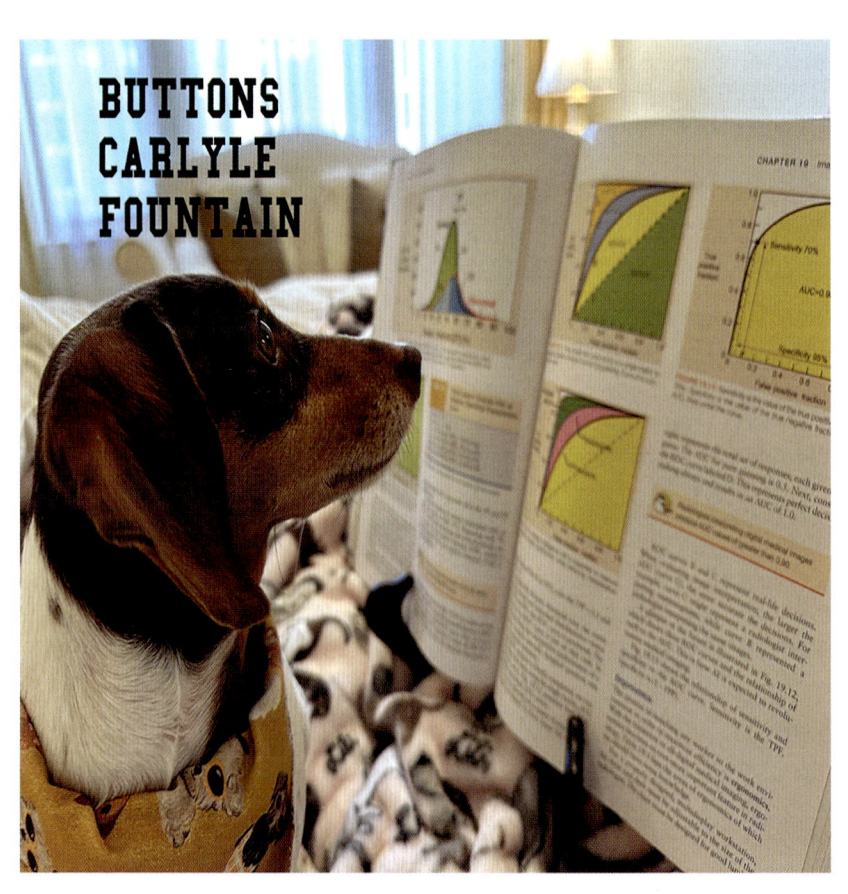

Stochastic Effects of Radiation

CHAPTER 36

OBJECTIVES

At the completion of this chapter, the student should be able to do the following:

1. Define the stochastic effects of radiation exposure.
2. Identify the radiation dose needed to produce stochastic effects.
3. Discuss the results of epidemiologic studies of populations exposed to radiation.
4. Explain the estimates of radiation risk.
5. Analyze radiation-induced leukemia and cancer.
6. Review the risks of low-dose radiation on fertility and pregnancy.

OUTLINE

Local Tissue Effects 482
  Skin 482
  Chromosomes 483
Life Shortening 483
Risk Estimates 484
  Relative Risk 484
  Excess Risk 485
  Attributable Risk 485
Radiation-Induced Malignancy 486
  Leukemia 486
  Cancer 488
Total Risk of Malignancy 491
  Nuclear Reactor Incidents 491
  Biologic Effects of Ionizing Radiation Report 491
Radiation and Pregnancy 493
  Effects on Fertility 493
  Irradiation In Utero 493
  Genetic Effects 496
Summary 497
Challenge Questions 497

481

DETERMINISTIC EFFECTS of radiation exposure are produced by high radiation doses. Stochastic effects of radiation exposure are the result of low doses delivered over a long period.

Radiation exposures experienced by personnel in digital imaging are low dose and low linear energy transfer (LET). In addition, patient radiation doses in digital imaging are delivered intermittently over long periods. Personnel radiation dose and patient radiation dose are delivered in a fractionated fashion.

The principal stochastic effects of low-dose radiation over long periods consist of radiation-induced malignancy and genetic effects. Life span shortening and effects on local tissues also have been reported as stochastic effects, but these are not considered significant. Radiation protection guides are based on suspected or observed stochastic effects of radiation and on an assumed linear, nonthreshold dose-response relationship.

This chapter reviews these stochastic effects and introduces the subject of risk estimation. Radiation effects during pregnancy are of considerable importance in digital imaging, and such effects are also discussed here.

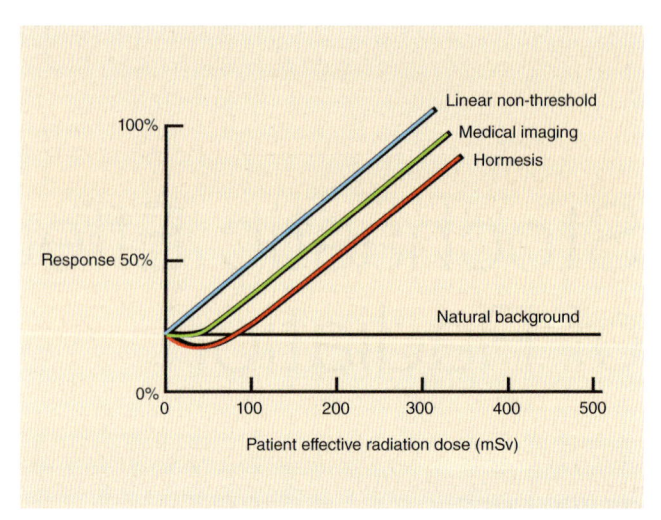

FIG. 36.1 The stochastic radiation dose-response relationship and that for radiation-induced hormesis. The presumed dose-response relationship for medical imaging patients is also shown.

TABLE 36.1 Minimum Population Sample Required to Show That the Given Radiation Dose Significantly Elevated the Incidence of Leukemia

Dose (mGy$_t$)	Population Size
50	6,000,000
100	1,600,000
150	750,000
200	500,000
500	100,000

The radiation exposures that we experience in digital imaging are low and of low LET; they are chronic in nature because they are delivered intermittently over long periods. Therefore, stochastic radiation effects are of particular importance (Fig. 36.1).

The principal stochastic effects are radiation-induced malignancy and genetic effects. Stochastic effects of radiation exposure exhibit an increasing **incidence** of response—not severity—with increasing dose. No dose threshold has been established for a stochastic response. The stochastic dose-response relationship is linear.

> Our radiation protection guides are based on the stochastic effects of radiation and on linear, nonthreshold radiation dose-response relationships.

Studies of large numbers of people exposed to a toxic substance require considerable statistical analyses. Such studies, called **epidemiologic studies**, are required when the number of persons affected is small.

Epidemiologic studies of people exposed to radiation are difficult because (1) the dose usually is not known but is presumed to be low, (2) the response cannot be definitely tied to the previous radiation exposure, and (3) the frequency of response is very low. Consequently, the results of radiation epidemiologic studies do not convey the statistical accuracy associated with observations of stochastic radiation effects.

Table 36.1 illustrates the difficulty of the problem. It shows the minimum number of persons who must be observed as a function of radiation dose if a definite link is to be established between an increase of leukemia and the radiation dose in question.

LOCAL TISSUE EFFECTS
Skin

In addition to the deterministic effects of erythema and desquamation and late-developing carcinoma, chronic irradiation of the skin can result in severe nonmalignant changes. Early radiologists who performed fluoroscopic examinations without protective gloves developed a very calloused, discolored, and weathered appearance to the skin of their hands and forearms. In addition, the skin would be very tight and brittle and sometimes would severely crack or flake.

This stochastic effect was observed many years ago in radiologists and is called **radiodermatitis**. The dose necessary to produce such an effect is very high. No such effects occur in the current practice of radiology.

Chromosomes

Irradiation of blood-forming organs can produce hematologic depression as a deterministic response or leukemia as a stochastic response. Chromosome damage in the circulating lymphocytes can be produced as both a deterministic and a stochastic response.

The types and frequency of chromosome aberrations have been described previously; however even a low dose of radiation can produce chromosome aberrations that may not be apparent until many years after radiation exposure. For example, individuals irradiated accidentally with rather high radiation doses continue to show chromosome abnormalities in their peripheral lymphocytes for as long as 20 years.

This stochastic effect presumably occurs because of radiation damage to the lymphocytic stem cells. These cells may not be stimulated into replication and maturation for many years.

LIFE SHORTENING

Many experiments have been conducted with animals after both acute and chronic radiation exposure showing that irradiated animals die young. Fig. 36.2, which has been redrawn from several such representative experiments, shows that the relationship between life shortening and dose is apparently linear and nonthreshold. When all animal data are considered collectively, it is difficult to attempt a meaningful extrapolation to humans.

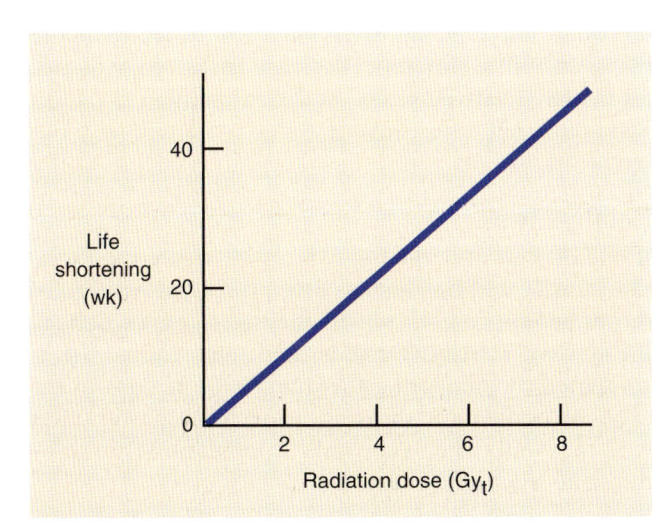

FIG. 36.2 In chronically irradiated animals, the relationship between the extent of life shortening and dose appears linear, nonthreshold. This graph shows the representative results of several such experiments with mice.

> At worst, humans can expect a reduced life of approximately 10 days for every 10 mGy_t.

The data presented in Table 36.2 were compiled by Cohen of the University of Pittsburgh and were extrapolated from various statistical sources of mortality. The expected loss of life in days is given as a function of occupation, disease, or other condition.

The results show that the most grievous risk is being male rather than female. Whereas the average life shortening caused by occupational accidents amounts to 74 days, for radiation workers, life is shortened by only 12 days.

> Radiology and radiography are safe occupations.

Radiation-induced life shortening is nonspecific; that is, no characteristic diseases are associated with it, and it does not include late malignant effects. It occurs simply as accelerated premature aging and death.

One investigator has evaluated the death records of radiographers who operated field x-ray equipment during World War II. These imaging systems were poorly designed and inadequately shielded, so radiographers

TABLE 36.2 Risk of Life Span Shortening as a Consequence of Occupation, Disease, or Various Other Conditions

Risky Condition	Expected Days of Life Lost
Being male rather than female	2800
Heart disease	2100
Being unmarried	2000
One pack of cigarettes a day	1600
Working as a coal miner	1100
Cancer	980
30 pounds overweight	900
Stroke	500
All accidents	435
Service in Vietnam	400
Motor vehicle accidents	200
Average occupational accidents	74
Speed limit increase from 55 to 65 mph	40
Radiation worker	12
Airplane crashes	1

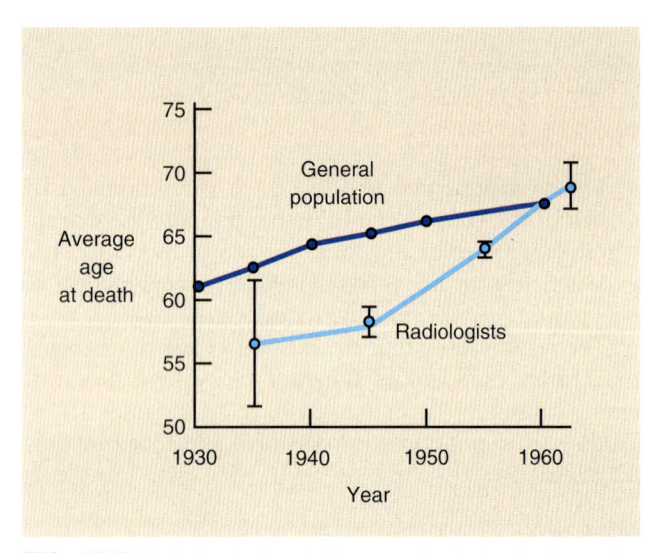

FIG. 36.3 Radiation-induced life-span shortening is shown for American radiologists. The age at death among radiologists was lower than that of the general population, but this difference has disappeared.

received higher-than-normal radiation exposures. There have been 7000 such radiographers studied, and no radiation effects have been observed.

An investigation of health effects from radiation exposure of American radiographers that began in 1982 has found no effects. This study was conducted as a mail survey that covered the work-related conditions of approximately 150,000 subjects.

Observations on human populations have not been totally convincing. No life-span shortening has been observed among atomic bomb survivors, although some received rather substantial radiation doses. Life-span shortening in radium watch-dial painters, x-ray patients, and other human radiation-exposed populations has not been reported.

American radiologists have been fairly extensively studied, and early radiologists appeared to have a reduced life span. Such research has many shortcomings, not the least of which is its retrospective nature. Fig. 36.3 shows the results obtained when the age at death for radiologists was compared with the age at death for the general population. Radiologists dying in the early 1930s were approximately 5 years younger than members of the general population who died at an average age. However this difference in age at death had shrunk to zero by 1965.

A more thorough study used two other physician groups as controls rather than the general population. Table 36.3 summarizes the results of this investigation. Physicians in the high-risk group observed in this study were members of the Radiological Society of North America; the low-risk groups consisted of members of the American Academy of Ophthalmology and Otolaryngology. Members of the American College of Physicians represented an intermediate-risk group.

TABLE 36.3 Death Statistics for Three Groups of Physicians

Died During	Median Age at Death	Age-Adjusted Deaths per 1000
1935–44		
RSNA	71.4	18.4
ACP	73.4	15.4
AAOO	76.2	13.0
1945–54		
RSNA	72.0	16.4
ACP	74.8	13.7
AAOO	76.0	11.9
1955–58		
RSNA	73.5	13.6
ACP	76.0	11.4
AAOO	76.4	10.6

ACP, American College of Physicians; *AAOO*, American Academy of Ophthalmology and Otolaryngology; *RSNA*, Radiological Society of North America.

A comparison of median age at death and age-adjusted death rates for these physician specialties demonstrates a significant difference in age at death during the early years of radiology.

RISK ESTIMATES

The deterministic effects of high-dose radiation exposure are usually easy to observe and measure. The stochastic effects are also easy to observe, but it is nearly impossible to associate a particular late response with a previous radiation exposure.

Consequently, precise dose-response relationships are often not possible to formulate, and we therefore resort to **risk estimates**. There are three types of risk estimates—relative, excess, and attributable risk; all of these represent different statements of risk and have different dimensions.

Relative Risk

If one observes a large population for stochastic radiation effects without having any precise knowledge of the radiation dose to which they were exposed, then the concept of **relative risk** is used. The relative risk is computed by comparing the number of persons in the exposed population showing a given stochastic effect with the number in an unexposed population who show the same stochastic effect.

Relative risk = Observed cases/Expected cases

A relative risk of 1.0 indicates no risk at all. A relative risk of 1.5 indicates that the frequency of a late response is 50% higher in the irradiated population than in the nonirradiated population. The relative risk for radiation-induced stochastic effects of particular importance observed in human populations is in the range of 1 to 2.

Occasionally, an investigation results in the identification of a relative risk of less than 1. This indicates that the radiation exposed population receives some protective benefit, which is consistent with the theory of **radiation hormesis**. However the usual interpretation of such studies is that the results are not statistically significant because of the small number of observations conducted or because the irradiated and control populations were not adequately identified.

> The theory of radiation hormesis suggests that very low radiation doses are beneficial.

Some evidence supports the principle of radiation hormesis. Radiation hormesis suggests that low levels of radiation, less than approximately 100 mGy_t, are good for you! Such low doses may provide a protective effect by stimulating molecular repair and immunologic response mechanisms.

Nevertheless, radiation hormesis remains a theory at this time, and until it has been proved, we will continue to practice ALARA—as low as reasonably achievable. An example of a reported dose-response relationship indicating radiation hormesis was shown in Fig. 32.7.

Question: In a study of radiation-induced leukemia after diagnostic levels of radiation, 227 cases were observed in 100,000 persons so irradiated. The normal incidence of leukemia in the United States is 150 cases per 100,000. Based on these data, what is the relative risk of radiation-induced leukemia?

Answer:
$$\text{Relative risk} = \frac{\text{Observed cases}}{\text{Expected cases}}$$
$$\frac{227}{100,000} \div \frac{150}{100,000} = 1.51$$
Or $227/150 = 1.51$

Excess Risk

Often, when an investigation of human radiation response reveals the induction of some stochastic effect, the magnitude of the effect is reflected by the excess number of cases induced. Leukemia, for instance, is known to occur spontaneously in nonirradiated populations. If the leukemia incidence in an irradiated population exceeds that which is expected, then the difference between the observed number of cases and the expected number would be **excess risk**.

> Excess risk = Observed cases − Expected cases

The excess cases in this instance are assumed to be radiation induced. To determine the number of excess cases, one must be able to measure the observed number of cases in the irradiated population and compare this with the number that would have been expected based on known population levels.

Question: There were 23 cases of skin cancer observed in a population of 1000 radiologists. The incidence in the general population is 0.5/100,000. How many excess skin cancers were radiation induced in the population of radiologists?

Answer: Excess cases = Observed cases − Expected cases
$$= \frac{23}{1000} - \frac{0.5}{100,000} = \frac{23}{1000} - \frac{0.005}{1000} \cong 23$$

Because none would be expected, all 23 cases represent excess radiation risk.

Attributable Risk

If at least two different dose levels are known, then it may be possible to determine the **attributable radiation risk**. In contrast to the relative risk, which is a dimensionless ratio, the attributable risk consists of units of cases/population/dose. The risk of the response is attributable to the radiation dose.

The attributable risk of total radiation-induced malignant disease has been determined by the National Academy of Science Committee on the Biologic Effects of Ionizing Radiation (BEIR). This value 8×10^{-2} Sv^{-1} is a considerable simplification of the results of many studies. The absolute risk of a fatal radiation-induced malignant disease is 5×10^{-2} Sv^{-1}. This is the risk coefficient used by radiation scientists to predict the stochastic radiation response in exposed populations (Table 36.4).

TABLE 36.4 Radiation-Induced Incidence and Mortality Attributable Risk Coefficients

Incidence: 8×10^{-2} Sv^{-1} (8/10,000/10 mSv)
Mortality: 5×10^{-2} Sv^{-1} (5/10,000/10 mSv)

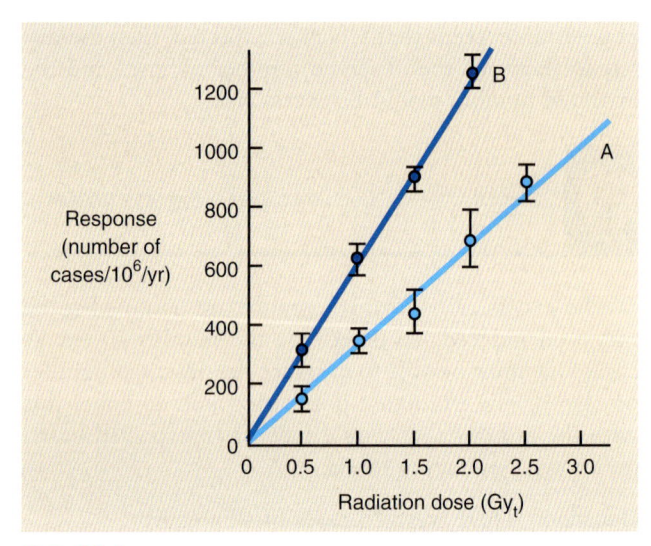

FIG. 36.4 The slope of the linear, nonthreshold dose-response relationship is equal to the attributable risk. A and B show the attributable risks of 3.4 and 6.2 cases per 10^6 persons/10 mGy$_t$/year, respectively.

To determine the attributable radiation risk, one must assume a linear dose-response relationship. If the dose-response relationship is assumed to be nonthreshold, then only one dose level is required. The value of the attributable radiation risk is equal to the slope of the dose-response relationship (Fig. 36.4). The error bars on each data point indicate the precision of the observation of response.

Question: The attributable risk for radiation-induced breast cancer is 5×10^{-2} Sv^{-1} for a 20-year at-risk period (actually it is much less than this). If 100,000 women receive 1 mSv during mammography, how many fatal cancers would be expected to be induced?

Answer:
$$5 \times 10^{-2} \text{ Sv}^{-1} = \frac{5}{100 \times \text{Sv}}$$
$$= \frac{5}{1000 \times 1 \text{ mSv}}$$
$$= 5 \text{ fatal cancers}$$

Question: There are approximately 300,000 American radiographers, and they receive an annual effective dose of 0.5 mSv. What is the expected number of annual deaths because of this occupational exposure?

Answer:
$$0.5 \text{ mSv} = \frac{5}{100 \times \text{Sv}}$$
$$= \frac{25}{10,000 \times 0.5 \text{ mSv}}$$
Therefore in 300,000 RTs
$= 7.5$ deaths from malignant disease

As we shall see in Chapter 41, the largest component of human-made radiation exposure is now CT. This patient radiation dose currently receives considerable newspaper discussion as harmful.

Question: Approximately 90 million patients per year are examined with CT, which requires an average patient effective radiation dose of 10 mSv. How many of these patients may die because of this radiation dose?

Answer:
$$\frac{5}{100 \times \text{Sv}} = \frac{25}{100,000 \times 10 \text{ mSv}}$$
$$\times 90,000,000$$
$$= 4500$$

However the natural incidence of death from malignant disease is approximately 20% or 18 million in an unexposed population of 90 million. Furthermore this type of discussion rarely includes an assessment of the number of lives saved by such examinations.

> Attributable radiation risk is the best risk assessment regardless of population.

Attributable risk is the metric most often used to estimate patient radiation risk. The units of attributable risk, number of cases/10^6 population/radiation dose, are the most descriptive units of radiation risk.

RADIATION-INDUCED MALIGNANCY

All the stochastic effects, including radiation-induced malignancy, have been observed in experimental animals, and based on these animal experiments, dose-response relationships have been developed. At the human level, these stochastic effects have been observed, but often, data are insufficient to allow precise identification of the radiation dose-response relationship. Consequently, some of the conclusions drawn regarding human responses are based in part on animal data.

Leukemia

When one considers radiation-induced leukemia in laboratory animals, there is no question that this response is real and that the incidence increases with increasing radiation dose. The form of the dose-response relationship is linear and nonthreshold. A number of human population groups have exhibited an elevated incidence of leukemia after radiation exposure—atomic bomb survivors, American radiologists, radiotherapy patients, and children irradiated in utero, to name a few.

Probably the greatest wealth of information that we have accumulated regarding radiation-induced leukemia in humans has been drawn from observations of

TABLE 36.5 Summary of the Incidence of Leukemia in Atomic Bomb Survivors

	Hiroshima	Nagasaki	Total
Total number of survivors in study	74,356	25,037	99,393
Observed cases	102	42	144
Expected cases	39	13	52

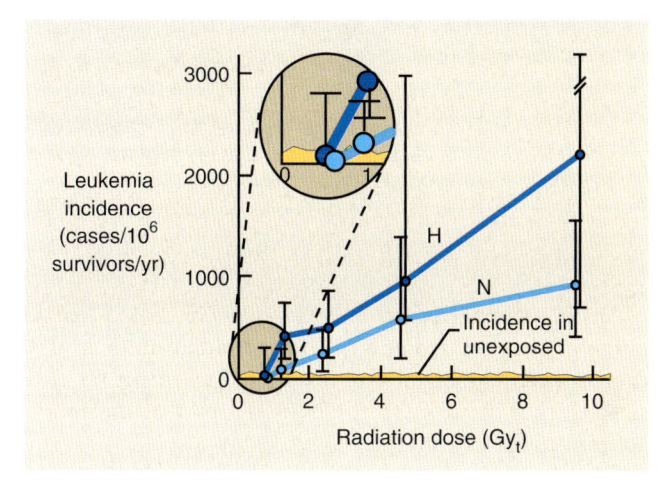

FIG. 36.5 Data from the atomic bomb survivors of Hiroshima (H) and Nagasaki (N) suggest a linear, nonthreshold dose-response relationship.

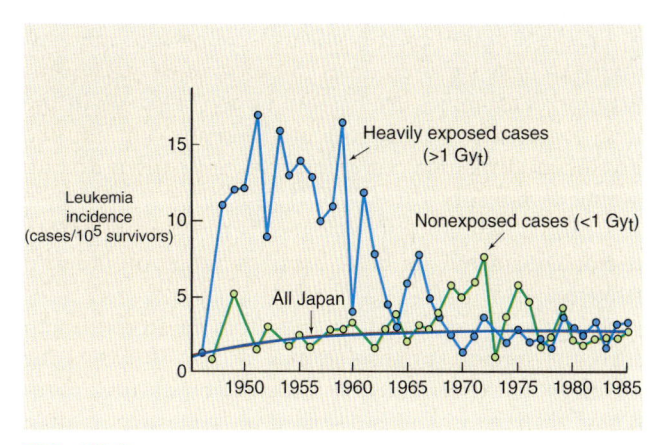

FIG. 36.6 The incidence of leukemia among atomic bomb survivors increased rapidly for the first few years, then declined to natural incidence by approximately 1975.

survivors of the atomic bombings of Hiroshima and Nagasaki. At the time of the bombings, approximately 300,000 people lived in those two cities.

Nearly 100,000 were killed from the blast and from the deterministic effects of radiation. Another 100,000 people received significant doses of radiation and survived. The remainder were unaffected because their radiation dose was less than 100 mGy$_t$.

After World War II, scientists of the Atomic Bomb Casualty Commission, now known as the Radiation Effects Research Foundation, attempted to determine the radiation dose received by each of the atomic bomb survivors in both cities. They estimated the dose to each survivor by considering not only distance from the explosion but also terrain, type of bomb, type of building construction if the survivor was inside, and other factors that might influence radiation dose.

A summary of the data obtained through these investigations is given in Table 36.5, and the data analysis is shown graphically in Fig. 36.5. After high radiation doses were delivered by these bombs, the leukemia incidence was as much as 100 times that in the nonirradiated population. Even though large error bars are seen at each dose increment, the response appears to be linear and nonthreshold.

If, however, one expands the data in the low-dose region (e.g., below 2 Gy$_t$), one could conclude that a threshold exists in the neighborhood of 500 mGy$_t$. Nevertheless, neither this information nor other available information is interpreted to support a threshold response at this time. Rejection of nonthreshold is a current hot topic in medical imaging.

> Radiation-induced leukemia follows a linear, nonthreshold dose-response relationship.

Fig. 36.6 demonstrates the temporal distribution of the onset of leukemia among atomic bomb survivors for the 40 years after the bombings. The data are presented as cases per 100,000 and include for comparison the leukemia rate in the population at large and in the nonexposed populations of the bombed cities.

A rather rapid rise in leukemia incidence reached a plateau after approximately 5 years. The incidence declined slowly for approximately 20 years, when it reached the natural level experienced by the nonexposed.

> Radiation-induced leukemia is considered to have a latent period of 4 to 7 years and an at-risk period of approximately 20 years.

The at-risk period is that time after irradiation during which one might expect the radiation effect to occur. The at-risk period for radiation-induced cancer is lifetime.

Data from atomic bomb survivors show without a doubt that radiation exposure to those survivors caused the later development of leukemia. It is interesting, however, to reflect on some additional aspects of these events.

Of the 300,000 total residents, 335 persons are estimated to have survived doses in excess of 6 Gy. The leukemia risk estimates are based on only 144 cases in the total exposed population. Acute leukemia and chronic myelocytic leukemia were observed most often among atomic bomb survivors.

Chronic lymphocytic leukemia is rare and therefore is not considered to be a form of radiation-induced leukemia.

Taken to the final analysis, data from the atomic bomb survivors support an absolute risk of 5×10^{-2} Sv^{-1} for mortality. The overall relative risk based on the total number of observed leukemia deaths (144) versus the number of expected leukemia deaths (52) is approximately 3:1.

By the second decade of radiology, reports of pernicious anemia and leukemia in radiologists began to appear. In the early 1940s, several investigators reviewed the incidence of leukemia in American radiologists and found it alarmingly high. These early radiologists functioned without the benefit of modern radiation protection devices and procedures, and many served as both radiation oncologists and diagnostic radiologists.

It has been estimated that some of these early radiologists received doses exceeding 1 Gy$_t$/year. Currently, American radiologists do not exhibit an elevated incidence of leukemia compared with other physician specialists.

A rather exhaustive study of mortality among radiologists in Great Britain during the period from the turn of the century to 1960 did not show an elevated risk of leukemia. The reasons for such a different experience between American and British radiologists are unknown.

> Studies of American radiographers consistently show no evidence of radiation induced leukemia.

In the 1940s and 1950s, particularly in Great Britain, it was common practice to treat patients who had ankylosing spondylitis with x-radiation. Ankylosing spondylitis is an arthritis-like condition of the vertebral column.

Patients cannot walk upright or move except with great difficulty. For relief, they would be given fairly high doses of radiation to the spinal column, and the treatment was quite successful. Patients who previously had been hunched over were able to stand and walk erect.

Such radiation oncology was a permanent cure and remained the treatment of choice for approximately 20 years until it was discovered that some who had been cured by radiation were dying from leukemia. Graphic results on the observations of these patients are shown in Fig. 36.7.

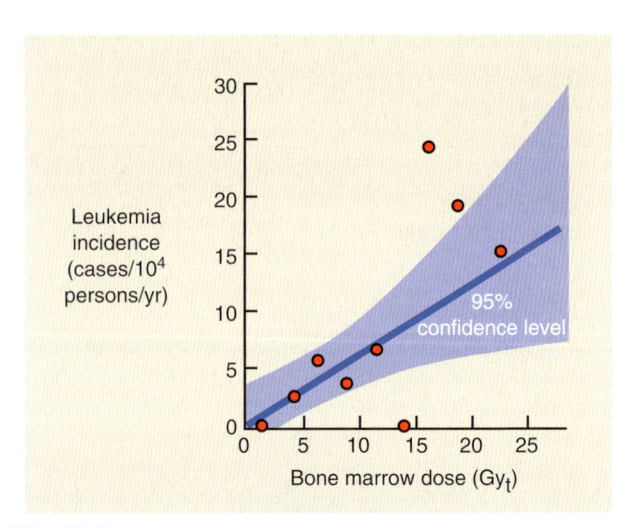

FIG. 36.7 Results of observations of leukemia in patients with ankylosing spondylitis treated with x-ray therapy suggest a linear, nonthreshold dose-response relationship.

During the period from 1935 to 1955, 14,554 male patients were treated at 81 different radiation oncology centers in Great Britain. A review of treatment records showed that the dose to the bone marrow of the spinal column ranged from 1 to 40 Gy.

Fifty-two cases of leukemia occurred in this population. When this incidence of leukemia is compared with that of the general population, the relative risk is 10:1.

Attributable risk can be obtained from these data by determining the slope of the best-fit line through the data points (see Fig. 36.7). Such an analysis yields a result of approximately 8×10^{-2} Sv^{-1}. If 95% confidence limits are placed on the data, one cannot rule out the possibility of a threshold dose at approximately 3 Gy$_t$.

Several studies have been designed to link leukemia incidence with environmental radiation. Natural background radiation levels increase in general with altitude and with latitude, but the range of levels observed is not sufficient to demonstrate a causal relationship with leukemia.

Other population groups that have provided evidence, both positive and negative, regarding the leukemia-inducing action of radiation include radium watch-dial painters, children receiving superficial x-ray treatment, and some additional adult radiation therapy groups.

Cancer

What has been discussed regarding radiation-induced leukemia also can be reported for radiation-induced cancer. We do not have similar quantities of human data regarding cancer as we do for leukemia. Nevertheless, it can be said without question that ionizing radiation can cause cancer.

The relative risks and absolute risks have been shown to be similar to those reported for leukemia. Many types of cancer have been implicated as radiation induced, and a discussion of the more important ones is in order.

> Approximately 20% of all deaths are caused by cancer; therefore any radiation-induced cancers are obscured.

It is not possible to link any case of cancer to a previous radiation exposure, regardless of its magnitude, because cancer is so common. Leukemia, on the other hand, is a relatively rare disease; this makes analysis of radiation-induced leukemia easier.

Thyroid cancer has been shown to develop in three groups of patients whose thyroid glands were irradiated in childhood. The first two groups, called the Ann Arbor series and the Rochester series, consisted of individuals who, in the 1940s and early 1950s, were treated shortly after birth for thymic enlargement. The thymus is a gland lying just below the thyroid gland that can enlarge shortly after birth in response to infection.

At these facilities, radiation was often the treatment of choice. After a dose of up to 5 Gy_t, the thymus gland would shrink so that all enlargement disappeared. No additional problems were evident until 20 years later, when thyroid nodules and thyroid cancer began to develop in some of these patients.

Another group included 21 children who were natives of the Rongelap Atoll in 1954; they were subjected to high levels of radioactive fallout during a hydrogen bomb test. The winds shifted during the test, carrying the fallout over an adjacent inhabited island rather than one that had been evacuated. These children received radiation doses to the thyroid gland from both external exposure and internal ingestion of an estimated 12 Gy_t.

If one computes the incidence of thyroid nodularity, considered preneoplastic, in these three groups and plots this incidence as a function of estimated dose, the result is that shown in Fig. 36.8. Admittedly, the error bars on the dose data and on the incidence levels are large.

> The implication of a linear, nonthreshold dose-response relationship for cancer is clear.

No radiation response has been observed in the 2 million people exposed to trace levels of radiation following the 1976 nuclear reactor incident at Three Mile Island or the nearly 100,000 persons exposed to radiation from the 1989 Chernobyl incident. No excess leukemia or cancer has been observed. A small increase in thyroid nodularity has been noted. The population

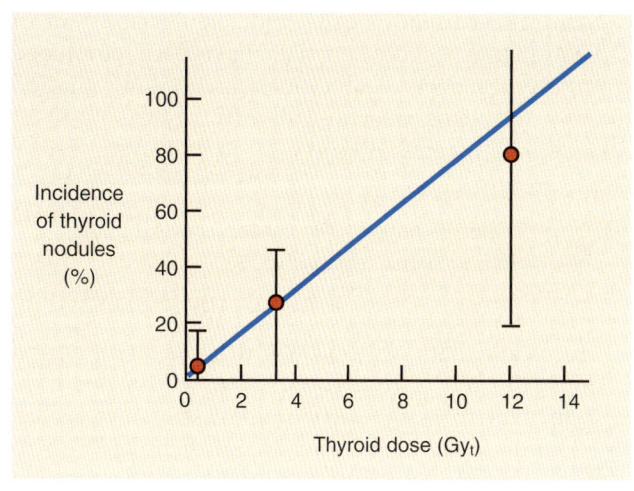

FIG. 36.8 Radiation-induced preneoplastic thyroid nodularity in three groups of persons whose thyroid glands were irradiated in childhood follows a linear, nonthreshold dose-response relationship.

of radiation doses from the 2011 Fukushima incident is even less. No radiation response is expected.

Two population groups have contributed an enormous quantity of data showing that radiation can cause **bone cancer**. The first group consists of radium watch-dial painters.

In the 1920s and 1930s, various small laboratories hired employees, most often female, who worked at benches painting watch dials with paint laden with radium sulfate. To prepare a fine point on the paintbrushes, the employees would touch the tip of the brush to the tongue. In this manner, substantial quantities of radium were ingested.

Radium salts were used because the emitted radiation, principally alpha and beta particles, would continuously excite the luminous compounds so the watch dial would glow in the dark. Current technology uses harmlessly low levels of tritium (^{3}H) and promethium (^{147}Pm) for this purpose.

> When ingested, the radium behaves metabolically similar to calcium and deposits in bone.

Because of radium's long half-life (1620 years) and alpha emission, these employees received radiation doses to bone of up to 500 Gy_t. Seventy-two bone cancers in approximately 800 persons have been observed during a follow-up period in excess of 50 years. Analysis of these data has disclosed an overall relative risk of 122:1. The attributable risk is equal to 1×10^{-2} Sv^{-1}.

Another population in whom excess bone cancer developed consisted of patients treated with radium salts for a variety of diseases, from arthritis to tuberculosis. Such treatments were common practice in many parts of the world until about 1950.

Skin cancer usually begins with the development of radiodermatitis. Significant data have been developed from several reports of skin cancer induced in radiation therapy recipients treated with orthovoltage (200 to 300 kVp) or superficial x-rays (50 to 150 kVp).

> Radiation-induced skin cancer follows a threshold dose-response relationship.

From these data, we conclude that the latent period is approximately 5 to 10 years, but we do not have enough data to assign attributable risk values. When the dose delivered to the skin was in the range of 5 to 20 Gy_t, the relative risk of developing skin cancer was 4:1. If the dose was 40 to 60 Gy_t or 60 to 100 Gy_t, the relative risks were 14:1 and 27:1, respectively.

In Chapter 18, some of the radiographic techniques used in mammography were discussed. The radiation dose to mammography patients is considered in a later chapter. Here we discuss the risk of radiation-induced **breast cancer**.

Controversy is ongoing regarding the risk of radiation-induced breast cancer, with implications for breast cancer detection by digital mammography. Concern over such risk first surfaced in the mid-1960s after reports were published of breast cancer developing in patients with tuberculosis.

Tuberculosis was for many years treated by isolation in a sanitarium. During the patient's stay, one mode of therapy was to induce a pneumothorax in the affected lung; this was done under fluoroscopy. Many patients received multiple treatments and up to several hundred fluoroscopic examinations.

Precise dose determinations are not possible, but levels of several gray would have been common. In some of these patient populations, the relative risk for radiation-induced breast cancer was shown to be as high as 10:1.

> Radiation-induced breast cancer exhibits a linear, nonthreshold dose-response relationship.

One such population exhibited no excess risk. This finding, however, was explained as a consequence of the fluoroscopic technique. In the positive studies, the patient faced away from the radiologist, toward the fluoroscopic x-ray tube, during exposure.

In the study that reported negative findings, patients were imaged while facing the radiologist so that the radiation beam entered posteriorly. The breast tissue was exposed only to the low-intensity beam that exited the patient.

Additional studies have produced results suggesting that radiation-induced breast cancer developed in patients treated with x-rays for acute postpartum mastitis. The dose to these patients ranged from 0.75 to 10 Gy_t. The relative risk factor in this population was approximately 3:1.

Radiation-induced breast cancer has also been observed among atomic bomb survivors. Through 1980, observations on nearly 12,000 women who received radiation doses to the breasts of 100 mGy_t or more showed a relative risk of 4:1.

In some of these studies, only one breast was irradiated. In nearly every such case, breast cancer developed only in the irradiated breast. These patients have now been followed for up to 40 years. Based on all available data regarding radiation-induced breast cancer, the best estimate for attributable risk is 6×10^{-2} Sv^{-1}.

Early in the 20th century, it was observed that approximately 50% of workers in the Bohemian pitchblende mines of Germany died of **lung cancer**. Lung cancer incidence in the general population was negligible by comparison. The dusty mine environment was considered to be the cause of this lung cancer. Now it is known that radiation exposure from **radon** in the mines contributed to the incidence of lung cancer in these miners.

Observations of American uranium miners active in the Colorado Plateau in the 1950s and 1960s have also shown elevated levels of lung cancer. The peak of this activity occurred in the early 1960s, when approximately 5000 miners were active in nearly 500 underground mines and 150 open-pit mines. Most of the mines were worked by fewer than 10 men; therefore, for such a small operation, one could expect a lack of proper ventilation.

The radiation exposure in these mines occurred because of the high concentration of uranium ore. Uranium, which is radioactive with a very long half-life of 10^9 years, decays through a series of radioactive nuclides by successive alpha and beta emissions, each accompanied by gamma radiation.

> Radon is an alpha-emitting radionuclide that adsorbs dust particles that lodge in the alveolar spaces of the lung.

One of the decay products of uranium is radon (^{222}Rn). This radionuclide is a gas that emanates through the rock to produce a high concentration in air. When breathed, radon can be deposited in the lung, where it undergoes an additional series of decay to a stable isotope of lead. During these subsequent decay actions, several alpha particles are released, resulting in a rather high local dose. Also, alpha particles are high-LET radiation and therefore have a high RBE (see Chapter 32).

To date, more than 4000 uranium miners have been observed, and they have received estimated doses to lung tissue as high as 30 Gy$_t$; on this basis, the relative risk was approximately 8:1. It is interesting to note that smoking uranium miners have a relative risk of approximately 20:1. Americans continue to smoke cigarettes less and less. One result of this trend is that radon exposure is now the leading cause of lung cancer—42,000 cases of lung cancer each year are considered to be radon induced.

Thorium dioxide (ThO$_2$) in a colloidal suspension known as **Thorotrast** was widely used in diagnostic radiology between 1925 and 1945 as a contrast agent for angiography. Thorotrast was approximately 25% ThO$_2$ by weight, and it contained several radioactive isotopes of thorium and its decay products. Radiation that was emitted produced a dose in the ratio of approximately 100:10:1 of alpha, beta, and gamma radiation, respectively.

The use of Thorotrast has been shown to be responsible for several types of carcinoma after a latent period of approximately 15 to 20 years. After extravascular injection, it is carcinogenic at the site of the injection. After intravascular injection, ThO$_2$ particles are deposited in phagocytic cells of the reticuloendothelial system and are concentrated in the liver and spleen. Its half-life and high alpha radiation dose have resulted in many cases of cancer in these organs.

TOTAL RISK OF MALIGNANCY

Based on many of these observations on human population groups after exposure to low-level radiation, and considering all the risk estimates taken collectively for leukemia and cancer, a number of simplified conclusions can be made. The overall attributable risk for **induction** of malignancy is approximately 8 cases/100 persons/Sv, with the at-risk period extending for 20 to 25 years after exposure.

The risk of **death** from radiation-induced malignant disease is 5 cases/100 persons/Sv. Expressed more simply, an effective dose of 10 mSv—a single CT scan—carries a risk of approximately 8/10,000 for malignant disease induction, half of whom will not survive.

Nuclear Reactor Incidents

To make these values somewhat more meaningful, we can consider the celebrated Three Mile Island incident in 1979. Approximately 2 million people resided within an 80-km radius of Three Mile Island, on the Susquehanna River in Pennsylvania.

Based on population statistics, one would expect to observe approximately 330,000 cancer deaths in these persons. During the total period of the radiation incident, the average dose to persons living within a 160-km radius was 15 µGy$_t$; to those within the 80-km radius, it was 80 µGy$_t$.

By applying 15 µGy$_a$ as the population dose, one can predict that the Three Mile Island incident will result in no more than two additional malignant deaths as a result of this population radiation exposure. Clearly this response is not detectable in the face of approximately 330,000 natural cancer deaths in this population.

> **Predicted Radiation-Induced Deaths at Three Mile Island**
> 2 × 10^{-6} people × 5 deaths/100 Sv × 15 × 10^{-6} Sv = 1.5 deaths

Seven years after the Three Mile Island nuclear reactor incident, in 1986, a considerably more serious accident occurred at the Chernobyl nuclear power plant in Ukraine, at that time part of the USSR. The Chernobyl reactor incident was a result of operator error and the reactor design, which was based on a graphite moderator not encased in a containment vessel, as are all boiling water or pressurized water nuclear reactors.

This design allowed for the dispersal of a highly radioactive cloud resulting in radioactive fallout over a large area of western USSR and Europe. Thirty-one workers died following acute radiation syndrome. An additional 30 heavily exposed residents near the facility also suffered early deaths.

It is not known at this time exactly the extent of late stochastic radiation effects, but an exposed population numbering approximately 5 million continues to be followed. Estimates of malignant disease range to the tens of thousands. Only thyroid cancer, which is easily treated, has been positively identified as a radiation response.

> Working as an offshore oilfield worker is far more hazardous than as a nuclear power plant worker.

The Fukushima nuclear disaster of March 2011 was the result of a magnitude 9.0 earthquake and tsunami. Unlike Three Mile Island and Chernobyl, Fukushima involved six nuclear reactors. All of the reactors suffered damage, and reactors 1, 2, and 3 contributed to high radiation exposures and radioactive fallout over a sizable population. All were boiling water reactors, but several containment vessels were breached.

Two reactor workers died from acute radiation injury and some 50 other ill patients were confirmed later as accident victims. The scale of the population exposure is similar to that of Chernobyl and will certainly be followed for decades. However, the population radiation dose is so small that stochastic effects are not likely.

Biologic Effects of Ionizing Radiation Report

A committee of the National Academy of Sciences has reviewed the data on stochastic effects of low-dose, low-LET radiation and has issued a document known

TABLE 36.6	Biologic Effects of Ionizing Radiation Report Estimated Excess Mortality From Malignant Disease in 100,000 People	
	Male	**Female**
Normal expectation	20,560	16,680
Excess cases		
Single exposure to 100 mGy$_t$	770	810
Continuous exposure to 10 mGy$_t$/year	2880	3070
Continuous exposure to 1 mGy$_t$/year	520	600

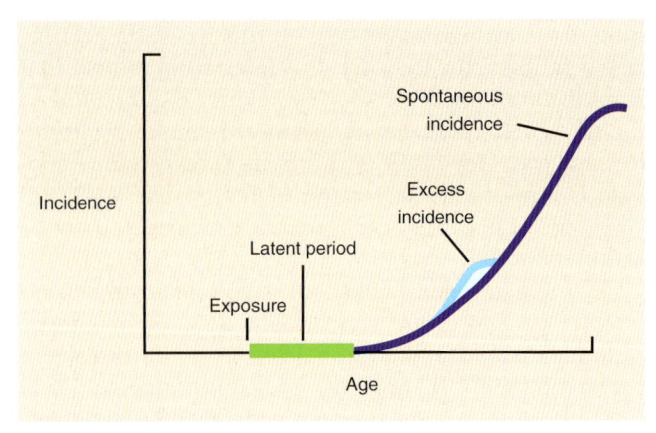

FIG. 36.9 Exposure at an early age can result in an excess bulge of cancer after a latent period.

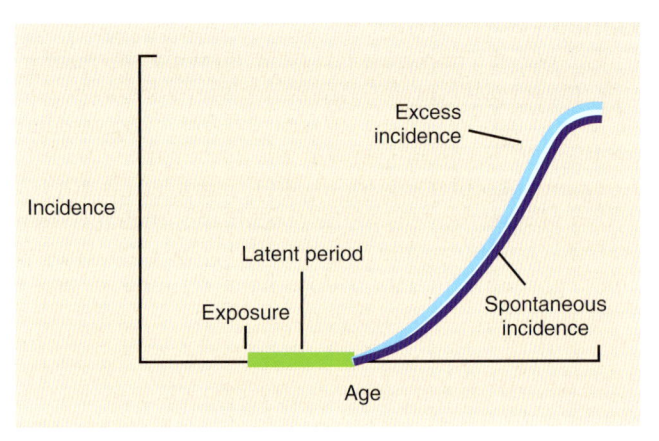

FIG. 36.10 The attributable risk model predicts that excess radiation-induced cancer risk is constant for life.

as the Biologic Effects of Ionizing Radiation (BEIR) Report. This report showed the results summarized in Table 36.6, which are considered authoritative.

BEIR Report authors examined three situations. First they estimated the excess mortality from a malignant disease after a one-time accidental exposure to 100 mGy$_t$; such a situation is highly unlikely in radiology. Second they considered the response to a dose of 10 mGy$_t$/year for life; this situation is possible in diagnostic radiology but is rare.

Finally they considered excess radiation-induced cancer mortality after a continuous dose of 1 mGy$_t$/year. This is still considerably higher than the experience of most radiologists and radiographers but can serve as a good upper limit of occupational radiation risk.

When a linear, nonthreshold dose-response relationship was assumed, these analyses showed an additional 800 cases of malignant disease death in a population of 100,000 after 100 mGy$_t$ and an additional 550 deaths after 1 mGy$_t$/year. These cases represent an addition to the normal incidence of cancer death, which is approximately 20,000 per 100,000 persons.

> The BEIR committee has further stated that because of the uncertainty in its analysis, less than 10 mGy$_t$ may not be harmful.

The BEIR committee also has analyzed available human data with regard to age at exposure, a limited time of expression of effects, and whether the response was **attributable** or **relative**. This requires additional definitions of these terms.

If one is irradiated at an early age and the response is limited in time, radiation-induced excess malignant disease appears as a bulge on the age-response relationship (Fig. 36.9). Childhood leukemia is a good example.

An attributable age-response relationship is shown in Fig. 36.10. Here the increased incidence of cancer is seen as a constant number of cases after a minimal latent period. Many subscribe to a relative age-response relationship, in which the increased incidence of cancer is proportional to the natural incidence (Fig. 36.11).

A 2022 report by the National Academies of Science, Engineering, and Medicine (NASEM) proposed activities in many areas, including radiology, for low-dose radiation research projects including radiology patients and personnel. NASEM identifies low radiation dose as less than 100 mGy$_t$, low radiation dose rate as less than 5 mGy$_t$/h.

> Low radiation dose < 100 mGy$_t$
> Low radiation dose rate < 5 mGy$_t$/h

Perhaps the best way to present these radiation risk data is to compare them with other known causes of death. As one might imagine, volumes of tables are available that analyze risk. This information is presented in a simplified form in Table 36.7.

Note that in these common situations, risk from radiation exposure is near the bottom of the list. Our actual occupational risk is even less because we use protective

CHAPTER 36 Stochastic Effects of Radiation

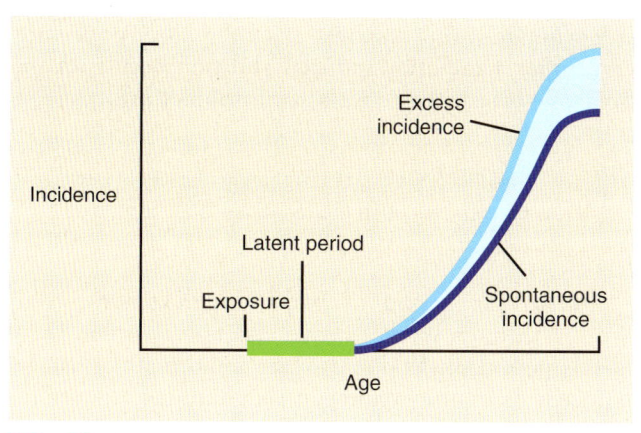

FIG. 36.11 The relative risk model predicts that excess radiation-induced cancer risk is proportional to the natural incidence.

TABLE 36.7	Average Annual Risk of Death From Various Causes
Cause	**Your Chance of Dying This Year**
All causes (all ages)	1 in 100
20 cigarettes per day	1 in 280
Heart disease	1 in 300
Cancer	1 in 520
All causes (25 years old)	1 in 700
Stroke	1 in 1200
Motor vehicle accident	1 in 4000
Drowning	1 in 30,000
Alcohol (light drinker)	1 in 50,000
Air travel	1 in 100,000
Radiation, 1 mSv	1 in 100,000
Texas Gulf Coast hurricane	1 in 4,500,000
Being a rodeo cowboy	1 in 6,200,000

apparel during fluoroscopy and because the radiation risk estimate assumes whole-body exposure.

RADIATION AND PREGNANCY

Since the first medical applications of x-rays, concern and apprehension have arisen regarding the effects of radiation before, during, and after pregnancy. Before pregnancy, the concern is interrupted fertility. During pregnancy, concern is directed to possible congenital effects in newborns. Postpregnancy concerns are related to suspected genetic effects. All these effects have been demonstrated in animals, and some have been observed in humans.

Effects on Fertility

The deterministic effect of high-level radiation on the interruption of fertility in both men and women was discussed earlier. Ample evidence shows that such an effect does occur and is radiation dose-related. The effects of low-dose, long-term irradiation on fertility, however, are less well defined.

Animal data in this area are lacking. Those that are available indicate that even when radiation is delivered at the rate of 1 Sv per year, no noticeable reduced fertility is noted.

> Low-dose, chronic irradiation does not impair fertility.

The health effects analysis of 150,000 American radiographers mentioned earlier has revealed no effect on fertility. The number of births that occurred during a 12-year sampling period equaled the number expected.

Irradiation In Utero

Irradiation in utero concerns the following two types of radiation exposures: that of the radiation worker and that of the patient. Recommended techniques and radiation control procedures associated with these exposed persons are considered fully in Chapters 41 and 42. Here we consider the biologic effects of such irradiation.

Substantial animal data are available to describe fairly completely the effects of relatively high doses of radiation delivered during various periods of gestation. Because the embryo is a rapidly developing cell system, it is particularly sensitive to radiation. With age, the embryo (and then the fetus) becomes less sensitive to the effects of radiation, and this pattern continues into adulthood.

After maturity has been reached, radiosensitivity increases with age. Fig. 36.12 summarizes the observed $LD_{50/60}$ in mice exposed at various times, showing this age-related radiosensitivity. Such findings are of particular concern because diagnostic x-ray exposure often occurs when pregnancy is unknown.

> All observations point to the first trimester during pregnancy as the most radiosensitive period.

The effects of ionizing radiation in utero are time-related and radiation dose related. They include prenatal death, neonatal death, congenital abnormalities, malignancy induction, general impairment of growth, genetic effects, and intellectual disability. Fig. 36.13 has been redrawn from studies designed to observe the effects of a 2-Gy_t dose delivered at various stages in utero in mice. The scale along the x-axis indicates the approximate comparable time in humans.

Within 2 weeks of fertilization, the most pronounced effect of a high radiation dose is prenatal death, which manifests as a spontaneous abortion. Observations in radiation therapy patients have confirmed this effect, but only after very high doses.

Based on animal experimentation, it would appear that this response is very rare. Our best estimate is that a 100-mGy$_t$ dose during the first 2 weeks will induce perhaps a 0.1% rate of spontaneous abortion. This occurs in addition to the 25% to 50% normal incidence of spontaneous abortions.

Fortunately, this response is of the all-or-none variety: Either a radiation-induced abortion occurs, or the pregnancy is carried to term with no ill effect.

> The first 2 weeks of pregnancy may be of least concern because the response is all or nothing.

During the period of **major organogenesis**, from Week 2 through Week 12, two effects may occur. Early in this period, skeletal and organ abnormalities can be induced. As major organogenesis continues, congenital abnormalities of the central nervous system may be observed if the pregnancy is carried to term.

If radiation-induced congenital abnormalities are severe enough, the result will be neonatal death. After a dose of 2 Gy$_t$ to the mouse, nearly 100% of fetuses suffered significant abnormalities. In 80%, this was sufficient to cause neonatal death.

Such effects are rare after diagnostic levels of radiation exposure and are essentially undetectable after radiation doses of less than 100 mGy$_t$. A dose of 100 mGy$_t$ during organogenesis is expected to increase the incidence of congenital abnormalities by 1% above the natural incidence. To complicate matters, an approximate 5% incidence of naturally occurring congenital abnormalities occurs in the unexposed population.

Irradiation in utero at the human level has been associated with childhood malignancy by several investigators. Perhaps the most complete study of this effect was conducted by Alice Stewart and coworkers in a project known as the Oxford Survey, a study of childhood malignancy in England, Scotland, and Wales.

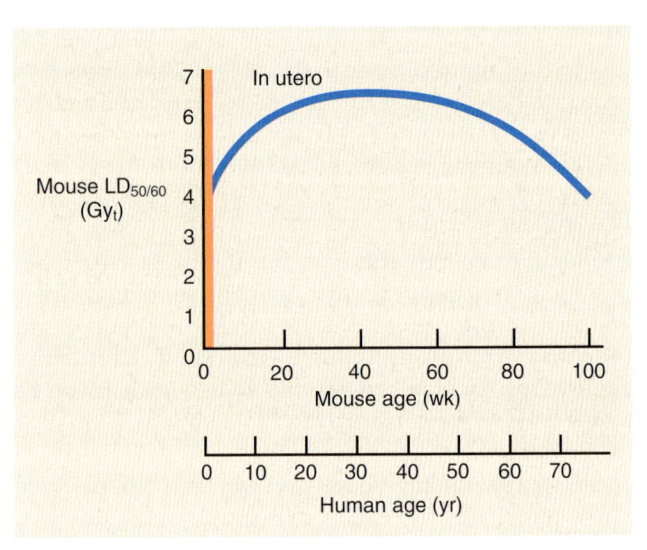

FIG. 36.12 LD$_{50/60}$ of mice in relation to age at the time of irradiation.

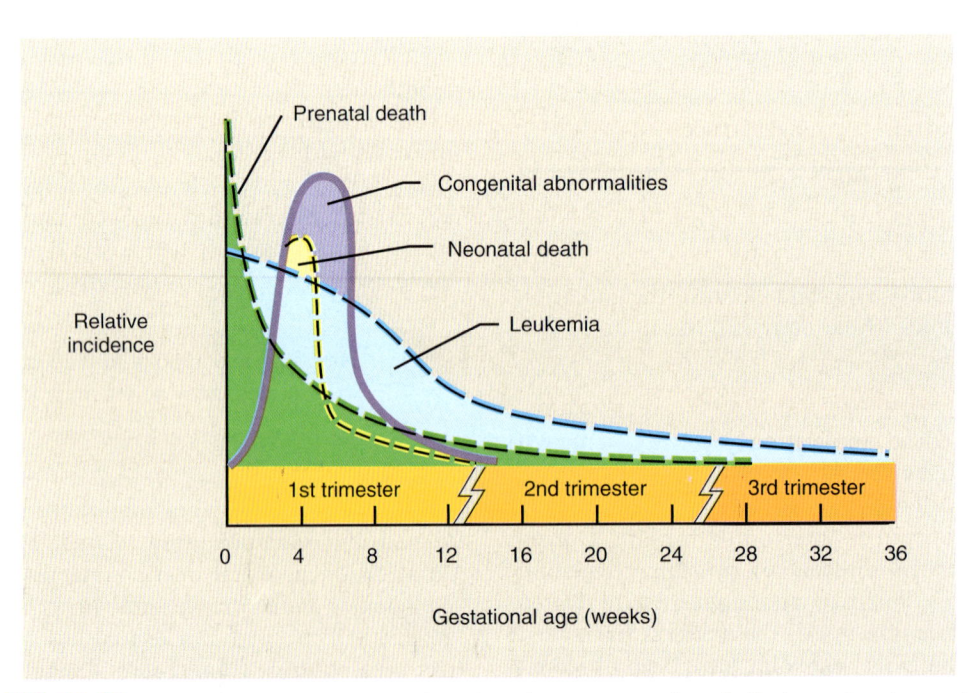

FIG. 36.13 After 2 Gy$_a$ are delivered at various times in utero, a number of effects can be observed.

TABLE 36.8	Relative Risk of Childhood Leukemia After Irradiation in Utero by Trimester
Time of X-Ray Examination	**Relative Risk**
First trimester	8.3
Second trimester	1.5
Third trimester	1.4
Total	1.5

TABLE 36.9	Summary of Effects After 100 mGy$_t$ In Utero		
Time of Exposure	**Type of Response**	**Natural Occurrence**	**Radiation Response**
0–2 weeks	Spontaneous abortion	25%	0.1%
2–10 weeks	Congenital abnormalities	5%	1%
2–15 weeks	Intellectual disability	6%	0.5%
0–9 months	Malignant disease	8/10,000	12/10,000
0–9 months	Impaired growth and development	1%	Nil
0–9 months	Genetic mutation	10%	Nil

Nearly every such case of childhood malignancy in these countries since 1946 has been investigated. Each case was first identified and then investigated by an interview with the mother, a review of the hospital charts, and a review of the physician records.

Each "case" of childhood malignancy was matched with a "control" for age, sex, place of birth, socioeconomic status, and other demographic factors. The control subject was a child who matched with the "case" in all respects, except that the control did not have cancer or leukemia. The Oxford Survey is being continued at this time and has now considered more than 10,000 cases and a similar number of matched control subjects.

Although the Oxford Survey has reviewed all malignancies, the findings of radiation-induced leukemia have been of particular importance. Table 36.8 shows the results of this survey in terms of relative risk.

> The relative risk of childhood leukemia after irradiation in utero is 1.5.

A relative risk of 1.5 for the development of childhood leukemia after irradiation in utero is significant. This indicates an increase of 50% over the nonirradiated rate. The number of cases involved, however, is small.

The incidence of childhood leukemia in the population at large is approximately 9 cases per 100,000 live births. According to the Oxford Survey, if all 100,000 had been irradiated in utero, perhaps 14 cases of leukemia would have resulted. Although these findings have been substantiated in several American populations, no consensus has been reached among radiobiologists that this effect after such low doses is indeed real.

Other effects after irradiation in utero have been studied rather fully in animals and have been observed in some human populations. An unexpected finding in the offspring of atomic bomb survivors is intellectual disability. Children of exposed mothers performed poorly on IQ tests and demonstrated poor scholastic performance compared with unexposed Japanese children.

These differences are marginal, yet significant. When assessment is based on test scores, measurable intellectual disability is apparent in approximately 6% of all children. A 100-mGy$_t$ dose in utero is expected to increase this incidence by an additional 0.5%.

> Radiation exposure in utero does retard the growth and development of the newborn.

Irradiation in utero, principally during the period of major organogenesis, has been associated with microcephaly (small head) and, as discussed, intellectual disability. Human data bearing on these effects have been obtained from patients irradiated medically, atomic bomb survivors, and residents of the Marshall Islands who were exposed to radioactive fallout in 1954 during weapons testing.

These effects, as well as intellectual disability, have been observed principally in those receiving doses in excess of 1 Gy$_t$ in utero. The lack of appropriate and sensitive tests of mental function makes it impossible to draw similar conclusions at doses below 1 Gy$_t$.

A summary of the effects of irradiation in utero is given in Table 36.9. Four responses of concern to radiology have been identified: spontaneous abortion, congenital abnormalities, intellectual disability, and childhood malignancy.

> Spontaneous abortion causes the least concern because it is an all-or-none effect.

Congenital abnormalities, intellectual disability, and childhood malignancy are of real concern, but it should be recognized that the probability of such a response after a fetal dose of 100 mGy$_t$ is nil. Furthermore 100 mGy$_t$ to the fetus very rarely occurs in radiology. It is essentially possible only during fluoroscopy and CT, not radiography or nuclear medicine.

The form of the dose-response relationship for each of these effects is unknown. However several appear to be linear and nonthreshold when based on doses greater than 1 Gy$_t$. When large experimental animal populations were acutely exposed, the minimum reported dose at which such effects were observed as statistically significant was approximately 100 mGy$_t$.

No evidence in humans or animals indicates that the levels of radiation exposure currently experienced occupationally and medically are responsible for any such effects on growth and development.

Although our efforts in protecting the unborn from the harmful effects of radiation are principally directed at diagnostic x-ray exposures, we also must be aware of similar hazards resulting from radioisotope examinations. For example, radioiodine is known to concentrate principally in the thyroid gland. After the administration of radioactive iodine, the dose to thyroid tissue will be several orders of magnitude higher than the whole-body dose because of this organ concentration effect.

The thyroid gland begins to function at approximately 10 weeks of gestation, and because radioiodine readily crosses the placental barrier from the mother's blood to the fetal circulation, radioiodine should be administered during pregnancy only in trace doses and before the 10-week gestation period begins. At any time thereafter, the hazard of such administration increases.

Genetic Effects

Unfortunately our weakest area of knowledge in radiation biology is the area of radiation genetics. Essentially all the data indicating that radiation causes genetic effects have come from large-scale experiments with flies or mice.

> We do not have any data that suggest that radiation-induced genetic effects occur in humans.

Observations of the atomic bomb survivors have shown no radiation-induced genetic effects, and descendants of survivors are now into the fourth generation. Other human populations have likewise provided only negative results. Consequently, in the absence of accurate human data, there is no choice but to rely on information from experimental laboratory studies.

In 1927, the Nobel Prize–winning geneticist H.J. Muller from the University of Texas reported the results of his irradiation of *Drosophila*, the fruit fly. He irradiated mature flies before procreation and then measured the frequency of lethal mutations among the offspring. The radiation doses used were hundreds of gray, but as

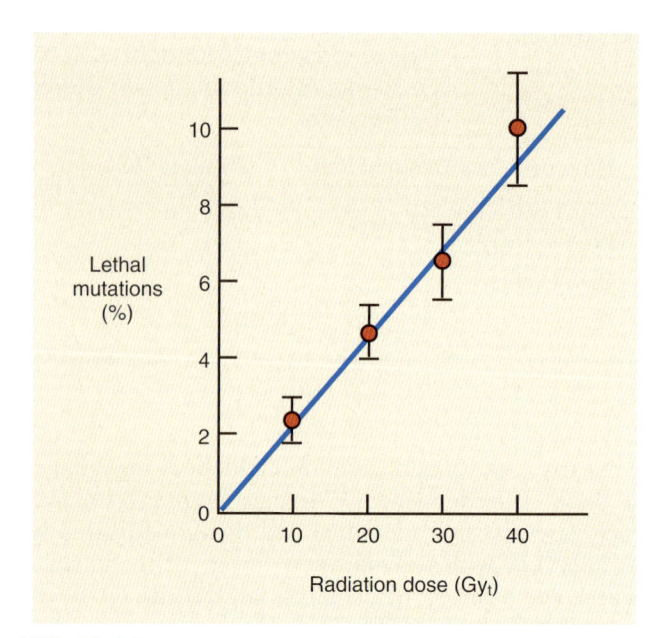

FIG. 36.14 Irradiation of flies by H.J. Muller showed the genetic effects to be linear, nonthreshold. Note that the doses were exceedingly high.

the data in Fig. 36.14 show, the dose-response relationship for radiation-induced genetic damage is unmistakably linear and nonthreshold.

Based on Muller's studies, other conclusions were drawn. Radiation does not alter the type of mutations but rather increases the frequency of those mutations that are observed spontaneously. Muller's data showed no dose rate or dose fractionation effects. Hence he concluded that such mutations were single-hit phenomena.

It was principally based on Muller's work that the National Council on Radiation Protection and Measurements in 1932 lowered the recommended occupational radiation dose limit and acknowledged officially for the first time the existence of nonthreshold radiation effects. Since then, all radiation protection guides have assumed a linear, nonthreshold dose-response relationship and have been based on the suspected genetic, as well as somatic, effects of radiation.

The only other experimental work of any significance is that of the Russells. Beginning in 1946, Lillian and Bill Russell began to irradiate a large mouse colony with radiation dose rates that varied from 0.01 to 900 mGy$_t$/min and total doses up to 10 Gy$_t$.

These studies are ongoing, and observations now have been reported on more than 8 million mice! The experiment requires the observation of seven specific genes that control readily recognizable characteristics, such as ear shape, coat color, and eye color.

The Russell data shows that a dose rate effect does exist; this would indicate that the mouse has the capacity to repair genetic damage. They have confirmed the linear, nonthreshold form of the dose-response relationship and have not detected any types of mutations that did not occur naturally.

TABLE 36.10	Additional Conclusions Regarding Radiation Genetics

- Radiation-induced mutations are usually harmful.
- Any dose of radiation, however small, to a germ cell results in some genetic risk.
- The frequency of radiation-induced mutations is directly proportional to dose so that a linear extrapolation of data obtained at high doses provides a valid estimate of low-dose effects.
- The effect depends on radiation protraction and fractionation.
- For most pre-reproductive life, the woman is less sensitive than the man to the genetic effects of radiation.
- Most radiation-induced mutations are recessive. These require that the mutant genes must be present in both the male and the female to produce the trait. Consequently, such mutations may not be expressed for many generations.
- The frequency of radiation-induced genetic mutations is extremely low. It is approximately 10^{-5} mutations/Gy_t/gene.

The average mutation rate per unit dose in the mouse is approximately 15 times that observed in the fruit fly. Whether an increased sensitivity exists in humans relative to the mouse is unknown.

> The doubling dose is that dose of radiation that produces twice the frequency of genetic mutations as would have been observed without the radiation.

From these experimental studies, the concept of the **doubling dose** has been developed. The genetic doubling dose in humans is estimated to lie in the range between 0.5 and 2.5 Gy_t.

So, what is the significance of all this in our daily practice? What is the significance for patients or for radiologists or for radiographers? First, it can be said with certainty that the incidence of radiation-induced genetic mutations after the levels of exposure experienced in digital imaging is essentially zero (Table 36.10).

Under nearly all such diagnostic exposures, no action is required; however, should a high radiation dose be experienced (e.g., in excess of 100 mGy_t), some protective action may be required. The prefertilized egg, in its various stages, exhibits a constant sensitivity to radiation; however it also demonstrates some capacity for the repair of genetic damage.

If repair occurs, it is rapid; therefore a delay in procreation of only a few days may be appropriate. In the male, in contrast, it might be prudent to refrain from procreation for a period of 60 days to allow cells that were in a resistant stage of development at the time of exposure to mature to functioning spermatids.

SUMMARY

The stochastic effects of radiation exposure occur a long time after exposure. Stochastic effects can result from high-dose, short-term exposure, but the concern in digital imaging involves low-dose exposures over time.

Many epidemiologic studies have reported positive results; however problems include the following: (1) the exact dose usually is not known, and (2) the frequency of observable response is low. With stochastic effects, the incidence of response is dose related and no dose threshold is evident.

Local tissues can be affected by low-dose radiation. Stochastic effects appear as nonmalignant changes in the skin. The skin shows a weathered, callused, and discolored appearance. Chromosome damage in circulating lymphocytes has been observed as stochastic effects of radiation exposure.

Because radiation dose-response relationships are not precise when stochastic effects of radiation exposure are observed, risk estimates are used to estimate radiation response in a population. Relative risk is calculated when the population's radiation dose is not known. Excess risk determines the magnitude of the stochastic effect as the difference between cases and control subjects. Attributable risk is most useful.

The effects of low-dose, long-term irradiation in utero can include the following: prenatal death, neonatal death, congenital abnormalities, malignancy, impaired growth, genetic effects, and intellectual disability. However, these abnormalities are based on doses greater than 1 Gy_t, with minimum reported doses in animal experiments at approximately 100 mGy_t. No evidence at the human or animal level indicates that the levels of radiation exposure currently experienced occupationally or medically are responsible for any such effects on fetal growth or development.

CHALLENGE QUESTIONS

1. Define or otherwise identify the following:
   a. Epidemiology
   b. In utero
   c. Attributable risk
   d. Thorotrast
   e. Major organogenesis
   f. The Oxford Survey
   g. H.J. Muller
   h. Genetic doubling dose
   i. Radon (^{222}Rn)
   j. Radium watch-dial painters
2. What population experienced radiation-induced cataracts?
3. What is the risk of life-span shortening for radiation workers?
4. What is the significance of the change in death statistics of American radiologists from the 1935 to

1944 time period to the 1955 to 1958 time period?
5. Approximately 300,000 radiographers are working in the United States, and their annual exposure is 0.5 mSv. If a 40-year working period is assumed, how many are likely to die from occupational radiation exposure?
6. What is the attributable risk when three cases of radiation-induced leukemia develop per year in 100,000 persons after an average dose of 20 mGy$_t$?
7. When should attributable risk be used as the preferable risk index?
8. Twenty million people in Scandinavia were exposed to an average of 7 μGy$_t$ as a result of Chernobyl. If an attributable risk of 10 cases/10^4/Gy$_t$/year over a 30-year period is assumed, how many malignancies will be induced?
9. What is the suspected reason why American radiologists have an elevated risk for leukemia?
10. Discuss the experience of radiation-induced leukemia in patients with ankylosing spondylitis.
11. Why was the thymus gland irradiated in the Ann Arbor and Rochester series? What were the late effects of the thymus irradiation?
12. Discuss the way that bone cancer developed in watch-dial painters in the 1920s and 1930s.
13. Explain the risk of radon gas to uranium miners.
14. During the period of the Three Mile Island incident, what was the average dose to persons living within a 200-km radius of the nuclear plant?
15. What are the effects on fertility caused by low-dose, long-term irradiation?
16. Is it true that most radiation-induced mutations are recessive?
17. In a population of 30,367 irradiated persons, 13 cases of leukemia developed; in a control population of 86,672 persons, 31 cases of leukemia developed. What was the relative risk?
18. What is the attributable risk if 32 cases of leukemia develop per year in 100,000 persons after an average dose of 20 mGy$_t$?
19. How many cases of radiation-induced leukemia are suspected to have occurred among atomic bomb survivors?
20. What is the difference between relative risk and excess risk?

The answers to the Challenge Questions can be found by logging on to our website at http://evolve.elsevier.com.

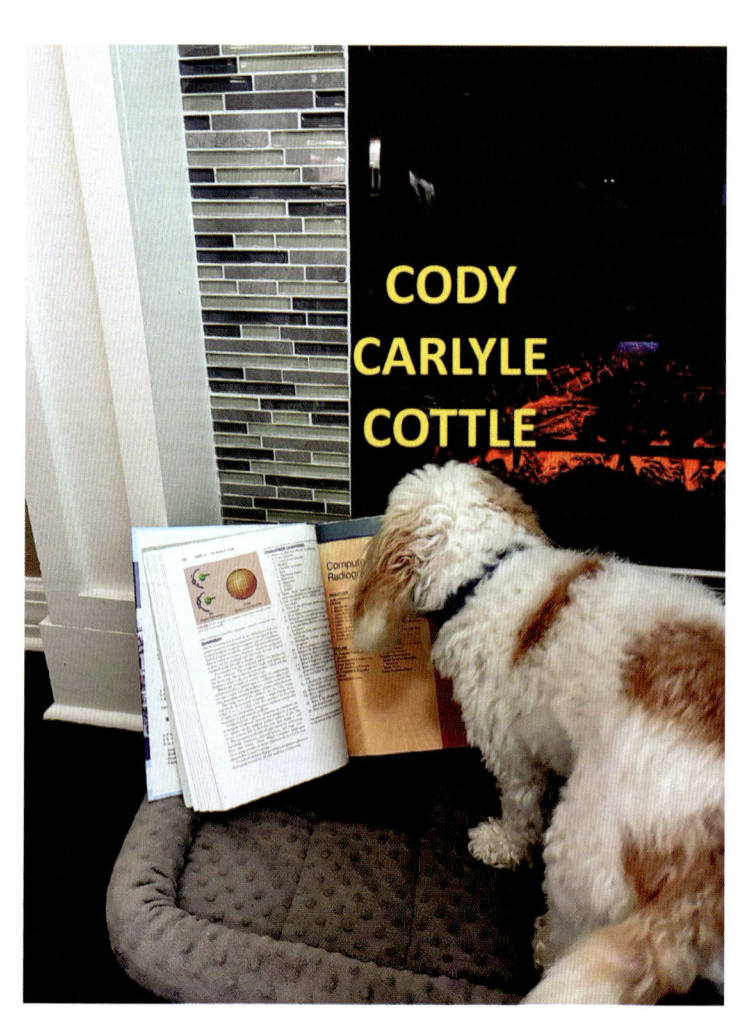

PART VIII

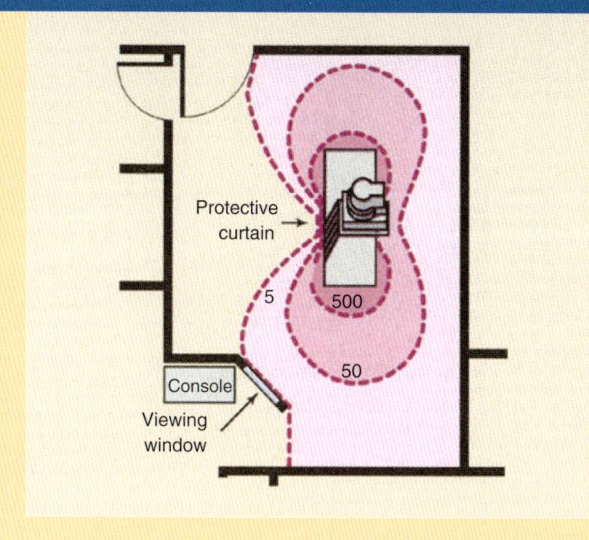

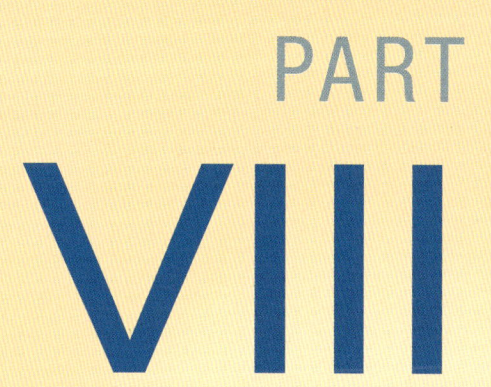

RADIATION PROTECTION

CHAPTER 37

Health Physics

OBJECTIVES

At the completion of this chapter, the student should be able to do the following:

1. Define health physics.
2. List the cardinal principles of radiation protection.
3. Explain the National Council on Radiation Protection and Measurements and the concept of dose limits.
4. Name the recommended dose limits for radiation workers and for the public.
5. Discuss the concept of ALARA (as low as reasonably achievable).
6. How do the three radiologic terrorism devices differ?

OUTLINE

Radiation and Health 501
Cardinal Principles of Radiation Protection 501
  Minimize Time 501
  Maximize Distance 503
  Use Shielding 504
Effective Dose 505
Radiologic Terrorism 507
Radiologic Devices 507
Radiation Protection Guidance 507
Radiation Detection and Measurement Equipment 508
Summary 508
Challenge Questions 508

IMMEDIATELY AFTER their discovery, x-rays were applied to the healing arts. It was recognized within months; however, that radiation could cause harmful effects.

The first American fatality that resulted from radiation exposure was Thomas Edison's assistant, Clarence Dally. Since that event, a great deal of effort has been devoted to developing equipment, techniques, and procedures to control radiation levels and reduce unnecessary radiation exposure to radiation workers and to the public.

The cardinal principles for radiation protection are simplified rules designed to ensure safety in radiation areas for occupational workers. In 1931 the first dose-limiting recommendations were made. Today the National Council on Radiation Protection and Measurements (NCRP) continuously reviews the recommended dose limits.

Providing radiation protection for workers and the public is the practice of **health physics**. Health physicists design equipment, calculate and construct barriers, and develop administrative protocols to maintain radiation exposures **as low as reasonably achievable (ALARA)**. That is the substance of this chapter.

The term *health physics* was coined during the early days of the Manhattan Project, the secret wartime effort to develop the atomic bomb. The group of physicists and physicians responsible for the radiation safety of persons involved in the production of atomic bombs were the first health physicists. Thus the health physicist is a radiation scientist who is concerned with the research, teaching, or operational aspects of radiation safety.

RADIATION AND HEALTH

At the turn of the millennium, the year 2000, the National Academy of Sciences identified the 20 greatest scientific and technical accomplishments of the 20th century. Medical imaging was number 14 on this list.

This is important to point out to our patients, many of whom remain wary of radiation. One never reads the word "radiation" in a newspaper or a magazine without the modifier "dangerous," "deadly," or "harmful."

> Health physics is concerned with providing occupational radiation protection and minimizing radiation dose to the public.

We practice ALARA in response to our acceptance of the linear nonthreshold (LNT) radiation dose-response relationship as the most representative for stochastic effects—cancer, leukemia, and genetic effects. Yet we should also recognize that we actually employ low levels of radiation in digital imaging.

Unquestionably the application of this radiation has had a major impact on our health and increasing longevity. If you had been born in the United States in 1900, your life expectancy was 47 years. During the first century of diagnostic x-ray imaging, life expectancy has soared (Fig. 37.1).

Nevertheless, because of LNT, we must continue to be aware of patient and occupational radiation dose and must take those steps necessary to implement ALARA.

CARDINAL PRINCIPLES OF RADIATION PROTECTION

All health physics activity in radiology is designed to minimize the radiation dose to patients (mGy_t) and the radiation exposure of personnel (mGy_a). Three cardinal principles of radiation protection developed for nuclear activities—**time, distance,** and **shielding**—were adopted early on for digital imaging. When these cardinal principles are observed, patient radiation dose and occupational radiation exposure can be minimized (Table 37.1).

Minimize Time

The radiation exposure of personnel is directly related to the duration of the exposure. If the time during which one is exposed to radiation is doubled, the exposure is also doubled, as follows:

> **EXPOSURE TIME**
> Exposure = Exposure rate × Exposure time

Question: A radiographer is exposed to 2.3 mGy_a/h during fluoroscopy. If the radiographer remains in that position for 36 minutes, what will be the total occupational radiation exposure?

Answer:
$$\text{Exposure} = 2.3 \text{ mGy}_a/\text{h} \times \frac{36 \text{ min}}{60 \text{ min/h}}$$
$$= 1.38 \text{ mGy}_a$$

Question: The parent of an infant patient is asked to remain next to the patient during fluoroscopy, where the radiation exposure level is 6 mGy_a/h. If the allowable daily radiation exposure is 0.5 Gy_a, how long may the parent remain (Fig. 37.2)?

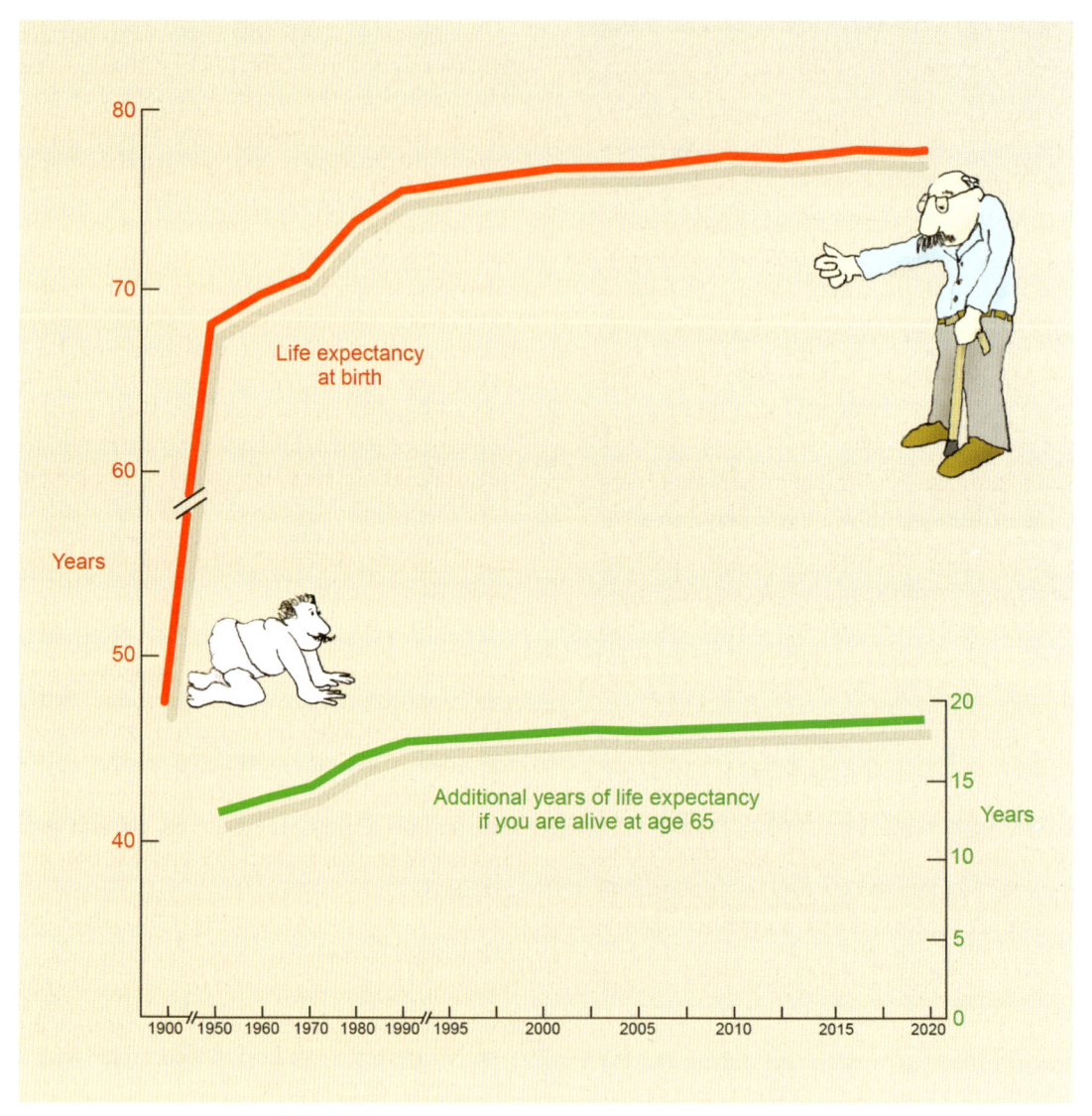

FIG. 37.1 Life expectancy as a function of year of birth.

TABLE 37.1	Cardinal Principles of Radiation Protection

- Keep the time of exposure to radiation as short as possible.
- Maintain as large a distance as possible between the source of radiation and the exposed person.
- Insert shielding material between the radiation source and the exposed person.

Answer: Time = Exposure ÷ Exposure rate
= 0.5 mGy$_a$ ÷ 6 mGy$_a$
= 1/12 hour
= 5 mintues

During radiography, the time of radiation exposure is kept to a minimum to reduce motion blur. During fluoroscopy, the time of radiation exposure also should be kept to a minimum to reduce patient radiation dose and personnel radiation exposure. This is an area of radiation protection that is not directly controlled by the radiographer.

Radiologists are trained to depress the fluoroscopic foot switch in an alternating fashion, sequencing **on-off** rather than continuously on during the course of the examination. A repeated up-and-down motion on the fluoroscopic foot switch permits a high-quality examination to be performed with considerably reduced patient radiation dose. Pulse-progressive fluoroscopy should be used (see Chapter 20).

The use of pulse-progressive fluoroscopy can reduce patient radiation dose considerably.

The **5-minute reset timer** on all fluoroscopes reminds the radiologist that a considerable amount

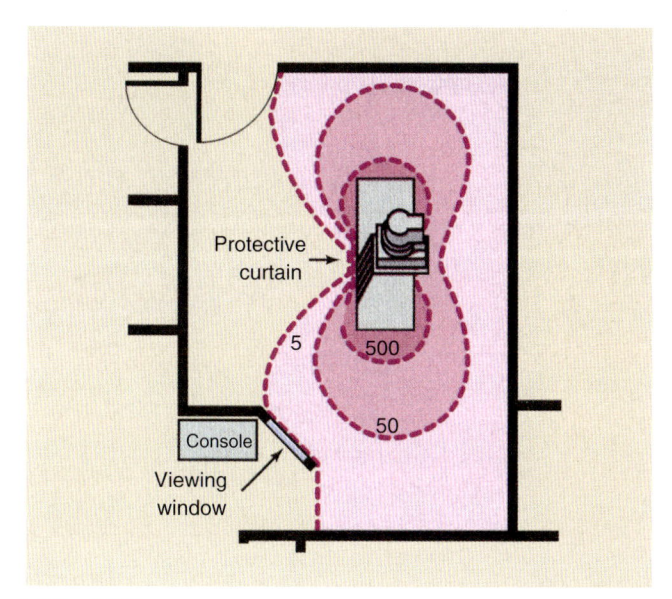

FIG. 37.2 Typical isoexposure contours during fluoroscopic examination (mGy$_a$/h).

of fluoroscopic time has elapsed. The timer records the amount of x-ray beam on time. Most fluoroscopic examinations take less than 5 minutes.

Only during difficult interventional radiology procedures should it be necessary to exceed 5 minutes of exposure time. A particular hazard lies in the use of mobile fluoroscopes in surgical suites where some physicians are less radiation conscious.

Question: A fluoroscope emits 42 mGy$_a$/min at the tabletop for every milliampere of operation. What is the patient radiation exposure in a barium enema examination that is conducted at 1.8 mA and requires 2.5 minutes of fluoroscopic x-ray exposure time?

Answer: Patient radiation exposure

$$= \left(\frac{42 \text{ mGy}_a}{\text{mA/min}}\right)(1.8 \text{ mA})(2.5 \text{ min})$$

$$= 189 \text{ mGy}_a$$

Maximize Distance

As the distance between the source of radiation and a person increases, radiation exposure decreases rapidly. This decrease in exposure is calculated using the inverse square law, which was discussed in Chapter 4.

> If the distance from the source exceeds five times the source diameter, it can be treated as a point source.

Most radiation sources are point sources. The x-ray tube target, for example, is a point source of radiation. The scattered radiation generated in a patient appears, however, to come not from a point source but rather from an extended area source. As a rule of thumb, even an extended source can be considered a point source at sufficient distance.

Earlier, when the square law was used to calculate exposure in radiographic technique, the following formula may have been used:

$$\frac{\text{New exposure}}{\text{Old exposure}} = \frac{\text{New distance squared}}{\text{Old distance squared}}$$

In this case, the radiation exposure from the x-ray tube was so varied that the exposure to the image receptor remained constant.

When the inverse square law is used in calculations for radiation protection, it is usual to calculate the dose received at a point with the radiation from the x-ray tube as the constant. Thus the formula becomes:

> **DISTANCE**
>
> $$\frac{\text{New exposure}}{\text{Old exposure}} = \frac{\text{New distance squared}}{\text{Old distance squared}}$$
>
> Note that the "distance" part of the equation is reversed. Assume a point source and apply the inverse square law.

Question: An x-ray tube has an output intensity of 26 mGy$_a$/mAs at 100-cm source-to-image receptor distance (SID) when operated at 70 kVp. What would be the radiation exposure 350 cm from the target?

Answer:

$$\frac{I_1}{I_2} = \frac{d_2^{\,2}}{d_1^{\,2}}$$

$$I_2 = I_1 \frac{d_1^{\,2}}{d_2^{\,2}}$$

$$= (26 \text{ mGy}_a/\text{mAs})\left(\frac{100 \text{ cm}}{350 \text{ cm}}\right)^2$$

$$= (26 \text{ mGy}_a/\text{mAs})(0.082)$$

$$= 2.1 \text{ mGy}_a/\text{mAs}$$

In radiography, the distance from a radiation source to a patient usually is fixed by the type of examination, and the radiographer is positioned behind a protective barrier.

During fluoroscopy, the radiographer can exercise good radiation protection procedures. Fig. 37.2 shows approximate radiation exposure levels at waist height during a **fluoroscopic** examination. The lines on the plot plan, called **isoexposure lines**, represent positions of equal radiation exposure in the fluoroscopy room. At the normal position, shielded by the protective curtain, for a radiologist or a radiographer, the exposure rate is approximately 1 to 5 mGy$_a$/h.

> During fluoroscopy, the radiographer should remain as far from the patient as practical.

During portions of the fluoroscopic examination, when it is not necessary for the radiographer to remain close to the patient, the radiographer should step back. Two steps back, the exposure rate is only approximately 50 μGy$_a$/h. This reduction in exposure does not follow the inverse square law because during fluoroscopy, the patient is an extended source of radiation due to scattered x-rays generated within the body.

Question: What is the approximate occupational exposure of a radiographer at a position where the exposure rate is 3 mGy$_a$/h, and farther back where the exposure rate is 0.2 mGy$_a$, during a fluoroscopic examination that lasts 4 minutes, 15 seconds?

Answer: Occupational exposure equals:
First position: (3 mGy$_a$/h)(4.25 min) (1 h/60 min) = 0.21 mGy$_a$
Second position: (0.2 mGy$_a$/h)(4.25 min) (1 h/60 min) = 0.014 mGy$_a$ = 14 μGy$_a$

Better yet, after taking two steps back to take advantage of "maximize distance," then take one step to the side and get behind the radiologist (Fig. 37.3)! This move results in additional shielding, and the exposure at that position will be zero. Besides, the radiologist is the one being paid the big bucks for this additional occupational radiation exposure!

Use Shielding

Positioning shielding between the radiation source and exposed persons greatly reduces the level of radiation exposure. Shielding used in diagnostic radiology usually consists of lead, although conventional building materials also are used.

The amount that a protective barrier reduces radiation intensity can be estimated if the half-value layer (HVL) or the tenth-value layer (TVL) of the barrier material is known. The HVL was defined and discussed in Chapter 9. The TVL is similarly defined as follows.

> One TVL is the thickness of the absorber that reduces the radiation intensity to one-tenth of its original value.

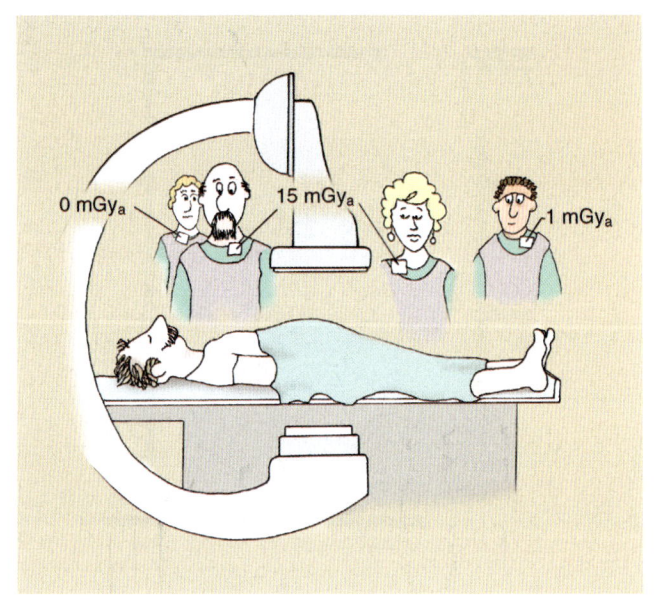

FIG. 37.3 Three positions for the technologist to assume during fluoroscopy and the approximate response of a collar-positioned occupational radiation monitor for a 5-minute procedure.

Table 37.2 shows approximate HVLs and TVLs for lead and concrete for diagnostic x-ray beams between 40 and 150 kVp.

Question: When operated at 80 kVp, an x-ray imaging system emits 36 μGy$_a$/mAs at an SID of 100 cm. How much shielding (concrete or lead) would be required to reduce the intensity to less than 2.5 μGy$_a$/mAs?

Answer: The amount of shielding in the first or second column of the following data reduces the beam intensity to the value in the third column. The last row is the answer.

Pb (mm)	Concrete (cm)	Beam intensity (μGya/mAs)
0	0	36
0.19	1.1	18
0.38	2.2	9.0
0.57	3.3	4.5
0.76	4.4	2.3

Question: An x-ray imaging system is used strictly for chest radiography at 125 kVp. The useful beam is always directed to a wall that contains 0.8-mm Pb shielding. How much additional shielding will be required if the workload doubles?

Answer: When the workload doubles, so does the exposure on the other side of the wall. From Table 37.2, it can be seen that 1 HVL, or 0.27-mm Pb, is necessary to reduce exposure to its original level.

CHAPTER 37 Health Physics

TABLE 37.2 Approximate Half-Value and Tenth-Value Layer of Lead and Concrete at Various X-ray Tube Potentials

Tube Potential (kVp)	HVL Lead (mm)	HVL Concrete (cm)	TVL Lead (mm)	TVL Concrete (cm)
40	0.03	0.33	0.06	1.0
60	0.11	0.64	0.34	2.2
80	0.19	1.1	0.64	3.6
100	0.24	1.5	0.80	5.1
125	0.27	2.0	0.90	6.4
150	0.28	2.2	0.95	7.1

HVL, Half-value layer; *TVL*, Tenth-value layer.

Another example of the application of shielding in radiology is the use of protective apparel. Protective aprons usually contain 0.5-mm Pb. This is approximately equivalent to 2 HVLs, which should reduce occupational exposure to 25%. Actual measurements show that such protective aprons reduce exposure to approximately 10% because scattered x-rays are incident on the apron at an oblique angle.

> 1 TVL = 3.3 HVLs

Usually the application of the cardinal principles of radiation protection involves the consideration of all three. The typical problem involves a known radiation level at a given distance from the source. The level of exposure at any other distance, behind any shielding, for any length of time can be calculated. The order in which these calculations are made makes no difference.

Question: The kVp of a radiographic imaging system rarely exceeds 100 kVp. The output intensity is 46 µGy$_a$/mAs at 100-cm SID. The distance to a desk on the other side of the wall to which the x-ray beam is directed is 200 cm. The wall contains 0.96-mm Pb, and 300 mAs is anticipated daily. If the exposure is to be restricted to 20 µGy$_a$/wk, how long each day may the desk be occupied?

Answer: Daily x-ray output at 100 cm =
(46 µGy$_a$/mAs)(300 mAs) = 13.8 mGy$_a$
Daily output at 200 cm =
(13.8) (100/200)^2 = 3.45 mGy$_a$
Daily output behind 0.96-mm Pb or 4 HVLs = 1.1 mGy$_a$
= 1100 µGy$_a$
Time allowed = 20 µGy$_a$/1100 µGy$_a$/wk
= 0.018 week = 43 minutes

However, this analysis does not take into account the x-ray beam attenuation by the patient, which is approximately 2 TVLs or 0.01. Therefore:

Daily output behind 0.96−mm Pb and the
patient = $(1100\ \mu Gy_a)(0.01) = 11\ \mu Gy_a$

$$\text{Today allowed} = \frac{20\ \mu Gy_a}{11\ \mu Gy_a/wk}$$

= 1.8 weeks (unlimited)

Question: Suppose an analysis shows that if an administrator remains at her desk for longer than 24 minutes each week, the occupational dose limit will be exceeded. How much additional protective lead would be required?

Answer: Full occupancy is 40 h × 60 min/h = 2400 min

$$\frac{24\ \text{min}}{2400\ \text{min}} = 0.01$$

That is, 2 TVLs or an additional 1.6-mm Pb.

Fig. 37.4 illustrates the use of these cardinal principles of radiation protection during a typical clinical situation.

EFFECTIVE DOSE

It is relatively easy to measure patient radiation dose during digital imaging. However digital imaging involves partial-body exposure. Radiographic images are collimated to the tissue of importance; therefore the total body is not exposed.

Radiation risk coefficients are based on total body radiation exposure, as for the atomic bomb survivors of Hiroshima and Nagasaki. When only part of the body is exposed, as in digital imaging, the risk of a stochastic radiation response is not proportional to the tissue dose but rather proportional to the **effective dose (E)**.

> Effective dose is the equivalent whole-body radiation dose following partial-body radiation exposure.

The equivalent whole-body radiation dose is the weighted average of the radiation dose to various organs and tissues. The NCRP has identified various tissues and organs and the relative radiosensitivity of each (Table 37.3).

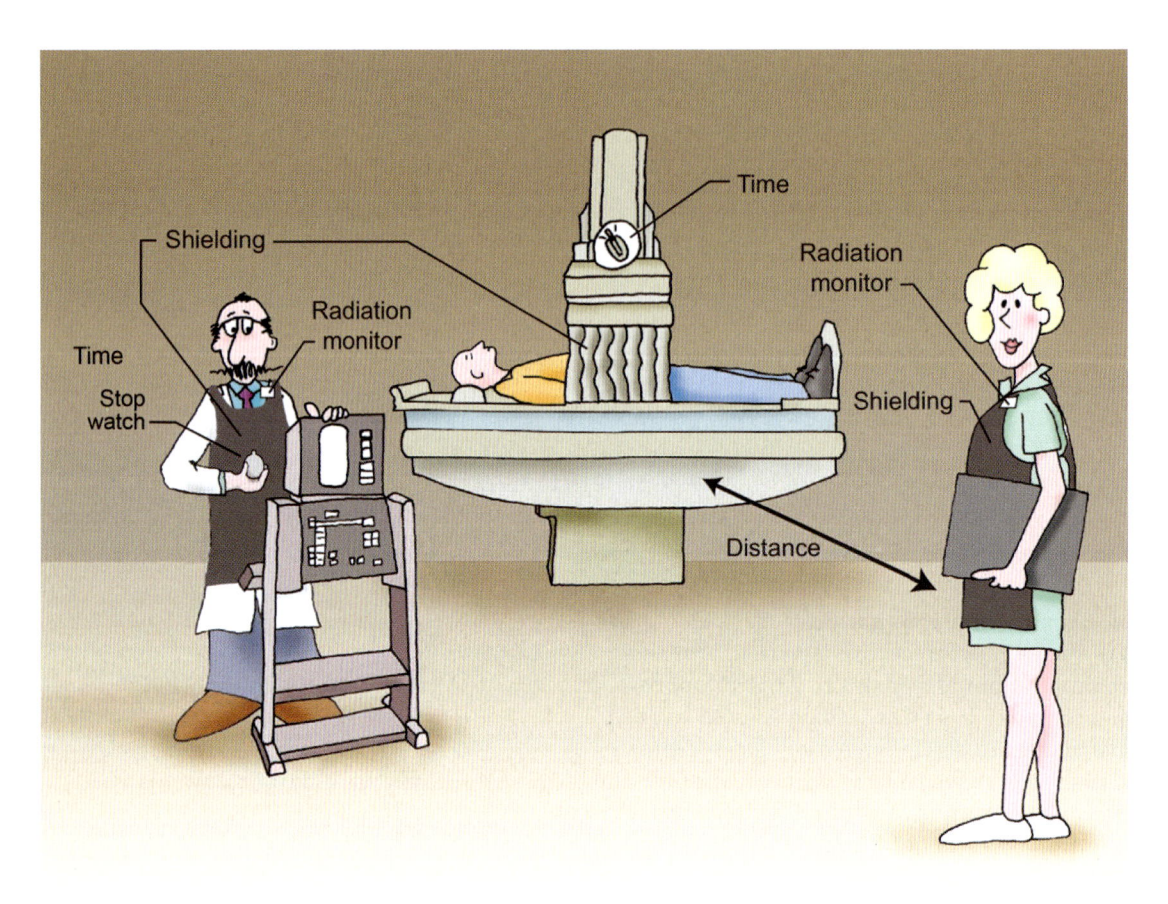

FIG. 37.4 Application of the cardinal principles of radiation protection in radiology.

Effective dose is the weighted average dose to each of the tissues in Table 37.3.

$E = \Sigma D_t W_t$
where D_t represents the radiation dose to a specific tissue and W_t is the sensitivity weighting factor for that tissue.

We receive essentially all of our occupational radiation exposure during fluoroscopy. During radiography and mammography, the radiographer is positioned behind a protective barrier, resulting in zero occupational radiation exposure.

During fluoroscopy, we position our occupational radiation monitor at the collar, as shown in Fig. 37.5, to estimate dose to the tissues of the head and neck. The tissues of the trunk of the body receive essentially zero dose; the protective apron does what it is designed to do.

Thus the estimation of effective occupational dose is shown in Table 37.4 for an occupational monitor response of 1 mSv. The result of this exercise is an occupational effective dose of 0.1 mSv.

TABLE 37.3	Weighting Factors for Various Tissues
Tissue	**Tissue Weighting Factor (W_t)**
Gonad	0.20
Active bone marrow	0.12
Colon	0.12
Lung	0.12
Stomach	0.12
Bladder	0.05
Breast	0.05
Esophagus	0.05
Liver	0.05
Thyroid	0.05
Bone surface	0.01
Skin	0.01

We assume the occupational effective dose to be 10% of the occupational radiation monitor dose.

TABLE 37.4	Occupational Effective Dose

An occupational radiation monitor records a dose of 1 mSv. What is the effective dose if the occupational dose is received during fluoroscopy when a protective apron is worn?

$E = \sum (D_i W_i)$
 $= (1)(0.05)$ thyroid
All other tissues receive essentially zero dose.
 $= 0.05 \text{ mSv} = 50 \text{ }\mu\text{Sv}$

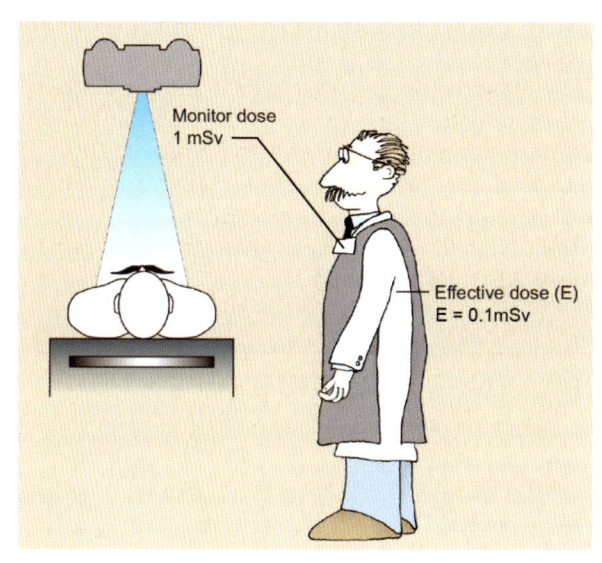

FIG. 37.5 Effective dose for occupational radiation exposure is based on the occupational radiation monitor.

Assuming an effective dose of 10% of the occupational monitor dose is conservative. In actuality, it is something less than 10%.

We will return to the concept of effective dose in Chapters 39 and 40. Be reminded that it is the effective dose that should be used for radiation risk estimation.

RADIOLOGIC TERRORISM

Emergency response to a radiologic incident conducted by terrorists, an exceptionally rare event, must be dealt with quickly and competently in order to save lives and limit property and environmental damage. Emergency responders are those individuals who must make the first decisions and take the first steps in the early stages of such an event.

The first emergency responders are likely to be police, fire, or emergency medical personnel. In the setting of a healthcare facility, radiographers may likely be the first emergency responders.

> Rescue and medical emergencies should be attended to before radiologic concerns are addressed.

The first task of emergency responders is to prevent injury and death and to attend to the medical needs of victims. Such immediate responses include limiting acute, high-intensity radiation exposure and limiting low-intensity radiation exposure that could result in late stochastic effects.

This is an ALARA exercise and will involve the application of the cardinal principles of radiation protection: reduce time of exposure, increase the distance from the source, and impose shielding between the source and the victim.

Radiologic Devices

The malevolent use of radiologic material by terrorists can be described as one of three devices: a radiation exposure device (RED), a radiologic dispersal device (RDD), and an improvised nuclear device (IND). Dealing with the effect of such devices requires specific response techniques for each.

> Being exposed to radiation does not make an individual radioactive.

An RED is a sealed source of radioactive material that directly exposes people. An RED will not disperse radioactive material; therefore radioactive decontamination of an RED is not required.

An RDD can be a bomb or a nonexplosive device that disperses radioactive contamination over a wide area. Although the radioactive contamination can be very troublesome, it is usually not life-threatening. It may be dispersed by hand in the form of powder, mist, or gas into a water supply or ventilation system.

An IND contains nuclear material that can produce a nuclear explosion. An IND is indeed a nuclear weapon; therefore it is unlikely to be the form of attack used by a terrorist. However, should an IND be employed, the death and devastation would be extreme.

Radiation Protection Guidance

Protection against exposure to external radiation, exposure from photon and particle radiation, and internal radioactive contamination transferred from surface radioactive contamination must be considered. This is accomplished by establishing boundaries for known levels of radiation exposure and radioactive contamination.

With the use of radiation monitoring instruments, an inner boundary is established at an exposure rate of 100 mGy$_a$/h. Inside this boundary, one should assume that levels of radioactive contamination are high until it is proved otherwise.

> Radioactive contamination is rarely life threatening.

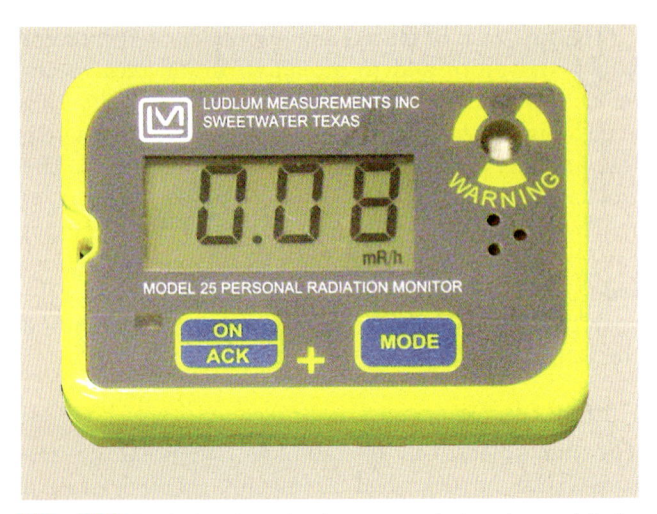

FIG. 37.6 Radiation detection instrument designed especially for radiologic terrorism. (Courtesy Ludlum Measurements, Inc.)

An outer boundary should be established when exposure exceeds 0.1 mGy$_a$/h or when radioactive contamination is detectable.

Radiation Detection and Measurement Equipment

Radiation detection equipment with appropriate and specific range capacity should be readily available to the first responder. It is recommended that such equipment be stored in the nuclear medicine laboratory and identified to all radiologic technologists and radiologists who might be pressed into emergency response.

> Radiologic terrorism can be addressed safely with an emergency responder's equipment kit.

The radiation detection apparatus should be capable of measuring radiation exposure levels to 500 mGy$_a$/h. Further it is recommended that such instruments should emit unambiguous alarms at 0.1, 100, and 500 mGy$_a$/h. (Such a specially designed instrument is shown in Fig. 37.6.) An additional instrument should be available that can be used to clearly detect the presence of alpha and beta radioactive contamination.

Emergency responders should have available standard protective coveralls and shoe covers to protect against radioactive contamination of the responder. Protective respiratory devices may be needed in the case of aerosol radioactive contamination. Decontamination of victims may be necessary, and an area should be cordoned off for such activity so that a contaminated-to-clean step-off pad is provided.

The radiation safety officer of a hospital should assign an individual to be responsible for establishing the emergency response equipment store and for seeing that adequate continuing education is provided for those who might be recruited to perform as emergency responders.

SUMMARY

Health physics is concerned with the research, teaching, and operational aspects of radiation protection. The three cardinal principles developed for radiation workers are as follows: minimize the time of radiation exposure, maximize distance from the radiation source, and use shielding to reduce radiation exposure. ALARA defines the principal concept of radiation protection.

The effective dose is that which should be used to estimate radiation risk to the patient or the radiology personnel. Assuming that effective dose is 10% of a collar-positioned monitor is conservative and results in the overestimation of stochastic response.

Radiologic terrorism is possible with three principal devices: RED, RDD, and IND.

CHALLENGE QUESTIONS

1. Define or otherwise identify the following:
   a. Health physics
   b. TVL
   c. NCRP
   d. Effective dose
   e. ALARA
   f. Tissue weighting factor (W_t)
   g. First responder
   h. Clarence Dally
   i. Manhattan Project
   j. LNT
2. Write the equation for the radiation dose as a function of time of exposure.
3. What is the function of the 5-minute reset timer on a fluoroscopy imaging system?
4. A fluoroscope emits 35 μGy$_a$/min at the tabletop for every mA of operation. What is the approximate patient entrance skin dose after a 3.2-minute fluoroscopic examination performed at 1.5 mA?
5. What are the three cardinal principles of radiation protection?
6. The output intensity of a radiographic unit is 42μGy$_a$/mAs. What is the total output after a 200-ms exposure at 300 mA?
7. At the exposure rate in Question 6, what is the approximate patient skin dose after a 3.2-minute fluoroscopic examination of 1.5 mA?
8. How can the three cardinal principles of radiation protection be best applied in digital imaging?
9. What exposure will a radiographer receive when exposed for 10 minutes at 4 m from a source with an intensity of 1 mGy$_a$/h at 1 m while wearing a protective apron equivalent to 2 HVLs?

10. What wartime effort coined the term *health physicist*?
11. The collar-positioned monitor of a fluoroscopist records 0.9 mSv over the course of a month. This represents approximately what effective dose?
12. Describe the change in longevity that occurred during the 20th century and the impact of ionizing radiation on that change.
13. How many HVLs equal a TVL?
14. What should first responders do in the event of a radiologic emergency?
15. Which one of the three types of terroristic radiologic devices is most life threatening?
16. At 80 kVp, the HVL in lead and concrete is approximately 0.2 mm and 1.0 cm, respectively. What is the HVL in soft tissue?
17. Where should the radiographer stand during fluoroscopy?
18. What is the use of an isoexposure line on an x-ray room drawing?
19. How much will patient radiation dose be reduced by selecting pulse-progressive fluoroscopy over continuous fluoroscopy?
20. What tissue weighting factor is proposed a reduction to 0.05 from 0.2?

The answers to the Challenge Questions can be found by logging on to our website at http://evolve.elsevier.com.

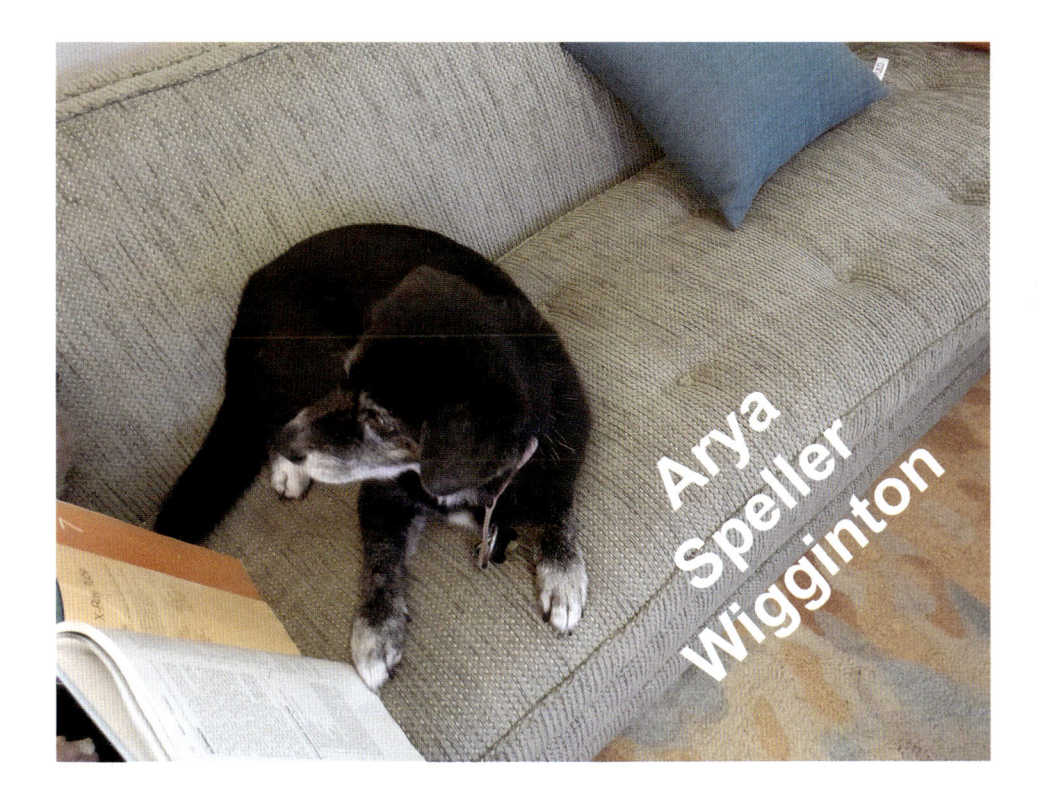

CHAPTER 38

Designing for Radiation Protection

OBJECTIVES

At the completion of this chapter, the student should be able to do the following:

1. State the leakage radiation limit for an x-ray tube.
2. List nine radiation protection features of a radiographic imaging system.
3. List nine radiation protection features of a fluoroscopic imaging system.
4. Discuss the design of primary and secondary radiation barriers.
5. Describe the three types of radiation dosimeters used in digital imaging.

OUTLINE

Radiographic Protection Features 511
  Protective X-ray Tube Housing 511
  Control Panel 511
  Source-to-Image Receptor Distance Indicator 511
  Collimation 511
  Positive-Beam Limitation 511
  Beam Alignment 511
  Filtration 511
  Reproducibility 512
  Linearity 512
  Operator Shield 512
  Mobile X-ray Imaging System 512

Fluoroscopic Protection Features 512
  Source-to-Skin Distance 513
  Primary Protective Barrier 513
  Filtration 514
  Collimation 514
  Exposure Control 514
  Bucky Slot Cover 514
  Protective Curtain 514
  Cumulative Timer 514

Design of Protective Barriers 514
  Type of Radiation 515
  Factors That Affect Barrier Thickness 516

Radiation Detection and Measurement 518
  Gas-Filled Detectors 519
  Scintillation Detectors 521
  Thermoluminescence Dosimetry 524
  Optically Stimulated Luminescence Dosimetry 525

Summary 525

Challenge Questions 526

CHAPTER 38 Designing for Radiation Protection

A NUMBER of features of modern x-ray imaging systems designed to improve image quality have been discussed in previous chapters. Many of these features are also designed to reduce patient radiation dose during digital examinations. For instance, proper beam collimation contributes to improved image contrast and is effective in reducing patient radiation dose.

More than 100 individual radiation protection devices and accessories are associated with modern digital imaging systems. Some are characteristic of either radiographic or fluoroscopic imaging systems, and some are mandated by federal regulation for all diagnostic x-ray imaging systems.

RADIOGRAPHIC PROTECTION FEATURES

Many radiation protection devices and accessories are associated with modern digital imaging systems. Two that are appropriate for all diagnostic digital imaging systems relate to the protective housing of the x-ray tube and to the control panel.

Protective X-ray Tube Housing

Every x-ray tube must be contained within a protective housing that reduces leakage radiation during use.

> Leakage radiation must be less than 1 mGy$_a$/h at a distance of 1 m from the protective housing.

Control Panel

The control panel must indicate the conditions of radiation exposure and must positively indicate when the x-ray tube is energized. These requirements are usually satisfied with the use of kVp and mA indicators. Sometimes visible or audible signals indicate when the x-ray beam is energized.

> X-ray beam-on must be positively and clearly indicated to the radiographer.

Source-to-Image Receptor Distance Indicator

A source-to-image receptor distance (SID) indicator must be provided. This can be as simple as a tape measure attached to the tube housing or as advanced as variously positioned laser lights.

> The SID indicator must be accurate to within 2% of the actual SID.

Collimation

Light-localized, variable-aperture rectangular collimators should be provided. Cones and diaphragms may replace the collimator for special examinations. Attenuation of the useful beam by collimator shutters must be equivalent to attenuation by the protective housing.

> The x-ray beam and the light beam must coincide to within 2% of the SID.

Question: Most radiographs are taken at an SID of 100 cm. How much difference is allowed between the projection of the light field and the x-ray beam at the image receptor?
Answer: 2% of 100 cm = 2 cm

Positive-Beam Limitation

Automatic, light-localized, variable-aperture collimators were required on all but special x-ray imaging systems manufactured in the United States between 1974 and 1994. These positive beam-limiting (PBL) devices are no longer required but continue to be a part of most new digital imaging systems. They must be adjusted so that with any image receptor size that is used and at all standard SIDs, the collimator shutters automatically provide an x-ray beam equal to the image receptor.

> The PBL must be accurate to within 2% of the SID.

Beam Alignment

In addition to proper collimation, each radiographic x-ray tube should be provided with a mechanism to ensure proper alignment of the x-ray beam and the image receptor. It does no good to align the light field and the x-ray beam if the image receptor is not also aligned.

Filtration

All general-purpose diagnostic x-ray beams must have a total filtration (inherent plus added) of at least 2.5 mm Al when operated above 70 kVp. Radiographic tubes operated between 50 and 70 kVp must have at least

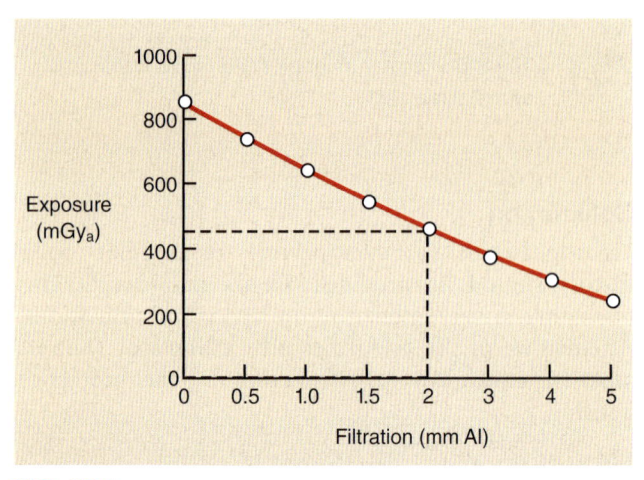

FIG. 38.1 Measurement of x-ray beam intensity as a function of added filtration results in a half-value layer of 2.0-mm Al.

1.5 mm Al. Below 50 kVp, a minimum of 0.5 mm Al total filtration is required.

> X-ray tubes designed for mammography have 30 μm Mo or 60 μm Rh filtration.

As was discussed in Chapter 9, it is not normally possible to examine and measure the thickness of each component of total filtration. An accurate measurement of half-value layer (HVL) is sufficient. If the HVL is equal to or greater than the values given in Table 9.3 at various kVp levels, total filtration is adequate.

Question: The following data are obtained on a three-phase digital imaging system operating at 70 kVp, 100 mA, 100 ms. Is the filtration adequate?

Added filtration (mm Al): 0 0.5 1.0 1.5 2.0 3.0 4.0 5.0

Exposure (mGy_a): 870 740 650 560 490 390 310 250

Answer: A plot of these data (Fig. 38.1) indicates an HVL of 2.0-mm Al. Table 9.3 shows that at 70 kVp, an HVL of 2.0-mm Al or greater is sufficient. The filtration is adequate.

Reproducibility

For any given radiographic technique, the output radiation intensity should be constant from one exposure to another. This is checked by making repeated radiation exposures with the same technique and observing the average variation in radiation intensity.

> The variation in x-ray intensity should not exceed +/- 5%.

Linearity

When adjacent mA stations are used, for example, 100 mA and 200 mA, and exposure time is adjusted to produce a constant mAs, the output radiation intensity should remain constant. When the exposure time remains constant, causing the mAs to increase in proportion to the increase in mA, radiation intensity should be proportional to mAs.

> The maximum acceptable variation in linearity is 10% from one mA station to an adjacent mA station.

This takes any inaccuracy in the exposure timer out of the analysis. Radiation intensity is expressed in units of mGy_a/mAs.

Operator Shield

It must not be possible to expose an image receptor while the radiographer stands unprotected outside a fixed protective barrier—usually the console booth. The exposure control should be fixed to the operating console and not to a long cord. The radiographer may be in the examination room during exposure, but only if protective apparel is worn.

Mobile X-ray Imaging System

A protective lead apron should be assigned to each mobile x-ray imaging system. The exposure switch of such an imaging system must allow the operator to remain at least 2 m from the x-ray tube during exposure. Of course, the useful beam must be directed away from the radiographer while positioned at this minimum distance.

FLUOROSCOPIC PROTECTION FEATURES

The features of fluoroscopic imaging systems that follow are intended primarily to reduce patient radiation dose. Usually when the patient radiation dose is reduced, personnel radiation exposure is reduced similarly.

The intensity of the x-ray beam at the tabletop of a fluoroscope should not exceed 20 mGy_a/min for each mA of operation at 80 kVp. If there is no optional high-level control, the intensity must not exceed 100 mGy_a/min during fluoroscopy. If an optional high-level control is provided, the maximum tabletop intensity allowed is 200 mGy_a/min.

> There is no limit on x-ray intensity when the image is recorded, as in cineradiography or videography.

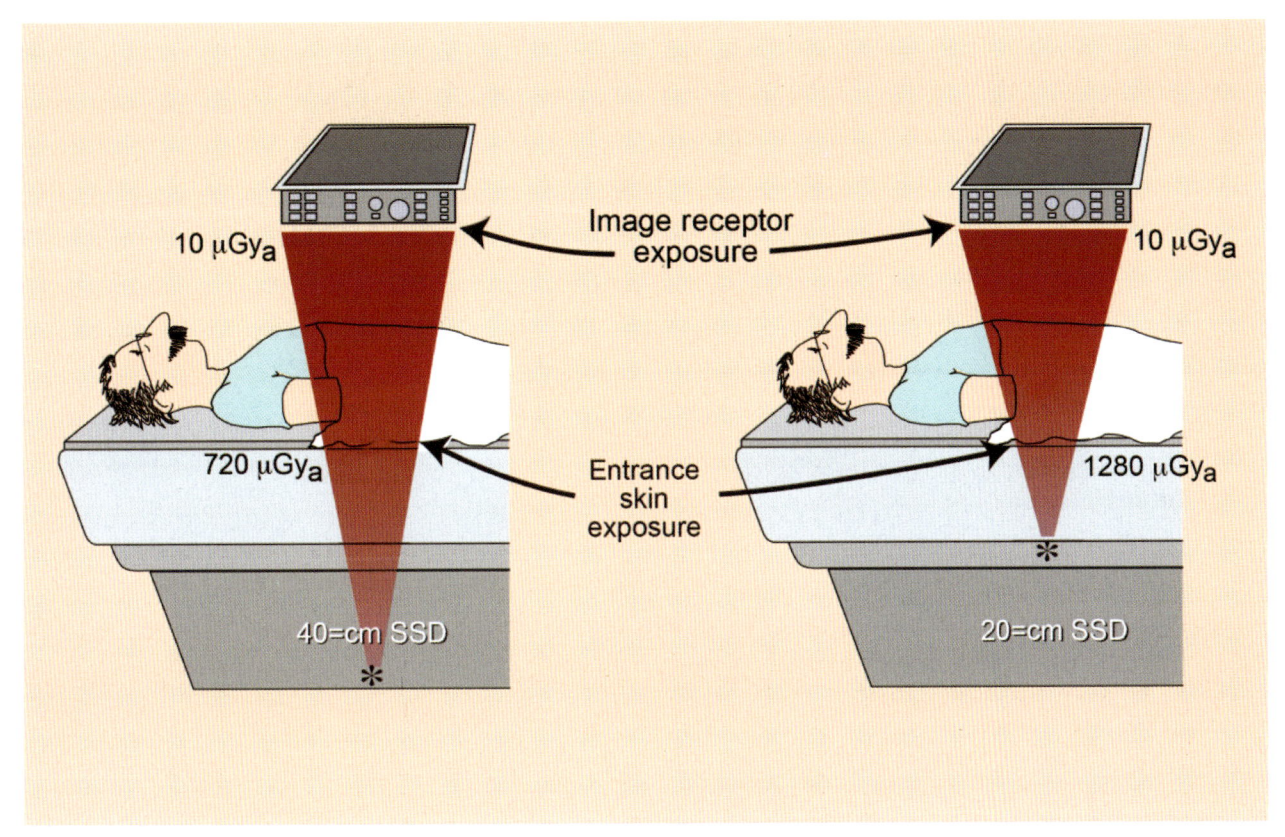

FIG. 38.2 Patient entrance skin exposure is considerably higher when the fluoroscopic x-ray tube is too close to the tabletop.

The overall stochastic risk to a patient depends on effective radiation dose, which is related to tissue radiation dose and to the volume of tissue exposed. Tissue radiation dose, which refers to the energy deposited locally, is the quantity that best reflects the potential for injury to that tissue as a deterministic effect.

Source-to-Skin Distance

One would think that increasing the distance between any x-ray tube and the patient would result in reduced patient radiation dose because of the increased distance. This is true; however, to maintain exposure to the image receptor, the mA must be increased to compensate for the increased distance. Because of the divergence of the x-ray beam, the entrance skin exposure (ESE) is reduced for the required exit dose as the source-to-skin (SSD) is increased.

> The SSD must be not less than 38 cm on stationary fluoroscopes and not less than 30 cm on mobile fluoroscopes.

Carefully review Fig. 38.2, where a 20-cm abdomen is 5 HVLs thick. If the fluoroscopic x-ray tube is moved from 40- to 20-cm SSD, the ESE is greatly increased. The exposure required at the image receptor is 10 µGy$_a$.

The ESE will be 22.5 mGy$_a$ and 40 mGy$_a$, respectively, solely because of the divergence of the x-ray beam—the inverse square law. Add the x-ray attenuation of 5 HVLs for each geometry, and the respective ESEs become 720 µGy$_a$ and 1280 µGy$_a$.

Question: At 40-cm SSD, the patient ESE is 1280 µGy$_a$. (A) What will be the patient ESE at 30 cm SSD? (B) What if the image receptor requires only 5 µGy$_a$ instead of 10 µGy$_a$? (C) What if it is a pediatric patient only 10 cm thick?

Answer: (A) $(40\,cm/30\,cm)^2 \times 1280\,\mu Gy_a = 0.56 \times 1280 = 717\,\mu Gy_a$

(B) $(5\,\mu Gy_a/10\,\mu Gy_a)^2 \times 717\,\mu Gy_a = 358\,\mu Gy_a$

(C) 10 cm = 2 HVL, ESE = 358 µGy$_a$/4 = 90 µGy$_a$

Primary Protective Barrier

The fluoroscopic image receptor assembly serves as a primary protective barrier and must be 2-mm Pb equivalent. It must be coupled with the x-ray tube and interlocked so that the fluoroscopic x-ray tube cannot be energized when the image receptor is in the parked position. This radiation protection feature is considered

TABLE 38.1 Minimum Half-Value Layer (HVL) Required to Ensure Adequate X-ray Beam Filtration

Minimum Half-Value Operating Kilovolt (kVp) Peak					
kVp	30	50	70	90	130
Minimum HVL (single phase)	0.3	1.2	1.6	2.6	3.6
Minimum HVL (three phase)	0.4	1.5	2.0	3.1	4.2

when computing protective barriers—walls, ceiling, floor—of the imaging suite.

Filtration

The total filtration of the fluoroscopic x-ray beam must be at least 2.5-mm Al equivalent. The tabletop, patient cradle, or other materials positioned between the x-ray tube and the tabletop are included as part of the total filtration. When the filtration is unknown, the HVL should be measured. The minimum HVL reported in Table 38.1 must be met so that adequate filtration can be assumed.

Collimation

Fluoroscopic x-ray beam collimators must be adjusted so that an unexposed border is visible on the image monitor when the image receptor is positioned 35 cm above the tabletop and the collimators are fully open. For automatic collimating devices, such an unexposed border should be visible at all heights above the tabletop. The collimator shutters should track with height above the tabletop.

Exposure Control

The fluoroscopic exposure control should be of the dead man type—that is, if the operator should drop dead or just release the pressure on either the hand or foot switch, the exposure would be terminated—unless, of course, they fall on the foot switch! The conventional foot pedal or pressure switch on the fluoroscopic image receptor satisfies this condition.

Bucky Slot Cover

During fluoroscopy, the Bucky tray is moved to the end of the examination table, leaving an opening in the side of the table approximately 5 cm wide at the gonadal level. This opening should be covered automatically with at least 0.25-mm Pb equivalent protective shielding.

Protective Curtain

A protective curtain or panel of at least 0.25-mm Pb equivalent should be positioned between the fluoroscopy

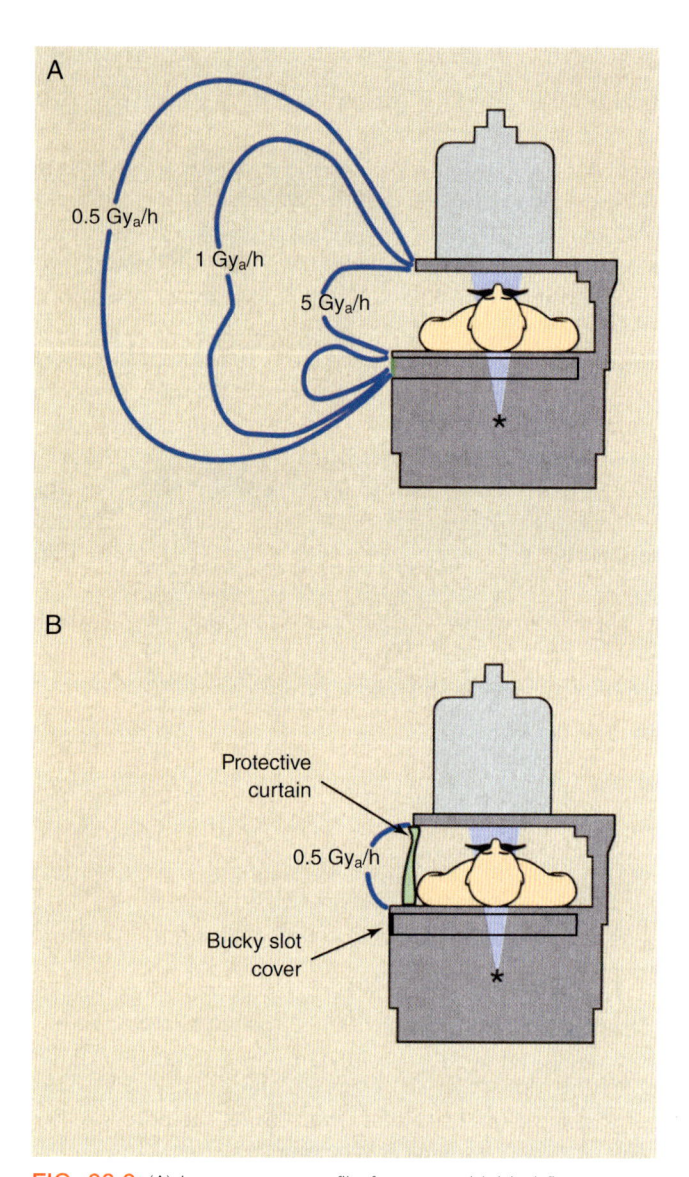

FIG. 38.3 (A) Isoexposure profile for an unshielded fluoroscope demonstrates the need for protective curtains and Bucky slot covers. (B) Isoexposure profile with these protective devices.

personnel and the patient. Fig. 38.3 shows the typical isoexposure distribution for a fluoroscope. Without the curtain and the Bucky slot cover, the exposure of radiology personnel is many times higher.

Cumulative Timer

A cumulative timer that produces an audible signal when the fluoroscopic time has exceeded 5 minutes must be provided. This device is designed to ensure that the radiologist is aware of the relative x-ray beam-on time during each procedure. The assisting radiographer should record total fluoroscopy beam-on time for each examination.

DESIGN OF PROTECTIVE BARRIERS

In designing a radiology department or an individual x-ray examination room, it is not sufficient to consider

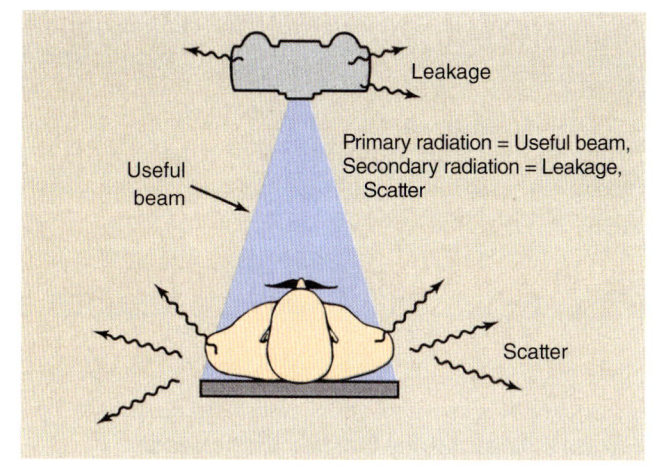

FIG. 38.4 Three types of radiation—the useful beam, leakage radiation, and scatter radiation—must be considered when the protective barriers of an x-ray room are designed.

only general architectural characteristics. Great attention must be given to the location of the x-ray imaging system in the examination room.

The use of adjoining rooms is also of great importance when the design is geared toward radiation safety. It is often necessary to include protective barriers, usually sheets of lead, in the walls of x-ray examination rooms. If the radiology facility is located on an upper floor, then it may be necessary to shield the floor as well.

A great number of factors are considered when a protective barrier is designed. This discussion touches only on the fundamentals and some basic definitions. Whenever new x-ray facilities are being designed or old ones renovated, a medical physicist must be consulted for assistance in the design of proper radiation shielding.

Type of Radiation

For the purpose of protective barrier design, three types of radiation are considered (Fig. 38.4). Primary radiation is the most intense and therefore the most hazardous and the most difficult to shield.

When a chest image receptor is positioned on a given wall, it is sometimes necessary to provide shielding directly behind the image receptor, in addition to that specified for the rest of the wall. Any wall to which the useful beam can be directed is designated a **primary protective barrier**.

> Primary radiation is the useful beam.

Lead bonded to drywall or wood paneling is used most often as a primary protective barrier. Such lead shielding is available in various thicknesses and is specified for architects and contractors in units of pounds per square foot (lb/ft^2).

TABLE 38.2 Lead and Concrete Equivalents for Primary Protective Barrier

LEAD			CONCRETE	
mm	in.	lb/ft^2	cm	in.
0.4	1/64	1	2.4	1 3/8
0.8	1/32	2	4.8	1 7/8
1.2	3/64	3	7.2	2 7/8
1.6	1/16	4	9.6	3 3/4

Concrete, concrete block, or brick may be used instead of lead. As a rule of thumb, 4 in. of masonry is equivalent to 1/16 in. of lead. Table 38.2 shows available lead thicknesses and equivalent thicknesses of concrete.

There are two types of secondary radiation: **scatter radiation** and **leakage radiation**. Scatter radiation results when the useful beam intercepts any object, causing some x-rays to be Compton scattered. For the purpose of protective shielding calculations, the scattering object can be regarded as a new source of radiation. During radiography and fluoroscopy, the patient is the single most important source of scatter radiation.

> The intensity of scatter radiation 1 m from the patient is approximately 0.1% of the intensity of the useful beam incident on the patient.

Question: The patient ESE is 4.1 mGy$_a$ for a kidney, ureter, and bladder (KUB) examination. What will be the approximate radiation exposure at 1 m from the patient? At 3 m from the patient?

Answer: At 1 m: 4.1 mGy$_a$ × 0.1% = 4.1 mGy$_a$ × 0.001 = 4.1 µGy$_a$
At 3 m: 4.1 µGy$_a$ × (1/3)^2 = 4.1 µGy$_a$ (1/9) = 0.46 µGy$_a$

Leakage radiation is the radiation emitted from the x-ray tube housing in all directions other than that of the useful beam. If the x-ray tube housing is designed properly, the leakage radiation will never exceed the regulatory limit of 1 mGy$_a$/h at 1 m. Although in practice, leakage radiation levels are much lower than this limit, 1 mGy$_a$/h at 1 m is used for protective barrier calculations.

Protective barriers designed to shield areas from secondary radiation are called **secondary protective barriers**. Secondary protective barriers are always less thick than primary protective barriers.

Often lead is not required for secondary protective barriers because the computation usually results in less than 0.4-mm Pb. In such cases, conventional gypsum board, glass, or lead acrylic is adequate.

TABLE 38.3	Equivalent Material Thicknesses for Secondary Barriers				
Lead Required (mm)	SUBSTITUTES			
	Steel (mm)	Glass (mm)	Gypsum (mm)	Wood (mm)
0.1	0.5	1.2	2.8	19
0.2	1.2	2.5	5.9	33
0.3	1.8	3.7	8.8	44
0.4	2.5	4.8	12	53

Many walls that are secondary protective barriers can be protected adequately with four thicknesses of 5/8-in. gypsum board. Operating console barriers are secondary protective barriers—the useful beam is never directed at the operating console booth. Four thicknesses of gypsum board and 1/2-in. plate glass may be all that is necessary. Sometimes glass walls 1/2- to 1-in. thick can be used as control booth barriers.

Table 38.3 gives equivalent thicknesses for secondary protective barrier materials.

Question: What percentage of the recommended 1-mSv/wk public dose limit will be incident on a control booth barrier located 3 m from the x-ray tube and the patient? Assume that the x-ray output is 30 µGy$_a$/mAs and that the weekly beam-on time is 5 minutes at an average 100 mA—a generous assumption.

Answer: From scatter radiation, the barrier will receive:

Total primary beam = 30 µGy$_a$/mAs × 10 mA × 5 min × 60 s/min
= 900,000 µGy$_a$

Scatter radiation = 900,000 µGy$_a$ × 1/1000 × (1/3)^2
= 10 µGy$_a$

From leakage radiation, the barrier will receive:

Leakage radiation at 1 m = 1 mGy$_a$ × 5/60 h
= 0.083 mGy$_a$
= 83 µGy$_a$

Leakage radiation = 83 µGy$_a$ (1/3)^2 = 9 µGy$_a$

Total secondary radiation
= 100 µGy$_a$ + 9 µGy$_a$
= 109 µGy$_a$ or

11% of the recommended dose limit

This analysis is representative of the clinical environment. The estimated radiation exposure occurs to the control booth barrier—not to the radiographer. The composition of the barrier and the additional distance reduce radiographer exposure even further. This is the reason why personnel radiation exposure during digital imaging is very low.

> Radiographers receive most of their occupational radiation exposure during fluoroscopy.

Factors That Affect Barrier Thickness

Many factors must be taken into consideration when the required protective barrier thickness is calculated. A thorough discussion of these factors is beyond the scope of this book; however, a definition of each is useful for an understanding of the problems involved.

The thickness of a barrier naturally depends on the distance between the source of radiation and the barrier. The distance is that to the adjacent occupied area, not to the inside of the wall of the digital imaging room.

A wall along which an digital imaging system is positioned probably requires more shielding than the other walls of the x-ray room. In such a case, the leakage radiation may be more hazardous than the scatter radiation or even the useful beam. It may be desirable to position the digital imaging system in the middle of the room because then no single wall is subjected to especially intense radiation exposure.

The use of the area that is being protected is of principal importance. If the area were a rarely occupied closet or storeroom, the required shielding would be less than if it were an office or laboratory that was occupied 40 h/wk.

This concept reflects the **time of occupancy factor**. Table 38.4 reports the occupancy levels of various areas,

TABLE 38.4	Levels of Occupancy of Areas That May Be Adjacent to X-ray Rooms, as Suggested by the National Council on Radiation Protection and Measurements
Occupancy	**Area**
Full	Work areas (e.g., offices, laboratories, shops, wards, and nurses' stations), living quarters, children's play areas, and occupied space in nearby buildings
Frequent	Corridors, restrooms, patient rooms
Occasional	Waiting rooms, stairways, unattended elevators, janitors' closets, outside areas

as suggested by the National Council on Radiation Protection and Measurements (NCRP).

An area that is occupied primarily by radiology personnel and patients is called a **controlled area**. The design limits for a controlled area are based on the recommended occupational dose limit; therefore, the barrier is required to reduce the exposure to radiology personnel in the area to less than 1 mSv/week.

> Design limits for a controlled area are based on the annual recommended occupational dose limit of 50 mSv/year.

An **uncontrolled area** can be occupied by anyone; therefore, the maximum exposure rate allowed is based on the recommended dose limit for the public of 1 mSv/year. This is equivalent to 0.02 mSv/week or 20 μSv/week, which is the design limit for an uncontrolled area. Furthermore, the protective barrier should ensure that no individual will receive more than 25 μSv in any single hour.

The shielding required for a digital imaging room depends on the level of radiation activity in that room. The greater the number of examinations performed each week, the thicker the shielding that is required.

This characteristic is called **workload** and is expressed in units of milliampere-minutes per week (mAmin/week). A busy, general-purpose digital imaging room may have a workload of 500 mAmin/week. Rooms in private offices have workloads of less than 100 mAmin/week.

Question: The plans for an urgent care facility call for two x-ray examination rooms. The estimated patient load for each room is 15 patients per day, and each patient will average three exposures at 80 kVp, 70 mAs. What is the projected workload of each room?

Answer: 15 patients/day × 5 days/week = 75 patients/week
75 patients/week × 3 exposures/pt = 225 exposures/week
225 exposures/week × 70 mAs/exposure = 15,750 mAs/week
15,750 mAs/week × 1 min/60 s = 262.5 mAmin/week

For combination radiographic/fluoroscopic imaging systems, usually only the radiographic workload needs to be considered for barrier calculations. When the fluoroscopic x-ray tube is energized, a primary protective barrier in the form of the fluoroscopic image receptor must intercept the useful x-ray beam. Consequently, the primary barrier requirements are always much less for fluoroscopic x-ray beams than for radiographic x-ray beams.

The percentage of time during which the x-ray beam is on and directed toward a particular protective barrier is called the **use factor** for that barrier. The NCRP recommends that walls be assigned a use factor of ¼ and the floor a use factor of 1.

> The use factor for secondary radiation is always 1.

Studies have shown these recommendations to be high and therefore very conservative. Many medical physicists suggest that primary barriers in fact do not exist. All barriers are secondary because the useful beam is always intercepted by the patient and the image receptor.

If a digital imaging room has a special design, other use factors may be assigned. A room designed strictly for chest radiography has one wall with a use factor of 1. All others have a use factor of zero for primary radiation and thus would be considered secondary radiation barriers. The ceiling nearly always is considered a secondary protective barrier.

> For a secondary barrier, leakage and scatter radiation are present 100% of the time that the x-ray tube is energized.

The final consideration in the design of an x-ray protective barrier is the energy of the x-ray beam. For protective barrier calculations, kVp is used as the measure of energy. Most modern digital imaging systems are designed to operate at up to 150 kVp. Most examinations, however, are conducted at an average of 70 to 80 kVp.

Usually constant operation is assumed at a kVp greater than that actually used: 100 kVp for general radiography, 30 kVp for mammography. Therefore it is more likely that the protective barrier will be too thick rather than too thin.

Alternatively, a workload distribution, as shown in Fig. 38.5, may be used. Workload distribution results in a more precise determination of required barrier thickness, but it is a considerably more difficult computation to perform.

Measurements of radiation exposure outside the x-ray examination room always result in radiation levels far less than those anticipated by calculation. The total beam-on time is always less than that assumed. The average kVp is usually closer to 75 kVp than to 100 kVp.

Calculations do not account for the fact that the patient and the image receptor always intercept the useful beam. Therefore although the calculations are

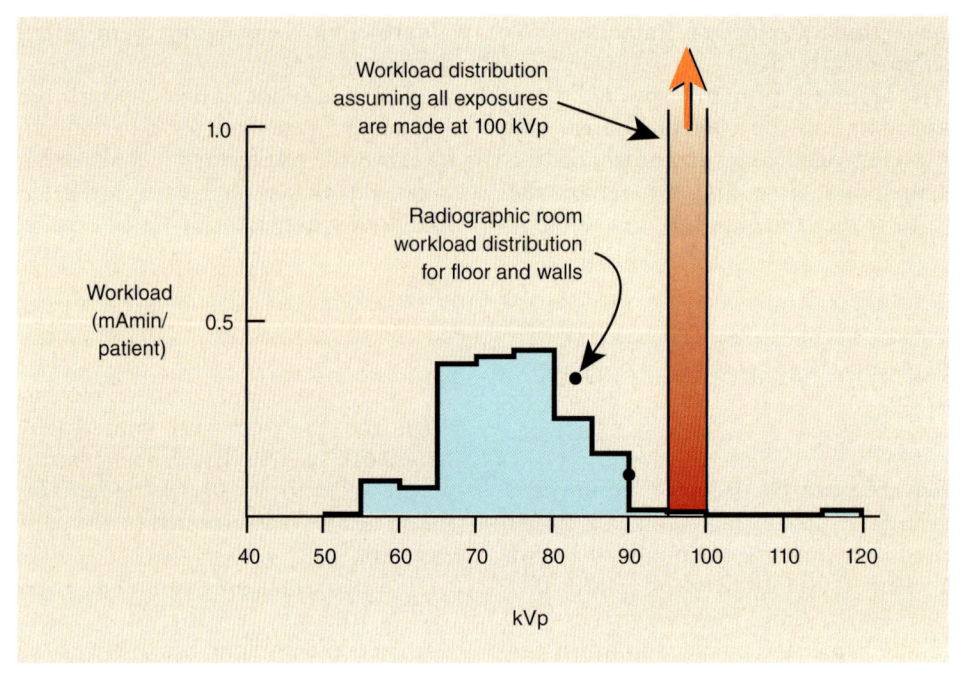

FIG. 38.5 Workload distribution of clinical voltage.

intended to result in a dose limit of 1 mSv/wk (20 µSv/wk) outside the x-ray room, rarely will the actual exposure exceed 1/10 of those dose limits. To confirm this for yourself, keep records for 1 week of kVp, mAs, and beam direction.

RADIATION DETECTION AND MEASUREMENT

Instruments are designed to detect radiation or to measure radiation, or to do both. Those designed for detection usually operate in the **pulse** or **rate mode** and are used to indicate the presence of radiation. In the pulse mode, the presence of radiation is indicated by a ticking, chirping, or beeping sound. In the rate mode, the instrument response usually is expressed in mGy_a/h.

Instruments designed to measure the intensity of radiation usually operate in the integrate mode. They accumulate the signal and respond with a total exposure (mGy_a or Gy_a).

> The measure of radiation intensity is called radiation dosimetry, and the radiation measuring devices are called radiation dosimeters.

The earliest radiation detection device was the photographic emulsion. Table 38.5 lists most of the currently available radiation detection and measurement devices, along with some of their principal characteristics and uses.

Previously film had two principal applications in diagnostic imaging: the making of a radiograph and occupational radiation monitoring of personnel (the film badge). Neither apply today.

The gas-filled radiation detector is used widely as a device to measure radiation intensity and to detect radioactive contamination. Thermoluminescence dosimetry (TLD) and optically stimulated luminescence (OSL) dosimetry are used for both patient and

TABLE 38.5	Radiation Detection and Measuring Device Characteristics and Uses
Device	**Characteristics—Uses**
Ionization chamber	Wide range, accurate, portable—survey for radiation levels 10 $µGy_a/h$
Proportional counter	Laboratory instrument, accurate, sensitive—assay of small quantities of radionuclides
Geiger-Muller counter	Limited to 1 mGy_a/h, portable—survey for low radiation levels and radioactive contamination
Thermoluminescence dosimetry	Wide range, accurate, sensitive—personnel monitoring, stationary, area monitoring
Optically stimulated luminescence dosimetry	Wide range, accurate, sensitive—personnel monitoring
Scintillation detection	Limited range, very sensitive, stationary or portable instruments—photon spectroscopy

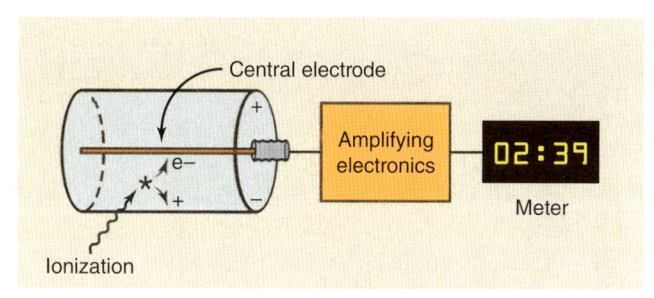

FIG. 38.6 The ideal gas-filled detector consists of a cylinder of gas and a central collecting electrode. When a voltage is maintained between the central electrode and the wall of the chamber, electrons produced in ionization can be collected and measured.

personnel radiation monitoring. Scintillation detection is the basis for the gamma camera, an imaging device used in nuclear medicine; it is also used in computed tomography (CT) and other digital imaging systems.

Gas-Filled Detectors

Three types of gas-filled radiation detectors are used: ionization chambers, proportional counters, and Geiger-Muller (GM) detectors. Although they differ in terms of response characteristics, each is based on the same principle of operation. As radiation passes through gas, it ionizes atoms of the gas. The electrons released in ionization are detected as an electrical signal that is proportional to the radiation intensity.

Consider an ideal gas-filled detector, as shown schematically in Fig. 38.6. It consists of a cylinder filled with air or any of a number of other gases.

Along the central axis of the cylinder, a rigid wire called the central electrode is positioned. If a voltage is impressed between the central electrode and the wall such that the wire is positive and the wall negative, then any electrons liberated in the chamber by ionization will be attracted to the central electrode.

These electrons form an electrical signal, either as a pulse of electrons or as a continuous electric current. This electric signal then is amplified and measured. Its size is proportional to the radiation intensity that caused it.

In general, the larger the chamber, the more gas molecules are available for ionization, and therefore the more sensitive is the instrument. Similarly, if the chamber is pressurized, then a greater number of molecules are available for ionization and even higher sensitivity results.

> The ionization of gas is the basis for gas-filled radiation detectors.

Radiation sensitivity is not the same as accuracy. A high level of accuracy means that an instrument can detect and precisely measure the intensity of a radiation field. Instrument accuracy is controlled by the overall electronic design of the device. Sensitivity is a "how low can you go" property (Fig. 38.7). Instruments with high sensitivity can measure very low radiation intensities.

If the voltage across the chamber of the ideal gas-filled detector is increased slowly from zero to a high level, the resulting electrical signal in the presence of fixed radiation intensity will increase in stages (Fig. 38.8). During the first stage, when the voltage is very low, no electrons are attracted to the central electrode. The ion pairs produced in the chamber recombine. This is known as the **region of recombination**, shown as stage R in Fig. 38.8.

As the chamber voltage is increased, a condition is reached whereby every electron released by ionization is attracted to the central electrode and collected. The voltage at which this occurs varies according to the design of the chamber, but for most conventional instruments, it occurs in the range of 100 to 300 V.

This portion of the gas-filled detector performance curve is known as the **ionization region**, indicated by I in Fig. 38.8. Ion chambers are operated in this region.

Several different types of ion chambers are used in digital imaging; the most familiar of these is the portable survey instrument (Fig. 38.9). This instrument is used principally for area radiation surveys. It can measure a wide range of radiation intensities, from 10 μGy_a/h to several thousand Gy_a/h.

The ion chamber is the instrument of choice for measuring radiation intensity in areas around a fluoroscope, around radionuclide generators and syringes, in the vicinity of patients with therapeutic quantities of radioactive materials, and outside of protective barriers. Other, more accurate ion chambers are used for precise calibration of the output intensity of digital imaging systems (Fig. 38.10).

Another application of a precision ion chamber is the dose calibrator (Fig. 38.11). These devices find daily use in nuclear medicine laboratories for the assay of radioactive material.

As the chamber voltage of the ideal gas-filled detector is increased above the ionization region, electrons of the filling gas released by primary ionization are accelerated more rapidly to the central electrode. The faster these electrons travel, the greater is the probability that they will produce additional ionization on their way to the central electrode. These additional ionizations result in additional electrons called secondary electrons.

Secondary electrons also are attracted to the central electrode and collected. The total number of electrons collected in this fashion increases with increasing chamber voltage. The result is a rather large electron pulse for each primary ionization. This stage of the voltage response curve is known as the **proportional region**.

520   PART VIII   Radiation Protection

Accuracy   Sensitivity

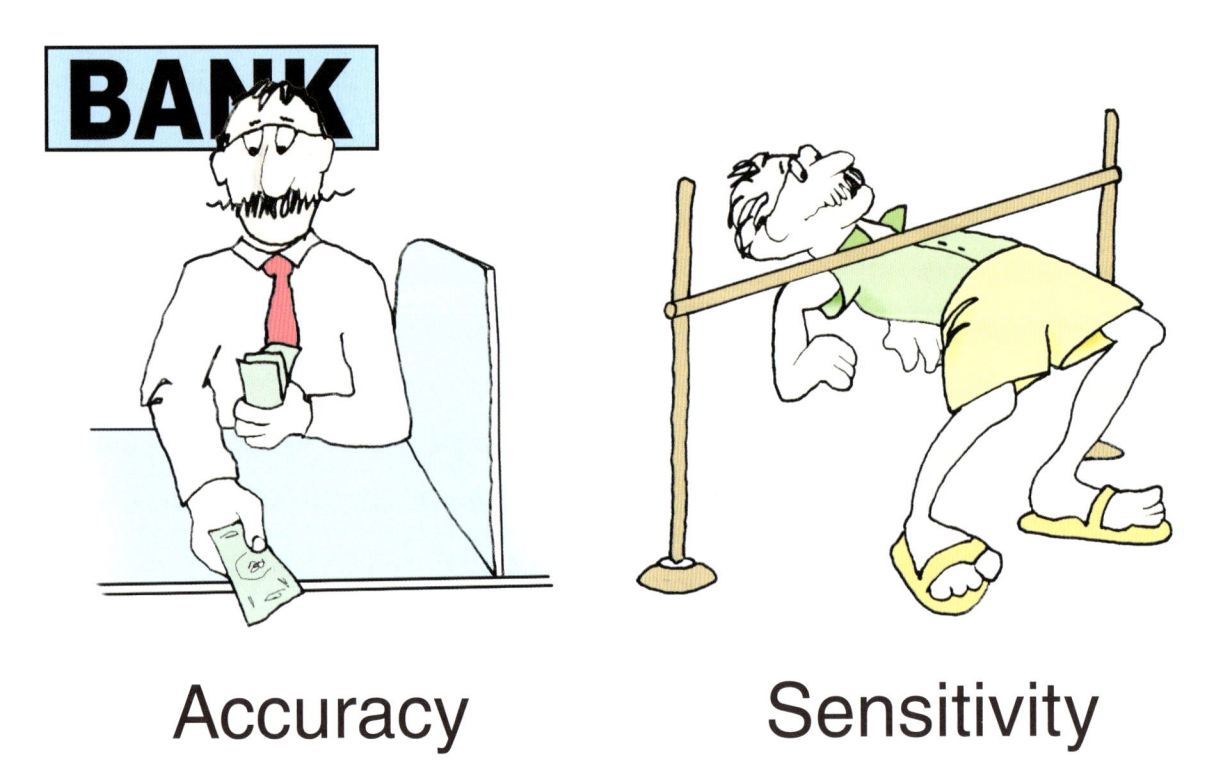

FIG. 38.7 A simple explanation of the difference between accuracy and sensitivity.

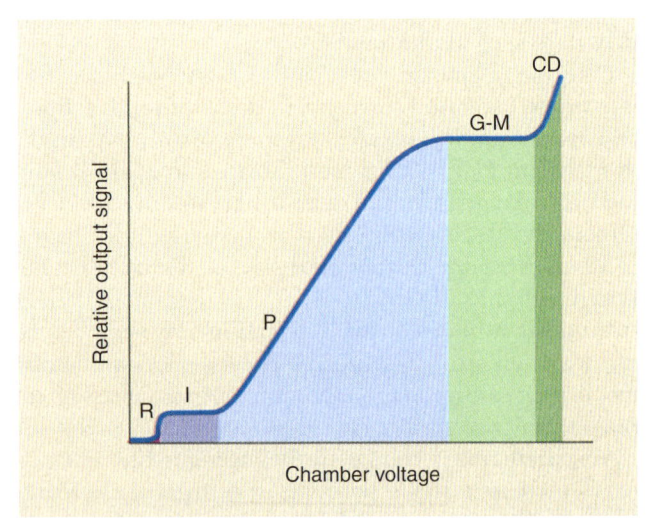

FIG. 38.8 The amplitude of the signal from a gas-filled detector increases in stages as the voltage across the chamber is increased.

> Proportional counters are sensitive instruments used primarily for the assay of small quantities of radioactivity.

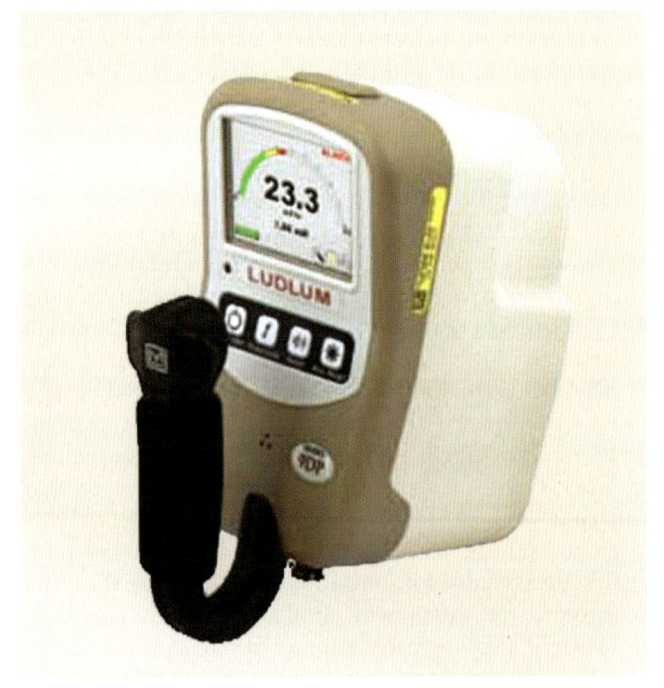

FIG. 38.9 This portable ion chamber survey instrument is useful for radiation surveys when exposure levels are in excess of 10 µGy$_a$/h. (Courtesy Ludlum Measurements, Inc.)

One characteristic of proportional counters that makes them particularly useful is their ability to distinguish between alpha and beta radiation. Nevertheless, proportional counters find few applications in clinical radiology.

The fourth region of the voltage response curve for the ideal gas-filled chamber is the **Geiger-Muller (G-M)**

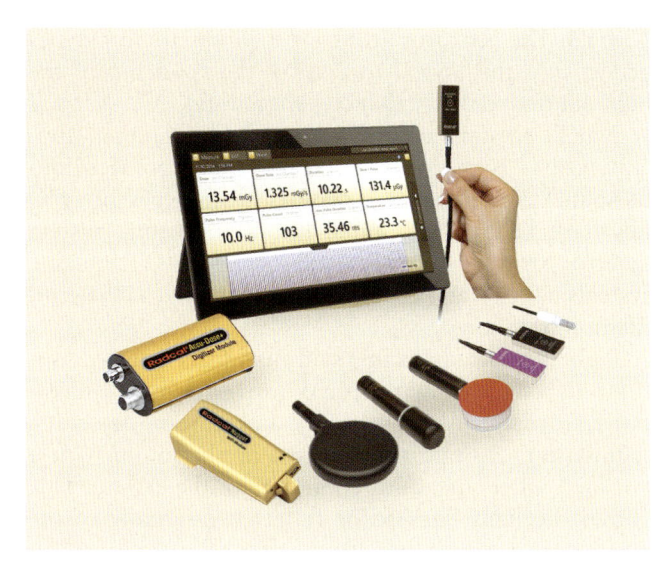

FIG. 38.10 This ion chamber dosimeter is used for accurate measurement of diagnostic x-ray beams. (Courtesy Patrick Pyers, Radcal Corp.)

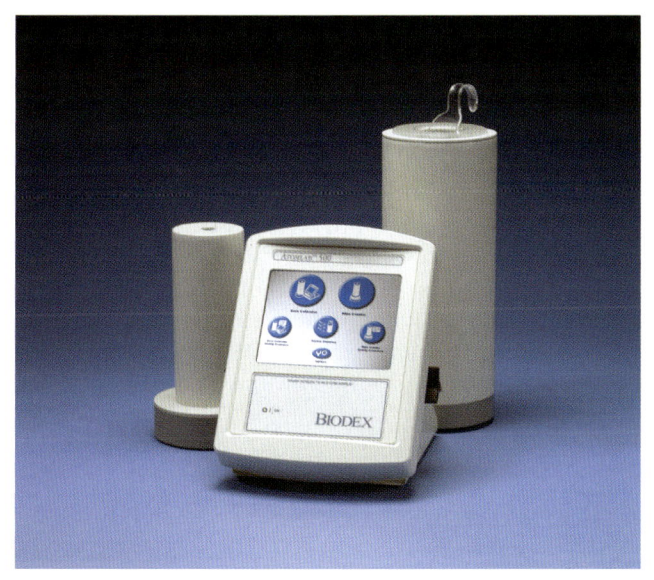

FIG. 38.11 This configuration of an ion chamber is called a dose calibrator. It is used in nuclear medicine to measure accurately quantities of radioactive material. (Courtesy Biodex Medical Systems, Inc.)

region. This is the region in which Geiger counters operate.

In the G-M region, the voltage across the ionization chamber is sufficiently high that, when a single ionizing event occurs, a cascade of secondary electrons is produced in a fashion similar to a very brief, yet violent, chain reaction. The effect is that nearly all molecules of the gas are ionized, liberating a large number of electrons. This results in a large electron pulse.

When sequential ionizing events occur soon after one another, the detector may not be capable of responding to a second event if the filling gas has not been restored to its initial condition. Therefore a **quenching agent** is added to the filling gas of the Geiger counter to enable the chamber to return to its original condition; subsequent ionizing events then can be detected.

> The minimum time between ionizations that can be detected is known as the resolving time.

Geiger counters are used for contamination control in nuclear medicine laboratories. As portable survey instruments, they are used to detect the presence of radioactive contamination on work surfaces and laboratory apparatus.

They are not particularly useful as dosimeters because they are difficult to calibrate for varying conditions of radiation. Geiger counters are sensitive instruments that are capable of detecting and indicating single ionizing events. If they are equipped with an audio amplifier and a speaker, one can even hear the crackle of individual ionizations.

The Geiger counter does not have a very wide range. Most instruments are limited to less than 1 mGy_a/h.

If the voltage across the gas-filled chamber is increased still further, a condition is reached whereby a single ionizing event completely discharges the chamber, as in operation in the G-M region. Because of the high voltage, however, electrons continue to be stripped from atoms of the filling gas, producing a continuous current or signal from the chamber.

In this condition of **continuous discharge**, the instrument is useless for the detection of radiation, and continued operation in this region results in damage. The region of continuous discharge is indicated as **CD** in Fig. 38.8.

Scintillation Detectors

Scintillation detectors are used in several areas of radiologic science. The scintillation detector is the basis for the gamma camera in nuclear medicine and is used in the detector arrays of CT imaging systems; it is the image receptor for several types of digital imaging systems.

Some types of material scintillate when irradiated; that is, they emit a flash of light immediately in response to absorption of an x-ray. The amount of light emitted is proportional to the amount of energy absorbed by the material.

Consider, for example, the two x-ray interactions diagrammed in Fig. 38.12. If a 50-keV x-ray interacts photoelectrically in the crystal, all the energy (50 keV) will reappear as light. If, however, that same x-ray interacts through a Compton scattering event in which only 20 keV of energy is absorbed, then a proportionately lower quantity of light will be emitted in the scintillation.

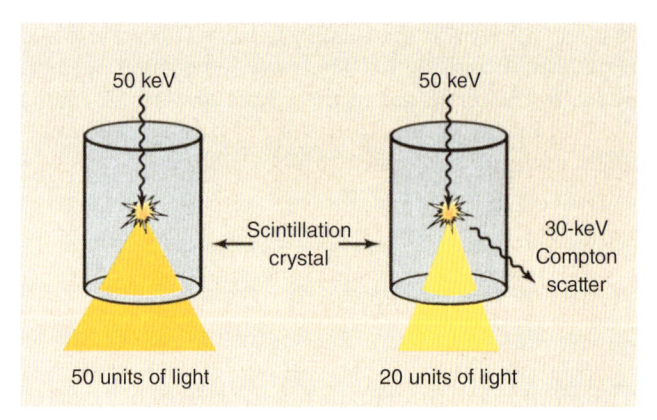

FIG. 38.12 During scintillation, the intensity of light emitted is proportional to the amount of energy absorbed in the crystal.

Only those materials with a particular crystalline structure scintillate. At the atomic level, the process involves the rearrangement of valence electrons into traps. The return of the electron from the trap to its normal position is immediate in scintillation and fluorescence. Phosphorescence is another form of delayed luminescence. Fluorescence and phosphorescence are luminescence processes involving outer shell electrons.

> Many different types of liquids, gases, and solids can respond to ionizing radiation by scintillation.

Scintillation detectors are used most often to indicate individual ionizing events and are incorporated into fixed or portable radiation detection devices. They can be used to measure radiation in the rate mode or the integrate mode.

Nearly all the noble gases can be made to respond to radiation by scintillation. Such applications are rare, however, because the detection efficiency is very low and the probability of interaction therefore is small.

Liquid scintillation detectors are used frequently in the research laboratory to detect low-energy beta emissions from carbon-14 (^{14}C) and tritium (^{3}H). Because they present a relatively harmless radiation hazard and are incorporated easily into biologic molecules, ^{14}C and ^{3}H are useful research radionuclides.

These radionuclides emit low-energy beta particles with no associated gamma rays. This makes them difficult to detect. With liquid scintillation counting, however, biologic molecules can be mixed with a liquid scintillation phosphor so that the beta emission interacts directly with the phosphor, causing a flash of light to be emitted. Liquid scintillation counters have nearly 100% detection efficiency for beta radiation.

By far, the most widely used scintillation phosphors are the inorganic crystals—thallium-activated sodium iodide (NaI:Tl) and thallium-activated cesium iodide (CsI:Tl). The activator atoms of thallium are impurities grown into the crystal to control the spectrum of the light emitted and to enhance its intensity.

NaI:Tl crystals are incorporated into gamma cameras; CsI:Tl is the phosphor that is incorporated into flat-panel digital image receptors. Both types of crystals have been incorporated into CT imaging system detector arrays. However, many of today's CT imaging systems use cadmium tungstate or a ceramic as the scintillation detector.

Light produced during scintillation is emitted isotopically; that is, with equal intensity in all directions. Consequently, when used as radiation detectors, scintillation crystals are enclosed in aluminum with a polished inner surface in contact with the crystal. This allows the light flash to be reflected internally to the one face of a crystal that is not enclosed, which is called the **window**.

Aluminum containment is also necessary to seal the crystal hermetically. A hermetic seal is one that prevents the crystal from coming into contact with air or moisture. This is necessary because many scintillation crystals are hygroscopic; that is, they absorb moisture. When moisture is absorbed, the crystals swell and crack. Cracked crystals are not useful because the crack produces an interface that reflects and attenuates the scintillation.

Fig. 38.13 shows the basic components of a single crystal–photomultiplier (PM) tube assembly representative of the type used in the portable survey instrument. The detector portion of the assembly is the NaI:Tl crystal contained in the aluminum hermetic seal. Coupled to the window of the crystal is a PM tube that converts light flashes from the scintillator into an electrical signal of pulses.

> **PHOTOMULTIPLIER TUBE GAIN**
> PM tube gain = g^n
> where dynode gain is g, and n is equal to the number of dynodes.

The PM tube is an electron vacuum tube that contains a number of elements. The tube consists of a glass envelope, which provides structural support for the internal elements and maintains the vacuum inside the tube.

The portion of the glass envelope that is coupled to the scintillation crystal is called the window of the tube. The crystal window and the PM tube window are sandwiched together with silicone grease, which provides optical coupling, so that the light emitted by the scintillator is transmitted to the interior of the PM tube with minimum loss.

As light passes from the crystal into the PM tube, it is incident on a thin metal coating called a **photocathode**,

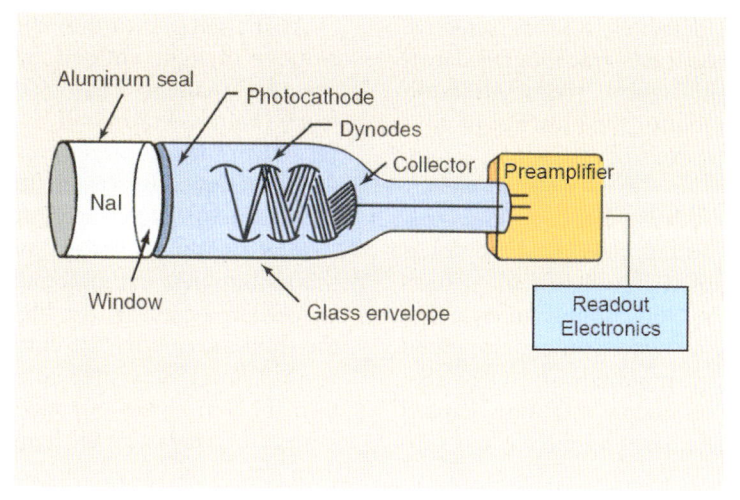

FIG. 38.13 Scintillation detector assembly characteristics of the type used in a portable survey instrument.

which consists of a compound of cesium, antimony, and bismuth. Electrons are emitted from the photocathode by a process called **photoemission**, which is similar to thermionic emission in the filament of an x-ray tube, except that the stimulus is light rather than heat.

> High sensitivity means that an instrument can detect very low radiation intensities.

The flash of light from the scintillation crystal therefore is incident on the photocathode and electrons are released by photoemission. The number of electrons emitted is directly proportional to the intensity of the light.

These photoelectrons are accelerated to the first of a series of plate-like elements called dynodes. Each dynode serves to amplify the electron pulse through secondary electron emission. For each electron incident on the dynode, several secondary electrons are emitted and directed to the next stage. Consequently, an electron gain occurs for each dynode in the PM tube.

> A photocathode is a device that emits electrons when illuminated.

The number of dynodes and the gain of each dynode determine the overall electron gain of the PM tube. PM tube gain is the dynode gain raised to the power of the number of dynodes.

> The dynode gain is the ratio of secondary electrons to incident electrons.

Question: An eight-stage PM tube (eight dynodes) has a dynode gain of three (three electrons emitted for each incident electron). What is the PM tube gain?

Answer: PM tube gain = $3^8 = 6561$

The last plate-like element of the PM tube is the collecting electrode or collector. The collector absorbs the electron pulse from the last dynode and conducts it to the preamplifier. The preamplifier provides an initial state of pulse amplification. It is attached to the base of the PM tube—a structure that provides support for the glass envelope and internal structures.

The overall result of scintillation detection is that a single-photon interaction produces a burst of light; this, in turn, produces photoelectron emission, which then is amplified to produce a relatively large electron pulse.

> The size of the electron pulse is proportional to the energy absorbed by the crystal from the incident photon.

It is this property of scintillation detection that promotes its use as an energy-sensitive device for gamma spectrometry that uses pulse height analysis. Through such an application, unknown gamma emitters can be identified and more sensitive radioisotope imaging can be accomplished by counting only those pulses with energy that represent total gamma-ray absorption.

Scintillation detectors are sensitive devices for x-rays and gamma rays. They are capable of measuring radiation intensities as low as single-photon interactions. This property of scintillation detectors results in their use as portable radiation detectors in much the same manner as Geiger counters are used.

A portable scintillation detector is more sensitive than a Geiger counter because it has much higher detection efficiency. For this application, the scintillation detector would be used to monitor the presence of contamination and perhaps low levels of radiation.

Thermoluminescence Dosimetry

Some materials glow when heated, thus exhibiting thermally stimulated emission of visible light, called **thermoluminescence**. In the early 1960s, John Cameron and coworkers at the University of Wisconsin experimented with some thermoluminescent materials and were able to show that exposure to ionizing radiation caused some materials to glow particularly brightly when subsequently heated.

> TLD is the emission of light by a thermally stimulated crystal following irradiation.

Radiation-induced thermoluminescence has been developed into a sensitive and accurate method of radiation dosimetry for personnel radiation monitoring and for measurement of patient radiation dose during diagnostic and therapeutic radiation procedures. Personnel and patient radiation monitoring are discussed later; however, at this time, it is important to discuss some of the basic principles of TLD (Fig. 38.14).

After irradiation, the TLD phosphor is placed on a special planchet for analysis in an instrument called a TLD analyzer. The temperature of the planchet can be controlled carefully. Directly viewing the planchet is a PM tube. The PM tube is the same type of light-sensitive and light-measuring vacuum tube that was described previously as a major component of scintillation detectors.

The PM tube–planchet assembly is placed in a chamber with a light-tight seal. The output signal from the PM tube is amplified and displayed.

As the temperature of the planchet is increased, the amount of light emitted by the TLD increases in an irregular manner. Fig. 38.15 shows the light output from lithium fluoride (LiF) as temperature increases. Several prominent peaks can be seen on the graph; each occurs because of a specific electron transition within the thermoluminescent crystals.

Such a graph is known as a **glow curve**; each type of thermoluminescent material has a characteristic glow curve. The height of the highest temperature peak and the total area under the curve are directly proportional to the energy deposited in the TLD by ionizing radiation. TLD analyzers are electronic instruments that are designed to measure the height of the glow curve or the area under the curve and relate this to radiation exposure or radiation dose through a conversion factor.

Many materials, including some body tissues, exhibit the property of radiation-induced thermoluminescence. Materials that are used for TLD, however, are somewhat limited in number and are principally types of inorganic crystals. LiF is the most widely used TLD material. It has an atomic number of 8.2 and therefore exhibits x-ray absorption properties similar to those of soft tissue.

LiF is relatively sensitive. It can measure doses as low as 50 μGy_t with modest accuracy, and at doses exceeding 100 mGy_t, its accuracy is very precise.

> LiF is a nearly tissue-equivalent radiation dosimeter.

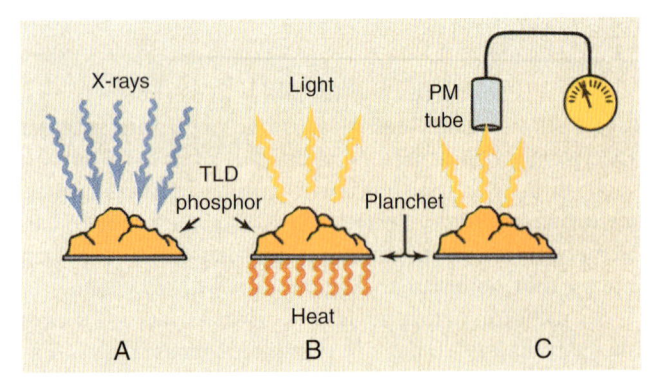

FIG. 38.14 Thermoluminescence dosimetry (*TLD*) is a multistep process. (A) Exposure to ionizing radiation. (B) Subsequent heating. (C) Measurement of the intensity of emitted light. *PM*, Photomultiplier.

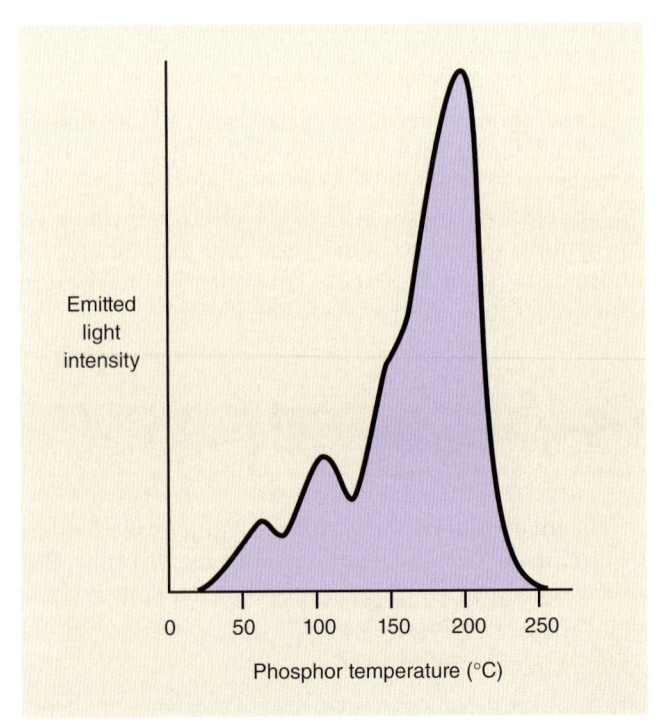

FIG. 38.15 Thermoluminescence glow curve for lithium fluoride (LiF).

TABLE 38.6 Some Thermoluminescent Phosphors and Their Characteristics and Uses

	Lithium Fluoride	Lithium Borate	Calcium Fluoride	Calcium Sulfate
Composition	LiF	$Li_2B_4O_7$:Mn	CaF_2:Mn	$CaSO_4$:Dy
Mass density ($\times 10^3 kg/m^3$)	2.64	2.5	3.18	2.61
Effective atomic number	8.2	7.4	16.3	15.3
Temperature of main peak (°C)	195	200	260	220
Principal use	Patient radiation dose	Research	Environmental monitoring	Environmental monitoring

Calcium fluoride (CaF_2) activated with manganese (CaF_2:Mn) has a higher effective atomic number (Z = 16.3) than LiF; this makes it considerably more sensitive to ionizing radiation. CaF_2:Mn can measure radiation doses of less than 10 μGy_t with moderate accuracy. Other types of TLDs are available. Table 38.6 lists some thermoluminescent phosphors and their principal characteristics and applications.

A particular advantage of TLD is size. The TLD can be obtained in several solid crystal shapes and sizes. Rectangular rods measuring 1 × 1 × 6 mm and flat chips measuring 3 × 1 mm are the most popular sizes. The TLD also can be obtained in powder form; this allows irradiation in nearly any configuration. TLDs are also available with the phosphor matrixed with Teflon or plated onto a wire and sealed in glass.

The TLD is reusable.

With irradiation, the energy absorbed by the TLD remains stored until released as visible light by heat during analysis. Heating restores the crystal to its original condition and makes it ready for another exposure.

The TLD responds proportionately to dose. If the dose is doubled, the TLD response also is doubled.

The TLD is rugged, and its small size makes it useful for monitoring doses in small areas, such as body cavities. The TLD does not respond to individual ionizing events; therefore it cannot be used in a rate meter type of instrument. The TLD is suitable only for integral dose measurements, but it does not give immediate results. It must be analyzed after irradiation for dosimetry results.

Optically Stimulated Luminescence Dosimetry

An additional radiation dosimeter especially adapted for personnel monitoring was developed by Landauer in the late 1990s (Fig. 38.16). The process is called **optically stimulated luminescence** (OSL) and is the principal type of occupational radiation dosimeter today. OSL uses aluminum oxide (Al_2O_3) as the radiation detector.

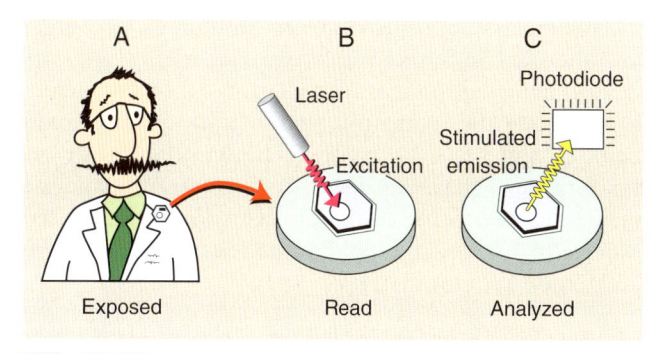

FIG. 38.16 Optically stimulated luminescence dosimetry is a multistep process. (A) Exposure to ionizing radiation. (B) Laser illumination. (C) Measurement of the intensity of stimulated light emission.

Irradiation of Al_2O_3 moves some electrons into an excited state. During processing, laser light stimulates these electrons, causing them to return to their ground state with the emission of visible light. The intensity of the visible light emission is proportional to the radiation dose received by the Al_2O_3.

The OSL process is not unlike TLD. Both are based on stimulated luminescence. However, OSL has several advantages over TLD, especially as applied to occupational radiation monitoring.

With a minimum reportable dose of 10 μGy_t, OSL is more sensitive than TLD. OSL has a precision of 10 μGy_t, which beats TLD. Other features of OSL include reanalysis for confirmation of dose, qualitative information about exposure conditions, wide dynamic range, and excellent long-term stability.

SUMMARY

Many radiation protection devices, accessories, and protocols are associated with digital imaging systems. This chapter discusses the radiation protection devices that are common to all radiographic and fluoroscopic imaging systems. Many of these devices are federally mandated; others exhibit features added by vendors.

Leakage radiation emitted by the x-ray tube during exposure must be contained by a protective x-ray tube housing. The limit of leakage must be no more than 1 mGy$_a$ per hour at a distance of 1 m from the housing. The control panel must indicate exposure by kVp and mA meters or visible and audible signals.

Great attention is given to the design of radiographic rooms, to the placement of x-ray imaging systems, and to the use of adjoining rooms. Two types of protective barriers are used: primary barriers and secondary barriers. Primary barriers intercept the useful x-ray beam and require the greatest amount of lead or concrete. Secondary barriers protect personnel from scatter and leakage radiation.

Dosimeters are instruments designed to detect and measure radiation. Four types of highly accurate devices are used to measure radiation. Gas-filled detectors include the ionization chamber, the proportional counter, and the GM counter. The scintillation detector is a very sensitive device that is used in nuclear medicine. Two other radiation detection devices used especially for occupational radiation monitoring are TLD and OSL dosimetry.

CHALLENGE QUESTIONS

1. Define or otherwise identify the following:
   a. TLD
   b. Use factor
   c. Diagnostic protective x-ray tube housing
   d. Glow curve
   e. Primary protective barrier
   f. X-ray linearity
   g. Secondary radiation
   h. Occupancy factor
   i. Geiger-Muller region
   j. Resolving time
2. What do audible and visible signals indicate on the radiographic control console?
3. List as many devices used for radiation protection on radiographic equipment as you can.
4. What is the result if the x-ray beam and the image receptor are not properly aligned?
5. What filtration is used for mammography equipment operated below 30 kVp?
6. How are reproducibility and linearity different when the intensity of the x-ray beam is measured?
7. What characteristics of fluoroscopic equipment are designed for radiation protection?
8. How can filtration be measured if the amount of inherent and added filtration is unknown?
9. Name the three types of radiation exposure that are of concern when protective barriers are designed.
10. List four factors that are taken into consideration when a barrier for a radiographic room is designed.
11. What is the difference between a controlled area and an uncontrolled area?
12. What are the units of workload for an x-ray examination room?
13. Explain the use factor as it relates to a protective barrier in an x-ray examination room.
14. Why is the use factor for secondary barriers always 1?
15. Name the three gas-filled dosimeters.
16. Discuss the properties of TLD that make it suitable for personnel monitoring.
17. Which modality of digital imaging uses scintillation detection as a radiation detector?
18. What are the two most widely used scintillation phosphors?
19. A PM tube has nine dynodes, each of which has a gain of 2.2. What is the overall tube gain?
20. Given the following conditions of operation, compute the weekly workload:
    a. 20 patients per day
    b. 3.2 films per patient
    c. 80 mAs per view on average

The answers to the Challenge Questions can be found by logging on to our website at http://evolve.elsevier.com.

Radiography/Fluoroscopy Patient Radiation Dose

CHAPTER 39

OBJECTIVES

At the completion of this chapter, the student should be able to do the following:

1. Define the differences between projection imaging, reflection imaging, and emission imaging.
2. Explain the use of entrance skin exposure, mean marrow dose, genetically significant dose, and tissue dose for patient radiation dose.
3. Identify the methods available for reducing patient radiation dose in fluoroscopy.
4. Describe effective dose and how it is used when describing patient radiation dose.
5. Relate the dose area product to the patient radiation dose.

OUTLINE

Patient Radiation Dose Descriptions 528
   Entrance Skin Exposure 530
   Mean Marrow Dose 532
   Genetically Significant Dose 532
   Tissue Dose 533

Fluoroscopic Patient Radiation Dose 534
   Dose Area Product 535
   Effective Dose 536
Summary 536
Challenge Questions 536

MEDICAL IMAGING has experienced considerable change since the turn of the millennium. From Roentgen's time through the 1970s, x-ray images were made by projecting the x-ray beam onto the patient. Those x-rays in the remnant beam produced the image. Emission imaging as in positron emission tomography and magnetic resonance imaging (MRI), and reflection imaging as in diagnostic ultrasound are now common digital imaging modalities.

Radiography, fluoroscopy, and computed tomography (CT) are examples of projection imaging. Radiography is still the most widely used, but it too has changed from screen-film radiography before the millennium to digital imaging today.

Over the past two or three decades, cost of living inflation in the United States has averaged approximately 4% per year. Health care increases at approximately 9% per year. Medical imaging increases at approximately 18% per year, principally due to radiography and advanced imaging modalities such as CT, MRI, and nuclear medicine, as shown in Fig. 39.1. This increase has been accompanied by an increase in average patient radiation dose, as discussed in Chapter 41.

Both radiography and fluoroscopy, as shown in Fig. 39.2, are imaging modalities that require an area x-ray beam projected onto a patient. Digital radiography currently dominates medical imaging. The principal modes of digital radiography are shown in Fig. 39.3, and it should be noted that no one digital imaging modality has emerged as the leader and is most likely to succeed.

PATIENT RADIATION DOSE DESCRIPTIONS

Patient radiation dose in radiography is expressed in one of four different ways, and the expression depends on the use of the numeric value of the dose estimate. Entrance skin exposure (ESE), mean marrow dose (MMD), genetically significant dose (GSD), and tissue dose are each important ways to express patient radiation dose.

Exposure of patients to x-rays is commanding increasing attention in our society for two reasons. First, the frequency of x-ray examination is increasing among all age groups. This indicates that physicians are relying more and more on x-ray diagnosis to assist them in patient care, even considering the newer imaging modalities.

This is to be expected. X-ray diagnosis is considered much more accurate now than in the past. More rigorous training programs required of radiologists and radiographers, and improvements in digital x-ray imaging systems allow for more difficult, but more substantive, x-ray examinations. Efficacy and diagnostic accuracy are much improved.

Second, concern among public health officials and radiation scientists is increasing regarding the risk of stochastic response that is associated with medical x-ray exposure. Deterministic response on superficial tissues after interventional radiology (IR) procedures is reported with increasing frequency.

The possible late effects of diagnostic x-ray exposure are of concern; therefore attention must be given to good radiation control practices. When a diagnosis

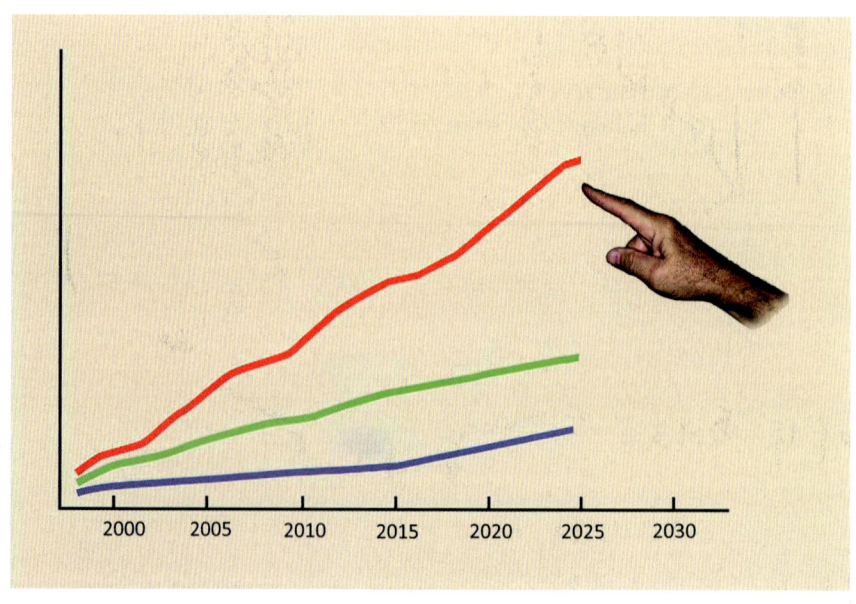

FIG. 39.1 The growth of the cost of medical imaging compared with healthcare costs and general inflation.

CHAPTER 39 Radiography/Fluoroscopy Patient Radiation Dose   529

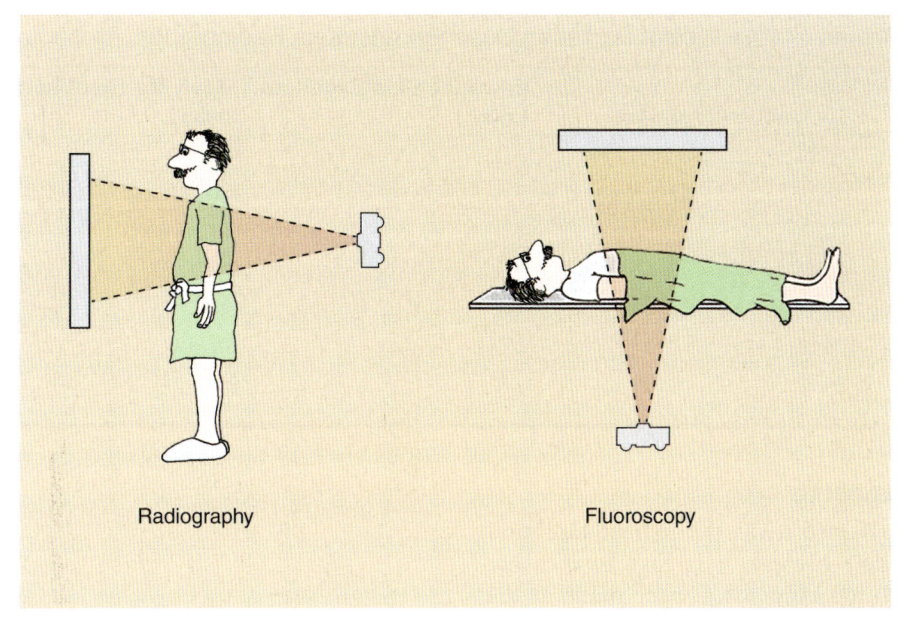

FIG. 39.2 The configuration for radiography and fluoroscopy, two projection x-ray imaging modalities.

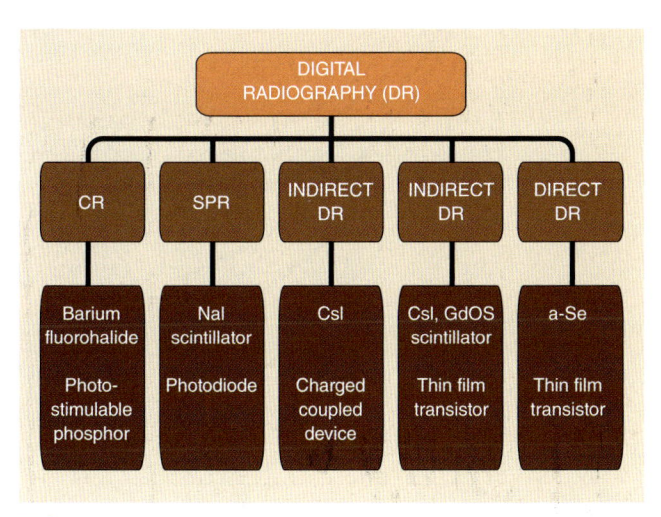

FIG. 39.3 The many digital radiographic imaging modes. *CR*, Computed radiography; *SPR*, scanned projection radiography.

can be obtained with a low radiation dose, or with an alternate imaging modality such as MRI or diagnostic ultrasound, it should be used because of reduced risk. This is in keeping with **ALARA** (as low as reasonably achievable).

To express patient radiation dose, one must first measure the output radiation intensity from the x-ray imaging system. Usually it is the medical physicist who makes this measurement of air KERMA (kinetic energy released in matter) expressed in units of mGy_a.

Patient radiation dose from diagnostic x-rays is reported in one of the following ways. Exposure to the entrance surface, or **entrance skin exposure (ESE)**, is reported most often because it is easiest to measure.

The dose to the **bone marrow** is important because bone marrow is the target organ believed responsible for radiation-induced leukemia. It is expressed as **mean marrow dose (MMD)**. Bone marrow dose cannot be measured directly; it is estimated from ESE.

The **gonadal dose** is important because of possible genetic responses to medical x-ray exposure. It is expressed as **genetically significant dose (GSD)**. The dose to the gonads can easily be measured or estimated.

> Patient radiation dose is expressed as ESE, MMD, and GSD.

Table 39.1 presents some representative values of entrance skin dose (ESD), MMD, and gonadal dose for various radiographic examinations. Note that these are only approximate values and should not be used to estimate patient radiation dose at any given medical imaging facility.

In any given medical imaging facility, actual doses delivered may be considerably different. Efficiency of x-ray production and image receptor (IR) speed are the most important variables.

> Patient radiation dose during fluoroscopy is too dependent on technique, equipment, and beam-on time to be estimated easily.

These values provide for relative dose comparisons among various radiologic examinations. Usually patient radiation dose in fluoroscopy must be measured and often it is measured during the examination with an integral DAP (**dose area product**) meter.

TABLE 39.1	Representative Patient Radiation Dose From Various Radiographic Procedures			
Examination	Technique (kVp/mAs)	Entrance Skin Exposure (mGy$_a$)	Mean Marrow Dose (mGy$_t$)	Gonadal Dose (mGy$_t$)
Skull	76/50	2.0	0.10	<1
Chest	110/3	0.1	0.02	<1
Cervical spine	70/40	1.5	0.10	<1
Lumbar spine	72/60	3.0	0.60	2.25
Abdomen	74/60	4.0	0.30	1.25
Pelvis	70/50	1.5	0.20	1.50
Extremity	60/5	0.5	0.02	<1

Entrance Skin Exposure

ESE most often is referred to as the patient radiation dose. It is used widely because it is easy to measure and reasonably accurate estimates can be made in the absence of measurements.

Thermoluminescence dosimeters (TLDs) and optically stimulated luminescence dosimeters (OSLs) are used most often during the examination. The size, sensitivity, and accuracy of these dosimeters make them very satisfactory patient radiation dose monitors.

A small grouping or pack of 3 to 10 TLDs or OSLs can be taped easily to the patient's skin in the center of the x-ray field. Because the response of these dosimeters is proportional to exposure and dose, they can be used to measure all levels experienced in digital imaging. With proper laboratory technique, the results of such measurements are accurate to within +/−5%.

> Three methods for estimating ESE are available in the absence of patient measurements.

The first method requires the use of a nomogram, such as that shown in Fig. 39.4. This figure contains a family of curves from which one can estimate the output intensity of a radiographic unit if the technique is known or assumed. The output intensity of different x-ray imaging systems varies widely, so the use of this nomogram method is only a good approximation.

Use of this nomogram first requires knowledge of the total filtration in the x-ray beam. This is usually available from the medical physics report, but if not, 3-mm Al is always a good estimate. Next, the kVp and mAs of the intended examination should be identified.

A vertical line rising from the value of total filtration should be drawn until it intersects with the kVp of the examination. From this intersection, a horizontal line is drawn to the left until it intersects the mGy$_a$/mAs axis. The resultant mGy$_a$/mAs value is the approximate output intensity of the radiographic unit. This value should be multiplied with the examination mAs value to obtain the approximate patient exposure.

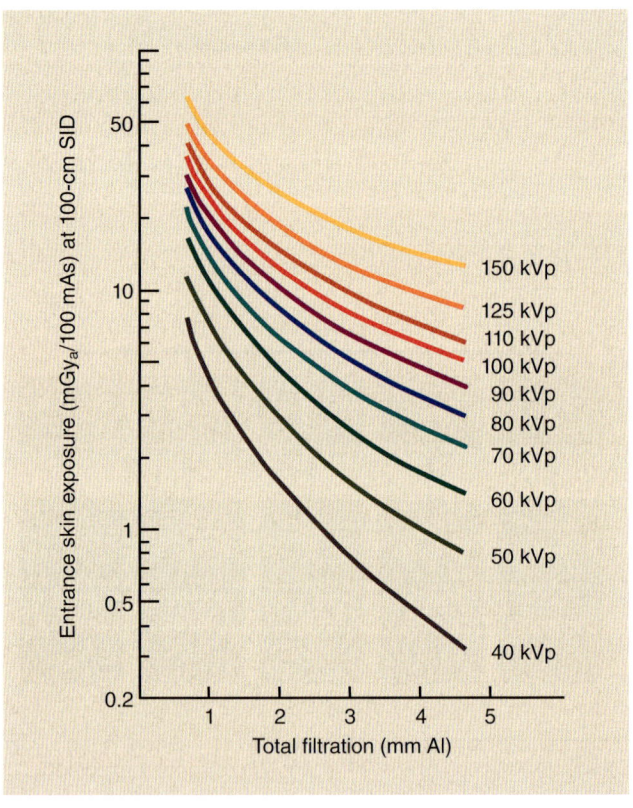

FIG. 39.4 This family of curves is a nomogram for estimating output x-ray intensity from a single-phase radiographic unit. SID, Source-to-image distance. (Courtesy John R. Cameron[†], University of Wisconsin.)

Question: With reference to Fig. 39.4, estimate the ESE from a lateral cervical spine image made at 66 kVp, 150 mAs, with a radiographic unit having 2.5-mm Al total filtration.

Answer: Estimate the intersection between a vertical line rising from 2.5-mm Al and a horizontal line through the 66-kVp curve. Extend the horizontal line to the y-axis and read 38 µGy$_t$/mAs.
38 µGy$_t$/mAs × 150 mAs = 5700 µGy$_t$ = 5.7 mGy$_a$

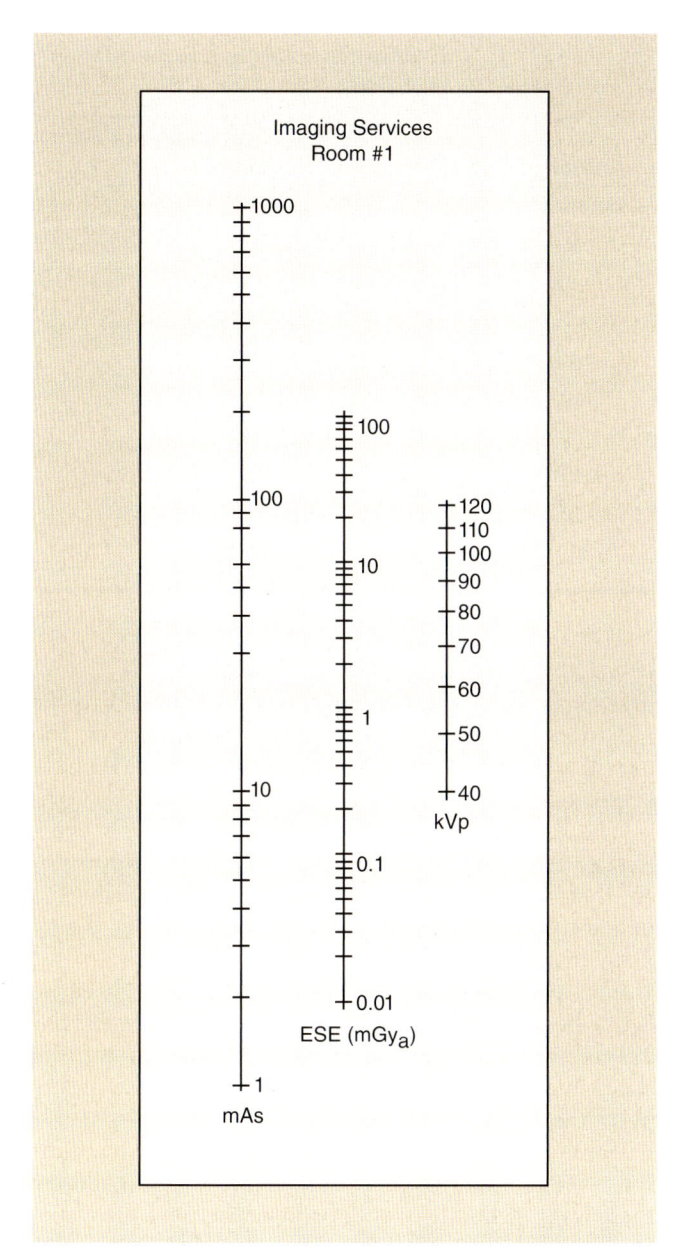

FIG. 39.5 This type of nomogram is very accurate but must be fashioned individually for each radiographic unit. *ESE*, Entrance skin exposure. (Courtesy Michael D. Harpen, University of South Alabama.)

condition. During the annual or special radiation control survey and calibration of an x-ray imaging system, the medical physicist measures this output intensity, usually in units of mGy$_a$/mAs at 80 cm—the approximate source-to-skin distance (SSD)—or at 100 cm—the source-to-image receptor distance (SID).

> At 70 kVp, radiographic output intensity varies from approximately 20–100 μGy$_a$/mAs at 80-cm SSD.

With this calibration value available, one would first make an adjustment for a different SSD by applying the inverse square law.

Question: The output intensity of a radiographic unit is reported as 37 μGy$_a$/mAs at 100-cm SID. What is the intensity at 75-cm SSD?

Answer: At 75-cm SSD, the intensity will be greater by $(100/75)^2 = (1.32)^2 = 1.7837$ μGy$_a$/mAs × 1.78 = 66 μGy$_a$/mAs.

With the ESE, one scales this according to the kVp and mAs of the examination. Output intensity varies according to the square of the ratio in terms of the change in kVp. Refer to Chapter 9 to review this relationship.

Question: The output intensity at 70 kVp and 75-cm SSD is 66 μGy$_a$/mAs. What is the output intensity at 76 kVp?

Answer: At higher kVp, the output intensity is greater by the square of the ratio of the kVp. $(76/70)^2 = (1.09)^2 = 1.18$ 66 μGy$_a$/mAs × 1.18 = 78 μGy$_a$/mAs

The final step in estimating ESE is to multiply the output intensity in mGy$_a$/mAs by the examination mAs value because these values are proportional.

Question: If the radiographic technique for an intravenous pyelogram calls for 80 mAs, what is the ESE when the output intensity is 78 μGy$_a$/mAs?

Answer: 78 μGy$_a$/mAs × 80 mAs = 6240 μGy$_a$ = 6.24 mGy$_a$

These steps can be combined into a single calculation, as illustrated in the following example.

Question: The output intensity for a radiographic unit is 45 μGy$_a$/mAs at 70 kVp and 80 cm. If a lateral skull digital image is taken at 66 kVp, 150 mAs, what will be the ESD at an 80-cm SSD? What would be the skin dose at a 90-cm SSD?

A better approach requires that a medical physicist construct a nomogram, such as that shown in Fig. 39.5 for each digital radiographic imaging system. A straight edge between any kVp and mAs value will cross the ESE scale at the correct mGy$_a$ value.

Question: Using the nomogram in Fig. 39.5, identify the ESE when a radiographic exposure is made at 66 kVp, 150 mAs.

Answer: When the line is drawn as instructed, it crosses the ESE scale at 10 mGy$_a$.

A third method for estimating ESE requires that one know the output intensity for at least one operating

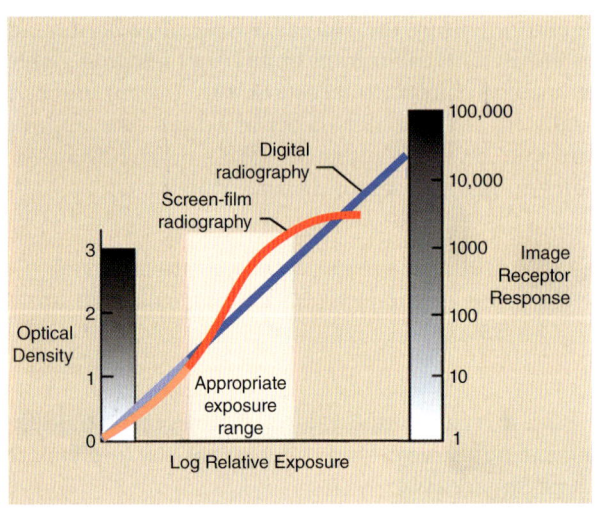

FIG. 39.6 Image receptor response for digital radiography helps to show why patient radiation dose can be reduced with digital imaging.

TABLE 39.2	Distribution of Active Bone Marrow in Adults
Anatomic Site	**Percentage of Bone Marrow**
Head	10
Upper limb girdle	8
Sternum	3
Ribs	11
Cervical vertebrae	4
Thoracic vertebrae	13
Lumbar vertebrae	11
Sacrum	11
Lower limb girdle	29
Total	**100**

Answer: At 80 cm SSD:

$$\text{Dose} = (45\ \mu Gy_a/mAs)\left(\frac{66\ kVp}{70\ kVp}\right)^2 (150\ mAs)$$

$$= 6000\ \mu Gy_a$$

$$= 6\ mGy_b$$

At 90 cm SSD:

$$\text{Dose} = (6000\ \mu Gy_a)\left(\frac{80}{90}\right)^2 = 4740\ \mu Gy_a$$

$$= 4.74\ mGy_a$$

The exit skin dose (ESD) is the easiest of the four measures of patient radiation dose to estimate or measure. When radiography is performed, one can measure the intensity of radiation to the entrance skin directly. And whatever the ESE value, the exit skin dose will be approximately 1% of the ESE.

> The half-value layer of x-rays in soft tissue is approximately 4 cm.

There are many reasons for patient radiation dose reduction using digital imaging techniques, but the main reason is the shape of the IR response function (Fig. 39.6). The linearity of the digital image receptor response function means that a lower dose is usually sufficient for good image quality.

Furthermore, the digital image receptor scales five orders of magnitude. With image postprocessing, we can visualize all five orders of magnitude.

Mean Marrow Dose

One of the risks of x-ray imaging is the induction of blood disorders such as leukemia, lymphoma, and myeloma. These stochastic responses are linked to the radiation dose to the stem cells of the bone marrow. The metric is the MMD, and many estimates of MMD have been made.

The hematologic effects of radiation are rarely experienced in diagnostic radiology. However, it is appropriate that we understand the concept of MMD, which is one measure of patient radiation dose during digital x-ray imaging procedures.

The MMD is the average radiation dose to the entire active bone marrow. For instance, if during a particular examination, 50% of the active bone marrow were in the primary beam and received an average dose of 250 μGy_t, the MMD would be 125 μGy_t.

Table 39.1 includes the approximate MMD in adults for various radiographic examinations. In children, these levels generally would be lower because the radiographic techniques used are considerably less. Table 39.2 shows the distribution of active bone marrow in the adult, and this gives some clue as to which diagnostic x-ray procedures involve exposure to large amounts of bone marrow.

In the United States, the MMD from diagnostic x-ray examinations averaged over the entire population is approximately 1 mGy_t/yr. Such a dose never results in the hematologic responses described in Chapter 35. However, it is a dose concept that is used to estimate, on a population basis, the risk of one late effect of radiation—leukemia.

Genetically Significant Dose

Measurements and estimates of gonad dose are important because of the suspected genetic effects of radiation. Although the gonad dose from diagnostic x-rays is low for each individual, this may have some significance in terms of population effects.

Similar to MMD, the GSD is an attempt to place a radiation dose value to our gene pool. In the United States, the GSD is estimated at 0.2 mGy$_t$/year. This is an insignificantly small radiation dose and not expected to cause any measurable radiation response.

> The population gonad dose of importance is the GSD, the radiation dose to the population gene pool.

The GSD is the gonad dose that, if received by every member of the population, would produce the total genetic effect on the population as the sum of the individual doses actually received. Thus it is a weighted-average gonad dose. It considers those persons who are irradiated and those who are not, with averaging of the results. The GSD can be estimated only through large-scale epidemiologic studies.

GENETICALLY SIGNIFICANT DOSE

$$GSD = \frac{\sum DN_X P}{\sum N_T P}$$

where Σ is the mathematical symbol meaning to sum or add values, D is the average gonad dose per examination, N_X signifies the number of persons receiving x-ray examinations, N_T is the total number of persons in the population, and P (progeny) is the expected future number of children per person.

Therefore for computational purposes, the GSD considers the age, sex, and expected number of children for each person examined with x-rays. It also acknowledges the various types of examinations and the gonad dose per examination type.

Estimates of GSD have been conducted in many different countries (Table 39.3). The estimate reported by the US Public Health Service is 0.2 mGy$_t$/year. Thus this is a genetic radiation burden over and above the existing natural background radiation level of approximately 1 mGy$_t$/year. The genetic effects of this total GSD, 1.2 mGy$_t$/year, are not detectable.

Tissue Dose

The various tissues and organs of the body have different sensitivity to radiation dose. One of the least radiation-sensitive tissues, as shown in Fig. 39.7 is the skin, and yet it is of primary concern.

Radiation-induced skin burns have appeared since the earliest days but are not now normally associated with radiography. For many years, reports of serious skin damage in the cardiac catheterization laboratory have been reported. More recently, IR has become implicated.

Radiographic tissue dose is very dependent on the technique used for the study, and therefore a range of values is possible for each type of study. Table 39.1 provides a start to such a table.

The newest radiographic imaging modality is digital radiographic tomosynthesis (DRT), introduced in 2011. Many think that this will replace a number of routine CT examinations. DRT (Fig. 39.8) is now regularly used for mammography as digital mammographic tomosynthesis (see Chapter 22).

DRT requires approximately the same patient radiation dose as digital radiography, and the image contrast is superior. DRT was not possible until the introduction of the digital image receptor.

TABLE 39.3 Genetically Significant Dose Estimated From Diagnostic X-Ray Examinations

Population	Genetically Significant Dose (mGy$_t$)
Denmark	0.22
Great Britain	0.12
Japan	0.27
New Zealand	0.12
Sweden	0.72
United States	0.20

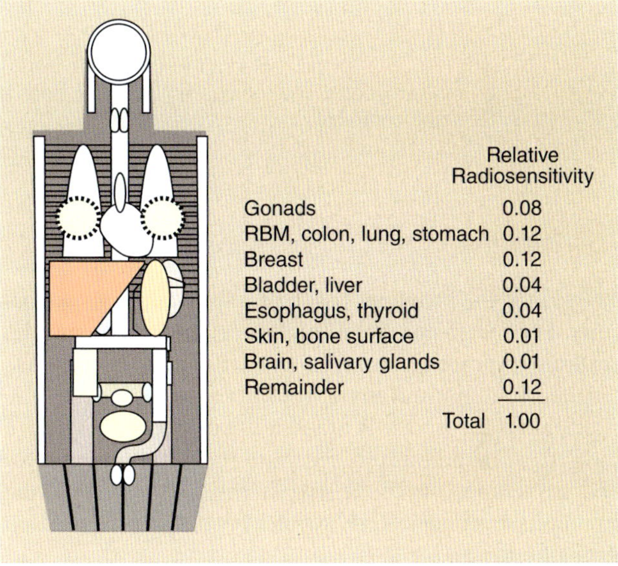

Relative Radiosensitivity
- Gonads 0.08
- RBM, colon, lung, stomach 0.12
- Breast 0.12
- Bladder, liver 0.04
- Esophagus, thyroid 0.04
- Skin, bone surface 0.01
- Brain, salivary glands 0.01
- Remainder 0.12
- Total 1.00

FIG. 39.7 This computer-generated anthropomorphic phantom identifies the various tissues and organs of the body and their relative radiation sensitivity. *RBM*, Red bone marrow.

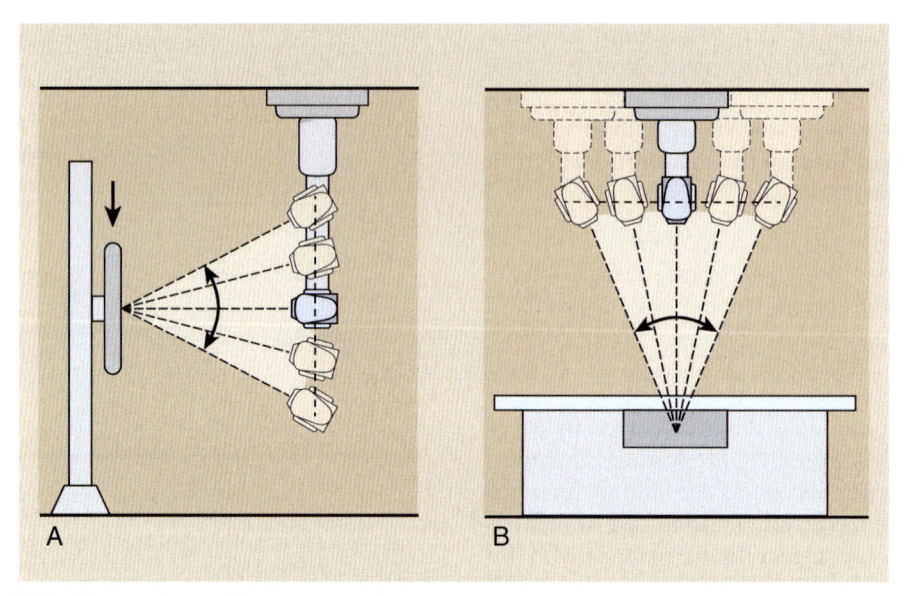

FIG. 39.8 Digital radiographic tomosynthesis involves several x-ray exposures at different angles to the image receptor. The total patient radiation dose is about that of a single digital radiograph with improved image contrast.

FLUOROSCOPIC PATIENT RADIATION DOSE

The skin is the principal tissue of importance in fluoroscopy. The increasing use of high-level fluoroscopy in the cardiology practice and in interventional radiology has resulted in many serious skin injuries.

ESE in fluoroscopy is much more difficult to estimate than that for radiography because the x-ray field moves and sometimes varies in size. If the field were of one size and stationary, ESE would be directly related to exposure time.

> For the average fluoroscopic examination, one can assume an ESE of 40 mGy$_a$/min.

Question: A fluoroscopic procedure requires 2.5 min at 90 kVp, 2 mA. What is the approximate ESE?

Answer: ESE = (40 mGy$_a$/min) (2.5 min) = 100 mGy$_a$

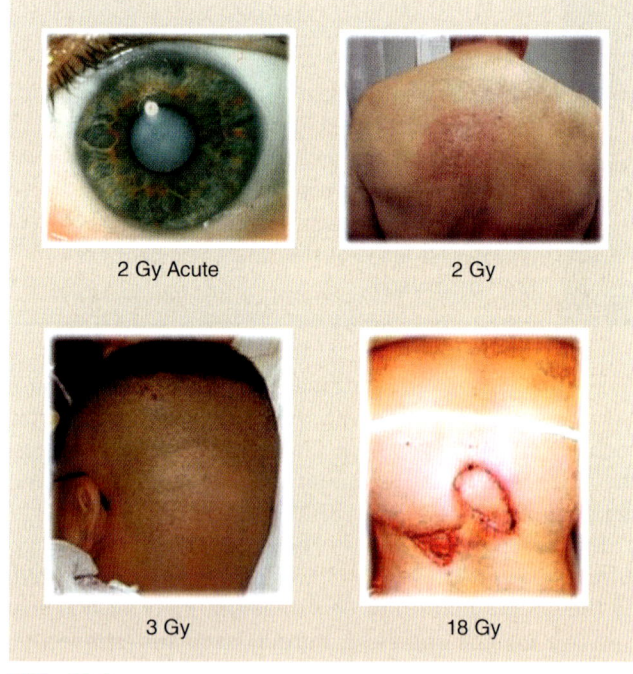

FIG. 39.9 Several reported fluoroscopic injuries and the related entrance skin dose.

What has been described for radiographic patient radiation dose applies equally well to fluoroscopic patient radiation dose. Furthermore, with the increasing processing power of digital fluoroscopy, the speed and capacity of such imaging is soaring.

Digital fluoroscopy has enabled ever faster and more complete energy subtraction and time interval difference image sequencing. The increasing use of pulse progressive fluoroscopy reduces this concern for patient radiation dose.

The Center for Devices and Radiation Health (CDRH) is an arm of the US Public Health Service. The CDRH considers that any skin dose exceeding 15 Gy$_t$ is a **sentinel event** and must be reported. A sentinel event is always followed by severe skin damage.

There are currently in excess of 500 such reported cases and Fig. 39.9 shows the appearance of some of the more recent. Essentially all are from the cardiac catheterization laboratory or the interventional radiology suite.

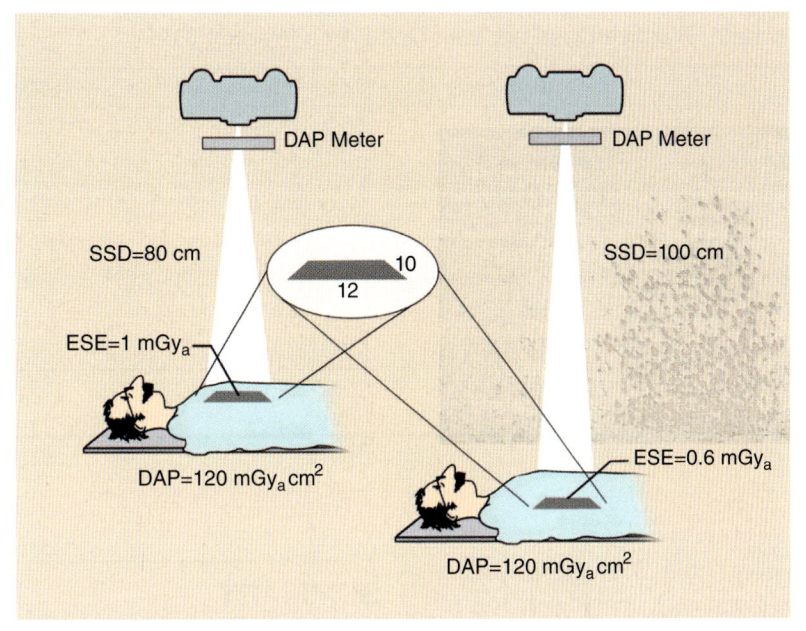

FIG. 39.10 The dose area product (*DAP*) is constant for a given field size regardless of source-to-skin distance (*SSD*) distance. *ESE*, Entrance skin exposure.

DOSE AREA PRODUCT

DAP is a quantity that reflects not only the patient radiation dose but also the amount of tissue irradiated; therefore it may be a better indicator of risk than dose. DAP is expressed in units of mGy$_a$-cm^2.

DAP increases with increasing radiation field size even if the dose remains unchanged. Smaller field size results in lower DAP and less risk because less tissue is exposed.

DAP meters are now common on most x-ray imaging systems and may be used to monitor radiation output from both radiographic and fluoroscopic imaging systems. Typically the DAP detector is positioned just after the x-ray beam collimator before the beam enters the patient.

The DAP detector is a transmission ionization chamber, parallel plate type, larger than the largest area x-ray beam. The ionization detected in the chamber is proportional to radiation dose and to the area of the x-ray beam.

The risk for injury to the skin where the x-ray beam enters the patient can be derived by dividing the DAP measurement by the area of the beam at the skin. Using DAP to monitor radiation intensity is a good way to implement radiation management procedures and keep the patient radiation dose low.

As we continue to estimate and record the radiation dose in the patient's medical record, DAP makes it easy. Whatever the DAP meter registers at the collimator position is the DAP at the patient entrance skin. Such a condition is true because the radiation dose decreases as the inverse square of the distance and the projected area increases as the square of the distance (Fig. 39.10).

Question: (a) A DAP meter registers 625 mGy$_t$-cm^2. If the SID = 70 cm, what is the patient DAP? (b) If the patient is moved closer to the x-ray source, SID = 50 cm, now what is the patient DAP?

Answer: (a) 625 mGy$_t$-cm^2; (b) 625 mGy$_t$-cm^2

What if a DAP meter registers 625 mGy$_t$-cm^2 and you do not know the patient thickness and therefore the SSD, and you do not know the size of the area exposed? Forget the SSD and estimate the x-ray beam size.

Question: What would be the patient radiation dose if you estimate a 10 × 10 cm field on the patient?

Answer: 10 × 10 cm = 100 cm^2
625 mGy$_t$-cm^2 / 100 cm^2 = 6.25 mGy$_t$
625 mGy$_t$-cm^2 / 625 cm^2 = 1 mGy$_t$

An even better but more difficult estimate of patient radiation dose for each particular projection is an estimate of effective dose (E). Recall that E = ΣDiWi, where DiWi is the product of radiation dose and tissue weighting factor. If one has a value for DAP, fluoroscopic or radiographic, one can estimate the effective dose from the conversion values shown in Table 39.4. Table 39.4 also shows the approximate effective dose per unit DAP.

TABLE 39.4 Approximate Effective Dose per Unit Dose Area Product (DAP)

Body Part	DAP (Gy$_t$-cm²)	E (mSv)	E/DAP (mSv/Gy$_t$-cm²)
Head	0.1–1	1–3	0.33
Chest	10–20	2–4	0.24
Abdomen	1–2	50–70	0.22
Pelvis	2–5	0.5–2	0.27
Intravenous pyelogram (6 images)	3–6	2.5	0.29
Hip	5–10	5–10	0.23
Coronary angiography	20–100	5–15	0.13
GI fluoroscopy	1–2	3–7	0.19

Some generalizations from Table 39.4 are in order. Conversion factors for head and neck imaging are lower than the trunk of the body because the tissue weighting factors are less. Conversion factors for posteroanterior (PA) examinations are less than anteroposterior examinations for the same reason, tissue weighting factors. In general, tissues with higher weighting factors are located anteriorly. The conversion factor range is 0.1 to 0.4 mSv/Gy$_t$-cm².

EFFECTIVE DOSE

Effective dose resulting from a radiographic procedure or especially a fluoroscopic procedure is very difficult to determine. The entrance skin dose is easy enough to measure; however, during fluoroscopy, the projection x-ray beam moves and therefore multiple organs can be irradiated for an unknown time.

Consider, for example, the PA chest radiographic examination. ESE for this examination is approximately 100 µGy$_a$. If one assumes an average tissue dose of half the entrance skin dose, 50 µGy$_t$, the effective dose is 0.014 mSv or 14 µSv, as follows.

Question: What is the patient effective dose following a PA chest examination if the average tissue dose is 50 µGy$_t$?

Answer: $E = \Sigma D_t W_t = 50 \times 0.12 = 6$ (lung)
$+ 50 \times 0.05 = 2.5$ (breast)
$+ 50 \times 0.05 = 2.5$ (esophagus)
$+ 50 \times 0.05 = 2.5$ (thyroid)
$= 13.5$ µSv (all other tissues receive zero radiation dose)

Effective dose is the patient radiation dose metric that is used to estimate stochastic radiation responses in populations.

SUMMARY

Patient radiation dose during radiography and fluoroscopy is expressed in several different ways. ESE is usually identified as the patient radiation dose because it is easy to express, compute, and measure.

TLDs and OSLs are the radiation monitors of choice for measuring patient radiation dose. By knowing the output intensity of at least one x-ray imaging technique and the SSD, the medical physicist can estimate the ESE for any patient examination.

For radiographic examination, a good starting assumption is 50 µGy$_t$/mAs. For fluoroscopic examination, assume 40 µGy$_t$/min.

Several methods are available to estimate effective dose (E) rather accurately for radiography. A similar estimate is very difficult during fluoroscopy because of changing field size and x-ray beam position.

CHALLENGE QUESTIONS

1. Define or otherwise identify the following:
    a. ALARA
    b. GSD
    c. ESE
    d. MMD
    e. DAP
    f. Sentinel event
    g. mGy$_t$-cm
    h. SSD
    i. DRT
    j. CDRH
2. How can the three cardinal principles of radiation protection best be applied in diagnostic radiology?
3. What estimate of patient radiation dose usually is measured and reported?
4. How does one use a radiation nomogram?

5. Estimate the ESE for a PA chest examination conducted at 110 kVp/mAs.
6. What factors are required to estimate the genetically significant dose (GSD)?
7. What does the symbol Σ mean?
8. How does one compute effective dose (E) for a radiographic examination?
9. Where is the DAP meter located during fluoroscopy?
10. Why does digital radiographic tomosynthesis produce higher-contrast images than digital radiography?
11. What is interventional radiology?
12. Why does progeny factor into the estimate of genetically significant dose?
13. What tissues have the highest radiation sensitivity?
14. Why is knowledge of gonadal radiation dose important?
15. What is the approximate half-value layer of diagnostic x-rays in soft tissue?
16. What is it about the digital image receptor response function that leads to lower patient radiation dose?
17. What is the approximate relationship between entrance skin dose and exit skin dose in digital imaging?
18. What is the best way to measure entrance skin exposure (ESE)?
19. What is the difference between projection imaging and emission imaging?
20. Discuss the stochastic responses of concern following digital imaging.

The answers to the Challenge Questions can be found by logging on to our website at http://evolve.elsevier.com.

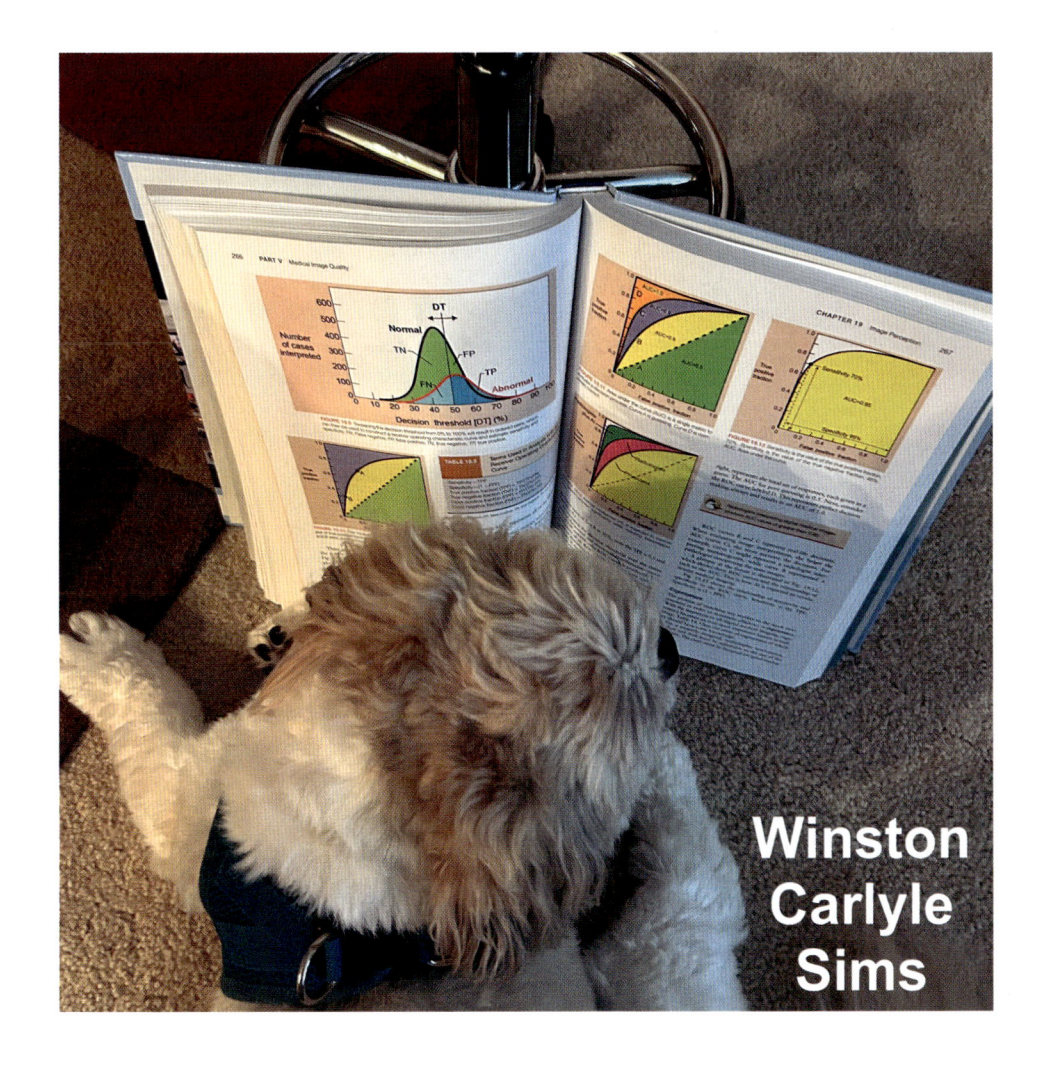

Winston Carlyle Sims

CHAPTER 40

Computed Tomography Patient Radiation Dose

OBJECTIVES

At the completion of this chapter, the student should be able to do the following:

1. Describe the x-ray beam shape and intensity during computed tomography.
2. Understand the principal advantages of the computed tomography image.
3. Define computed tomography dose index and its relationship to patient radiation dose.
4. Describe how computed tomography dose index is obtained and by whom.
5. Define dose length product and its relationship to computed tomography dose index.
6. Understand the concept of size-specific dose.
7. Show how to compute effective dose for a given patient examination.

OUTLINE

Computed Tomography Dose Delivery 540
 Patient Radiation Dose Distribution 540
 Radiation Dose Profile 541
 Computed Tomography Output Intensity 542

Computed Tomography Dose Index 543
 Dose Length Product 544
 Size-Specific Dose Estimates 545
 Effective Dose 545
 Summary 546
 Challenge Questions 547

CHAPTER 40 Computed Tomography Patient Radiation Dose

COMPUTED TOMOGRAPHY (CT) is an x-ray imaging modality unlike that of radiography or fluoroscopy. With CT, the x-ray beam is incident on all entrance skin circling the patient, resulting in a near-uniform radiation dose throughout the section of the patient being imaged. Review Chapter 21 for the history and x-ray beam movement during CT.

X-ray tomography was first demonstrated in the 1930s by several different investigators (Fig. 40.1). The principle purpose for tomography is to increase image contrast. This is accomplished by blurring overlying and underlying tissues so that those tissues in the fulcrum plane of rotation are emphasized.

Conventional tomography has disappeared with the introduction of digital imaging. The first digital imaging modality was CT, which has superior contrast resolution. Unfortunately it also results in high patient radiation dose that is increasing on a population basis because of overutilization and therefore is the cause of considerable concern. The past 10 years has seen a halt to further increase.

The x-ray beam emitted during CT is not an area beam but rather a cone beam (Fig. 40.2), and this contributes to the improved image contrast. The cone beam results in more scatter radiation rejection than an area beam and that results in better image contrast. Now, with the introduction of the digital image receptor in the

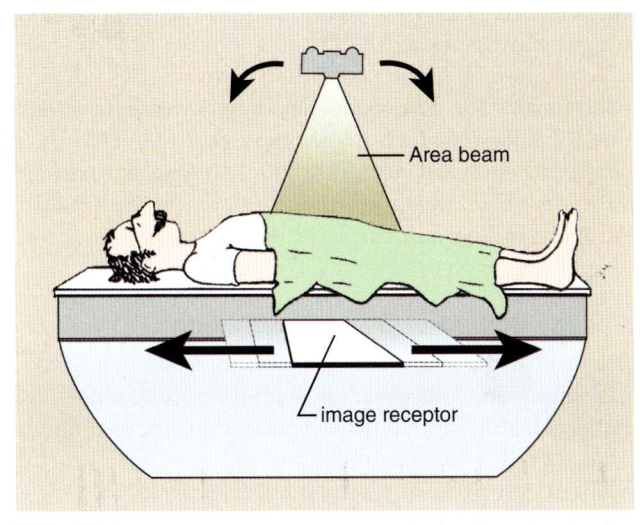

FIG. 40.1 Conventional x-ray tomography involves the simultaneous movement of x-ray tube and image receptor to improve the image contrast.

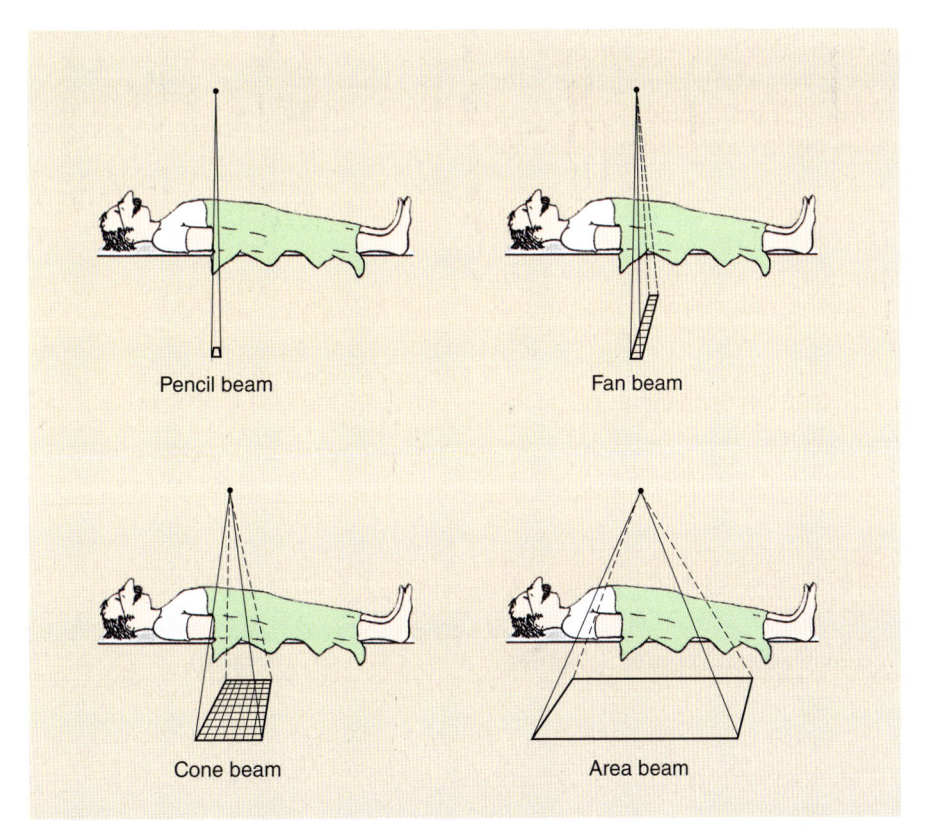

FIG. 40.2 Compared to the area x-ray beams of radiography and fluoroscopy, the CT x-ray beam is described as a cone.

year 2000, digital radiographic tomosynthesis is possible and may indeed replace many CT examinations.

COMPUTED TOMOGRAPHY DOSE DELIVERY

An important consideration in CT imaging, as with any x-ray procedure, is not only the entrance skin exposure (ESE) but also the distribution of dose to internal organs and tissues during imaging. On the basis of ESE, CT results in a higher dose than other digital imaging procedures. The ESE delivered by a series of contiguous CT slices is much higher than that delivered by a single radiographic view. Table 40.1 shows approximate values for ESE, mean marrow dose, and gonadal dose. A typical radiographic head or body examination, however, often involves several CT procedures.

Patient Radiation Dose Distribution

Because of the increasing use of multislice helical CT, CT must be considered a high-dose procedure. US Public Health Service data suggest that approximately 15% of all x-ray examinations are now CT, yet CT accounts for 50% of total patient effective dose.

> The CT tissue dose is approximately equal to the average fluoroscopic dose.

As was pointed out in Chapter 21, CT differs in many important ways from other x-ray examinations. A radiograph can be likened to a photograph taken with a flash in that the patient is "floodlighted" with x-rays to directly expose the image receptor through a large area x-ray beam.

On the other hand, CT exposes the patient with a restricted cone beam of x-rays. This difference in radiation delivery also means that the dose distribution from CT is different from that in radiographic procedures. Radiographic and fluoroscopic doses are high at the entrance surface and very low at the exit surface.

The CT dose is nearly uniform throughout the imaging volume for a head examination, as seen in Fig. 40.3.

The CT central axis radiation dose is approximately 50% of the ESE for body CT.

Part of the dose efficiency of CT is attributable to the precise collimation of the x-ray beam. Scatter radiation increases patient radiation dose and reduces image contrast. Because CT uses a cone-shaped x-ray beam rather than an area beam, scatter radiation is reduced significantly and contrast resolution is improved. Thus a larger percentage of the x-ray beam contributes usefully to the image and increases image contrast.

The precise collimation used in CT means that only a well-defined volume of tissue is irradiated for each imaging procedure. The ideal x-ray beam for CT would have sharp boundaries. No overlap between adjacent images would be seen. Thus the dose delivered to a patient from a series of ideal contiguous CT images should be the same as that from a single slice.

> It is essential that CT collimators be monitored periodically for proper adjustment.

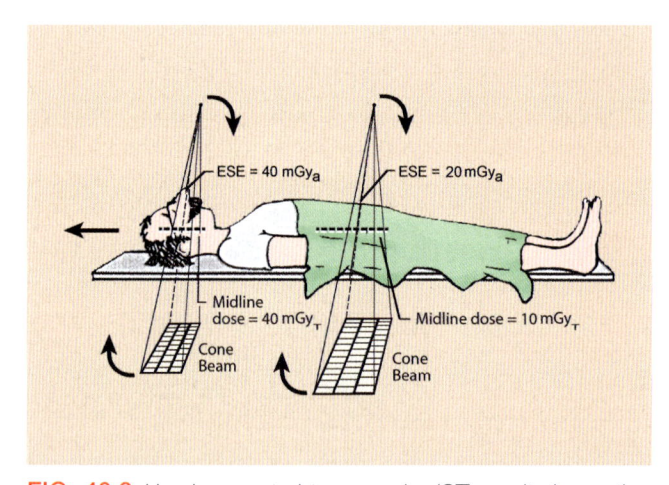

FIG. 40.3 Head computed tomography (CT) results in a rather uniform patient radiation dose of approximately 40 mGy$_t$. For body CT, the approximate dose is 20 mGy$_t$. *ESE*, Entrance skin exposure.

TABLE 40.1 Representative Patient Radiation Dose from CT X-ray Procedures

Examination	Technique (kVp/mAs)	Entrance Skin Exposure (mGy$_a$)	Mean Marrow Dose (mGy$_t$)	Gonad Dose (mGy$_t$)
CT head	125/300	40	0.2	0.5
CT pelvis	125/400	20	0.5	20
CT chest	110/200	10	0.6	0.5
CT abdomen	120/300	15	0.5	10

CT, Computed tomography.

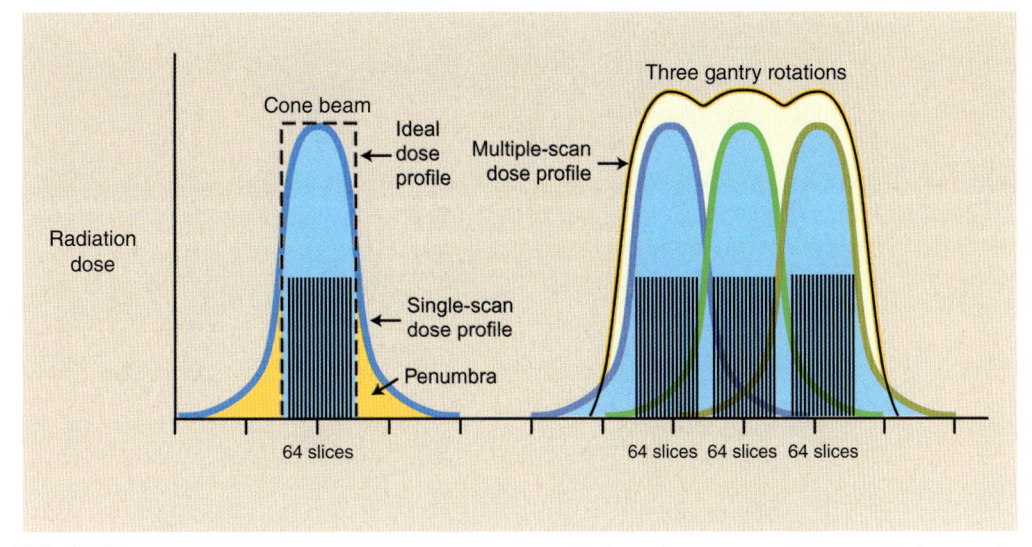

FIG. 40.4 Patient dose distribution in step-and-shoot multislice spiral computed tomography is complicated because the profile of the x-ray beam cannot be made sharp.

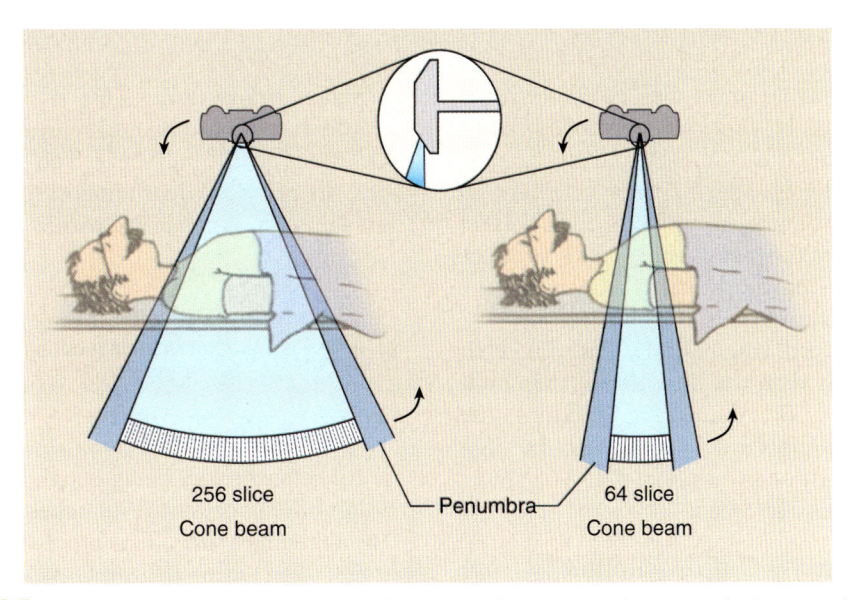

FIG. 40.5 Patient radiation dose is lower with higher multislice computed tomography because the beam penumbra is less for a given imaged anatomy.

Fig. 40.4 illustrates, however, why this ideal situation cannot be attained in practice. The size of the focal spot of the x-ray tube blurs the sharp boundaries of the section. Also the x-ray beam is not precisely parallel, and some spreading occurs as the beam crosses the image field.

Radiation Dose Profile

Multislice helical CT results in a lower patient radiation dose than step-and-shoot CT because fewer tails are seen on the dose profile for a given volume of tissue. The dose profile tail is called **penumbra**.

A 64-slice helical CT imaging system will result in a slightly lower patient radiation dose than fewer slices because a lower contribution is made from the penumbra for the same volume of tissue (Fig. 40.5). Additional patient dose saving occurs when the same beam width is imaged with combined pixel rows (Fig. 40.6) because the mA can be reduced without compromising image noise and therefore image contrast is improved.

> The higher the multislice value, the lower the patient radiation dose will be.

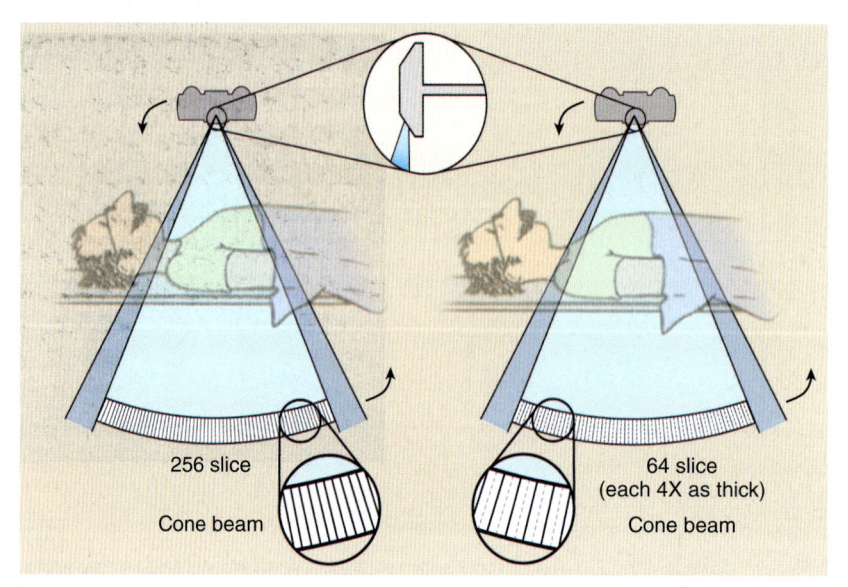

FIG. 40.6 When four detector rows are combined for the same beam width, the patient radiation dose will be lower.

Because the CT x-ray beam is well collimated, the area of irradiation can be precisely controlled. Thus radiosensitive organs such as the eyes and the gonads can be avoided selectively. Specific area shielding as protection from the primary x-ray beam in CT is of little use. Not only does the metal from shields produce artifacts in the image, but the rotational scheme of the x-ray source greatly reduces their effectiveness.

Patient radiation dose during helical CT is somewhat more difficult to assess than the dose during step-and-shoot CT. At a pitch of 1.0:1, the patient radiation dose is approximately the same. At a higher pitch, the dose is reduced compared with conventional CT. At a lower pitch, the patient dose is increased.

Computed Tomography Output Intensity

As with any radiographic procedure, many factors influence CT patient radiation dose. For CT imaging, a generalization is possible.

> **COMPUTED TOMOGRAPHY PATIENT DOSE**
>
> $$\text{Patient dose} = k \frac{IE}{\sigma^2 w^3 h}$$
>
> where k is a conversion factor, I is a beam intensity in mAs, E is average beam energy in keV ($\approx$ ½ kVp), σ is a system noise, w is pixel size, and h is beam width.

Note that, as with radiography, the patient dose is proportional to the x-ray beam intensity. It is also directly proportional to the average beam energy. Other factors are variables that are unique to CT imaging.

Sigma (σ) is noise. This is equivalent to quantum mottle in radiography and represents random statistical variations in CT numbers. The w stands for the pixel size, the principal determinant of spatial resolution. The last factor, h, is the beam width.

> A reduction in the noise or beam width, while other factors remain constant, increases patient radiation dose.

All other factors being equal, a low-noise, high-resolution CT image results in higher patient radiation dose. The challenge with CT, as indeed with all x-ray imaging, is not so much to deliver fantastically good resolution and low noise (because this could be achieved at the cost of very high patient dose) but to use the x-ray beam efficiently, producing a quality image at a reasonable patient radiation dose.

This expression for patient radiation dose in CT is rarely used. It is presented here just to show the parameters that affect CT radiation intensity. The concepts of computed tomography dose index (CTDI) and dose length product (DLP) that follow are important and are regularly employed.

Essentially all CT imaging systems today are third generation—both the x-ray source and the detector array image receptor rotate about a common axis (Fig. 40.7). The detector array is three dimensional, as seen in Fig. 40.8, and therefore intercepts something less than an area x-ray beam. The prepatient collimators define the cone beam, and the predetector collimators further reject scatter radiation, thereby improving image contrast.

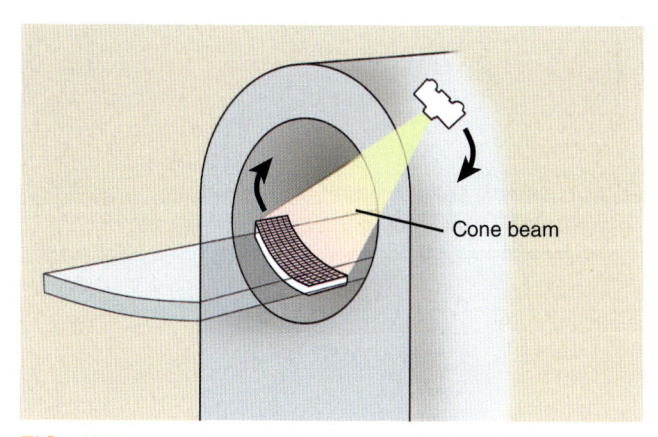

FIG. 40.7 Current computed tomography imaging systems are third-generation types, having a detector array that intercepts what is termed a *cone beam*.

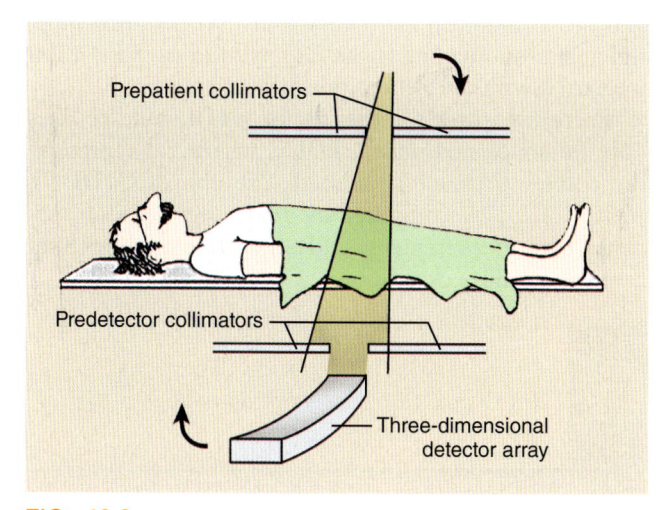

FIG. 40.8 The detector array for multislice, helical computed tomography is three dimensional, having several rows of individual detector cells.

The CT technologist normally selects an anatomical section for imaging, and the console computer automatically selects the kVp and mA. Current CT imaging systems have dose modulation (Fig. 40.9). Dose modulation is like automatic exposure control in radiography and automatic brightness stabilization in fluoroscopy. Dose modulation varies the kVp, mA, or both during imaging, depending on the body thickness at that particular position of the scan. This feature results in an additional 30% to 50% reduction in patient radiation dose.

COMPUTED TOMOGRAPHY DOSE INDEX

Whereas radiographic patient radiation exposure is measured in mGy_a/mAs and that for fluoroscopy in mGy_a/min, there is no simple metric for CT radiation exposure. When one inserts a radiation dosimeter into the CT x-ray beam, the response is in the 10 to 50 mGy_a/s range. This, however, is not how the CT x-ray beam intensity is defined.

During manufacture, a sampling of CT imaging systems will be selected for precise radiation dosimetry using either a 16-cm or 32-cm-diameter cylinder, or both, with a series of holes drilled peripherally and on the central axis (Fig. 40.10). The radiation measurements are made with an ionization chamber called a *pencil dosimeter* (Fig. 40.11). When the pencil dosimeter is inserted into a hole for measurement, the remaining holes are plugged with the test object plastic material.

These measurements result in nearly uniform radiation dose in the 32-cm test object, which represents the adult body. There is a cupping effect on radiation dose distribution with the 16-cm test object, which represents the adult head and the pediatric patient.

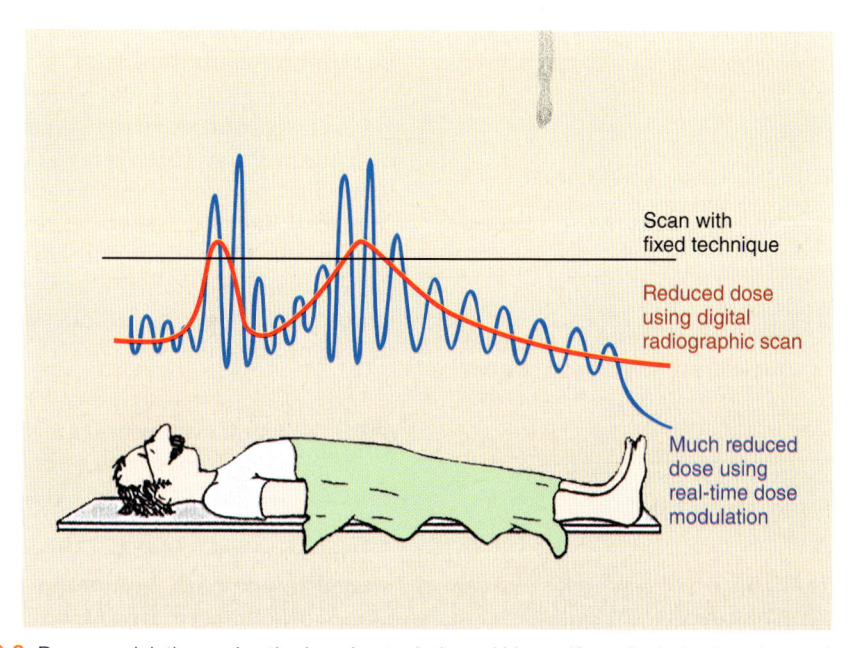

FIG. 40.9 Dose modulation varies the imaging technique, kVp and/or mA, during imaging and results in substantial patient radiation dose reduction.

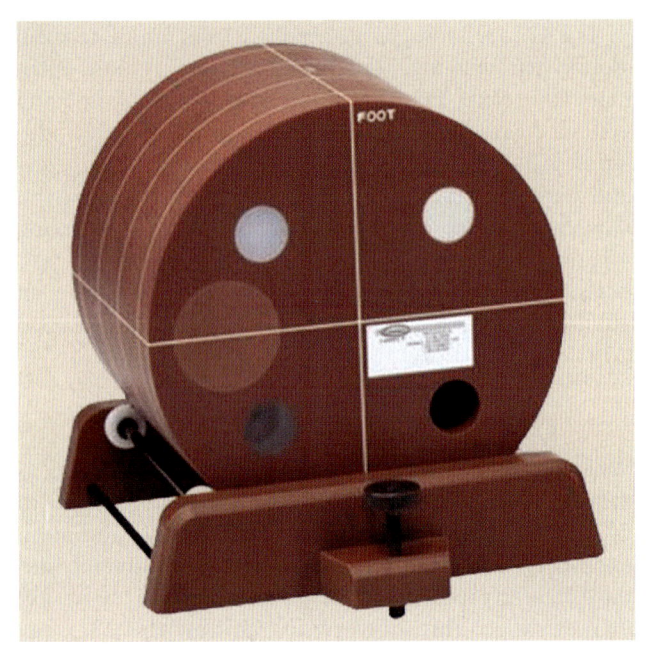

FIG. 40.10 Computed tomography radiation dose is measured using either a 32-cm or a 16-cm cylindrical test object. Image quality factors are also evaluated. The result of the measurement is computed tomography dose index. (Courtesy Pamela Durden, Gammex.)

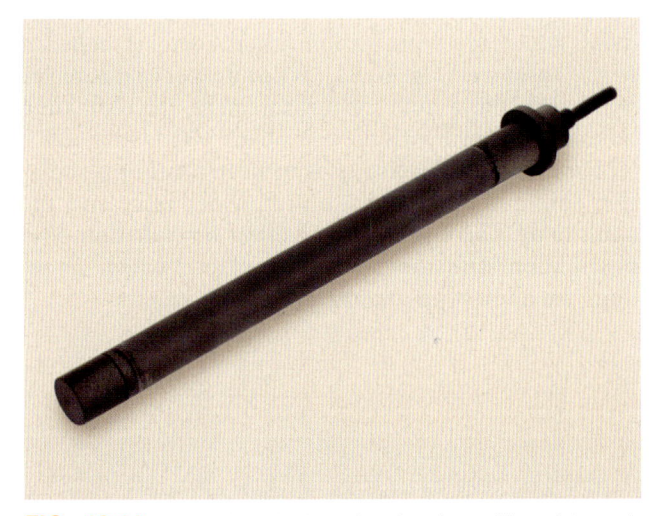

FIG. 40.11 A pencil ionization chamber is positioned in each hole of the test object and the response used to express computed tomography dose index. (Courtesy Thomas Kraus, CNMC Co. Inc.)

The slice thickness is the nominal width of the dose profile, regardless that we would prefer to have it present as a square wave.

> The penumbra beyond the nominal beam width contributes to patient radiation dose during multislice helical CT.

Multislice helical CT involves many rotations and therefore the summation of many x-ray beam intensities

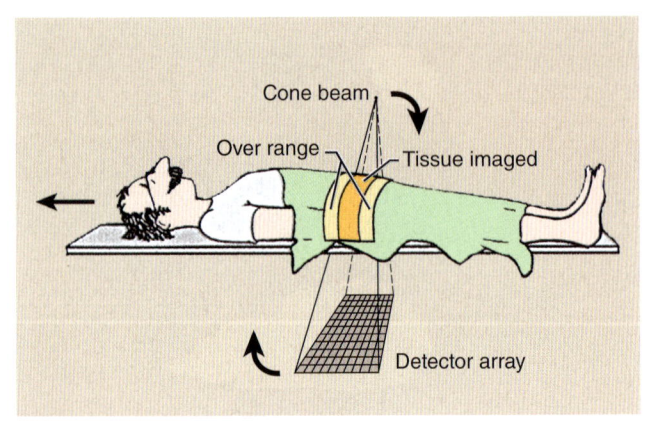

FIG. 40.12 Overranging is necessary for multislice helical CT imaging but can substantially increase patient radiation dose.

and the x-ray beam penumbra. The average of the multiple rotation imaging is the CTDI, and this is the value measured with the pencil ionization chamber.

There are several measures of CTDI, but we need only be concerned with $CTDI_{vol}$, where vol represents the volume of tissue irradiated. The unit of $CTDI_{vol}$ is mGy_t. $CTDI_{vol}$ is computed by averaging the peripheral pencil dose measurements and comparing them with the central axis dose as follows.

> $CTDI_{vol} = 1/3\ CTDI_{center} + 2/3\ CTDI_{periphery}$
> Therefore $CTDI_{vol}$ is a weighted average of the test object measurements.

DOSE LENGTH PRODUCT

A new metric is required to properly describe patient radiation dose in CT. With multislice helical CT, more than a single rotation is usually engaged. Suppose the x-ray beam width is 16 cm.

If the CT pitch is 1, the patient will move 16 cm during each rotation. Actually something more than 32 cm of tissue will have been irradiated because of the x-ray beam dose penumbra and because of **overranging**.

If three helical revolutions are made with a 16-cm-wide beam, the patient will have moved 48 cm during the examination. Actually, tissue on either side of the imaged tissue must be irradiated, even though that tissue is not imaged.

> Patient movement is somewhat more than the tissue imaged because of overranging.

The irradiated but not imaged tissue data that is needed to compute, by interpolation, the edges of the tissue to be imaged are shown in Fig. 40.12. The precise value of additional patient radiation dose due to

TABLE 40.2	Representative CTDI$_{vol}$ and DLP Values for Normal-Sized Adults During Routine CT Examinations			
Anatomy	CTDI$_{vol}$ (mGy$_t$)	DLP (mGy$_t$-cm)	16-cm Test Object	32-cm Test Object
Head (15 cm)	60	30	900	450
Chest (30 cm)	30	15	900	450
Abdomen (25 cm)	40	20	1000	500
Pelvis (25 cm)	40	20	1000	500
Brain (perfusion)	440	220	2400	1200

CT, Computed tomography; *CTDI*, computed tomography dose index; *DLP*, dose length product.

overranging is very dependent on the examination technique but can easily approach 50%.

This combination of output radiation intensity, CTDI$_{vol}$, and the volume of tissue imaged is called **DLP**, and it has units of mGy$_t$-cm. CTDI$_{vol}$ is a measure of the output intensity of the CT imaging system. DLP is an attempt to better address the extent of patient radiation dose.

Table 40.2 presents some average values for CTDI and DLP for several types of examinations. These are expressed as determined from either the 16-cm test object or the 32-cm test object.

SIZE-SPECIFIC DOSE ESTIMATES

In 2011 the American Association of Physicists in Medicine (AAPM) issued a very detailed report to better define patient radiation dose in pediatric and adult body CT examinations. The AAPM effort started as an attempt to better identify pediatric CT radiation dose in response to the **Image Gently** initiative. Image Gently is a continuing educational program developed by several medical imaging societies to apply ALARA principles to pediatric imaging.

The concern is that both CTDI$_{vol}$ and DLP are very much determined by imaging parameters such as kVp, mA, rotation time, and CT pitch. Both CTDI$_{vol}$ and DLP are independent of patient size and therefore not truly representative of the actual pediatric patient radiation dose.

Patient radiation dose is very much dependent on patient size. If one relies only on CTDI$_{vol}$ and DLP from either the 16- or 32-cm test object measurements, then patient radiation dose can be underestimated considerably.

To engage the size-specific dose estimate (SSDE), the CT technologist measures the lateral and anteroposterior (AP) dimensions from a representative transverse image (Fig. 40.13). These data are then used to compute an effective diameter for that patient and that anatomic section.

This discussion is meant to simply introduce the concept of SSDE. The mathematics are fairly stout. Only the medical physicist or CT technologist can be expected to engage this exercise to estimate patient radiation dose more accurately.

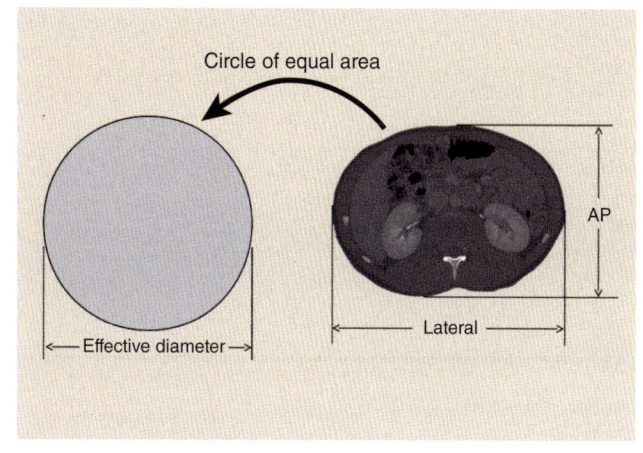

FIG. 40.13 Patient-effective diameter is obtained from lateral and AP measurements observed on a transverse image.

Rather large tables for estimating effective diameter are given in AAPM Report No. 204. That value of effective diameter is then used to better determine CTDI for that individual patient, rather than, as described earlier, for a 16- or 32-cm test object. Table 40.3 is an example of average effective diameter as a function of patient age.

EFFECTIVE DOSE

Effective dose (E) was introduced in Chapter 37. It is essentially the whole-body equivalent of the actual partial body radiation dose received during digital imaging.

This dose metric is that which is used to evaluate risk in populations exposed to radiation. It is that dose which is used to describe stochastic radiation responses.

Consider, for example, the relationship between patient radiation dose and effective dose in CT (Fig. 40.14). CT examination of the pelvis results in a rather uniform dose of 20 mGy$_t$ to the tissues of the abdomen. Other tissues are not irradiated because the x-ray beam is collimated. The effective dose for this examination is 7.4 mSv.

CT patient radiation dose is not delivered to the whole body—just an anatomical region. The effective dose is that dose which, if delivered to the entire body, would have the same risk of stochastic response as the actual risk from the partial body radiation dose.

TABLE 40.3 Effective Diameter as a Function of Age

Patient Age (Years)	Effective Diameter (cm)
0.0	11.2
0.5	13.4
1.0	15.1
1.5	15.9
2.0	16.8
2.5	17.3
3.0	17.6
3.5	17.9
4.0	18.1
5.0	18.5
7.0	19.6
9.0	20.9
11	22.4
13	24.1
15	26.0
17	28.1

Question: What is the effective dose if a CT examination results in a tissue dose of 20 mGy_t to the abdomen and pelvis?

Answer:
$E = \Sigma(D_t W_t)$
$= (20\ mGy_t)(0.2)$ gonads
$+ (20\ mGy_t)(0.12)$ colon
$+ (20\ mGy_t)(0.05)$ liver.
All other organs listed in Table 37.3 receive essentially zero radiation dose.
$= 4\ mGy_t$ gonads
$+ 2.4\ mGy_t$ colon
$+ 1.0\ mGy_t$ liver
$= 7.4\ mSv$

> Effective dose in CT depends on the various tissues irradiated and the age of the patient.

Consequently CT effective dose is dependent on the part of the body examined and the age of the patient. Table 40.4 is a summary of conversion factors that allow the estimation of E from DLP for several anatomic sites and various age groups.

CT protocols that register the kVp and mA for a given patient examination are poor metrics for reporting patient radiation dose. CTDI and DLP should be reported for each CT examination. This information is readily available from the dose page of each examination (Fig. 40.15).

Typical CT doses range from 30 to 50 mGy_t during head imaging and from 20 to 40 mGy_t during body imaging. These values are only approximate and vary widely, depending on the type of CT imaging system and the examination technique used. The effective dose for each examination is approximately 10 mSv.

SUMMARY

Unlike radiography and fluoroscopy, computed tomography uses a cone beam rather than an area beam. Such use of a cone beam requires over ranging which includes a dose penumbra adding to the patient radiation dose profile.

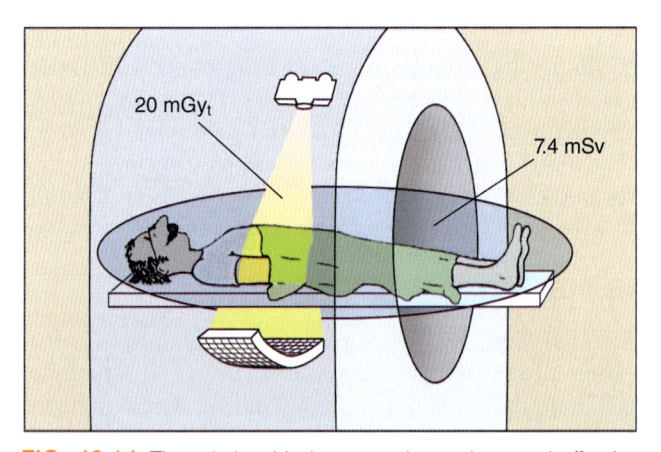

FIG. 40.14 The relationship between tissue dose and effective dose during computed tomography.

TABLE 40.4 Conversion from Dose Length Product to Effective Dose (mSv/mGy$_t$-cm)

	Newborn	1-Year-Old	5-Year-Old	10-Year-Old	Adult
Head and neck	0.013	0.0085	0.0057	0.0042	0.0031
Head	0.011	0.0067	0.0040	0.0032	0.0021
Neck	0.017	0.012	0.011	0.0079	0.0059
Chest	0.039	0.026	0.018	0.013	0.014
Abdomen/pelvis	0.049	0.030	0.020	0.015	0.015
Trunk	0.044	0.028	0.019	0.014	0.015

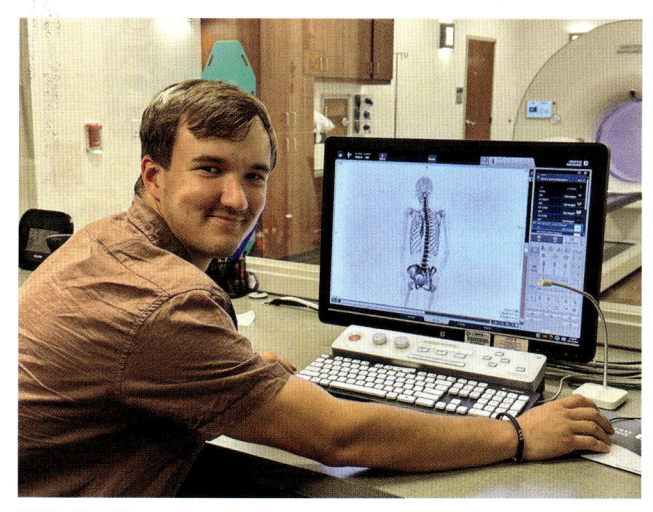

FIG. 40.15 This total body PET/CT used ^{18}F sodium fluoride. The CT parameters and patient dose report are on screen right. Ct parameters on the EXPLORER total body PET/CT at University of California, Davis, USA. (Courtesy Hugo Currie, Australian National University, Australia.)

CT patient radiation dose is expressed by the automatically generated computed tomography dose index. Dose modulation during the examination reduces patient radiation dose significantly.

Dose length product is a new metric used to properly describe CT patient radiation dose. When combined with size specific dose estimates the dose length product is converted to patient effective dose.

CHALLENGE QUESTIONS

1. Define or otherwise identify the following:
   a. Pencil radiation dosimeter
   b. DLP
   c. ESE
   d. Effective diameter
   e. Beam width
   f. Interpolation
   g. Overranging
   h. SSDE
   i. AAPM
   j. CTDI$_{vol}$

2. What information is presented on the CT dose page at the end of a report?
3. What are the two most important dose metrics in CT?
4. Patient age is one important characteristic required for computing patient radiation dose. What is the other characteristic, and why is it important?
5. What effect does x-ray beam collimation have on CT image quality?
6. What are the different uses for the 16- and 32-cm CT test objects?
7. What does the symbol (σ) mean? How does it affect image quality when summing detector rows?
8. What is Image Gently all about? Why is it particularly important in CT?
9. What is penumbra, and how does it affect patient radiation dose and image quality?
10. What precisely do the prepatient and predetector collimators do for image quality and for patient radiation dose?
11. What type of x-ray beam is used for CT?
12. What new imaging modality competes with CT?
13. What is dose modulation, and how does it affect patient radiation dose and image quality?
14. How do we compute CTDI$_{vol}$ from center and peripheral dose measurements?
15. What are the units used for CTDI$_{vol}$ and for DLP?
16. Why is it necessary for the CT technologist to measure the lateral and AP dimensions of a patient from CT images?
17. What is the use of effective diameter in computing CT patient radiation dose?
18. Define effective dose (E).
19. Why are kVp and mAs not appropriate for computing patient radiation dose in CT?
20. What steps are required to compute effective dose from DLP?

The answers to the Challenge Questions can be found by logging on to our website at http://evolve.elsevier.com.

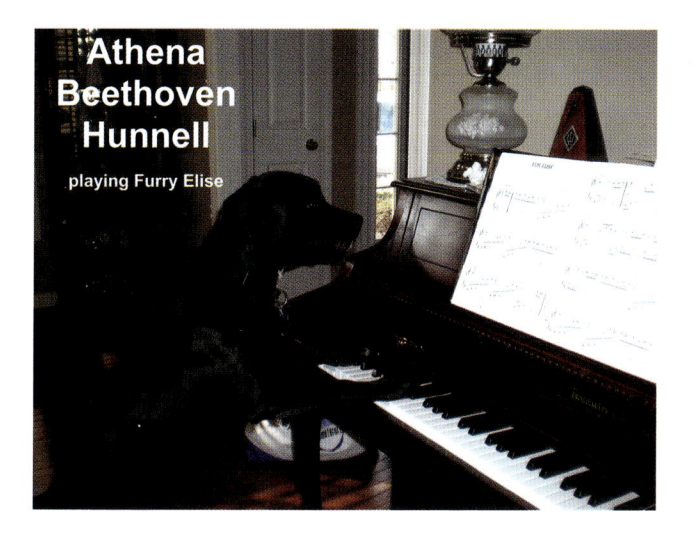

CHAPTER 41

Patient Radiation Dose Management

OBJECTIVES

At the completion of this chapter, the student should be able to do the following:

1. Indicate three ways that patient radiation dose can be reported.
2. Discuss ALARA principles applied to patient radiation dose management.
3. Discuss factors that affect patient radiation dose.
4. Describe the recommended management procedures for the pregnant patient.
5. Describe the intensity and distribution of radiation dose in mammography and computed tomography.
6. Explain when gonad shields should be used.

OUTLINE

Patient Radiation Dose in Special Examinations 549
   Mammography 549
   Extremity Radiography 550
Reduction of Unnecessary Patient Radiation Dose 550
   Unnecessary Examinations 550
   Repeat Examinations 551
   Radiographic Technique 551
Specific Area Shielding 552
The Pregnant Patient 553
   Radiobiologic Considerations 553
   Patient Information 554
Patient Radiation Dose Trends 556
Summary 558
Challenge Questions 558

CHAPTER 41 Patient Radiation Dose Management

ALL MEDICAL health physics activity is directed in some way toward minimizing the radiation exposure of radiologic personnel and the radiation dose to patients during x-ray examination. Radiation exposure of radiologists and radiographers is measured with the use of occupational radiation monitors. Patient radiation dose usually is estimated by conducting simulated x-ray examinations with human phantoms and test objects.

If radiation control procedures are adopted, occupational radiation exposure and patient radiation dose can be kept acceptably low. Health physicists subscribe to ALARA—keep radiation exposure **as low as reasonably achievable**. Radiographers follow this guide as well.

Exposure of patients for x-ray examination is commanding increasing attention in our society for two reasons.

First, the frequency of x-ray examination is increasing among all age groups. This indicates that physicians are relying more and more on digital imaging to assist them in patient care, even considering the newer imaging modalities.

This is to be expected. Digital imaging is considered much more accurate now than previous imaging modalities. More rigorous training programs required of radiologists and radiographers and improvements in diagnostic x-ray imaging systems allow for more difficult, but more substantive, x-ray examinations. Efficacy and diagnostic accuracy are much improved.

Second, concern among public health officials and radiation scientists continues regarding the risk that is associated with medical x-ray exposure. At present, acute effects on superficial tissues following interventional radiology procedures are in decline.

The possible late effects of diagnostic x-ray exposure are of concern; therefore attention must be given to good radiation control practices. When a diagnosis can be obtained with a low radiation dose, or with an alternate imaging modality such as MRI or diagnostic ultrasound, it should be used because of reduced risk. This is in keeping with **ALARA**.

We dealt with radiographic and fluoroscopic patient radiation dose in Chapter 39. In the following discussion, we concentrate on additional special x-ray examinations and special situations. What follows can also be applied to general radiography and fluoroscopy.

PATIENT RADIATION DOSE IN SPECIAL EXAMINATIONS

Mammography

Because of the considerable application of x-rays for an examination of the female breast and concern for the induction of breast cancer by radiation, it is imperative that we have some understanding of the radiation doses involved in such examinations.

> Mammography has improved with the addition of digital breast tomosynthesis (DBT).

An entrance skin exposure (ESE) of approximately 8 mGy_a/view is normal in mammography. Increasing the x-ray tube potential much beyond 28 kVp degrades image quality; therefore further dose reduction by technique manipulation is unlikely.

Radiographic grids are used in some mammography examinations. Grid ratios of 4:1 and 5:1 are most popular. The contrast enhancement produced by the use of such grids is significant, but so is the increase in patient radiation dose. Patient radiation dose is increased by approximately two times with the use of such grids compared with the nongrid technique.

The values stated for patient radiation dose in mammography can be misleading. Because of the low x-ray energies used in mammography, the dose falls off very rapidly as the x-ray beam penetrates the breast. If the ESE for a craniocaudad view is 8 mGy_a, the dose to the midline of the breast may be only 1.0 mGy_t because of the rapid attenuation of the low kVp x-ray beam.

Fortunately it is known that the risk of an adverse biologic response from mammography is small. Certainly it is nothing about which a patient should be concerned.

Mammography has been very successful in reducing mortality from breast cancer, while the incidence of breast cancer in a growing population remains unchanged at approximately 1 in 8 females. The incidence of breast cancer in men is approximately 1 in 800. Before mammography, we experienced a 50% mortality rate from breast cancer. It is currently 5%.

However, any possible response is related to the average radiation dose to glandular tissue and not to skin exposure. Glandular dose (D_g) varies in a complicated way, with variations in x-ray beam energy and intensity but averages approximately 15% of the ESE.

> Glandular dose is approximately 15% of the ESE.

Specification of an ESE can be misleading when one considers a two-view examination, such as that used for screening (Fig. 41.1). Consider an examination that consists of craniocaudad and mediolateral oblique views, each of which produces an ESE of 8 mGy_a.

It would be incorrect to describe this total examination procedure as resulting in an ESE of 16 mGy_a. Skin exposures from different projections cannot be added.

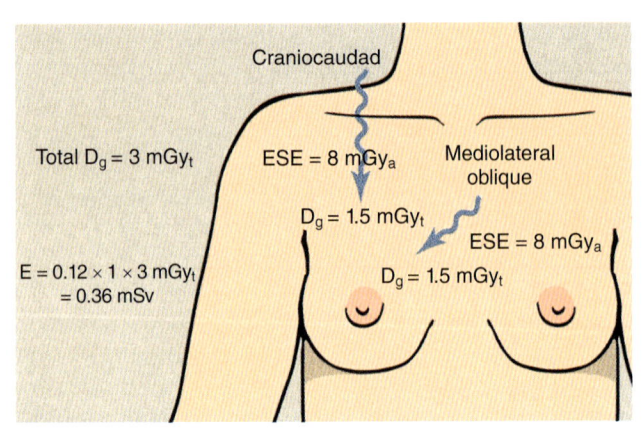

FIG. 41.1 Two mammographic exposures result in a total glandular dose that is the sum of the individual glandular doses. *ESE*, Entrance skin exposure.

We must specify the skin dose for each view or attempt to estimate the total glandular dose.

Total glandular dose can be estimated by approximating that the contribution from each view will be 15% of the ESE. Consequently, the total D_g would be the sum of (0.15 × 8 mGy$_a$ = 1.2 mGy$_t$) as the contribution from each of the craniocaudad and mediolateral oblique views. Therefore the total D_g would be 2.4 mGy$_t$.

> Mammography glandular dose should not exceed 1 mGy$_t$/view or 3 mGy$_t$/view when a grid is used.

From this discussion, it would seem that patient dose in mammography can be considerably reduced if the number of views is restricted. The axillary view should not be done routinely. For screening programs, no more than two views per breast are advisable. DBT is being incorporated into screening mammography with the result of reduced patient radiation dose and improved diagnosis.

Extremity Radiography

Extremity radiography is a special x-ray examination, but it is not one high on the list of patient radiation dose concerns. Radiographic technique is low, less than 60 kVp and less than 100 mAs, and therefore of no concern for a harmful skin response.

There is relatively little bone marrow in the extremities, and the x-ray examination is often of a joint and not a long bone. Consequently, there is little contribution to mean marrow dose. There is no gonadal irradiation and therefore no contribution to the genetically significant dose.

REDUCTION OF UNNECESSARY PATIENT RADIATION DOSE

The radiographer has considerable control over many sources of unnecessary patient radiation dose. Unnecessary patient radiation dose is defined as any radiation dose that is not required for the patient's well-being or for proper management and care. Reduction of unnecessary patient radiation dose is the ultimate ALARA.

Unnecessary Examinations

The radiographer has practically no control over what some consider the largest source of unnecessary patient radiation dose (i.e., the unnecessary x-ray examination). This is almost exclusively the radiologist's or the clinician's responsibility. Radiographers can help by asking whether the patient has had a previous x-ray examination. If so, perhaps those images should be obtained for review before any other steps are taken.

Unfortunately, this source of unnecessary patient radiation dose presents a serious dilemma for the radiologist and the clinician. Many x-ray examinations are requested when it is known that the yield of helpful information may be extremely low or nonexistent. When such an examination is performed, the benefit to the patient in no way compensates for the patient radiation dose.

If the examination is not performed, however, the clinician and the radiologist may be criticized severely if management of the patient's condition results in failure. Even though the examination in question would have contributed little, if anything, to effective patient management, the radiologist may even be sued. In such situations, the radiologist is caught between the proverbial "rock and a hard place."

> Routine x-ray examinations should not be performed when there is no medical indication.

Substantial evidence shows that such examinations are of little benefit because they are not cost-effective and the disease detection rate is very low. Examples of such cases are discussed in the following sections. General screening by chest x-ray examination has not been found to be effective.

> Better methods of tuberculosis testing than chest x-ray examination are currently available.

Some x-ray screening in high-risk groups (e.g., medical and paramedical personnel), in service personnel posing a potential community hazard (e.g., food handlers, teachers), and in special occupational groups (e.g., miners, workers having contact with beryllium, asbestos, glass, or silica) may be appropriate.

Chest x-ray examinations should not be performed for routine hospital admission when no clinical indication of chest disease is indicated. Among patients who might be candidates for such examination are those admitted to the pulmonary service.

Chest and lower back x-ray examinations as part of a preemployment physical examination are not justified because the knowledge gained about previous injury or disease through this approach is nil.

Many physicians and healthcare organizations promote annual or biannual physical examinations. Certainly when such an examination is conducted on an asymptomatic patient, it should not include x-ray examination, especially fluoroscopic examination.

Computed tomography (CT) has replaced radiography as the first line of digital imaging. This overutilization, especially in the emergency department, must be controlled because of the population effective dose.

Some facilities now offer whole-body multislice helical CT screening to the public for self-referral. Until evidence reveals a significant disease detection rate, this should not be done. The patient radiation dose is too high.

Every radiologist is aware of the Appropriateness Criteria reports of the American College of Radiology (ACR). The radiographer should also be so aware. In addition to identifying the most appropriate imaging modality, these reports provide relative patient radiation dose levels.

Repeat Examinations

During the 20th century of screen-film imaging, a measurable source of unnecessary patient radiation dose was the repetition of studies because of unacceptable image quality. The frequency of repeat examinations in the typical hospital facility at that time has been estimated to range as high as 10% of all examinations. Examinations with the highest repeat rates included lumbar spine, thoracic spine, chest, and abdomen.

Some repeat examinations were performed because of equipment malfunction. However, most were caused by radiographer error. Studies of causes of repeat examinations have shown that improper positioning and poor radiographic technique resulting in an image that was too light or too dark were primarily responsible for repeats.

> It should never be necessary to repeat a digital imaging examination.

In this 21st century of digital imaging, critique has shifted to individual workstations throughout the department, with radiographers reviewing images before transfer to radiologists for interpretation. Misuse of the software allows radiographers to erase an image that should be recorded as a repeat. But wait, the problem gets worse.

Postprocessing software allows an unprincipled radiographer to digitally mask an image to hide the lack of primary beam collimation. The radiologist is unaware that the image was not properly collimated.

This potential source of unnecessary patient radiation dose is actually rather small, certainly less than 1 mSv. However, such a situation must be avoided because more often than not it occurs during pediatric imaging. This places the responsibility on education programs and on the quality control radiographer.

Proper collimation is essential to good radiographic technique. Positive beam limitation does not prevent the radiographer from reducing field size still further through collimation. With the use of collimation, not only is the patient effective dose reduced, but image quality is also improved with enhanced contrast resolution because scatter radiation is reduced.

Proper collimation also affects the appropriate use of specific area shields. If an improperly collimated beam extends over the specific area shield, the automatic exposure control (AEC) can be driven to higher patient radiation dose.

Radiographic Technique

In general, the use of a high-kVp technique results in reduced patient radiation dose. Increasing the kVp is always associated with a reduction in mAs to obtain an acceptable radiation exposure of the image receptor; this, in turn, results in reduced patient radiation dose.

This dose reduction occurs because the patient radiation dose is linearly related to the mAs but is related to approximately the square of the kVp. An area of radiography for which a high-kVp technique is widely accepted is an examination of the chest.

Question: A lateral skull radiograph is obtained at 64 kVp, 80 mAs, and results in an ESE of 4 mGy$_a$. If the tube potential is increased to 74 kVp (15% increase) and the mAs is reduced by half, to 40 mAs, the image receptor exposure will remain the same. What will be the new ESE?

Answer:
$$\text{ESE} = (4 \text{ mGy}_a)\left(\frac{40 \text{ mAs}}{80 \text{ mAs}}\right)\left(\frac{74 \text{ kVp}}{64 \text{ kVp}}\right)^2$$
$$= (4 \text{ mGy}_a)(0.5)(1.34)$$
$$= 2.68 \text{ mGy}_a$$

Of course, the radiologist must be the final judge of radiographic quality. In the current digital imaging world, much more technique latitude is possible because of postprocessing image-reconstruction algorithms.

> Digital radiography can be conducted at higher kVp, resulting in lower patient radiation dose.

Many digital image receptors are currently available for radiography, as discussed in Chapters 11 to 14. A single type of digital image receptor has not yet been found acceptable to all. We are still evaluating. The radiation dose necessary to produce a quality image should be kept in mind when evaluating image receptors.

SPECIFIC AREA SHIELDING

When an upper extremity or the breast is examined, especially with the patient in a seated position, care should be taken that the useful beam does not intercept the gonads. Position the patient lateral to the useful beam and provide a protective apron as a shield.

X-ray examinations result in partial-body exposure, although most radiation protection guides and radiation response information are based on whole-body exposure. The partial-body nature of the x-ray examination has previously been controlled by proper beam collimation and the use of specific area shielding.

The use of specific area shielding, usually 0.5-mm Pb equivalent contact shield, is indicated when a particularly sensitive tissue or organ is near the useful beam. The lens of the eye, the breasts, and the gonads were frequently shielded from the secondary radiation beams—scatter radiation and leakage radiation.

A few years ago, specific area shielding became a topic of discussion in many radiology and medical physics journals. Convincing arguments were made resulting in our current understanding of the use of specific area shields.

The benefit of specific area shields, especially gonadal shields, is that they reduce dose to approximately 50%. However, we now accept that no gonadal radiation dose has resulted in a genetic effect. Multiple studies of the atomic bomb survivors have shown no genetic effect at the human level following several generations.

The improper use of specific area shields carries two negative effects. Incidentalomas have been missed which would have resulted in different patient management and a better patient outcome had that area not been shielded.

A frequent and measurably worst result of specific area shields is when the radiographic, fluoroscopic, or CT x-ray beam interacts with the specific area shield. That automatically drives the automatic exposure control (AEC) or automatic brightness stabilization (ABS) resulting in much higher radiation dose.

Following much journal discussion, in 2019 the American Association of Physicists in Medicine (AAPM) followed by the American College of Radiology (ACR) proclaimed in official documents that we should abandon specific area shielding. Except for some special situations, this abandonment is now in effect universally.

The most familiar specific area shield to patients is that used in the dentist office. The recommendation and the universally applied procedure is to drape a protective lead apron, including a neck shield, on the patient during dental radiography. When using such shielding, we totally understand that the dental x-ray beam is well collimated with a cone and that the x-ray beam is rarely directed to the trunk of the body.

The reduction in the patient effective dose by using a dental patient protective apron is clearly miniscule. We continue this procedure because it is in keeping with ALARA and it may improve the examination by calming the patient.

Lens shields can be small and shaped or simply cut from an abandoned lead apron. The most frequent use of lens shields is during a CT of the head. Such use is questionable because the useful beam must not come into contact with the shield. Such contact will produce severe image artifacts. The use of lens shields does reduce the tissue radiation dose from scatter radiation.

> Do not allow the useful x-ray beam to intercept a specific area shield.

Breast shields are contact shields that are recommended for use during scoliosis examinations. Such examinations often consist of an anteroposterior (AP) projection, which subjects juvenile breasts to primary beam x-irradiation. Shield positioning by the radiographer is critical. If the breast shield intercepts any part of the useful x-ray beam, it could trigger the AEC system to increase technique and thereby increase patient radiation dose.

However, the posteroanterior (PA) projection is equally satisfactory because magnification is of little importance and breast shields are not necessary. The PA projection results in a breast dose of only approximately 1% of the AP projection.

> An incidentaloma is an unanticipated finding not related to a suspected abnormality.

The use of gonadal shielding in the newborn intensive care unit (NBICU) should be approached with caution and perhaps avoided totally. Radiographic technique is so reduced in the NBICU that patient radiation dose is very small and the occurrence of incidentalomas is higher.

The tissue weighting factors (Wt) for these patient areas are low: 0.08 for gonads and 0.05 for breast. Eye lens do not have an assigned weighting factor because

TABLE 41.1	Gonadal Shielding

- Gonadal shielding should be considered for all patients, especially children and those who are potentially reproductive. As an administrative procedure, this would include all patients younger than 40 years of age and perhaps even older males.
- Gonadal shielding should be used when the gonads are near the useful beam.
- Proper patient positioning and beam collimation should not be relaxed when gonadal shields are in use.
- Make sure gonadal shielding does not interfere with the AEC or ABS.
- Gonadal shielding should be used only when it does not interfere with obtaining the required diagnostic information.

ABS, Automatic brightness stabilization; *AEC*, automatic exposure control.

the suspected radiation dose response, cataracts, is a deterministic response with a dose threshold of 2 Gy_t. Table 41.1 lists some primary points regarding gonadal shielding.

THE PREGNANT PATIENT

Two situations in diagnostic radiology require particular care and action. Both are associated with pregnancy. Their importance is obvious from both a physical and emotional standpoint.

Radiobiologic Considerations

The severity of the potential response to radiation exposure in utero is both time related and dose related, as was discussed in Chapter 36. Unquestionably, the period most sensitive to radiation exposure occurs before birth. Furthermore, the fetus is more sensitive early in pregnancy than late in pregnancy. As a general rule, the higher the radiation dose, the more severe will be the radiation response.

A grave misunderstanding is that the most critical time for irradiation is during the first 2 weeks, when it is most unlikely that the expectant mother knows of her condition. In fact, this is the time during pregnancy when such irradiation is least hazardous. Pregnancies fail during this period for reasons other than exposure to radiation.

The most likely biologic response to irradiation during the first 2 weeks of pregnancy is resorption of the embryo and therefore no pregnancy. No other response is likely.

No concern has been expressed over the possibility of induction of congenital abnormalities during the first 2 weeks of pregnancy. Such a response has not been demonstrated in experimental animals or in humans after any level of radiation dose.

The time from approximately the 2nd week to the 10th week of pregnancy is the period of major organogenesis. During this time, the major organ systems of the fetus are developing. If the radiation dose is sufficiently high, congenital abnormalities may result.

Early in organogenesis, the most likely congenital abnormalities are associated with skeletal deformities. Later in this period, neurologic deficiencies are more likely to occur.

During the second and third trimesters of pregnancy, the responses previously noted are unlikely. The results of numerous investigations strongly suggest that if a response occurs after radiation exposure during the latter two trimesters, the principal response would be the appearance of malignant disease during childhood. These radiation responses during pregnancy require a very high radiation dose before the risk of occurrence is significant.

> No such responses during pregnancy occur at less than 250 mGy_t.

Such dose levels are highly unlikely, yet they are possible with patients who receive multiple x-ray examinations of the abdomen or pelvis. These dose levels are essentially impossible as an occupational radiation exposure for radiographers or radiologists. No other significant responses have been reported after irradiation in utero.

As one might imagine, virtually no information is available at the human level to construct dose-response relationships for irradiation in utero. However, a large body of data on animal irradiation, particularly that in rats and mice, serves as the basis from which such relationships can be estimated. The statements that follow, although attributed to human exposure, represent estimates based on extrapolation from animal studies.

After an in utero radiation dose of 2 Gy_t, it is nearly certain that each of the effects noted previously will occur. However, the likelihood is small that an exposure of this magnitude would be experienced in digital imaging.

Spontaneous abortion after irradiation during the first 2 weeks of pregnancy is unlikely at radiation doses less than 250 mGy_t. The precise nature of the dose-response relationship is unknown, but a reasonable estimate of the risk suggests that 0.1% of all conceptions would be resorbed after a dose of 100 mGy_t.

> The incidence of spontaneous abortion in the absence of radiation exposure is estimated to be in the 25% to 50% range.

In the absence of radiation exposure, approximately 5% of all live births exhibit a manifest congenital abnormality. A 1% increase in congenital abnormalities is estimated to follow a 100 mGy_t fetal dose, with a proportionately lower increase at lower doses. The likelihood is also very small at 100 mGy_t.

The induction of a childhood malignancy after irradiation in utero is difficult to assess. Risk estimates are even lower than those reported for spontaneous abortion and congenital abnormalities. The best approach to assessing risk of childhood malignancy is to use a relative risk estimate.

During the first trimester, the relative risk of radiation-induced childhood malignancy is in the range of 5 to 10; it drops to approximately 1.4 during the third trimester. The overall relative risk is accepted to be 1.5—a 50% increase over the naturally occurring incidence.

Attributable risk is also a very helpful assessment method for any population group. Attributable risk provides a numerical value to those in the group with a response that could have been radiation induced.

Patient Information

Safeguards against accidental irradiation early in pregnancy present complex administrative problems. This situation is particularly critical during the first 2 months of pregnancy, when such a condition may not be suspected and when the fetus is particularly sensitive to radiation exposure. After 2 months, the risk of irradiating an unknown pregnancy becomes small because the patient is usually aware of her condition.

If the state of pregnancy is known, then under some circumstances, the radiologic examination should not be conducted. One should never knowingly examine a pregnant patient with x-rays unless a documented decision to do so has been made. When such an examination does proceed, it should be conducted with all of the previously discussed techniques for minimizing patient radiation dose.

When a pregnant patient must be examined, the examination should be done with precisely collimated beams and carefully positioned specific area shields. The use of high-kVp technique is most appropriate in such situations. There are administrative protocols that can be used to ensure that we do not knowingly expose pregnant patients; these vary from complex to simple.

The most direct way to ensure against the irradiation of an unsuspected pregnancy is to institute **elective booking**. This requires that the radiologist or radiographer determine the time of the patient's previous menstrual cycle. X-ray examinations in which the fetus is not in or near the primary beam may be allowed, but they should be accompanied by carefully positioned, specific area shielding. Understand that improperly positioned, the specific area shield coupled with improper collimation can drive the AEC to higher patient radiation dose.

Ideally, the referring physician should be responsible for determining the menstrual cycle and for withholding the examination request if there is any question about its necessity. This may require a radiologist-sponsored educational program that can be conducted easily at regularly scheduled medical staff meetings.

> An alternative procedure is to have the patient indicate her menstrual cycle.

In many diagnostic imaging departments, the patient must complete an information form before undergoing examination. These forms often include questions such as "Are you or could you be pregnant?" and "What was the date of your last menstrual period?" Fig. 41.2 is an example of such a simple, yet effective questionnaire for protecting against the irradiation of a pregnant patient.

If neither elective booking nor the request form seems appropriate for a digital imaging service, an equally successful method is to post signs of caution in the waiting room. Such signs could read "Are you pregnant or could you be? If so, please inform the radiographer," "Warning—special precautions are necessary if you are pregnant," or "Caution—if there is any possibility that you are pregnant, it is very important that you inform the radiographer before you have an x-ray examination."

> We fulfill our responsibility to the pregnant patient by posting signs in the waiting room.

Fig. 41.3 is a helpful poster that is available from the Center for Devices and Radiological Health. Such a posting satisfies our responsibility to the patient and to the healthcare facility.

It has been estimated that less than 1% of all females referred for x-ray examination are potentially pregnant. However, if a pregnant patient escapes detection and is irradiated, what is the subsequent responsibility of the radiology service to the patient? What should be done?

The first step is to estimate the fetal dose. The medical physicist should be consulted immediately and requested to estimate the fetal dose. If a preliminary review of the examination techniques used (i.e., type of examination, kVp, and mAs) determines that the dose may have exceeded 10 mGy_t, a more complete dosimetric evaluation should be conducted.

Table 41.2 presents representative fetal dose levels for many examinations. With knowledge of the types of examinations performed and the techniques and apparatus used, the medical physicist can accurately determine the fetal dose. Test objects and dosimetry materials are available to ensure that this determination can be made with confidence.

Once the fetal dose is known, the referring physician and the radiologist should determine the stage of gestation at which x-ray exposure occurred. With this information, only two alternatives are possible: Allow the patient to continue to term or terminate the pregnancy.

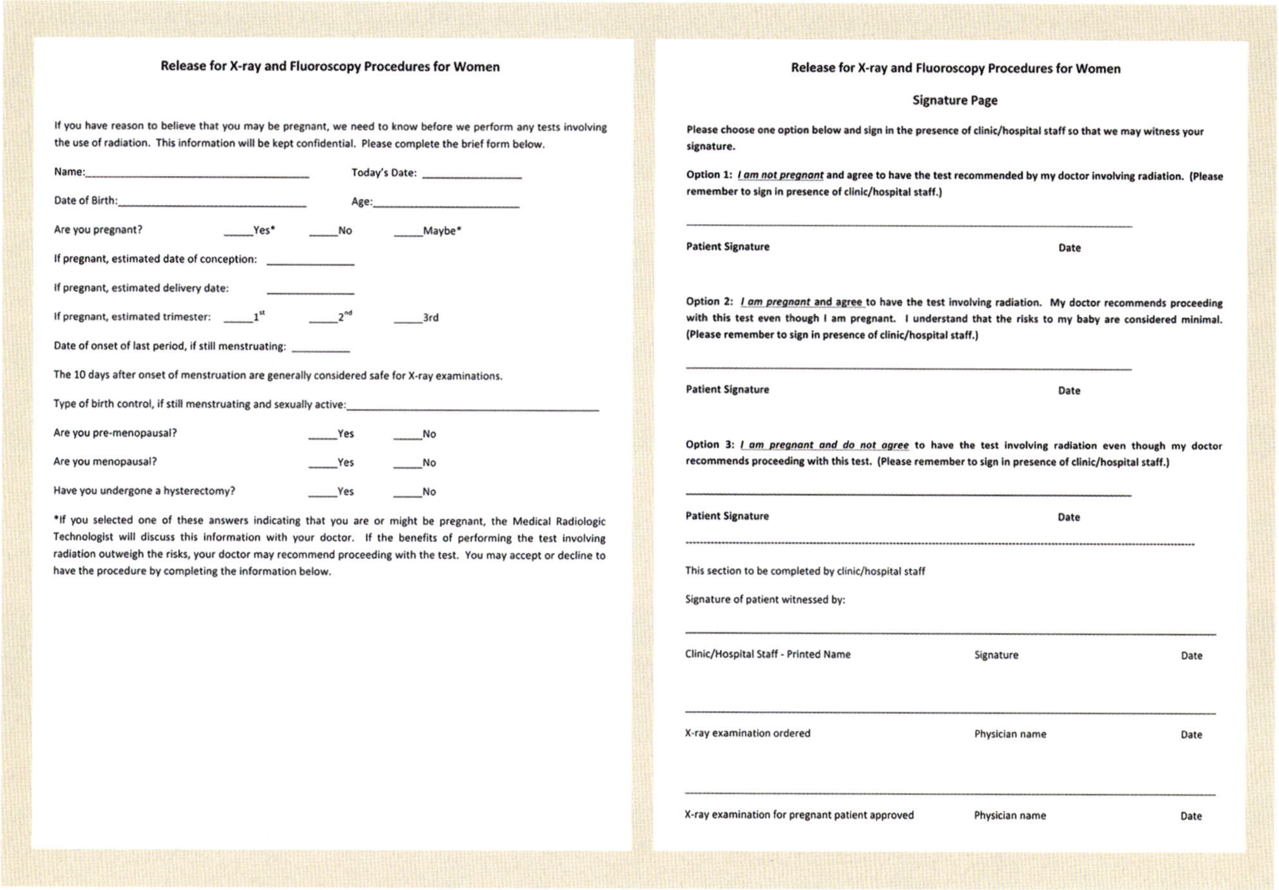

CHAPTER 41   Patient Radiation Dose Management   555

FIG. 41.2 X-ray examination consent form for females of childbearing age.

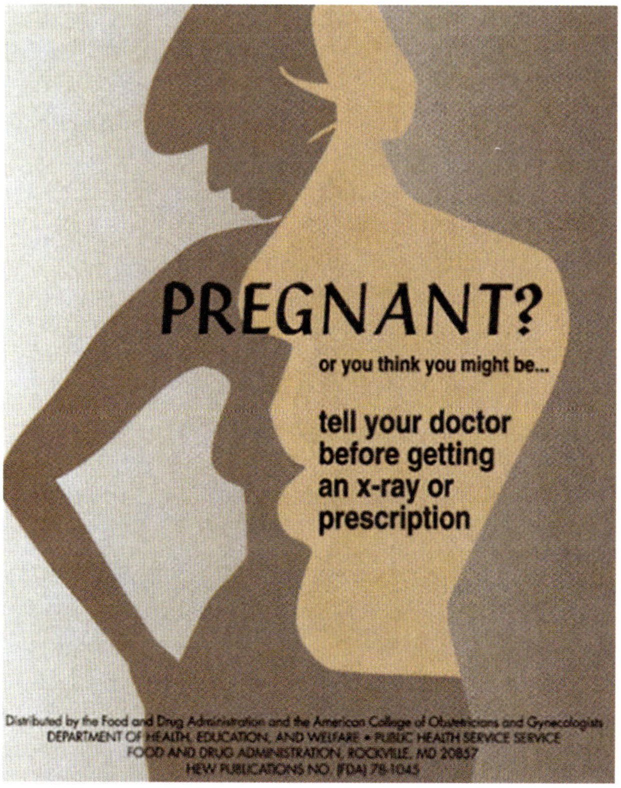

FIG. 41.3 Wall posters with warnings about radiation and pregnancy are available from the Center for Devices and Radiological Health. (Courtesy of Center for Devices and Radiological Health.)

TABLE 41.2	Representative Entrance Exposures and Fetal Doses for Digital Radiographic Examinations	
Examination	**Entrance Skin Exposure (mGy$_a$)**	**Fetal Dose (mGy$_t$)**
Skull (lateral)	0.70	0
Cervical spine (AP)	1.10	0
Shoulder	0.90	0
Chest (PA)	0.10	0
Thoracic spine (AP)	1.80	0.01
Cholecystogram (PA)	1.50	0.01
Lumbosacral spine (AP)	2.50	0.80
Abdomen or KUB (AP)	2.20	0.770
IVP	2.10	0.60
Hip	2.20	0.50
Wrist or foot	0.05	0

AP, Anteroposterior; *IVP*, intravenous pyelogram; *KUB*, kidneys, ureters, bladder; *PA*, posteroanterior.

556 PART VIII Radiation Protection

> Recommendation for abortion after digital imaging x-ray exposure essentially is never indicated.

Because the natural incidence of congenital anomalies is approximately 5%, no such effects can reasonably be considered a consequence of digital imaging radiation doses. Manifest damage to the newborn is unlikely at fetal radiation doses less than 250 mGy$_t$, although some suggest that lower doses may cause mental developmental abnormalities.

In view of the available evidence, a reasonable approach is to apply a 100 to 250-mGy$_t$ rule. If less than 100 mGy$_t$, a therapeutic abortion is not indicated unless additional risk factors are involved. If greater than 250 mGy$_t$, the risk of latent injury may justify a therapeutic abortion, but that dose level to the fetus is never attained.

Between 100 and 250 mGy$_t$, the precise time of irradiation, the emotional state of the patient, the effect an additional child would have on the family, and other social and economic factors may be considered carefully.

Fortunately, experience with such situations has shown that fetal doses have been consistently low. The fetal dose rarely exceeds 50 mGy$_t$ even after a series of x-ray examinations.

PATIENT RADIATION DOSE TRENDS

The National Council on Radiation Protection and Measurements (NCRP) issues scientific reports on various aspects of radiation control, including patient radiation dose. An earlier NCRP report included data to construct the pie chart shown earlier in Fig. 1.3. Note that our average annual dose was 3.6 mSv and medical imaging contributed 0.6 mSv to that total dose.

The current NCRP pie chart is shown in Fig. 41.4. This figure shows no change in natural background radiation exposure as expected, but the change in digital x-ray imaging exposure is exceptional. In 1990,

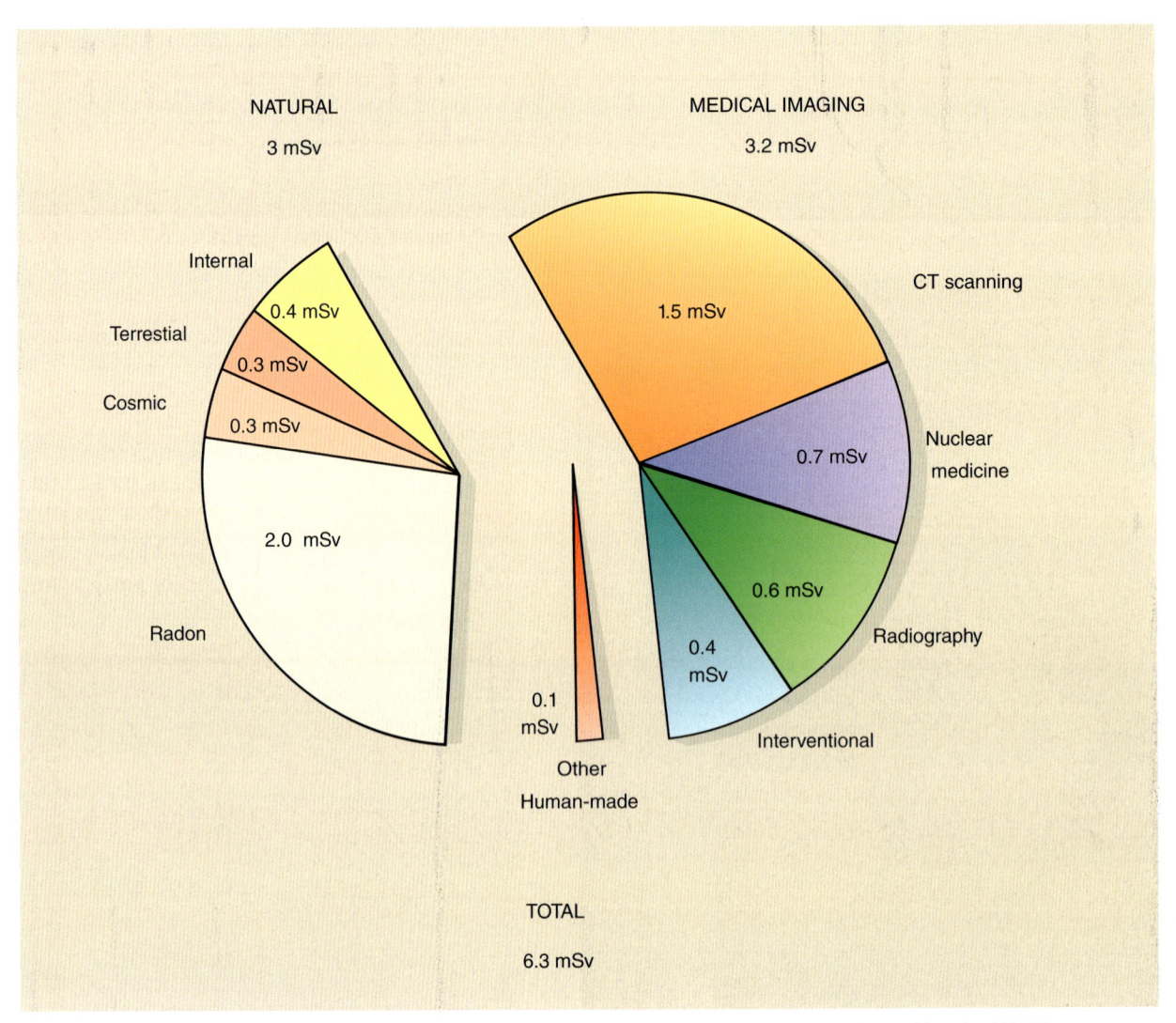

FIG. 41.4 Radiation dose to the population of the United States in 2008 as estimated by the NCRP. (Courtesy Fred Mettler, University of New Mexico.)

medical imaging resulted in average patient radiation dose of 0.6 mSv; currently, it is 3.2 mSv! That is cause for concern.

The past few decades have seen an exceptional increase in the use of advanced diagnostic imaging techniques, including CT, magnetic resonance imaging (MRI), diagnostic ultrasound, and nuclear medicine. There are many reasons for this—inappropriate utilization, physician ownership, and public demand. This increased utilization has resulted in significant increases in patient radiation dose, except for MRI and diagnostic ultrasound, which use nonionizing radiation.

Fig. 41.5 is NCRP data showing the increasing utilization of four medical imaging modalities. The contribution from CT is high but has been brought under control in the past few years with dose reduction techniques.

This increase in patient radiation dose requires that radiographers and radiologists exercise more control over medical imaging. In acknowledging ALARA, we must be more aware of appropriateness criteria for diagnostic imaging and gain more control over unnecessary x-ray imaging.

With digital x-ray imaging, we are in a better position to automatically estimate the patient effective dose for each x-ray examination and record that to a continuing patient radiation dose file. We monitor our occupational radiation exposure for life; we will be instituting protocols to do the same for patient medical radiation dose.

The ACR has made a major contribution to patient radiation dose management with the establishment of the Dose Registry. This voluntary program solicits patient dose data from imaging facilities with the intention of using the data to implement ALARA imaging instructions.

The ACR has also developed the ACR Appropriateness Criteria, which are evidence-based guidelines to assist referring physicians in making the most appropriate imaging decision for a specific clinical condition.

Using these guidelines helps to enhance quality patient care and management of patient radiation dose. There are approximately 250 different clinical conditions covered by these reports and more appear regularly.

Each report includes a table, such as that shown in Table 41.3. Each appropriateness criteria report recommends a number of different imaging modalities as appropriate for that patient's condition. Furthermore, each imaging modality will have a numerical score indicating its level of appropriateness.

Because there is a wide range of radiation dose associated with different diagnostic procedures, a relative radiation level (RRL) indication is included in each

TABLE 41.3 Relative Radiation Level

RRL	Adult Effective Dose Estimate (mSv)	Pediatric Effective Dose Estimate (mSv)
0	0	0
☢	<0.1	<0.03
☢☢	0.1–1	0.03–0.3
☢☢☢	1–10	0.3–3
☢☢☢☢	10–30	3–10
☢☢☢☢☢	30–100	10–30

RRL, Relative radiation level.

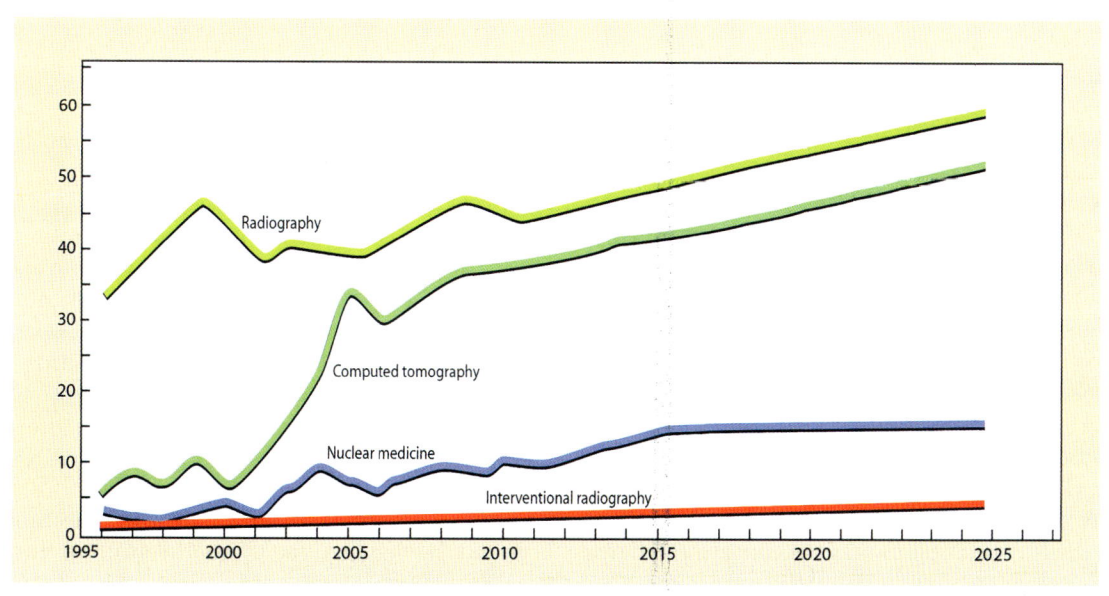

FIG. 41.5 Relative frequency of these four imaging modalities over the past 30 years.

TABLE 41.4	Imaging Modalities According to Relative Radiation Level
0	Diagnostic Ultrasound, MRI
☢	Chest radiographs, extremity radiographs
☢☢	Mammography, pelvis/abdomen radiographs
☢☢☢	Nuclear medicine scans, abdomen/chest CT
☢☢☢☢	CT with/without contrast, SPECT, PET
☢☢☢☢☢	CT angiography, TIPS, PET-CT

CT, Computed tomography; *MRI*, magnetic resonance imaging; *PET*, positron emission tomography; *SPECT*, single-photon emission computed tomography; *TIPS*, transjugular intrahepatic portosystemic shunt placement.

Appropriateness Criteria report. The RRLs are based on the range of effective dose indicated by the number of radiation symbols.

Patients in the pediatric age group are at inherently higher risk from radiation exposure, both because of organ radiosensitivity and longer life expectancy. Consequently, the RRL dose estimate ranges for pediatric examinations are lower as compared with those specified for adults.

Each recommended imaging modality also has attached to it the appropriate number of radiation symbols, so that the referring physician knows the relative radiation intensity of each imaging modality. Diagnostic ultrasound and magnetic resonance imaging are assigned zero because no ionizing radiation is involved.

A partial list of imaging modalities and the appropriate number of radiation symbols assigned to each is shown in Table 41.4. Radiography is lowest and positron emission tomography (PET)-CT highest in the order.

SUMMARY

Patient radiation dose from diagnostic x-rays usually is recorded in one of the following three ways: (1) ESE, (2) mean marrow dose, or (3) gonadal dose. Thermoluminescence dosimeters and optically stimulated luminescence dosimeters are the monitors of choice for patient radiation dose. By knowing the output intensity of at least one x-ray technique and the source-to-skin distance, the medical physicist can estimate the ESE for any patient examination. For fluoroscopic examination, a good general assumption for the ESE is 40 mGy$_a$/min.

Patient radiation dose can be reduced easily by eliminating unnecessary examinations and by ensuring proper radiographic technique and patient positioning. The radiobiology of pregnancy requires particular attention to the pregnant patient. By posting the waiting room and the examination room with educational signs, we meet our responsibility to the pregnant patient.

CHALLENGE QUESTIONS

1. Define or otherwise identify the following:
   a. ALARA
   b. Fetal dose limit
   c. Major organogenesis
   d. Elective booking
   e. Genetically significant dose
   f. Penumbra
   g. Specific area shielding
   h. Entrance skin exposure
   i. CT beam width
   j. Mean marrow dose
2. What is the embryo's response to irradiation above 250 mGy$_t$ during the first 2 weeks after conception?
3. During the fetal period of major organogenesis, what radiation responses are possible?
4. What procedure should be followed if a patient is examined and subsequently discovers that she is pregnant?
5. List five procedures that could result in a measurable fetal dose.
6. How can the three cardinal principles of radiation protection best be applied in diagnostic radiology?
7. What estimate of patient radiation dose usually is measured and reported?
8. How does one use a radiation nomogram?
9. Estimate the entrance skin exposure for a PA chest image conducted at 110 kVp/2 mAs.
10. What factors are required to estimate the genetically significant dose?
11. What radiation dose description is most important for x-ray digital mammography?
12. What is the effective dose range for adult CT angiography?
13. How does the term dose distribution affect specification of patient radiation dose in x-ray imaging?
14. According to the ACR Appropriateness Criteria, what imaging modalities are associated with no ionizing radiation?
15. Name a screening x-ray examination that should not be performed regularly.
16. Estimate the fetal dose after an AP abdominal image is conducted at 76 kVp/40 mAs.
17. What does the symbol Σ mean?
18. Approximately what percentage of the ESE is D$_g$ for mammography?
19. What is the approximate contribution of CT to total patient radiation dose?
20. What is the approximate fetal dose after a 3.5-min barium enema fluoroscopic examination?

The answers to the Challenge Questions can be found by logging on to our website at http://evolve.elsevier.com

Occupational Radiation Dose Management

CHAPTER 42

OBJECTIVES

At the completion of this chapter, the student should be able to do the following:

1. Discuss the units and concepts of occupational radiation exposure.
2. Discuss ways to reduce occupational radiation exposure.
3. Explain occupational radiation monitors and where they should be positioned.
4. Discuss personnel radiation monitoring reports.
5. List the available thicknesses of protective apparel.

OUTLINE

Occupational Radiation Exposure 560
- Interventional Radiology 560
- Mammography 561
- Computed Tomography 561
- Surgery 561
- Mobile Radiology 562

Radiation Dose Limits 562
- Whole-Body Dose Limits 562
- Dose Limits for Tissues and Organs 565
- Public Exposure 566
- Educational Considerations 566

Reduction of Occupational Radiation Exposure 566

Occupational Radiation Monitoring 567
- Where to Wear the Occupational Radiation Monitor 568
- Occupational Radiation Monitoring Report 569
- Protective Apparel 570
- Pregnant Radiographer/Radiologist 571
- Management Principles 572

Summary 574

Challenge Questions 575

RADIATION DOSE is measured in units of gray (Gy_t). Radiation exposure expressed as air KERMA (kinetic energy released in matter) is also measured in gray (Gy_a). When the exposure is to radiographers and to radiologists, the proper unit is the sievert (Sv).

The sievert is the unit of effective dose; it is used for radiation protection purposes. Although exposure, dose, and effective dose have precise and different meanings, they often are used interchangeably in radiology because they have approximately the same numeric value following whole-body exposure.

When properly used, exposure (Gy_a) refers to radiation intensity in air. Patient radiation dose and tissue dose (Gy_t) measure the radiation energy absorbed as a result of x-ray exposure during digital imaging. Effective dose (Sv) identifies the biologic effectiveness of the radiation energy absorbed. This unit is applied to occupationally exposed persons and to population exposure. Radiation regulations are expressed in sievert.

OCCUPATIONAL RADIATION EXPOSURE

Although the recommended dose limit for radiologic personnel is 50 mSv/year, experience has shown that considerably lower exposures than this are routine. The occupational radiation exposure of radiologic personnel engaged in general x-ray activity normally will not exceed 1 mSv/year.

Radiologists usually receive slightly higher radiation exposures than radiographers. This is because the radiologist receives most occupational exposure during fluoroscopy and is usually closer to the radiation source—the patient—during such procedures. Table 42.1 reports the results of an analysis of the annual occupational radiation exposure of a very large population of radiologic personnel. Clearly, the radiation exposures are low.

Interventional Radiology

Unquestionably, the highest occupational exposure of diagnostic x-ray personnel occurs during fluoroscopy and mobile radiography. During radiography, the radiologist is rarely present and the radiographer is behind the console protective barrier.

TABLE 42.1 Occupational Radiation Exposure of Radiologic Personnel

Exposure Category	Value
Average whole-body dose	0.7 mSv/year
Those receiving less than the minimum detectable dose	53%
Those receiving <1 mSv/year	88%
Those receiving >50 mSv/year	0.05%

> Scatter radiation from the patient is the source of occupational radiation exposure during fluoroscopy.

During fluoroscopy, both the radiologist and the radiographer are exposed to relatively high levels of radiation. However, personnel exposure is related directly to the x-ray beam-on time. With care, personnel exposures can be kept as low as reasonably achievable (ALARA).

Question: A barium enema examination requires 2.5 min of fluoroscopic x-ray beam time. If the radiographer is exposed to 2.5 Gy_a/h, what will be the occupational radiation exposure?

Answer:
$$\text{Exposure} = \text{Exposure rate} \times \text{Time}$$
$$= 2.5\ Gy_a/h \times 2.5\ \text{min}$$
$$= 2.5\ Gy_a/h \times 0.0147\ h$$
$$= 0.1\ mGy_a$$

Remote fluoroscopy results in low personnel exposures because personnel are not in the x-ray examination room with the patient. With some fluoroscopes, the x-ray tube is over the table and the image receptor (IR) under the table. This geometry offers some advantage in terms of image quality, but personnel exposures are higher because secondary radiation (scatter and leakage) levels are higher. The entrance skin is the highest intensity of secondary radiation during any digital imaging procedure.

This condition should be kept in mind during mobile radiography and C-arm fluoroscopy. It is best to position the x-ray tube under the patient during C-arm fluoroscopy (Fig. 42.1).

Personnel engaged in interventional radiology procedures often receive higher exposures than do those in general radiologic practice because of longer

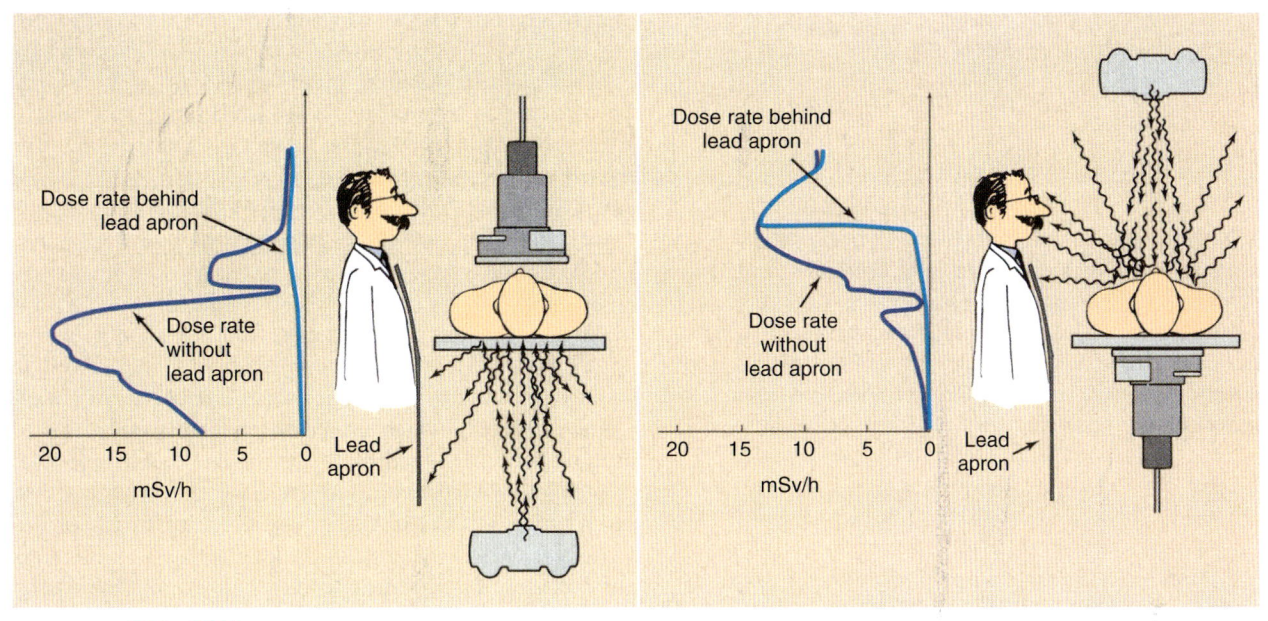

FIG. 42.1 Scatter radiation during portable fluoroscopy is more intense with the x-ray tube over the patient. (Courtesy Stephen Balter, Columbia University Medical Center.)

fluoroscopic x-ray beam-on time. The frequent absence of a protective curtain on the image-intensifier tower and the use of image capture also contribute to higher personnel exposure.

> Extremity occupational monitoring must be provided for interventional radiologists.

Extremity exposure during interventional radiology procedures may be significant. Even with protective gloves, exposure of the forearm can approach the recommended dose limit of 500 mSv/year if care is not taken. Without protective gloves, excessive hand exposures are possible.

Mammography

Personnel exposures associated with mammography are low because the low kVp of the examination results in less scatter radiation from the patient. Usually a long exposure cord and a conventional wall or window wall are sufficient to provide adequate radiation protection.

Rarely does a room that is used strictly for mammography require protective lead shielding. Dedicated mammography x-ray units have personnel protective barriers made of leaded glass, leaded acrylic, and even plate glass as an integral component. Usually such barriers are totally adequate.

Computed Tomography

Personnel exposures in computed tomography (CT) facilities are low. Because the CT x-ray beam is finely collimated and only secondary radiation is present in the examination room, radiation levels are low compared with those experienced in fluoroscopy.

Fig. 42.2 shows the isoexposure profiles for the horizontal and vertical planes of a multislice helical CT imaging system. These data are given as μGy_a/360-degree rotation, and they show that personnel can be permitted to remain in the room during imaging. However, protective apparel should always be worn when you remain in the CT examination room.

Question: It is necessary for a CT technologist to remain in the CT room at midtable position during a 20-rotation examination. What would be the occupational exposure if no protective apron were worn?

Answer: From Fig. 40.2, we may assume an exposure of 1 μGy_a/scan.
Occupational exposure = 1 μGy_a/scan × 20
= 20 μGy_a
= 0.02 mGy_a

Of course, with a protective apron, the trunk of the body would receive essentially zero exposure.

Surgery

Nursing personnel and others working in the operating room and in intensive care units are sometimes exposed to radiation from mobile x-ray imaging systems and C-arm fluoroscopes. Although these personnel are often anxious about such exposures, many studies have shown that their occupational radiation exposure is near zero and certainly is no cause for concern.

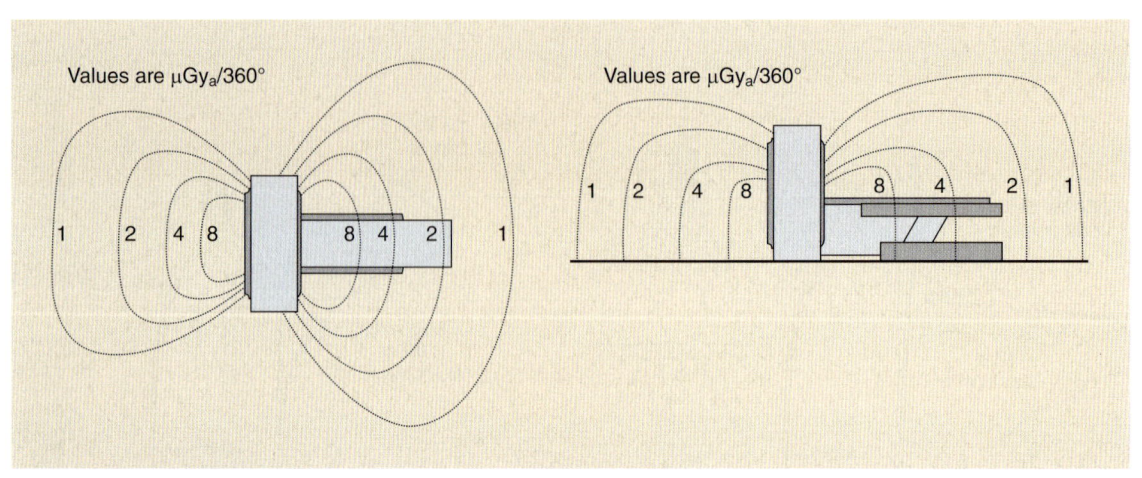

FIG. 42.2 Isoexposure profiles (in μGy$_a$/360 degrees) in horizontal and vertical planes for multislice computed tomography.

It usually is not necessary to provide occupational radiation monitors for such personnel. Depending on the room size and personnel positioning, such personnel may be required to wear protective apparel.

Mobile Radiology

When fixed protective barriers are not available, such as during mobile examination, the mobile x-ray imaging system is equipped with an exposure cord long enough to allow the radiographer to leave the immediate examination area. The radiographer should wear a protective apron for each such mobile examination.

Occupational radiation monitors are not necessary during mobile radiography for personnel who are not directly involved in the examination. Personnel who regularly operate or are in the immediate vicinity of a C-arm fluoroscope should wear an occupational radiation monitor in addition to protective apparel. During C-arm fluoroscopy, the x-ray beam may be on for a relatively long time, and the beam can be pointed in virtually any direction.

It should never be necessary for radiologic personnel to exceed 50 mSv/year. In smaller hospitals, emergency centers, and private clinics, occupational exposures rarely exceed 5 mSv/year. As Table 42.1 reported, average exposures in most facilities are less than 1 mSv/year.

RADIATION DOSE LIMITS

A continuing effort of health physicists has been the description and identification of occupational radiation dose limits. For many years, a maximum permissible dose (MPD) was specified. The MPD was the minimum dose of radiation not expected to produce significant radiation response.

At radiation doses less than the MPD, no responses should occur. At the level of the MPD, the risk is not zero, but it is small—lower than the risk associated with other occupations and reasonable in light of the benefits derived. The concept of MPD is now obsolete and has been replaced by **recommended dose limits**.

> Low radiation dose is less than 100 mGy$_t$. Low radiation dose rate is less than 5 mGy$_t$/h.

A 2022 report by the National Academies of Science, Engineering and Medicine (NASEM) proposed activities in many areas, including radiology for low-dose radiation research projects dealing with radiology patients and personnel. NASEM identifies low radiation dose as less than 100 mGy$_t$ and low radiation dose rate as less than 5 mGy$_t$/h.

Whole-Body Dose Limits

To establish recommended dose limits, the National Council on Radiation Protection and Measurements (NCRP) assessed risk on the basis of data from reports of the National Academy of Sciences and the National Safety Council (Table 42.2).

State and federal government agencies routinely adopt these recommended dose limits as law. Current dose limits are prescribed for various organs as well as for the whole body and for various working conditions. If one received the recommended dose limit each year, the lifetime risk would not exceed 1 in 10,000 per year.

> Recommended dose limits imply that if received annually, the risk of death would be less than 1 in 10,000.

The value 1 in 10,000 represents the approximate risk of death for those working in safe industries. The dose limits recommended by the NCRP ensure that

TABLE 42.2 Fatal Accident Rates in Various Industries

Industry	Rate (per 10,000 per Year)
Trade	0.4
Manufacture	0.4
Service	0.4
Government	0.9
Radiation workers	0.9
All groups	0.9
Transport	2.2
Public utilities	2.2
Construction	3.1
Mining	4.3
Agriculture	4.4

radiation workers have the same risk as those in safe industries.

Question: Suppose all 300,000 American radiographers receive the annual whole-body dose limit (50 mSv) this year. How many would be expected to die prematurely?

Answer: (300,000)(1/10,000) = 30

But, of course, they actually receive approximately 0.5 mSv/year; therefore the expected mortality is as follows:

(300,000)(1/10,000)(0.5 mSv/year ÷ 50 mSv/year) = 0.3; less than 1!

Particular care is taken to ensure that no radiation worker receives a radiation dose in excess of the recommended dose limit. That dose limit is specified only for occupational exposure. It should not be confused with radiation dose received as a patient.

> Although patient radiation dose should be ALARA, there is no patient dose limit.

The first occupational dose limit, 500 mSv/week, was recommended in 1902. The current occupational dose limit is 1 mSv/week. Through the years, a downward revision of the recommended dose limit has occurred. The history of these continuing recommendations is given in Table 42.3 and is shown graphically in Fig. 42.3.

In the early years of radiology, the dose limit consisted of a single value that was considered the safe working level for whole-body exposure. It was based primarily on the known acute response to radiation exposure and presumed that a threshold radiation dose existed.

Currently the recommended dose limit is specified not only for whole-body exposure but also for partial-body exposure, organ exposure, and exposure of the general population, again excluding medical radiation dose as a patient and exposure from natural sources (Table 42.4). The dose limits included in Table 42.4 were published by the NCRP first in 1987 and refined in 1993.

They replaced the previous MPDs, which had been in effect since 1959. These recommended dose limits have been adopted by state and federal regulatory agencies and are now the law of the United States.

The basic annual recommended radiation dose limit is 50 mSv/year. The radiation dose limit for the lens of the eye is 150 mSv/year and that for other organs is 500 mSv/year.

The cumulative whole-body radiation dose limit is 10 mSv times age in years. The dose limit during pregnancy is 5 mSv, but once pregnancy has been declared, monthly exposure should not exceed 0.5 mSv.

> Current recommended radiation dose limits are based on the linear, nonthreshold dose-response relationship.

In practice, at least in digital imaging, it is seldom necessary to exceed even one-tenth the appropriate dose limit. However, because the basis for the dose limit assumes a linear, nonthreshold dose-response relationship, all unnecessary radiation exposure should be avoided.

Occupational radiation exposure is described as effective dose in units of millisievert. This scheme has been adopted to afford enhanced precision in radiation protection practices.

The effective dose concept accounts for different types of radiation because of their varying relative biologic effectiveness. Effective dose also considers the relative radiosensitivity of various tissues and organs.

These are particularly important considerations when a protective apron is worn. Wearing a protective apron reduces radiation dose to many tissues and organs to near zero. Therefore effective dose is much less than that recorded by a collar-positioned occupational radiation monitor.

> Effective dose (E) = Radiation weighting factor (W_r) × Tissue weighting factor (W_t) × Absorbed dose

As can be seen in Table 42.5, the radiation weighting factor (W_r) is equal to 1 for the types of radiation used

PART VIII Radiation Protection

TABLE 42.3 Historical Review of Dose Limits for Occupational Exposure

Year	Recommendation	Approximate Daily Dose Limit (μSv)	Source
1902	Dose limited by fogging of a photographic plate after 7-min contact exposure	100,000	Rollins
1915	Lead shielding of tube needed (no numeric British Roentgen Society exposure levels given)		
1921	General methods to reduce exposure		British X-ray and Radium Protection Committee
1925	"It is entirely safe if an operator does not receive every 30 days a dose exceeding 1/100 of an erythema dose."	2000	Mutscheller
1925	10% of SED per year	2000	Sievert
1926	One SED per 90,000 working hours	400	Dutch Board of Health
1928	0.000028 of SED per day	1750	Barclay and Cox
1928	0.001 of SED per month 5R per day permissible for the hands	1500	Kaye
1931	Limit exposure to 0.2 R per day	2000	Advisory Committee on X-ray and Radium Protection of the United States
1932	0.001 of SED per month	300	Failla
1934	5R per day permissible for the hands	50,000	Advisory Committee on X-ray and Radium Protection of the United States
1936	0.1 R per day	1000	Advisory Committee on X-ray and Radium Protection of the United States
1941	0.02 R per day	200	Taylor
1943	200 mR per day is acceptable	2000	Patterson
1959	5 rem per year, 5 (N-18) rem cumulative	200	National Council on Radiation Protection and Measurements
1987	50 mSv per year, 10 × N mSv cumulative	200	National Council on Radiation Protection and Measurements
1991	20 mSv per year	80	International Commission on Radiation Protection

SED, Skin erythema dose.

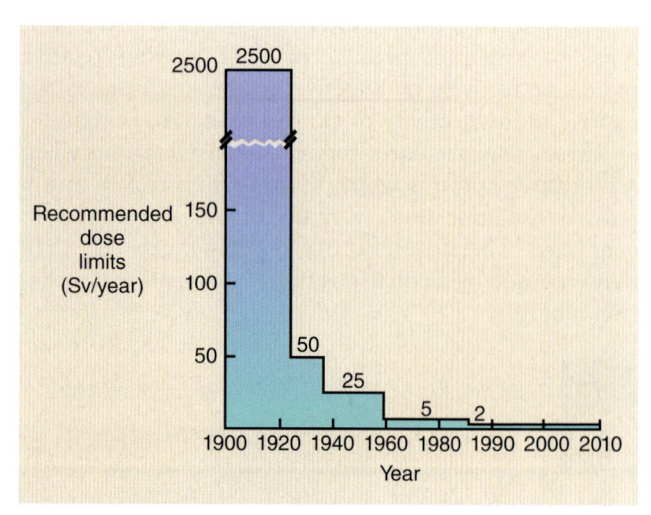

FIG. 42.3 Dose limits over the years.

in digital imaging. The value of W_r for other types of radiation depends on the linear energy transfer of that radiation.

The tissue weighting factor (W_t) accounts for the relative radiosensitivity of various tissues and organs. Tissues with a higher value of W_t are more radiosensitive. These are shown in Table 42.6. Practical implementation of these dose limits and weighting factors does not change our previous approach.

> The recommended radiation dose limit is sufficiently high that it rarely, if ever, is exceeded in digital imaging.

TABLE 42.4	Dose Limits Recommended by the National Council on Radiation Protection and Measurements

A. Occupational exposures
  1. Effective dose
     a. Annual: 50 mSv
     b. Cumulative: 10 mSv × age
  2. Equivalent annual dose for tissues and organs
     a. Lens of the eye: 150 mSv
     b. Thyroid, skin, hands, and feet: 500 mSv
B. Public exposures (annual)
  1. Effective dose, frequent exposure: 1 mSv
  2. Equivalent dose for tissues and organs
     a. Lens of eye: 15 mSv
     b. Skin, hands, and feet: 50 mSv
C. Education and training exposures (annual)
  1. Effective dose: 1 mSv
  2. Equivalent dose for tissues and organs
     a. Lens of eye: 15 mSv
     b. Skin, hands, and feet: 50 mSv
D. Embryo-fetus exposures
  1. Total equivalent dose: 5 mSv
  2. Equivalent dose in 1 month: 0.5 mSv
E. Negligible individual dose (annual): 0.01 mSv

TABLE 42.5	Weighting Factors for Various Types of Radiation

Type of Energy Range	Radiation Weighting Factor (W_r)
X- and gamma rays, electrons	1
Neutrons, energy <10 keV	5
10–100 keV	10
>100 keV to 2 MeV	20
>2–20 MeV	10
>20 MeV	5
Protons	2
Alpha particles	20

With a collar-positioned occupational radiation monitor, a change in procedure is necessary to estimate effective dose. Because essentially all of our radiation exposure occurs during fluoroscopy and the trunk of the body is shielded by a lead apron, the response of the occupational radiation monitor overestimates the effective dose.

A conversion factor of 0.1 should be applied to the collar monitor-reported value to estimate effective dose. If a protective apron is not worn (e.g., by a radiographer who does no fluoroscopy), then the monitor response may be considered the effective dose.

TABLE 42.6	Weighting Factors for Various Tissues

Tissue	Tissue Weighting Factor (W_t)
Active bone marrow	0.12
Colon	0.12
Lung	0.12
Stomach	0.12
Bladder	0.05
Breast	0.05
Esophagus	0.05
Liver	0.05
Thyroid	0.05
Gonad	0.02
Bone surface	0.01
Skin	0.01

Dose Limits for Tissues and Organs

The whole-body dose limit of 50 mSv/year is an effective dose, which considers the weighted average to various tissues and organs. In addition, the NCRP has identified several specific tissues and organs with specific recommended dose limits.

Some organs of the body have a higher dose limit than the whole-body dose limit. The dose limit for the skin is 500 mSv/year.

This limit is not normally of concern in digital imaging because it applies to nonpenetrating radiation such as alpha and beta radiation and very soft x-rays. Radiographers exclusively engaged in mammography or nuclear medicine are highly unlikely to sustain radiation exposure to the skin in excess of 10 mSv/year.

Interventional radiologists often have their hands near the primary fluoroscopic x-ray beam; therefore extremity exposure may be of concern. The dose limit for the extremities is the same as that for the skin—500 mSv/year.

These radiation levels are quite high and under normal circumstances should not even be approached. For certain occupational groups, such as interventional radiologists and nuclear medicine technologists, extremity occupational personnel monitors should be provided.

> Extremity occupational personnel monitors are worn on the wrist or the finger.

Because radiation is known to produce cataracts, a dose limit is specified for the lens of the eye. This dose limit is 150 mSv/year, and it should never be approached, much less exceeded, in digital imaging. The response of a collar-positioned occupational radiation monitor can be used as the lens dose.

Public Exposure

Individuals in the general population are limited to 1 mSv/year. For hospital workers who are not radiology employees but who may regularly visit x-ray rooms, the recommended dose limit is 1 mSv/year.

> The recommended radiation dose limit for nonoccupationally exposed persons is 1 mSv/year.

This value of 1 mSv/year is the dose limit that medical physicists use when computing the thickness of protective barriers. If a barrier separates an x-ray examining room from an area occupied by the general public, the shielding is designed so that the annual exposure of an individual in the adjacent area cannot exceed 1 mSv/year.

If the adjacent area is occupied by radiation workers, the shielding must be sufficient to maintain an annual exposure level less than 10 mSv/year. This approach to shielding derives from the (10 mSv × age) cumulative recommended dose limit.

Radiation exposure of the general public or of individuals in this population is measured rarely because this process is not necessary. Most radiology personnel do not receive even this level of exposure.

Educational Considerations

Several special situations are associated with whole-body occupational dose limits. Students younger than 18 years of age may not receive more than 1 mSv/year during the course of their educational activities. This is included in and is not added to the 1 mSv permitted each year as a nonoccupational exposure as a member of the general public.

Consequently student radiographers younger than 18 years of age may be engaged in x-ray imaging, but their exposure must be monitored and must remain below 1 mSv/year. Because of this, it is general practice not to accept applicants into radiography educational programs unless their 18th birthday is within sight.

In keeping with ALARA, even more changes in recommended dose limits are on the way. The International Commission on Radiological Protection has issued several recommendations, including an annual whole-body recommended dose limit of 20 mSv. Such a reduction is currently under consideration in the United States.

REDUCTION OF OCCUPATIONAL RADIATION EXPOSURE

The radiographer can do much to reduce occupational radiation exposure. Most exposure control procedures do not require sophisticated equipment or especially rigorous training, but simply a conscientious attitude regarding the performance of assigned duties. Most equipment characteristics, technique changes, and administrative procedures designed to minimize patient radiation dose also reduce occupational radiation exposure.

In diagnostic radiology, at least 95% of the radiographer's occupational radiation exposure comes from fluoroscopy and mobile radiography. Attention to the cardinal principles of radiation protection (time, distance, and shielding) and ALARA are the most important aspects of occupational radiation control.

During fluoroscopy, the radiologist should minimize x-ray beam-on time. This can be done through careful technique, which includes intermittent activation of fluoroscopic views rather than one long period of x-ray beam-on time.

Most fluoroscopes have the capacity to image using pulse-progressive x-ray beam time. Pulse-progressive fluoroscopy should be used whenever appropriate and that is most of the time. As the radiographer, be aware that if the fluoroscopist is not a radiologist, you may understand patient radiation management better than the fluoroscopist. Do not hesitate to speak up and recommend pulse-progressive mode if constant fluoroscopic mode is being used. Failure to do so in several situations has resulted in severe patient radiation skin burns.

It is a common radiation protection practice to maintain a log of fluoroscopy time by recording x-ray beam-on time with the 5-minute reset timer. If a dose area product (DAP) meter is available, record the DAP for each fluoroscopic procedure. Recording these patient radiation dose measures is the responsibility of the radiographer.

During fluoroscopy, the radiographer should step back from the table when their immediate presence and assistance are not required. The radiographer also should take maximum advantage of all protective shielding, including apron, curtain, and even the radiologist. If the radiologist should question your move behind them, reply "That's what Bushong told me to do!"

> Each mobile x-ray unit should have a protective apron assigned to it.

The radiographer should wear a protective apron during all mobile examinations and should maintain maximum distance from the x-ray source. The primary beam should never be pointed at the radiographer or other nearby personnel.

> The exposure cord on a portable x-ray unit must be at least 2 m long.

Always wear the protective apron during mobile radiography. Even though the distance from the x-ray source is 2 m and from the patient is 3 m, the leakage and scatter radiation is measurable. Try this. Put on protective lead gloves, and hold a hand phantom over an IR in front of your protective apron during a mobile x-ray examination. You will image the phantom hand!

During radiography, the radiographer is positioned behind a control booth barrier. Such barriers usually are considered secondary barriers because the primary x-ray beam is never pointed in that direction. Control booth barriers intercept only leakage and scatter radiation. Consequently, leaded glass and leaded gypsum board are often unnecessary for such barriers.

> The useful beam should never be directed toward the operating console.

Other work assignments in digital imaging, such as scheduling and filing, result in essentially no occupational radiation exposure.

Occupational Radiation Monitoring

The level of occupational radiation exposure to radiologists and radiographers depends on the type and frequency of activity in which they are engaged. Determining the exposure of radiation they receive requires a program of occupational radiation monitoring. Occupational radiation monitoring refers to procedures instituted to estimate the amount of radiation received by individuals who work in a radiation environment.

> Occupational radiation monitoring is required when there is any likelihood that an individual will receive more than one-tenth of any recommended dose limit.

Most digital imaging personnel must be monitored; however it usually is not necessary to monitor diagnostic radiology secretaries and file clerks. Furthermore, it usually is not necessary to monitor operating room personnel, except perhaps those routinely involved in cystoscopy and C-arm fluoroscopy.

> The occupational radiation monitor offers no protection against radiation exposure!

The occupational radiation monitor simply measures the quantity of radiation to which the monitor was exposed; therefore it is simply an indicator of radiation exposure to the wearer. Basically two types of personnel monitors are used in diagnostic radiology: thermoluminescence dosimeters (TLDs) and optically stimulated luminescence (OSLs) dosimeters.

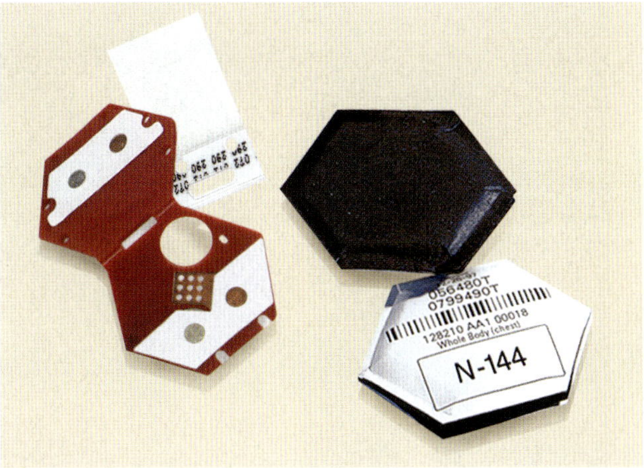

FIG. 42.4 Representative radiation monitors. In many, metal filters are incorporated to help identify the type of radiation and its energy. (Courtesy Linda Bosy, Landauer, Inc.)

Regardless of the type of monitor used, it is essential that it be obtained from a certified laboratory. In-house processing of radiation monitors should not be attempted. Fig. 42.4 presents a view of two typical occupational radiation monitors.

Film badges came into general use during the 1940s and were used widely in diagnostic radiology until late in the 20th century. Film badges are specially designed devices in which a film similar to dental radiographic film is sandwiched between metal filters inside a plastic case.

The sensitive material of the TLD monitor (Fig. 42.5) is lithium fluoride in crystalline form, either as a powder or more often as a small chip approximately 3 mm square and 1 mm thick. When exposed to x-rays, the TLD absorbs energy and stores it in the form of excited electrons in the crystalline lattice.

When heated, these excited electrons fall back to their normal state with the emission of visible light. The intensity of visible light is measured with a photomultiplier tube or photodiode and is proportional to the radiation dose received by the lithium fluoride crystal. This sequence was described in Chapter 37.

The TLD occupational radiation monitor offers several advantages over film. It is more sensitive and more accurate than a film badge occupational radiation monitor. Properly calibrated TLD monitors can measure exposure as low as 50 µGy$_a$. The TLD monitor does not suffer from loss of information after it is exposed to excessive heat or humidity.

> TLD occupational radiation monitors can be worn for intervals up to 1 year.

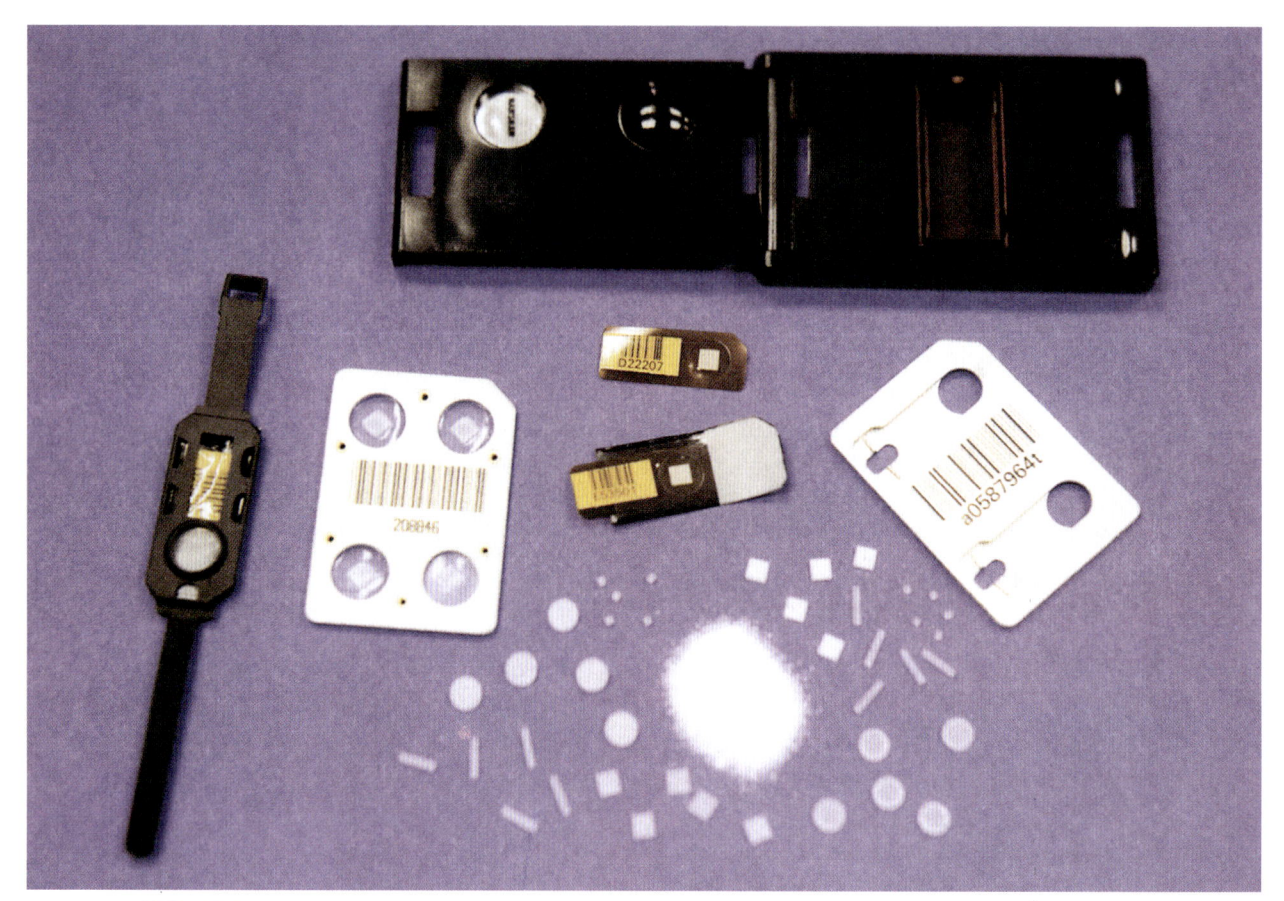

FIG. 42.5 Thermoluminescence dosimeters are available as chips, disks, rods, and powder. These are used for area and environmental radiation monitoring, and especially for occupational radiation monitoring. (Courtesy Bicron Electronics.)

OSL dosimeters (Fig. 42.6) are worn and handled just as TLDs are, and they are approximately the same size. OSL dosimeters have one advantage over TLDs. They are more sensitive, measuring as low as 10 μGy$_a$.

Where to Wear the Occupational Radiation Monitor

Much discussion and research in health physics have gone into providing precise recommendations about where a radiographer should wear the occupational radiation monitor. Official publications of the NCRP offer suggestions that have been adopted as regulations in most states.

Many radiographers wear their personnel monitors in front at the waist or chest level because it is convenient to clip the badge over a belt or a shirt pocket. If the radiographer is not involved in fluoroscopic procedures, these locations are acceptable.

> If the radiographer participates in fluoroscopy, the occupational radiation monitor should be positioned on the collar above the protective apron.

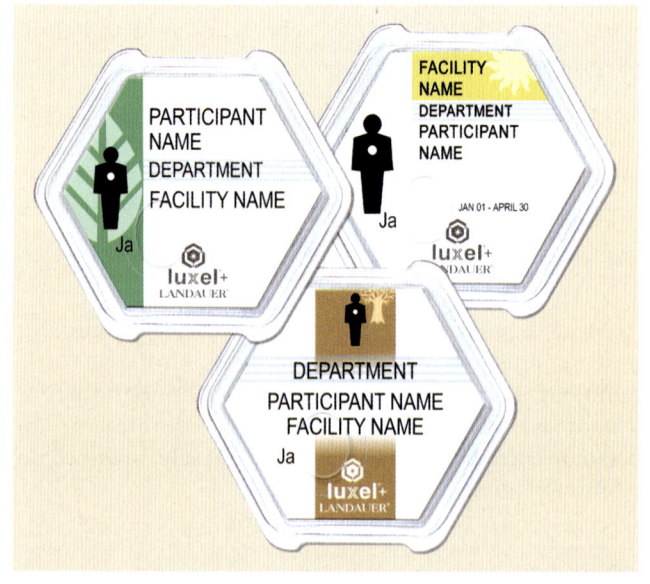

FIG. 42.6 Optically stimulated luminescence dosimeters. (Courtesy Linda Bosy, Landauer, Inc.)

The recommended dose limit of 50 mSv/year refers to the effective dose. It has been shown that during fluoroscopy, when a protective apron is worn, exposure to the collar region is approximately 20 times greater than that to the trunk of the body beneath the protective

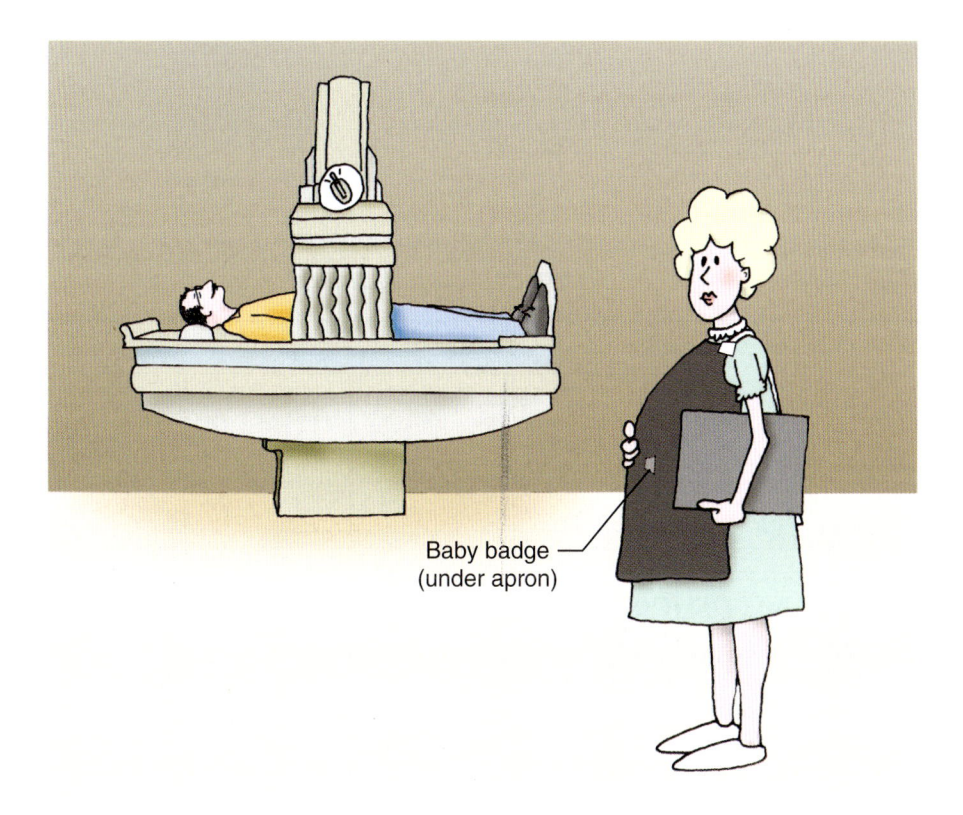

FIG. 42.7 When the radiographer is pregnant, a second "baby badge" should be positioned under the protective apron.

apron. So if the occupational radiation monitor is worn beneath the protective apron, it will record a falsely low exposure, usually zero, and will not indicate what could be excessive exposure to unprotected body parts.

In some clinical situations (e.g., during pregnancy and with extremity monitoring), it may be advisable to wear more than one radiation monitor. The abdomen should be monitored during pregnancy. During fluoroscopy and portable examinations, the pregnant radiographer should wear the additional abdominal monitor under the lead apron (see Fig. 42.7). The extremities should be monitored during interventional procedures when the radiologist's hands are in close proximity to the useful x-ray beam. Nuclear medicine technologists should wear extremity monitors when handling millicurie quantities of radioactive material.

Occupational Radiation Monitoring Report

State and federal regulations require that results of the occupational radiation monitoring program be recorded in a precise fashion and maintained for review. Annual, quarterly, monthly, or weekly monitoring periods are acceptable.

The occupational radiation monitoring report must contain a number of specific items of information (Fig. 42.8). These various items are identified in the headers of each column.

Exposure data that must be included on the form include current exposure and cumulative annual exposure. Separate radiation monitors, such as extremity monitors or fetal monitors, are identified separately from the whole-body monitor.

Occasionally, if occupational exposure involves low energy radiation, the dose to the skin might be greater than the dose of penetrating radiation. In such cases, the skin dose is separately identified. Areas on the report are provided for neutron radiation exposure to accommodate nuclear reactor and particle accelerator workers.

> Lifetime occupational radiation exposure must be recorded.

When a radiographer changes employment, the total radiation exposure history must be transferred to the records of the new employer. Consequently, when one leaves a job, one should automatically receive a report of the total radiation exposure history at that facility. Such a report should be given automatically; if it is not, it must be requested.

When an occupational radiation monitoring program is established, the supplier of the monitor should be informed of the type of radiation facility involved. This information influences the method of calibration of monitors and **control monitors**.

The control monitor should never be stored in or adjacent to a radiation area. It should be kept in a

SAMPLE HOSPITAL
ATTN: RSO
4242 MAIN STREET
SMALLVILLE, MA 01432

Received Date / Reported Date	2014-05-30 / 2014-06-03
Page	1 of 4
Analytical Work Order / QC Release	1415095001 / NHE
Copy / Version	0 / 1

NVLAP LAB CODE 100518-0**

LANDAUER®
Landauer, Inc., 2 Science Road
Glenwood, Illinois 60425-1586
www.landauer.com
Telephone: (708) 755-7000
Facsimile: (708) 755-7016
Customer Service: (800) 323-8830
Technical: (800) 438-3241

Radiation Dosimetry Report

Account: 709008 Subaccount: 1431640 Series: CST

**No NVLAP accreditation is available from NVLAP for thermal neutron or X type dosimeters. When exposure results are reported for thermal neutrons or X type dosimeters, this report contains data that are not covered by the NVLAP accreditation.

Participant Number	Name		Dosimeter	Use	Rad. Type	Rad. Quality	Dose Equivalent (mrem) for Periods Shown Below — DDE-Deep Dose Equivalent LDE-Lens Dose Equivalent SDE-Shallow Dose Equivalent												Inception Date	Serial Number
							Period Shown Below			Quarter to Date			Year to Date			Lifetime to Date				
	ID Number	Birth Date					DDE	LDE	SDE	DDE	LDE	SDE	DDE	LDE	SDE	DDE	LDE	SDE		
For Monitoring Period:							2014-05-01 to 2014-05-31			QUARTER 2			2014			LIFETIME				
	Average Control Dose		Pa				5	5	5											
01067	Halpert, Jim		Pa	COLLAR	*P		10	10	10										2005/03	6794392C
	000-11-2222	1979-10-20		ASSIGNED			10	10	10	12	12	12	12	12	12	12	12	12		
				NOTE			Participant active in other account(s) or subaccount(s)													
For Monitoring Period:							2014-06-01 to 2014-06-30			QUARTER 2			2014			LIFETIME				
00CST	CONTROL		Ja	CNTRL																7254728C
	Control Dose Used		Ja				22	22	22											
	CONTROL		Pa	CNTRL																7254729C
	Control Dose Used		Pa				22	22	22											
	CONTROL		Ta	CNTRL																7254730C
	Control Dose Used		Ta				22	22	22											
01068	Beesly, Pam		Pa	COLLAR			M	M	M										2005/03	7254731C
	1111-22-3333	1974-05-07		ASSIGNED			M	M	M	M	M	M	M	M	M	M	M	M		
				NOTE			Participant active in other account(s) or subaccount(s)													
01069	Reynolds, Malcolm		Pa	COLLAR	P		18	18	18										2014/06	7254733C
	222-33-4444	1971-03-27		ASSIGNED			5	18	18	8	30	34	8	30	34	8	30	34		
				NOTE			Assigned dose based on EDE2 Calculation													
				NOTE			Participant active in other account(s) or subaccount(s)													
01070	White, Walter		Pa	COLLAR	P		1078	1078	1078										2008/01	7254734C
	333-44-5555	1956-03-07		NOTE			Imaging indicates an irregular exposure. Dosimeter reprocessed, second read agrees with reported dose.													
				ASSIGNED			1078	1078	1078	2092	2123	2124	2092	2123	2124	2092	2123	2124		
				NOTE			Participant active in other account(s) or subaccount(s)													

* - Standard background control rate used for control subtraction

This report must not be used to claim product certification, approval, or endorsement by NVLAP, NIST, or any agency of the federal government.

FIG. 42.8 The occupational radiation monitoring report must include the items of information shown here. (Courtesy Linda Bosy, Landauer, Inc.)

distant room or office. After processing, the response of the control monitor is subtracted from each individual monitor. In this way, the report for each individual monitor represents only the occupational radiation exposure.

> The control monitor measures background exposure during transportation, handling, and storage.

All monitors should be returned to the supplier together and in a timely fashion so they can be processed together. Lost or inadvertently exposed monitors must be evaluated, and an estimate of true exposure should be made by the medical physicist.

Protective Apparel

The operating console usually is positioned behind fixed protective barriers during digital imaging procedures. During fluoroscopy or mobile radiography, digital imaging personnel are in the examination room and near the x-ray source.

> Protective apparel must be worn during fluoroscopy and mobile radiology.

Protective gloves and aprons are available in many sizes and shapes. These usually are constructed of lead-impregnated vinyl. Some protective garments are impregnated with tin or other metals because other metals have some advantages over lead as a shielding material in the digital imaging x-ray energy range.

Normal thicknesses for protective apparel are 0.25, 0.5, and 1 mm of lead equivalent. The garments themselves are much thicker than these dimensions, but they provide shielding equivalent to these thicknesses of lead (Table 42.7). Protection of at least 0.25-mm Pb is required; 0.5-mm Pb is normal.

Maximum exposure reduction is obtained with the 1-mm lead equivalent garment, but an apron of this material can weigh as much as 12 kg (25 lb). The wearer could be exhausted by the end of the fluoroscopy schedule just from having to wear the protective apron. X-ray

TABLE 42.7 Some Physical Characteristics of Protective Lead Aprons

Equivalent Thickness (mm Pb)	Weight (kg)	PERCENTAGE X-RAY ATTENUATION		
		50 kVp	75 kVp	100 kVp
0.25	1–5	97	66	51
0.50	3–7	99.9	88	75
1.00	5–12	99.9	99	94

attenuation at 75 kVp for 0.25-mm lead equivalent and 1-mm lead equivalent is 66% and 99%, respectively.

The 0.5-mm lead equivalent protective aprons represent a workable compromise between unnecessary weight and desired protection.

Protective aprons for interventional radiology should be of the wrap-around type. During these procedures, a lot of personnel movement can occur, and some personnel, such as anesthesiologists, may even have their backs to the radiation source.

When not in use, protective apparel must be stored on properly designed racks. If they are continually folded or heaped in the corner, cracks can develop. At least once a year, aprons and gloves should be imaged with x-rays to ensure that no such cracks appear. If fluoroscopy is not available, high-kVp radiography (e.g., 120 kVp/10 mAs) may be used.

> Radiation protective eyewear, leaded glasses, is not necessary.

If the radiographer or the radiologist feel safer and more comfortable with protective glasses, that is OK. The response of the lens of the eye to radiation exposure is cataract formation on the posterior of the lens. However, such radiation response is deterministic in nature with a radiation dose threshold above 2 Gy_t. That will never happen in today's interventional radiology.

During fluoroscopy, all personnel should remain as far from the patient as possible, keeping the front of the apron facing the radiation source, usually the patient, at all times. The radiographer should take a step or two backward from the table when their presence is not required. After stepping back, step sideways behind the radiologist to take advantage of the additional shielding.

The radiologist should use the dead man foot switch sparingly and pulse-progressive mode frequently. Naturally, when x-ray beam-on time is high, the radiation exposure to patient and personnel will be proportionately high.

Many patients referred for x-ray examination, including infants, older adults, and the incapacitated, are not physically able to support themselves. Mechanical immobilization devices should be available for such patients. Otherwise, a relative or a friend who accompanies the patient should be asked to help.

> Radiology personnel should never hold patients.

When it is necessary to have another person hold the patient, protective apparel must be provided to that person. An apron and gloves are necessary, and the holder should be positioned and instructed carefully, so that they are not exposed to the useful beam. Because the holder is often the mother of a child patient, be sure to ask whether she could be pregnant.

Pregnant Radiographer/Radiologist

When a radiographer becomes pregnant, she should notify her supervisor. The pregnancy then is **declared**, and the recommended dose limit becomes 0.5 mSv/month. The supervisor then should review her previous radiation exposure history because this facilitates decisions regarding what protective actions are necessary.

The recommended dose limit for the fetus is 5 mSv for the period of pregnancy—a dose level that most radiographers will not reach regardless of pregnancy. Although some may receive doses that exceed 5 mSv/year, most receive less than 1 mSv/year.

This usually is indicated with the personnel occupational radiation monitoring device positioned at the collar above the protective apron. Exposure at the waist under the protective apron normally does not exceed 10% of these values; therefore, under normal conditions, specific protective action is not necessary.

Most lead protective aprons are 0.5-mm lead equivalent. These provide approximately 90% attenuation at 75 kVp, which is sufficient. One-millimeter lead equivalent protective aprons are available, but such thickness is not necessary, particularly in view of the additional weight of the apron. Back problems during pregnancy constitute a greater hazard than radiation exposure.

The length of the apron need not extend below the knees, but wrap-around aprons are preferred during pregnancy. If necessary, a special effort should be made to provide an apron of proper size because of its weight.

> The pregnant radiographer should be provided with a second personnel monitoring device.

An additional occupational radiation monitor should be positioned under the protective apron at waist level. The exposure reported on this second monitor should be maintained on a separate record and identified as exposure to the fetus.

Do not allow the monitors to be switched and the record confused. Try color coding—red for the collar badge (red neck!) and yellow for the waist badge (yellow belly!). Additional or thicker lead aprons normally are not necessary (see Fig. 42.8).

Experience with the use of an additional monitor shows consistently that exposures to the fetus are zero. Suppose, for instance, that a pregnant radiographer wearing a single radiation monitor at collar level receives 1 mSv during the 9-month period. The dose at waist level under a protective apron would be less than 10% of the collar dose, or 0.1 mSv. This is the dose to the monitor; the dose to the fetus is near zero.

Attenuation by maternal tissues overlying the fetus reduces the dose to the fetus to approximately 30% of the abdominal skin dose, or 30 µSv. Consequently, when normal protective measures are taken, it is nearly impossible for a radiographer even to approach the fetal dose limit of 5 mSv.

Management Principles

It should be clear that the probability of a harmful effect after any occupational radiation exposure in digital imaging is highly unlikely. A biologic response is expected very rarely and has not been observed in radiologic personnel for the past 50 years or so.

Nevertheless it is essential for the director of radiology to incorporate three steps into the radiation protection program: new employee training, periodic in-service training, and counseling during pregnancy.

The initial step in any administrative protocol involving pregnant employees involves orientation and training. During these orientation discussions, all female employees should be instructed as to their responsibility regarding pregnancy and radiation.

Each radiographer should be provided with a copy of the facility radiation protection manual and other appropriate materials. This material might include a one-page summary of doses, responses, and proper radiation control working habits (see Table 40.7).

The new employee then should read and sign a form (see Fig. 42.9) to indicate that instruction in this area of radiation protection has been provided. An important point to be made by signing this document is that the female employee will notify her supervisor voluntarily when she is pregnant or suspects she is pregnant.

Every well-run radiology service maintains a regular schedule of in-service training. Usually this training is conducted at monthly intervals, but sometimes it occurs more often. At least twice each year, such training should be devoted to radiation protection, and

---

New Employee Notification

This is to certify that _____, a new employee of this radiologic facility, has received instructions regarding mutual responsibilities should she become pregnant during this employment.

In addition to personal counseling by _____, she has been given to read several documents dealing with pregnancy in diagnostic radiology. Furthermore, the additional reading material that follows is available in the departmental office:

1. *Review of NCRP radiation dose limit for embryo and fetus in occupationally-exposed women,* NCRP Report No 53, Washington, DC, 1977, National Council on Radiation Protection and Measures.
2. *Medical radiation exposure of pregnant and potentially pregnant women,* NCRP Report No 54, Washington, DC, 1977, National Council on Radiation Protection and Measures.
3. Wagner, LK et al: *Exposure of the pregnant patient to diagnostic radiation,* Philadelphia, 1985, JB Lippincott.
4. *The effects on populations of exposure to low levels of ionizing radiation,* Washington, DC, 1990, National Academy of Sciences.

I understand that should I become pregnant and I decide to declare my pregnancy, it is my responsibility to inform my supervisor of my condition so that additional protective measures can be taken.

_____   _____
Supervisor   Employee

_____
Date

FIG. 42.9 Form for new employee notification.

TABLE 42.8 Pregnancy in Diagnostic Radiology

HUMAN RESPONSE TO LOW-LEVEL EXPOSURE

Life-span shortening	1 day/mGy$_t$
Cataracts	None <2 Gy$_t$
Leukemia	1 cases/10^6/mGy$_t$/year
Cancer	0.2 cases/10^4/mGy$_t$
Genetic effects	Doubling dose = 0.5 Gy$_t$
Death from all causes	0.2 deaths/10^4/mGy$_t$

EFFECTS OF IRRADIATION IN UTERO

0–14 days	Spontaneous abortion: 25% natural incident; 0.1% increase/100 mGy$_t$
2–10 weeks	Congenital abnormalities: 5% natural incidence; 1% increase/100 mGy$_t$
2nd–3rd trimester	Cell depletion: no effect at <0.5 Gy$_t$
	Latent malignancy: 4:10,000 natural incidence; 0.6:10,000/mGy$_t$
0–9 months	Genetic effects: 10% natural incidence; 5 × 10^{-8} mutations/mGy$_t$

PROTECTIVE MEASURES FOR THE PREGNANT RADIOGRAPHER

Two occupational radiation monitors
Dose limit: 5 mSv/9 mo, 0.5 mSv/month

---

a portion of these sessions should be directed at the potentially pregnant employee.

The material to be covered in such sessions is outlined in Table 42.8. Although it is good to review doses and responses, it is probably more appropriate to emphasize radiation control procedures. These, of course, affect the radiation safety of all radiographers—not only pregnant radiographers.

> A review of occupational personnel monitoring records is particularly important.

A helpful procedure is to post the most recent radiation monitoring report for all to see. The year-end report should be initialed by each radiographer, and the director of radiology should ensure that radiographers understand the nature and magnitude of their annual exposure.

Through such training, radiologic personnel will realize that their occupational radiation exposure is minimal—usually at less than 10% of the recommended dose limit.

> The effective occupational radiation dose limit is 50 mSv/year.
> Environmental background radiation is approximately 1 mSv/year.
> Occupational exposures are closer to the latter than the former.

The director of radiology takes the next action when the radiographer declares her pregnancy. First the director should counsel the employee after reviewing her radiation exposure history and considering any future modifications to her schedule that may be appropriate.

> Under no circumstance should termination or an involuntary leave of absence occur as a consequence of pregnancy.

In all likelihood, a review of the employee's previous radiation exposure history will show a low exposure profile. Those who wear the radiation monitor positioned at the collar, as recommended, and who are heavily involved in fluoroscopy, may receive an exposure greater than 5 mSv/year. However, such employees are protected by lead aprons, so that exposure to the trunk of the body normally would not exceed 500 µSv.

During this review of occupational radiation exposure, it is appropriate to emphasize that the recommended dose limit during pregnancy is 5 mSv and 0.5 mSv/month. Furthermore, it should be shown that this dose limit refers to the fetus and not to the radiographer. The level of 5 mSv to the fetus during gestation is considered an absolutely safe radiation exposure level.

> An alteration in work schedule because of reported occupational radiation exposure is not required.

For radiographers involved in radiation oncology, nuclear medicine, or ultrasonography, similar consultation and level of modification as previously discussed are appropriate. In radiation oncology, the pregnant radiographer may continue their normal workload but should be advised not to participate in brachytherapy applications.

Acknowledgment of Radiation Risk During Pregnancy

I, _____, do acknowledge that I have received counseling from _____ regarding my employment responsibilities during my pregnancy.

It is clear to me that there is a vanishingly small probability that my employment will in any way adversely affect my pregnancy. The reading material listed below has been made available to me to demonstrate that the additional risk during my pregnancy is much less than that for most occupational groups. I further understand that, although I may be assigned to low-exposure duties and provided with a second radiation monitor, these are simply added precautions and do not in any way convey that any assignment in this department is especially hazardous during pregnancy.

1. *Review of NCRP radiation dose limit for embryo and fetus in occupational-exposed women,* NCRP Report No 53, Washington, DC, 1977, National Council on Radiation Protection and Measures.
2. *Medical radiation exposure of pregnant and potentially pregnant women,* NCRP Report No 54, Washington, DC, 1977, National Council on Radiation Protection and Measures.
3. Wagner, LK et al: *Exposure of the pregnant patient to diagnostic radiation,* Philadelphia, 1985, JB Lippincott.
4. *The effects of populations of exposure to low levels of ionizing radiation,* Washington, DC, 1990, National Academy of Sciences.

_____   _____
Supervisor   Employee

_____
Date

FIG. 42.10 Form for acknowledgment of radiation risk during pregnancy.

In nuclear medicine, the pregnant technologist should handle only small quantities of radioactive material. She should not elute radioisotope generators or inject millicurie quantities of radioactive material.

Ultrasound technologists normally are not classified as radiation workers. However, a sizable number of ultrasound patients are nuclear medicine patients and therefore become a potential source of exposure to the ultrasonographer. This situation presents a remote risk because the quantity of radioactivity used is so low.

Finally, the pregnant radiographer should be required to read and sign a form (Fig. 42.10) that attests to the fact that she has been given proper attention to the subject and that she understands that the level of risk associated with her employment is much less than that experienced by nearly all occupational groups.

A 2022 report by the National Academies of Science, Engineering and Medicine (NASEM) proposed activities in many areas including radiology for low-dose radiation research projects including radiology patients and personnel. NASEM identifies low radiation dose as less than 100 mGy$_t$ and low radiation dose rate as less than 5 mGy$_t$/h.

SUMMARY

Dose limits are recommended by the NCRP for various organs, the whole body, and various working conditions, so that the lifetime risk from occupational radiation exposure does not exceed one death in 10,000 per year.

The NCRP recommends a cumulative whole-body dose limit of 10 mSv times age in years. The dose limit during pregnancy is 5 mSv. However, in digital imaging, it is seldom necessary to exceed one-tenth the appropriate dose limit.

Occupational radiation exposure is measured in millisieverts, and the description of such exposure is effective dose (E). Effective dose accounts for type of radiation and the relative radiosensitivity of tissues and organs.

Although the dose limit for occupational workers is 50 mSv/year, most radiologic personnel receive less than 0.5 mSv/year. Radiologists may receive a higher dose if engaged in a heavy fluoroscopy schedule.

Because 95% of occupational exposure comes from fluoroscopy and mobile radiography, the radiographer

should follow these guidelines for reducing occupational radiation exposure:
- During mobile radiography, wear an apron, maintain maximum distance from the source, and never direct the primary beam toward oneself or others.
- During fluoroscopy, step back from the table if not needed, and use shielding, including an apron, a curtain, a Bucky slot cover, and the radiologist.
- During radiography, stand behind the control booth and never direct the primary beam toward the control booth barrier.

Personnel monitoring is required when there is any likelihood that an individual will receive more than one-tenth the occupational radiation dose limit. The various available personnel radiation monitors include TLD and OSL dosimeters. The OSL is very sensitive and accurate and may be worn for up to 1 year. For general use, the radiographer should wear the personnel monitor at waist or chest level; however, during fluoroscopy, the monitor is worn on the collar outside the protective apron.

Radiographers and radiology personnel should never be used to hold patients during an x-ray examination.

The radiobiology of pregnancy requires particular attention to the pregnant radiographer and the pregnant patient. The pregnant radiographer should be provided with a second radiation monitoring device to be worn under the protective apron at waist level.

CHALLENGE QUESTIONS

1. Define or otherwise identify the following:
   a. NCRP
   b. ALARA
   c. Tissue weighting factor (W_t)
   d. Extremity monitor
   e. Personnel monitor
   f. Units of x-radiation output intensity
   g. Recommended extremity dose limit
   h. Effective dose
   i. Recommended lens dose limit
   j. OSL
2. What is the dose limit for diagnostic radiology personnel?
3. During what two examinations can occupational radiation exposure be high?
4. What does the value 10^{-4} year^{-1} mean with regard to the NCRP recommended dose limits?
5. How do some radiation occupational groups such as nuclear medicine technologists monitor their extremity doses?
6. What is the whole-body occupational dose limit for radiography students younger than 18 years of age?
7. State the management protocol for the pregnant radiographer.
8. What information regarding radiation protection should be covered in regularly scheduled in-service training classes?
9. What exposure will a radiographer receive while wearing a protective apron equivalent to 2 HVLs and exposed for 10 minutes at 4 m from a source with intensity of 1 mGy$_a$/h at 1 m?
10. The collar-positioned monitor of a fluoroscopist records 0.9 mSv during a month. This represents approximately what effective dose (E)?
11. What is the required length of the exposure cord on the mobile radiographic unit?
12. When must occupational radiation monitoring be provided?
13. Describe the design of occupational radiation monitors. How are they to be worn, and where on the body are they placed?
14. List the exposure data that must be included in the personnel monitoring report.
15. What is an appropriate thickness for protective apparel?
16. What procedure is used for holding patients during an x-ray examination?
17. Describe the features of OSL that make it particularly effective for occupational radiation monitoring.
18. What is the dose limit for the lens of the eye and the requirement for protective eyewear?
19. What is the approximate protective value of an occupational radiation monitor?
20. Describe an appropriate radiation protection program for nursing and surgical personnel.

The answers to the Challenge Questions can be found by logging on to our website at http://evolve.elsevier.com.

Index

Page numbers followed by *f* indicate figures, *t* indicate tables, and *b* indicate boxes

A

AART. *See* American Registry of Radiologic Technologists
Abacus, example of, 379*f*
ABCC. *See* Atomic Bomb Casualty Commission
Abdomen
 histogram, 253*f*
 imaging of, radiographic techniques in, 306
 serial radiography of, aluminum step-wedge in, 151*f*
 subject contrast, 346*b*
Abdominal imaging, 122
Abdominal structure, visualization of, 306
Abortion
 recommendation for, 556*b*
 spontaneous, incidence of, 553*b*
Absolute risk, 485, 485*t*
Absorbed dose (Gyt), 14
Absorption, 164
 blur, 243
 differential, 160–164, 160*b*, 160*f*
 examples of, 62, 63*f*
AC. *See* Alternating current
Acceleration, 27, 27*b*
Accreditation test objects, 286*f*
ACR. *See* American College of Radiology
ACR-AAPM-SIIM Technical Standard, 365, 365*t*
Action/reaction, Newton's third law, 28*b*
Active bone marrow, distribution of, 532*t*
Active matrix array (AMA)
 thin-film transistor (AMA-TFT), photomicrograph of, 186*f*
 use of, 186*f*
Active-matrix liquid crystal displays, 358
 pixel of, cross-sectional rendering of, 354*f*
Acute radiation lethality, 466–470, 466*b*, 467*b*, 467*t*
 latent period of, 467
 manifest illness in, 467–468, 468*b*
 nonlinear threshold dose-response relationship of, 469*b*
 prodromal period of, 467
Acute radiation syndrome, 467
ADA (computer language), 386
ADC. *See* Analog-to-digital conversion
Added filtration, 149*b*, 207, 207*f*
 sources of, 149
Address, in computer, 388, 388*b*
Address drivers, 186
Adenine, 433
Adenine-thymine, 434*b*, 435
Adipose tissue, 262
Adults, active bone marrow in, 532*t*
Advanced interventional fluoroscopic equipment, 302*f*
AEC. *See* Automatic exposure control
Age, radiation and, 444, 444*f*
Air, Z values of, 163–164
Air kerma (kinetic energy released in matter) (Gya), 14, 14*b*
Air-gap technique, 230–231, 230*f*
 disadvantage, 230*b*
 usage of, 230*f*
ALARA. *See* As low as reasonably achievable
Algebra, 20–21, 20*b*
Algorithm, 385
Alkali metals, 36
Alpha emission, 46
 radioactive decay, 45–46, 46*f*
Alpha particles, 49*b*
 beta particles differ from, 50
 emission of, 46*b*
 energy of, lost of, 50
 helium nucleus, equivalent to, 49–50

Alpha particles *(Continued)*
 particulate radiation, 49
 travel, 50
Alpha radiation, ionization accompanied by, 50
Alternating current (AC), 75–76
 conversion, rectification of, 101*b*
 intensity of, changes in, 88*b*
 representation of, 78*f*
 transformers, operation of, 101
 voltage/current in (magnitude change), transformer (usage), 88
 waveform for, 77
Alternating electric current, 54–55
ALU. *See* Arithmetic/logic unit
Aluminum
 electron configuration of, 40–41
 plastic fiber, contrast, 222
Aluminum step-wedge, usage of, 151*f*
AMA. *See* Active matrix array
Ambient light, 355
American Association of Physicists in Medicine Task Group Report 18 (AAPM TG 18), 370, 370*b*
 pattern, half-moon targets, half-16 area, 373, 373*f*
 TG 18-AD pattern (usage), 372, 372*f*
 TG 18-AFC pattern (usage), 374, 375*f*
 TG 18-CH anatomic image, 374, 375*f*
 TG 18-CX pattern, 374, 374*f*, 375*f*
 TG 18-PX pattern, 374, 374*f*, 375*f*
 TG 18-QC test pattern, 371, 371*f*, 374–375
 TG 18-UN/TG 18-UNL patterns, 373, 374*f*
American College of Radiology (ACR)
 in patient radiation dose management, 557
 radiologic/fluoroscopic accreditation test objects, 286*f*
American Registry of Radiologic Technologists (AART), 15
Amorphous selenium (a-Se), 183, 187, 187*b*
 as image receptor capture, 187*f*
 use of, 198
Ampere, equation for, 203*b*
Amplitude, 54–55
 definition of, 55*b*
 of high voltage transformer, 100–101
Anabolism, 431
Analog
 digital, contrast between, 381*f*
 term, use of, 380, 380*f*
Analog-to-digital conversion (ADC), 178*b*
Analog-to-digital converter, 294–295
Anaphase, of mitosis, 436
Anatomically programmed radiography (APR), 210
 microprocessors, incorporation of, 210, 210*f*
 principle of, 210
Anatomy
 compression of, 216*b*
 description of, spatial frequency and, 191
 thickness, increase, 217*f*
Angiography, 275, 294
Animal glycogen, 432–433
Ankylosing spondylitis
 leukemia, observations, 488
 patients, 488
Ann Arbor series, thyroid cancer, 489
Annihilation radiation, 159
Annotation, 357
Anode
 focal-spot blur in, 240
 of x-ray tube, 116–123, 116*b*
 angle of, 122*b*
 cooling chart, 126–127, 127*f*
 dissipation of, by radiation, 124*f*

Anode *(Continued)*
 electrical conductor, 116–117
 high-capacity, 117, 120*f*
 layered, 118*f*
 line-focus principle in, 120, 120*b*, 120*f*
 rotating, 112, 112*f*, 117, 117*f*
 stationary, 116, 117*f*
 stem of, 118
 target, 117
 thermal dissipater in, 117
Anode heat, 131, 131*b*
Antennas, 61
Anteroposterior abdominal examination, fixed kilovolt peak technique for, 345*t*
Anteroposterior pelvis examination, variable kilovolt peak technique, 346*t*
Anteroposterior view, blacked-out spine, 255*f*
Anthropomorphic phantom, for radiation sensitivity, 533*f*
Antibodies, 432
Antigen, 432
Aperture diaphragm, 218
 fixed lead opening, design of, 219*f*
Aperture ratio, 353
Application programs, 383, 383*b*
APR. *See* Anatomically programmed radiography
Area shielding, 552–553
Arithmetic/logic unit (ALU), 386
 performance of, 387
Array processor, 314
Arterial access, 299–300
Arteriography, risks of, 301
Artifacts, 248
 reduction, imaging plate performance (documentation form), 249*f*
 tomosynthesis and, 335–336
Artificial intelligence (AI)
 algorithm, 421, 421*f*
 benefits, 401*t*
 concepts, 396–399
 deep learning (DL), 400–401
 ethics and, 402–404
  algorithmic bias, 403
  cognitive bias, 403–404
  representativeness bias, 403
 imaging workflow, 401–402
 machine learning (MI)
  supervised learning, 400
  unsupervised learning, 400
 RSNA website, 402*f*
 as a service, 398*t*
 vectors, 396–398
Artificially produced permanent magnets, availability of, 80
As low as reasonably achievable (ALARA), 197, 445, 528–529
 in personnel exposure, 560, 563*b*
 practice, 485
ASCC. *See* Automatic Sequence Controlled Calculator
Assemblers, 383
Asthenic patients, 345
Atansoff, John, 379*b*
Atomic Bomb Casualty Commission (ABCC), 487
Atomic bomb survivors, 487
 Hiroshima and Nagasaki, 487*f*
 leukemia, incidence (summary), 487*t*
 observations, 495
Atomic configurations, 42*f*
 tungsten, 132*f*
Atomic mass, determination of, 43
Atomic mass numbers, 38
 not equal, 43*b*
 in whole number, 43

576

Atomic mass units (amu), 38
Atomic nomenclature, 43–44
Atomic number
  dependence on, 161–162, 161f
  effective atomic number, 242–243
  increase in, 46, 138
  of tungsten, 117b
Atomic progression, scheme of, 41
Atomic structure, 38–43, 38b
Atoms, 3
  combinations of, 45, 45f
  composition, 39f
  definition of, 35b
  electrically neutral, 39, 39b
  electron configuration of, 39
  empty space, 38
  fundamental particles of, 37–38, 37b
  Greek, 35
  indivisible, considered, 35
  ionization, 39b, 40f
  mass, not equal, 43b
  smallest particle of element, 45b
  symbols, represented by, 36f
Atrophy, 444, 470b
Attenuation, 164
  definition of, 146b
  examples of, 62
  exponential, 164, 164b, 165f
Audio files, 388
Audio input device, 392
Audio noise, 234
Automatic brightness control (ABC), 275
  x-ray tube mA in, 281
Automatic control x-ray systems, automation level of, 209b
Automatic exposure, techniques for, 209–210
Automatic exposure control (AEC), 95, 99–100, 99f, 209
  clinical operation of, 99
  devices, 270
    relative position of, 270f
  exposure chart, construction factors, 209t
  mammographic imaging system, 270
  mode, for radiographs, 99
  sensors, position for, 210f
  600 mAs safety override for, 210
  use of, 99
  x-ray imaging system installed in, 99
Automatic exposure systems, in fluoroscopy, 285
Automatic radiation field recognition, 253b
Automatic Sequence Controlled Calculator (ASCC), 379
Automatic variable-aperture collimator, 219
Autotransformer, 89f, 95–98
  definition of, 89b
  design of, 95b
  diagram for, 96f
  iron core in, 89
  primary connections, 96
  size of, 89
Autotransformer law, equation for, 96b
Axial tomography, 306

B
Babbage, Charles, 379
Backlight, LED and, 355, 355b
Backscatter radiation, 155
Baking soda, 45
Ball-throwing machine
  distribution, example of, 134f
  ejection, observation (bar graph example), 134f
Bandpass, 285, 285b
Bar graph, example, 134f
Bar magnet, magnetic dipoles in, 79–80
Bar pattern
  of increasing spatial frequency, 321f
  modulation of, 192
Barcode readers, 391
Barium (Ba)
  atomic number of, 41
  isotopes in, 43, 44b
  list of, 46–47
  usage of, 41
Barium fluorobromide (BaFBr)
  atomic numbers, 172
  use of, 198
Barium fluorohalide with europium (BaFBr:Eu or BaFI:Eu), 172

Barrier thickness
  distance, 516–518
  factors, 516–518
Barriers, protective, 12–13, 12f
Basal cells, 470, 470f
Base quantities, 24
Baseline mammogram, 262
BASIC. See Beginners All-purpose Symbolic Instruction Code
Basic input/output system (BIOS), 387
Beam, useful, 567b
Beam penetrability, 203
Beam-splitting mirror, 283
Becquerel (Bq), 14–15, 14b
Beginners All-purpose Symbolic Instruction Code (BASIC), 385
Berners-Lee, Tim, 391
Berry, Clifford, 379b
Beta emission, 46
  electron created by, 46
  occurrence of, 46–47
  result, 46
Beta particles, 49, 50b
  alpha particles, differ from, 49
  contrast to, 50
  emitted, 49–50
  particulate radiation, 49–50
  release of, 44
Biangular targets, 120
Biannual physical examinations, 551
Bilateral wedge filter, usage of, 149
Binary notation, 382t
Binary number system, 380b
  decimal number, relationship with, 382t
  organization of, 380, 382t
Biologic Effects of Ionizing Radiation (BEIR) Committee, 491–493
  analysis, uncertainty, 492b
  estimated excess mortality, 492t
  low dose, low-LET radiation, 491–492
Biologic tissue, ionizing radiation on, 49
BIOS. See Basic input/output system
Bismuth germanate ($Bi_4Ge_3O_{12}$), 315
Bit, 383b, 388
Blurred-ripple artifact, 335, 335b, 338f
Body
  composition of, 430–434, 431t
  habitus, 345
    states, 345f
  molecular composition of, 431–434, 431t
  tissues and organs of, 438–439, 438t, 439t
  trunk, scanned projection radiograph, 184f
Bohr, Niels, 37
Bohr atom, 37
Bohr model, 54
Bone
  atomic number of, 161–162
  cancer, 489
    radium salts, 489
  marrow, dose, importance in, 529
Bootstrap, 384
  program, 387
  operating system, loading by, 384
Bowel, double exposure, 249f
"Bow-tie" filter, 149, 150f
Breast
  anatomy, 262–263
  architecture, 263f
  DRI in, 337–339, 338f
  examination, intervals for, 262t
  self-examinations, American Cancer society recommendations, 262
  shields, 552
  tissue
    differential absorption, enhancement, 265
    types of, 263b
Breast cancer, 261, 490
  development of, 261b
  incidence of, 263f
  mortality, reduction, 261
  risk of, 261–262
  factors, 262t
Bremsstrahlung radiation, 133–134
  diagnostic range, 138b
  emission spectrum, extension of, 136f
  production of, 133f
  result, 133f
  spectrum, 135–136
    change in, 138
    shape of, 136

Bremsstrahlung radiation (Continued)
  x-rays
    low- energy, 134
    production, 265
    suppressed, 268f
    suppression, 268f
Bright edge artifact, 339, 339f
Brightness gain, 278b, 279
Bucky, Gustave, 10, 221
Bucky factor (B), 223, 223b
  equation, 223b
  increase, 223
Bucky slot cover, fluoroscopic protection, 514, 514f
Bucky tray, film-loaded cassette (insertion), 219–220
Bus, in CPU, 386
Bytes, 388

C
C (computer language), 386
C++ (computer language), 386
C-arm support system, in x-ray tube, 112, 113f
CAD. See Computer-aided detection
Cadmium tungstate ($CdWO_4$), 315
Calcium tungstate ($CaWO_4$), 9
Camera lenses, 283
Cancer, 488–491
  absolute risks, 489
  bone cancer, 489
  breast cancer, 490
  latent period, early age, exposure, 492f
  lung cancer, 490
  radiation-induced, 446b, 489b
  relative risks, 488
  skin cancer, 490
  thyroid cancer, 489
Candela (lumens per steradian), 351
Candela per meter squared (nit), 351
Capacitor discharge generator, 106, 106b
Capture element, 183
Carbohydrates, 432, 432f, 433b
Carbon (C)
  atomic mass of, 41–43
  biologically active, 49f
  combination of, 45
  fiber couches, 93b
  importance, 41–43
  ionization, x-ray, 40f
  occurring radioisotope, 48
Carotid CT scan, reconstruction of, 319f
Catabolism, 431
Catheters, 300, 300b, 300f
Cathode
  focal-spot blur in, 240–241
  of x-ray tube, 114–116, 114b
Cathode ray tube (CRT)
  principal parts of, 283f
  soft copy and, 353
Cathode rays, 6–7
  properties of, 36–37
CCD. See Charge-coupled device
CD-ROM (compact disc-read-only memory), 389
Ceiling support system, in x-ray tube, 112, 113f
Cell
  function of, 435–436
  proliferation of, 435–436, 436b
  theory, 431
  type, radiation and, 438t
Cell-cycle effects, 462, 462b
Cell lethality, 457
Cell-survival kinetics, 457–462, 458b, 458f
Cellular membranes, 435b
Cellular radiobiology, 456–464
Central electrode, 519
Central nervous system (CNS) death, 467
Central nervous system (CNS) syndrome, 467
Central processing unit (CPU), 386
  components of, 386–390
  examples, 386f
Central ray, 122
  x-ray beam, 226
Centripetal force, 41, 41b
Cervical spine, histogram, 253f
Cesium iodide (CsI), 183, 315
  amorphous silicon, 185–187, 186b, 186f
  CCD, 185
    indirect process, 185b
  crystals, 277, 278f

Cesium iodide (CsI) *(Continued)*
  phosphor
    DR image receptor, 186*f*
    scintillation light, 185
  use of, 187, 198
Characteristic x-rays, 157
  discrete spectrum/emission spectrum, 134*b*
  production of, 133
    K-shell electron ionization and, 132*f*
  radiation, 131–133, 133*b*
  spectrum, 135
  of tungsten, effective energies and, 133*t*
Charge-coupled device (CCD), 176–177, 183, 290–292, 291*f*, 292*b*
  advantages of, medical imaging, 292*t*
  cesium iodide (CsI), 185
    indirect process, 185*b*
  cross-sectional view of, 291*f*
  dynamic range, 185
  image contrast, usage of, 185
  lens-coupling system for, 291*f*
  light-sensing element, 184
  manner in, 291*f*
  radiation
    linear response to, 185
    response to, 185*f*
  response to light of, 292*f*
  sensitivity, 185, 185*b*
  in television monitoring, 283*f*
  tiled CCD, design, 185*f*
Charged particle
  circular/elliptical path of, 79*f*
  magnetic field of, 79
  motion of, magnetic field (creation), 79*b*
Charges, steady flow of, production of, 84
Chemical agents, radiosensitivity and, 444–445
Chemical element, 38
Chemical energy, 4
Chemical symbol (X), positioned, 45
Chernobyl, 466
Chest, 151*f*
  board, positioned, 515
  DRT in, 339, 340*f*
  scanned projection radiography, components, 184*f*
  subject contrast, 346*b*
Chest radiography
  bilateral wedge filter in, usage of, 149
  cathode in, 122
  simulated, 253*f*
  source-to-image receptor distance, 211*f*
  stimulation, characteristics, 253*f*
  trough filter in, usage of, 149
Childhood leukemia
  incidence, 495
  relative risk, irradiation in utero, 495*b*, 495*t*
Childhood malignancy, 494
Chlorine atom, ionized, 45
Chromatid
  deletion of, 478
  stickiness of, 478
Chromosome aberrations
  kinetics of, 478–479, 478*f*, 479*b*
  radiation-induced, 451, 452*f*, 476*b*
  types and frequency, 483
Chromosome hit, 478
Chromosomes, local tissue effects, 483
Chronic lymphocytic leukemia, 488
Chronically irradiated animals, 483*f*
Circular effective focal spot, 120–121
Classical physics, 407*b*, 412
Client, of network, 361–362
Clinical digital radiographic tomosynthesis, characteristics of, 335*t*
Clinical tolerance, 470
Clinical voltage, workload distribution, 518*f*
Clone PC, creation of, 387
Cloning, 458
Closed-core transformer, 89, 89*f*
Closed iron core, usage of, 88*f*
Coast time, x-ray tube, 119
COBOL. *See* COmmon Business Oriented Language
Codon, 435*b*
Coherent scattering, 154–155, 154*f*, 155*b*
  relative frequency of, 162
Cold anode, radiographic techniques in, 124*b*
Collection element, 183
Collimated multiple fields, problems, 257*f*
Collimation, 13, 214, 511
  application of, 9
  fluoroscopic protection, 514

Collimation *(Continued)*
  objective artifacts, 253–254
  proper, 253*b*
Collimator, filtration, requirement, 221
Color LCD, monochrome LCD and, 353
Colossus (computer), 379
Commission Internationale de l'Éclairage (CIE), human vision and, 351
COmmon Business Oriented Language (COBOL), 385
Compact disc (CD), 388
  drive, 388
  example, 388*f*
Compass
  in Earth, reaction of, 83*f*
  usage of, 83
Compensating filters, 149, 150*f*, 207–208
Compilers, 383
Complementary metal-oxide semiconductor (CMOS) technology, 387
Complete grid cutoff, 228*f*
Compound, 45*b*
Compression
  advantages of, 269*t*
  importance, 268
  mammographic imaging system, 268–269
  principles, 269*f*
Compton effect, 155*b*
Compton interaction, occurrence of, 172
Compton processes, 215*t*
Compton scattering, 155–156, 155*b*, 155*f*, 156*t*
  contribution, 215*f*
Computed radiography (CR), 169–181
  background radiation, 251*f*
  cassettes sensitivity, 250
  components and optical path of, 177*f*
  computer control, 177–178
  image noise in, sources of, 180*t*
  image plate
    example, 250*f*
    residual glue, appearance, 248*f*
  image receptor, 171–176, 171*b*, 173*f*
    response function of, 178–179
    sizes, 255*t*
  images
    gray levels of, 179, 179*b*
    radiographic technique, use of, 179*f*
  mechanical features of, 176
  plates
    came apart, 250*f*
    usage, 251*f*
  steps, example, 174*f*, 175*f*
  terms, 172*t*
  workload, 180, 181*f*
Computed radiography (CR) reader, 176–178, 176*f*
  computer complement to, 178*f*
  drive mechanisms, 177*f*
  mechanical features of, 176
  optical features of, 176–177, 176*b*
Computed tomography (CT), 8, 332, 540–543
  array processor in, 314
  collimation, 315
  collimators, monitored, 540*b*
  components of, 313*f*
  computer in, 314, 314*b*
  contrast resolution in, 322–323, 328–329, 329*f*
  couch incrementation in, 329
  data acquisition rate in, 326–327
  detector array in, 314–316
  dose delivery for, 540–543, 540*t*
  examination, 320*f*
  focal-spot size in, 314
  gantry in, 314–316
  generations of, 307–309, 308*b*, 309*b*
  image characteristics in, 316–320
  image matrix, 317, 317*f*
  image quality, 320–325
    phantom in, 323*f*
  image reconstruction in, 318–319, 318*f*
    four-pixel matrix, 318*f*
  imaging system
    components of, 313*f*
    design in, 313–316
    x-ray beams, 308*f*
  imaging technique in, 325–327
  laser localizer in, 329
  linearity in, 324–325, 325*f*, 328
  MTF curves for, 321*f*, 322*f*
  multiplanar reformation in, 319–320, 319*b*
  multislice detector array in, 325–326
  noise in, 324, 328

Computed tomography (CT) *(Continued)*
  numbers, 317–318, 317*b*
  occupational radiation exposure in, 561
  operating console in, 313–314, 313*b*, 314*f*
  operation, principles of, 306–307, 306*b*
  output intensity of, 542–543, 542*b*, 543*f*, 544*f*
  patient radiation dose in, 538–547
  precise collimation in, 540
  quality control, 327–329
  reconstruction time in, 314
  section sensitivity profile for, 313, 313*f*
  slice thickness in, 329
  slip-ring technology in, 316, 316*f*
  spatial resolution in, 320–322, 320*b*, 321*b*
  test object, 328*f*
  translation, 306
  uniformity in, 325, 328
  x-ray tube in, 314
Computed tomography dose index, 543–544, 543*f*, 544*b*, 544*f*, 545*t*
Computer-aided detection (CAD), 252, 334*b*, 335
Computer-assisted automatic exposure systems, electronic exposure timer, use of, 209
Computer-assisted diagnosis (CADx), 397–398
Computers
  application programs, 383
  architecture of, 380–390
  capacity
    increase in, 392*f*
    requirement of, calculation, 363
  communications, 390
  components, 386–390
  configuration, 383
  defined, 380*b*
  development of, 379
  evolution, timeline for, 381*f*
  hexadecimal number system, 384*b*, 385*t*
  history of, 379–380
  language of, 380–386
  large-scale integration (LSI), 380
  memory, 387
  operating system, loading of, 384
  output devices, 389–390, 390*b*
  program, 383, 383*b*
  speed, increase in, 392*f*
  system software, 384
  very large scale integration (VLSI), 380
Concrete, tube potentials, half-value and tenth-value layer, 505*t*
Conducting wire, modifying, 75
Conduction, 31, 123–124, 124*f*
Conductor
  definition of, 74*b*
  electric charge of, concentration of, 73*b*
  electric resistance of, 75*f*
Cones, 218, 276, 419
Conic filter, 150*f*
Connective tissues, 438
  patterns, 262
Contact, electrification by, 70
Contact shield, 552
Continuous ejection spectrum, 135*b*
Continuum, 54
Contrast
  agents, 164
  examinations, 164
  image subtraction and, 358*b*
  loss, 256*f*
  media, 300
  perception, 276, 421*b*
  resolution, DF through, 295*b*
Contrast improvement factor, 222–223, 223*b*
  equation of, 222*b*
Contrast resolution, 190*b*, 194–197, 234, 281*t*, 285, 421
  in computed tomography, 322–323, 323*b*, 328–329, 329*b*
    test objects for, 328*f*
  limitation of
    image noise and, 197*b*
    SNR and, 197
  preservation of, 198*b*
  use of, 347
Control grid, 284
Control monitor, 570*b*
  storage of, 570*b*
Control panel, 511, 511*b*
Control unit, 386
  central processing unit, relationship with, 386*f*, 387*f*
Controlled area, 517
Convection, 31, 123–124, 124*f*

Conventional fluoroscopy, imaging chain in, 289f
Conventional tomography, results, 307f
Conversion factor, 279, 279b, 286f
Coolidge, William D., 10, 10b
Copper plates, usage, 84
Cormack, Alan, 306
Cornea, 276, 418
Cosine law, 351–352, 352b
    importance of, 352
Cosmic rays, 5
Couch incrementation, in computed tomography, 329
Couches, floating, 93–94
Coulomb's law, 72
    equation of, 72b
Coupling element, 183
Covalent bonds, 45
CPU. See Central processing unit
CR. See Computed radiography
Crookes tube, 6–7, 7f
    electric potential in, 58
    modifications of, 113
    Snook transformer and, 9
Crossed grid, 225, 225b, 225f
    advantage of, 225b
    efficiency, 225
Crossing over, 438
Cross-linking, 450, 450f
CRT. See Cathode ray tube
CT. See Computed tomography
CT angiography (CTA), 312–313
Cumulative timer, 514
Current
    intensity of, changes in, 88b
    transformer law effect on, 88b
Current Procedural Terminology (CPT codes), 365
Curvilinear detector array, in third-generation CT imaging system, 309
Cylinders, 218
Cytogenetic damage, 451
Cytogenetic effects, 475–479, 476f
Cytogenetics, 475b
Cytoplasm, 434–435
Cytosine, 435
Cytosine-guanine, 434b, 435

D

Dally, Clarence, 9
Dalton, John, 35–36
Dalton atom, 35–36
Data acquisition
    modes of, interaction among, 362f
    rate, in computed tomography, 326–327
Data files, 388
Data interpolation, 310–311
Data lines, 186
Death, average annual risk, 493t
Decimal number system, origin of, 381f
Decimals, 19, 19b
Decision threshold, 422, 423f
Deep learning (DL), 400–401
Dense anatomy (contrast loss), digital radiography (underexposure), 254f
Deoxyribonucleic acid (DNA), 433, 433b, 433f
    base bonding in, 434
    double-helix configuration of, 434, 434f
    genetic code of, 451f
    molecular structure of, 431, 434f
    radiation effects on, 451–452, 452b, 452f
    radiation response of, 452, 452b
    as target molecule, 457b
    types of damage to, 452, 452f
Deposited energy, 429
Derived quantities, 24
Desquamation, 470
Destructive pathology, 346–347
Detail, 347, 347b
Detective quantum efficiency (DQE), 198–199
    digital image receptor and, 198
    as function of x-ray energy, 200f
    higher, 194
    measurement of, 198b
    relative value of, 198–199
Detector array, 314–316
16-detector array, 312f
Deterministic effect, 430
    cause of, 451
Deterministic radiation responses, 445, 445b, 445t
Deutsches Institut für Normung (DIN) 2001, 369
DF. See Digital fluoroscopy
Diagnostic imaging systems, x-ray production in, 60

Diagnostic mammography, 262
Diagnostic radiology, pregnancy in, 573t
Diagnostic ultrasound, electromagnetic spectrum and, 58b
Diagnostic x-ray beams
    ion chamber dosimeter, 521f
    partial-body exposure of, 466b
Diagnostic x-ray imaging, 442b
Diagnostic x-ray tubes, classification of, 117f
Diagnostic x-rays
    imaging, 442
    LET of, 442b
    RBE of, 442b
Diamagnetic materials, 80
Diaphragm, 9
Differential absorption, 160–164, 160b, 160f
    characteristics of, 163t
    dependence
        on atomic number of, 161–162, 161f, 162b
        on mass density, 162–164, 162b, 163f, 163t
Diffuse nonconductor, electrification in, 73
Diffuse reflections, 372f
    evaluation, TG 18-AD pattern (usage), 372, 372f
Digital
    analog, contrast between, 381f
    term, use of, 380
Digital breast tomosynthesis (DBT), 332
Digital chest radiograph, simulation, 253f
Digital display device, 368–376
    correction, signal interpolation and, 356
    matrix size of, 357
    spatial resolution and, improvement of, 353b
    viewing angle of, 352
        illumination and image contrast, reduced, and, 352f
Digital display device quality control, 371–374
    display noise, 374
    display resolution, 374
    geometric distortion, 371
    luminance response, 372–374, 372b, 373b
    reflection, 372, 372b
Digital fluoroscopy imaging system, 289–290, 290f
    advantages of, 289b
    operating console for, 290f
    remotely controlled, 290f
    x-ray tube, 289b
Digital image
    components of, 383
    contrast, dose and, 198b
    inversion, 357, 357f
    with PACS network, combining, 366f
    with Picture Archiving and Communication System (PACS) network, 358f
    postprocessing of, 357t
        operator manipulation and, 357b
    preprocessing, 356
    receptors
        correction, signal interpolation and, 356
        response of, 199f
        spatial resolution and contrast maintenance and, 199f
    viewing, 350–359
Digital imaging, 400b, 401b
    advantage of, 194
    contrast resolution in, preservation of, 198b
    postprocessing and, 194–197
    spatial resolution in, 192
    systems
        dynamic range of, 194, 195f
        spatial resolution in, pixel size limitation and, 192
Digital Imaging and Communications in Medicine (DICOM)
    format, 362
    National Electrical Manufacturers Association Digital Imaging and Communications in Medicine (NEMA-DICOM), 369
Digital mammography (DM), 263b, 337b, 393b
    contrast resolution quality, 263b
    spatial resolution limitation, 263b
Digital Mammography Imaging Study Trial (DMIST)
    contrast resolution, 264b
    design, 263
    findings of, 263
    results of, 196
Digital medical image
    postprocessing, 356
    preprocessing, 356
Digital medical imaging systems, dynamic range of, 195t
Digital radiographic technique, 189–201

Digital radiographic tomosynthesis (DRT), 306, 307f, 332–333, 332b, 334b, 533, 534f
Digital radiography (DR), 171b, 182–188, 183b, 552b
    advance in, 306
    dose reduction with, 199t
    electronic preprocessing, failure of, 250f
    image receptors
        availability, 253
        classification scheme for, 248f
        debris, 248f
        irradiation, 250
        with pixel failure, 248b
        sizes, 255t
    images
        artifacts, classification scheme for, 248f
        production, CsI phosphor light, 186b
        receptors, CsI phosphor, 186f
    organizational scheme for, 183f
    patient dose in, 198b
    tiled CCD design, 184f
    underexposure, impact, 254f
Digital subscriber lines (DSLs), 391
Digital subtraction angiography (DSA), 294–295, 295b, 298f
    image formation of, 295–299
Digital system, values, 380f
Digital video discs (DVDs), 388
Dipolar field, 79
Direct current (DC), 75
    representation of, 77f
    waveform for, 76–77
Direct digital radiography, 187
Disaccharides, 432–433
Discrete emission spectrum shift, 139f
Discrete spectrum, 134b
Display evaluation, TG 18-CH anatomic image, 375f
Display noise, 374
    assessment, TG 18-AFC pattern (usage), 374, 375f
Display resolution, 374
    TG 18-CX pattern, 374, 374f, 375f
Dissociation, 453b
Distance, 145–146
    equation, 503b
    impact of, 206
    maximize, 503–504, 503b, 504b
    radiation protection, principles of, 501
    x-ray intensity and, relationship of, 145b
Distortion
    depends on, 238b
    geometric factor, 238–239, 238b, 238f
    shape distortion, 238b
Distribution, example of, 134f
DM. See Digital mammography
DMIST. See Digital Mammography Imaging Study Trial
DNA. See Deoxyribonucleic acid
Dose
    creep, technique creep and, 198b
    reduction with digital radiography, 199t
Dose area product (DAP), 535–536, 536t
Dose equivalent, 571
Dose index, of computed tomography, 543–544, 543f, 544b, 544f
    measurement of, 544
Dose length product, 544–545, 544b, 544f
Dose limit, 562–566
    educational considerations in, 566
    effective occupational, 573b
    historical review of, 564t
    lens, 563
    National Council on Radiation Protection and measurements, recommended by, 564f, 565t
    for organs, 565–566
    public exposure and, 566
    recommended
        annually, 562b
        in diagnostic radiology, 564b
        linear, nonthreshold dose-response relationship, 563b
    for skin, 565–566
    for tissues, 565–566
Dose modulation, 543, 543f
Dose-response relationships, 445–447
    constructing, 446–447, 447f
    for cytogenetic damage, 479b
    medical radiation and, 446, 446b
    for radiation hormesis, 447, 447f
    for single-hit aberrations, 478f
Dosimeters, 518b

Dosimetry, 518b
Double-contrast examination, 164
Double-helix configuration, of DNA, 434, 434f
DQE. *See* Detective quantum efficiency
Drosophila, irradiation, 496
DRT. *See* Digital radiographic tomosynthesis
DSA. *See* Digital subtraction angiography
Dual-filament cathode, in focal spots, 114f
Dual-focus x-ray tube, 116f
Dual-slice imaging, demonstration of, 325
Dual-source multislice helical computed tomography imaging system, 326f
Duct tissue, patterns, 262
Dumb terminal, 390
Duodecimal system, 380
Duty cycle, 290
Dynamic range, 194
   of digital medical imaging systems, 195t
   gray shades and, 194b
Dynode gain, 523b

E

Eckert, J. Presper, 379
Edge enhancement, 358
   impact, 261
Edge response function (ERF), 320
Edison, Thomas A., 9, 9f
   fluoroscope, 275, 418b
Effective atomic number, 242–243
Effective diameter, 545, 546t
Effective dose, 505–507, 505b, 506b, 536, 563b
   in computed tomography, 545–546, 546b, 546f, 546t
   occupational effective dose, 507t
   occupational radiation exposure, 506, 507f
   radiologic technologist, 505–507
   Sievert (Sv), 14, 14b, 15f
   whole-body dose, equivalent, 505
Effective occupational radiation dose limit, 573b
Egan, Robert, 261
Einstein, Albert, 4–5, 156
Elective booking, 554
Electric charge
   attraction/repulsion of, 72
   concentration, 73b
   distribution of, uniformity in, 73
   positive/negative units in, 70
   potential energy in, 74
   units of, 71
Electric circuits, 75–77
   elements, symbol and function of, 76t
   types of, 75–77
Electric current (electricity), 69–90
   applications of, 75–76
   data transfer, 390
   direction of, importance of, 74
   electrons, flow of, 75
   induction, magnetic field intensity in, 86b
   measurement of, 75
   occurrence of, 74
   reduction of, 75b
Electric fields, radiation of, 73f
Electric ground, 70
Electric motor, components of, 86
Electric potential, 74
   measurement of, 75, 84b
   unit of, 74b
   as voltage, 74
Electric power, 77
   equation, 77b
Electric resistance, increasing, 75b
Electric states, 76t
Electrical conductor, anode as, 116–117
Electrical energy, 4
   conversion, 72
   x-ray imaging system conversion, 71f
Electrification
   creation of, 70b
   example of, 71
   intensity of, 72
Electrified copper wire, cross section of, 73f
Electrodynamics, 74–77, 74b
Electroluminescence, 354
Electromagnetic energy, 4, 53–68
   amplitude, 54–55
   attenuation, 62b
   energy, state of, 54
   frequency and wavelength in, inversely proportional, 57
   properties of, 54
   quantum, 54

Electromagnetic energy *(Continued)*
   velocity, 54–55
   wave equation usage, 56–57
   wave model of, usage, 61–62
Electromagnetic induction, 86, 86b
   motor, 118, 119f
Electromagnetic radiation, 5, 50, 50t
   distance from source and, 62–64
   field theory of (Maxwell's), 83
   intensity of, inverse relation to square of distance, 62–63
   matter with, interaction of, 61
   visualization of, 65f
Electromagnetic spectrum, 57–60
   definition of, 57b
   investigation of, 58
   orders of magnitude of, 58f
   ranges of, precise, 58
Electromagnetic wave equation, 57b
Electromagnetism, 83–90
Electromagnets
   closed iron core in, 88f
   definition of, 85b
   magnetic field lines of, 85f
   method for usage of, 81f
Electromechanical devices, 86–87
Electron arcing, 125b
Electron beam, 282
Electron cloud, x-rays emission in, 60
Electron flow, reversal of, impact of, 101
Electron gun, 282
Electron optics, 278
Electron transition, 157
Electronic computer, 379
   development of, 379
Electronic medical record (EMR), 363–364, 364f
Electronic Numerical Integrator and Calculator (ENIAC), 379, 380f
Electronic preprocessing, failure of, 250f
Electronic programs, 361–367, 361t
Electronic timers, 99
Electrons, 36–37, 36f
   acceleration, 130
   arrangement, 39–41, 40b
      shell notation of, 41
   during beta emission, 46
   beta particles, contrast to, 49
   binding energy, 41–43, 42f
      for tungsten, 132f
   characteristics of, 36–37
   configuration, complexity of, 39
   direction, oscillation in, 77
   electric charges and, association of, 70
   flow of, 76b
   orbits, into "shell", 38
   spin, 79
   target interactions, 130–134
   transfer of, example of, 72f
Electrostatic charge, 97b
   concentration of, 74f
   measurement of, 205b
Electrostatic focusing lenses, 278
Electrostatic grids, 282
Electrostatic laws, 71–74
Electrostatics, 70–74, 70b
Elements
   characteristics of, 43t
   chemical properties of, 43
   Dalton perspective of, 36, 36f
   identification, 35
   in natural state, 43
   periodic table of, 36, 37f
   protocol for representing, 44f
   rarity of, 45
Emergency department, 339–340, 551
Emergency responders, 507
Emulsion, 264
Encode, term, 383b
Endocrine glands, 432
Endoplasmic reticulum, 434
Energy, 3–5, 3b, 29–30, 30b, 60f, 66–67
   absorption, 62
   continuum, 54
   definition of, 4b
   law of conservation of, 66
   levels (orbits), 37
   mass and, 67f
   reflection, 62f
Energy subtraction, 297, 297b
   temporal subtraction *versus*, 295t
Energy thermometer scales temperature, 32f

ENIAC. *See* Electronic Numerical Integrator and Calculator
Entrance skin exposure (ESE), 529, 529b, 531b, 532b, 549
   for digital image receptor, 229t
   elevation, 513f
   estimating of, 530b
   fluoroscopic injuries and the related, 535f
   result of, 144
   specification of, 549
Environmental radiation, 249b
Enzymes, 432
Epidemiologic studies, 482
Epilation, 471
Epithelium, 438
Erase, CR step, 175f
ERF. *See* Edge response function
Ergonomically designed digital image workstation, 355f
Ergonomics, 355, 424, 424t
Erythema, 470
Erythrocytes, 474
ESE. *See* Entrance skin exposure
Europium (Eu), presence of, 172
Examinations, repeat examinations, 551, 551b
Excess risk, 485, 485b
Experimental mammalian cell lines, 461t
Exponential attenuation, 164, 164b, 165f
Exposed matter, 5
Exposure
   control, fluoroscopic protection, 514
   CR step, 173
   distance, impact of, 206
   events in, sequence of, 174f
   factors, 203–206, 203t
   rate, in fluoroscopy, 285
   timers for, 98–100
Exposure technique
   automatic, 209–210
   factors, 345
Exposure time, 204–206
   calculation, 204b
   constant, 204
   units of, relationship among, 204t
External components, of x-ray tube, 112–114, 113f
External magnetic field, impact of, 80f
External radiation, exposure, 507
Extinction time, 105, 290
Extrafocal radiation, reducing, 123f
Extrafocal x-rays, 123f
Extrapolation, 310
   values of, estimating, 311f
Extrapolation number, 461, 461b
Extremities
   dose limit of, 565–566
   monitoring, 569
Extremity radiography, 550
Eyes, response of, 351

F

Falling load generator, 97–98, 106, 107f
   design, 205–206
Fan beam, disadvantage of, 308
Faraday, Michael, 86
   law, 86, 86b
   schematic description of, 86f
Fatal accident rates, 563t
Fatal radiation-induced malignant disease, absolute risk, 485
Fatty acid, 432
Ferromagnetic core, 89
Ferromagnetic materials, 81
   magnetic dipoles in, random orientation of, 80f
   magnetic lines of induction, attraction of, 83f
   removal of, 83
Ferromagnetic objects, magnet creation, 82b
Fertility
   low-dose, chronic irradiation on, 493b
   radiation effects on, 493
Fertilization, radiation dose, 493
Fiberoptics, 283f
Fibrous tissue, 262
Field, 54
   size, 215–216, 215b
Field of view (FOV), 317
Filament, 114
Filament circuit, 97, 97f
Filament current
   increase, 115
   saturation current in, 116f

Filament transformer, 98
  generator component, 100b
File, term, use of, 388
Fill factor, 186, 186f, 353
Film
  badges, 567
  emulsions surface, 264
Filter, addition of, 149
Filtered back projection (FBP), 318, 334
Filtration, 146, 207–208, 511–512, 512b, 512f
  added, 207–208, 207f
    effect of, 138, 138b
  added filtration, 149
  application of, 9
  fluoroscopic protection, 514
  inherent, 148–150, 207
  mammographic imaging system, 267
  selective usage of, 149f
  total filtration, components of, 149f
  types of, 148–150, 207
Firmware, 387
First trimester, radiosensitivity during, 494b
First-generation CT imaging systems, 307–308
Five-Pin American College of Radiology Accreditation Phantom, characteristics of, 325t
Five-pin test object, of American Association of Physicists in Medicine, 324f
5-minute reset timer, 502–503
Fixation time, 421
Fixed kilovolt peak technique, for anteroposterior abdominal examination, 345t
Fixed-kVp radiographic technique, 209
Flash drive, 388–389, 389b, 389f
Flat Panel Display Measurement (FPDM), 369
Flat panel displays, 390
Flat panel image display, 293–294, 294b
Flat panel image receptor (FPIR), 292–293
  in digital fluoroscopy, advantages of, 293t
  fluoroscopy, in magnetic steering, 293f
Flatfielding, 250, 250b, 356
  preprocessing, 251f
Flickering, 284
Flies, irradiation (Muller), 496f
Floor-to-ceiling support system, in x-ray tube, 112, 113f
Fluorescence, 7, 354
Fluorescent screen, 284
Fluoroscope, 9, 9f, 275b
  5-minute reset timer, 502–503
Fluoroscopic couches, 93–94
Fluoroscopic examination, isoexposure contours, 503f
Fluoroscopic image
  monitoring of, 281–285, 283b
  quality of, kVp and mA on, 277
  television monitoring system in, 281
Fluoroscopic protection
  Bucky slot cover, 514
  collimation, 514
  cumulative timer, 514
  exposure control, 514
  features, 512–514, 512b
  filtration, 514
  primary protective barrier, 513–514, 514t
  source-to-skin distance, 513
Fluoroscopic technique, 276–277
Fluoroscopy, 8, 274–287
  automatic exposure systems in, 285
  configuration for, 529f
  contrast sensitivity, 420–421, 421b
  exposure rate in, 285
  human vision in, 276f
  illumination in, 275, 276f, 418, 418f
  occupational radiation exposure in, 560–562
  overview of, 275
  patient radiation dose in, 529b, 533, 534b
  position for, 570
  protective apparel for, 570–571, 570b
  quality control, 285
  scatter radiation during, 561f
  special demands of, 275–276, 418–421
  visual physiology in, 418–420, 419b, 419f
  visual physiology of, 276
  x-ray beams of, 539f
Flux gain, 278, 278b, 286f
Focal spot
  change in, 207b
  circular effective, 120–121
  definition of, 120f
  diaphragm in, 123f
  line-focus principle in, 120, 120b

Focal spot (Continued)
  selection of, 116
  shape of, 121f
  targets in, 120, 121f
Focal-spot blur, 240–241, 240b
  cause of, 240f
  example of, 241f
  production of, 303f
Focal-spot cooling algorithms, 315
Focal-spot size, 206–207
  changes in, 123f
  in computed tomography, 314
  controlling, 116f
  heel effect in, 122
  mammographic imaging system, 266
  National Electrical Manufacturers Association in, 121
  nominal, compared with maximum acceptable dimensions, 121t
Focused grid
  manufacture, difficulty, 225
  misalignment, 227t
Focusing cup, 114, 115f
Foot phantom
  digital images of, 199f
  screen-film radiographs of, 198
    overexposure and underexposure of, 198f
Force, 28b
  imaginary lines of, 80f
Foreshortening, 347, 348f
FORmula TRANslation (FORTRAN), 384, 384b
FORTRAN. See FORmula TRANslation
Four-pixel matrix, 318f
Four-slice helical CT scan, 326f
  changes of, in slice thickness, 326f
4% voltage ripple, 106
14% voltage ripple, 106
Fourth generation computers, 380
Fourth-generation CT imaging system, 309, 309f
FOV. See Field of view
Fovea centralis, 276, 419
FPDM. See Flat Panel Display Measurement
FPIR. See Flat panel image receptor
Fractionation, 443
Fractions, 18–19, 18b
Free radical, 453
Frequency, 55–57, 56f
  definition of, 55–57
  rate of, 55
  representation of, 55–57
  velocity and, relationship of, 56f
  wave parameters, 56
  wavelength and, inversely proportional, 56b
Friction, electrification by, 70
Frontal sinuses, radiographs of, 219
Fulcrum plane, 333f
Full-field size, comparison, 216
Full-wave rectification, 103, 103f, 105b
  circuit of, 104f
  voltage waveform for, 208–209
Full-wave-rectified waveforms, 139
Full-wave-rectified x-ray imaging systems, diodes (presence), 103–104, 103b, 103f
Full width at half maximum (FWHM), 313, 313f
Fundamental particles, 37–38, 37b
  characteristics of, 38t
FWHM. See Full width at half maximum

G
G_1 phase, of cell cycle, 462
Gadolinium oxysulfide (GdOS), 183
  DR image receptor, increase in, 187
Gain, images, 356
Galvani, Luigi, 84
Gametogenesis, 472
Gamma rays, 50, 50b
  emission of, 60
  energy, x-rays and, 60
  existence of, 50
  photons, 50
  production inside nucleus, 60f
  x-rays and, 60b
Gantry
  collimation in, 315
  in computed tomography, 314–316, 315b, 316f
  detector array in, 314–316
  high-frequency generator in, 316
  high-speed rotors in, 314
  of multislice helical computed tomography imaging system, 316f
  rotation time, changing pitch and, 312t

Gantry (Continued)
  x-ray tube in, 314
Gas, ionization, 519b
Gas-filled detectors, 519–521, 519b, 520b, 521b, 522b
  components, 519f
  signal, amplitude, 519f
Gastrointestinal (GI) death, 467
Gastrointestinal (GI) syndrome, 468
Geiger-Muller counter, 518t
Genetic cells, 436
Genetic effects, 496–497, 496b
  radiation-induced, 446b
Genetically significant dose (GSD), 529, 529b, 532–533, 533b, 533t
Geometric distortion, 371
Geometric factors, 235–241, 235b, 236f
Germ cells, 433, 472, 472f
Gigabyte (GB), bytes, equivalence, 388
Glandular dose (Dg), 549, 549b
  mammographic exposure, 550b, 550f
  variation of, 549
Glandular tissue, 262
  radiation sensitivity, 263b
Glass
  enclosure, in x-ray tube, 113–114
  opaque, 62
  surface of, roughened, 62
  transparent, 62
Glass envelope, 282
"Glitterblende", 10
Glucose, 433
Glycerol, 432
Glycogen, 432–433
Gonad dose, 529
Gonad shields, 552, 552b, 553t
Gonadal shielding, 12
Gonads, effects on, 471–473, 472b
Granulocytes, 474
Graph, 22–23, 22f, 23f, 23t
Gravitational field, 54
Gravity, 3
Gray (Gy_t), 14b
Grayscale
  dynamic range and, 196f
  rendering of, postprocessing and, 195f
  visibility of, 194
Grayscale display function (GSDF), 369
Greek atom, 35
Grenz rays, 471
Grid ratio, 221
  definition of, 221f
  equation of, 222b
  increase, 228
Grid-controlled tubes, 114
Grids, 114
  aluminum/plastic fiber, usage, 222
  Bucky factor values, 223t
  cutoff, 223–224
    equation, 224b
    types, 223–226, 224f
  focused, 225, 225f, 226b
  frequency, 222
    equation of, 222b
    increase, 222
  mammographic imaging system, 269–270
  off-level grid, 227
  oscillating, 226
  patient dose, 228–231
  problems, 226–228, 226b
  radiographic technique, change, 229t
  reciprocating grid, 226
  selection, 228–231, 229b
    clinical consideration in, 230t
    factors, 229b
  strip, 221
  types, 223–226, 223f
  upside-down grid, 228
GSD. See Genetically significant dose
GSDF. See Grayscale display function
Guanine, 433
Guard timer, 98
Guidewires, 300, 300b

H
Half-life
  concept of, 48
  radioactive, 46b, 47–48
Half-value layer (HVL), 48, 94, 146–147, 148f
  determination of, 146–147
    data in, example of, 147f

Half-value layer (HVL) *(Continued)*
  experimental arrangement for, 147*f*
  methods for, 146–147
    steps in, 147*b*
  increase, added filtration to, 149
  knowledge, 504
    requirement of, 146–147
  measurement, 512
  tube potentials, 505*t*
Half-wave rectification, 103, 103*f*
  result, 208*b*
Half-wave rectified generator, 208
Half-wave-rectified circuits, diodes (presence), 103, 103*f*
Half-wave-rectified waveforms, 139
Halogens, 36
Hard copy, 352–353
Hard drives, 388, 389*f*
  compared with CDs and flash drives, 389
Hardware, use of, 380
Header, 393
Headhunter tip, 300
Health, radiation and, 501, 501*b*
Health physics, 499–509
Heart, volume-rendering display of, 320*f*
Heat, 30–32, 30*b*
Heat (thermal energy), 4
  production of, 133
Heat capacity, 118
Heat dissipation, rate of, 124
Heel effect, 241, 241*f*, 242*t*
  in focal spot size, 122, 122*b*
  mammographic imaging system, 268, 268*f*
  posteroanterior chest images of, 122*f*
  response, 251*f*
  results, 121*f*
Helical computed tomography, 310*f*
Helical pitch ratio, 311
Helium nucleus, alpha particle and, 49–50
Hematologic death, 467
Hematologic effects, 474–475, 474*b*
Hematologic syndrome, 467
Hemopoietic cell survival, 475, 475*b*, 476*f*
Hemopoietic system, 474–475, 474*b*, 475*f*
Hexadecimal number system, 384*b*, 385*t*
High-capacity x-ray tubes, 117
High-contrast line, separated by interspace, 191*f*
High-dose fluoroscopy, 471, 471*t*
  skin effects resulting from, 446*b*
High-energy electrons, output phosphor with, interaction of, 278
High-frequency generation results, 209*b*
High-frequency generator, 105–106, 209
  characteristics of, 106*t*
  in gantry, 316
  inverter circuit of, 105, 105*f*
  voltage waveform of, 105*f*
High-frequency grids, usage, 226
High-frequency operation, efficiency, 140*f*
High-LET radiation, 457
High-mAs, usage, 235*b*
High melting point, of tungsten, 117*b*
High-quality image, 234
High-ratio grids
  effectiveness, 222*f*
  positioning latitude, decrease, 225*b*
High sensitivity, 523*b*
High-speed rotors, 314
High-transmission cellular (HTC) grid, mammographic design, 270, 270*f*
High-voltage generation, 208–209
  characteristics of, 208*t*
  mammographic imaging system, 264
  types, 208
High-voltage generator, 94, 100–109, 314
  components of, 100*b*
  cutaway view of, 100*f*
High-voltage generator power (kW), 108*b*
High-voltage transformer, 100–101
  generator component, 100*b*
  primary side of, 98
  step-up transformer, 100–101
  voltage induced in, 101*f*
Highlighting, 358
Hinck, Vincent, 300
Hiroshima, atomic bombings, 486–487
  survivors, 487*f*
Histogram
  analysis errors, sampling, 255*f*
  definition of, 252*b*
  example of, 252*f*
  image, 252–253

Histogram *(Continued)*
  samples, 253*f*
  values, discrete plot, 252
Hits, 457*b*
Hoff, Ted, 380
Holes, 101
Hollerith, Herman, 379
Homeostasis, 431
Hooke, Robert, 431
Horizontal resolution, 285
Horizontal retrace, 284
Hormesis, 445
Hormones, 432
Horsepower (hp), 29
Hospital, variation of power distribution in, 95
Hot-cathode x-ray tube, 10
Hounsfield, Godfrey, 306
Hounsfield unit (HU), 317
Housing cooling chart, 127
Human cell, 434–438, 434*f*, 462
Human genome, 479–480
Human-made radiation, 5
Human radiation, response, 429–430, 429*b*, 429*f*, 430*t*
Human vision
  Commission Internationale de l'Éclairage (CIE) and, 351
  fluoroscopy in, 276*f*, 418, 419*f*, 420*f*, 421*f*
  photometric response curves for, 351*f*
  range of, 276*f*, 418*f*
Human visual system, window and level adjustment and, 357
Humans
  biology, 427–440
  fibroblasts, after irradiation, 462*f*
  irradiation in utero, 494
  populations, observations, 484
  radiation exposure, estimated level of, 557*f*
  reduced life of, 483*b*
HVL. *See* Half-value layer
Hybrid subtraction, 295, 299*f*
Hydrogen (H₂)
  atoms, combination of, 45
  oxygen and, combination of, 45
Hydrogen peroxide, 453*b*
  formation, 454*b*
Hydroperoxyl formation, 454*b*
Hypersthenic patients, 345
Hypertext Markup Language (computer language), 386
Hyposthenic patients, 345

I

Illuminance, 351
Illuminance, levels, 370*t*
Illumination, in fluoroscopy, 275, 276*f*, 418, 418*f*
Image acquisition, 202–212
Image contrast
  loss of, 355*f*
  scatter radiation, effect, 216–218, 217*b*, 218*f*
  sharpness, 347, 347*b*
  visibility of, 347, 347*b*
    measurement, of using contrast resolution, 347
Image files, 388
Image-forming x-rays, transmission of, 197*f*
Image intensification, 277–281
  multifield, 279–281
Image intensifier, in brightness gain, 278–279
Image-intensifier tube, 277–279, 285*b*
  25/17/12, 280*f*
  charge-coupled device in, 283*f*
  modes of operation with, 279*f*
  television camera tubes in, 283*f*
  veiling glare in, 280*f*
  in x-ray beam, converting, 278*f*
Image noise, 155, 160, 179
  contrast resolution and, 197*b*
  sources of, in computed radiography, 180*t*
Image perception, 418, 418*b*
Image-quality factors, 345, 347–348, 347*b*
Image receptor (IR), 171, 244, 551
  artifacts, 248–249, 248*f*
  atomic number and K-shell binding energy for, 199*t*
  debris, 248*f*
  digital, response of, 199*f*
  exposure, factors, 143*t*
  raw x-ray beam exposure, 251*f*
  response curve, example of, 180*f*
  response function of, 178–179

Image receptor (IR) *(Continued)*
  response of, 197–198
    for screen-film radiography, 532*f*
  sizes, 255*t*
  of tomosynthesis, 334
  x-ray beam incident on, 200*f*
  x-rays, impact, 214
Image reconstruction, of tomosynthesis, 334–335, 335*t*
Image resolution, pixel values in, 321–322
Images
  appearance difference of, MTF curves and, 194*f*
  archiving, interaction among, 362*f*
  degradation, rarity, 228
  flip, 357
  foreshortening, 347, 348*f*
  interpretation, teleradiology and, 362
  lag, 356
  luminance, 353–354
  magnification, 357
  pre-fetching from archive, 362
  processing
    activities, digital imaging and, 195
    interaction among, 362*f*
  storage, requirement, determination of, 363
  subtraction, 357–358
  visualization, pan, scroll, and zoom, 358
Imaging
  characteristics of, 178–180
  contrast loss, 256*f*
  modalities, digital file sizes, 251*t*
Imaging plate (IP), 173, 173*f*
  lead backing, 173
  use of, 175*b*
Imaging systems
  characteristics of, 206–209
  contrast resolution, 321*f*, 322*f*
  spatial resolution for, 191*b*
  spatial frequency and, 193*b*
Impact printers, 390
Improvised nuclear device (IND), 507
In-service training, 572
In utero
  effects, summary, 495*t*
  irradiation, 493–496
  radiation exposure, 495*b*
In vitro irradiation, 450*b*
In vivo irradiation, 450*b*
Incident x-ray, 154
Inclined object, lateral position, 239*f*
IND. *See* Improvised nuclear device
Induction
  electrification by, 70–71
  magnetic lines, attraction of, 83*f*
Induction motor
  electromagnetic, 118, 119*f*
  parts of, 87*f*
  power, 87*b*
Inertia, Newton's first law, 27*b*
Informatics communication, 364–365, 365*f*
Infrared laser beam, PSP interaction with, 174*f*
Infrared light, photons in, 59
Inherent filtration, 148, 207
Initiation time, 105
Inkjet printers, 390
Input hardware, 391, 391*b*
Input phosphor, 277
  in image-intensifier tube, 278–279
Insulator, definition of, 74*b*
Integrated circuits (ICs), use of, 380
Integrated services digital network (ISDN), 391
Intelligent terminal, 390
Interlace, 284
Internal components, of x-ray tube, 114–123
Internally deposited radionuclides, 5
International Classification of Diseases (ICD codes), 365
International System (SI) units, 13*t*, 14
Interphase, 436, 436*f*
  death, 444, 444*b*
Interpolation, 250*b*
  algorithms, 310–311
  estimation of, 311*f*
Interpreters, 383
Interrogation time, 290
Interrupterless transformer, 9
Interspace material, 221
  primary beam x-rays, transmission, 222
Interventional procedures, types of, 294–299
Interventional radiologist, extremity monitoring for, 561*b*

Interventional radiology, 275, 288–304
　arteriography, risks of, 301
　catheters, 300, 300b, 300f
　contrast media in, 300
　control room in, 301
　digital subtraction angiography, 294–295
　equipment in, 302–303
　focal-spot blur, production of, 303f
　guidewires in, 300, 300b
　high-frequency generators in, 303
　image display of, 293–294
　image receptors, 290–293, 303b
　occupational radiation exposure in, 560–562
　patient couch in, 303, 303f
　patient preparation and monitoring in, 300–301
　patient radiation dose in, 303
　personnel in, 301–302
　principles of, 299–301
　procedures, difficult, 503
　protective aprons, wrap-around type, 571
　spatial resolution, 289b
　suite, 301–304
　　layout of, 301f
　　procedures conducted in, 295t
　x-ray tube, specifications for, 302t
Intracellular repair, combined processes of, 444b
Inverse square law, 62–64, 63b, 63f, 145, 351–352
　application of, 62–64
　　parameters, 63b
Inverter circuit, DC power feed, 264
Iodinated contrast agent, 164
Iodine (I)
　decay, 46f
　　calculation of, 47
　half-life of, 47–48, 47f
　usage of, 41
Ion chamber, 519
　configuration, 521f
　dosimeter, 521f
　survey instrument, 520f
Ion pair, 5
Ionic bonds, 45
Ionization, 5b, 5f, 39b, 40f, 453b
　chamber, 518t
　potential, 41–43
　region, 519
Ionized electron, 39
Ionizing radiation, 5, 49–51, 49t, 60
　human responses to, 430
　sources of, 5–6, 6f
　types of, 49, 50t, 51f
IP. See Imaging plate
IR. See Image receptor
Iris, 276, 418–419
Irradiated matter, 5
Irradiation
　biologic response to, 553
　of macromolecules, 450–452, 450f
　mice, LD$_{50/60}$, 494f
Irradiation in utero, 493–496
　animal data, 493
　effects, observations, 494f
　Oxford survey, 494
ISDN. See Integrated services digital network
Isobar, 44, 44b
Isobaric radioactive transitions, 44
Isochromatids, 478
Isoexposure contours, 503f
Isoexposure lines, 503–504
Isomer, 44, 44b
Isotone, 44
　constant value, 44
Isotopes, 38, 44t
　description of, 41–43

J
Java (computer language), 386
Jones, Mason, 294
Joule per coulomb, 74, 84b
J-tip, for guidewires, 300
Jukeboxes, 389, 389f
Jump drive/stick, 389b

K
K absorption edge, 298b
Karyotypes, normal, 477, 477b, 477f
Kidneys, ureters, and bladder (KUB), radiographic technique for, exposure calculation in, 144
Kilobyte (kB), bytes, equivalence, 383, 388

Kilogram (kg), 14, 24–25
Kilovolt peak (kVp), 9, 144–145, 203
　adjustment of, 96–97
　barrier thickness, factor, 517
　beam energy and, 203b
　change in, 137b, 137f
　effect of, 137–138
　half-value layer and, relationship of, 148t
　impact, 97b, 148
　increase in, 137–138
　　diagnostic range, 138b
　meter for, placement of, 96–97
　x-ray intensity and, relationship of, 144b
Kinetic energy, 4, 30b
　calculation of, 130b
　conversion of, 131f
　definition of, 130b
　equation, 130b
　guillotine, representation, 4f
　magnitude in, determination of, 130
　mass/velocity, proportion of, 130f
Kinetic energy released in matter (air kerma), 14, 14b
Knee, histogram, 253f
K-shell binding energy, 157, 157t
K-shell electron
　binding energy of, 41–43
　ionization of, 132f
K x-rays, 132
　relative intensity of, 135

L
Lambda (λ), wavelength symbol, 55
Large-scale integration (LSI), 380
L-arm, 112
Laser beam, diameter of, impact of, 173, 173b
Laser localizer, in computed tomography, 329
Latent image, stimulation of, 174f
Latent period, of acute radiation lethality, 467
Lateral decentering, 227
Lateral dispersion, 284
Law of Bergonie and Tribondeau, 442, 442t
Law of conservation, matter/energy, 66
Layered anode, components of, 118f
LCDs. See Liquid crystal displays
Lead, tube potentials, half-value and tenth-value layer, 505t
Lead aprons, physical characteristics of, 571t
Lead bar patterns, imaging of, 193f
Leakage radiation, 113, 113f
　definition, 515
　level, 511b
Leibniz, Gottfried, 379
Length, standard unit of, 24
Lens
　dose limit for, 563
　shields, 552
Leonard, Charles L., 9
LET. See Linear energy transfer
Lethal dose$_{50/60}$ (LD$_{50/60}$), 468–469, 468b, 469t
Leukemia, 486–488
　incidence
　　atomic bomb survivor, 487f
　　elevated, population sample, 482t
　　summary, 487t
　observations, results, 488f
　radiation-induced, 446b, 489b
　radiologists, 488
Life expectancy, 502f
Life span shortening, 484
　radiation dose and, 483f
　radiation-induced life span shortening, 484f
　risk, 483t
Light
　amplifier tube, 10
　beam, SID and, 511b
　data transfer, 390
　localization, 219
　speed of, 65
　　calculation, 54
　wavelengths of, reflection of, 61
Light-emitting diode (LED), 354
Light-emitting diode display, 354–356, 355b
　ambient light and, 355
　backlight and, 355, 355b
　symbol for, 355f
Light field, mirror, 208f
Light stimulation-emission, 173–176
Lighting, modern, illuminance in, 352t
Light-localizing variable-aperture collimators, 149, 511

Lightning
　electrification discharge, 70–71
　source of, 72f
Like charges, repulsion of, 71b, 72
Limiting resolution, 321
Line compensator, voltage measurement, 95
Line noise, 356
Line pair
　pattern, imaging of, 193f
　spatial frequency and, 191f
　　relationship of, 190
Linear dose-response relationships, 445–446, 446f
Linear energy transfer (LET), 442, 443f, 443t
　description of, 41–43
　target theory and, 457, 458f
Linear interpolation, 311b
Linear nonthreshold dose-response relationship, 447
　for cancer, 489b
　slope of, absolute risk, 486f
Linearity, 512
　in computed tomography, 324–325, 325f
　test objects for, 328f
　maximum acceptable variation, 512b
Line-focus principle, 120, 120b, 120f
Lipids, 432, 432f
Liquid crystal displays (LCDs), 353–354, 390
　ambient light and, 355
　display characteristics of, 353
　grayscale definition and, 354
　image luminance of, 353–354
　　measurement, aperture ratio and, 353b
　inefficiency of, 353
　off-perpendicular viewing of, image contrast and, 355f
Liquid crystals, orientation of, 353f
Local tissue damage, 470–474
Local tissue effects, 482–483
　chromosomes, 483
　skin, 482–483
Lodestone, 77
Logarithmic scale, 158, 159f
Logic function, 382
LOGO (computer language), 386
Long bone, cross section (radiographs), 217
Lossless compression, 251
Low-contrast CT test object, 329f
Low-contrast objects, resolution of, 323
Low-energy x-rays, contribution of, 146
Lower extremities, aluminum step-wedge in, usage of, 151f
Low-kVp, usage, 235b
Low-LET radiation, 457
L-shell x-rays, absorption, 264–265, 265b
Lumbar spine radiography, beam collimation (requirement), 216f
Lumen, 351
　photometric unit and, 351b
Lumens per steradian (candela), 351
Luminance, 351
　intensity, 351, 351f
　meter, 370, 370b
　nonuniformity, 373
　response, 372–374, 372b, 373b
　　measurement, luminance patches (examples), 372–373, 373f
　uniformity
　　assessment, TG 18-UN/TG 18-UNL patterns, 373, 374f
　　quantitative evaluation, 373–374
Luminescence, 354
Luminous flux, 351
Lung cancer, 490
L x-rays, 132
Lymphocytes, 474
Lysosomes, 435

M
Machine learning (Ml)
　supervised learning, 400
　unsupervised learning, 400
Macromolecules, 431, 431b
　cross-linking of, 450, 450f
　irradiation of, 450–452, 450f
　macromolecular synthesis of, 450–451, 450b, 451b, 451f
　main-chain scission of, 450, 450f
　point lesions in, 450, 450b, 450f
Macros, writing, 386
Magnetic dipole, 79
Magnetic domain, 79

Magnetic field
    imaginary lines of, 82f
    intensification of, 85
    intensity of, 85
Magnetic field induction
    charge of, motion in, 85b
    moving charged particle in, 79f
    spinning charged particle in, 79f
Magnetic field lines
    closed loops, 79b
    concentration of, 85f
    from concentric circles, 85f
Magnetic force
    lines of, demonstration of, 82f
    proportionality of, 83b
Magnetic induction, 82–83
Magnetic laws, 81–82
Magnetic moment, 79
Magnetic permeability, 80b
Magnetic resonance imaging (MRI), 10
Magnetic states, 82t
Magnetic susceptibility, 81b
Magnetism, 77–83
    physical laws of, comparison of, 81
    understanding, difficulty, 77–83
Magnetite, discovery of, 77
Magnets
    baby, 82f
    field strength, SI unit of, 83b
    movement of, 86
    poles, 82
    types of, 80
Magnification, 357
    geometric factor, 235–238, 235b, 237f
    mammography, 270, 270b
    minimization, 237b
        clinical situations, 238
    radiography, 210–211
        principle, 211f
Magnification factor (MF), equation of, 211b, 237b
Magnification mode results, 281t
Magnification radiography, 235
Magnitude, 25
Main-chain scission, 450, 450f
Major kV$_p$, label for, 96–97
Male gametogenesis, 473b
Malignancy, total risk, 491–493
Malignant disease, BEIR Committee, estimated excess mortality, 492t
Mammalian cells, irradiation of, 461t, 463b
Mammographer, 271f, 272
Mammographic imaging system, 263–270
    automatic exposure control, 270
    compression, 268–269
    filtration, 267
    focal-spot size, 266
    grid, 269–270
    heel effect, 268f
    high-voltage generation, 264
    magnification mammography, 270, 270b
    target composition, 264–265
Mammographic technique chart, 266t
Mammography, 247–257, 259–273, 271b, 549–550, 549b
    baseline, 262
    basis for, 261–263
    dedicated system, 265t
    diagnostic, 262
    digital, 263b
    imaging, dedicated system, 264f
    low-ratio grids, usage, 229
    occupational radiation exposure in, 561
    quality control, 270–271
    screen-film, 270
    screening, 262
    soft tissue radiography, 261
    spatial resolution and, 193
    types of, 262
    x-ray tube, 122
        circular focal spot, pinhole camera images, 266f
        double banana shaped focal spot, 266f
        focal spot characteristics, 266
Manifest illness, 467–468, 468b
Mark I (computer), 379
Marshall Islands, atomic bomb survivors, and residents, 495
Mask mode, 295, 296f
    digital fluoroscopy, 296f
Mass
    definition of, 3, 3b

Mass (Continued)
    inequality, 43
Mass, standard unit of, 24–25
Mass density
    dependence on, 162–164, 162b, 163f, 163t
    of materials important to radiologic science, 163t
    no large differences in, 324f
    tissue, 242, 243f
Mass-energy equivalence, 4–5, 5b
Maternal tissue, attenuation by, 572
Matter, 3–5, 3b, 66–67
    centuries of discovery, 35–37
    characteristic of, 3
    classification of, 80b
    electric states of, 76t
    irradiated, 5
    law of conservation of, 66
    magnetic states of, 82t
    size, varies, 35f
    structure of, 34–52
    visible light with, interaction of, 61–62
    x-ray interactions with, 153–167
Mauchly, John, 379
Maxillary sinuses, radiographs, 220f
Maximum intensity projection (MIP), 319
    reconstruction of, 319f
Maximum permissible dose (MPD), 562
Maximum x-ray energy, 136b
Maxwell, James Clerk, 54
Mean lethal dose, 461, 463t
Mean marrow dose (MMD), 529b, 532
Mean survival time, 469–470, 469f
Measurement, standard units of, 14, 23–26
    length, 24
    mass, 24–25, 25f
    time, 25
    units, 25–26, 25b, 31t
Mechanical support
    in anode, 116–117
    in protective housing, 113
Medical flat panel digital display devices
    color LCDs and, 353
    sizes of, 354t
Medical image descriptors, 233–246
    definitions of, 234–235
    resolution/noise/speed, relationship, 235f
    rules, 235b
Medical image quality, 234
Medical images
    digital file size for, 363t
    signal-to-noise ratio and, 197
Medical imaging, 284b, 528
    computer applications, 390–393
    computer science, 377–394
    development of, 8–10, 10b
    growth of the cost, 528f
    systems, spatial resolution for, 192t
    team, 15
Medical physicist, 271–272, 272b, 272t
Medical radiation exposure, levels of, 6
Megabyte (MB), bytes, equivalence, 388
Meiosis, 436–438, 437b, 437f
Memory
    archival form of, 388b
    computer component, 387
    location, sequence of, 388
    storage, 388b
    working storage, 387b
Mendeleev, Dmitri, 36
Messenger RNA, 433
Metabolism, 431, 431b
Metal enclosure, in x-ray tube, 113–114
Metal filters, in estimation of the x-ray energy, 567
Metaphase, of mitosis, 436, 436b
Metastable electrons, ground state, 172, 172f
Mice, irradiation, LD50/60, 494f
Microcalcifications, deposits, 262
Microcomputer processing speeds, 386
Microprocessor, 126b, 386
    for exposure timers, 99b
Microwave radiation, 59
    interaction of, 61
Milk of Magnesia, 78f
Milliamperage (mA)
    change in, 137b, 137f
    effect of, 136–137
Milliampere seconds (mAs), 143–144
    equation, 144b
    equivalent exposures of, 205b
    exposure, equation, 203b, 204b
    measurement of, 144b

Milliampere seconds (mAs) (Continued)
    x-ray exposure time and, 204b
    x-ray quantity and, proportionality of, 145b
Milliamperes (mAs), 203–204
    calculation, 205t
    change in, 137f
    control of, 97–98
    effect of, 136–137
    equation for, 203b
    meter for, 98f
    selector switch, voltage delivery, 98
    timers for, 99
Milligray in air (mGy$_a$), x-ray beam intensity measurement, 143
Minification gain, 278–279, 279b, 286f
Minimum x-ray wavelength, 136b
Minor kVp, label for, 96–97
MIP. See Maximum intensity projection
MIPS (millions of instructions per second), 386
Misregistration artifacts, 297, 298f
Mitochondria, 435
Mitosis, 436, 437f
Mobile radiography, SID level of, 145
Mobile radiology
    occupational radiation exposure in, 562
    protective apron for, 570–571
Mobile x-ray imaging systems, 94b, 512
Mobile x-ray unit, protective apron in, 566b
Modern physics, 407b, 407f
Modulation data, plot of, 193f
Modulation transfer function (MTF), 192–194
    construction of, lead bar patterns and, 193f
    curve, 321f, 322f
        characterization of, 200f
        photographs and, association of, 194f
        result of, 193f
    determining, 328
    graphic representation of, 320
    plot of, in image fidelity, versus spatial frequency, 321f
    ratio, 321
    view of, 192b
Molecular imaging, 431
Molecular radiobiology, 449–455, 450b
Molecules, 3, 45b
    smallest particle of compound, 45b
Molybdenum (Mo)
    K-characteristic x-rays, 265
    target element, use of, 139
    as targets in x-ray tube, 41
    x-ray emission spectrum for, 265f
        unfiltered, 267, 268f
Momentum, 29, 29b, 29f
Monochrome LCD, color LCD and, 353
Monoenergetic x-ray beam, 162
Monosaccharides, 432–433
Motherboard, 388
Motion blur, 243, 243b
    reduction
        exposure time, impact of, 204b
        procedures, 244t
Moving charged particle, in magnetic field induction, 79f
Moving grid, 225–226
    installation, 227f
    mechanisms, success, 228
MPD. See Maximum permissible dose
MPR. See Multiplanar reformation
MRI. See Magnetic resonance imaging
MTF. See Modulation transfer function
Muller, H.J., 496
    irradiation, of flies, 496f
Multidetector array, components of, 315f
Multifield image intensification, 279–281, 280b
Multihit chromosome aberrations, 478, 478f
Multiplanar reformation (MPR), 319–320, 319b
Multiple CCDs, assembly of, 185
Multiple digital images, partitioning of, 254b
Multislice computed tomography
    isoexposure profiles in, 562f
    patient radiation dose and, 541f
Multislice detector array, 325–326, 326b
Multislice helical computed tomography, 309–313, 544
    features of, 327t
    high-voltage generator in, 316f
    image data in, 311f
    imaging systems, 316f
        gantry of, 316f
    interpolation algorithms in, 310–311, 311f
    multidetector array, 326
    pitch, 311–313, 312f

Multislice helical computed tomography
(Continued)
  sensitivity profile in, 313, 313f
  x-ray tubes in, 314
multislice spiral computed tomography, 541f
Multislice value, 541b
Multi-target, single-hit model, 459–461, 460f, 461b, 461f, 461t
Muscle, 438
Myelography, 294

N

Nagasaki, atomic bombings, 486–487
  survivors, 487f
National Council on Radiation Protection and Measurements (NCRP), 496
  dose limits recommended by, 565t
  on patient radiation dose trends, 556–558
National Electrical Manufacturers Association (NEMA)
  in focal spot size, 121
  standard imaging and interface format and, 362
National Electrical Manufacturers Association Digital Imaging and Communications in Medicine (NEMA-DICOM), 369
National Institute of Standards and Technology (NIST), luminance measurement, 370
Natural environmental radiation in United States, 7f
Natural magnet, example of, 80
Natural response level, 445–446
NCRP. *See* National Council on Radiation Protection and Measurements
Near-range photometers, 370, 371f
Nervous tissue, 438
Network, PACS and, 361–362, 361b
Neuroangiography, 294
Neurons, 438
Neutrons, 37
  in atoms, 39f
  nucleons, 38
  in nucleus, 38f
New employee notification, form for, 572f
New employee training, 572, 572f
Newton, 24–25
Newton's laws of motion, 27–28, 27b, 27f, 407
Nickel-cadmium (NiCd) battery, use of, 106
Niobium, superconducting material, 75
Nit (candela per meter squared), 351
Noble gases, 36
Noise, 234–235, 234b
  in computed tomography, 324, 324b
  sources of, 197
Nominal focal spot size, maximum acceptable dimensions and, comparison of, 121t
Nomogram
  accuracy of, 531f
  curve, 530f
  for x-ray beam intensity estimation, 143f
Nonionizing radiation, 49
Nonlinear dose-response relationships, 446, 446f
Nonoccupationally exposed persons, dose limit for, 566b
North pole, 82
N-type semiconductors, 101
Nuclear arrangement, characteristics of, 44t
Nuclear energy, 4
Nuclear reactor incidents, 491
Nuclear structure, defined, 37, 38f
Nucleic acids, 433
Nucleolus, 434
Nucleons, 38
Nucleotides, 433–434
Nucleus, 37, 434
  components, 38, 38f
  electrons revolve in, 41f
  projectile electron, passage of, 133
Nuclide, 45–46
Number systems, 21–22, 21f, 21t
Numeric prefixes, 13, 13t

O

Object artifacts, 252–254
  alignment, 254
  collimation and partition, 252–254
  image histogram, 252–253
Object organ, computed tomography examination of, 320f
Object-oriented programming (OOP), 386

Object-to-image receptor distance (OID), 237
  minimization, 270
Objective lens, 283
Objects
  foreshortened image, 239f
  inclination of, 239f
  lateral position, 239
  magnification of, 237f
  position, 238
  shape, 243, 243f
  size, reduction, spatial frequency and, 190–192
  thickness, 238f
Occupancy, levels, 516t
Occupancy factor, time, 516–517
Occupational effective dose, 507t
Occupational radiation, 562
  dose limits, historical review for, 564t
  dose management, 559–575
  monitoring report for, 569–570, 569b, 570f
Occupational radiation exposure, 560–562
  in computed tomography, 561
  effective dose, 506, 507f
  in fluoroscopy, 560, 561f
  in interventional radiology, 560–561
  in mammography, 561
  management principles for, 572–574, 573b
  in mobile radiology, 562
  of radiologic personnel, 560t
  reduction of, 566–574
  in surgery, 561–562
Occupational radiation monitoring, 504f, 567–568, 567b
  where to wear, 568–569, 568b
OER. *See* Oxygen enhancement ratio
Oersted, Hans, 84
  experiment, 84f
Off-center grid, 227–228
  off-focus grid, combination, 228, 228f
Off-focus grid, 227f, 228
Off-focus radiation, 123, 219
Off-level grid, 227, 227f
Offset images, 356
Offset voltage, 356
Offshore oilfield worker, work of, 491b
Ohm's law, 75
  equation, 75b
OID. *See* Object-to-image receptor distance
100% voltage ripple, 106
1% voltage ripple, 106
Oogonia, 472
OOP. *See* Object-oriented programming
Open collimator, components, 208f
Operating console, 94–95, 95f
  circuit diagram for, 96f
  computer technology basis of, 94–95
Operating system, 383
  loading of, 384
Operator shield, 512
Optical density (OD), distance, impact of, 206b
Optically stimulated luminescence (OSL), 173
  dosimeters, 568, 568f
  dosimetry, 518–519
Orbital electrons, projectile electron avoidance of, 133
Orbits (energy levels), 37
  "shells" grouped into, 38
Organic free radical formation, 454b
Organic molecules, 431
Organs, 438–439, 439t
  dose limit for, 565–566
  systems, 438, 438b
Orthovoltage x-rays, 470
Oscillating grid, 226
OSL. *See* Optically stimulated luminescence
Outer shell electrons, 40b
  energy level of, change in, 131
  filling, 131b
Output devices, 389–390, 390b
Output hardware, 390b
Output intensity, for computed tomography, 542–543, 542b
Output phosphor, 278, 278b
  in image-intensifier tube, 279f
Output x-ray intensity, nomogram for estimating, 530f
Ovaries, radiation response of, 472–473, 473t
Overranging, 544, 544f
Ovum, 472
Oxford survey, 494
Oxygen (O_2)
  atoms, combination of, 45

Oxygen (O_2) *(Continued)*
  effect, radiation and, 443–444
  hydrogen and, combination of, 45
Oxygen enhancement ratio (OER), 443, 443b, 444f, 464b

P

PA chest radiography, 149
PACS. *See* Picture archiving and communication system
Pair production, 66, 159, 159b, 159f
Parallel grid, 223–224, 224b
  optical density, decrease, 224f
Paramagnetic materials, 81
Partial grid cutoff, 227f
Partial volume averaging, 319
Particle accelerators, 37
Particle model, quantum theory, 65–66
Particles, 60–66
Particulate radiation, 49–50
Partition, object artifacts, 253–254
Pascal (computer language), 385
Pascal, Blaise, 379
Pathology
  appearance, 346b
  classification of, 347t
  constructive, 346–347
  destructive, 346–347
  of patients, 346–347
Patient-image optimization, 343–349
Patient radiation dose, 228–229, 336–340, 337b, 338f, 339f, 340f
  computed tomography, 538–547, 542b
  considerations, 197–200
  descriptions of, 528–534
  detector rows, combined, 542f
  distribution, in CT, 540–541, 540b, 540f, 541f
  expression of, 528
  increase, high-ratio grids, impact, 222f
  management, 548–558
  reduction, 543f
    collimation, impact, 214b
    limitation of, 198b
  in special examination, 549–550
  trends of, 556–558, 556f
  unnecessary, reduction, 550–552
Patient-supporting examination couch, 93
Patients
  artifacts, 348
  characteristics of, 180
  composition, 345t, 346, 346t
  couch movement, divided by x-ray beam width, 312f
  detail, 347
  distortion, 347, 347b
  factors, 345–347, 345b
  holding of, 571
  pathology, 346–347, 347t
  positioning, 209b, 244, 347b
    accuracy in, requirement of, 209b
  primary x-rays, interaction, 218f
  thickness, 216, 216b, 217f, 242, 345–346, 345b, 345t, 346t
  tissue, off-focus radiation in, 123
  x-rays, exit, 221
PBL. *See* Positive-beam-limiting
Pencil ionization chamber, 544f
Penetrability
  changes in, 147
  x-ray beam and, description of, 146
Penguin, 398b–399b
Penumbra, 541, 544b
Peptide bonds, 431
Periodic table of elements, 36, 37f
Permanent magnets
  availability of, 80
  design, developments in, 81f
Pernicious anemia, radiologists, 488
Personal computer (PC), 380
Phosphor, 354
Phosphorescence, 354
Photocathode, 277, 277b, 523b
Photodiodes (PDs), 174
Photodisintegration, 159–160, 160b, 160f
Photoelectric absorption
  in iodine, bone, and muscle, 298f
  x-ray energy, 262b
Photoelectric effect, 156–159, 156b, 156f, 158f, 158t
  Compton interactions and, 162f
  contribution, 215f

Photoelectric effect *(Continued)*
    features of, 159*t*
Photoelectric x-ray interactions, occurrence of, 172
Photoelectron, 156
Photoemission, 277
Photographic emulsion, 518*t*
Photometric quantities, 351–352, 352*t*
Photometric response curve, 351*f*
Photometric units, 351, 352*t*
    lumen and, 351*b*
Photometry, 351
Photomultiplier tube gain, 522*b*
Photon energy
    calculation of, 66
    frequency and, proportionality of, 58*b*, 65*b*
    inverse proportion to wavelength photon, 66
    third power of (1/E)³, 157
Photons, 50, 54–57
    frequency of, calculation of, 57
    interaction, with matter, 61*b*
    mass in, absence of, 54–57
    radiation, intensity loses, 49–50
    types of energy in, 57
Photopic vision, 276, 420
Photospot camera, 283
Photostimulable luminescence (PSL), 172, 172*b*
    infrared laser beam, interaction with, 174*f*
    signal production in, 174
Photostimulable phosphor (PSP)
    imaging plate and, 173
    processing with, stimulation portion of, 175
    screen
        cross-section, 172, 172*f*
        housing, 173
    stimulation of, with laser light, 175
        monochromatic, 176*f*
    x-ray interaction with, 172*f*
Phototimers, AEC devices, 270
Physicians, death statistics, 484*t*
Physician's viewing console, 314
Physics, 17–33
    mathematics for radiologic science, 18–23
    mechanics, 26–32
        acceleration, 27, 27*b*
        energy, 29–30, 30*b*
        heat, 30–32, 30*b*
        momentum, 29, 29*b*, 29*f*
        Newton's laws of motion, 27–28, 27*b*, 27*f*
        power, 29, 29*b*
        velocity, 26–27, 26*b*, 27*f*
        weight, 28–29, 28*b*
        work, 29, 29*b*
    standard units of measurement, 23–26
Picture archiving and communication system (PACS), 360–367
    components of, 361, 393
    electronic medical record and, 363, 364*f*
    film file room replacement and, 366
    hospital space and, cost of, 363*b*
    implementation of, 361, 361*b*
    informatics communication and, 364, 365*f*
    medical information organizations, 365
    networks and, 361–362, 361*b*
        digital images with, combining, 366*f*
        interaction of, 362*f*
    radiologic technologist responsibilities, 365–366
    storage system and, 363, 363*b*, 364*f*
    workstations, 361
        image transfer and, 362
Picture element, 317
Pigtail catheters, 300
Pitch, 311–313
    changing, tissue imaged with, 312*t*
    increasing, 311
    patient couch movement, divided by x-ray beam width, 312*f*
Pixel
    cell of information, 317
    computed tomography numbers in, 317–318
    control, TFT and, 353
    cross-sectional rendering of, 354*f*
    face, portion of, 186
    information, 393
    shift, 358
    values of, in image noise, 324
Pixel size, 317*b*
Planck, Max, 65
Planck's constant, 22, 65–66
Planck's equation, equivalent, 66*b*
Planck's quantum equation, 65*b*
Planck's quantum theory, 65
Plant starches, 432–433

Plotters, 390
Pluripotential stem cell, 474
P-n junction semiconductor, solid-state diodes in, 101, 102*f*
Pneumoencephalography, 294
Point lesions, 450, 450*b*, 450*f*
Point mutations, 452, 453*f*
Poles, 82
Polyenergetic x-ray beam, 162
Polysaccharides, 432–433
Portable fluoroscopy, scatter radiation during, 561*f*
Portable x-ray unit, exposure cord in, 566*b*
Positive-beam limitation, 511, 511*b*
Positive-beam-limiting (PBL) devices, 219
Positive beta particles (positrons), 50
Positron, 159
Positrons (positive beta particles), 50
Posterior-anterior (PA) chest radiography, effective dose for, 536
Posteroanterior (PA) chest examination, x-ray imaging system with, impact of, 145
Posteroanterior chest images, of heel effect, 122*f*
Postinjection image, 297*f*
Postmenopausal breasts, characterization, 262
Postprocessing, 194–197
    annotation and, 357
    of digital images, operator manipulation and, 357*b*
    digital radiographic image, 356
    gray shades and, visualization, 196*b*
    use of, 195*f*
Potential energy, 4, 30*b*, 30*f*
    guillotine, representation, 4*f*
Potter, Hollis E., 226
Potter-Bucky diaphragm, 306
Potter-Bucky grid, 10
Pound, 24–25
Power, 29, 29*b*, 108
Power of ten, 382*t*
Power of two, 382*t*
Power rating, 108–109, 108*b*
Predetector collimator, 316
    multislice helical computed tomography imaging systems, 316*f*
Predicted radiation-induced deaths, 491*b*
Preemployment physical examination, 551
Preferred detent position, 112
Pregnancy
    counsel for, 573
    diagnostic radiology in, 573*t*
    form for acknowledgement of radiation risk during, 574*f*
    radiation and, 493–497, 493*b*
    termination or an involuntary leave of absence during, 573*b*
Pregnant patient, 553–556, 553*b*
    collimated beams, 554
    elective booking in, 554
    irradiation, biologic response to, 553–556
    patient information, 554–556, 554*b*
    post signs in, 554
    questions for, 554
    radiobiologic considerations in, 553–556
    radiographic examinations, entrance exposures and fetal doses, 555*t*
    recommendation for abortion in, 556*b*
    wall posters, for radiation in, 555*f*
    x-ray and fluoroscopy consent, 555*f*
Pregnant technologist/radiologist, 571–572, 571*b*
    "baby monitor" position of, 569*f*
Preinjection mask, 297*f*
Preneoplastic thyroid nodularity, incidence, 489
Prepatient collimator, 315–316
    multislice helical computed tomography imaging systems, 316*f*
Preprocessing, 249–250
    actions, 356
    automation of, 356*b*
    calibration techniques of, 356
    digital image, 356*b*
    digital radiographic image, 356
Prereading kVp meter, use of, 97
Primary beam x-rays, 221
Primary connections, 96
Primary memory, 387
Primary protective barrier
    concrete equivalents, 515*t*
    fluoroscopic protection, 513–514, 514*f*
Primary side, 98
Primary x-rays
    attenuation, 224
    patient interaction, 218*f*

Primordial follicles, 472
Principal quantum number, 40
Printers, as output device, 390
Processor, 386*b*
Prodromal period, of acute radiation lethality, 467
Program files, 388
Programming languages, 385*t*
Projectile electron
    avoidance of, 133
    maximum energy of, 136*f*
Projection imaging, characteristics of, 528, 528*f*, 529*f*
Projections, data, for DRT, 334
Proper collimation, 551
Prophase, of mitosis, 436
Protective apparel, 12, 570–571, 570*b*
Protective apron, wrap-around type, 570–571
Protective barrier
    design of, 514–518
    window in, requirement of, 94
Protective curtain, 514, 514*f*
Protective housing, in x-ray tube, 113, 113*b*, 113*f*
Protective lead aprons, physical characteristics of, 571*t*
Protective x-ray tube housing, 511
Protein synthesis, 431, 435, 435*f*
Proteins, 431, 431*b*, 432*f*
Protons, 37
    in atoms, 39*f*
    nucleons, 38
    in nucleus, 38*f*
    number of, 43
Protraction, 443
PSL. *See* Photostimulable luminescence
PSP. *See* Photostimulable phosphor
P-type semiconductors, 101
Pulse mode, 518
Pulse-progressive fluoroscopy, 291*f*
Pupin, Michael, 9
Purines, 433
Pyrimidines, 433

Q

QC. *See* Quality control
QC radiologic technologist, 272
QCD. *See* Quantum chromodynamics
Quality control (QC)
    digital display device, 371–374
    of fluoroscopy, 285
    by radiologic technologist, 374–375, 374*b*
    test objects and tools, design, 192
Quality control, in DRT, 336, 336*f*
Quality control team, 271–272, 271*f*
Quantum, 54
    theory, particle model, 65–66
Quantum chromodynamics (QCD), 37
Quantum computers
    algorithms, 413–414
    applications, 414–415
    classical physics, 412
    fault-tolerant qubit, 414, 415*f*
    IBM Q System, 412*f*
    probability density function, 412–413, 414*f*
    types of, 415*t*
    unit of information, 412–413
Quantum entanglement, 409–412
Quantum mechanics
    quantum entanglement, 409–412
    quantum superposition, 409
    quantum tunneling, 409
    Solvay Conference, 407*b*
    subatomic particle, 409
    uncertainty principle, 408–409
    wave-particle duality, 408
Quantum mottle, 234

R

Radiation, 5*b*, 123, 124*f*
    barriers, protective, 12–13, 12*f*
    collimation, 13
    control, emphasis, 10
    deterministic effects of, 466*f*, 466*t*
    direct and indirect effects of, 454, 454*b*
    doubling dose, 497*b*
    educational considerations in, 566
    effect modification, 463–464, 463*f*
    filtration, 13
    genetics, conclusions, 497*t*
    gonadal shielding, 12
    health and, 501, 501*b*

Radiation *(Continued)*
  hormesis, 485, 485*b*
  injury, 10, 10*b*
  intensity, integrate mode, 518
  internal source of, 50
  inverse relation to square of distance, 63
  lethal effects of, 458
  measurement of, 146
    characteristics and uses, 518*t*
  monitoring instruments, 507
  monitors for, 567*f*
  pregnancy and, 493–497
  protection, 10–13, 10*b*
    ten commandments of, 12*t*
  protection guides, 482*b*
  public exposure on, 566
  safety regulation, 474
  sources, point sources, 503
  stochastic effects of, 481–498
  types, 515–516, 515*b*, 515*f*, 516*b*, 517*b*
    weighting factors of, 565*t*
  wall posters, warning for, 555*f*
Radiation detection
  accomplishment in, 309
  apparatus, 508
  characteristics and uses, 518*t*
  instrument, design, 508*f*
  measurement, 518–526
    equipment, 508, 508*b*
  pulse or rate mode, 518
Radiation doses, 180*b*, 180*f*, 560–562
  limits of, 562–566
  profile, 541–542
Radiation Effects Research Foundation (RERF), 487
Radiation exposure, 143
  determination of, 209
  in utero, 495*b*
Radiation exposure device (RED), 507
Radiation-induced breast cancer, observations, 490*b*
Radiation-induced cancer risk (excess)
  absolute risk model, 492*f*
  relative risk model, 493*f*
Radiation-induced chromosome aberrations, 451, 452*f*
Radiation-induced chromosome damage, 436*b*
Radiation-induced congenital abnormalities, 494
Radiation-induced death, 469*f*
Radiation-induced leukemia
  latent period, and at-risk period, 487*b*
  non-threshold dose-response relationship, linear, 487*b*, 487*f*
Radiation-induced life span shortening, 484*f*
Radiation-induced malignancy, 486–491
Radiation-induced preneoplastic thyroid nodularity, 489*f*
Radiation-induced skin cancer, threshold dose response relationship, 490*b*
Radiation intensity, line-focus principle in, 121
Radiation protection
  cardinal principles of, 501–505, 502*t*
    application of, 506*f*
  designing for, 510–526
  filtration, 511–512, 512*b*
  guidance, 507–508, 507*b*
  mobile x-ray imaging system, 512
  operator shield, 512
  reproducibility, 512, 512*b*
  time, distance, and shielding, principles, 501
Radiation quality, 94, 94*b*, 203
  change of, 209*b*
Radiation quantity, 94*b*, 203
  control of, 205
  impact of milliamperes, 204*b*
Radiation risk
  coefficients, 505
  estimates, 484–486
  form for acknowledgment of, 574*f*
Radiation Safety Officer, 508
Radiation weighting factor (WR), 442
Radio
  experimentation of, 58
  reception, electromagnetic induction in, 87*f*
Radioactive decay, 45–46, 48*ba*
  by alpha emission, 46
  law, 47
  results, 46*b*
Radioactive disintegration, 45–46
Radioactive half-life, 47–48, 47*b*, 48*b*
Radioactive material, gamma rays emission in, 60

Radioactivity, 45–49, 46*b*
  becquerel (Bq), 14–15, 14*b*
  estimated, 48*f*
Radiobiology, 430*b*
  fundamental principles of, 441–448
Radiofrequency (RF), 54, 59
  data transfer, 390
  electromagnetic spectrum and, 59
  emissions, 59
  importance of, 60
Radiograph
  making, factors, 245*t*
  obtaining, equipment arrangement for, 307*f*
  radiolucency, 346*f*
Radiographers, frequency selection of, 101
Radiographic artifacts, 247–257
  image receptor, 248–249
Radiographic cones/cylinders, 219*f*
  x-ray beam production, 219*f*
Radiographic contrast, 242
Radiographic examination, entrance exposures and fetal doses for, 555*t*
Radiographic grids, 221–223, 221*b*, 221*f*
  crossed grid, 225, 225*b*
  focused grid, 225, 225*f*
  in mammography examination, 549
  moving grid, 225–226
  photoelectric effect/Compton scattering, contribution, 215*f*
  strip, 221–223
  usage, disadvantage, 229
Radiographic image
  contrast, control of, 195*f*
Radiographic noise, 234, 234*b*
Radiographic procedures
  effective dose for, 536
  patient radiation dose from, 530*t*
Radiographic protection features, 511–512
Radiographic quality
  image, tools for improved, 244–245
  image receptors, 244
  technique factors, 244, 244*b*
Radiographic rating chart, 125–126, 125*f*
Radiographic technique, 551–552
Radiography, 8
  configuration for, 529*f*
  patient radiation dose from, 527–537
  screen-film, MTF and, 193
  x-ray beams of, 539*f*
Radioisotopes, 46–47
  artificially produced, 46
  decay, 45–46
  elements in, 45
  radioactivity of, 47
Radiologic devices, 507, 507*b*
Radiologic dispersal device (RDD), 507
Radiologic imaging, 401, 404*f*
Radiologic personnel, occupational radiation exposure, 560*t*
Radiologic science
  atomic number of materials important to, 158*t*
  concepts of, 1–16
  mathematics for, 18–23
    algebra, 20–21, 20*b*
    decimals, 19, 19*b*
    fractions, 18–19, 18*b*
    graphing, 22–23, 22*f*, 23*f*, 23*t*
    number systems, 21–22, 21*f*, 21*t*
    significant figures, 19–20, 19*b*
  numeric prefixes, 13, 13*t*
  special quantities of, 14*t*
  summary of, 15
  terminology for, 13–15
Radiologic technologist, 294*f*
  deaths, records, 484
  effective dose, 505–507
  example of, 73*f*
Radiologic technology, safety, 483*b*
Radiologic terrorism, 507–508, 507*b*
  radiation detection instrument, 508*f*
Radiologist, 271, 271*b*, 271*f*
Radiology
  dates in, 11*t*
  radiation protection, principles, application, 506*f*
Radiology Information System (RIS), 362
Radiolucency, 346
  relative degrees of, 346*t*
Radionuclides, 45–46
  internally deposited, 5
Radiopacity, 346

Radiopaque, 62
  structure of, 63*f*
Radioprotective agents, 445
Radioresistant cells, 461*b*
Radiosensitivity
  age and, 444, 444*f*
  biologic factors that affect, 443–445
  chemical agents and, 444–445
  fractionation and, 443
  hormesis and, 445
  linear energy transfer and, 442, 443*f*
  oxygen effect and, 443–444
  physical factors that affect, 442–443
  protraction and, 443
  recovery and, 443*b*, 444
  relative biologic effectiveness and, 442–443, 442*b*
  of tissues and organs, 438*t*
Radiosensitizers, 444
Radium, 489*b*
  salts, 489
RadLex, 365, 402*f*
Radon, 5, 490*b*
RAID. *See* Redundant array of independent discs
RAM. *See* Random access memory
Random access memory (RAM), 387
Raster pattern, electron beams in, 284, 284*f*
Rate mode, 518
Rating charts, 125–127
Raw x-ray beam, exposure to, 356*f*
Read, CR step, 175*f*
Read-only memory (ROM), 387
  chips, variations in, 387
  information in, 387
Receiver operating characteristic (ROC) curves, 421*f*, 422–424, 422*b*, 422*f*, 422*t*, 423*b*, 423*f*, 423*t*, 424*f*
Reciprocal translocations, 478, 478*f*
Reciprocating grid, 226
Recombination, region of, 519
Reconstruction time, 314
Recovery, 443*b*, 444
  in multi-target, single-hit model, 461–462, 462*b*
Rectification, 101*b*
Rectifiers, 101, 102*b*, 102*f*
RED. *See* Radiation exposure device
Red goggles, 277*f*, 419*f*
Reduction division, 437*b*
Redundant array of independent discs (RAID), 389
Reflection, 61, 372, 372*b*
Refraction, 59
  prism, 59*f*
Region of interest (ROI), 358
  viewing, 314
Registers, 387
Relative biologic effectiveness, 442–443, 442*b*, 463*b*
Relative radiation level (RRL), 557–558, 557*t*
Relative risk, 484–485, 484*b*
  investigation results, 485
Relativity, 66*b*
Remnant x-rays, 217
Repair mechanism, 444
Repeat examinations, 551, 551*b*
Reproducibility, 512
RERF. *See* Radiation Effects Research Foundation
Resistance, decreasing, 74
Resolution
  contrast resolution, 234
  uniformity evaluation, TG 18-PX pattern, 374, 374*f*, 375*f*
Retina, light in, 276*b*, 419*b*
Rhodium (Rh)
  K-characteristic x-rays, 264–265
  target element, use of, 139
  target x-ray tube, emission spectrum, 266*f*
  x-ray tube usage, 264–265
Ribonucleic acid (RNA), 433
Ribosomes, 435
Ring artifacts, occurrence of, 309
Ripple, reduced, 139, 140*b*
RIS. *See* Radiology Information System
Risk
  absolute risk, 485
  estimates, 484–486
  excess risk, 485
  relative risk, 484–485
RNA. *See* Ribonucleic acid
Roadmapping, 299
  neurovascular image, 299*f*
Rochester series, thyroid cancer, 489
Rods, 276, 419

Roentgen, 471
 first x-ray examination, 7, 8f
 original properties of x-rays, 7t
ROI. See Region of interest
ROM. See Read-only memory
Rongelap Atoll, fallout, 489
Rotating anode x-ray tube, 117–118, 117f
 appearances of, comparison of, 119f
 electromagnetic induction motor in, 118b, 119f
 exposure times in, 118b
 principal parts of, 112f, 118
Rotor, in glass or metal enclosure, 118
Rutherford, Ernest, 37

S

S phase, DNA during, 451f
Saccharides, 432–433
Samei, Ehsan, 183
SAR. See Slice acquisition rate
Saturation current, 116, 116f
Scanned projection radiography, 183–184
 components of, 184f
 development of, 183
 example, 184f
 obtaining, 184f
Scanners, data translation with, 391
Scapula, projection/elongation, foreshortening of, 348f
Scatter radiation, 213–232, 560b
 control of, 216–221
 effect of, 216–218, 217b, 218f
 increase, x-ray beam field size (increase), 215
 intensity, 515b
 kVp, impact, 214–216, 215b
 production of, 214–216, 214b, 214f
 reduction, cones, impact, 220f
 relative intensity, increase, 217f
 secondary radiation, type, 515
 transmission, decrease, 229f
Scatter x-ray beam, energy level and, 199b
Scattered x-ray, angle of, 217
Scintillation detectors, 521–524, 522b, 522f, 523b
 assembly, characteristics, 523f
 x-ray detection efficiency in, 315
Scotopic response curve, 351f
Scotopic vision, 276, 420
Screen-film
 image receptor, characteristic curve, 178f
 radiograph, dynamic range of, 194–197
 response of, 199f
Screen-film mammography, 270
 modulation transfer function and, 193f
 quality control (QC) procedures, 270
 results of, 196f
Screen-film radiography
 activity sequence, 171f
 image receptor responses for, 532f
 MTF curve, representative of, 193
 spatial resolution, determination of, 197b
Screening mammography, 262
SCRs. See Silicon-controlled rectifiers
Second (s), 14–15
Second-generation CT imaging systems, 308, 308f
Secondary barriers
 equivalent material thickness, 516t
 use factor, 517
Secondary connections, 96
Secondary memory, 388
Secondary protective barrier, 515
 walls, protection, 515
Secondary radiation, types, 515
Section sensitivity profile (SSP), 313f
Seldinger, Sven Ivar, 299
Seldinger needle, 299
Selectable added filtration, examples, 207f
Self-rectified, 103
Semiconduction, demonstration of, 74
Semiconductor, 101
 definition of, 74b
Sensitivity (speed), of CCD, 185, 185b
Sensitivity profile, 313, 313f
Sentinel event, 534
Serial radiography, aluminum step-wedge in, usage of, 151f
Shaded surface display (SSD), 319
 computer-aided design in, 319–320
Shaded surface image, during virtual colonoscopy reconstructed, 319f
Shaded volume display (SVD), 319
Shell-type transformer, 89, 89f
"Shells" (electron orbits), 38
 electron exist in, 38

"Shells" (electron orbits) *(Continued)*
 maximum electrons per, 39b, 40t
 notation, 41
Shielding
 equation, 505b
 radiation protection, principles of, 501
 use of, 504–505, 504b
Shockley, William, 74, 379
SID. See Source-to-image receptor distance
Sievert (Sv), 15f
Sigma, 542
Sigmoid type, of radiation dose-response relationship, 446
Signal, amplitude, 519f
Signal interpolation, 356
Signal plate, 282
Signal-to-noise ratio (SNR), 197
 increase of, 197
Significant figures, 19–20, 19b
Silicon-controlled rectifiers (SCRs), 105
Silicon photodiodes, active matrix array, 186f
SIMMS. See Single in-line memory modules
Sine waves
 association of, 55f
 existence of, 54
 identical, 55, 55f
 wavelengths, different, 56, 56f
Single-frequency operation, efficiency, 140f
Single-hit chromosome aberrations, 477–478, 477f, 478b
Single in-line memory modules (SIMMS), 387
Single phase, 126b
Single phase high-voltage generator, 208
Single-phase power, 104
Single-phase radiographic unit, x-ray intensity, estimating of, 530f
Single-target, single-hit model, 458–459, 458f, 459b, 459f, 460f
Sinusoidal fashion, 54
Sinusoidal variation, examples of, 54
Size-specific dose estimates, 545, 546f
Skin
 cancer, 490
 dose limit of, 565–566
 effects on, 470–471, 470b, 471f
 local tissue effects, 482–483
Skin erythema dose, 471
Slice acquisition rate (SAR), 326–327, 326b
Slice thickness, in computed tomography, 329
 test object for, 328f
Slip-ring technology, 316, 316f
Slip rings, brushes and, 316f
Slow scan, 176
SMPTE. See Society of Motion Picture and Television Engineers
Snook, H.C., 9
Snook transformer, Coolidge tube, 9
SNR. See Signal-to-noise ratio
Society of Motion Picture and Television Engineers (SMPTE), 369
 pattern, 369
Sodium (Na), chlorine (Cl) and, combination of, 45
Sodium bicarbonate (NaHCO$_3$), 45
Sodium chloride (NaCl), 45
Sodium iodide (NaI), 183, 315
Soft copy, 352–353
 viewing, cathode ray tube and, 353
Soft tissue
 radiography, 261
  edge enhancement, 261
 Z values of, 163–164
Software
 manipulations, sequence, 384f
 use of, 380
Software artifacts, 249–252
 image compression, 250–252
 preprocessing, 249–250
Solenoid
 definition of, 85b
 magnetic field lines of, 85f
Solid-state diodes, 101–102, 102f
Solid-state drive (SSD), 389
Solid-state laser, wavelength light of, 175–176
Solid-state radiation detectors, 100, 100f
Solid-state semiconductor diodes, 354–355
Somatic cells, 436
Sound
 speed of, wavelength calculation of, 57
 wave equation usage, 57
Source data entry devices, 391
Source-to-image receptor distance (SID), 531
 change in, compensation for, 145
 increase in, 145b

Source-to-image receptor distance (SID) *(Continued)*
 indicator, 511, 511b
 x-ray intensities at, 143–146
 in x-ray tube, 112
Source-to-skin distance, 513, 531
 effect, 513b
 increase, 513
Source-to-tabletop distance (STD) indicator, 228
South pole, 82
Space charge, 116
 effect, 97, 116
Spatial distortion, 239
Spatial frequency, 190–192, 320b
 blurring, quality control test objects and tools, 193
 concept, representation of, 191f
 for CT imaging systems, 320–321
 expression of, 190b
 increase, 193
 line pair and, 191f
  relationship of, 190
 representation, calculation of, 193
 and size, relationship between, 192t
Spatial resolution, 190–194, 234, 234b, 266b, 281, 281t, 285, 320b, 421
 ability of, 190b
 compromise, 269b
 computed tomography, 328, 328b
  test object in, 328f
 determination of, 197b
 in digital imaging, 192
 in digital mammography, 337b
 improvement, 261
 in interventional radiology, 289b
 measurement, representation, 190f
 for medical imaging systems, 192t
 pixel size, limitation of, 192b
Spatial uniformity, 325
Special examination, patient radiation dose in, 549–550
Special quantities, 14t, 24
Speed, 235, 236f
Sperm, 472
Spermatid, 472
Spermatocyte, 472
Spermatogonia, 472
Spermatogonial stem cells, 473
Spermatozoa, 472
Spindle fibers, 436
Spindles, 436
Spine, imaging, computed radiography plates, 256f
Spinning charged particle, in magnetic field induction, 79f
Spiral computed tomography, 319f
Split-dose irradiation, 461, 462f
Spontaneous abortion, 495b
 incidence of, 553b
Spot-film kVp, fluoroscopic and, for common examination, 277t
SPSs. See Storage phosphor screens
Square law, 145b
 derivation of, 206b
 equation, 206b
SSD. See Shaded surface display
SSP. See Section sensitivity profile
Standard deviation, noise, 324
Standard units of measurement, 23–26
 length, 24
 mass, 24–25, 25f
 time, 25
 units, 25–26, 25b, 31t
Starches, 432–433
Stationary anode x-ray tube, 116, 117f
Stationary objects, kinetic energy (absence), 130
Stators, 87
 in glass or metal enclosure, 118
Stem cells, 438, 438b
 pluripotential, 474
Step-down transformer, 88
Step-up transformer, 88
Step-wedge filter, application of, 150
Steradian, 351f
Stewart, Alice, 494
Stickiness, 478
Stimulation, CR step, 173–176, 174f
Stochastic effect, 430
 cause of, 452
 of radiation, 481–498, 482f
Stochastic radiation responses, 445, 445b, 445t
Stop-and-shoot artifact, 339, 340f
Storage
 batteries, use of, 105
 memory, archival form, 388b
 system, 363, 363b, 364f

Index

Storage phosphor screens (SPSs), 172, 173f
  appearance of, 172
  mechanical stability of, 172
  phosphors, incorporation of, 173f
Subatomic particles, ionization of, 49
Subject contrast, 242–243, 242b
  anatomical thickness, impact, 242f
  tissue mass density, variation (impact), 242, 243f
Subject factors, 241–244, 242t
Sublethal damage, 461
Sublethal radiation damage, 444
Substances, 35, 36f
Subtracted image, 296b
Superconducting materials, rise in critical temperature for, 76f
Superconductivity, 75
  discovery of, 84
Superconductor, electrical resistance of, 75f
Supervised learning, 400
Supporting tissues, 438
Surgery, occupational radiation exposure in, 561–562
SVD. *See* Shaded volume display
Sweep angle, for DRT, 333b, 333f, 334, 334f
Synchronous timers, 99
System board, 388
System software, 384

T

Target, 117, 282
  angles, focal spot size in, 120
  assembly, 282
  characteristics of, 118t
  composition mammographic imaging system, 264–265
  of television camera tube, 281f
Target atomic number, increase in, 138b
Target-characteristic radiation, 267b
Target number, 461
Target theory, 457, 458f
Technique creep, 198
Telecommunications, 390
Teleradiology, 362–363, 362b, 390–393, 390b, 393b
  remote transmission and, 362
  support, 252
Television camera, 281
  tube, 282b
    conducts electrons, 282f
    in image-intensifier tube, 283f
Television designers, objective of, 285
Television field, 284
Television frame, 284
Television image, 284
Television monitoring system, 281
Television picture tube, 283–284, 283b
  principal parts of, 283f
Telophase, of mitosis, 436
Temperature conversion, 31b
Temperature scales, 31b, 31f
Temporal subtraction, energy subtraction *versus*, 295t
Ten, power of, 382t
Tenth-value layer
  known, 504
  tube potentials, 505t
Terabyte (TB), bytes, equivalence, 388
Terminal, input/output device, 390
Terrestrial radiation, 5
Tesla (magnet field strength), 83b
Testes, radiation response of, 473, 473t
"The Technical Standard for Electronic Practice of Medical Imaging", 365
Thermal conductivity, of tungsten, 117b
Thermal cushion, to dissipate heat, 113
Thermal dissipater, in anode, 117
Thermal energy (heat), 4
  measurement of, in heat units, 126
Thermal radiation, 31
Thermionic emission, 97b, 114, 277
  in space charge, 116b
Thermionic television camera, 281
Thermoluminescence dosimeter, 530, 567, 568f
Thermoluminescence dosimetry (TLD), 518–519, 524–525, 524f
Thick objects, distortion, increase, 238f
Thin-film transistor (TFT), 183
  digital radiography (DR) image receptor photomicrograph, 186f
Third generation computers, 380
Third-generation CT imaging systems, 308f, 309, 309f
  curvilinear detector array in, 309
  principal disadvantages of, 309

Third-generation CT imaging systems *(Continued)*
  ring artifacts in, 309f
  in rotate-only mode, 308f
Thomson, J.J., 36–37, 154
Thomson atom, 36–37
Thoriated tungsten, 114
Thorium dioxide (ThO$_2$), colloidal suspension, 491
Thorotrast, 491
Three-dimensional image, in maximum intensity projection reconstruction, 319f
Three-dimensional multiplanar reformation, 319
Three Mile Island, 466, 491
  predicted radiation-induced deaths, 491b
Three phase/high frequency, 127b
Three-phase operation, efficiency of, 140f
Three-phase power, 104–105, 105f
  forms, 209
  results, 209b
Three-phase/six-pulse power/twelve-pulse power (contrast), 139
Threshold dose, 461, 461b, 462b
Threshold-type dose-response relationship, 470
Thrombocytes, 474
Thrombocytopenia, 475
Thymine, 433
Thyroid cancer, 489
Thyroid nodularity, incidence, 489
Tiled CCD, design, 184f
Time
  equation, 501b
  minimize, 501–503, 502b
  radiation protection, principles of, 501–505
  standard unit of, 25
Time-interval difference (TID) mode, 295–296, 297b, 297f
Timer circuit, 98
Time of occupancy factor, 516–517
Time-varying analog signal, 178
Tissue radiation dose, 530t, 533, 533f
Tissues, 438–439, 438t, 439t
  compression, 217f
  computed tomography numbers in, 318t
  dose limit for, 565–566
  imaged, with changing pitch, 312t
  mass density, 242, 243f
  maternal tissues, attenuation by, 572
  slice, thickness of, 314
  weighting factors for, 506t, 565t
Titanium, superconducting material, 75
TLD. *See* Thermoluminescence dosimetry
Tomography, results, 307f
Tomosynthesis, 331–341, 333f
  artifacts, 335–336
  digital radiographic, 332–333, 332b, 334b
  image receptor, 334
  image reconstruction, 334–335, 335t
  patient radiation dose, 336–340, 337b, 338f, 339f, 340f
  quality control, 336, 336f
  x-ray source, 333–334
Tomosynthesis Mammographic Imaging Screening Trial (TMIST), 338
Total beam filtration, 267b
Total filtration
  components of, 149f
  equation of, 221b
Total projectile electrons, calculation, 205b
Tracks (CD rings), 388
Transbrachial selective coronary angiography, 294
Transfemoral angiography, 294
Transfer RNA, 433
Transformer, 9, 88–89
  intensity of, changes in, 88b
  law
    effect of, 88b
    equation, 88b
  operation of, 101
  type of, 89f
  usage of, 88
Transistor, development of, 379
Transitional elements, 41
Translation, 306
Transmission
  examples of, 62, 63f
  speed of, 390
Transverse images, reconstruction of, 310f
Trough filter, 150f
  usage of, 149, 150f
Truncation artifacts, 335, 335f, 336f
Tuberculosis
  testing, 550b
  treatment, 489

Tungsten (W)
  alloying, 117
  anatomic configuration for, 132f
  atomic number in, 117b
  binding energies for, 132f
  high melting point in, 117b
  K-characteristic x-rays, usefulness of, 132b
  L-shell x-rays, value (absence), 265b
  target x-ray tube, 41
    emission spectrum, molybdenum/rhodium filtration, 267f
    usage, 267
    x-ray emission spectrum, 267f
  thermal conductivity, 117b
  thoriated, 114
  vaporization of, 114b
  x-ray emission spectrum of, 135f
Tuning fork, vibration of, 55
Turns ratio, of high-voltage transformer, 100
20-20-20 rule, 424
Two, power of, 382t

U

U-arm, 112
Ultrasound, production of, 58
Ultraviolet, location in electromagnetic spectrum, 59
Uncontrolled area, 517
Unfiltered Mo beam, x-ray emission, 267
  spectrum, 268f
Uniformity, in computed tomography, 325, 325b, 328
  test object in, 328f
Units
  radiologic, 13–15
  system of, 25–26, 25b, 31t, 54
UNIVersal Automatic Computer (UNIVAC), 380
Unlike charges, attraction of, 71b, 72
Unnecessary examination, 550–551, 550b
Unnecessary patient radiation dose, reduction of, 550–551
Unrectified voltage, 102–103, 102f
Unshielded fluoroscope, isoexposure profile, 514f
Unsupervised learning, 400
Upside-down grid, 228
Uranium miners, lung cancer, 490–491
US Food and Drug Administration (USFDA) designations, 396
Use factor, barrier thickness, factor, 517

V

Variable-aperture collimator, light localization collimator, 219
  schematic, 220f
Variable-aperture light-localizing collimator, Al equivalent, 207
Vectors
  advanced techniques, 397
  efficient data representation, 397
  facilitates ML, 397
  measure similarity, 396
  nature of vectors, 396
  performance calculations, 397
  represent data, 396
  scalability and performance, 397
  universality and interoperability, 397
Veiling glare, 279, 280f
Velocity, 26–27, 26b, 27f, 54–55
  electromagnetic radiation, 54b
  frequency and, relationship of, 56f
  wave parameters, 56
  wavelength and frequency in, inversely proportional, 56b
Vertical chest Bucky, AEC sensor position, 210f
Vertical resolution, 285
Vertical retrace, 284
Very large-scale integration (VLSI), 380
Vessels, opacification of, 294
Video Electronics Standard Association (VESA), 369
Video files, 388
Video frame, from raster pattern, 284f
Video monitoring, rate of, 284b
Video signal
  creating, 282f
  progressive mode of, 293f
Video system, in conventional fluoroscopy, 293, 293b, 294f
Vidicon television camera, 282f
  principal parts of, 282f
  three variations of, 281f

Vigorous compression, 268
  advantages of, 269t
  used in x-ray mammography, 268b
Virtual assistance, 398
Virtual grids, 226, 226b, 270b
Virtual personal assistants (VPAs), 397t
Visible light, 58–59
  electromagnetic spectrum, 59
  identification of, by wavelength, 60b
  importance of, 60
  matter, interaction with, 62
  measurement of, 61–62
  spectrum, extension of, 61
  wave behavior of, 61b
  wave model, 61–62
  wave nature of, 61–62, 61f
Visible-light photons
  behavior, 60–61
  travel of, 58–59
  x-radiation and, photon of, 60
Visual accommodation, 419
Visual acuity, 276, 420
Visual adaption, 419
Visual programming (computer language), 386
Visual search, 421, 421f
Voice-recognition systems, 392
Volt (V), electric potential unit, 74b
Voltage, 74, 75b
  measurement, line compensator use for, 95
  ripple, 106–108, 106b, 107f
Voltage rectification, 101–104, 101b, 102f
Voltage ripple, 208b
Voltage waveform, impact of, 139–140
Voltaic pile, 84f
  battery, precursor of, 84
Volume imaging, 325
Volume-rendering display, of heart, 320f
Voxel size, 317b

W

Wagner/Archer method, 14
The Wall Street Journal, 408f
WANTED sign, 409, 410f
Water, 431
  radiolysis of, 452–454, 453b, 453f
Water bath image, in noise, 324
Water-soluble salts, formation of, 36
Watt (W), 29, 108–109
  electric power, 77
  equivalence of, 77b
Wave equation, 57b
  electromagnetic wave equation, 57b
  simple mathematical formula of, 56–57
  usage, 56–57
Wave model, visible light, 61–62
Wave parameters, 56
Wave-particle duality, 60–61
Waveform, 76–77
Wavelength, 55–57, 60f
  calculation of, 57
  definition of, 56
  different, of sine waves, 56f
  frequency and, inversely proportional, 56b
  representation of, 55–57
  velocity and, frequency, relationship of, 56f
  wave parameters, 56
Waves, 60–66
Wedge filter, 150f
  usage of, 149, 150f
Weight (Wt), 28–29, 28b
Weighting factors
  of types of radiation, 565t
  for various tissues, 565t
Wet squares analogy, 459
White light
  photons in, 59
  prism refraction and, 59f
Whole-body dose limits, 562–565
Whole-body multislice helical CT screening, 551
Window
  in glass envelope, 282
  level adjustment and, 357
  of x-ray tube, 113
Wirth, Nicklaus, 385
Women, childbearing age, x-ray and fluoroscopy consent, 555f
Words, 383
Work, 29, 29b
Workload
  characteristic, 517

Workload *(Continued)*
  distribution, clinical voltage, 518f
World wide web, creation of, 391
Wrist images, signal intensity, 256f
Wurlitzer jukebox, optical disc jukebox, 389f

X

Xeromammography, 261
"X-light", 7, 8f
X-radiation, photon of, 60
X-ray absorption, efficiency, measurement of, DQE and, 198b
X-ray beams, 9b
  alignment, 511
  aperture diaphragm, 218–219
  attenuation of, added filtration in, 149
  collimation of, 214
    result, 215f
  energy
    filtration (impact), 138
    fixed, 204b
  field size, increase, 215
  filter in, addition of, 149
  filtration
    addition of, 146b
    types, 207–208
  half-value life in, determination of, 146–147
    methods in, 146–147
  intensity
    estimation of, nomogram for, 143f
    measurement, 512f
  penetrability of, 203
    changes in, 147, 147b
  quality of
    change in, 140t
    determination, use of kVp for, 97b
    increasing kVp in, 148b
  quantity of, change in, 140t
  raw, exposure to, 356f
  restrictors, 218–221, 218f, 220b
  SID and, 511b
  used in CT imaging, 308
  variable aperture collimator, 219
X-ray detection efficiency, 315
X-ray emission, 142–152
X-ray emission spectrum, 134–136
  effect of kVp on, 137–138
  effect of mA and mAs on, 136–137
  factors affecting, 136–140
  shape, factors in, 137f
  size/position, factors, 136t
  target material, impact of, 138–139
  variation in, 135f
  voltage waveform, effect on, 139–140
X-ray energy, 146–148
  function of, detective quantum efficiency and, 200f
  gamma rays and, 60
  maximum, 136f
X-ray imaging system, 70, 71f, 91–110
  chest radiography, impact, 219
  circuits of, 109f
  electrical energy conversion in, 71f
  filtration in, 146
  summary in, 109
  synchronous timers in, 99
  types of, 93, 93f
X-ray-induced image-forming signal, result of, 174f
X-ray intensity, 143–146, 143b
  calculation of, 145–146
  distance, 145–146
    relationship, equation of, 145b
  equation, 144b
  kVp
    increase in, 138
    proportion of, 144b
  kVp^2 and, proportion of, 144b
  mAs and, 205b, 206b
    proportion of, 144b
X-ray linear attenuation coefficients, computed tomography numbers in, 318t
X-ray photon
  electromagnetic energy quantum, 54b
  energy, bundle of, 65b
X-ray production, 129–141
X-ray projection tomography, 539–540, 539f
X-ray quality
  compensating filters, 149
  factors of, 147–148, 148t, 203t
  filtration
    adding, 148

X-ray quality *(Continued)*
  increasing, 148b
  types of, 148–150
  half-value layer and, 146–147
  kVp in, impact of, 148
  x-ray beam penetrability and, 146
  zero filtration, 147
X-ray quantity
  definition of, 143
  distance, square of, proportion, 145b
  equation, 144b
  factors of, 143, 203t
X-ray source, for DRT, 333–334
X-ray targets
  characteristics of, 118t
  material, impact of, 138–139
X-ray tube, 94, 111–128
  anode in, 116–123
    rotating, 112, 112f, 117f
    stationary, 116, 117f
  C-arm support system in, 112
  cathode in, 114–116, 114f
  ceiling support in, 112
  central ray, 122
  coast time, 119
  current
    adjustment of, 115b
    control of, 97, 115f
    monitoring of, 98
  effect of added filtration on, 138f
  excessive heat and, 124b
  exposure, product of, 97b
  external components of, 112–114, 113f
  failure, 123–125, 124f
  filament in, 114
  floor-to-ceiling support system in, 112
  focusing cup in, 114, 115f
  glass or metal enclosure in, 113–114, 113b
  grid-controlled tubes in, 114
  heat dissipation in, 120f
  for helical computed tomography, 315, 316f
  housing, tilt, 267f
  internal components of, 114–123
  in interventional radiology, 302
    specifications for, 302t
  motion, 333–334, 333f, 334f
  movement of, 310f
  off-focus radiation, 123
  protective housing of, 113, 113f
  rating charts, 125–127
  target, 130–134
  travel, 333f
  voltage
    applied to, 104b
    increase in, 139f
X-rays
  attenuation, 164
  behavior of, 61b
  circuits of, 109, 109f
  Compton-scattered, 155
  discovery of, 6–8
  emission of, 60
  examination room
    plan drawing of, 94f
    purpose of, 93
  examinations, types of, 8
  existence of, 50
  features of, 7–8
  gamma rays and, 60b
  for high-quality radiograph, 60
  image receptor exposure in, 143t
  interactions with matter, 153–167
  internal scatter radiation in, 279
  K x-rays, 132
  L x-rays, 132
  off-focus radiation, 123
  percent interaction, photoelectric/Compton processes, 215t
  photoelectric absorption of, 160
  production outside nucleus, 60f
  room, design, 517
  short wavelengths of, 154
  types of, 65, 65t
  voltages, 9

Z

Z-axis coverage, 327b
Z-axis resolution, improving, 311
Zinc calcium sulfide, 9
Zinc plates, usage, 84